# Photographic Atlas of Anatomy

# Photographic Atlas of Anatomy

Ninth Edition

**Prof. Dr. med. Dr. med. h.c. Johannes W. Rohen**
Anatomisches Institut I
University of Erlangen-Nürnberg
Erlangen, Germany

**Chihiro Yokochi, MD**
Professor Emeritus, Department of Anatomy
Kanagawa Dental College
Yokosuka, Kanagawa, Japan

**Prof. Dr. med. Elke Lütjen-Drecoll**
Anatomisches Institut II
University of Erlangen-Nürnberg
Erlangen, Germany

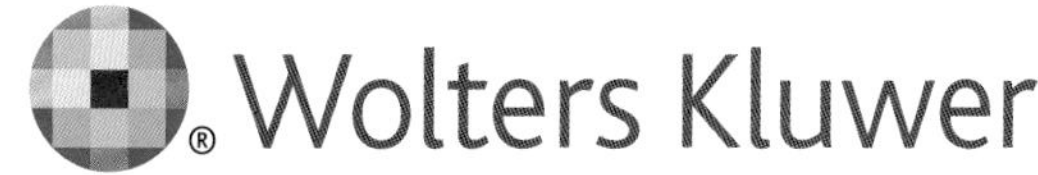


Philadelphia • Baltimore • New York • London
Buenos Aires • Hong Kong • Sydney • Tokyo

*Acquisitions Editor:* Crystal Taylor
*Development Editors:* Greg Nicholl (freelance), Amy Millholen
*Editorial Assistant:* Parisa Saranj
*Marketing Manager:* Phyllis Hitner
*Production Project Manager:* Alicia Jackson
*Designers (Germany):* Stephanie Gay, Bert Sender
*Creative Director:* Larry Pezzato
*Manufacturing Coordinator:* Margie Orzech
*Prepress Vendor:* <TK>

Ninth Edition



Georg Thieme Verlag KG
Rüdigerstrasse 14, D-70469 Stuttgart
Germany
www.thieme.de

Wolters Kluwer
Two Commerce Square
2001 Market Street
Philadelphia, PA 19103



9 8 7 6 5 4 3 2 1

Printed in China

---

**Library of Congress Cataloging-in-Publication Data**

ISBN-13: 978-1-9751-5134-8
ISBN-10: 1-9751-5134-8

Cataloging-in-Publication data available on request from the Publisher.

---



LWW.com

# Preface

Profound knowledge of the structures of the human body is of fundamental importance for the physician as well as for all those involved in the diagnosis and treatment of human diseases. Ultimately this knowledge can be only acquired through the dissection of the human body. Previous and currently available anatomical atlases usually contain schematic or semi-schematic graphics. They can usually only show reality to a limited extent and often lack the third dimension (i.e., the spatial impression). Photographs of anatomical specimens have two decisive advantages: In the first place, they reproduce the reality of the object and thus its proportions and spatial dimension much more accurately and realistically than the usually simplified "beautiful" graphics of the usual atlases. Second, they correspond to what students actually see in the dissection lab. Students can therefore orientate themselves during the preparation exercises directly on the photos in our atlas. The new order of the chapters in the atlas also follows the order in which the structures are very often taught in the dissection lab. It thus corresponds to the structure of most anatomical textbooks. Even though diagnostics today is increasingly based on the use of imaging techniques, the physician still needs the experience gained on the anatomical specimen for the evaluation of the corresponding images and the further treatment steps derived from them. Producing the high-quality preparations in this atlas not only required a lot of time, but also comprehensive anatomical knowledge. They were therefore prepared with the help of dedicated colleagues from anatomy and surgical disciplines at various topographic levels. Our special thanks go to Prof. S. Nagashima, Prof. K. Okamoto, and Dr. M. Takahashi (Japan), some of whom have been working in the Institute of Anatomy in Erlangen for a long time, as well as to Dr. G. Lindner-Funk (now Nuremberg, Germany), Dr. M. Rexer (now Klinikum Neumarkt), R. M. McDonnell (now Dallas, USA), and J. Bryant (Erlangen, Germany).

The new individual muscle and liver preparations were produced by the students Khann Nguyen, Ramona Witt, Anne Jacobsen, and Alexander Mocker under the supervision of Prof. Bremer (Erlangen, Germany) in the EMPTY course. A number of excellent natural bone preparations for macro photography were provided by Mr. H. Sommer (SOMSO company, Coburg, Germany). For this we would like to thank him very much. All photos of the preparations, including the photographs newly produced in this edition, were produced with great technical skill by our long-standing employee, Mr. M. Gößwein. For this ninth edition, too, the equipment with photos and graphics of the specimens has been further optimized by adding new illustrations or replacing older illustrations with new ones. We would like to thank our long-standing colleague, Mr. J. Pekarsky, for the colored and three-dimensional drawings, which were also renewed in this ninth edition and produced in close adaptation to the anatomical preparations. For the drawings in the new Appendix, we would like to thank Ms. A. Gack. It is also an important didactic concern of this atlas to make it easier for students to learn systematically about the great variety of anatomical structures and to make the positional relationships of the structures understandable. For this reason, we have retained in this edition the principle of presenting the individual structures of the topographical representation in the individual regions. Knowledge of the individual structures and the regional relationships is also required in order to be able to diagnostically assess the structures represented by imaging procedures in the clinic. The MRI and CT images were provided by Prof. M. Uder (Radiological Institute, Erlangen University Hospital) and Prof. A. Heuck (Radiological Institute of the University of Munich-Pasing) as well as by PD Dr. G. Wieners (Charité Berlin), Prof. H. Rupprecht (Neumarkt Hospital), and Prof. A. Herrlinger (Fürth Hospital), for which we would also like to express our sincere thanks. We owe the clinical images of the retina to Prof. Mardin (University Eye Hospital Erlangen). We would also like to express our special thanks to Prof. M. Uder and his staff. They have not only produced new MRI images for this new edition, but have also made sure that the sectional planes of specimen and MRI images correspond to each other to a large extent. This considerably increases the clarity and understanding of anatomical structures as well as clinical references of our photographic atlas. Our sincere thanks also go to the staff of the Thieme Verlag, where this atlas has fortunately found a new "home"—above all to Ms. S. Bartl for her committed and careful editorial work on the texts and illustrations for this new edition; without her tireless efforts, this edition would not be available in this quality. We would like to thank Dr. J. Neuberger warmly for his program planning support and efficient coordination of the numerous "threads," which had to be pulled sensibly on the way to this ninth edition. We would like to thank Ms. L. Diemand for the planning and supervision of the production. For this new edition, numerous contents have been newly compiled. Together with the new design of the pages, this was a great challenge for the layout designers Stephanie Gay and Bert Sender (Bremen), which they mastered brilliantly! Finally, we would like to thank again all scientists, students, staff and helpers, as well as the staff of the publishers Igaku-Shoin, Tokyo, Japan, and Wolters Kluwer, USA, for their manifold support.

August 2020

Johannes W. Rohen
Chihiro Yokochi
Elke Lütjen-Drecoll

# General Anatomy and Musculoskeletal System

## 1 General Anatomy



## 2 Trunk



## 3 Upper Limb

## 4 Lower Limb

# Internal Organs

## 5 Thoracic Organs



## 6 Abdominal Organs



## 7 Retroperitoneal Organs

# Head, Neck, and Brain

## 8 Head and Neck



## 9 Brain and Sensory Organs

## Appendix: Additional Resources

# 1 General Anatomy

## General Anatomy and Musculoskeletal System

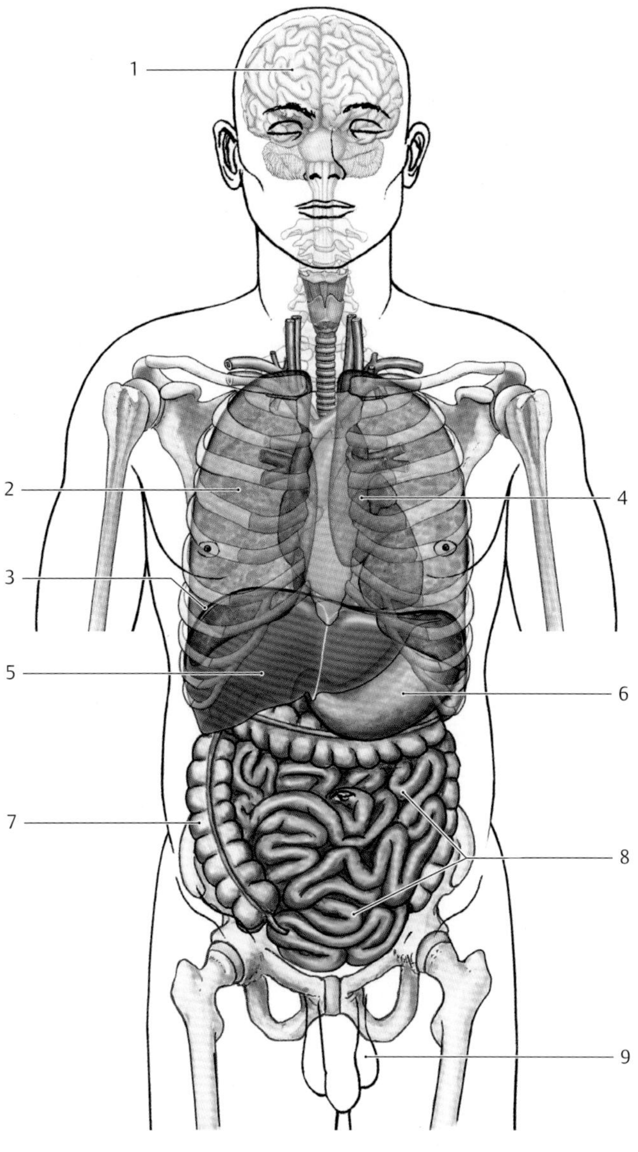


Fig. 1.1 **Position of the internal organs of the human body** (anterior aspect). The main cavities of the body and their contents.

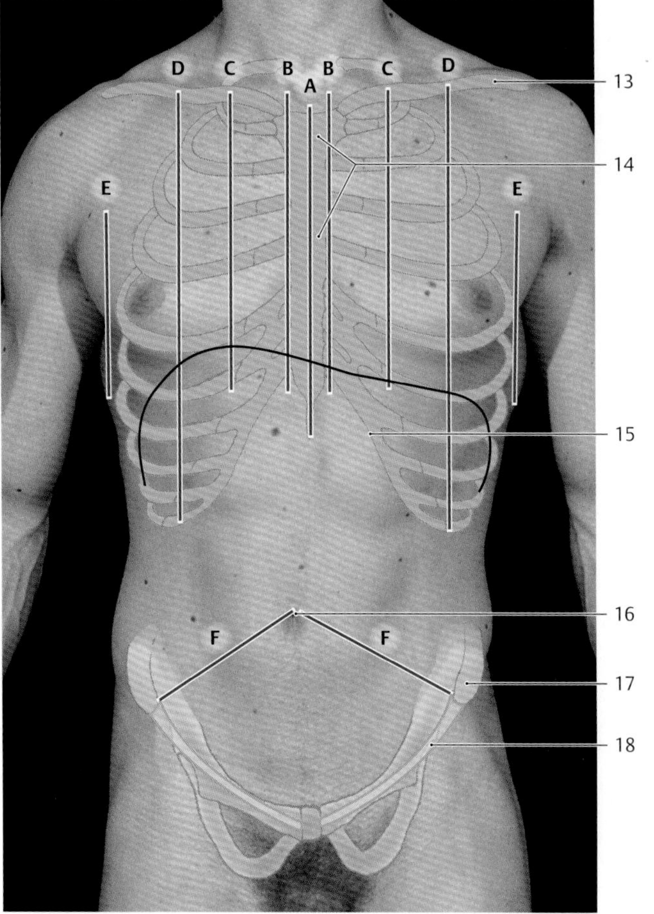


Fig. 1.2 **Regional lines at the anterior side of the human body.**

**Regional lines:**
A = Anterior median line
B = Sternal line
C = Parasternal line
D = Midclavicular line
E = Anterior axillary line
F = Umbilical-pelvic line

1 Brain
2 Lung
3 Diaphragm
4 Heart
5 Liver
6 Stomach
7 Colon
8 Small intestine
9 Testis
10 Kidney
11 Ureter
12 Anal canal
13 Clavicle
14 Manubrium sterni
15 Costal arch
16 Umbilicus
17 Anterior superior iliac spine
18 Inguinal ligament
19 Scapular spine
20 Spinous processes
21 Iliac crest
22 Coccyx and sacrum

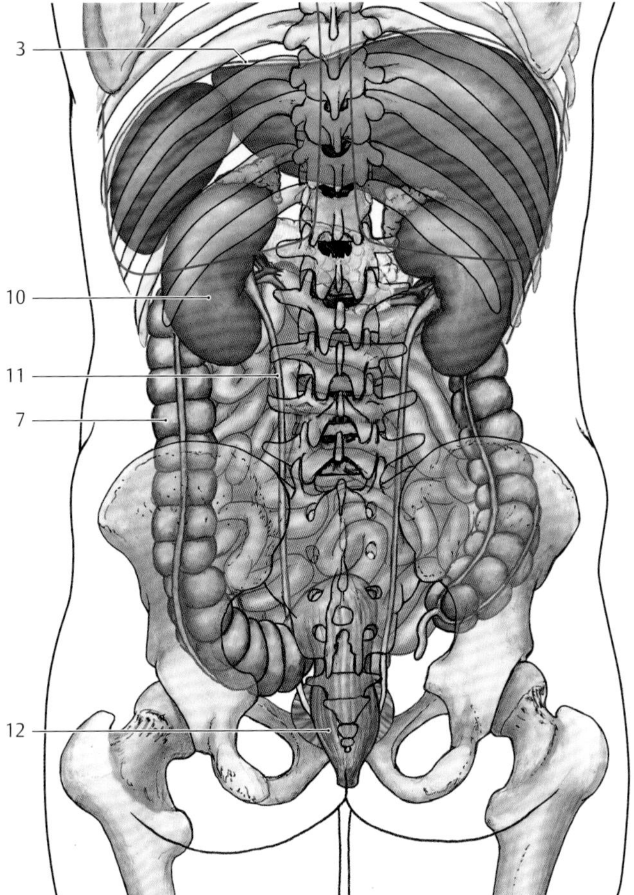


Fig. 1.3 **Position of the internal organs of the human body** (posterior aspect).

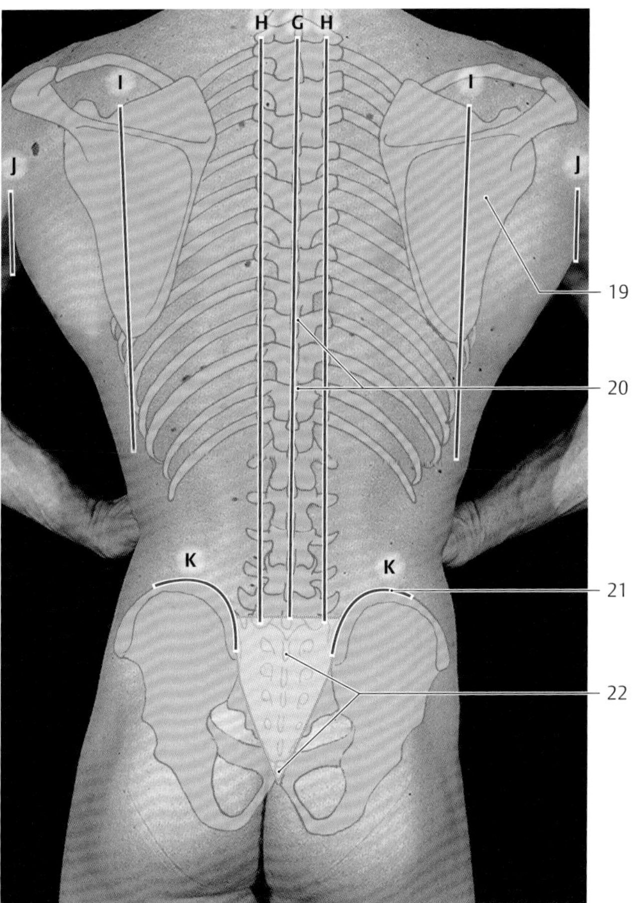


Fig. 1.4 **Regional lines at the posterior side of the human body.**

**Regional lines:** G = Posterior median line
H = Paravertebral line
I = Scapular line
J = Posterior axillary line
K = Iliac crest

The bones of the skeletal system are palpable through the skin at different points. This enables physicians to localize the internal organs. On the **anterior (ventral) side**, the clavicle, sternum, ribs, and intercostal spaces, in the pelvic area, the anterior iliac spine and the symphysis are palpable. For better orientation, several **lines of orientation** are indicated in Figure 1.2 (anterior side of the body) and Figure 1.4 (posterior side of the body). By means of these lines, the heart and the position of the vermiform process can be localized.

At the **posterior (dorsal) side** of the body, the posterior spines of the vertebral column, the ribs, the scapula, the sacrum, and the iliac crest are palpable. Lines of orientation to localize the kidneys, for example, are the paravertebral line and the lower ribs.

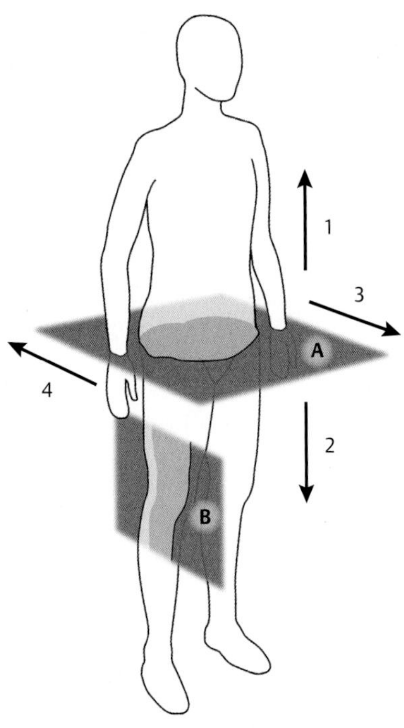


**Fig. 1.5 Planes of the body.**
A = Horizontal or axial or transverse plane
B = Sagittal plane (at the level of the knee joint)

**Directions:**

1 = Cranial
2 = Caudal
3 = Anterior (ventral)
4 = Posterior (dorsal)

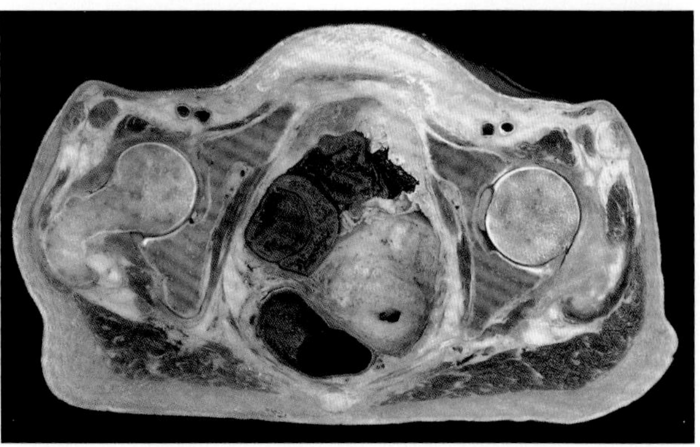

**Fig. 1.6 Horizontal section through the pelvic cavity and the hip joints.**

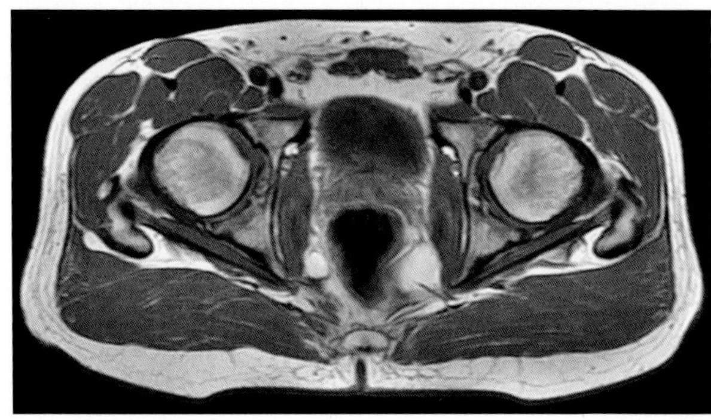

**Fig. 1.7 MRI scan through the pelvic cavity and the hip joints** (horizontal or axial or transverse plane). (Heuck A, et al. MRT-Atlas des muskuloskelettalen Systems. Stuttgart, Germany: Schattauer, 2009.)

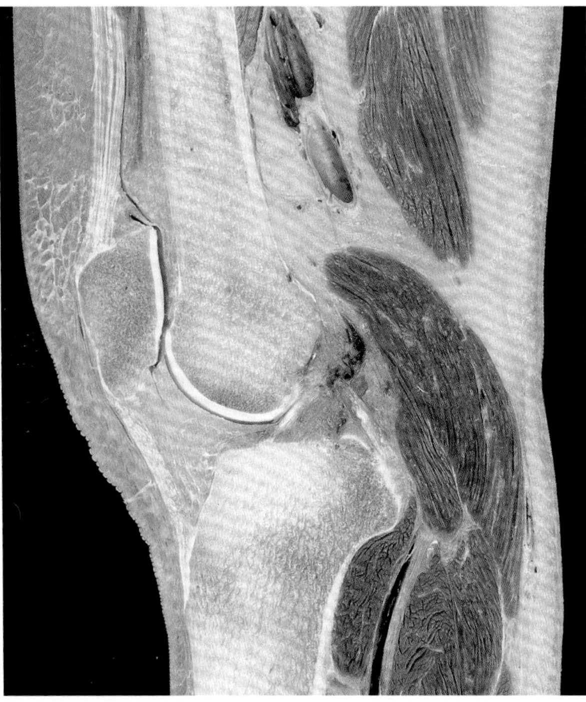

**Fig. 1.8 Sagittal section through the knee joint.**

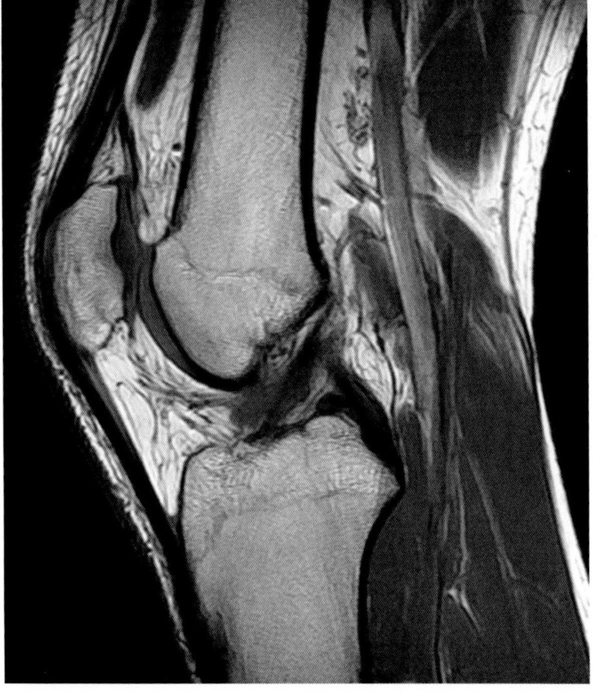

**Fig. 1.9 MRI scan through the knee joint** (sagittal plane). (Heuck A, et al. MRT-Atlas des muskuloskelettalen Systems. Stuttgart, Germany: Schattauer, 2009.)

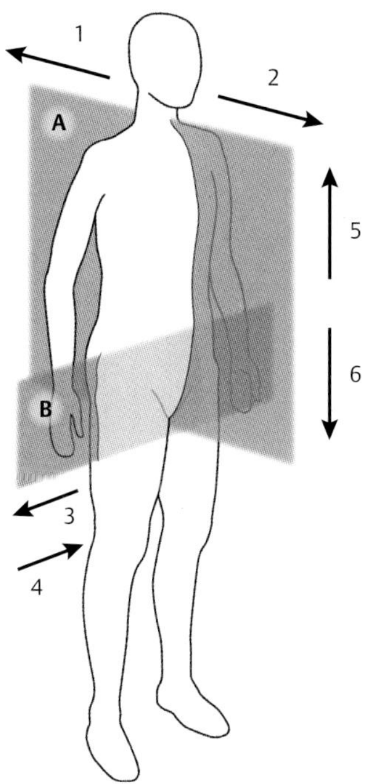


Fig. 1.10 **Planes of the body.**
A = Midsagittal or median plane
B = Frontal or coronal plane (through the pelvic cavity)

**Directions:**

1 = Posterior (dorsal)
2 = Anterior (ventral)
3 = Lateral
4 = Medial
5 = Cranial
6 = Caudal

**Radiological terminology:**

Horizontal section = axial or transverse plane
Frontal plane = coronal plane
Sagittal section = sagittal plane

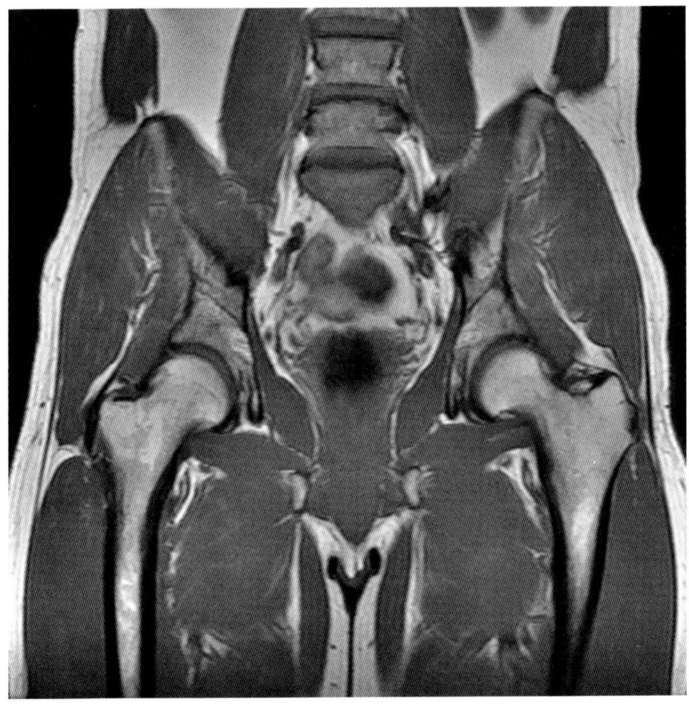

Fig. 1.11 **MRI scan through the pelvic cavity and the hip joints** (frontal or coronal plane). (Heuck A, et al. MRT-Atlas des muskuloskelettalen Systems. Stuttgart, Germany: Schattauer, 2009.)

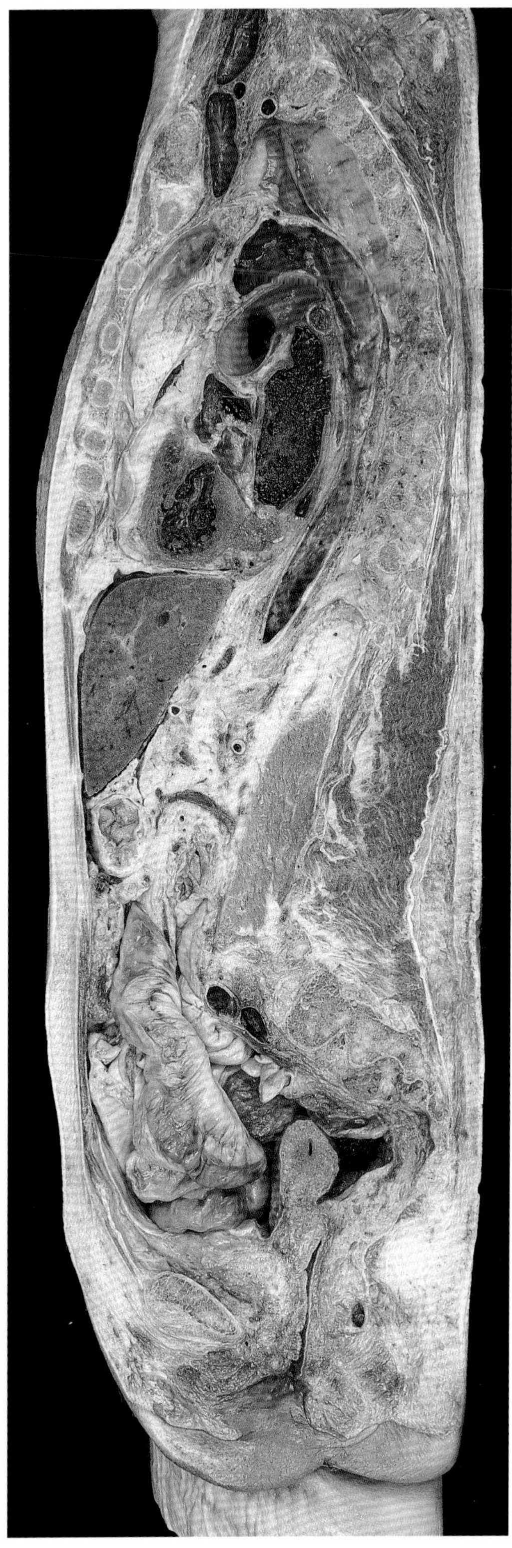

Fig. 1.12 **Median section through the trunk of a female.**

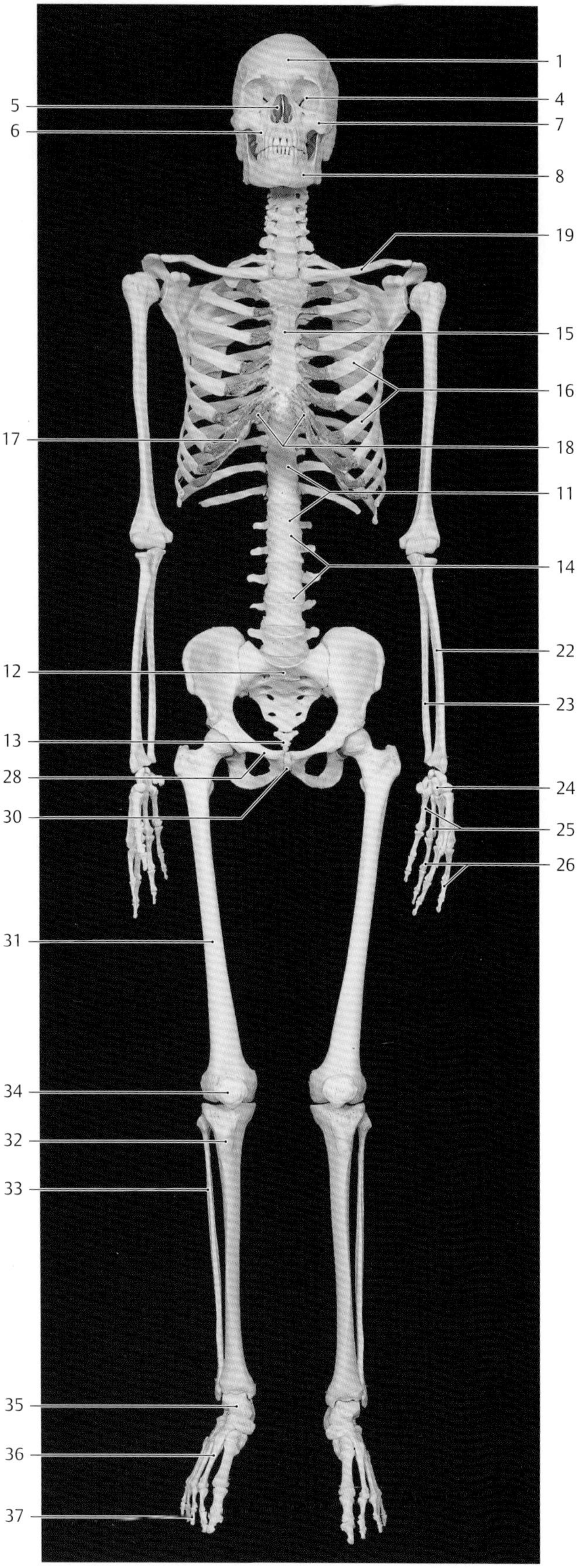


Fig. 1.13 **Skeleton of a female adult** (anterior aspect).

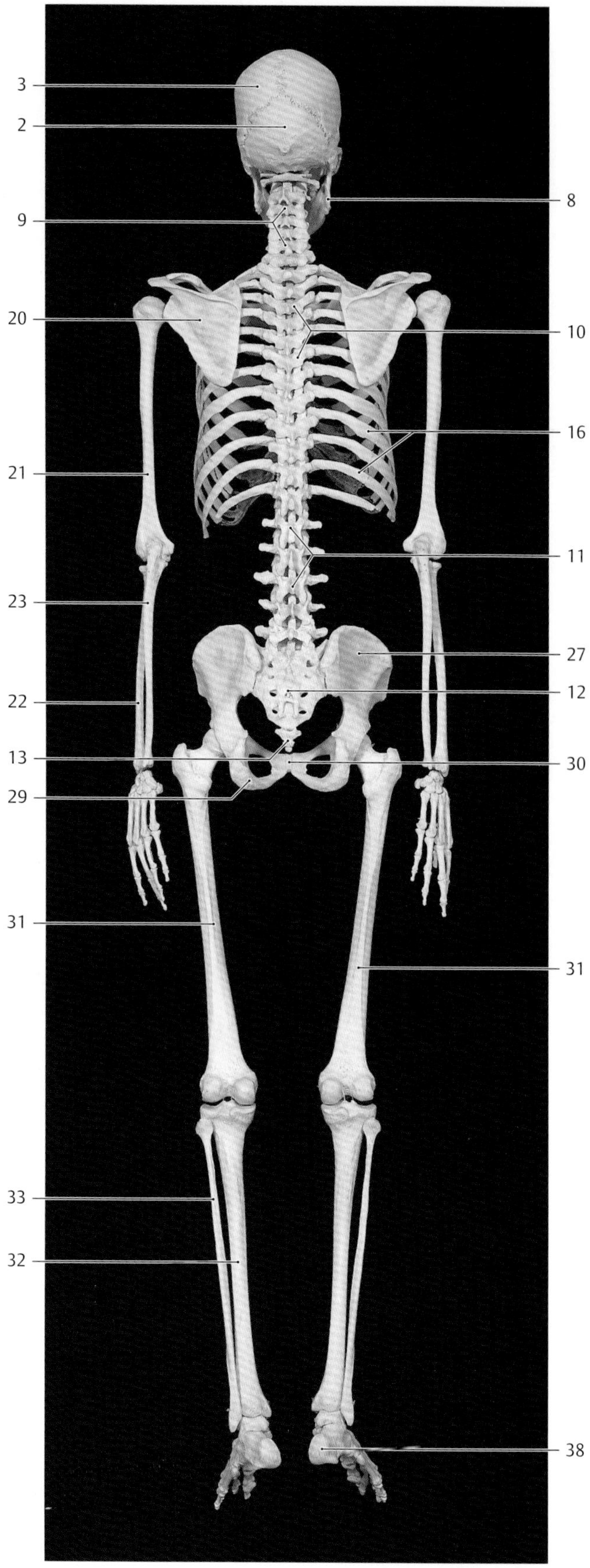

Fig. 1.14 **Skeleton of a female adult** (posterior aspect).

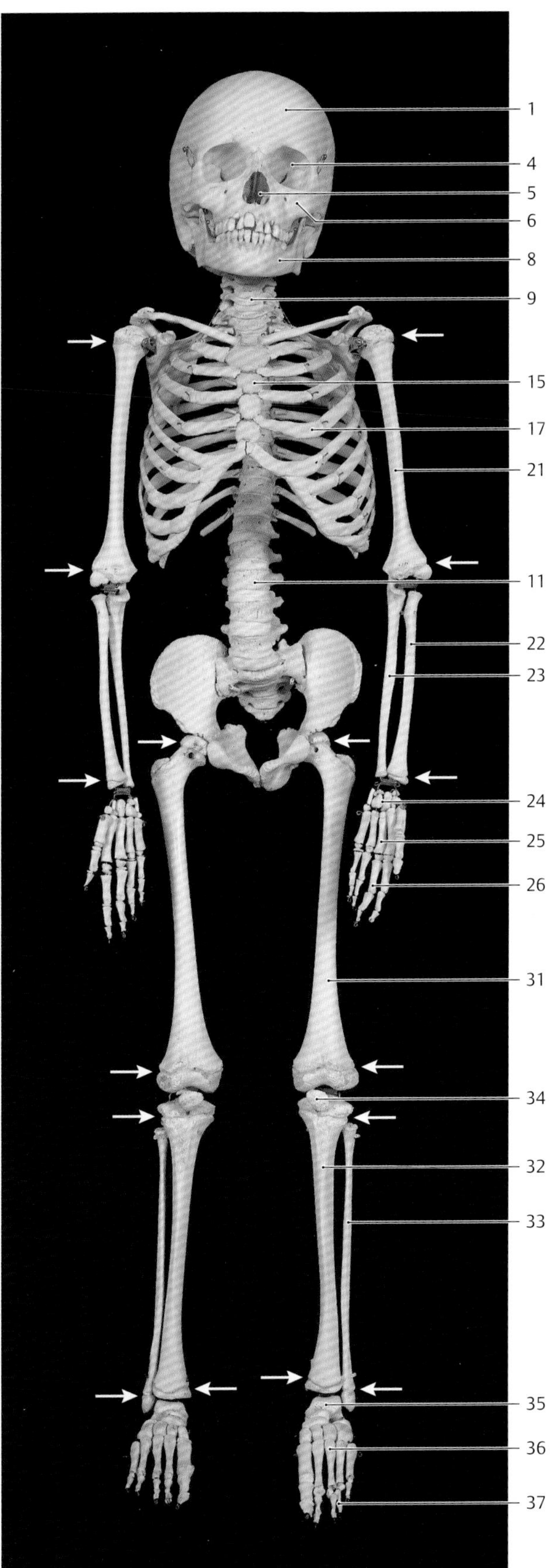


Fig. 1.15 **Skeleton of a 5-year-old child** (anterior aspect).
The zones of the cartilaginous growth plates are seen (arrows). In contrast to the adult, the ribs show a predominantly horizontal position.

**AXIAL SKELETON**

**Head**

1 Frontal bone
2 Occipital bone
3 Parietal bone
4 Orbit
5 Nasal cavity
6 Maxilla
7 Zygomatic bone
8 Mandible

**TRUNK AND THORAX**

**Vertebral column**

9 Cervical vertebrae
10 Thoracic vertebrae
11 Lumbar vertebrae
12 Sacrum
13 Coccyx
14 Intervertebral discs

**Thorax**

15 Sternum
16 Ribs
17 Costal cartilage
18 Infrasternal angle

**APPENDICULAR SKELETON**

**Upper limb and shoulder girdle**

19 Clavicle
20 Scapula
21 Humerus
22 Radius
23 Ulna
24 Carpal bones
25 Metacarpal bones
26 Phalanges of the hand

**Lower limb and pelvis**

27 Ilium
28 Pubis
29 Ischium
30 Pubic symphysis
31 Femur
32 Tibia
33 Fibula
34 Patella
35 Tarsal bones
36 Metatarsal bones
37 Phalanges of the foot
38 Calcaneus

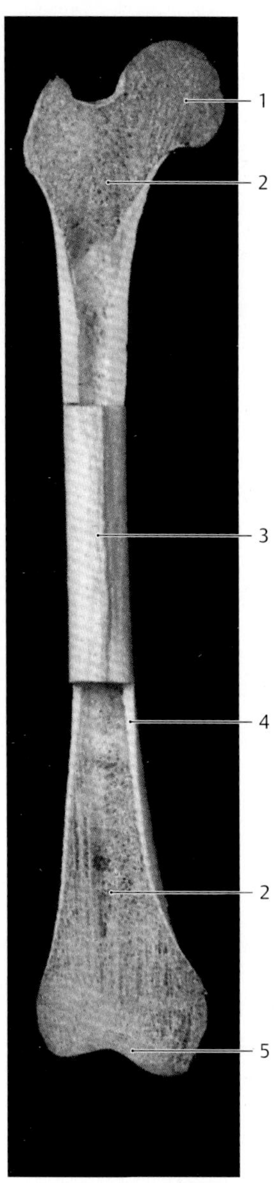


Fig. 1.16 **Femur of the adult.** Coronal section of the proximal and distal epiphyses displaying the spongy bone and the medullary cavity.

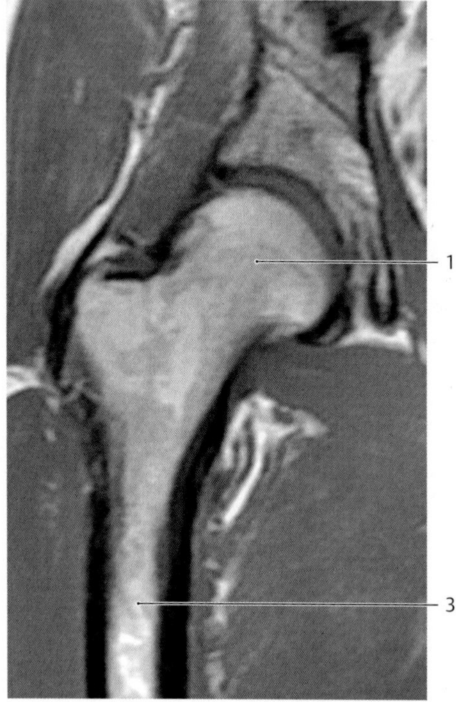


Fig. 1.17 **MRI scan of the right femur and hip joint** (coronal section). (Heuck A, et al. MRT-Atlas des muskuloskelettalen Systems. Stuttgart, Germany: Schattauer, 2009.)

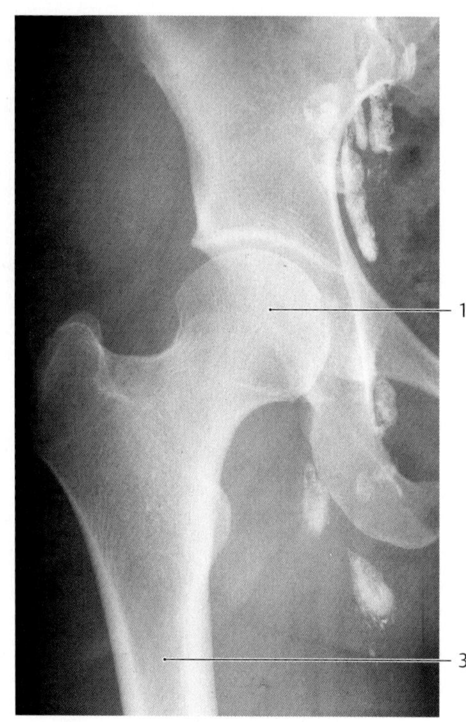


Fig. 1.18 **X-ray of the right femur and hip joint** (antero-posterior direction). (Courtesy of Prof. Uder, Institute of Radiology, University Hospital Erlangen, Germany.)

1 Head of the femur
2 Spongy bone
3 Diaphysis of the femur
4 Compact bone
5 Articular cartilage

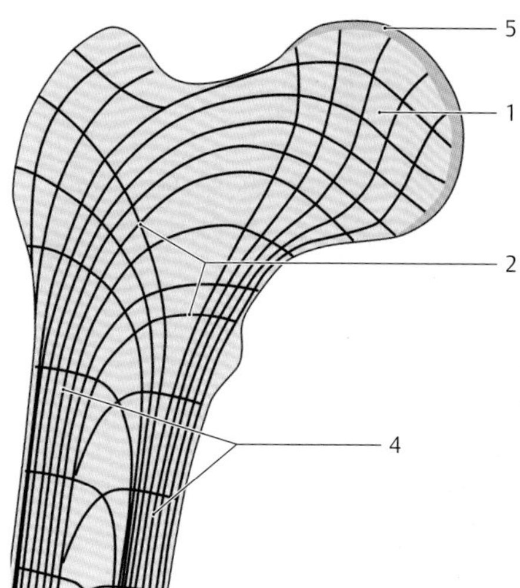


Fig. 1.19 **Three-dimensional representation of the trajectorial lines of the femoral head.**

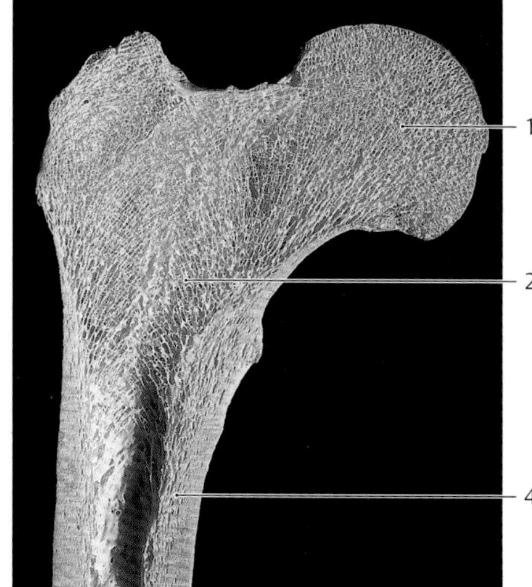


Fig. 1.20 **Coronal section through the proximal end of the adult femur** showing the characteristic structure of the spongy bone.

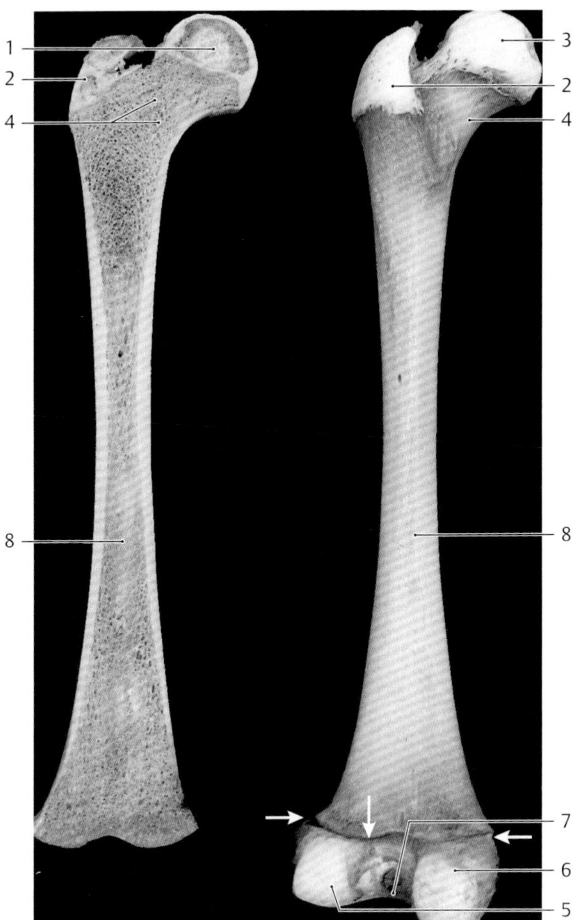

**Fig. 1.21 Ossification of the femur** (coronal section [left]; posterior aspect of femur [right]). The ossification of the bones of the limbs starts within the ossification centers of the primary cartilagenous bones. Here, the medullary cavity develops. The ossification process of limb bones is not finished at birth (see Figs. 1.22 and 1.23). Arrows = distal epiphysis.

1 Ossification center in the head of the femur
2 Greater trochanter
3 Head of the femur
4 Neck of the femur
5 Lateral condyle
6 Medial condyle
7 Intercondylar notch
8 Diaphysis

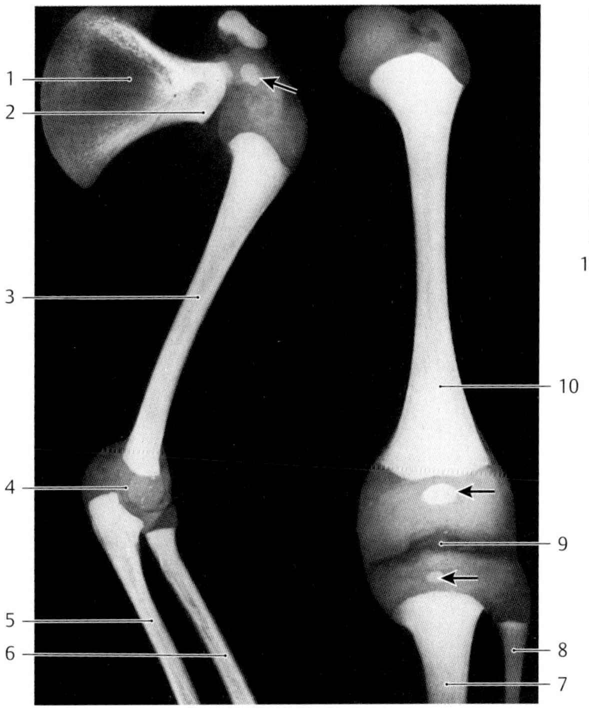

1 Scapula
2 Shoulder joint
3 Humerus
4 Elbow joint
5 Ulna
6 Radius
7 Tibia
8 Fibula
9 Knee joint
10 Femur

**Fig. 1.22 X-ray of the upper and lower limb of a newborn child** (upper limb [left], lower limb [right]). Arrows = ossification centers.

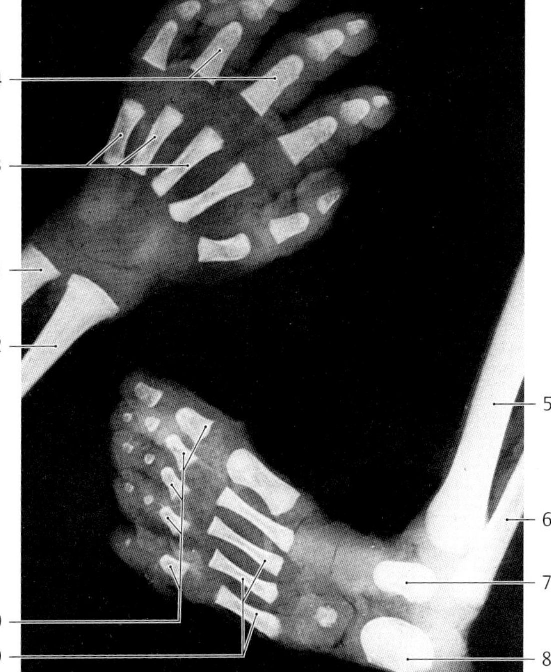

1 Ulna
2 Radius
3 Metacarpal bones
4 Phalanges of the hand
5 Tibia
6 Fibula
7 Talus
8 Calcaneus
9 Metatarsal bones
10 Phalanges of the foot

**Fig. 1.23 X-ray of hand and foot of a newborn.** Ossification of the joints has not yet been achieved. Wrist and tarsal bones are still more or less cartilaginous.

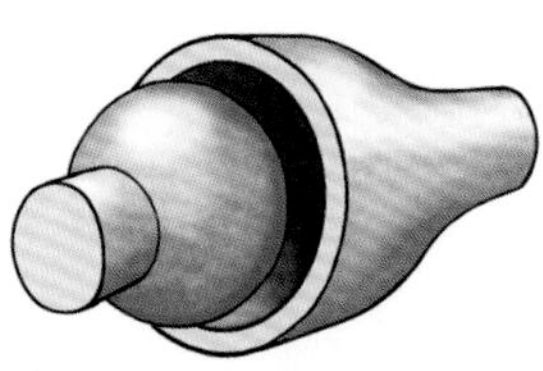

Fig. 1.24 **Ball-and-socket joint** (e.g., shoulder joint). This type of joint has three axes of movement.

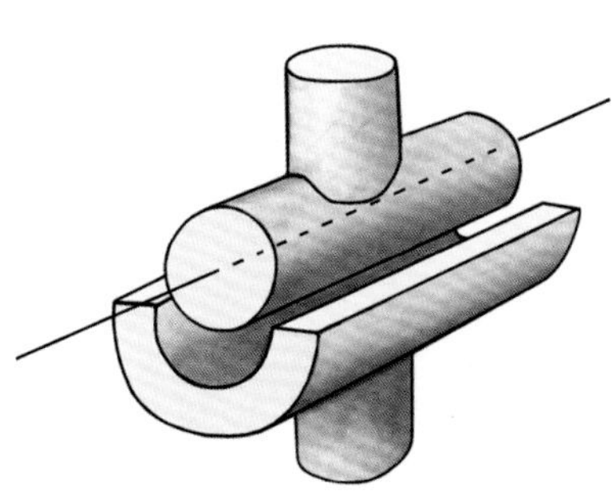

Fig. 1.25 **Hinge joint,** monoaxial (e.g., humero-ulnar joint).

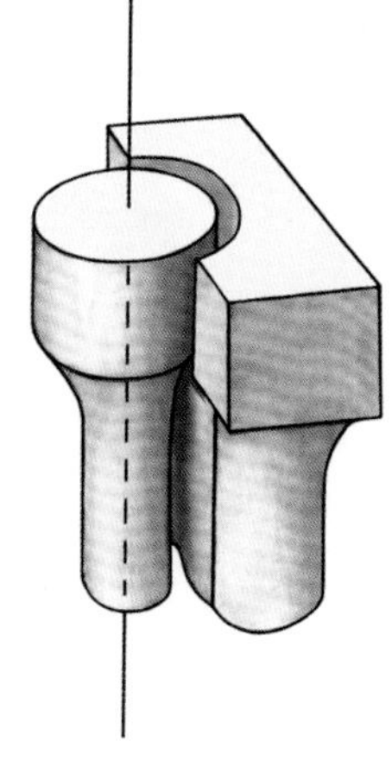

Fig. 1.26 **Pivot joint,** monoaxial (e.g., radio-ulnar joint).

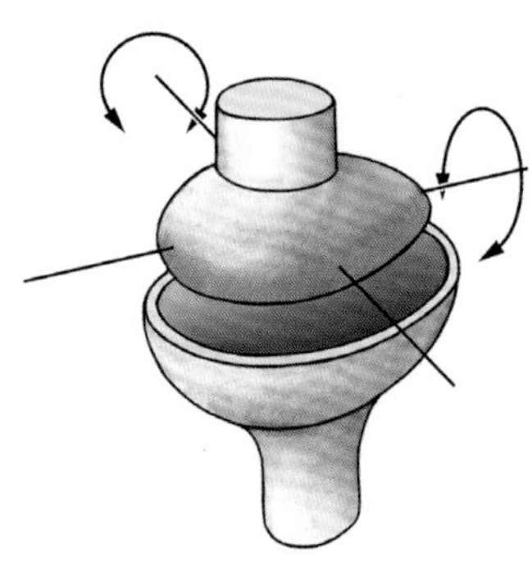

Fig. 1.27 **Condyloid joint,** biaxial (e.g., radiocarpal joint of hand).

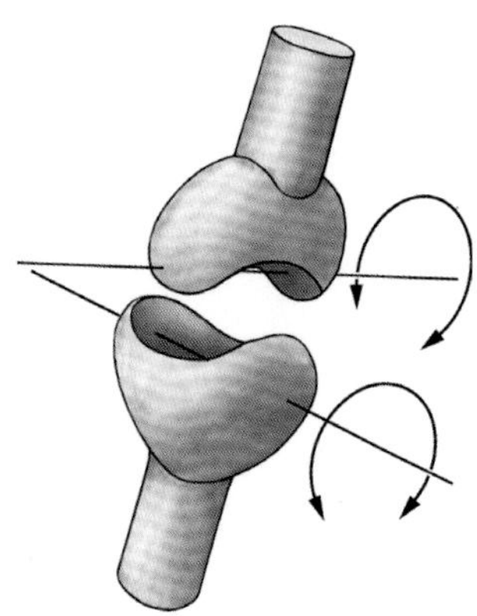

Fig. 1.28 **Saddle joint,** biaxial (e.g., carpometacarpal joint of thumb).

Joints exhibit a variety of functions. In general, mobility becomes reduced in the direction from proximal to distal. For example, the hip joint is multiaxial, the knee joint is biaxial, and the joints of toes and fingers are monaxial.

The number of articulating bones increases in the direction from proximal to distal: There are only two bones articulating in the shoulder joint but three in the elbow joint, four in the wrist joint, and five in the finger joints. So the range of motion of a singular joint becomes reduced, but the variety of individual positions is increasing.

A Ball-and-socket-joint
B Hinge joint
C Pivot joint
D Condyloid joint
E Saddle joint

1 Humerus
2 Radius
3 Ulna
4 Metacarpo-phalangeal joint
5 Joints of fingers

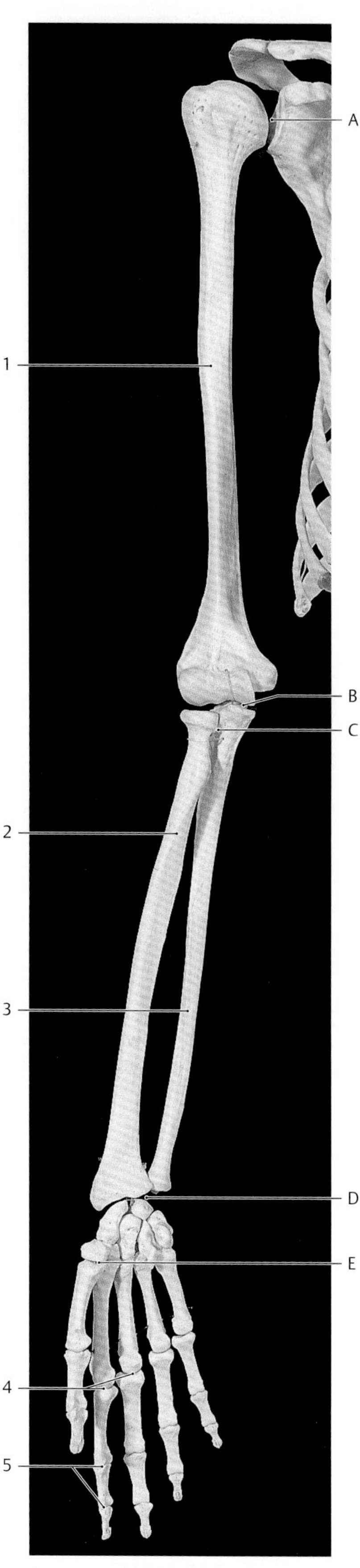


Fig. 1.29 **Skeleton of the arm and shoulder girdle** (anterior aspect).

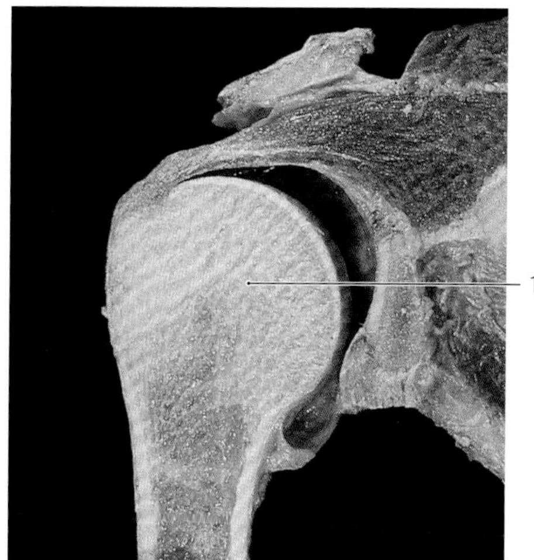


**Fig. 1.30 Shoulder joint** as an example of a multiaxial ball-and-socket joint (coronal section).

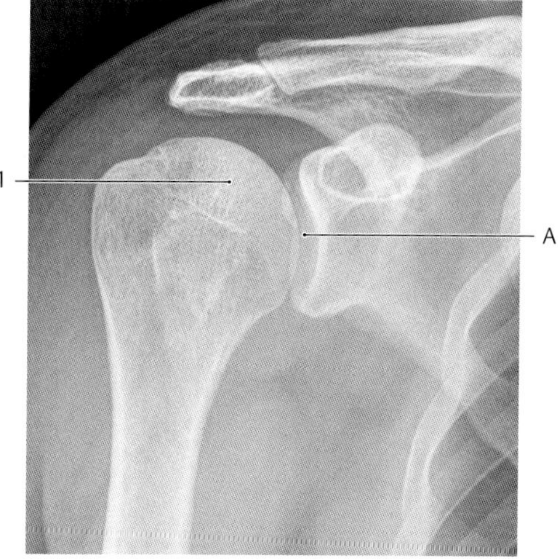


**Fig. 1.31 X-ray of a shoulder joint.** (Courtesy of Prof. Uder, Institute of Radiology, University Hospital Erlangen, Germany.)

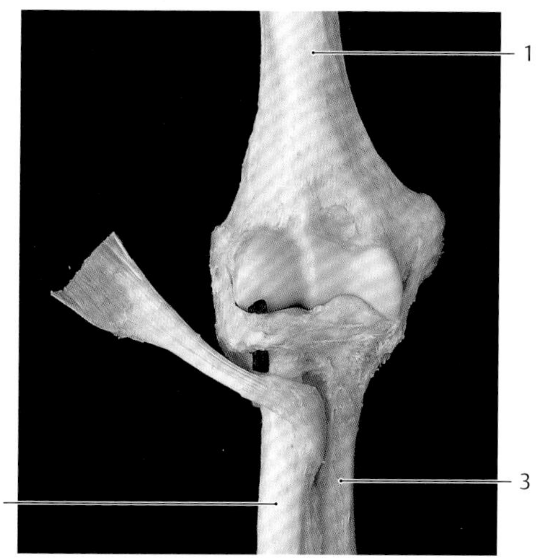


**Fig. 1.32 Elbow joint with ligaments** as an example of a hinge joint (monaxial humero-ulnar joint).

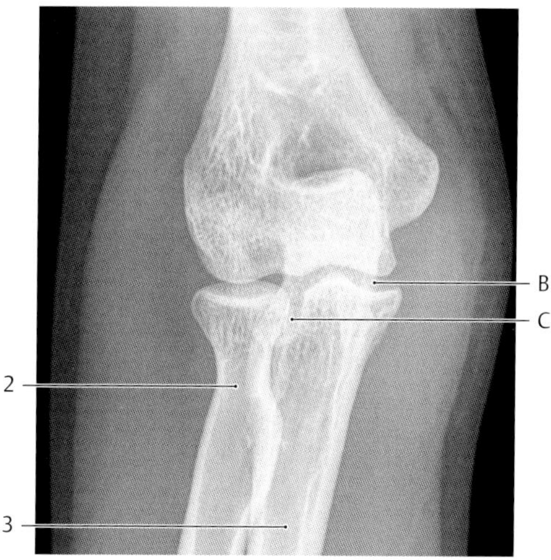


**Fig. 1.33 X-ray of an elbow joint.** (Courtesy of Prof. Uder, Institute of Radiology, University Hospital Erlangen, Germany.)

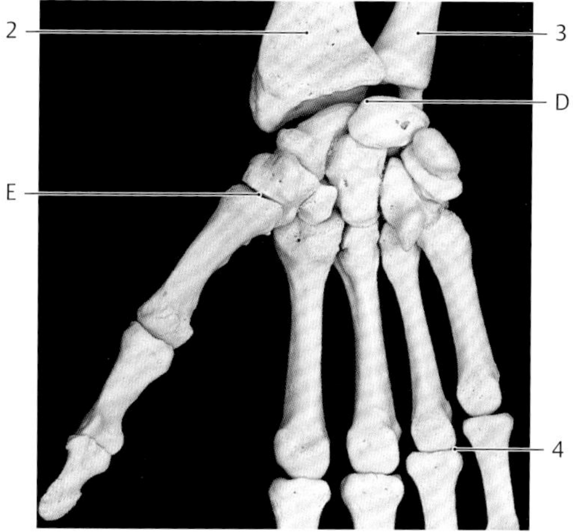


**Fig. 1.34 Wrist joint** as an example of a condyloid joint; carpometacarpal joint of the thumb as an example of a saddle joint.

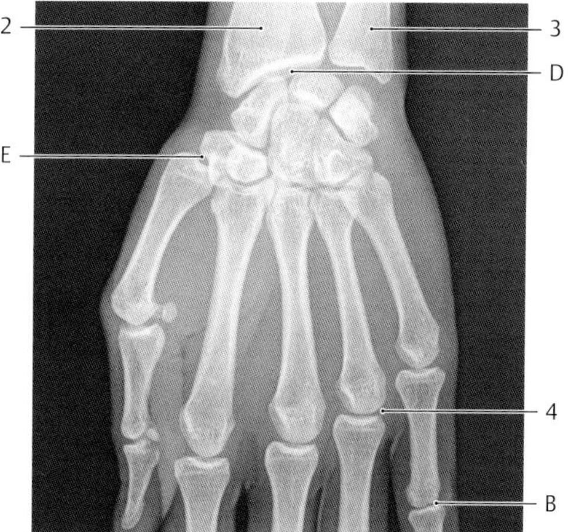


**Fig. 1.35 X-ray of a wrist joint.** (Courtesy of Prof. Uder, Institute of Radiology, University Hospital Erlangen, Germany.)

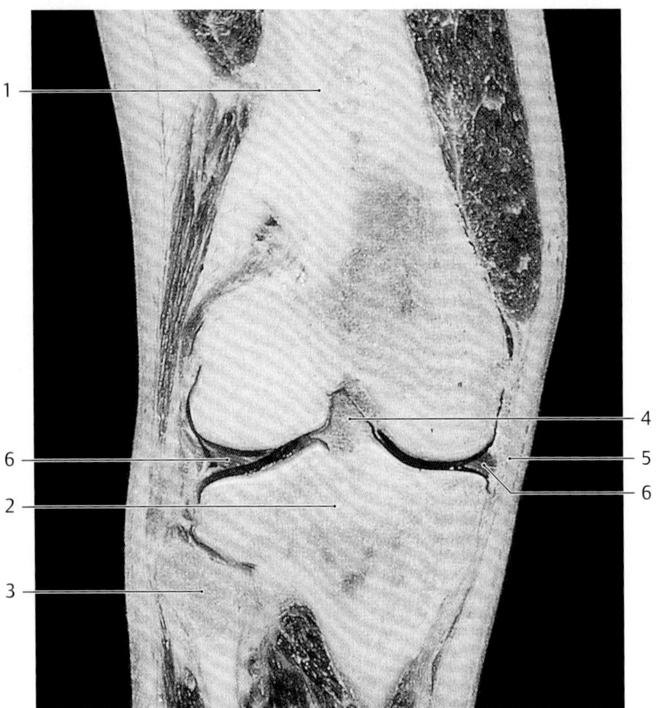


Fig. 1.36 **Coronal section through the knee joint** (anterior aspect of the right joint in extension).

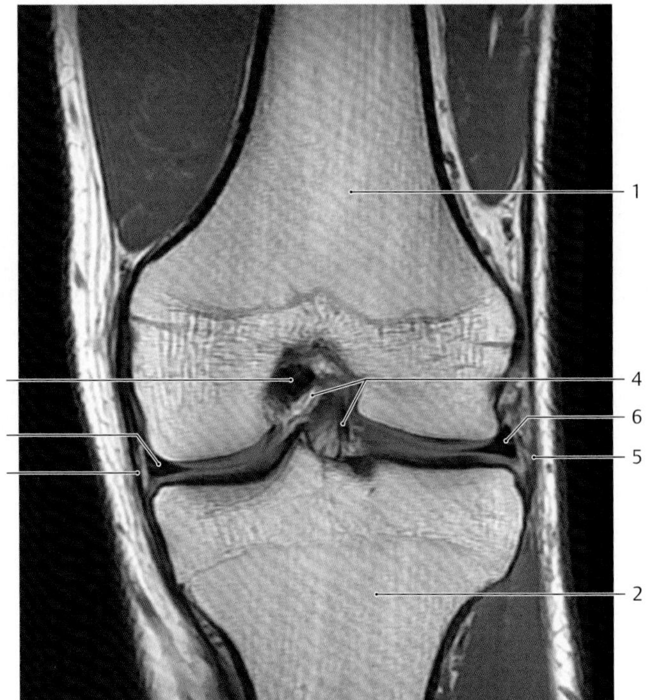


Fig. 1.37 **Coronal section through the knee joint** (MRI scan). (Heuck A, et al. MRT-Atlas des muskuloskelettalen Systems. Stuttgart, Germany: Schattauer, 2009.)

1 Femur
2 Tibia
3 Fibula
4 Cruciate ligaments
5 Collateral ligaments
6 Menisci

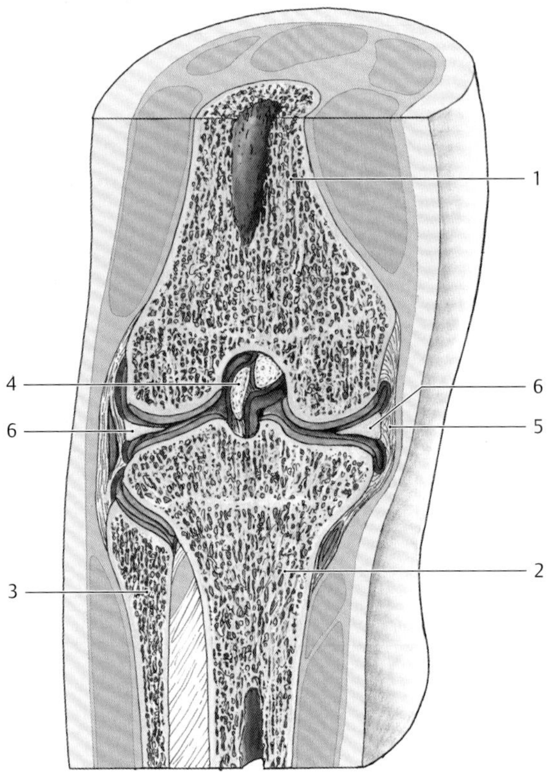


Fig. 1.38 **Schematic drawing of the knee joint** as an example of a synovial joint, characterized by a joint cavity enclosed by a joint-capsule (red) containing synovial fluid. Blue = articular cartilage.

**Joints** are places of articulation allowing movements between bones. Synovial joints are characterized by a joint cavity enclosed by a joint capsule containing synovial fluid, which is produced by the articular capsule. The kind of movements depends not only on form and structure of the articulating bones but also on ligaments incorporated into the articular capsule. In some synovial joints, fibrocartilagenous articular discs develop, when the articulating surfaces of the bones are incongruous.

---

The human body possesses **a great variety of muscles**. The architecture of the muscles depends on the functional systems in which they are involved, i.e., the kind of movements, the form of the joints with their specific ligaments, etc. The movements themselves vary to a great extent individually.

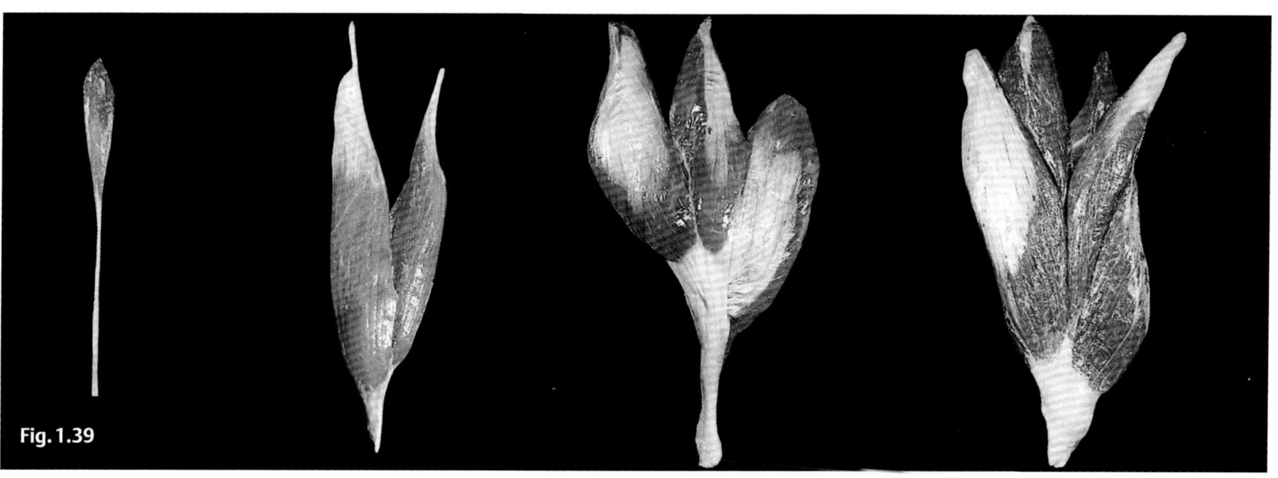


**Fusiform** (palmaris longus) | **Bicipital** (biceps brachii) | **Tricipital** (triceps surae, gastrocnemius, and soleus) | **Quadricipital** (quadriceps femoris)

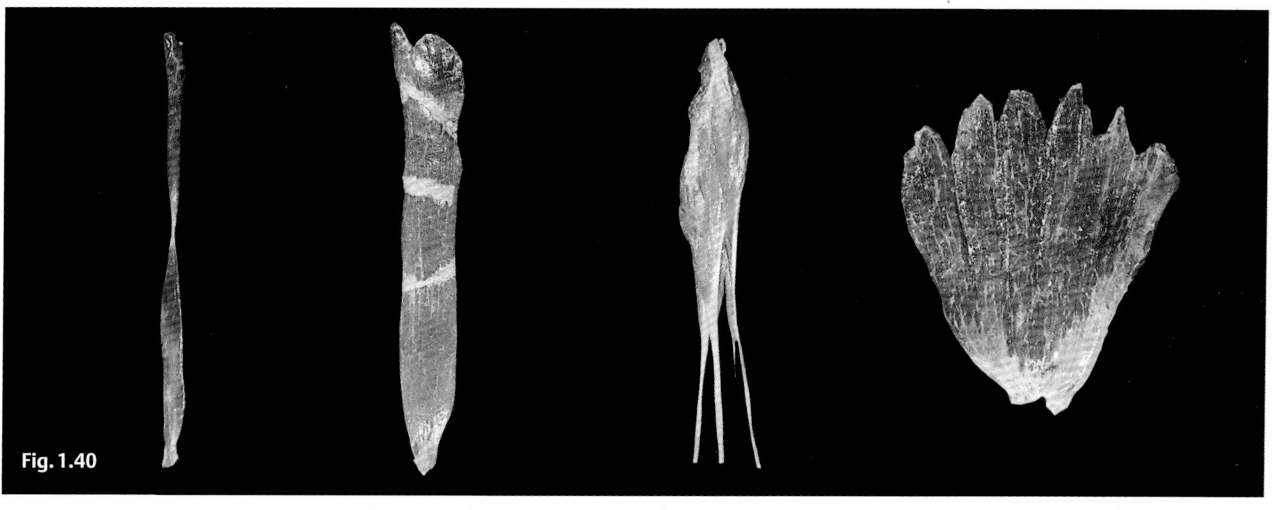


**Digastric** (omohyoideus) | **Multiventral** (rectus abdominis) | **Multicaudal** (flexor digitorum prof.) | **Serrated** (serratus anterior)

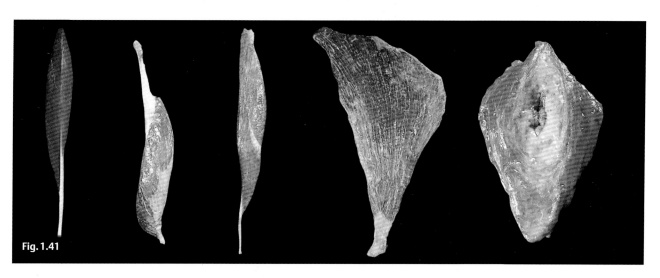


**Bipennate** (tibialis anterior) | **Unipennate** (semimembranosus) | **Semitendinous** (semitendinosus) | **Broad, flat muscle** (latissimus dorsi) | **Ring-like** (sphincter ani externus)

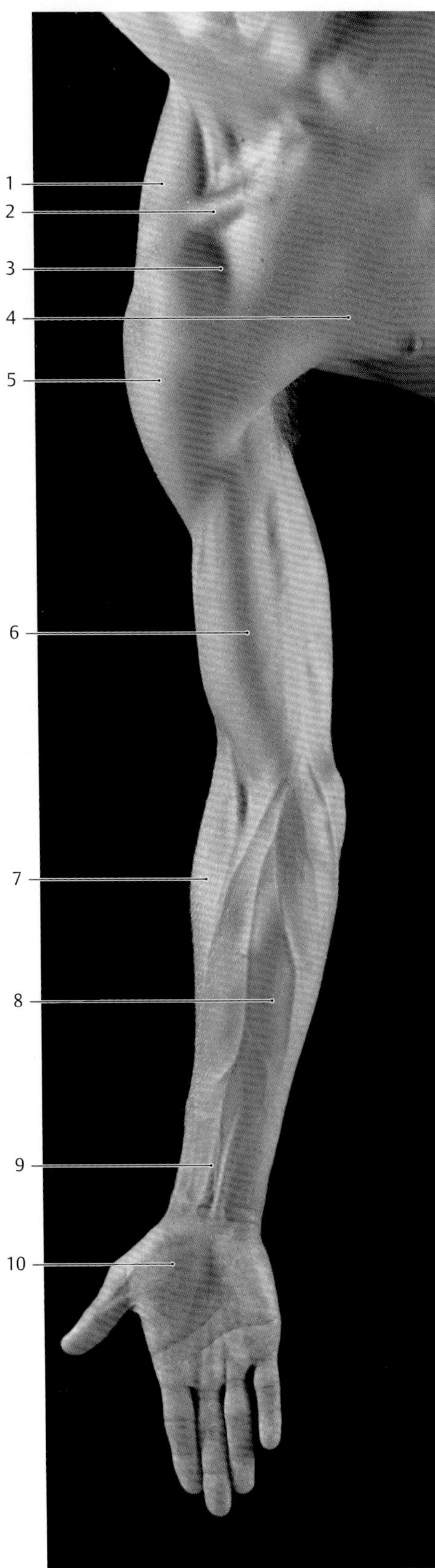


Fig. 1.42 **Surface anatomy of the upper limb.** (right side, anterior aspect).

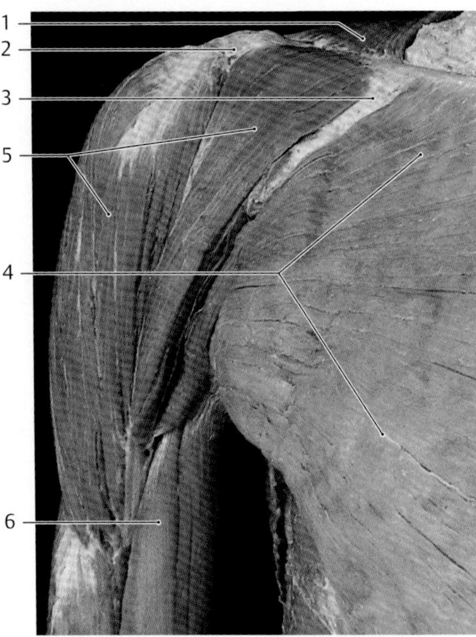


Fig. 1.43 **Muscles of shoulder and arm,** superficial layer (right side, anterior aspect).

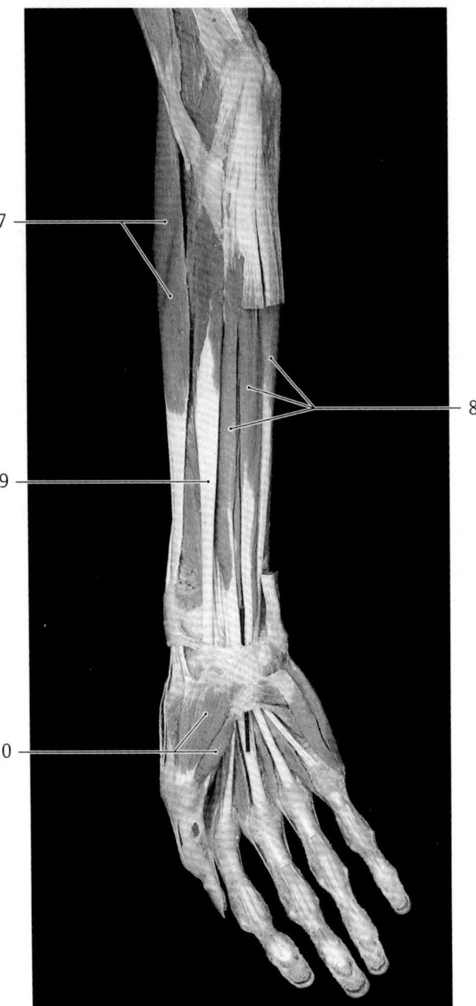


Fig. 1.44 **Flexor muscles of forearm and hand,** superficial layer (right side, anterior aspect).

1 Trapezius muscle
2 Clavicle
3 Deltopectoral triangle
4 Pectoralis major muscle
5 Deltoid muscle
6 Biceps brachii muscle
7 Brachioradialis muscle
8 Flexor digitorum superficialis muscle
9 Tendon of flexor carpi radialis
10 Thenar muscles

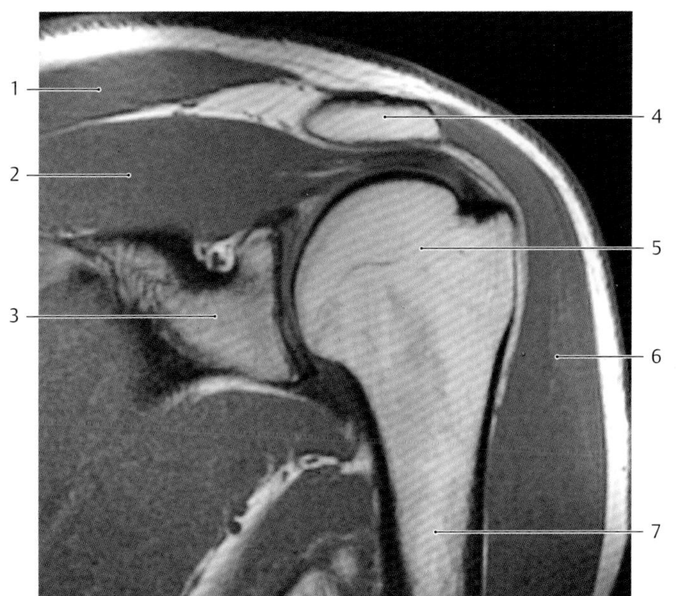


Fig. 1.45 **Frontal section through the shoulder joint** (MRI scan). (Heuck A, et al. MRT-Atlas des muskuloskelettalen Systems. Stuttgart, Germany: Schattauer, 2009.)

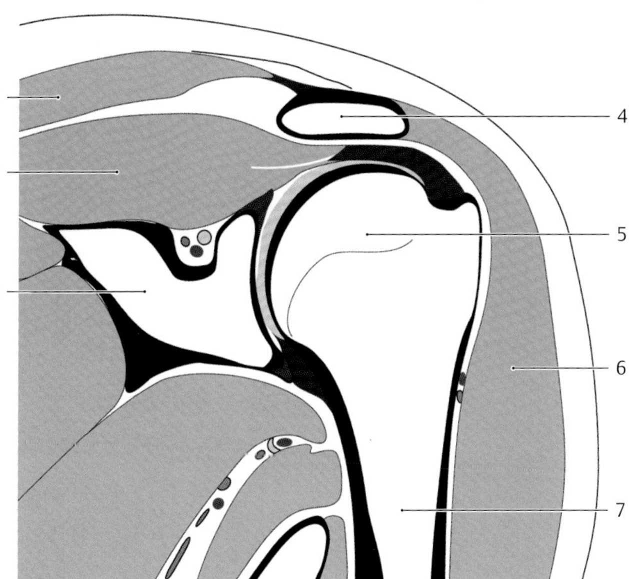


Fig. 1.46 **Frontal section through the shoulder joint** (schematic drawing of the MRI scan on the left). (Heuck A, et al. MRT-Atlas des muskuloskelettalen Systems. Stuttgart, Germany: Schattauer, 2009.)

Joints are moved by muscles. The highly differentiated movements are coordinated by special groups of muscles (synergists). Their counterparts are called antagonists. Movements can only be carried out harmoniously if the contraction of the **synergists** are supported by a corresponding dilatation of the **antagonists**. This interaction is controlled by the nervous system. In order to carry out certain directions of movements, often the tendons of muscles have to be directed by ligaments. At those places, the tendons often develop synovial sheaths, e.g., at the wrist joint or at the fingers.

1 Trapezius muscle
2 Supraspinatus muscle
3 Scapula
4 Acromion
5 Head of humerus
6 Deltoid muscle
7 Humerus
8 Biceps brachii muscle
9 Brachialis muscle
10 Brachioradialis muscle
11 Radius
12 Ulna
13 Triceps brachii muscle

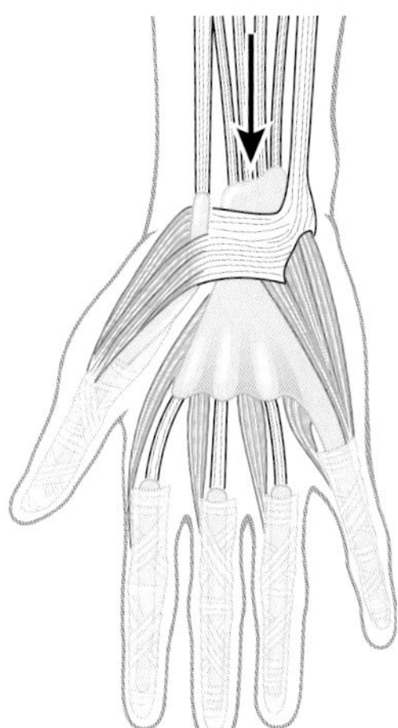

Fig. 1.47 **Synovial sheaths of flexor tendons** (palmar aspect of the right hand). The flexor retinaculum protects the flexor tendons passing through the carpal tunnel (arrow).

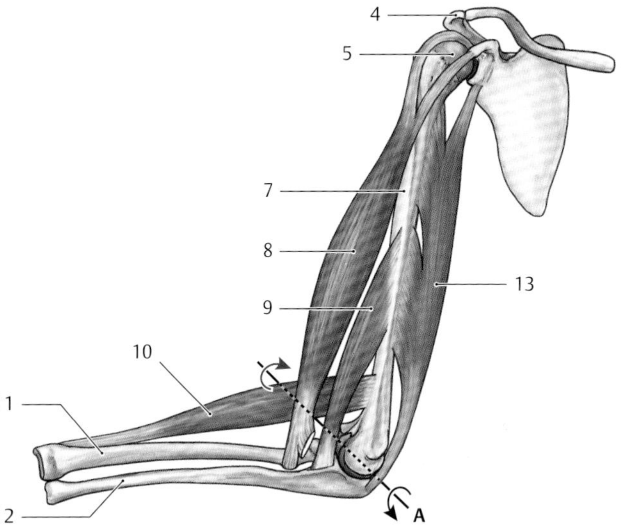


Fig. 1.48 **Diagram illustrating the position of the flexor and extensor muscles of the arm** and their effect on the elbow joint. A = axis of humero-ulnar joint; arrows = direction of movements; red = flexion; black = extension.

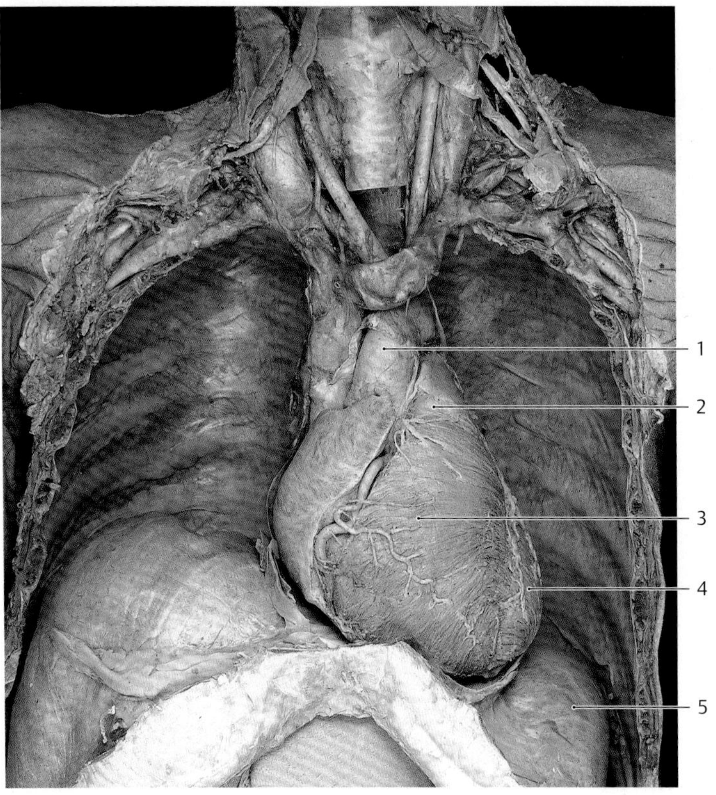


Fig. 1.49 **Heart and related vessels in situ** (anterior aspect). Anterior thoracic wall, pericardium, and epicardium have been removed.

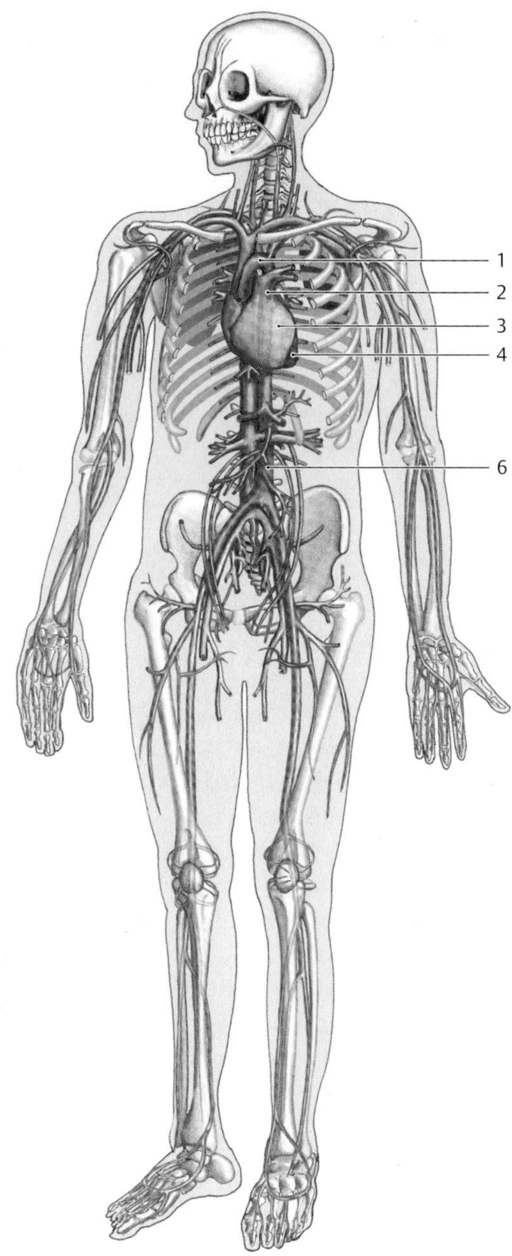


1 Aorta
2 Pulmonary artery
3 Right heart
4 Left heart
5 Diaphragm
6 Abdominal aorta

Fig. 1.51 **Organization of the circulatory system with the heart in the center** (anterior aspect). Red = arteries; blue = veins.

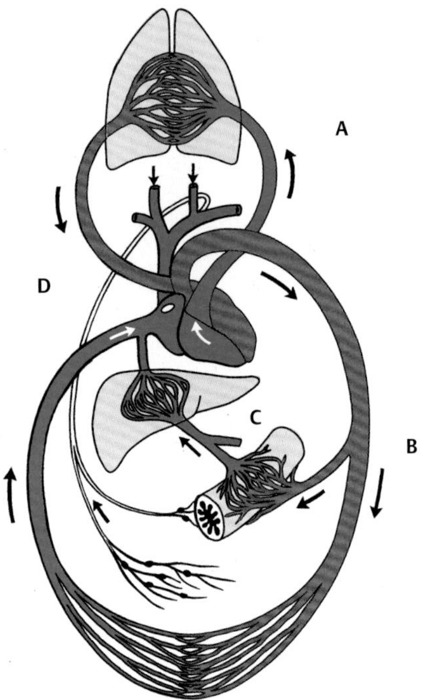


Fig. 1.50 **Organization of the circulatory systems in the human body.** The center of this system represents the heart. Red = arteries; blue = veins.

A = Pulmonary circulation C = Portal circulation
B = Systemic circulation D = Lymphatic circulation

The center of the circulatory system is the heart, which is situated in the thoracic cavity and in contact with the diaphragm. In the right ventricle, the venous blood is collected and pumped through the pulmonary artery and into the lung where the blood is oxygenated. The veins of the lung transport the blood to the left ventricle, where it is pumped through the aorta and its branches (arteries) in the human body. Arteries and veins mostly run parallel. The venous blood from the intestine reaches the liver via the portal vein (portal circulation).

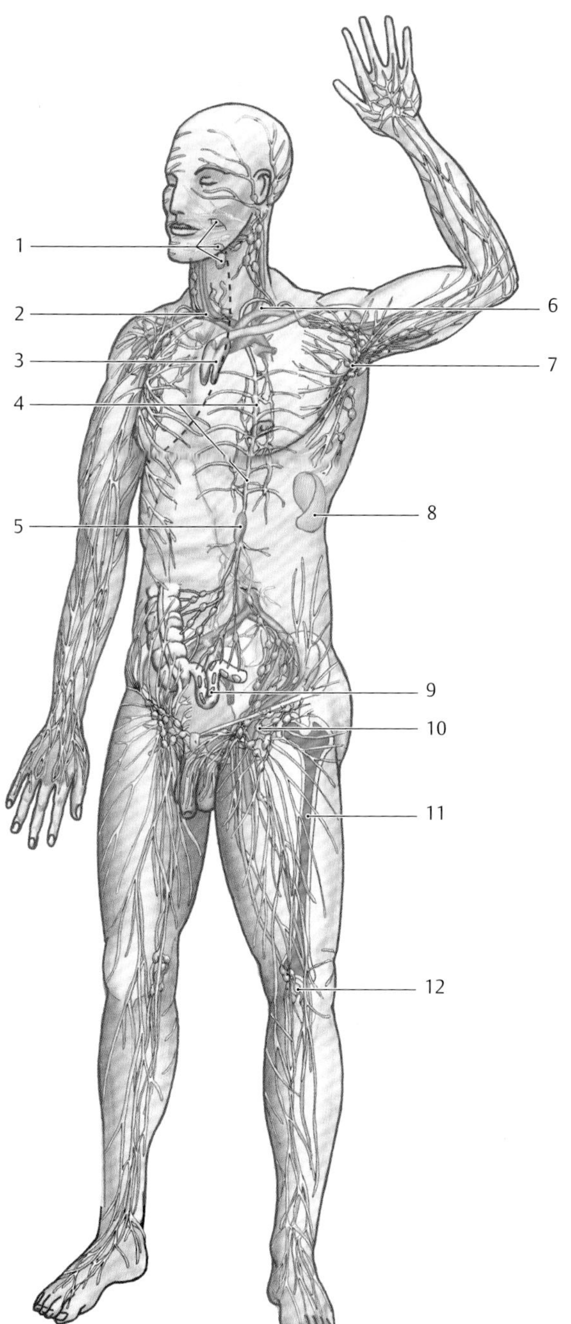


Fig. 1.52 **Organization of the lymphatic system** (anterior aspect). Course of the main lymphatic vessels and location of the most important lymph nodes in the body. Red line = border between the lymphatic vessels draining to the left and right venous angles.

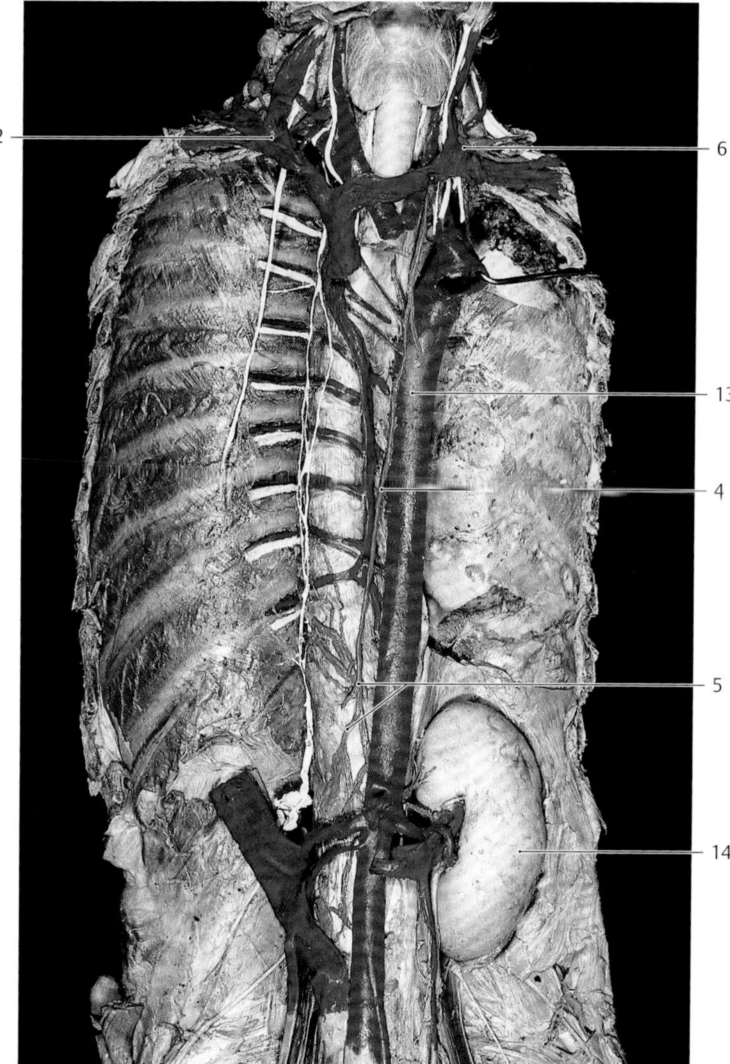


Fig. 1.53 **Major lymph vessels of the trunk** (green). Blue = veins; red = arteries; white = nerves.

1 Tonsils and submandibular lymph nodes
2 Right venous angle
3 Remnants of the thymus gland
4 Thoracic duct
5 Cisterna chyli
6 Left venous angle with drainage form the thoracic duct
7 Axillary lymph nodes
8 Spleen
9 Lymph nodes of the intestinal tract
10 Inguinal lymph nodes
11 Bone marrow
12 Lymph nodes of the popliteal fossa
13 Aorta
14 Left kidney

Lymphatic vessels originate in the tissue spaces (lymph capillaries) and unite to form larger vessels (lymphatics). These resemble veins but have a much thinner wall, more valves, and are interrupted by lymph nodes at various intervals. Large groups of lymph nodes are located in the inguinal and axillary regions, deep to the mandible and sternocleidomastoid muscle, and within the root of the mesentery of the intestine. The lymphatic vessels of the right half of the head and neck, the right thorax, and the right upper limb drain toward the right venous angle; those of the rest of the body, toward the left venous angle. The border between both is indicated by the red line in Figure 1.52.

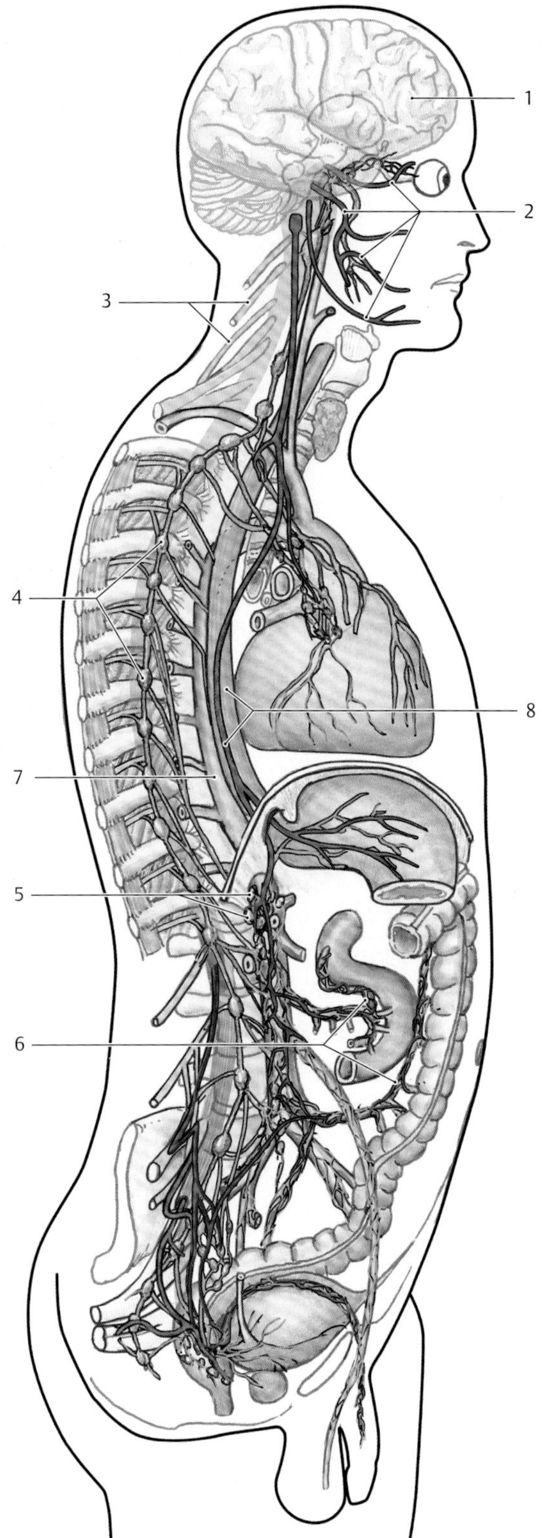


Fig. 1.54 **Diagram illustrating the localization of the three functional portions of the nervous system** (brain, spinal cord and autonomic nervous system). Yellow and green = sympathetic system; red = parasympathetic system.

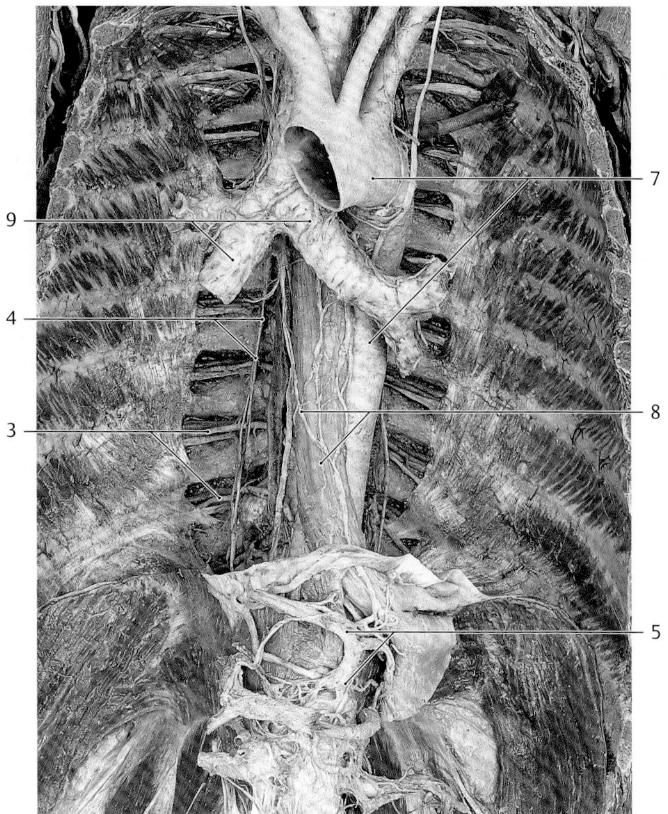


Fig. 1.55 **Posterior part of the trunk.** The solar plexus with its connection to the vagus nerve and the sympathetic trunk has been dissected.

1 Cerebrum
2 Cranial nerves
3 Spinal nerves
4 Sympathetic trunk
5 Solar plexus
6 Nervous plexus of the autonomic system
7 Aorta
8 Vagus nerve and esophagus
9 Bifurcation of trachea

The nervous system can be divided into three functionally distinct parts:

1. The cranial part, which comprises the great sensory organs and the brain.
2. The spinal cord, which shows a segmental structure and serves predominantly as a reflex organ.
3. The autonomic nervous system, which controls the involuntary functions (subconscious control) of organs and tissues. The autonomic part of the nervous system forms many delicate plexuses near or within the organs. At certain places these plexuses contain aggregations of nerve cells (prevertebral and intramural ganglia).

The spinal nerves leave the spinal cord at regular intervals.The ventral rami of the spinal nerves form the cervical and brachial plexus, which innervates the upper extremity, and the ventral rami of the lumbar and sacral spinal nerves form the lumbosacral plexus, which innervates the pelvis and genital organs and the lower extremity.

# 2 Trunk

## General Anatomy and Musculoskeletal System

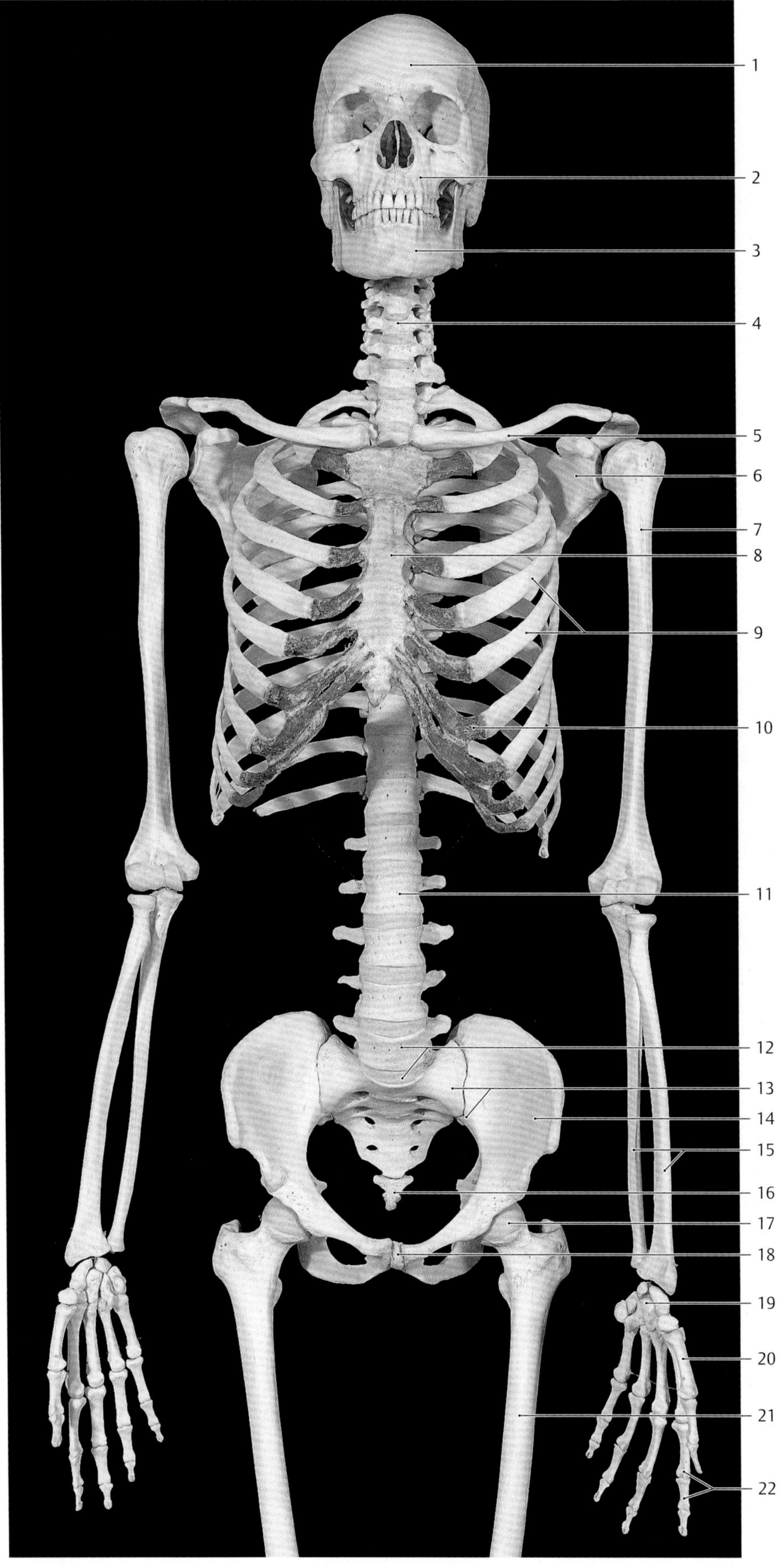


1 Frontal bone
2 Maxilla
3 Mandible
4 Cervical vertebrae
5 Clavicle
6 Scapula
7 Humerus
8 Sternum
9 Ribs
10 Costal cartilage
11 Lumbar vertebrae
12 Lumbar vertebra (L5) and promontory
13 Sacrum
14 Hip bone
15 Radius and ulna
16 Coccyx
17 Head of femur
18 Pubic symphysis
19 Carpal bones
20 Metacarpal bones
21 Femur
22 Phalanges

Fig. 2.1 **Skeleton of the trunk** with head, vertebral column, thorax, pelvis, and upper limb (anterior aspect).

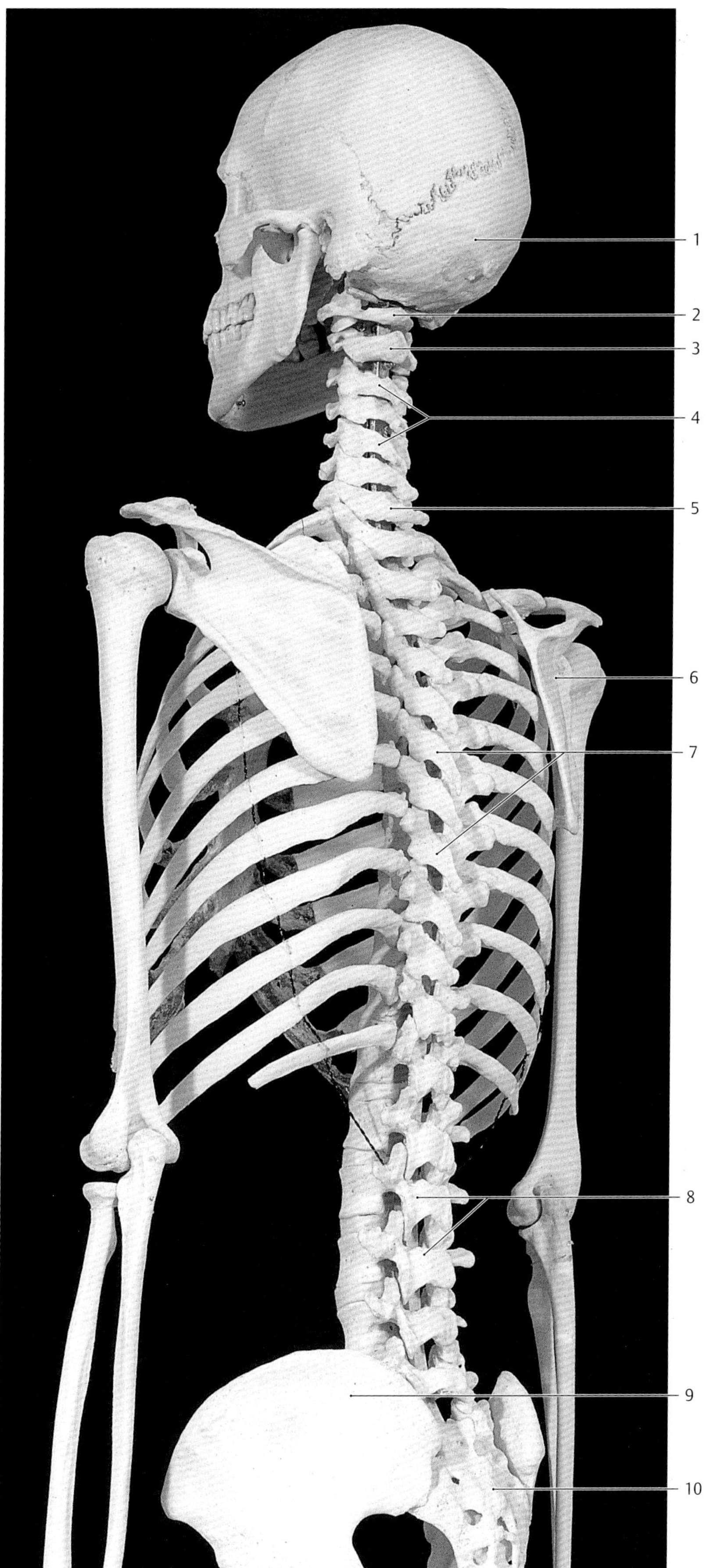


1 Occipital bone
2 Atlas
3 Axis
4 Cervical vertebrae
5 Vertebra prominens (C7)
6 Scapula
7 Thoracic vertebrae
8 Lumbar vertebrae
9 Hip bone
10 Sacrum

Fig. 2.2 **Skeleton of the trunk** with head, vertebral column, thorax, pelvis, and shoulder girdle (oblique-posterior aspect).

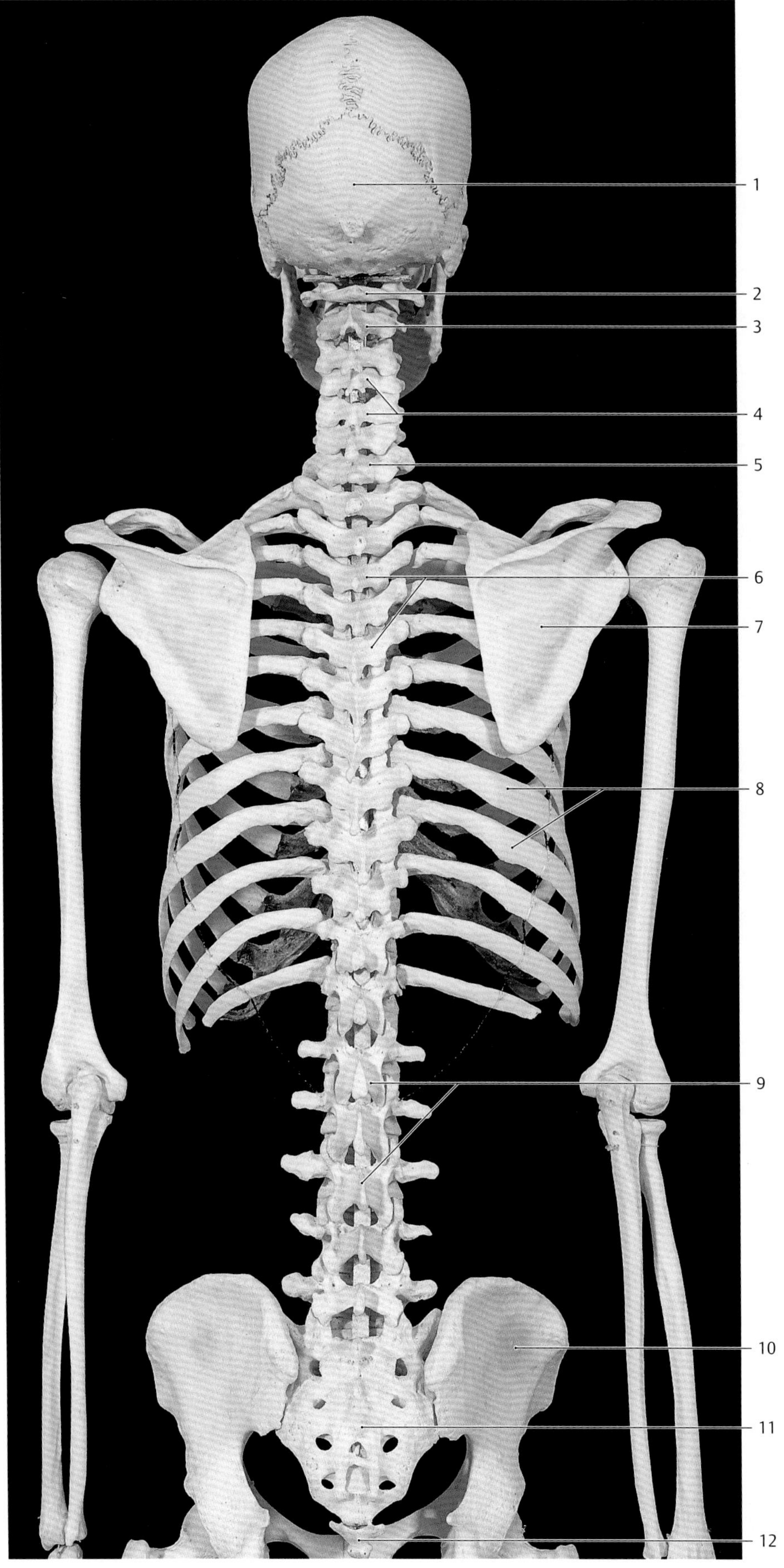


1 Occipital bone
2 Atlas
3 Axis
4 Cervical vertebrae (C4 and C5)
5 Vertebra prominens (C7)
6 Thoracic vertebrae (T3 and T5)
7 Scapula
8 Ribs 8 and 9
9 Lumbar vertebrae (L1 and L3)
10 Hip bone
11 Sacrum
12 Coccyx

Fig. 2.3 **Skeleton of the trunk** with head, vertebral column, thorax, pelvis, and shoulder girdle (posterior aspect). Note how the spine is connected to the occipital bone and to the hip bone.

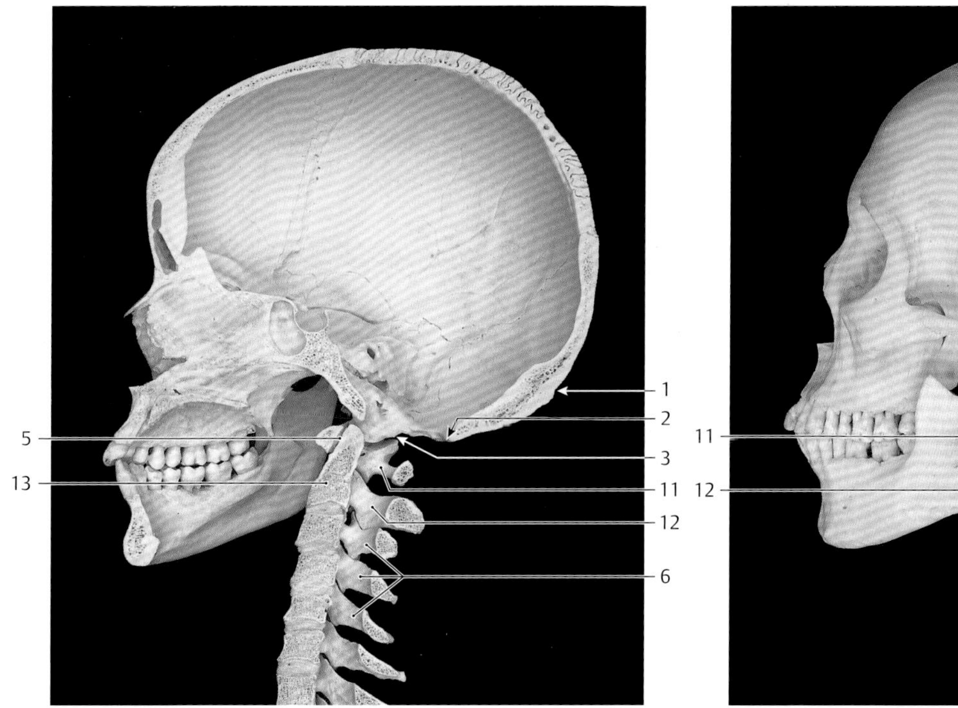


Fig. 2.4 **Cervical vertebral column in relation to the head** (midsagittal section, medial aspect).

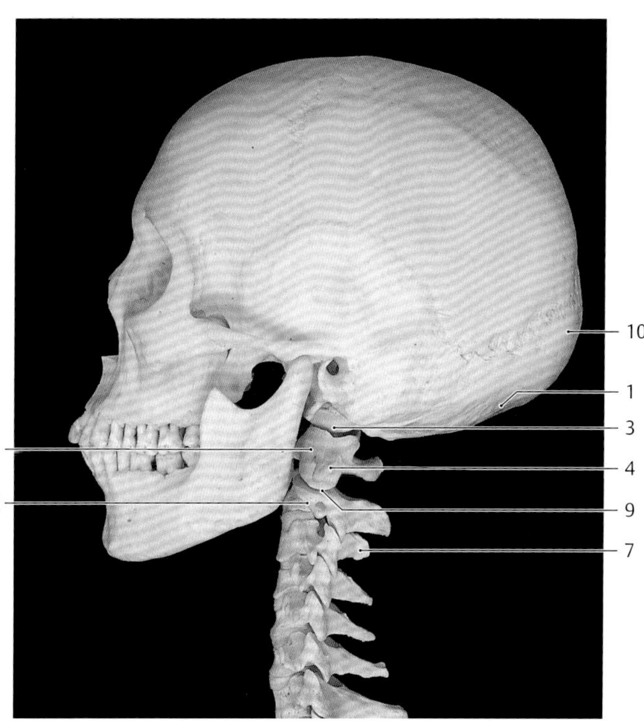


Fig. 2.5 **Atlas and axis in relation to the head** (lateral aspect).

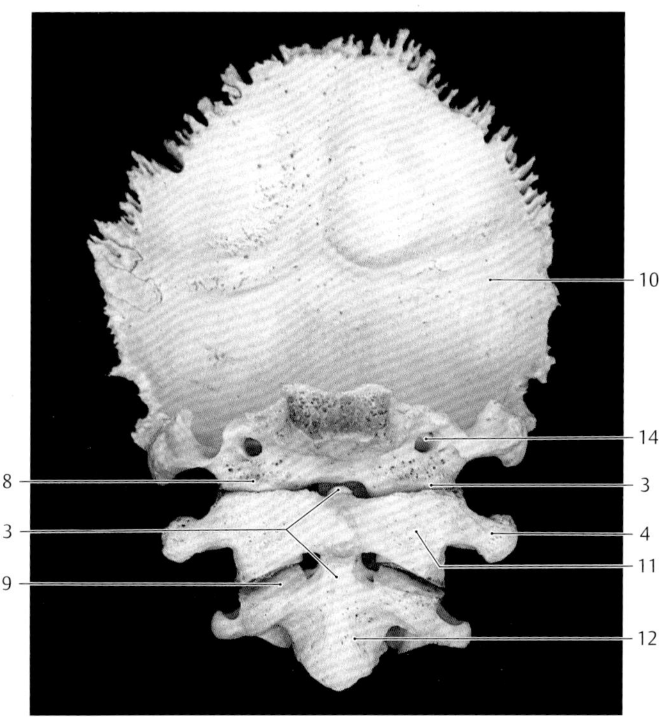


Fig. 2.6 **Occipital bone, atlas, and axis** (anterior aspect).

Fig. 2.7 **Occipital bone, atlas, and axis** (left lateral aspect).

1 External occipital protuberance
2 Foramen magnum
3 Atlanto-occipital joint
4 Transverse process of atlas
5 Median atlanto-axial joint
6 Vertebral canal
7 Spinous process of third cervical vertebra
8 Occipital condyle
9 Lateral atlanto-axial joint
10 Occipital bone
11 Atlas
12 Axis
13 Dens of axis
14 Hypoglossal canal
15 Spinous process of axis

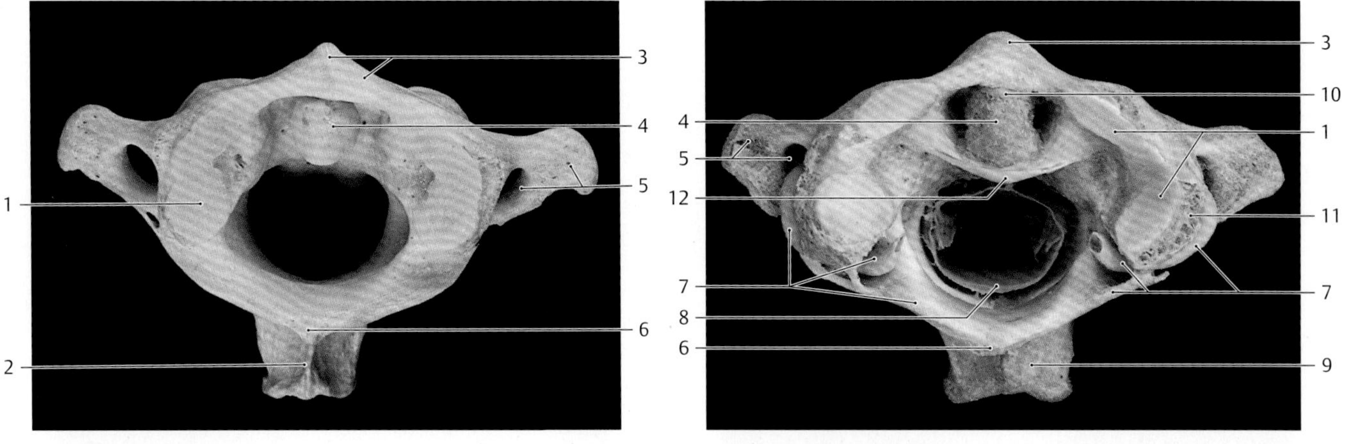


Fig. 2.8 **Atlas and axis** (from above).

Fig. 2.9 **Median atlanto-axial joint and transverse ligament of atlas** (from above). Dens of axis partly severed.

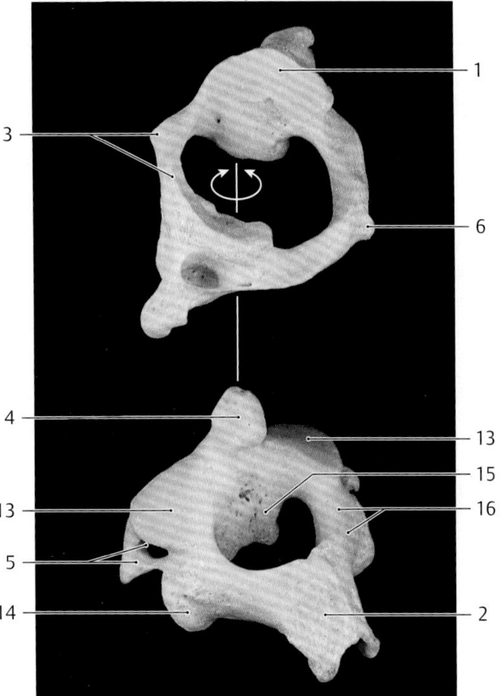


Fig. 2.10 **Atlas and axis** (left oblique postero-lateral aspect, demonstrating the articulation of the dens of axis with the atlas [arrows]).

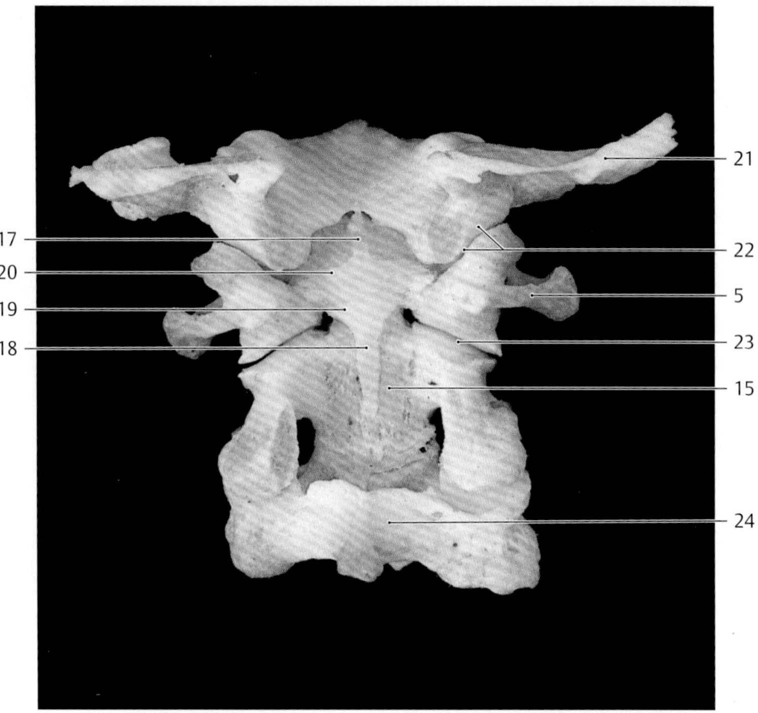


Fig. 2.11 **Atlanto-occipital and atlanto-axial joints** (posterior aspect). Posterior part of occipital bone, posterior arch of atlas, and axis have been removed to show the cruciform ligament.

1 Superior articular facet of atlas
2 Spinous process
3 Anterior arch of atlas with anterior tubercle
4 Dens of axis
5 Transverse foramen and process
6 Posterior tubercle of atlas
7 Posterior arch of atlas and vertebral artery
8 Dura mater
9 Spinous process of axis
10 Median atlanto-axial joint (anterior part)
11 Articular capsule of atlanto-occipital joint
12 Transverse ligament of atlas
13 Superior articular facet of axis
14 Inferior articular process
15 Body of axis
16 Pedicle and lamina of axis
17 Superior longitudinal band of cruciform ligament } Cruciform ligament
18 Inferior longitudinal band of cruciform ligament } Cruciform ligament
19 Transverse ligament of atlas
20 Alar ligaments
21 Occipital bone
22 Atlanto-occipital joint
23 Lateral atlanto-axial joint
24 Third cervical vertebra (C3)

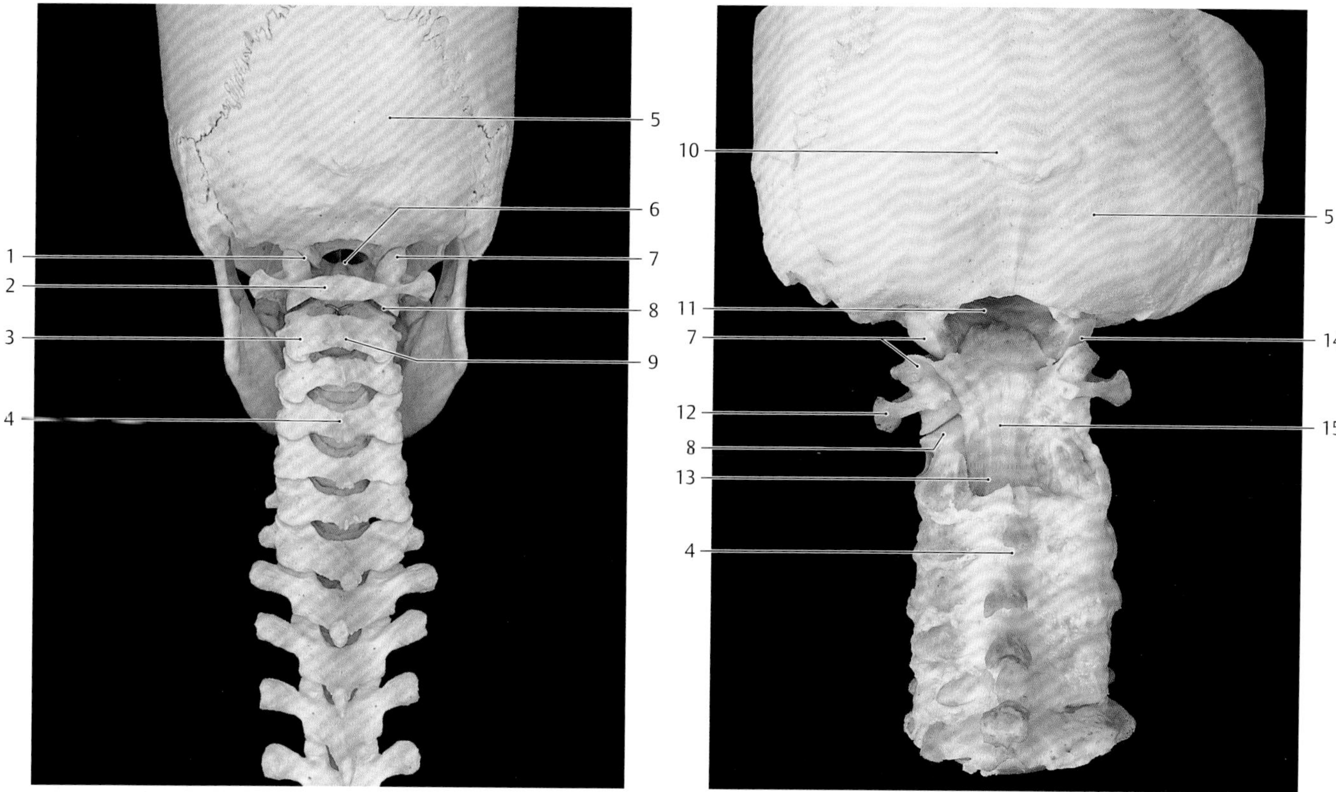


**Fig. 2.12 Cervical vertebral column and skull** (posterior aspect). Note the location of the atlanto-occipital and atlanto-axial joints.

**Fig. 2.13 Cervical vertebral column and skull with ligaments** (posterior aspect). Posterior arches of atlas and axis have been removed to show the tectorial membrane.

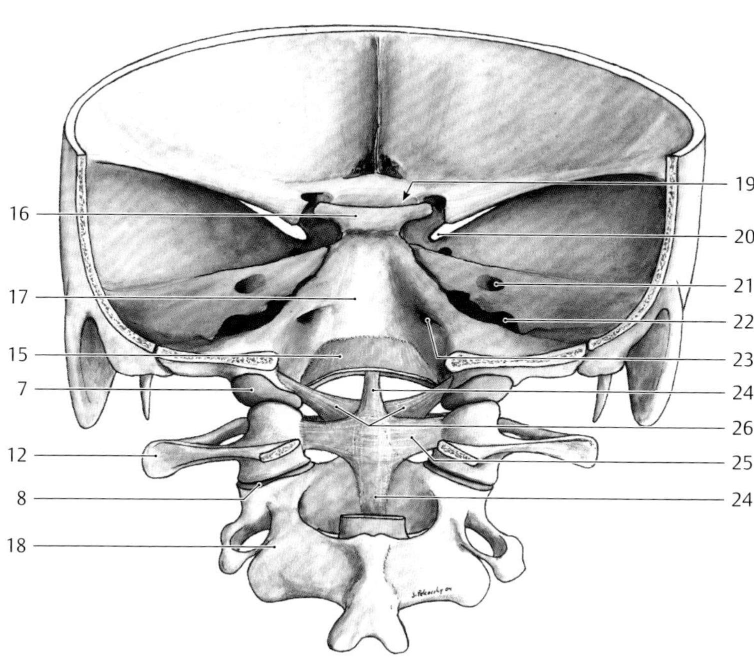


**Fig. 2.14 Atlanto-occipital and atlanto-axial joints with ligaments** (posterior aspect). Posterior part of occipital bone and posterior arch of atlas have been removed to show the cruciform ligament.

1 Superior articular facet
2 Posterior tubercle of atlas
3 Vertebral arch of axis
4 Spinous process of cervical vertebra
5 Occipital bone
6 Dens of axis
7 Atlanto-occipital joint
8 Lateral atlanto-axial joint
9 Spinous process of axis
10 External occipital protuberance
11 Foramen magnum
12 Transverse process of atlas
13 Posterior longitudinal ligament
14 Occipital condyle
15 Tectorial membrane
16 Dorsum sellae
17 Clivus
18 Axis
19 Sella turcica
20 Superior orbital fissure
21 Internal acoustic meatus
22 Jugular foramen
23 Hypoglossal canal
24 Superior and inferior longitudinal bands of cruciform ligament } Cruciform ligament
25 Transverse ligament of atlas }

26 Alar ligaments

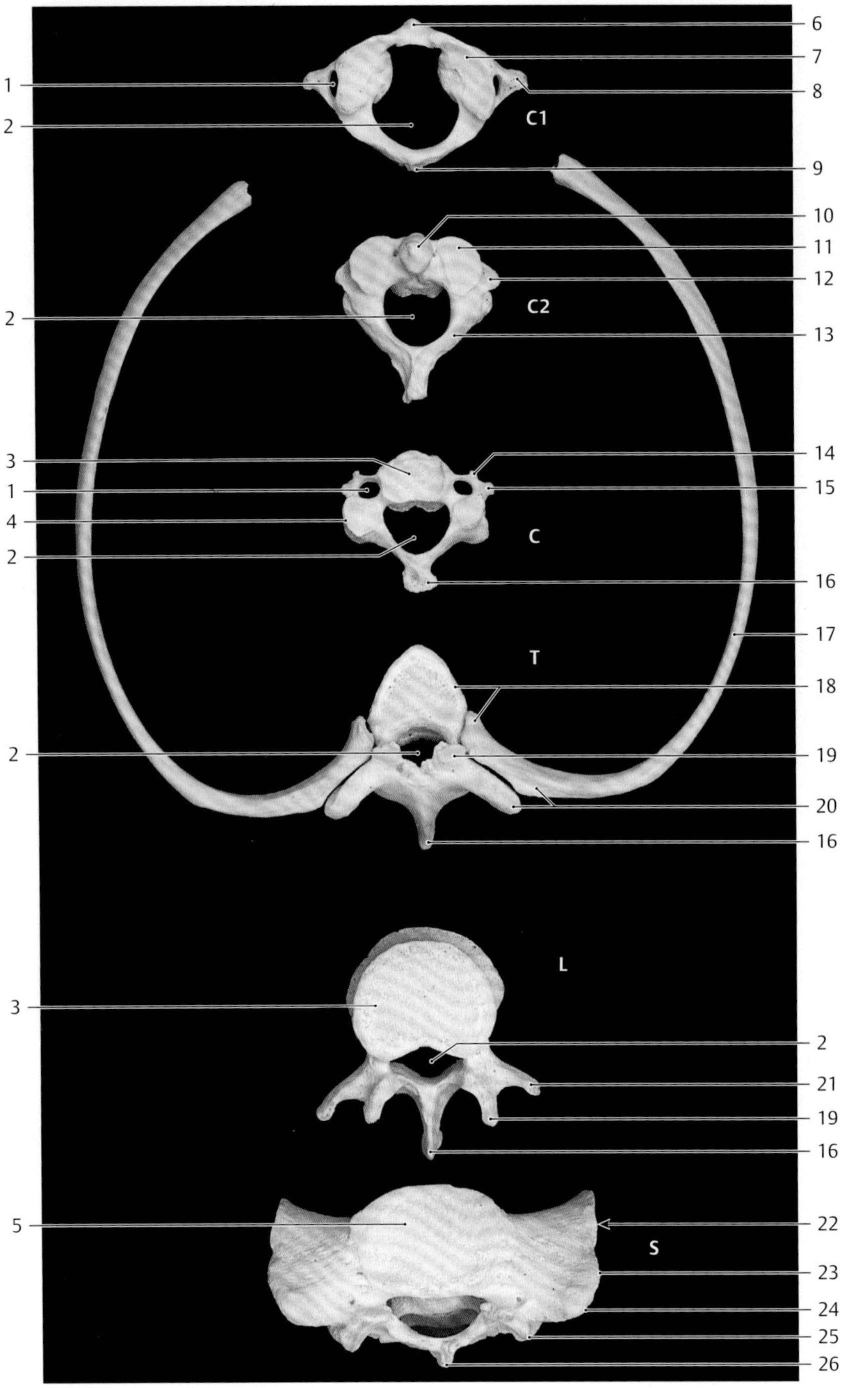

Fig. 2.15 **Representative vertebrae from each region of the vertebral column** (superior aspect). From top to bottom: atlas (C1), axis (C2), cervical vertebra (C), thoracic vertebra (T), lumbar vertebra (L), and sacrum (S).

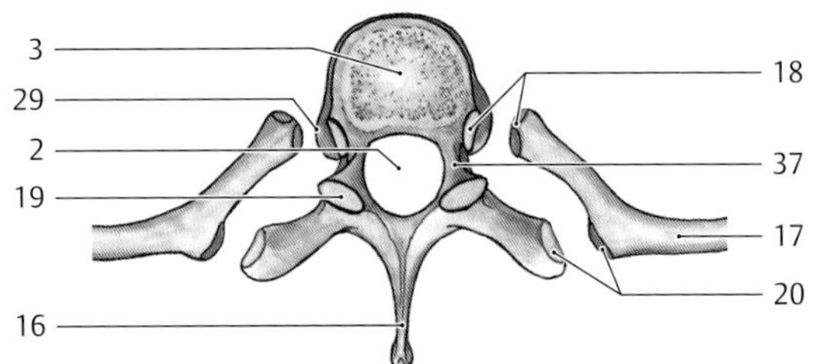


Fig. 2.19 **General organization of ribs and vertebrae.**

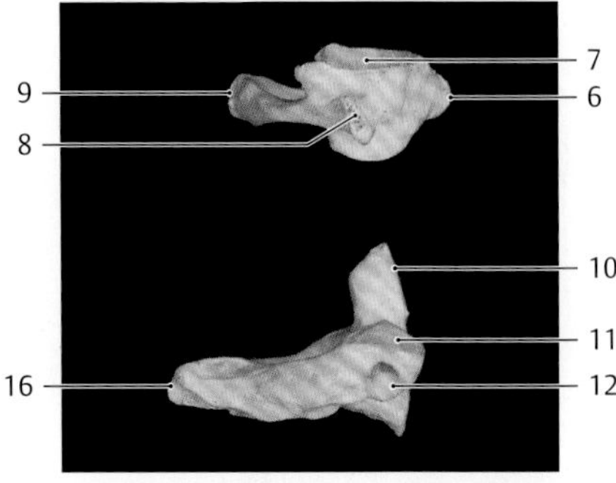


Fig. 2.16 Atlas (C1) and Axis (C2).

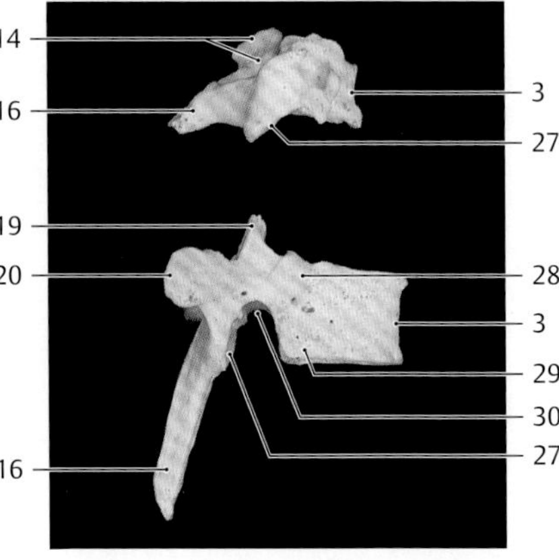


Fig. 2.17 Typical cervical (C) and thoracic vertebrae (T).

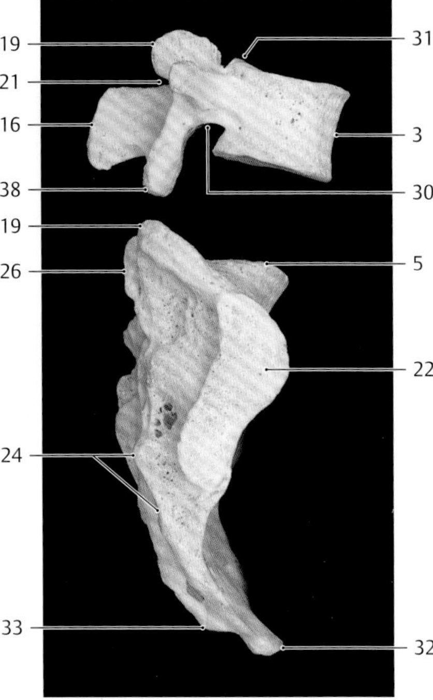


Fig. 2.18 Typical lumbar vertebra (L) and sacrum (S).

**Representative vertebrae from each region of the vertebral column** (lateral aspect, ventral surface on the right).

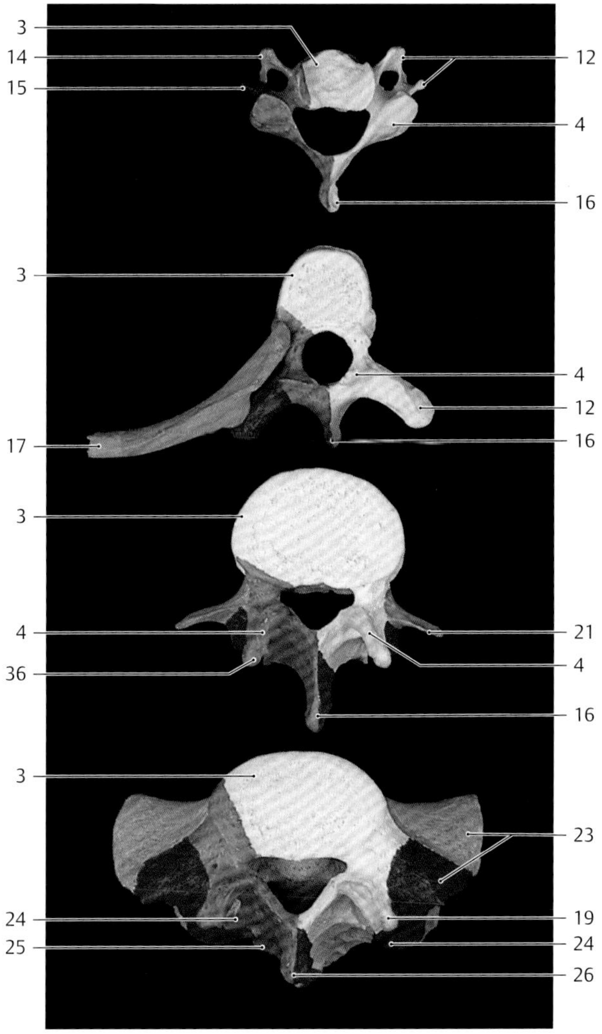


Fig. 2.20 **General characteristics of the vertebrae.** Typical cervical, thoracic, and lumbar vertebrae and sacrum.

Green = Ribs or homologous processes
Red = Muscular processes (transverse and spinous processes)
Orange = Laminae and articular processes
Yellow = Articular facets

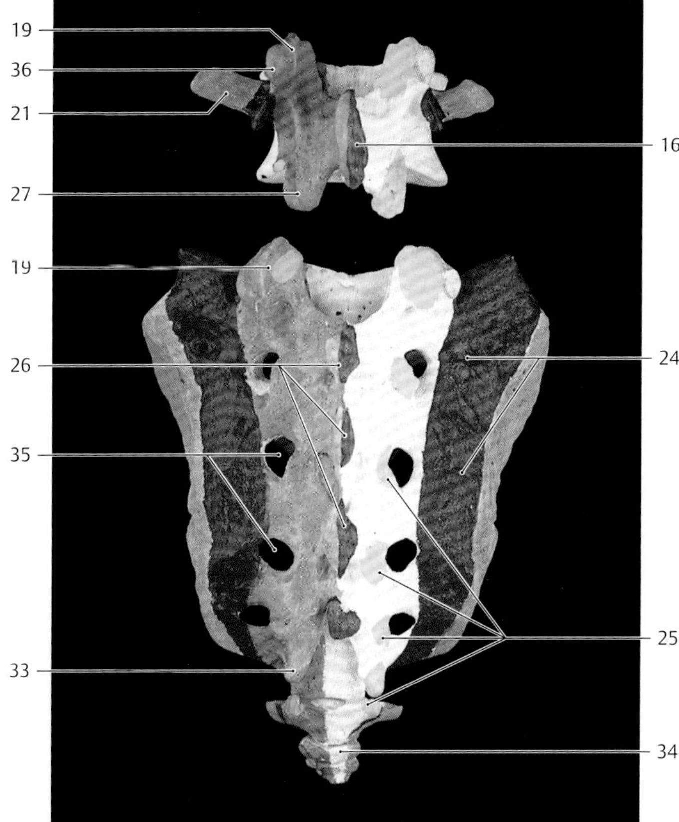


Fig. 2.21 **General characteristics of lumbar vertebrae and sacrum** (posterior aspect). Transformation of the spinal processes into the sacrum.

1 Foramen transversarium
2 Vertebral foramen
3 Body of vertebra
4 Superior articular facet
5 Base of sacrum
6 Anterior tubercle of atlas
7 Superior articular facet of atlas
8 Transverse process
9 Posterior tubercle of atlas
10 Dens of axis
11 Superior articular surface
12 Transverse process
13 Arch of vertebra
14 Anterior tubercle of transverse process
15 Posterior tubercle of transverse process
16 Spinous process
17 Shaft of rib
18 Body of vertebra and head of rib articulating with each other (costovertebral joint)
19 Superior articular process
20 Transverse process and tubercle of rib articulating with each other (costotransverse joint)
21 Costal process
22 Auricular surface
23 Lateral part of sacrum
24 Lateral sacral crest
25 Intermediate sacral crest
26 Median sacral crest
27 Inferior articular process
28 Superior demifacet for head of rib
29 Inferior demifacet for head of rib
30 Inferior vertebral notch
31 Superior vertebral notch
32 Apex of the sacrum
33 Sacral cornu
34 Coccyx
35 Dorsal sacral foramina
36 Mammillary process
37 Pedicle
38 Inferior articular process

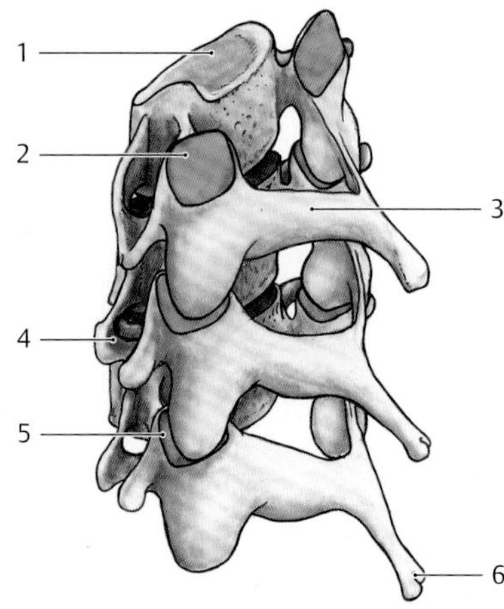


Fig. 2.22 **Cervical vertebrae** (lateral aspect). Blue = articular facets.

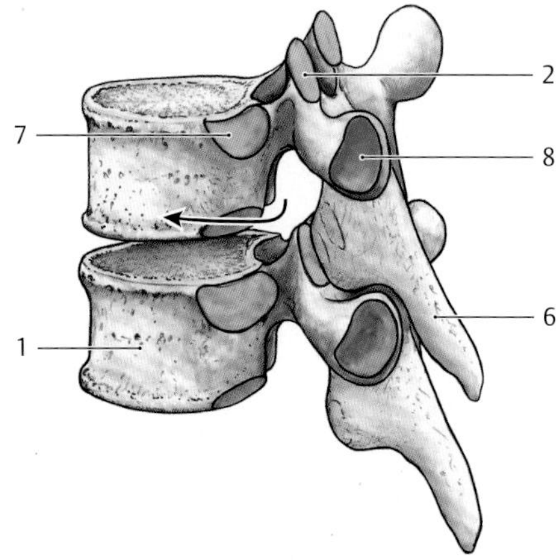


Fig. 2.23 **Thoracic vertebrae** (lateral aspect). Blue = articular facets; arrow = exit of spinal nerves through the intervertebral foramen.

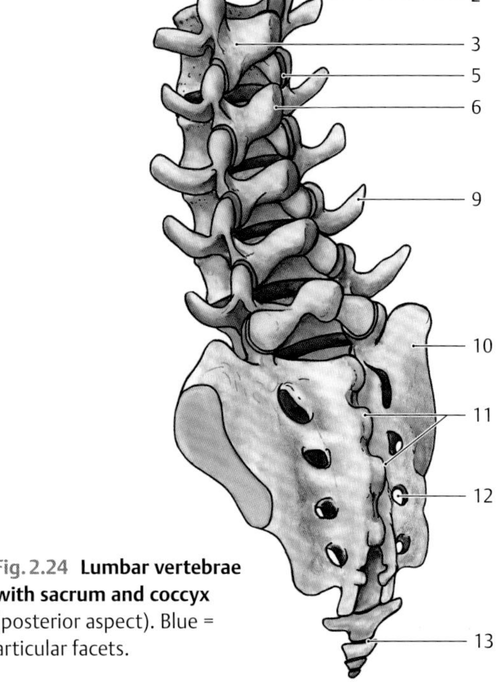


Fig. 2.24 **Lumbar vertebrae with sacrum and coccyx** (posterior aspect). Blue = articular facets.

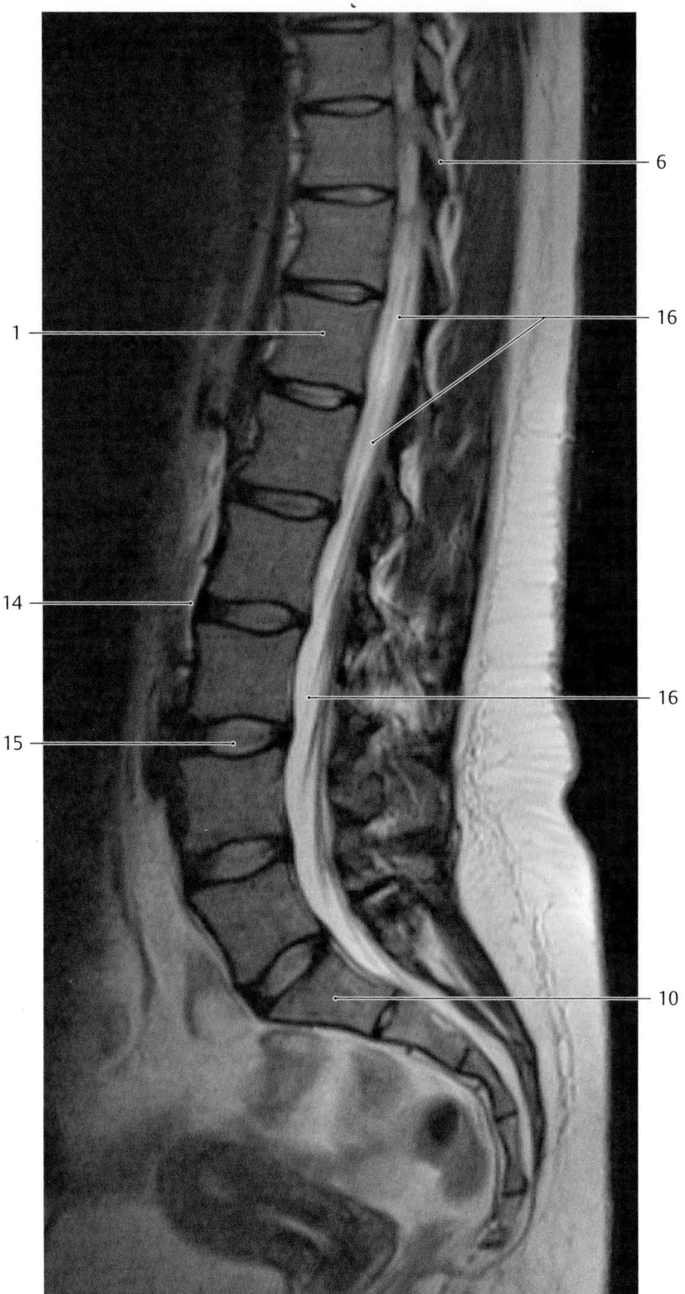


Fig. 2.25 **Paramedian section through the vertebral column with pelvic cavity** (MRI scan). (Courtesy of Prof. Uder, Institute of Radiology, University of Erlangen, Germany.)

1 Body of vertebra
2 Superior articular facet
3 Vertebral arch
4 Transverse process of vertebra
5 Zygapophysial joint
6 Spinous process
7 Superior articular facet of articulation with head of ribs
8 Transverse process with articular facet of costotransverse joint
9 Costal process of lumbar vertebra
10 Sacrum
11 Median sacral crest
12 Dorsal sacral foramina
13 Coccyx
14 Anterior longitudinal ligament
15 Intervertebral disc
16 Vertebral canal

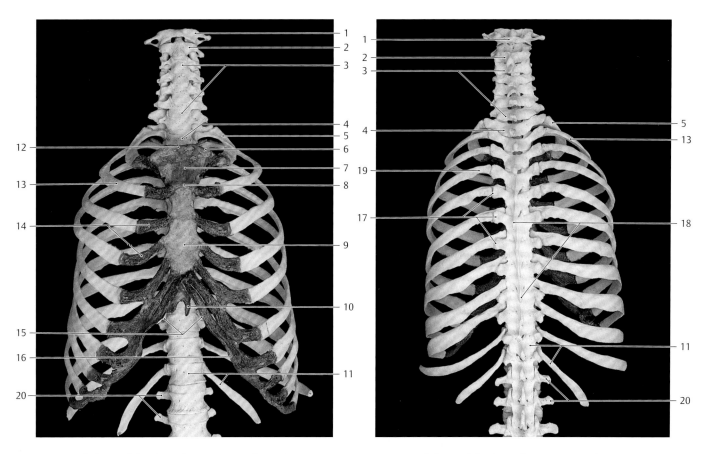

Fig. 2.26 **Skeleton of the thorax** (anterior aspect).

Fig. 2.27 **Skeleton of the thorax** (posterior aspect).

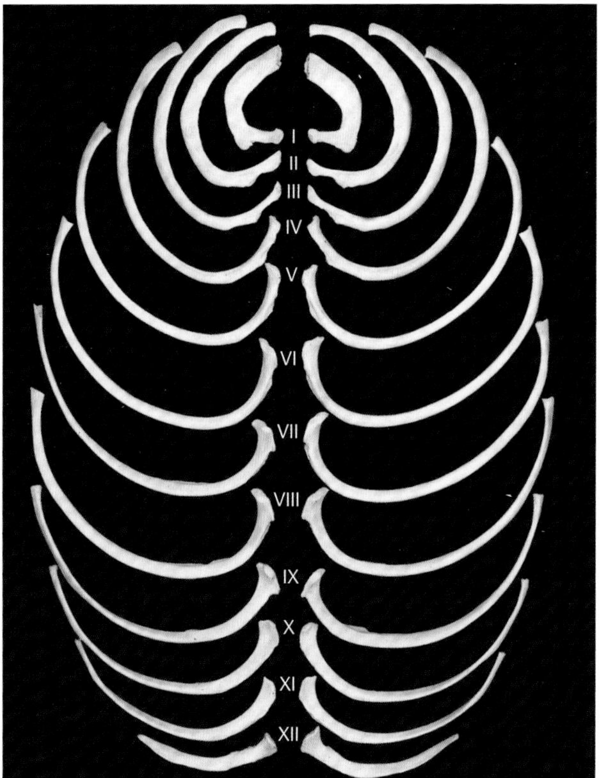


Fig. 2.28 **Disarticulated skeleton of the thorax.** The twelve ribs (I–XII) are arranged in a craniocaudal direction.

1 Atlas
2 Axis
3 Cervical vertebrae
4 First thoracic vertebra
5 First rib
6 Facet for clavicle and clavicular notch
7 Manubrium sterni
8 Sternal angle
9 Body of sternum
10 Xiphoid process
11 Twelfth thoracic vertebra and rib
12 Jugular notch
13 Second rib
14 Costal cartilages
15 Infrasternal angle
16 Costal arch
17 Costotransverse joints between the transverse processes of thoracic vertebrae and the tubercles of the ribs
18 Spinous processes
19 Costal angle
20 Costal processes of lumbar vertebrae

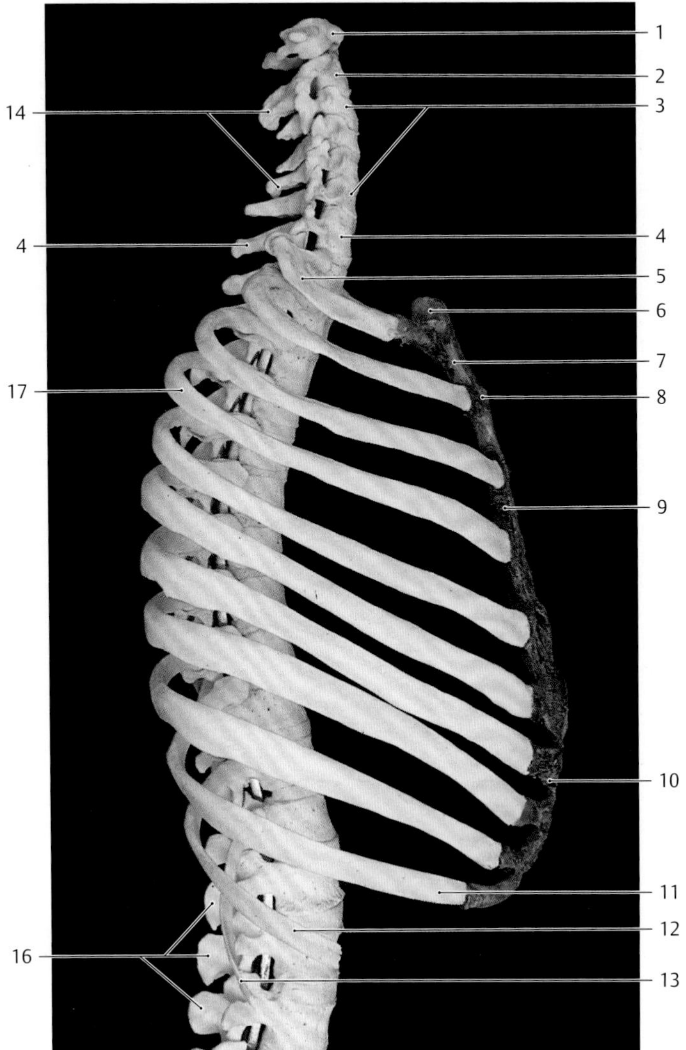


Fig. 2.29 **Skeleton of the thorax** (right lateral aspect).

1 Atlas
2 Axis
3 Cervical vertebrae
4 Vertebra prominens (C7)
5 First rib
6 Facet for clavicle
7 Manubrium sterni
8 Sternal angle
9 Body of sternum
10 Costal arch
11 Tenth rib
12 Eleventh rib
13 Twelfth rib
14 Spinous processes of cervical vertebrae
15 Spinous processes of thoracic vertebrae
16 Spinous processes of lumbar vertebrae
17 Costal angle
18 Intervertebral foramina
19 Intervertebral discs
20 Cervical curvature
21 Thoracic curvature
22 Lumbar curvature
23 Sacrum
24 Coccyx

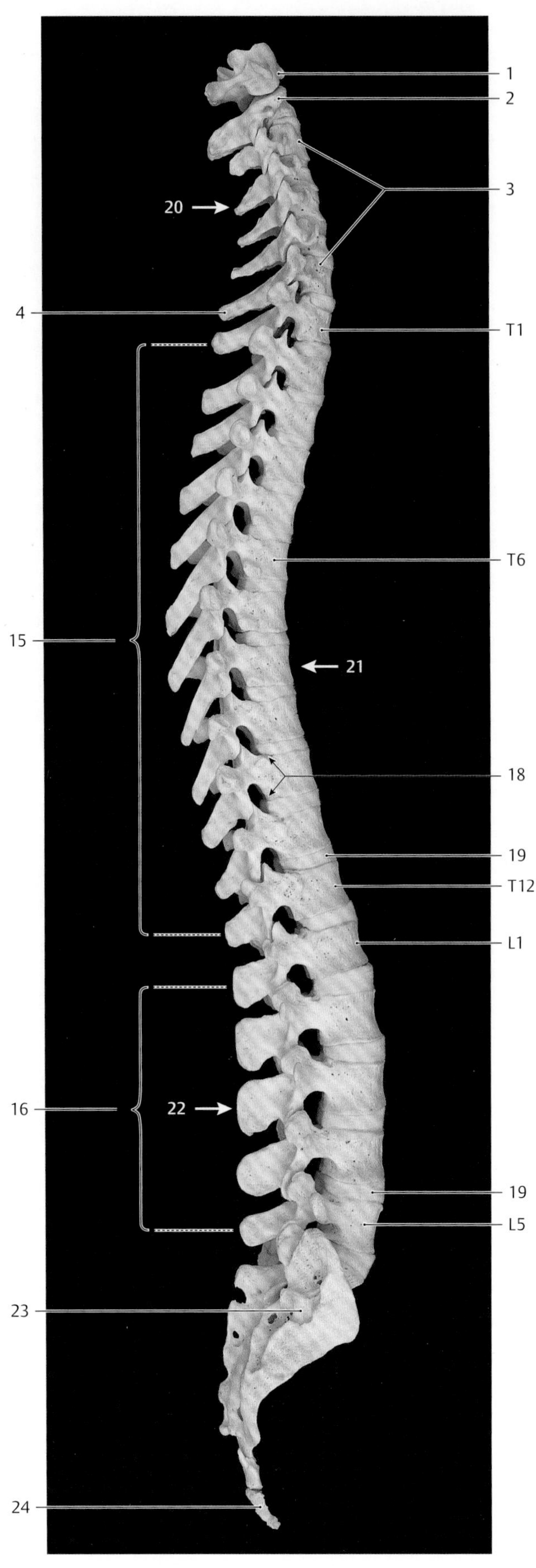


Fig. 2.30 **Vertebral column** (right lateral aspect). T1, T6, and T12 = first, sixth, and twelfth cervical vertebrae; L1 and L5 = first and fifth lumbar vertebrae.

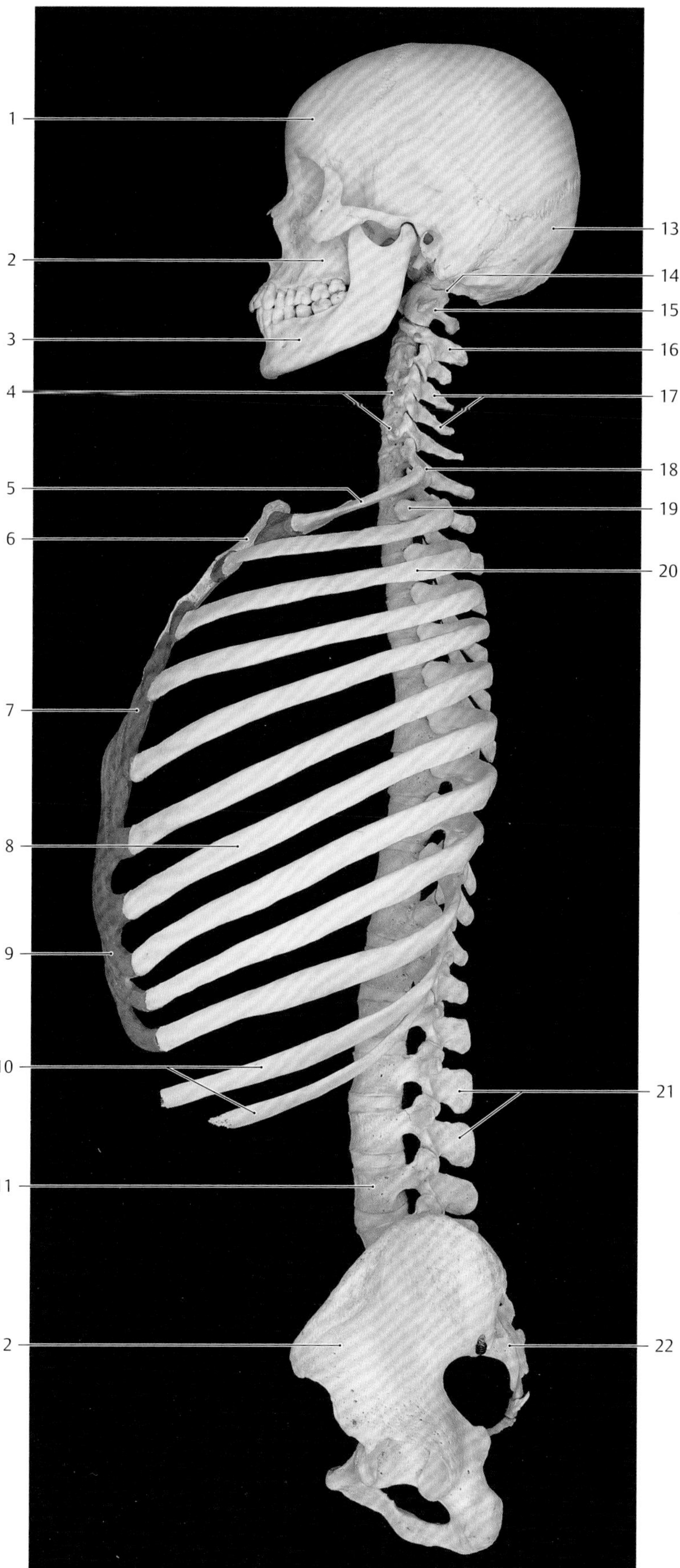


Fig. 2.31 **Vertebral column and thorax in connection with head and pelvis** (lateral aspect).

1 Frontal bone
2 Maxilla
3 Mandible
4 Bodies of cervical vertebrae
5 First rib
6 Manubrium of sternum
7 Sternum (corpus sterni)
8 Seventh rib (last of the true ribs)
9 Costal arch
10 Floating ribs (costae fluctuantes)
11 Body of fourth lumbar vertebra
12 Pelvis
13 Occipital bone
14 Atlanto-occipital joint
15 Atlas
16 Axis
17 Spinous processes of cervical vertebrae (C4, C5)
18 Costotransverse joint of first rib
19 Head of second rib
20 Third rib
21 Spinous processes of lumbar vertebrae (L2, L3)
22 Sacrum

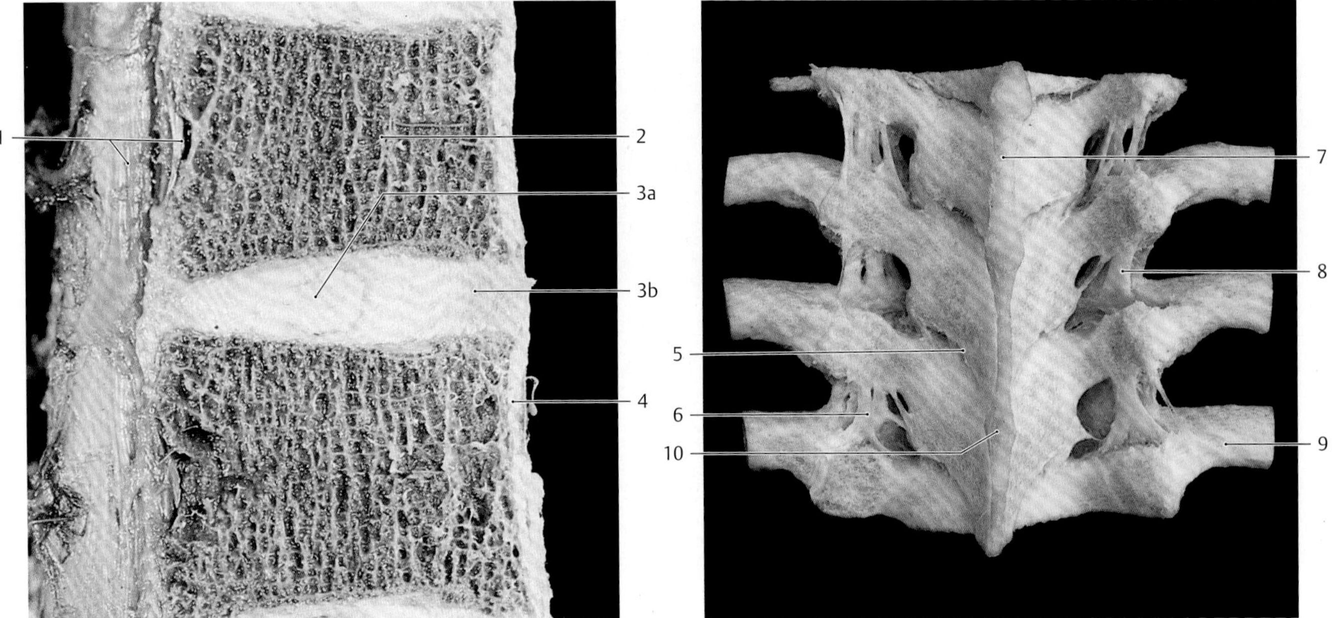


Fig. 2.32 **Median sagittal section through the bodies of lumbar vertebrae,** showing the intervertebral discs, each of which consists of an outer laminated portion and an inner core.

Fig. 2.33 **Ligaments of the thoracic vertebrae** (posterior aspect).

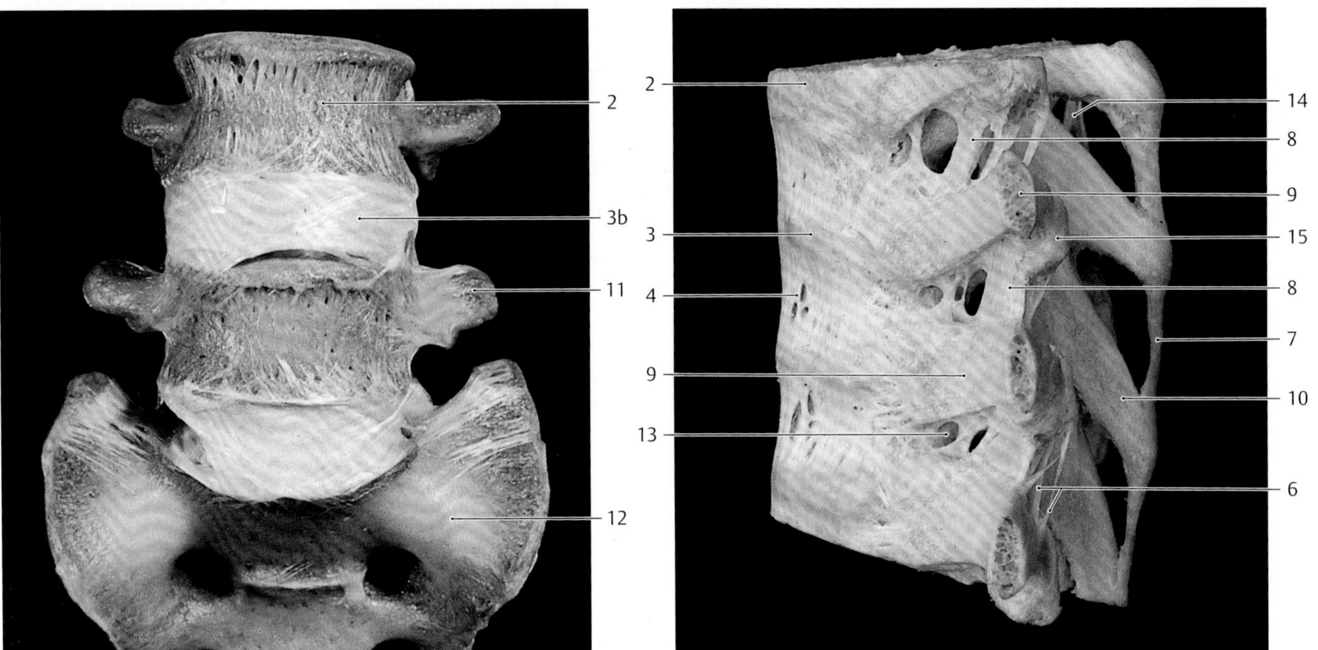


Fig. 2.34 **Two caudal lumbar vertebrae and sacrum with their intervertebral discs** (anterior aspect). Anterior longitudinal ligament removed.

Fig. 2.35 **Ligaments of the thoracic vertebrae** (left lateral aspect).

1 Posterior longitudinal ligament and spinal dura mater
2 Body of vertebra
3 Intervertebral disc
 (a) Inner core (nucleus pulposus)
 (b) Outer portion (anulus fibrosus)
4 Anterior longitudinal ligament
5 Ligamentum flavum
6 Intertransverse ligament
7 Supraspinous ligament
8 Superior costotransverse ligament
9 Rib
10 Spinous process
11 Costal process of lumbar vertebra
12 Sacrum
13 Intervertebral foramen
14 Interspinous ligament
15 Transverse process of thoracic vertebra

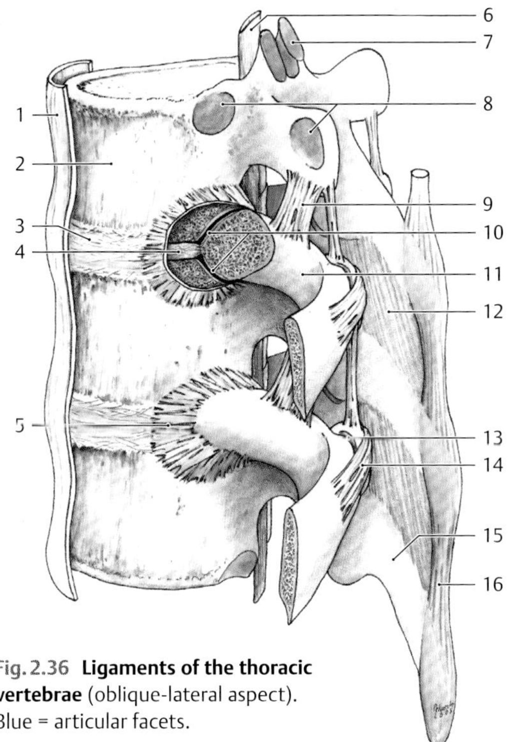


Fig. 2.36 **Ligaments of the thoracic vertebrae** (oblique-lateral aspect). Blue = articular facets.

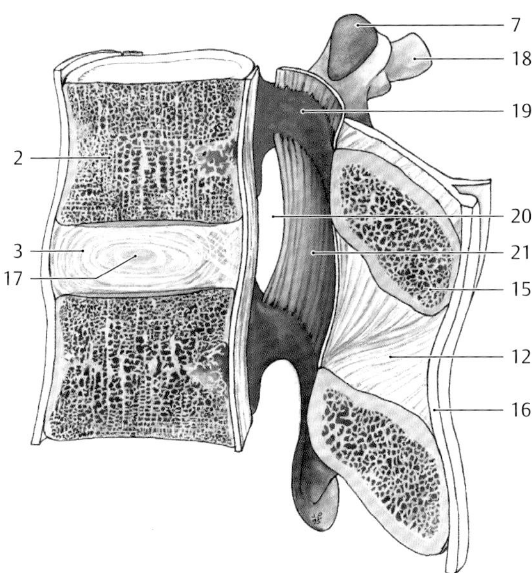


Fig. 2.37 **Ligaments of the lumbar vertebrae** (median sagittal section). Blue = articular facets.

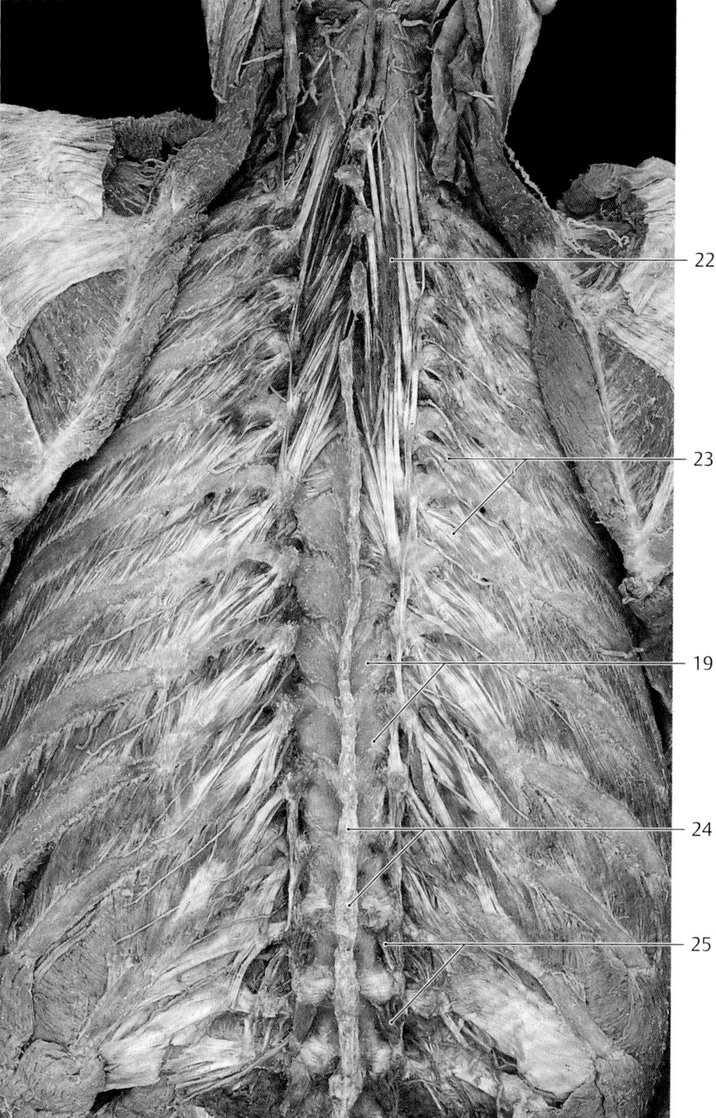


Fig. 2.38 **Vertebral column and ribs** (posterior aspect). Muscles of the back have been widely removed to display the ligaments.

1 Anterior longitudinal ligament
2 Body of vertebra
3 Intervertebral disc
4 Intra-articular ligament
5 Radiate ligament
6 Posterior longitudinal ligament
7 Superior articular facet
8 Articular facets of joint of head of rib and costotransverse joint
9 Superior costotransverse ligament
10 Joint of head of rib
11 Rib
12 Interspinal ligament
13 Costotransverse joint
14 Lateral costotransverse ligament
15 Spinous process
16 Supraspinal ligament
17 Nucleus pulposus
18 Costal process
19 Vertebral arch
20 Intervertebral foramen
21 Intertransverse ligament
22 Semispinalis cervicis muscle
23 Levatores costarum muscles
24 Spinous processes of lumbar vertebrae and supraspinal ligaments
25 Intertransversarii muscles

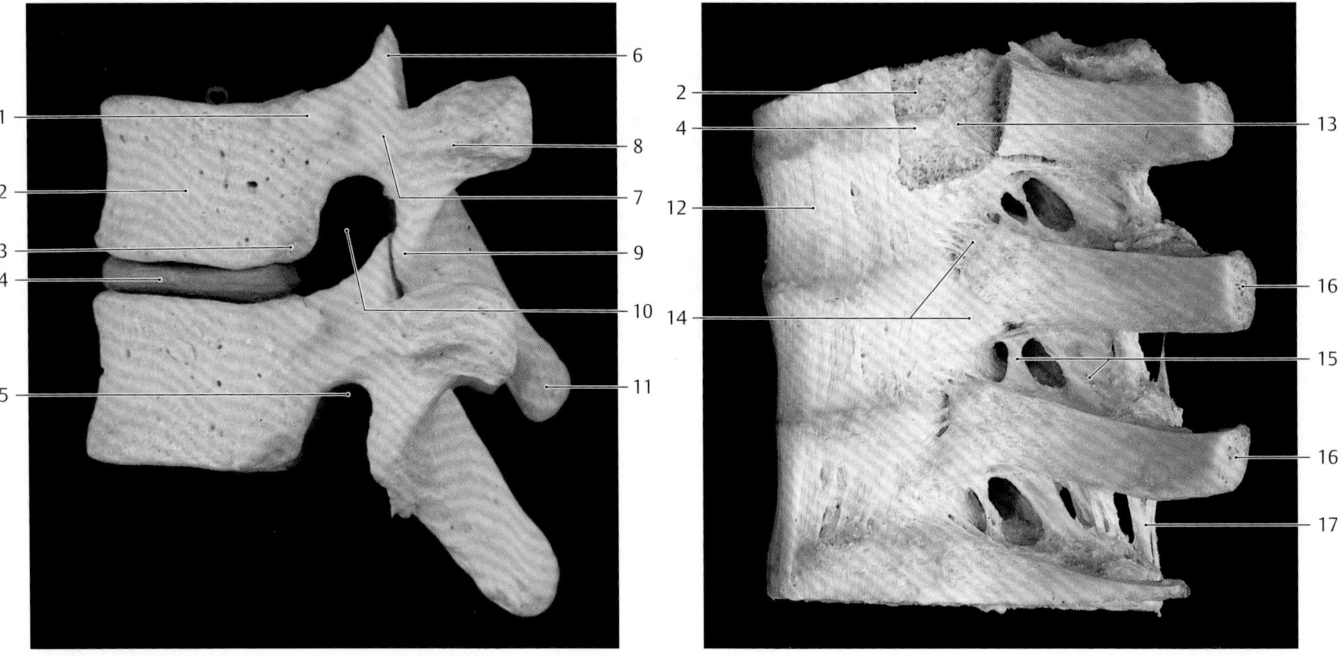


Fig. 2.39 **Two thoracic vertebrae** (left lateral aspect).

Fig. 2.40 **Ligaments of thoracic vertebrae and costovertebral joints** (left antero-lateral aspect).

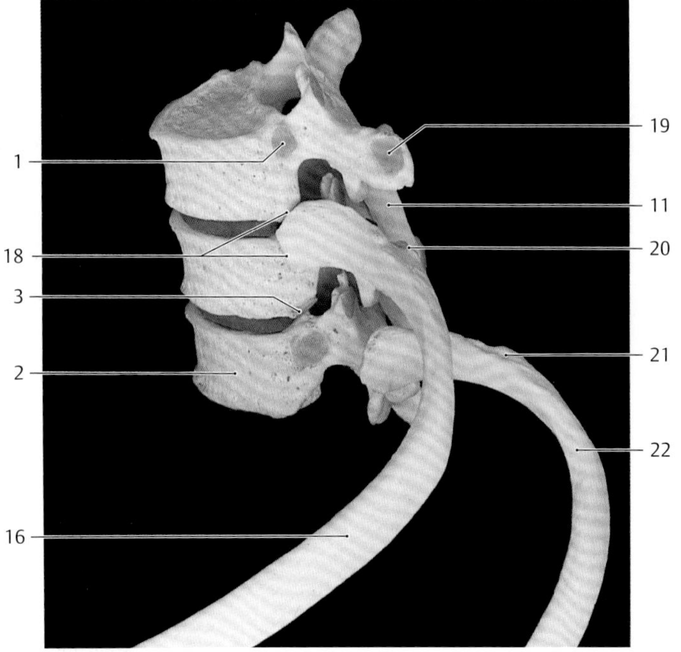


Fig. 2.41 **Costovertebral joints** (lateral aspect).

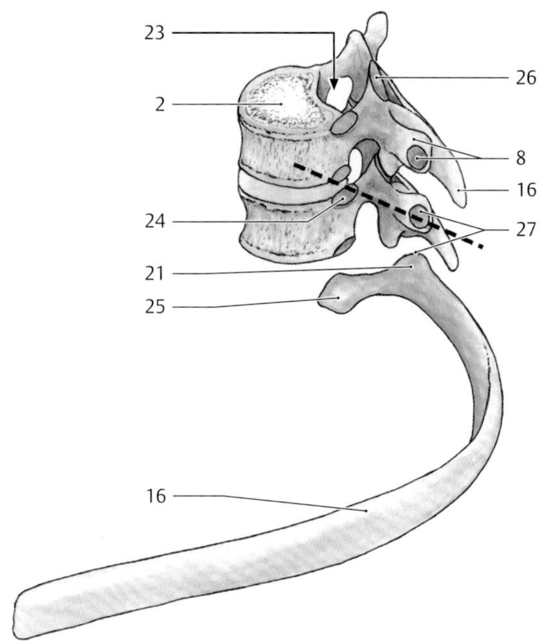


Fig. 2.42 **Costovertebral joints** (lateral aspect). Two thoracic vertebrae with an articulating rib (separated). Axis of movement indicated by dashed line. Blue = articular facets.

1 Superior demifacet for head of rib
2 Body of vertebra
3 Inferior demifacet for head of rib
4 Intervertebral disc
5 Inferior vertebral notch
6 Superior articular facet and superior articular process
7 Pedicle
8 Transverse process and facet for tubercle of rib
9 Inferior articular process
10 Intervertebral foramen
11 Spinous process
12 Anterior longitudinal ligament
13 Intra-articular ligament
14 Radiate ligament
15 Superior costotransverse ligament
16 Body of rib
17 Intertransverse ligament
18 Articulation of head of rib with two vertebrae
19 Angle of costotransverse joint (articular facet)
20 Costotransverse joint
21 Tubercle of rib
22 Costal angle of rib
23 Vertebral canal
24 Inferior facet of articulation with head of rib
25 Head of rib
26 Superior articular process
27 Facets of articulation with costotransverse joint

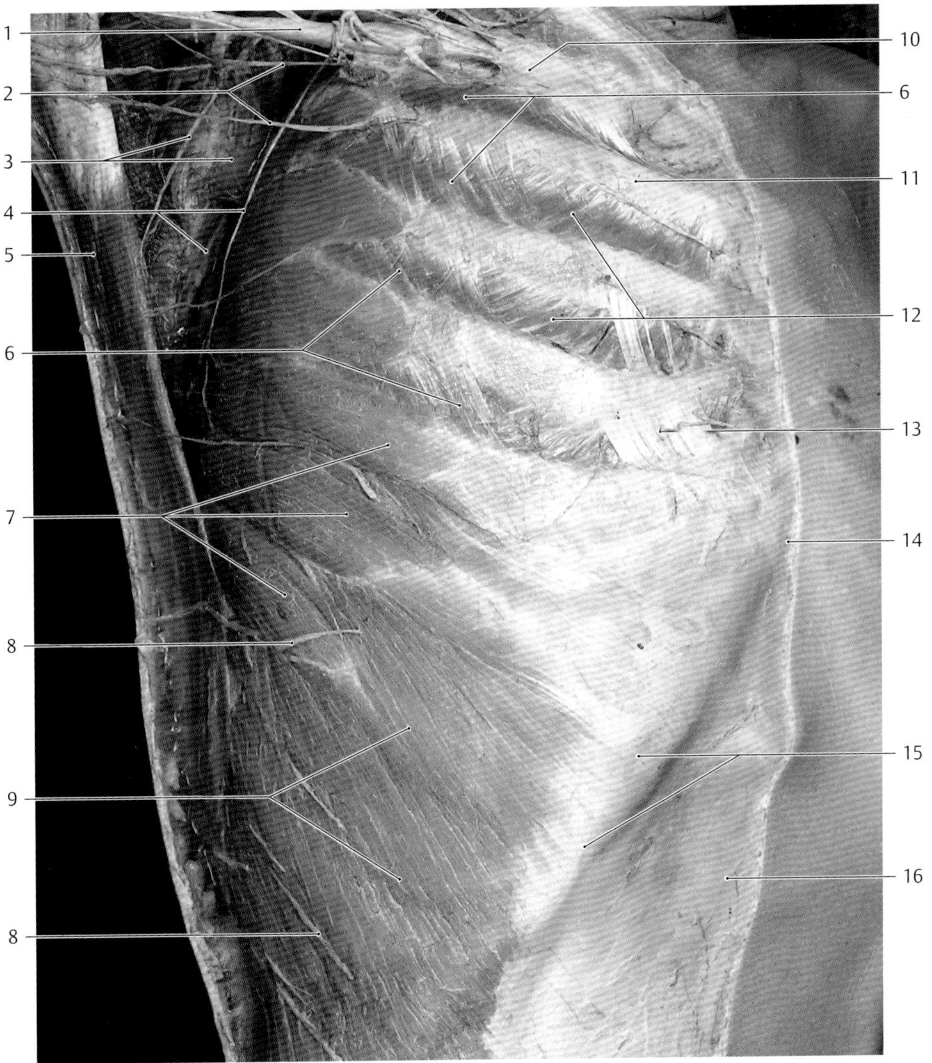


1 Axillary vein
2 Intercostobrachial nerves
3 Subscapularis muscle and thoracodorsal nerve
4 Long thoracic nerve, lateral thoracic artery and vein
5 Latissimus dorsi muscle
6 External intercostal muscles
7 Serratus anterior muscle
8 Lateral cutaneous branches of intercostal nerves
9 External abdominal oblique muscle
10 Clavicle (divided)
11 Second rib (costochondral junction)
12 Internal intercostal muscles
13 External intercostal membrane
14 Position of xiphoid process
15 Costal arch or margin
16 Anterior layer of rectus sheath

Fig. 2.43 **Muscles of the thorax,** superficial layer (lateral aspect). Upper limb elevated. Pectoralis major and minor muscles have been removed.

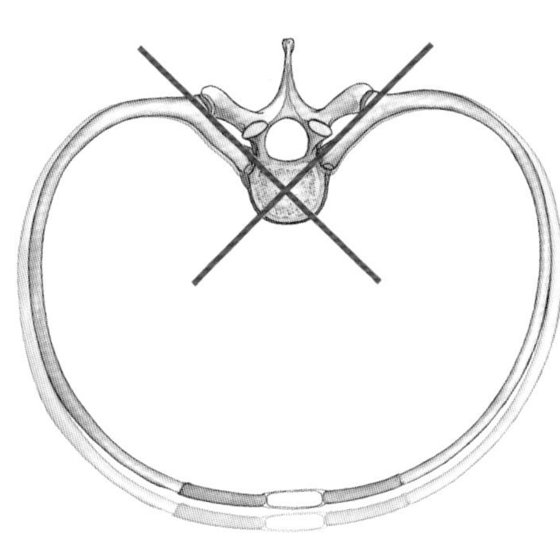

Fig. 2.44

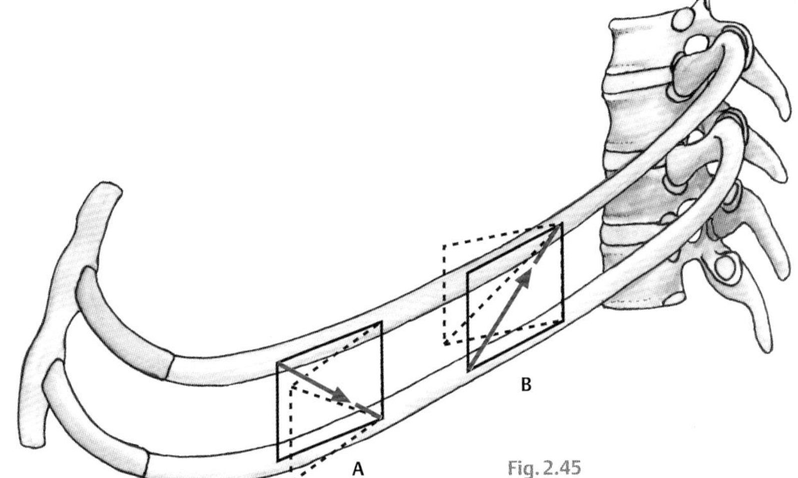


Fig. 2.45

Figs. 2.44 and 2.45 **Effect of intercostal muscles on the costovertebral and costotransverse joints.** Axes of movement indicated by red lines; direction of movements indicated by red arrows.

A = Action of internal intercostal muscles (expiration)
B = Action of external intercostal muscles (inspiration)

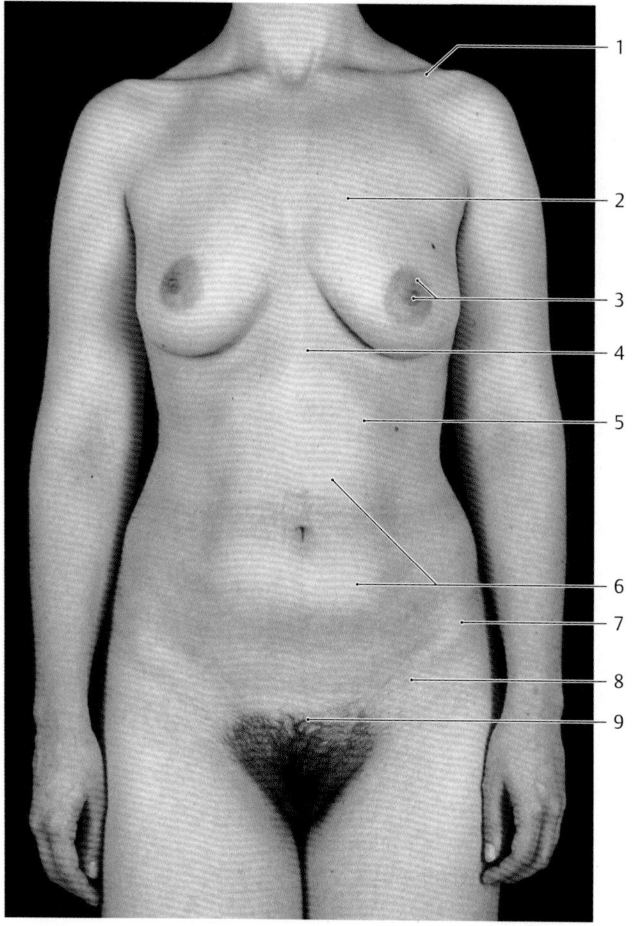


1 Clavicle
2 Pectoralis major muscle
3 Areola and nipple
4 Infrasternal angle
5 Costal arch
6 Rectus abdominis muscle
7 Anterior superior iliac spine
8 Inguinal ligament
9 Mons pubis
10 External abdominal oblique muscle
11 Spermatic cord
12 Deltoid muscle
13 External intercostal muscle
14 Internal abdominal oblique muscle
15 Transverse abdominal muscle
16 Pectoralis minor muscle
17 Anterior serratus muscle
18 Linea alba
19 Biceps brachii muscle
20 Coracobrachialis muscle
21 Latissimus dorsi muscle

**Fig. 2.46 Surface anatomy of the anterior body wall in the female.** Note the differences of hairiness between the regions.

◂ **Labels for Figure 2.47 only:**

1 Anterior cervical region
2 Sternocleido-mastoid region
3 Omoclavicular triangle
4 Lateral cervical region
5 Infraclavicular fossa
6 Axillary region
7 Clavipectoral triangle
8 Deltoid region
9 Presternal region
10 Inframammary region
11 Mammary region
12 Pectoral region
13 Epigastric region
14 Hypochondriac region
15 Umbilical region
16 Lateral abdominal region
17 Inguinal region
18 Pubic region
19 Urogenital region
20 Femoral triangle
21 Anterior median line
22 Sternal line
23 Parasternal line
24 Mammillary line (medioclavicular line)
25 Axillary line
26 Horizontal plane at the level of the inferior thoracic aperture
27 Horizontal plane at the level of the anterior superior iliac spine

**Fig. 2.47 Regions and regional lines of the anterior body wall in the female.**

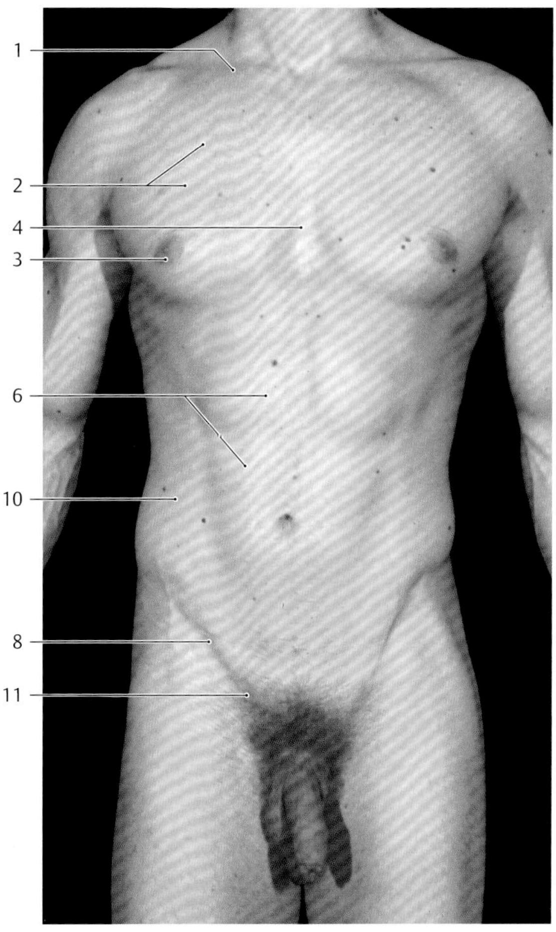


Fig. 2.48 **Surface anatomy of the anterior body wall in the male.** Localization and structure of the muscles can be identified.

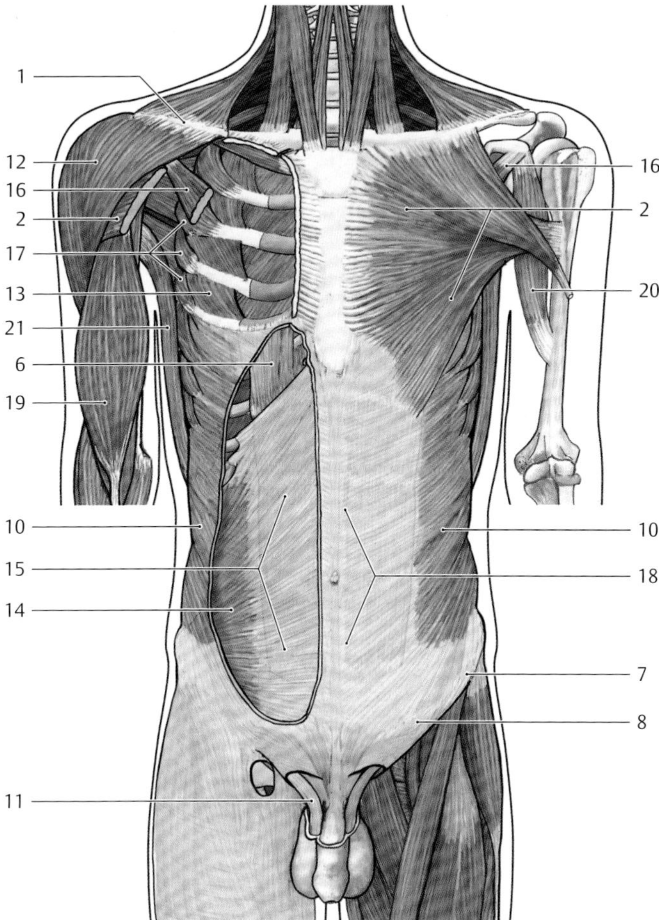


Fig. 2.49 **Muscles of the anterior body wall.**

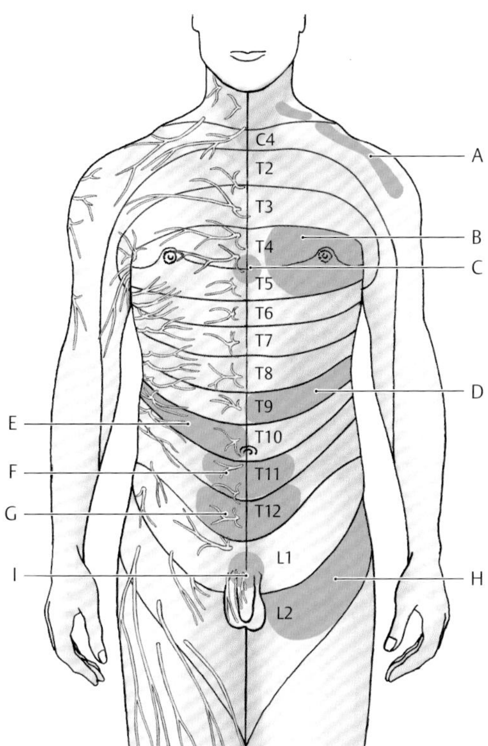


**Head's zones**

A = Diaphragm (C4)
B = Heart (T3–T4)
C = Esophagus (T4–T5)
D = Stomach (T8)
E = Liver, gallbladder (T9–L1)
F = Small intestine (T10–L1)
G = Colon (T11–L1)
H = Kidney, testis (T10–L1)
I = Urinary bladder (T11–L1)

Fig. 2.50 **Segments of the anterior body wall.** Head's zones are indicated.

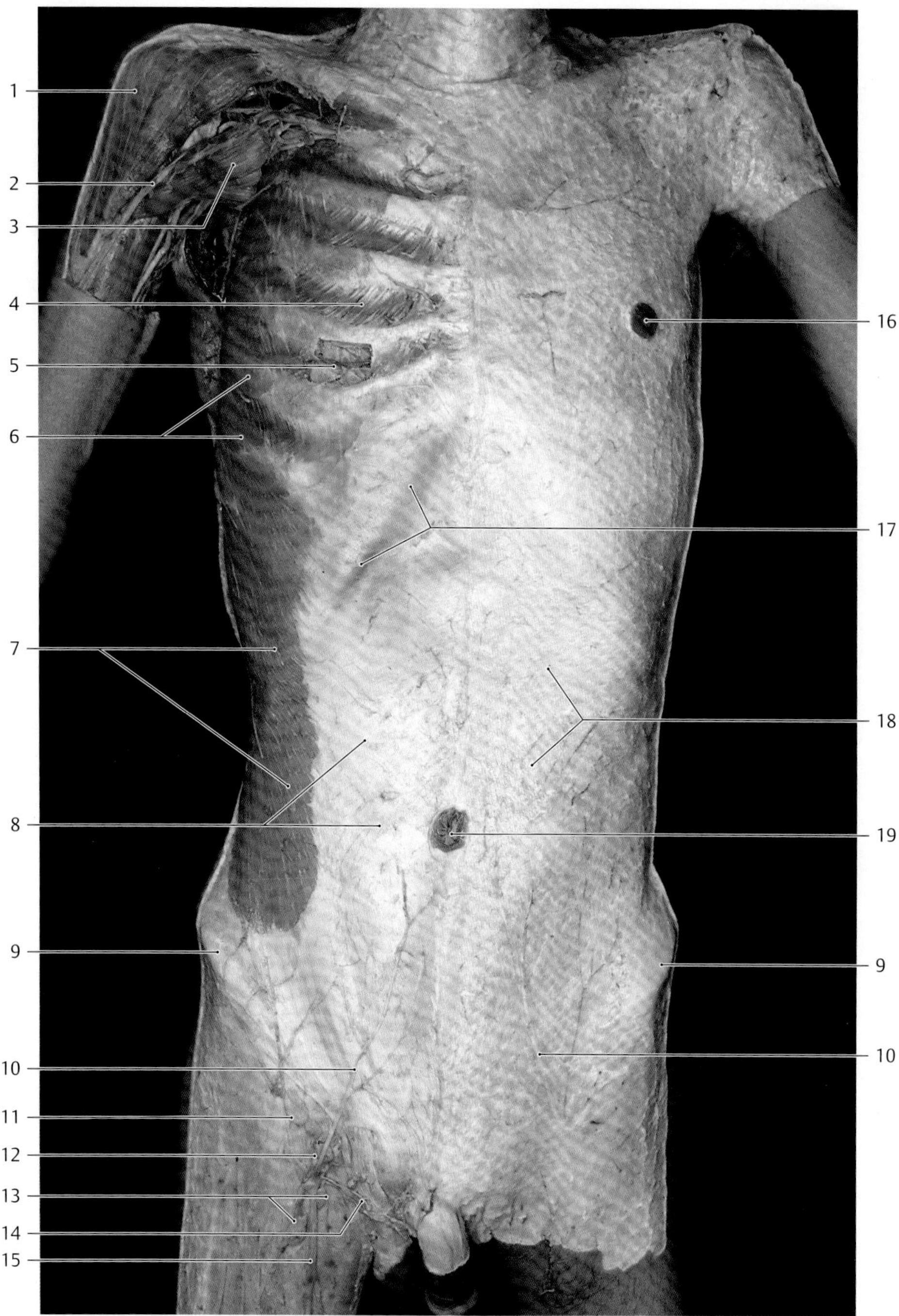


**Fig. 2.51 Thoracic and abdominal walls** (anterior aspect). Right pectoralis major and minor muscles are divided. Muscles of thoracic and abdominal walls on the right side are displayed.

1 Deltoid muscle
2 Cephalic vein
3 Pectoralis major muscle (divided)
4 Internal intercostal muscle
5 Intercostal artery and vein (intercostal space, fenestrated)
6 Serratus anterior muscle
7 External abdominal oblique muscle
8 Anterior layer of rectus sheath
9 Iliac crest
10 Superficial epigastric vein
11 Superficial circumflex iliac vein
12 Saphenous opening
13 Superficial inguinal lymph nodes
14 Superficial external pudendal veins
15 Great saphenous vein
16 Nipple
17 Costal margin
18 Subcutaneous fatty tissue
19 Umbilicus

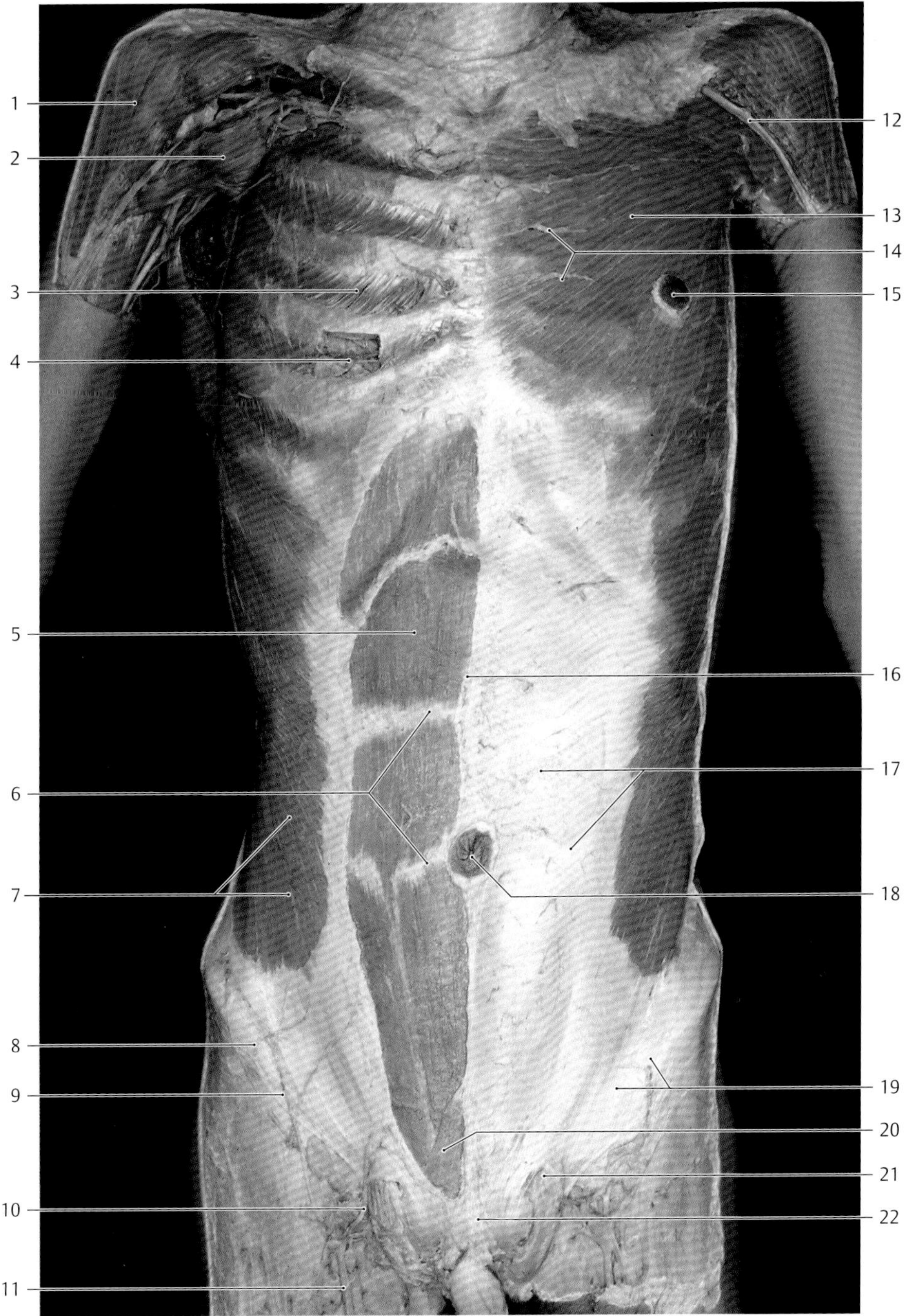


Fig. 2.52 **Thoracic and abdominal walls** (anterior aspect). Right pectoralis major and minor muscles and anterior layer of rectus sheath have been removed on the right side.

1 Deltoid muscle
2 Pectoralis major muscle (divided)
3 Internal intercostal muscle
4 Intercostal artery and vein
5 Rectus abdominis muscle
6 Tendinous intersections
7 External abdominal oblique muscle
8 Anterior superior iliac spine
9 Superficial circumflex iliac vein
10 Superficial epigastric vein
11 Great saphenous vein
12 Cephalic vein
13 Pectoralis major muscle
14 Anterior cutaneous branches of intercostal nerves
15 Nipple
16 Linea alba
17 Anterior layer of rectus sheath
18 Umbilicus
19 Inguinal ligament
20 Pyramidal muscle
21 Superficial inguinal ring and spermatic cord
22 Fundiform ligament of penis

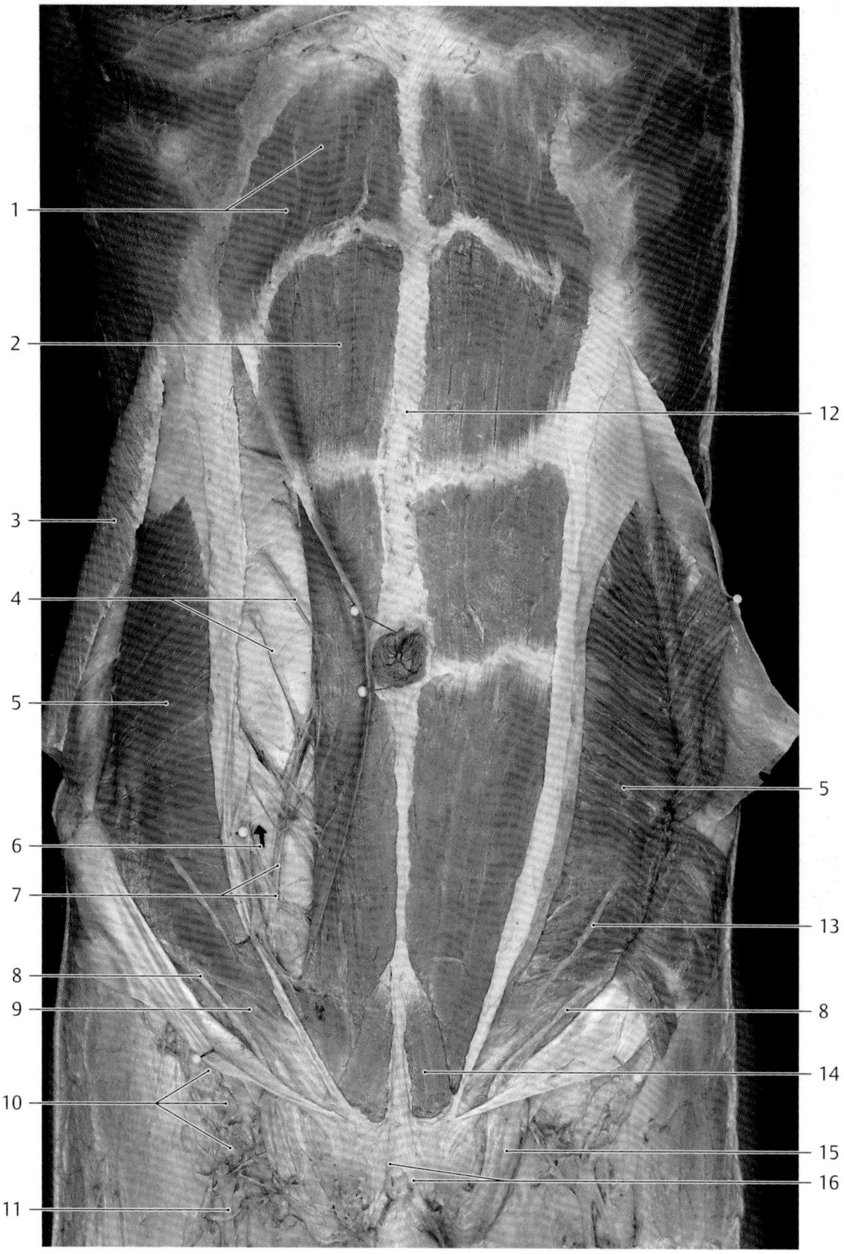

1 Costal margin
2 Rectus abdominis muscle
3 External abdominal oblique muscle (reflected)
4 Thoraco-abdominal (intercostal) nerves with accompanying vessels
5 Internal abdominal oblique muscle
6 Arcuate line (arrow)
7 Inferior epigastric artery and vein
8 Ilio-inguinal nerve
9 Position of deep inguinal ring
10 Superficial inguinal lymph nodes
11 Great saphenous vein
12 Linea alba
13 Iliohypogastric nerve
14 Pyramidal muscle
15 Spermatic cord
16 Fundiform ligament of penis

**Fig. 2.53 Thoracic and abdominal walls** (anterior aspect). External abdominal oblique muscle has been divided and reflected on both sides. The right rectus muscle has been reflected medially to display the posterior layer of rectus sheath. Arrow = location of arcuate line.

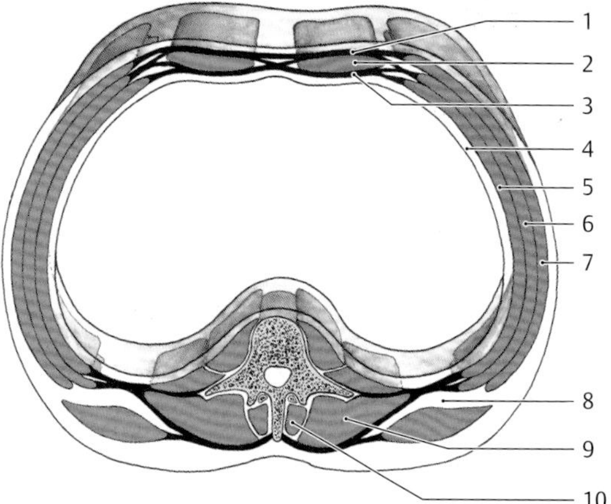


1 Anterior layer of rectus sheath
2 Rectus abdominis muscle
3 Posterior layer of rectus sheath
4 Transversalis fascia
5 Transverse abdominal muscle
6 Internal abdominal oblique muscle
7 External abdominal oblique muscle
8 Thoracolumbar fascia with superficial and deep layer
9 Lateral column of erector spinae muscle
10 Medial column of erector spinae muscle

**Fig. 2.54 Horizontal section through the trunk,** superior to arcuate line (inferior aspect).

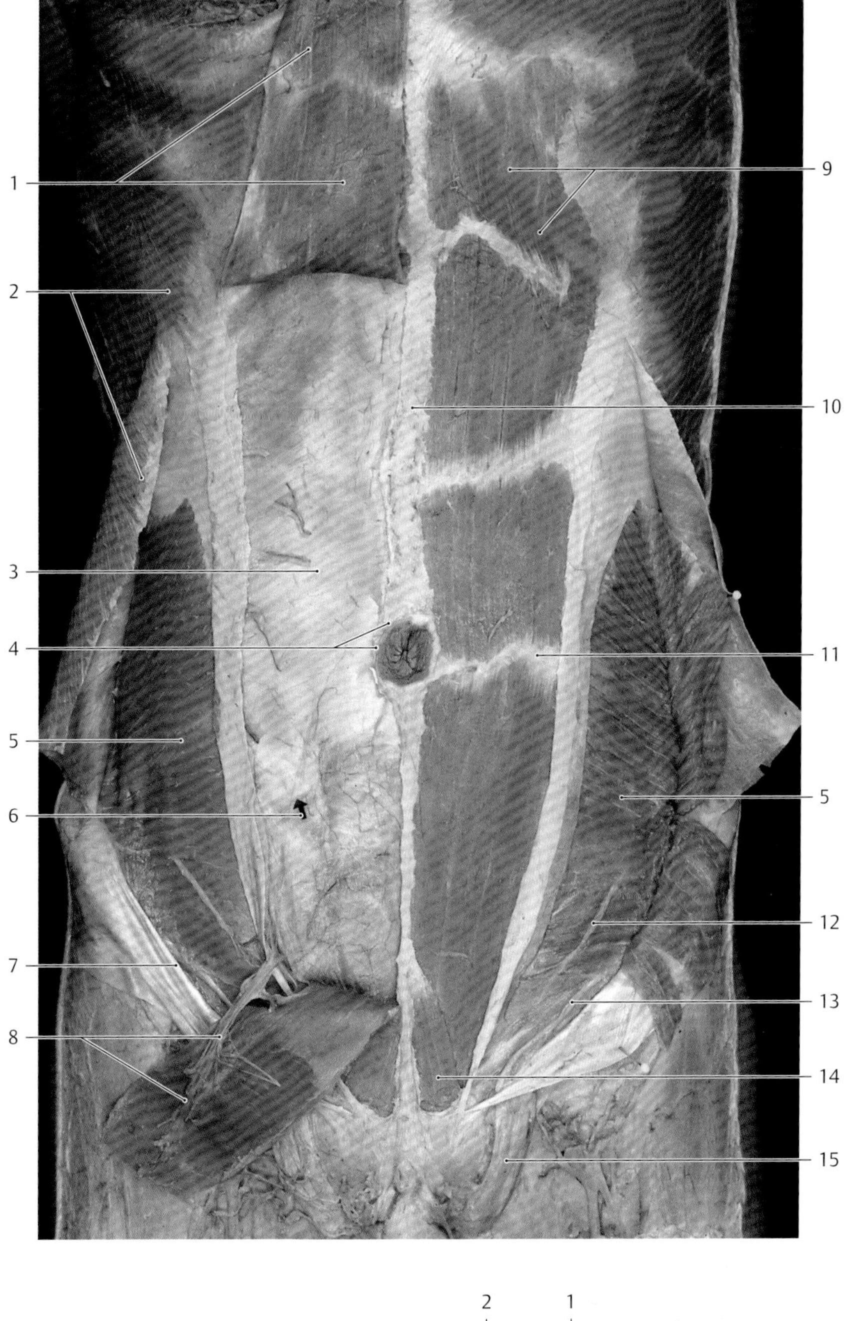


1 Rectus abdominis muscle (reflected)
2 External abdominal oblique muscle (divided)
3 Posterior layer of rectus sheath
4 Umbilical ring
5 Internal abdominal oblique muscle
6 Arcuate line (arrow)
7 Inguinal ligament
8 Inferior epigastric artery and vein and rectus abdominis muscle (divided and reflected)
9 Costal margin
10 Linea alba
11 Tendinous intersection
12 Iliohypogastric nerve
13 Ilio-inguinal nerve
14 Pyramidal muscle
15 Spermatic cord

Fig. 2.55 **Thoracic and abdominal walls** (anterior aspect). External abdominal oblique muscle has been divided and reflected on both sides. The right rectus muscle has been cut and reflected to display the posterior layer of rectus sheath. Arrow = location of arcuate line.

1 Linea alba
2 Rectus abdominis muscle
3 Epidermis
4 Fascia of external abdominal oblique muscle (green)
5 External abdominal oblique muscle
6 Internal abdominal oblique muscle
7 Transverse abdominal muscle
8 Transversalis fascia (green)
9 Peritoneum

Fig. 2.56 **Transverse sections through the abdominal wall. a** superior and **b** inferior to arcuate line. Notice the difference in the structure of the rectus sheath in both sections.

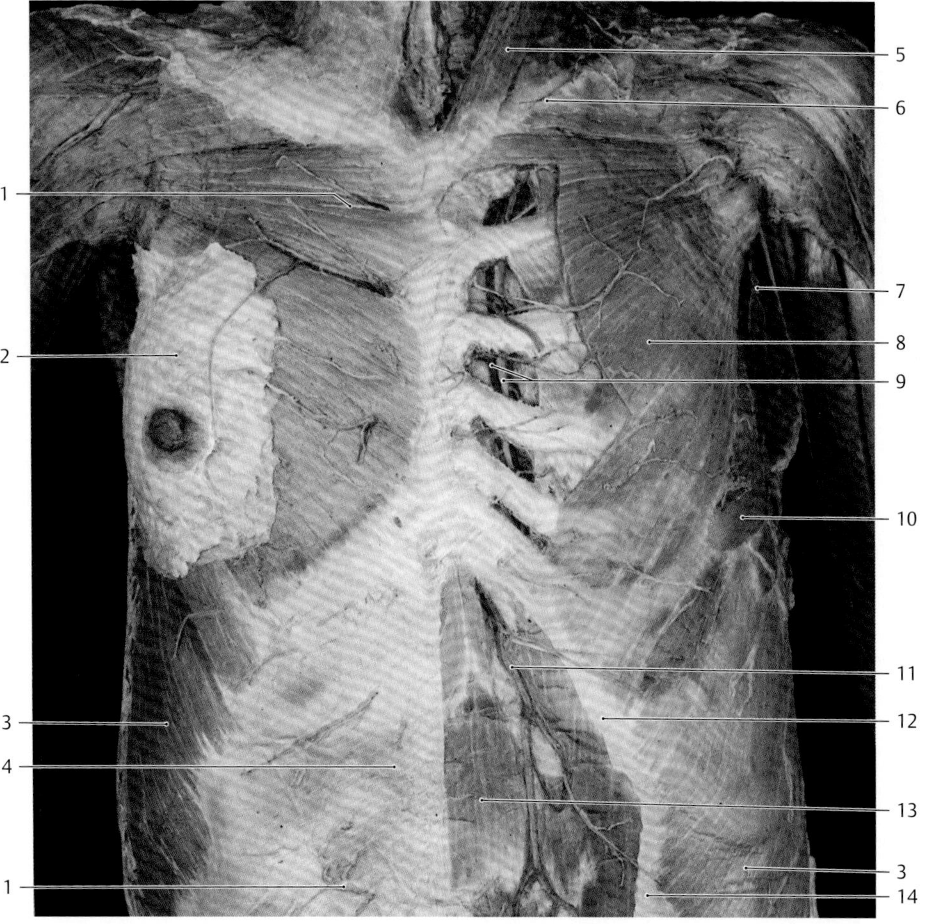


1 Anterior perforating branches of intercostal nerve
2 Mammary gland
3 External abdominal oblique muscle
4 Rectus sheath (anterior layer)
5 Sternocleidomastoid muscle
6 Clavicle
7 Lateral thoracic artery and vein
8 Pectoralis major muscle
9 Internal thoracic artery and vein
10 Serratus anterior muscle
11 Superior epigastric artery and vein
12 Costal margin
13 Rectus abdominis muscle
14 Cut edge of the anterior layer of the rectus sheath
15 Subclavian artery
16 Highest intercostal artery
17 Internal thoracic artery
18 Musculophrenic artery
19 Superficial epigastric artery
20 Deep circumflex iliac artery
21 Superior epigastric artery
22 Inferior epigastric artery
23 Superficial circumflex iliac artery

**Fig. 2.57 Thoracic and abdominal walls** (anterior aspect). Dissection of the internal thoracic artery and vein. Left pectoralis major muscle partly removed. Anterior lamina of the rectus sheath on the left side has been removed.

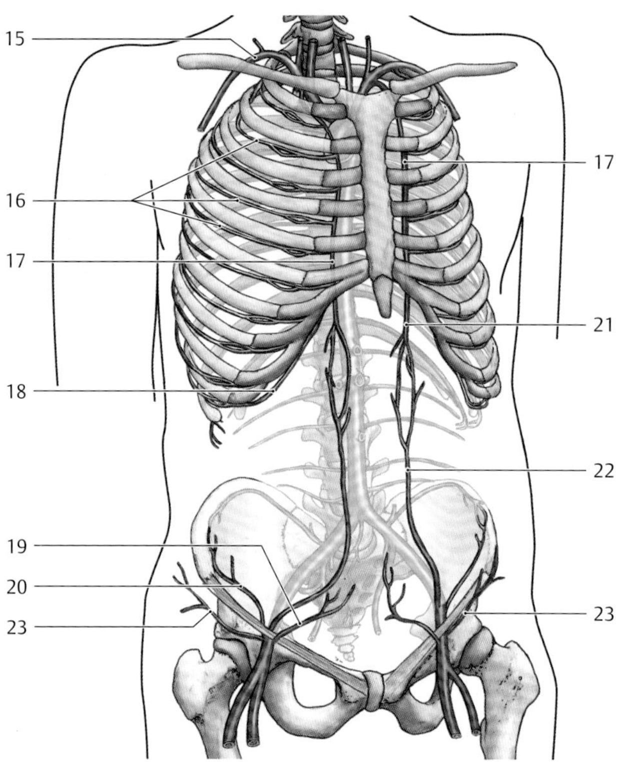


**Fig. 2.58 Main arteries of thoracic and abdominal walls** (anterior aspect). The superior and inferior epigastric arteries anastomose with each other in the area of the anterior rectus sheath.

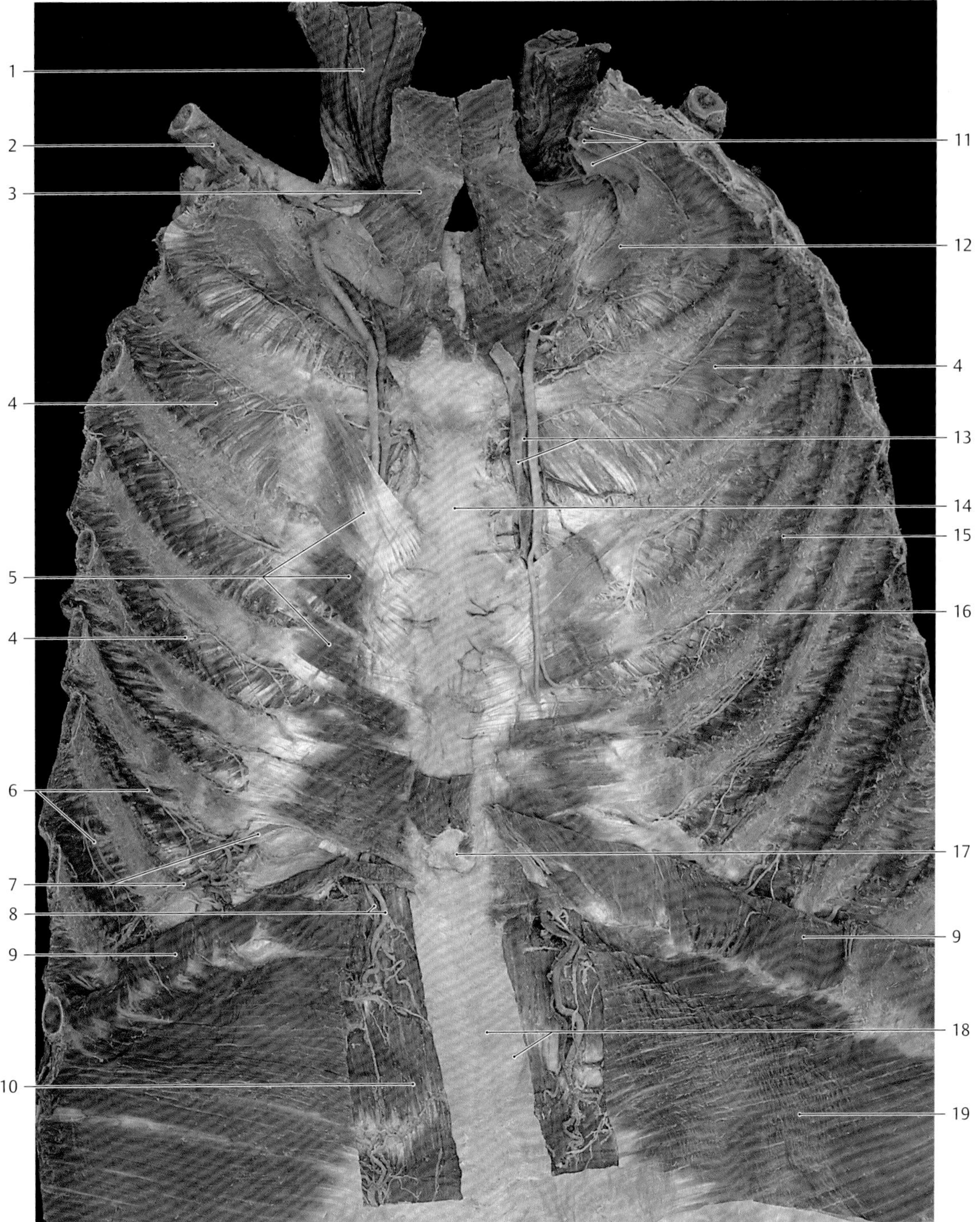


Fig. 2.59 **Anterior thoracic wall** (posterior aspect). Diaphragm partly removed, posterior layer of rectus sheath fenestrated on both sides.

1 Sternocleidomastoid muscle (divided)
2 Clavicle
3 Sternothyroid muscle
4 Internal intercostal muscle
5 Transversus thoracis muscle
6 Intercostal arteries and nerves
7 Musculophrenic artery
8 Superior epigastric artery and vein
9 Diaphragm (divided)
10 Rectus abdominis muscle
11 Subclavian artery and brachial plexus
12 First rib
13 Internal thoracic artery and vein
14 Sternum
15 Innermost intercostal muscle
16 Intercostal artery and vein
17 Xiphoid process
18 Linea alba and posterior layer of rectus sheath
19 Transverse abdominal muscle

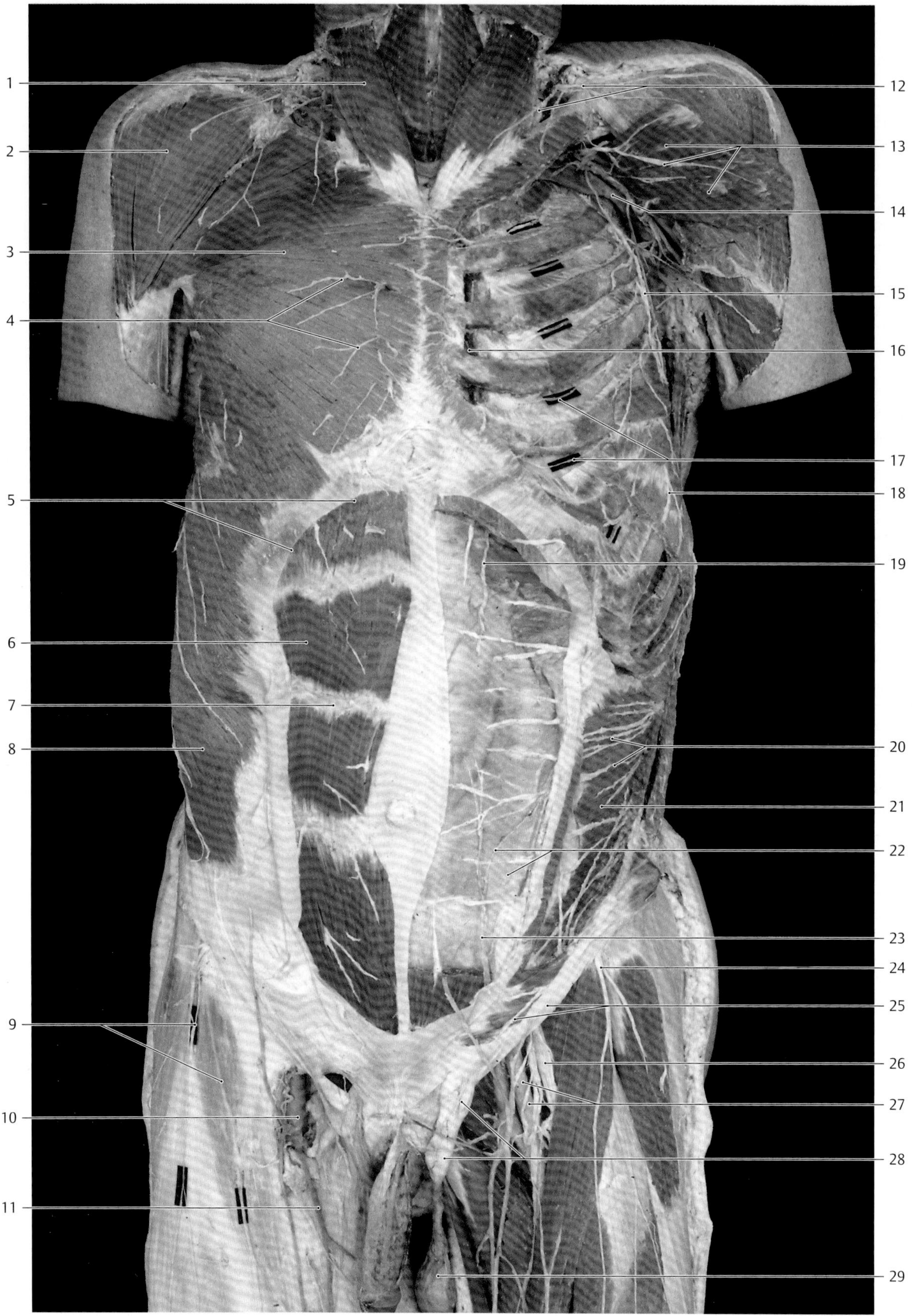


**Fig. 2.60 Thoracic and abdominal walls with vessels and nerves** (anterior aspect). Right side = superficial layers; left side = deeper layers. Pectoralis major and minor muscles and the external and internal intercostal muscles on the left side have been removed to display the intercostal nerves. The anterior layer of the rectus sheath, the left rectus abdominis muscle, and the external and internal abdominal oblique muscles have been removed to show the thoraco-abdominal nerves within the abdominal wall.

1 Sternocleidomastoid muscle
2 Deltoid muscle
3 Pectoralis major muscle
4 Anterior cutaneous branches of intercostal nerves
5 Cut edge of anterior layer of rectus sheath
6 Rectus abdominis muscle
7 Tendinous intersection
8 External abdominal oblique muscle
9 Lateral femoral cutaneous nerve
10 Femoral vein
11 Great saphenous vein
12 Medial supraclavicular nerves
13 Pectoralis minor muscle (reflected) and medial pectoral nerves
14 Axillary vein
15 Long thoracic nerve and lateral thoracic artery
16 Internal thoracic artery
17 Intercostal nerves
18 Lateral cutaneous branches of intercostal nerves
19 Superior epigastric artery
20 Thoraco-abdominal (intercostal) nerves
21 Transverse abdominal muscle
22 Posterior layer of rectus sheath
23 Inferior epigastric artery
24 Lateral femoral cutaneous nerve
25 Inguinal ligament and ilio-inguinal nerve
26 Femoral nerve
27 Femoral artery
28 Spermatic cord
29 Testis
30 Posterior intercostal arteries
31 Internal abdominal oblique muscle
32 Lateral cutaneous branch of intercostal nerve
33 Dorsal branch of spinal nerve
34 Latissimus dorsi muscle
35 Deep muscles of the back (medial and lateral tract)
36 Anterior layer of rectus sheath
37 Posterior layer of rectus sheath
38 Thoracolumbar fascia
39 Spinal cord
40 Aorta
41 Ventral root of spinal nerve
42 Dorsal root of spinal nerve

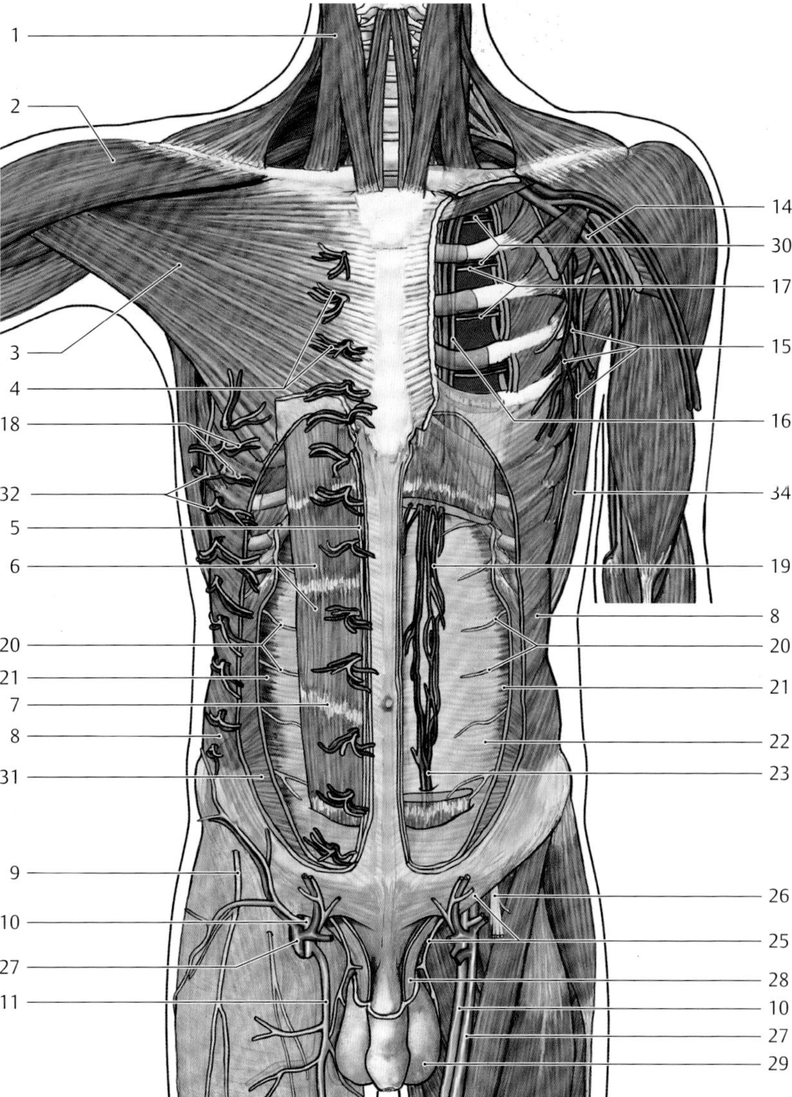


**Fig. 2.61 Thoracic and abdominal walls with vessels and nerves** (anterior aspect). Right side = superficial layers; left side = deeper layers. Note the segmental organization of the blood vessels and nerves.

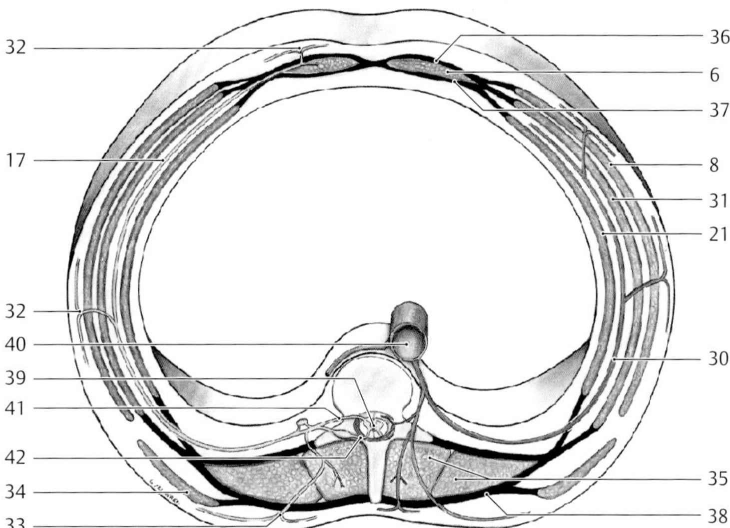


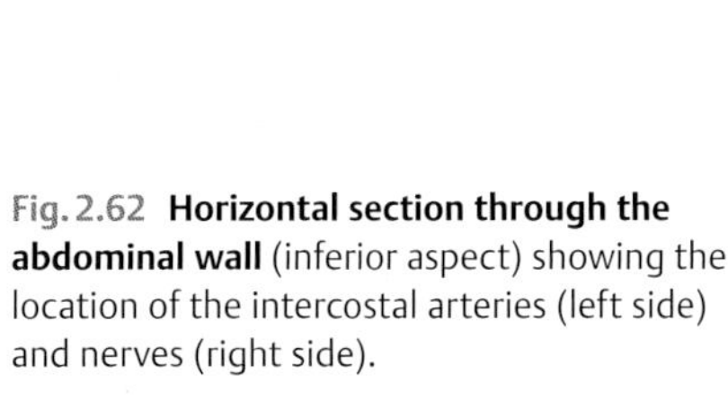

**Fig. 2.62 Horizontal section through the abdominal wall** (inferior aspect) showing the location of the intercostal arteries (left side) and nerves (right side).

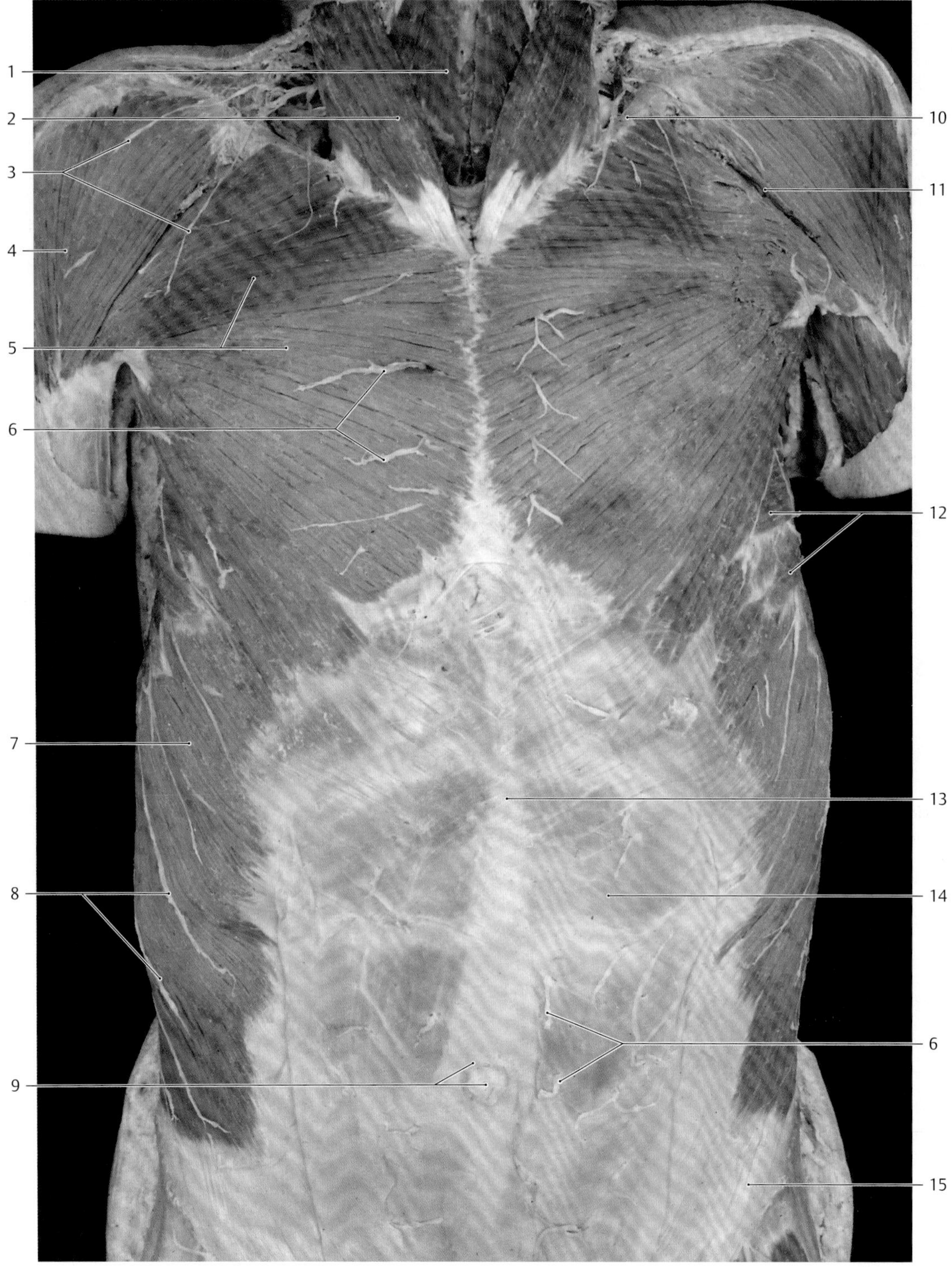


Fig. 2.63 **Thoracic and abdominal walls with superficial muscles** (anterior aspect). The fascia of the pectoralis major muscle and the abdominal wall have been removed; the anterior layer of the sheath of the rectus abdominis muscle is displayed.

1 Sternohyoid muscle
2 Sternocleidomastoid muscle
3 Supraclavicular nerves (branches of cervical plexus)
4 Deltoid muscle
5 Pectoralis major muscle
6 Anterior cutaneous branches of intercostal nerves
7 External abdominal oblique muscle
8 Lateral cutaneous branches of intercostal nerves
9 Umbilicus and umbilical ring
10 Clavicle
11 Cephalic vein
12 Serratus anterior muscle
13 Linea alba
14 Sheath of rectus abdominis muscle (anterior layer)
15 Inguinal ligament

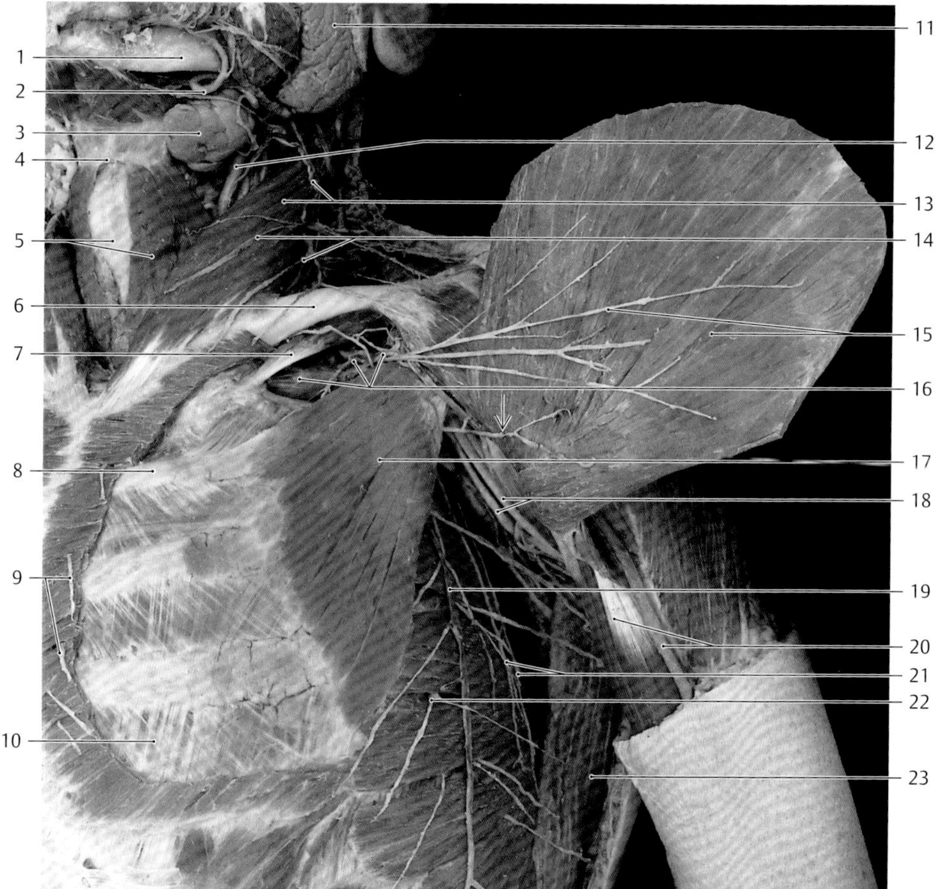

Fig. 2.64 **Thoracic wall** (anterior aspect). Left pectoralis major muscle has been divided and reflected. Note the connection of the cephalic vein with the subclavian vein. Arrow = medial pectoral nerve.

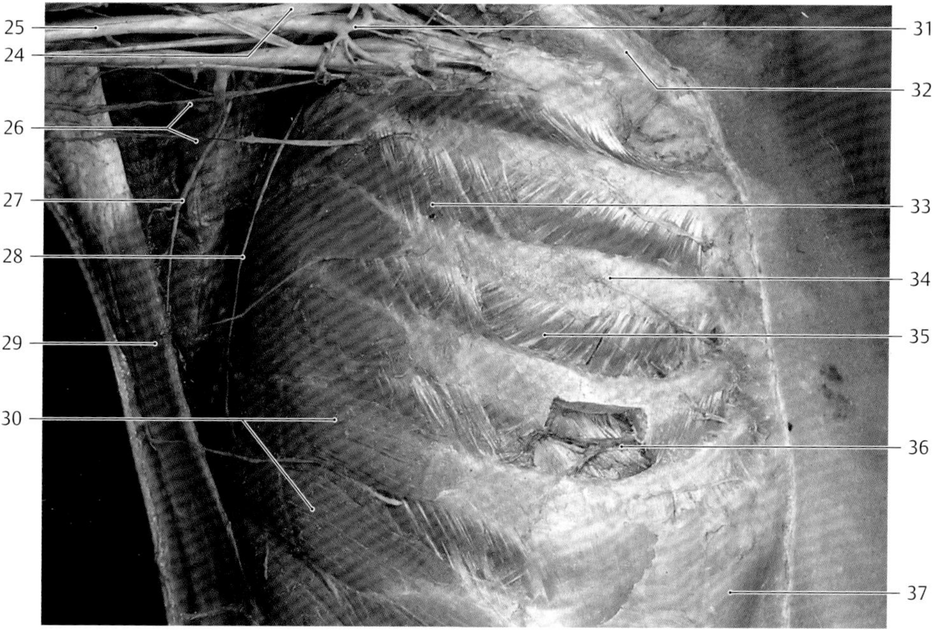

Fig. 2.65 **Thoracic wall** (lateral aspect). Pectoralis major and minor muscles have been removed. A section of the fourth rib has been cut and removed to display the intercostal vessels and nerve.

1 Mandible
2 Facial artery
3 Submandibular gland
4 Hyoid bone
5 Thyroid cartilage and sternohyoid muscle
6 Clavicle
7 Subclavius muscle
8 Second rib
9 Anterior cutaneous branches of intercostal nerves
10 External intercostal membrane
11 Parotid gland
12 External carotid artery
13 Sternocleidomastoid muscle and cutaneous branches of cervical plexus
14 Supraclavicular nerves
15 Pectoralis major muscle and lateral pectoral nerves
16 Thoraco-acromial artery and subclavian vein
17 Pectoralis minor muscle
18 Median and ulnar nerve
19 Thoraco-epigastric vein
20 Cephalic vein and long head of biceps brachii muscle
21 Lateral thoracic artery and long thoracic nerve
22 Lateral cutaneous branches of intercostal nerve
23 Latissimus dorsi muscle
24 Median nerve
25 Axillary artery
26 Intercostobrachial nerves
27 Thoracodorsal nerve
28 Long thoracic nerve
29 Latissimus dorsi muscle
30 Serratus anterior muscle
31 Thoraco-acromial artery
32 Clavicle
33 External intercostal muscle
34 Third rib
35 Internal intercostal muscle
36 Anterior intercostal artery and vein, and intercostal nerve
37 Costal arch or margin

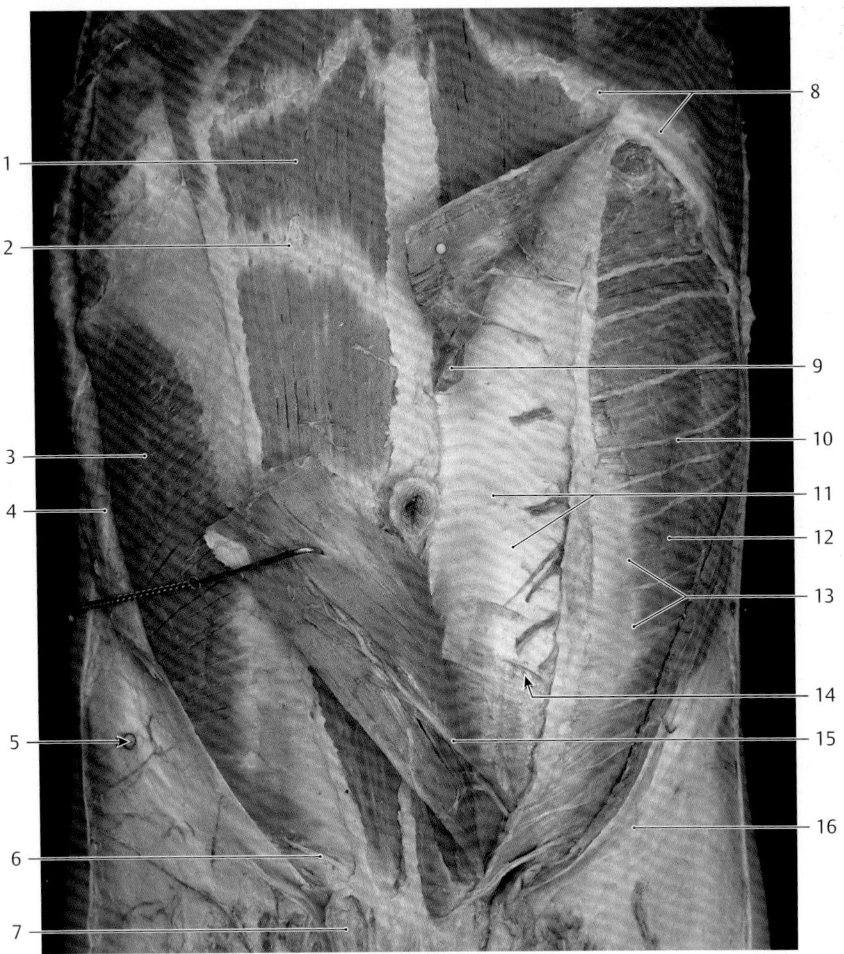


1 Rectus abdominis muscle
2 Tendinous intersection
3 Internal abdominal oblique muscle
4 External abdominal oblique muscle (reflected)
5 Anterior superior iliac spine
6 Ilio-inguinal nerve
7 Spermatic cord
8 Costal margin
9 Superior epigastric artery
10 Thoraco-abdominal (intercostal) nerves
11 Posterior layer of rectus sheath
12 Transverse abdominal muscle
13 Semilunar line
14 Arcuate line
15 Inferior epigastric artery
16 Inguinal ligament

Fig. 2.66 **Abdominal wall with vessels and nerves** (anterior aspect). The left rectus abdominis muscle has been divided and reflected to display the inferior epigastric vessels. The left internal abdominal oblique muscle has been removed to show the thoraco-abdominal nerves.

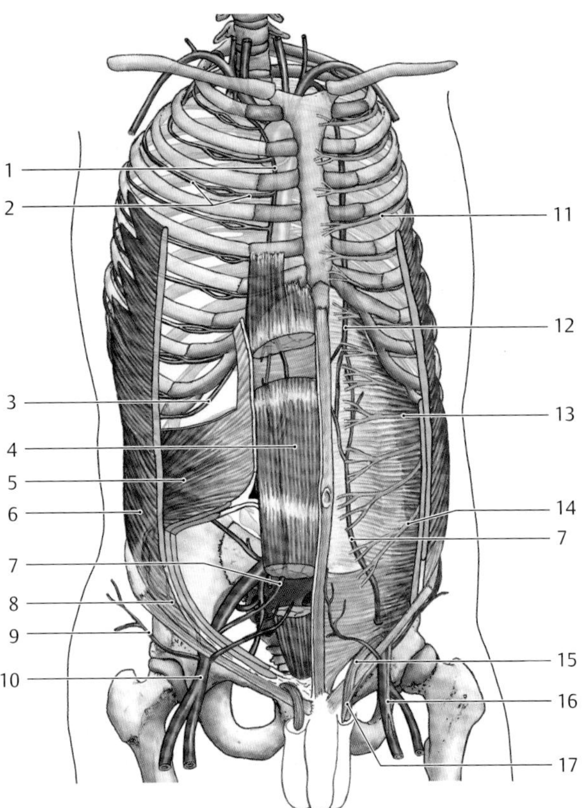


1 Internal thoracic artery
2 Intercostal artery
3 Musculophrenic artery
4 Rectus abdominis muscle
5 Internal abdominal oblique muscle
6 External abdominal oblique muscle
7 Inferior epigastric artery
8 Deep circumflex iliac artery
9 Superficial circumflex iliac artery
10 Femoral artery
11 Intercostal nerve
12 Superior epigastric artery
13 Intercostal nerve
14 Iliohypogastric nerve (L1)
15 Spermatic cord
16 Femoral branch of genitofemoral nerve
17 Genital branch of genitofemoral nerve

Fig. 2.67 **Thoracic and abdominal walls with arteries and nerves** (anterior aspect).

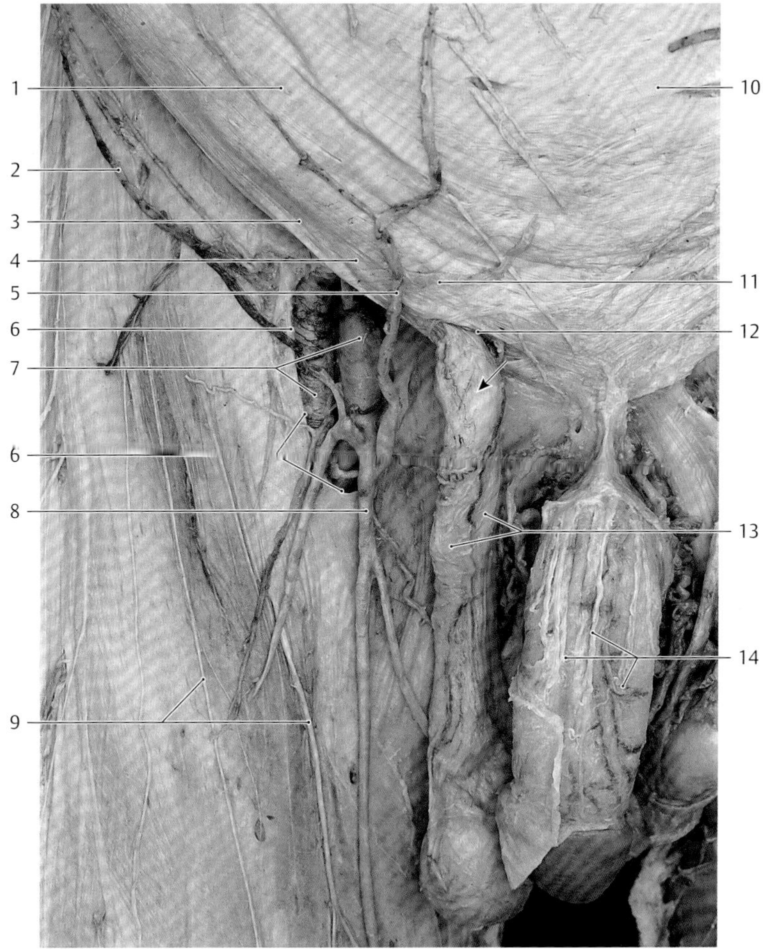


Fig. 2.68 **Inguinal canal in the male,** right side (superficial layer, anterior aspect). There is a small inguinal hernia (arrow).

1 Aponeurosis of external abdominal oblique muscle
2 Superficial circumflex iliac vein
3 Inguinal ligament
4 Lateral crus of inguinal ring
5 Superficial epigastric vein
6 Saphenous opening
7 Femoral artery and vein
8 Great saphenous vein
9 Anterior cutaneous branches of femoral nerve
10 Anterior layer of rectus sheath
11 Intercrural fibers
12 Superficial inguinal ring
13 Spermatic cord and genital branch of genitofemoral nerve
14 Penis with dorsal nerves and deep dorsal vein of penis
15 Aponeurosis of external abdominal oblique muscle (divided and reflected)
16 Internal abdominal oblique muscle
17 Ilio-inguinal nerve
18 Anterior cutaneous branches of iliohypogastric nerve
19 Superficial external pudendal veins

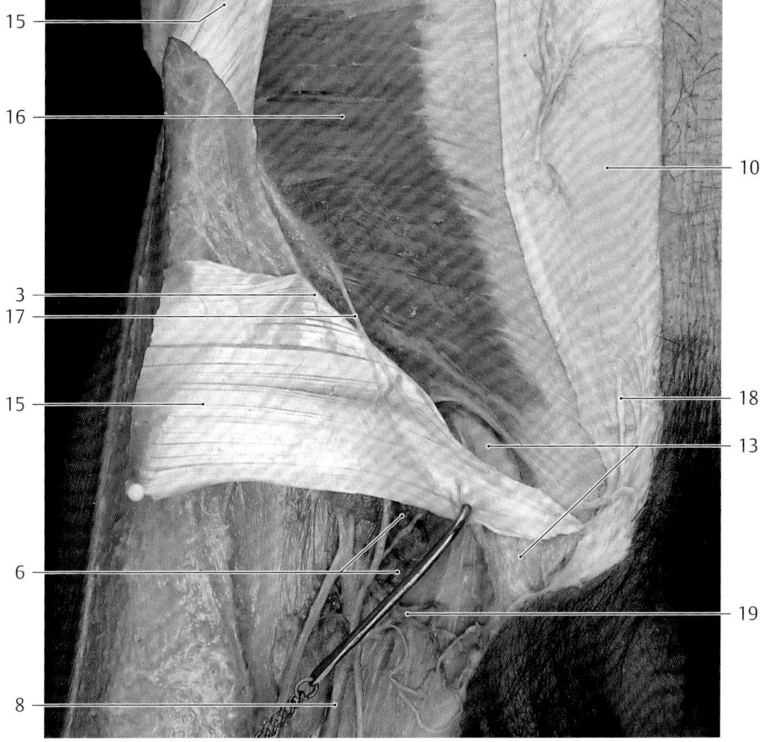


Fig. 2.69 **Inguinal canal in the male,** right side (superficial layer, anterior aspect). The external abdominal oblique muscle has been divided to display the inguinal canal.

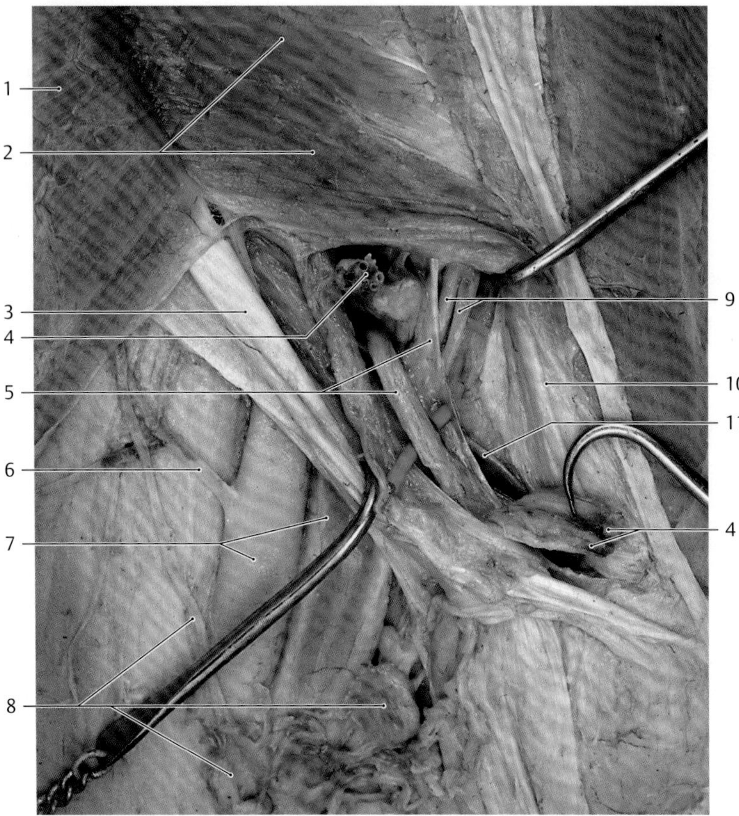


Fig. 2.70 **Inguinal canal in the male,** right side (deep layer, anterior aspect). Spermatic cord with exception of ductus deferens (probe) has been divided and reflected.

1 Internal abdominal oblique muscle (reflected)
2 Transverse abdominal muscle
3 Inguinal ligament
4 Spermatic cord with the exception of the ductus deferens (divided and reflected)
5 Ductus deferens and interfoveolar ligament
6 Superficial circumflex iliac artery
7 Femoral artery and vein
8 Superficial inguinal lymph nodes and inguinal lymph vessel
9 Inferior epigastric artery and vein
10 Falx inguinalis or conjoint tendon (cut)
11 Pubic branch of inferior epigastric artery
12 Iliacus muscle
13 Ureter
14 Ductus deferens (in situ)
15 Femoral nerve
16 Spermatic cord with ductus deferens and external spermatic fascia
17 Cremaster muscle
18 Internal spermatic fascia
19 Tunica vaginalis testis
20 Testis and epididymis
21 Rectum
22 Anterior layer of rectus sheath
23 Intercrural fibrae
24 Urinary bladder
25 Superficial inguinal ring
26 Saphenous opening with great saphenous vein
27 Deep dorsal vein of penis
28 Penis
29 Glans penis
30 Rectus abdominis muscle
31 Deep inguinal ring
32 Pampiniform venous plexus and testicular artery
33 Fascia lata and sartorius muscle
34 Anterior superior iliac spine
35 Inferior epigastric artery
36 Lateral femoral cutaneous nerve
37 Ilioinguinal nerve
38 Suspensory ligament of penis
39 Sartorius muscle
40 External abdominal oblique muscle
41 Dartos fascia and scrotal skin
42 Ductus deferens
43 Vaginal process
44 Peritoneum

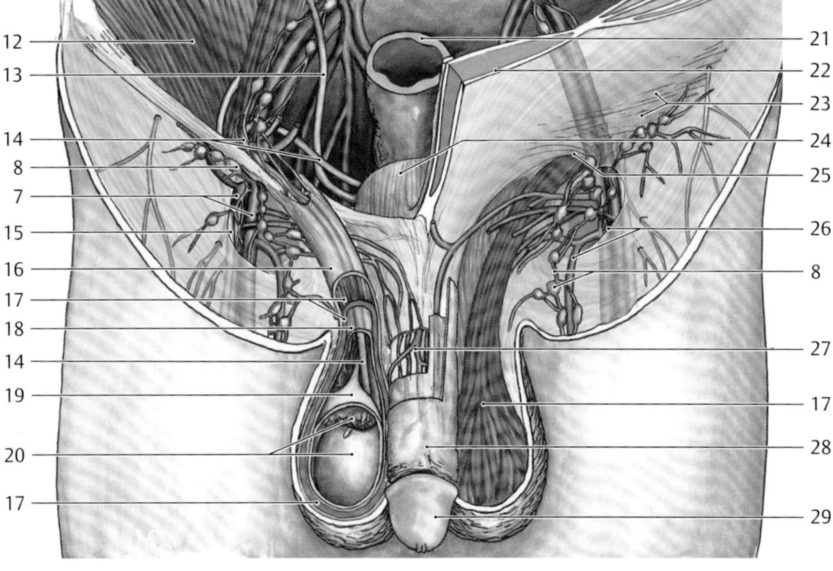


Fig. 2.71 **General characteristics of lower part of anterior abdominal wall and inguinal canal.** Inguinal hernias (Figs. 2.71–2.73) either follow the course of the inguinal canal (indirect inguinal hernia) or push through the abdominal wall via the superficial inguinal ring (direct inguinal hernia). Femoral hernias occur just below the inguinal ligament. The examination of the inferior epigastric vessels (9) can help to assess the type of hernia.

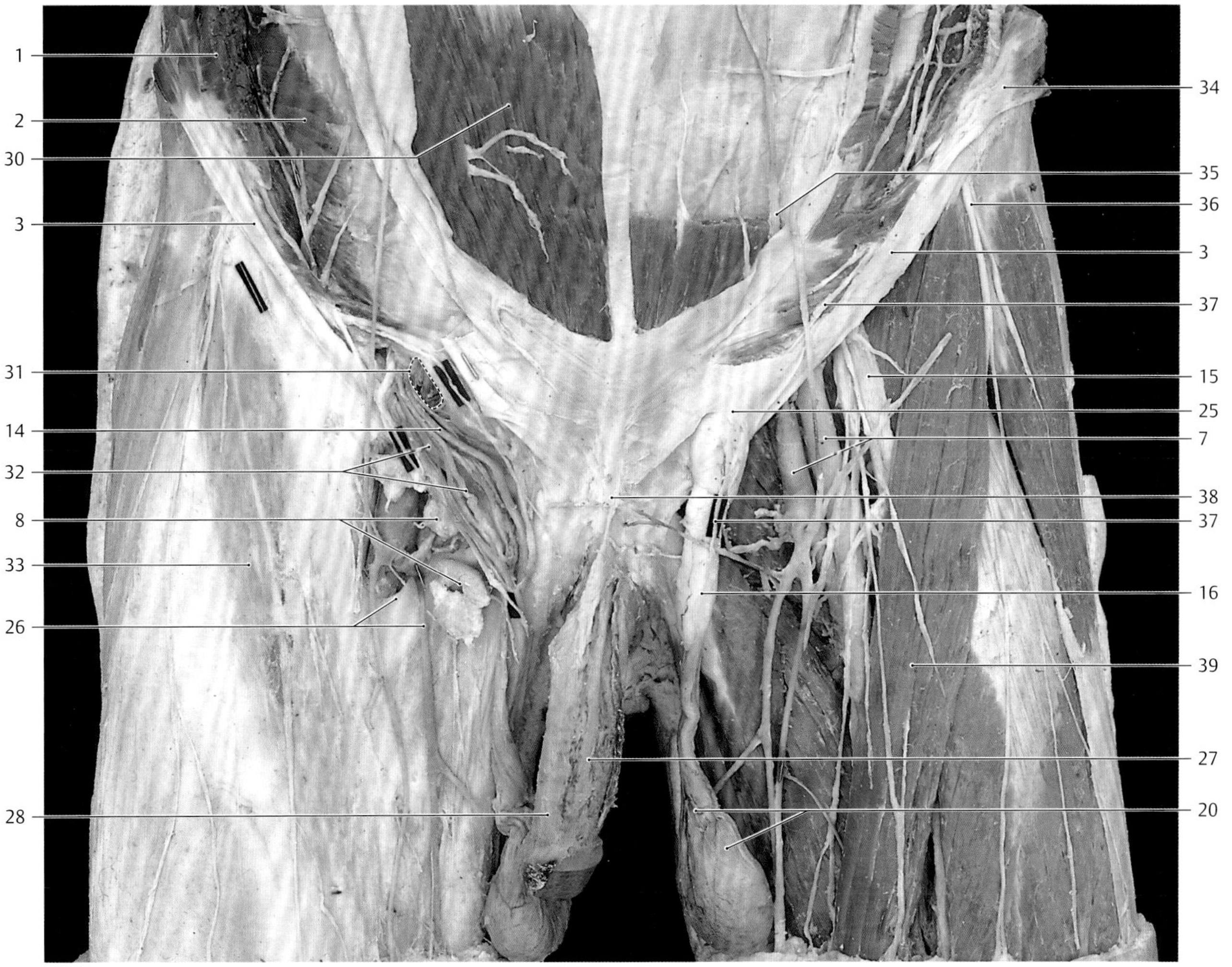

**Fig. 2.72 Inguinal and femoral regions in the male** (anterior aspect). On the right, the spermatic cord was dissected to display the ductus deferens and the accompanying vessels and nerves. The fascia lata on the left side has been removed.

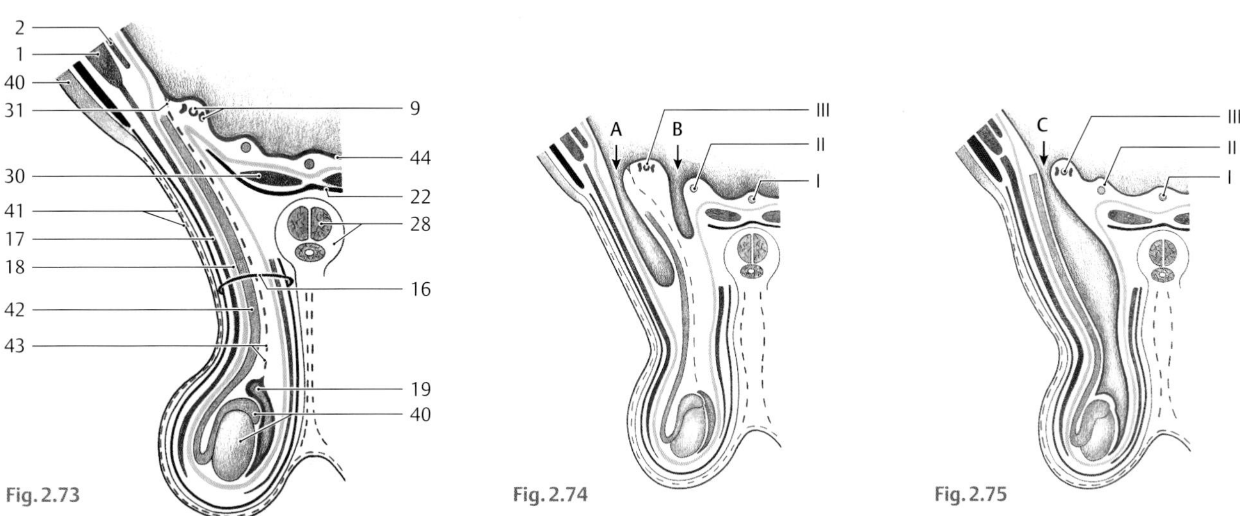


**Figs. 2.73–2.75 Layers of spermatic cord and types of hernias.** Left = normal situation. Middle = location of acquired inguinal hernias: A = indirect inguinal hernia; B = direct inguinal hernia. Right = congenital indirect inguinal hernia (C); the vaginal process remained open.

I = Median umbilical fold containing urachus chord
II = Medial umbilical fold with remnants of umbilical artery
III = Lateral umbilical fold with inferior epigastric artery and vein

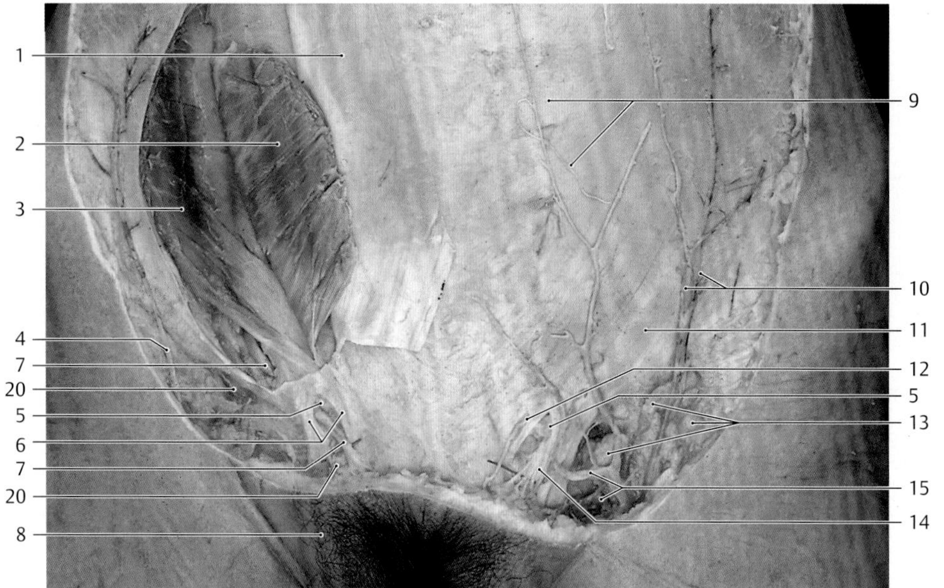


**Fig. 2.76 Inguinal region in the female** (anterior aspect). Left side = superficial layer; right side = external and internal abdominal oblique muscles divided and reflected.

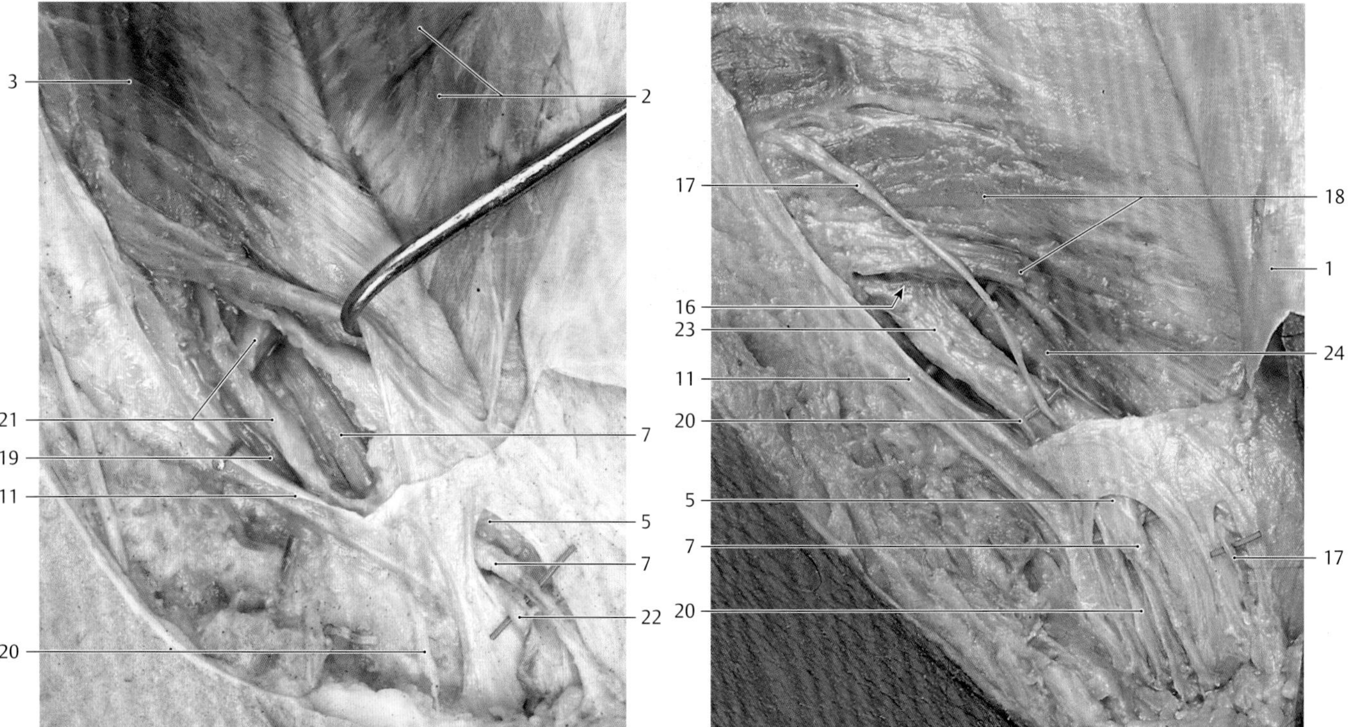


**Fig. 2.77 Inguinal canal in the female,** right side (anterior aspect). The external abdominal oblique muscle has been divided and reflected to display the ilio-inguinal nerve and the round ligament.

**Fig. 2.78 Inguinal canal in the female,** right side (anterior aspect). The external and internal abdominal oblique muscles have been divided and reflected to show the content of the inguinal canal.

1 Aponeurosis of external abdominal oblique muscle
2 Internal abdominal oblique muscle (divided and reflected)
3 Transverse abdominal muscle
4 Superficial circumflex iliac artery and vein
5 Superficial inguinal ring with fat pad
6 Medial and lateral crural fibers
7 Round ligament (ligamentum teres uteri)
8 Labium majus pudendi
9 Anterior layer of rectus sheath
10 Superficial epigastric artery and vein
11 Inguinal ligament
12 Cutaneous branch of ilio-inguinal nerve
13 Superficial inguinal lymph nodes
14 Entrance of round ligament into the labium majus
15 External pudendal artery and vein
16 Position of deep inguinal ring
17 Ilio-inguinal nerve
18 Internal abdominal oblique muscle
19 Pubic branch of inferior epigastric artery
20 Genital branch of genitofemoral nerve
21 Fat pad of inguinal canal
22 Ilio-inguinal nerve
23 Sheath of round ligament (inguinal canal)
24 Transversalis fascia

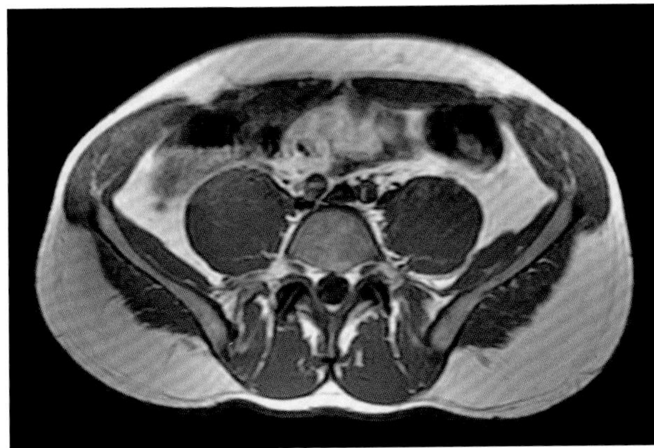

Fig. 2.79 **Horizontal section through the trunk at the level of the pelvic crest** (inferior aspect, MRI scan). (Heuck A, et al. MRT-Atlas des muskuloskelettalen Systems. Stuttgart, Germany: Schattauer, 2009.)

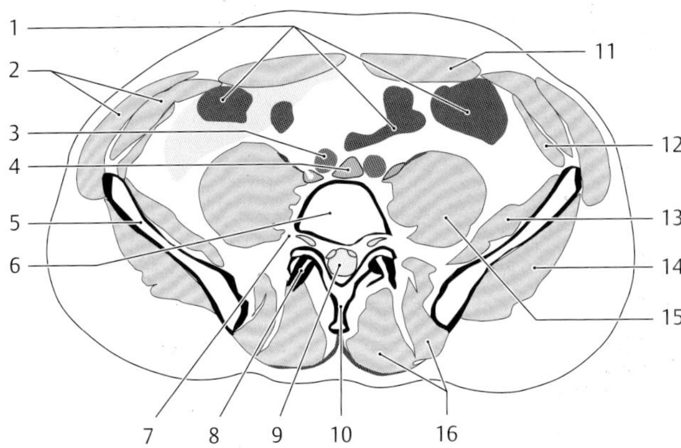


Fig. 2.80 **Horizontal section through the trunk** (schematic; see corresponding sections in Figs. 2.79 and 2.81). (Heuck A, et al. MRT-Atlas des muskuloskelettalen Systems. Stuttgart, Germany: Schattauer, 2009.)

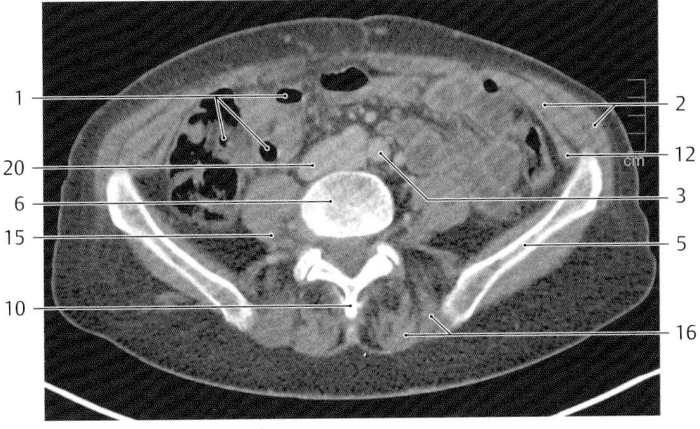


Fig. 2.81 **Horizontal section through the trunk** at the level of fourth lumbar vertebra (inferior aspect, CT scan). (Courtesy of Prof. Uder, Institute of Radiology, University Hospital Erlangen, Germany.)

1 Intestine
2 External and internal abdominal oblique muscles
3 Common iliac artery
4 Common iliac vein
5 Iliac bone
6 Body of lumbar vertebra
7 Lumbar spinal nerve
8 Zygapophyseal joint
9 Vertebral canal
10 Spinous process (L5)
11 Rectus abdominis muscle
12 Transverse abdominal muscle
13 Iliacus muscle
14 Gluteus medius muscle
15 Psoas major muscle
16 Erector spinae muscle
17 Quadratus lumborum muscle
18 Ureter
19 Abdominal aorta
20 Inferior vena cava
21 Descending colon

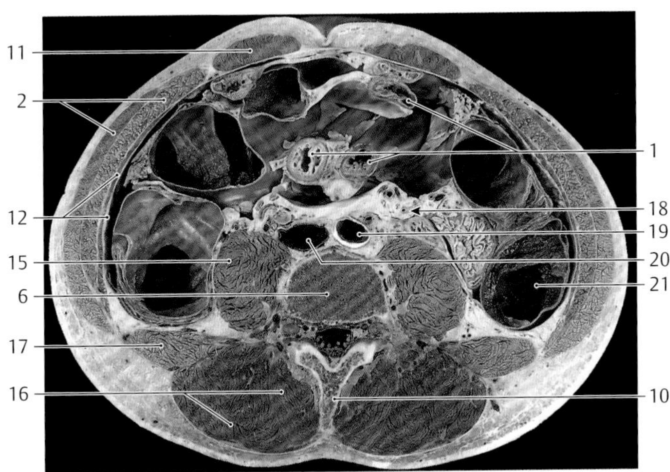


Fig. 2.82 **Horizontal section through the trunk** at the level of the umbilicus, superior to arcuate line (inferior aspect).

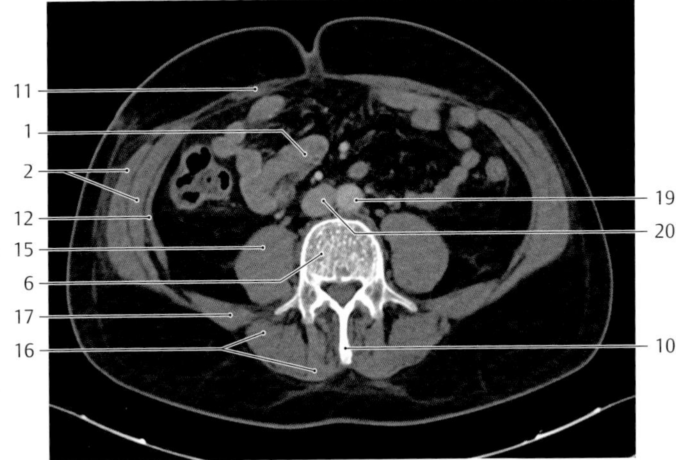


Fig. 2.83 **Horizontal section through the trunk at the level of the umbilicus** (inferior aspect, CT scan). (Courtesy of Prof. Uder, Institute of Radiology, University Hospital Erlangen, Germany.)

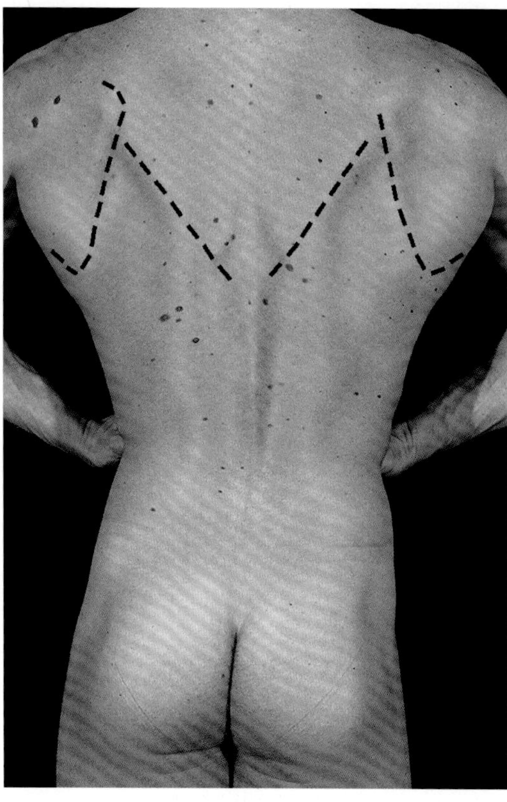

Fig. 2.84 **Back of a strong man.** Borderlines indicate the scapula and the trapezius muscle.

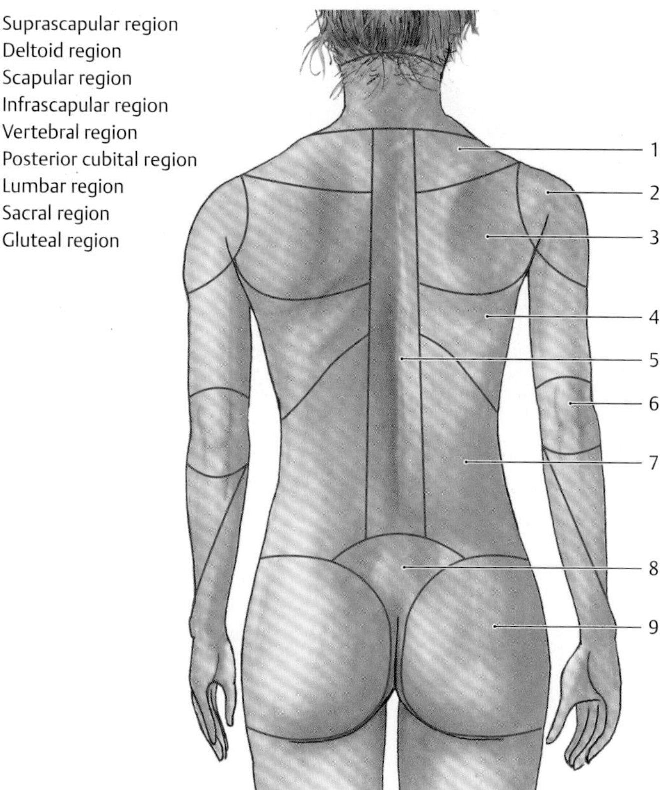


Fig. 2.85 **Regions of the back in the female.**

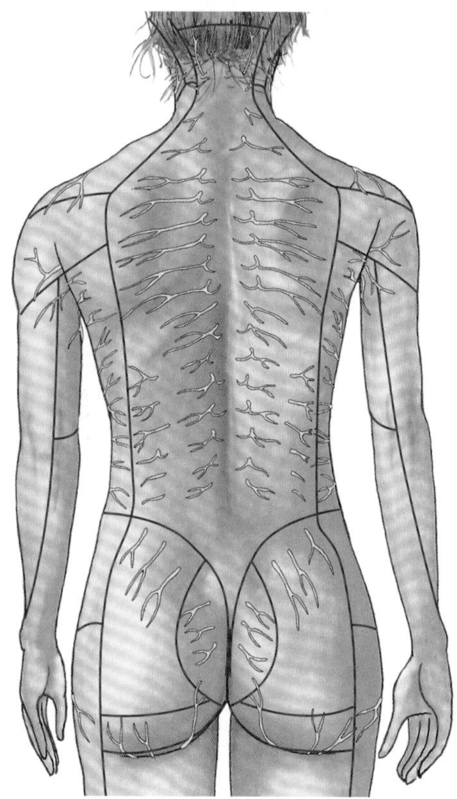

Fig. 2.86 **Innervation of the back.** The dorsal branches of the spinal nerves display a segmental arrangement. The segmental innervation regions of the back are indicated.

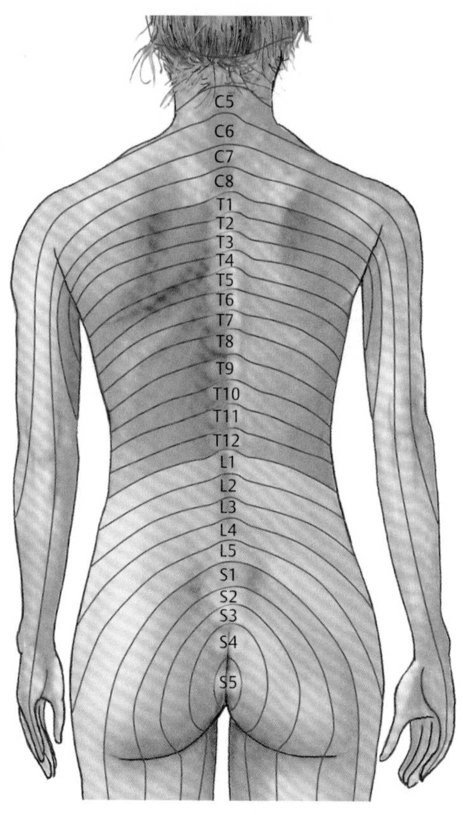


Fig. 2.87 **Segmental arrangement of the back.** Cervical (C1–C8; only shown are C5–C8), thoracic (T1–T12), lumbar (L1–L5), and sacral (S1–S5) segments are colored different.

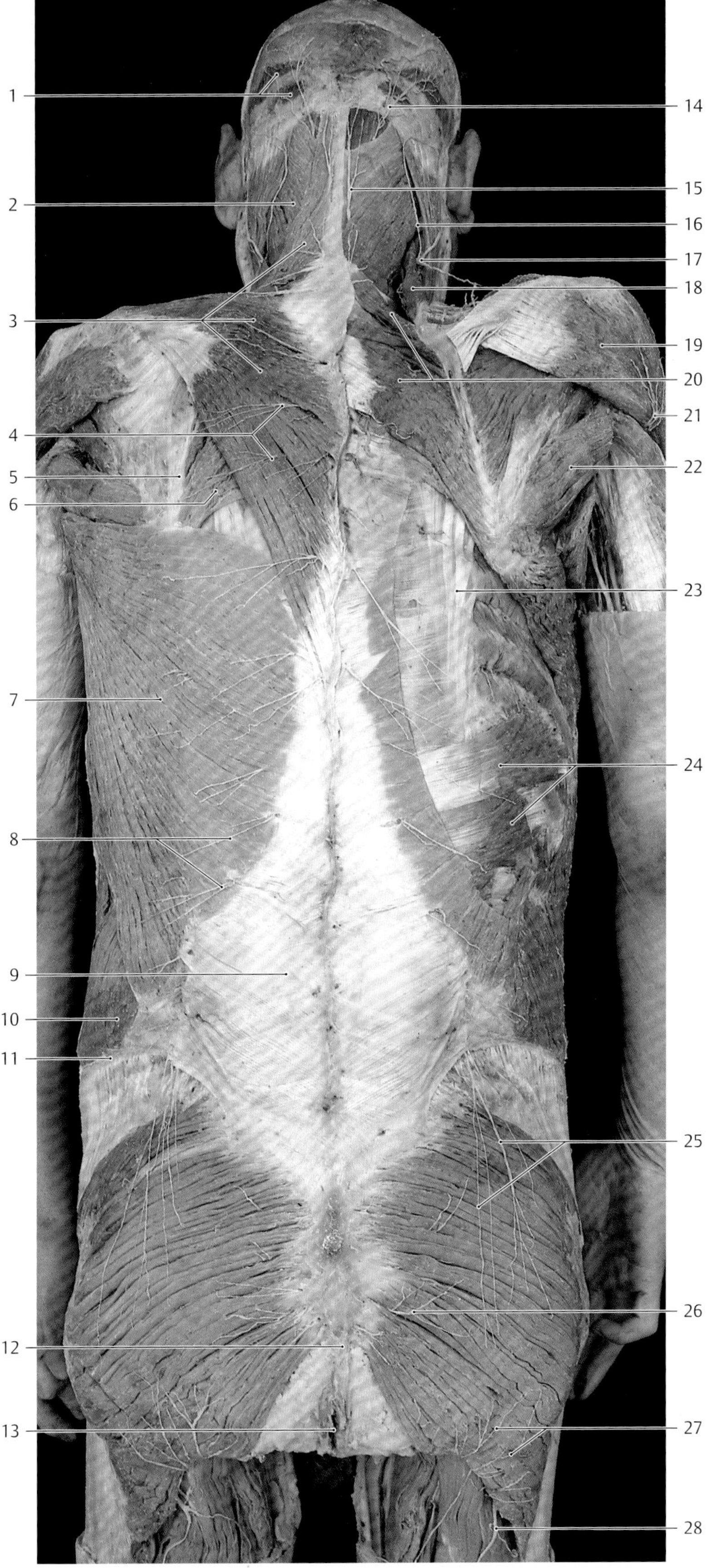


Fig. 2.88 **Innervation of the back** (superficial [left] and deeper [right] layers). Right trapezius and latissimus dorsi muscles have been removed.

1 Occipital belly of occipitofrontalis muscle
2 Splenius capitis muscle
3 Trapezius muscle
4 Medial cutaneous branches of dorsal rami of spinal nerves
5 Medial margin of scapula
6 Rhomboid major muscle
7 Latissimus dorsi muscle
8 Lateral cutaneous branches of dorsal rami of spinal nerves
9 Thoracolumbar fascia
10 External abdominal oblique muscle
11 Iliac crest
12 Last coccygeal vertebra
13 Anus
14 Greater occipital nerve
15 Third occipital nerve
16 Lesser occipital nerve
17 Cutaneous branches of cervical plexus
18 Levator scapulae muscle
19 Deltoid muscle
20 Rhomboid major and minor muscles
21 Upper lateral cutaneous nerve of arm (branch of axillary nerve)
22 Teres major muscle
23 Iliocostalis thoracis muscle
24 Serratus posterior inferior muscle
25 Superior cluneal nerves
26 Middle cluneal nerves
27 Inferior cluneal nerves
28 Posterior femoral cutaneous nerve

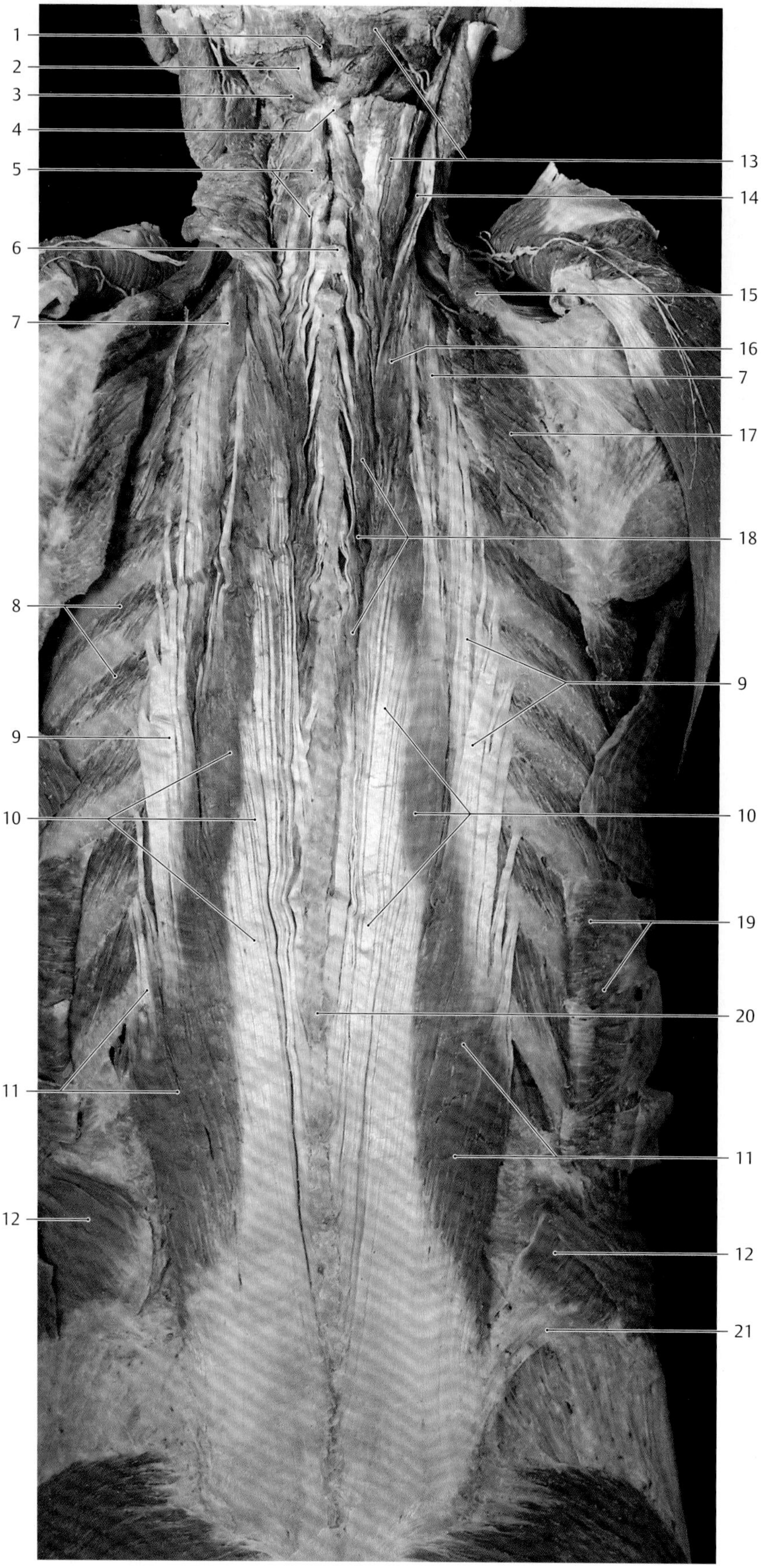

1 Rectus capitis posterior minor muscle
2 Rectus capitis posterior major muscle
3 Obliquus capitis inferior muscle
4 Spinous process of axis
5 Semispinalis cervicis muscle
6 Spinous process of seventh cervical vertebra
7 Iliocostalis cervicis muscle
8 External intercostal muscles
9 Iliocostalis thoracis muscle
10 Longissimus thoracis muscle
11 Iliocostalis lumborum muscle
12 Internal abdominal oblique muscle
13 Semispinalis capitis muscle (divided)
14 Longissimus capitis muscle
15 Levator scapulae muscle
16 Longissimus cervicis muscle
17 Rhomboid major muscle
18 Spinalis thoracis muscle
19 Serratus posterior inferior muscle (reflected)
20 Spinous process of second lumbar vertebra
21 Iliac crest
22 Mastoid process

**Fig. 2.89 Muscles of the back.** Dissection of the erector spinae muscle (lateral column of the intrinsic back muscles).

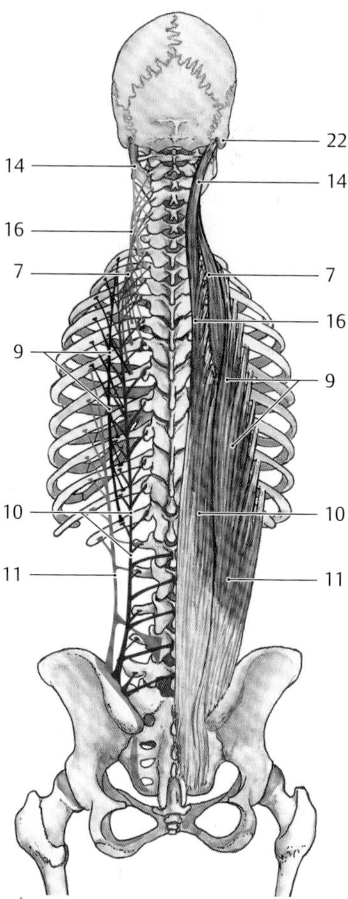


**Fig. 2.90 Origin and insertion of erector spinae muscle** (sacrospinal system).

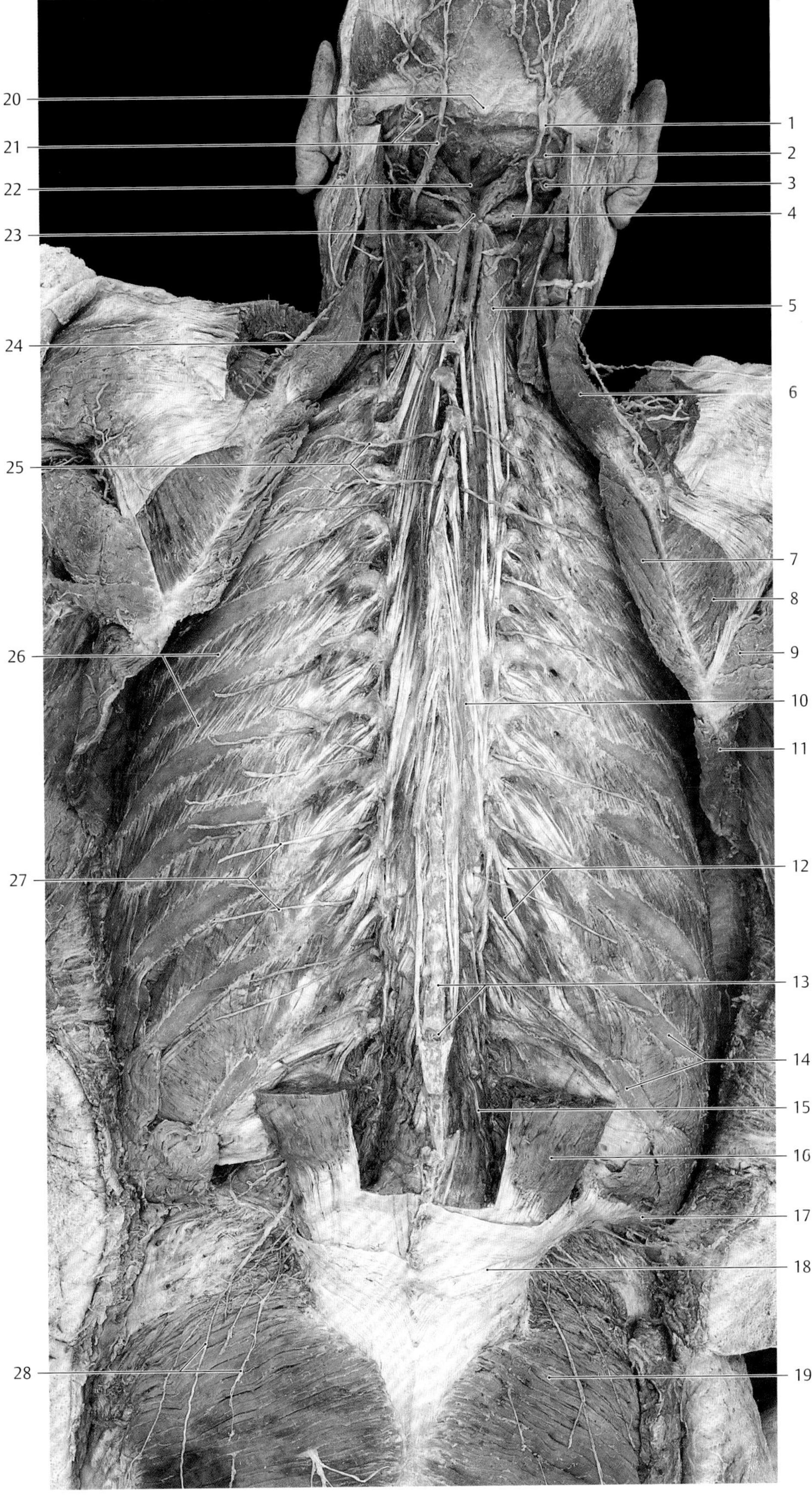


1 Rectus capitis posterior minor muscle
2 Rectus capitis posterior major muscle
3 Obliquus capitis superior muscle
4 Obliquus capitis inferior muscle
5 Semispinalis cervicis muscle
6 Levator scapulae muscle
7 Rhomboid major muscle
8 Scapula with infraspinatus muscle
9 Teres major muscle
10 Spinalis muscle
11 Latissimus dorsi muscle
12 Levatores costarum muscles
13 Spinous processes of lumbar vertebrae
14 Ribs (T11, T12)
15 Multifidus muscle
16 Longissimus and iliocostalis muscles (cut)
17 Iliac crest (lumbar triangle)
18 Thoracolumbar fascia
19 Gluteus maximus muscle
20 External occipital protuberance
21 Occipital artery and greater occipital nerve (C2)
22 Posterior tubercle of atlas
23 Spinous process of axis
24 Spinous process of seventh cervical vertebra (vertebra prominens)
25 Medial branches of dorsal branches of spinal nerves
26 External intercostal muscles
27 Lateral branches of dorsal branches of spinal nerves
28 Superior cluneal nerves

Fig. 2.91 **Muscles of the back.** Dissection of the deeper layer of the intrinsic back muscles. Longissimus and iliocostalis muscles have been cut.

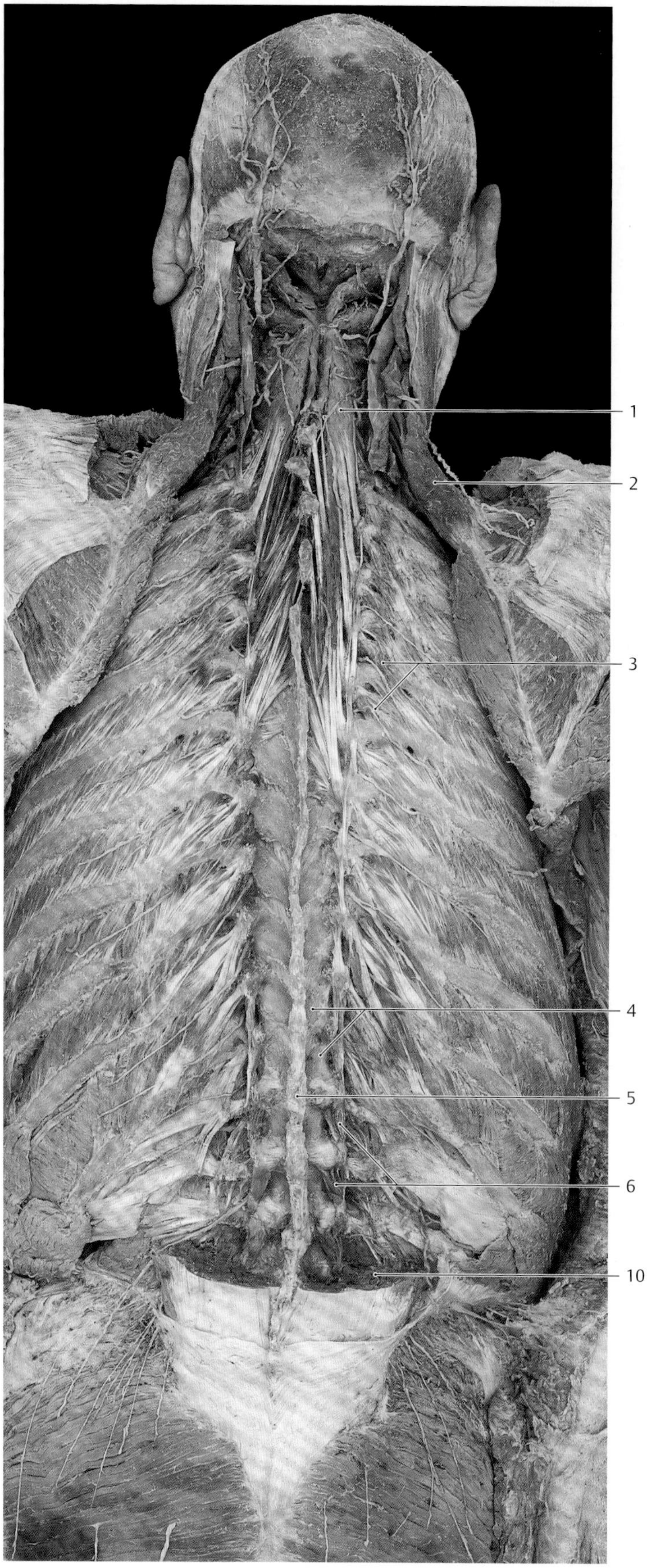

Fig. 2.92 **Muscles of the back** (deepest layer). Dissection of neck muscles, deep layer of back muscles (semispinalis cervicis and levatores costarum muscles), and ligaments connected to the spine and ribs.

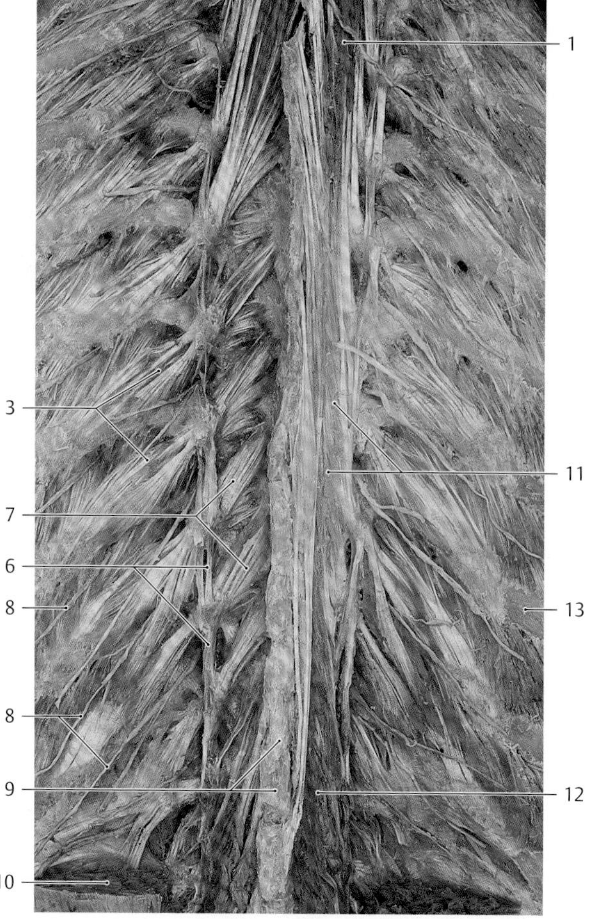


Fig. 2.93 **Muscles of the back** (deepest layer). Lumbar region (higher magnification).

1 Semispinalis cervicis muscle
2 Levator scapulae muscle
3 Levatores costarum muscles
4 Vertebral arches of lumbar vertebrae
5 Supraspinal ligaments
6 Intertransverse lumbar muscles
7 Lumbar rotator muscles
8 Cutaneous branches of spinal nerves
9 Lumbar interspinal muscles
10 Longissimus and iliocostalis muscles (cut)
11 Spinal muscle of the back
12 Multifidus muscle
13 Tenth rib (T10)

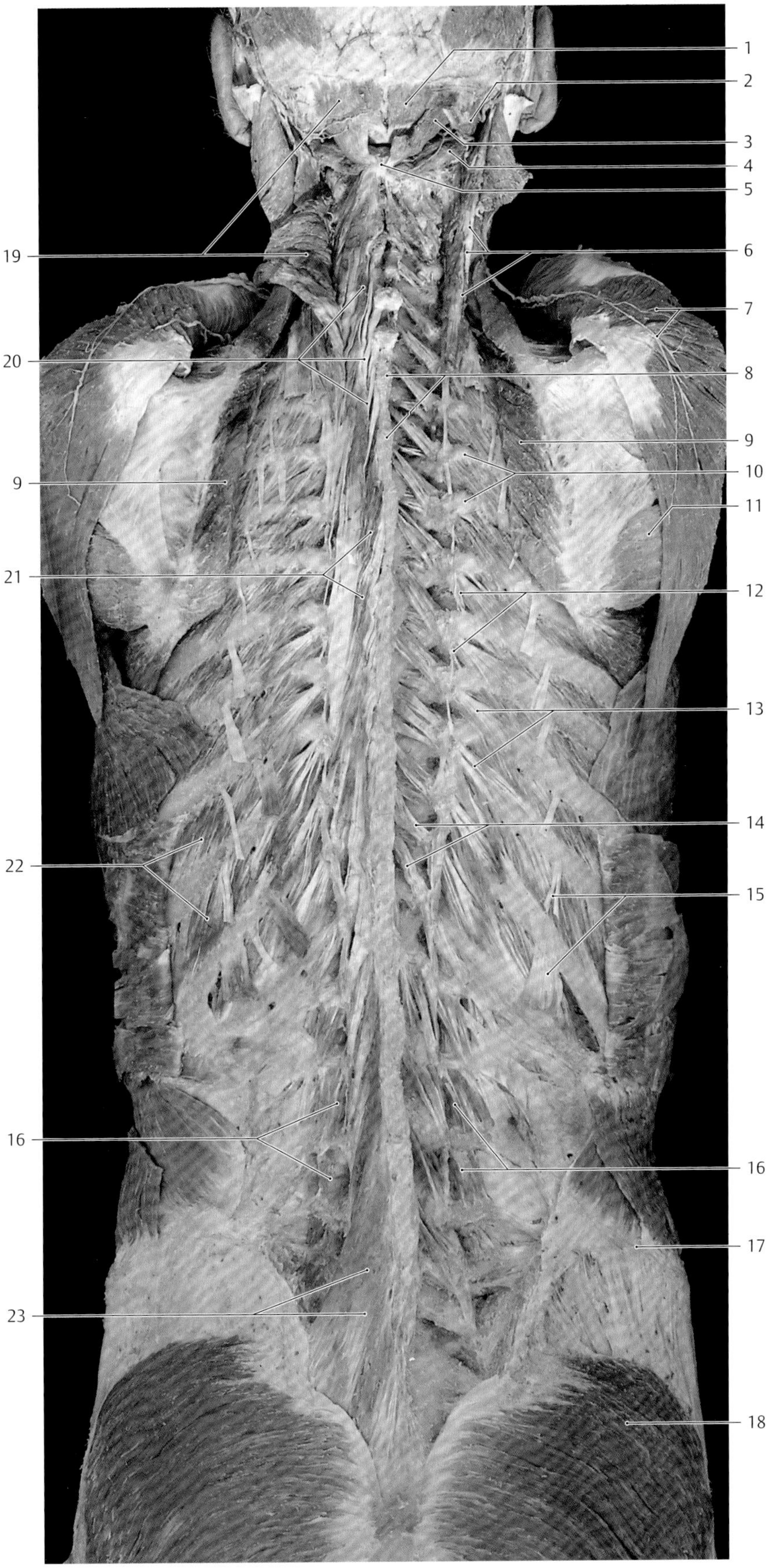

1 Rectus capitis posterior minor muscle
2 Obliquus capitis superior muscle
3 Rectus capitis posterior major muscle
4 Obliquus capitis inferior muscle
5 Spinous process of axis
6 Longissimus capitis muscle
7 Trapezius muscle (reflected) and accessory nerve (CN XI)
8 Spinous processes
9 Rhomboid major muscle
10 Transverse processes of thoracic vertebrae
11 Teres major muscle
12 Intertransverse ligaments
13 Levatores costarum muscles
14 Rotatores muscles
15 Tendons of iliocostalis muscle
16 Intertransversarii laterales lumborum muscles
17 Iliac crest
18 Gluteus maximus muscle
19 Semispinalis capitis muscle
20 Semispinalis cervicis muscle
21 Semispinalis thoracis muscle
22 External intercostal muscles
23 Multifidus muscle
24 Posterior cervical intertransversarii muscles
25 Spinalis thoracis muscle

Fig. 2.94 **Muscles of the back.** Transversospinal muscles, deepest layer on the right, where all parts of semispinalis and multifidus muscles have been removed.

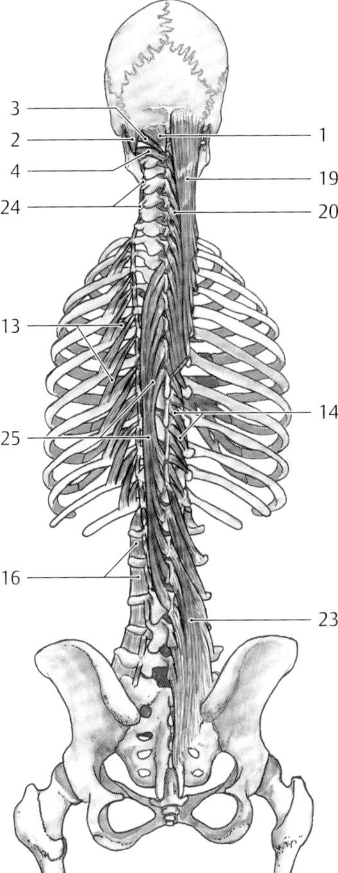


Fig. 2.95 **Origin and insertion of erector spinae muscle, medial column** (transversospinal and intertransversal system).

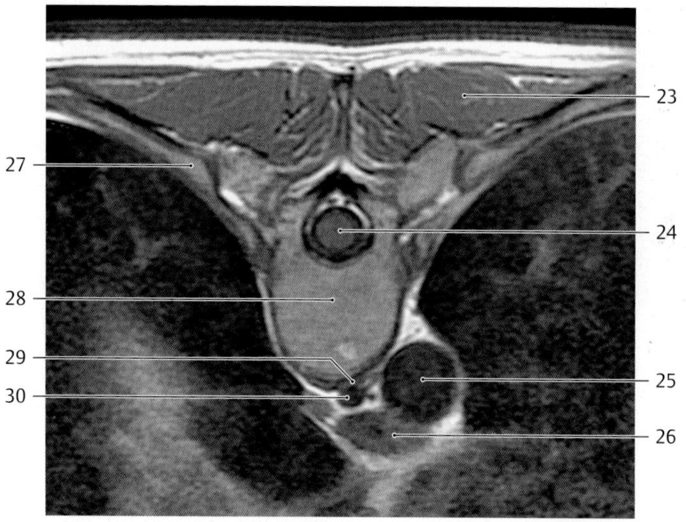


Fig. 2.96 **Horizontal section through the posterior part of the thoracic wall** (MRI scan). (Heuck A, et al. MRT-Atlas des muskuloskelettalen Systems. Stuttgart, Germany: Schattauer, 2009.)

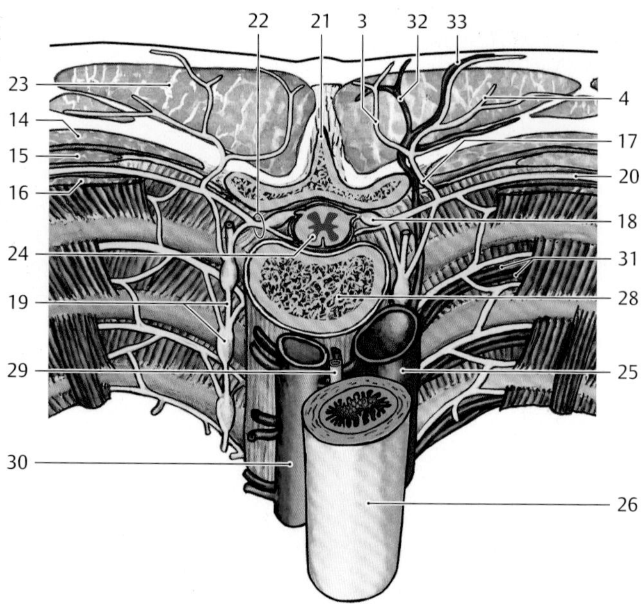


Fig. 2.98 **Horizontal section through the anterior and posterior parts of the thoracic wall.** Position and branches of spinal nerves and vessels in one thoracic segment are shown.

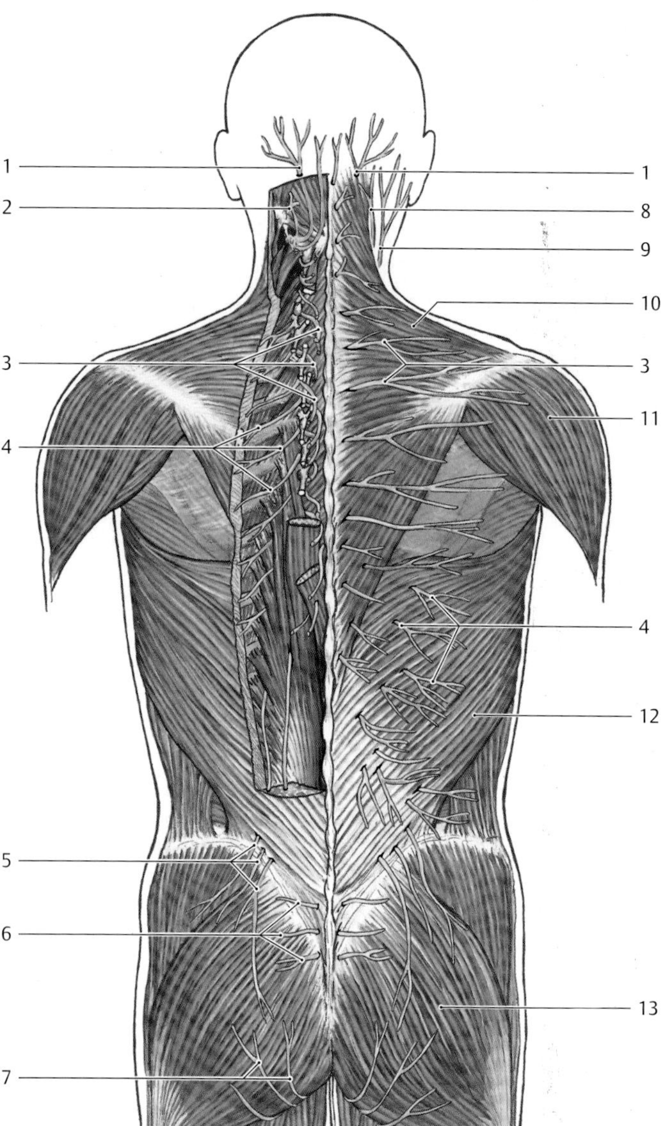


1 Greater occipital nerve (C2)
2 Suboccipital nerve (C1)
3 Medial branches of dorsal rami of spinal nerves
4 Lateral branches of dorsal rami of spinal nerves
5 Superior cluneal nerves (L1–L3)
6 Middle cluneal nerves (S1–S3)
7 Inferior cluneal nerves (derived from branches of the sacral plexus, ventral rami)
8 Lesser occipital nerve
9 Great auricular nerve
10 Trapezius muscle
11 Deltoid muscle
12 Latissimus dorsi muscle
13 Gluteus maximus muscle
14 External intercostal muscle
15 Internal intercostal muscle
16 Innermost intercostal muscle
17 Dorsal ramus of spinal nerve
18 Spinal nerve and spinal ganglion
19 Sympathetic trunk with ganglion
20 Intercostal nerve
21 Spinous process
22 Intervertebral foramen
23 Longissimus thoracis muscle
24 Spinal cord
25 Aorta
26 Esophagus
27 Body of rib
28 Thoracic rib
29 Thoracic duct
30 Azygos vein
31 Posterior intercostal artery and vein
32 Posterior (dorsal) branch of the spinal nerves
33 Cutaneous branch

Fig. 2.97 **General characteristics of the innervation of the back.** Distribution of dorsal branches of spinal nerves. Note the segmental arrangement of the innervation of the dorsal part of the trunk.

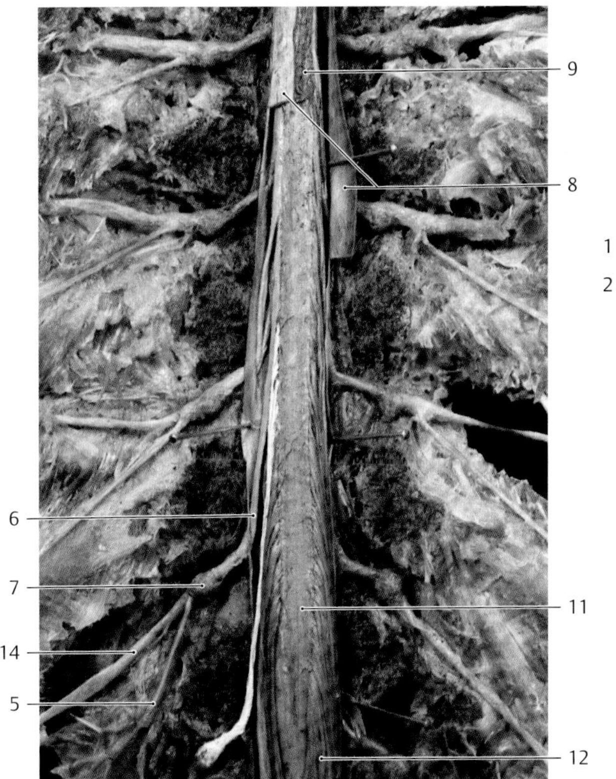


Fig. 2.99 **Lumbar part of spinal cord** (posterior aspect). Note the relation between the nervous and muscular segments.

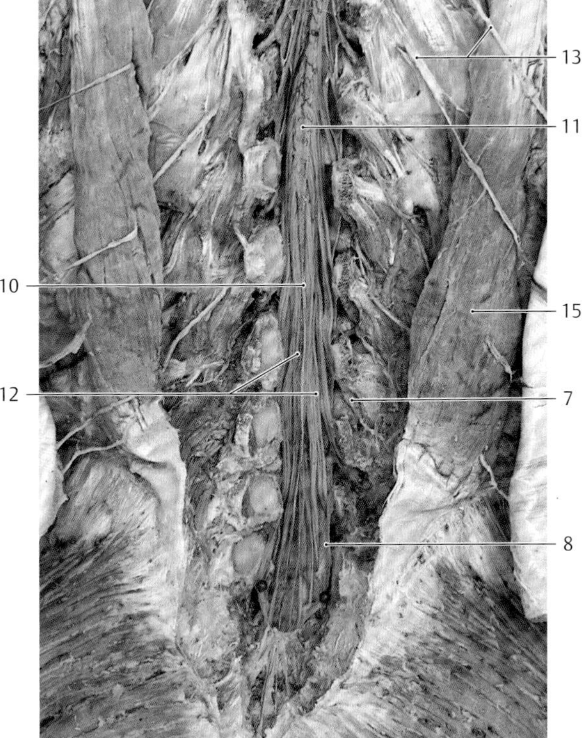


Fig. 2.100 **Terminal part of spinal cord** (posterior aspect). The dura mater has been removed.

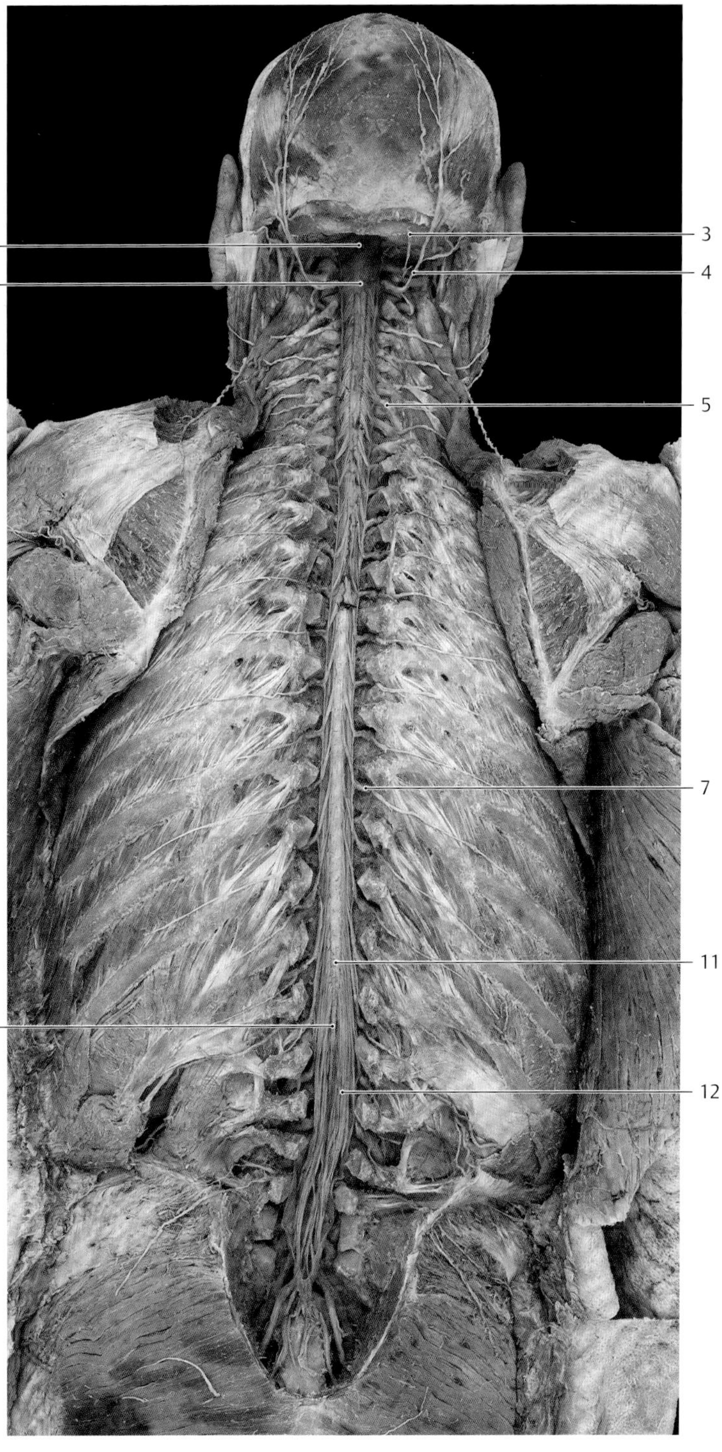


Fig. 2.101 **Spinal cord with spinal nerves and meningeal coverings.** The vertebral canal has been opened. Longissimus dorsi and iliocostal muscles have been removed.

1 Cerebellomedullary cistern
2 Medulla oblongata
3 Third cervical nerve (C3)
4 Greater occipital nerve (C2)
5 Dorsal primary ramus
6 Dorsal roots
7 Spinal ganglion
8 Spinal dura mater
9 Spinal arachnoid mater
10 Filum terminale
11 Conus medullaris
12 Cauda equina
13 Lateral branch of dorsal ramus of spinal nerve
14 Ventral ramus of spinal nerve (intercostal nerve)
15 Iliocostalis muscle

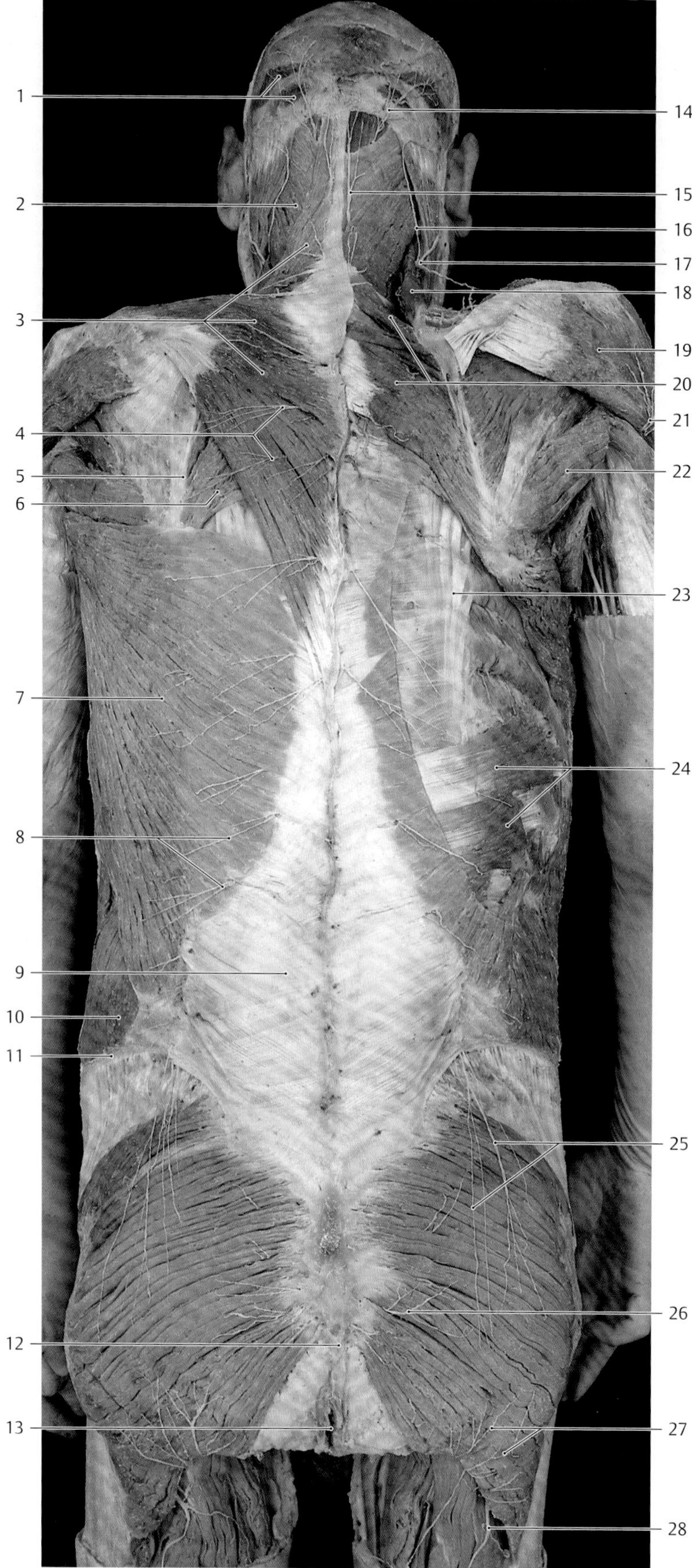


1 Occipital belly of occipito-frontalis muscle
2 Splenius capitis muscle
3 Trapezius muscle
4 Medial cutaneous branches of dorsal rami of spinal nerves
5 Medial margin of scapula
6 Rhomboid major muscle
7 Latissimus dorsi muscle
8 Lateral cutaneous branches of dorsal rami of spinal nerves
9 Thoracolumbar fascia
10 External abdominal oblique muscle
11 Iliac crest
12 Last coccygeal vertebra
13 Anus
14 Greater occipital nerve
15 Third occipital nerve
16 Lesser occipital nerve
17 Cutaneous branches of cervical plexus
18 Levator scapulae muscle
19 Deltoid muscle
20 Rhomboid major and minor muscles
21 Upper lateral cutaneous nerve of arm (branch of axillary nerve)
22 Teres major muscle
23 Iliocostalis thoracis muscle
24 Serratus posterior inferior muscle
25 Superior cluneal nerves
26 Middle cluneal nerves
27 Inferior cluneal nerves
28 Posterior femoral cutaneous nerve

Fig. 2.102 **Innervation of the back** (superficial [left] and deeper [right] layers). Right trapezius and latissimus dorsi muscles have been removed.

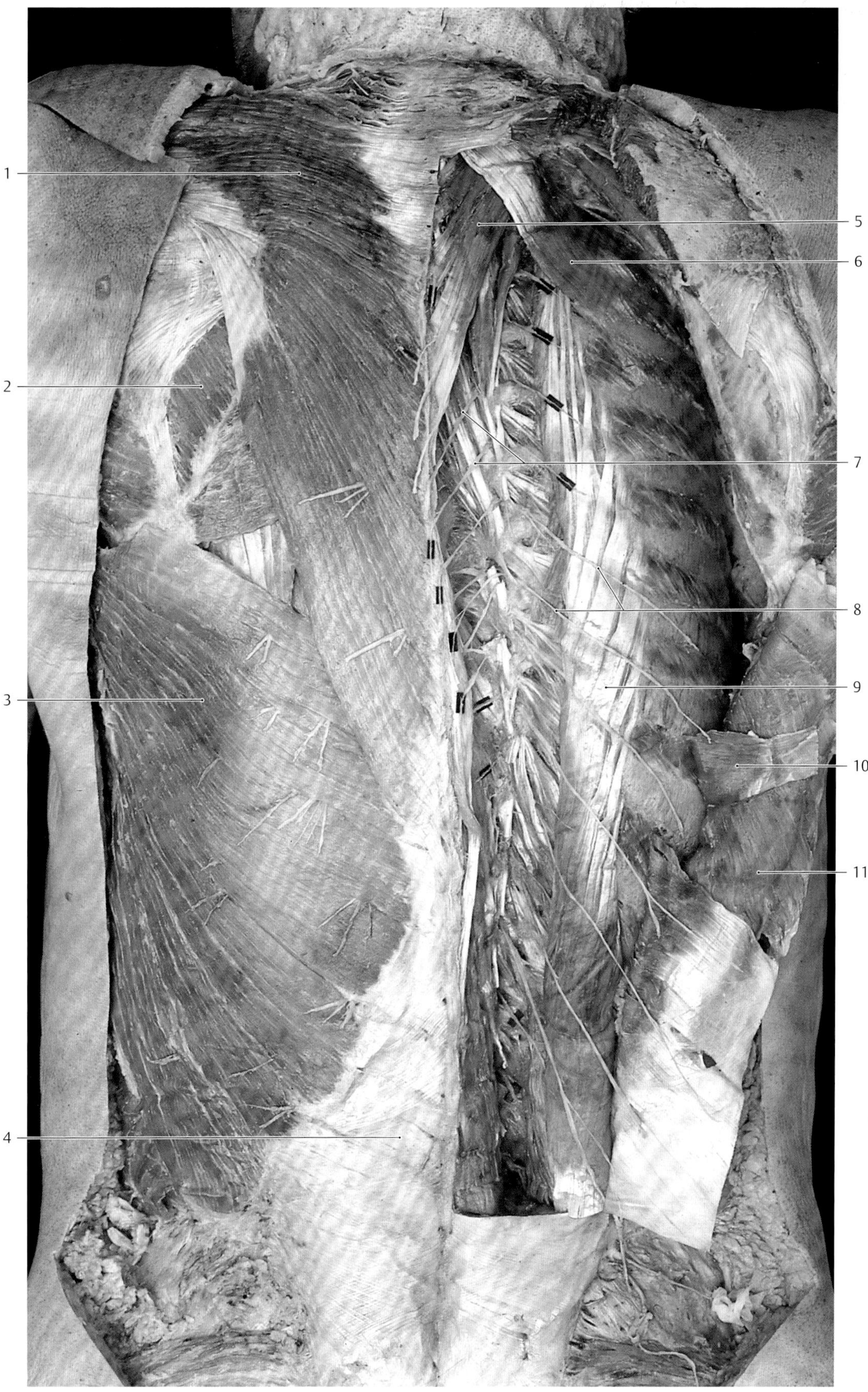


1 Trapezius muscle
2 Infraspinatus muscle
3 Left latissimus dorsi muscle
4 Thoracolumbar fascia
5 Splenius cervicis muscle
6 Serratus posterior superior muscle
7 Medial branches of dorsal rami of thoracic spinal nerves
8 Lateral branches of dorsal rami of thoracic spinal nerves
9 Iliocostalis muscle
10 Serratus posterior inferior muscle
11 Latissimus dorsi muscle (reflected)

Fig. 2.103 **Innervation of the back.** Dissection of the dorsal branches of the spinal nerves. On the right, the longissimus thoracis muscle has been removed and the iliocostalis muscle laterally reflected.

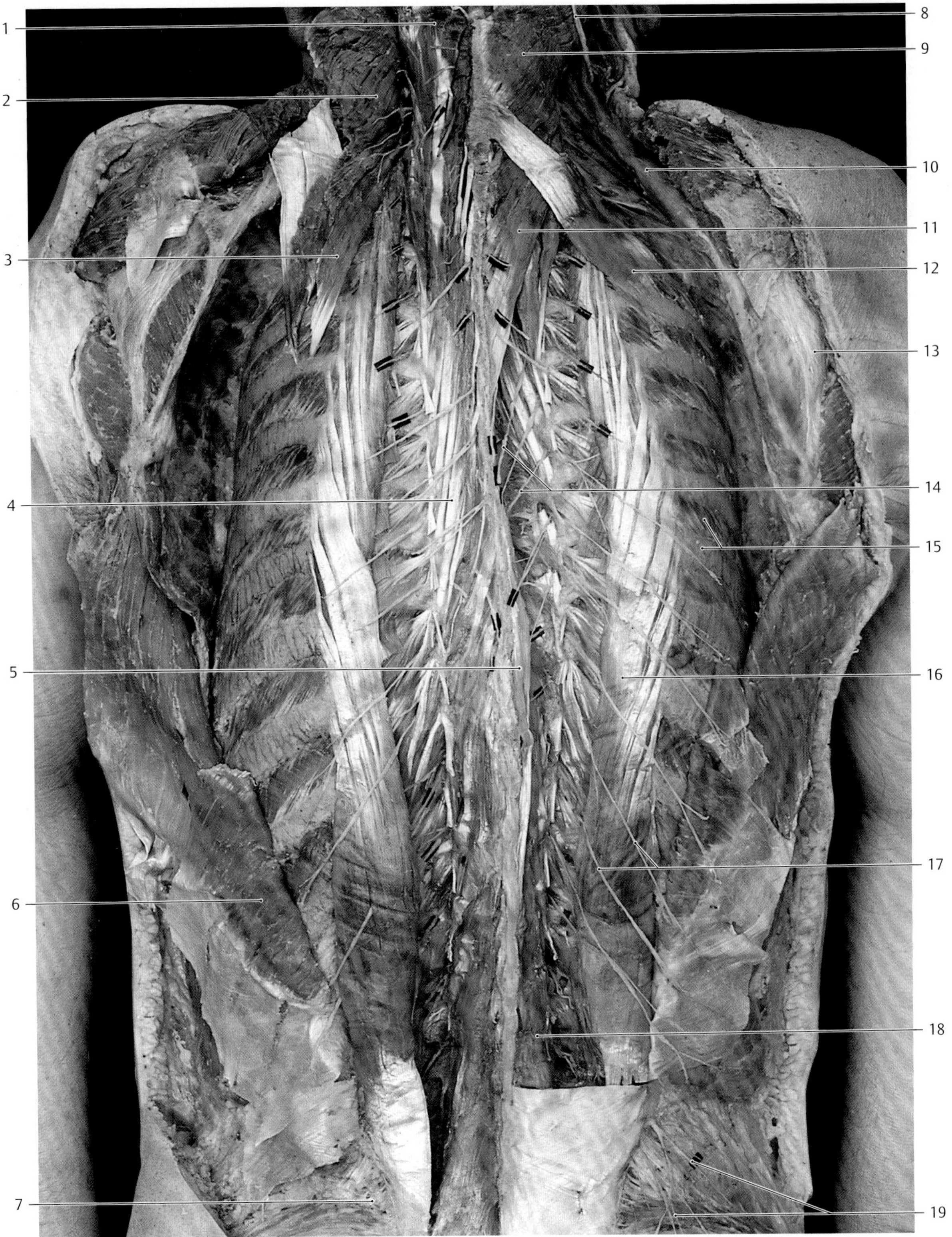


Fig. 2.104 **Innervation of the back** (deeper layer). Dissection of the medial and lateral branches of the dorsal rami of the spinal nerves. The iliocostalis muscle has been laterally reflected.

1 Semispinalis capitis muscle
2 Left splenius capitis muscle (cut and reflected)
3 Left splenius cervicis muscle (cut and reflected)
4 Semispinalis thoracis muscle
5 Spinalis thoracis muscle
6 Latissimus dorsi muscle (reflected)
7 Iliac crest
8 Lesser occipital nerve
9 Splenius capitis muscle
10 Levator scapulae muscle
11 Splenius cervicis muscle
12 Serratus posterior superior muscle
13 Scapula
14 Medial branches of dorsal rami of spinal nerves
15 Rib and external intercostal muscle
16 Iliocostalis thoracis muscle
17 Lateral branches of dorsal rami of spinal nerves
18 Multifidus muscle
19 Superior cluneal nerves

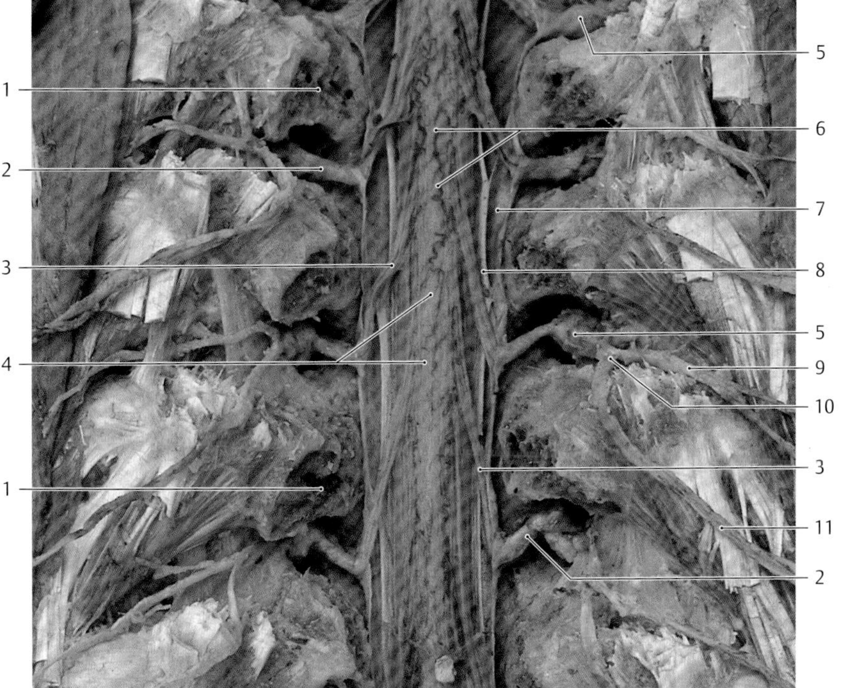


Fig. 2.105 **Thoracic part of spinal cord** (posterior aspect). Vertebral canal and dura mater have been opened.

1 Arch of vertebra (divided)
2 Spinal nerve with meningeal coverings
3 Dorsal roots of thoracic spinal nerves
4 Spinal cord (thoracic portion)
5 Spinal ganglia with meningeal coverings
6 Pia mater with blood vessels
7 Dura mater (opened)
8 Denticulate ligament
9 Lateral branch of dorsal ramus of spinal nerve
10 Dorsal ramus of spinal nerve (dividing into a medial and lateral branch)
11 Medial branch of dorsal ramus of spinal nerve
12 Spinal dura mater
13 Spinal nerves of sacral segments
14 Filum terminale

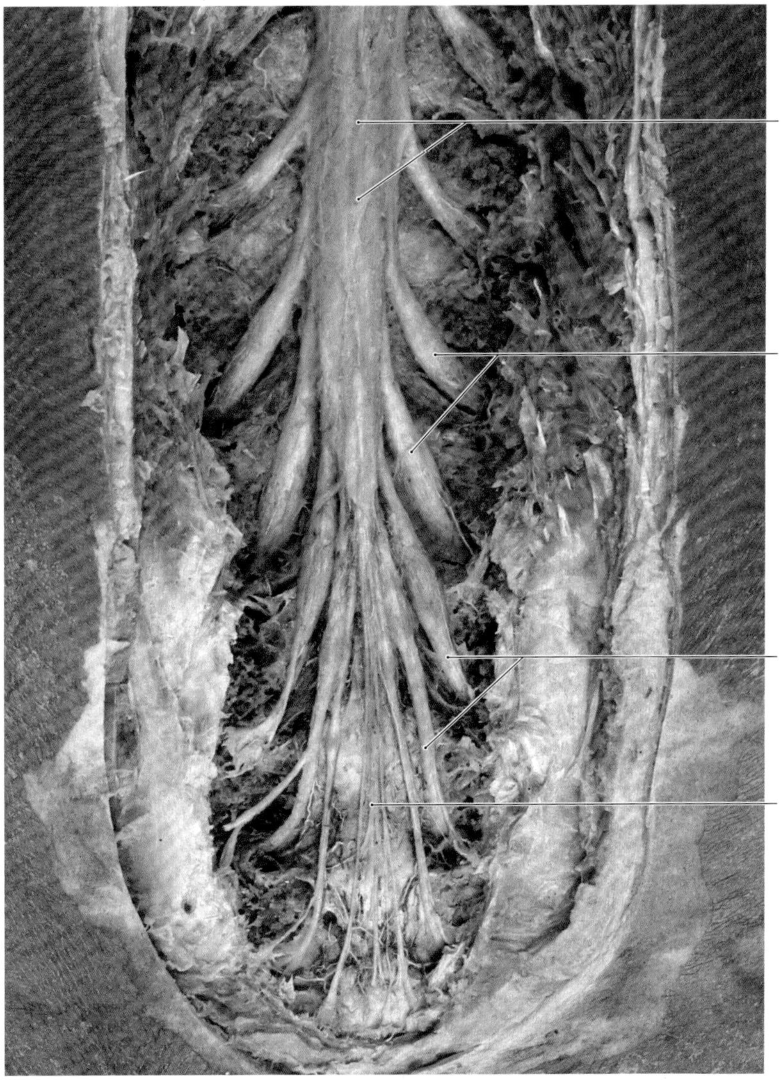

Fig. 2.106 **Terminal part of spinal cord with dura mater** (posterior aspect). Dorsal part of sacrum has been removed.

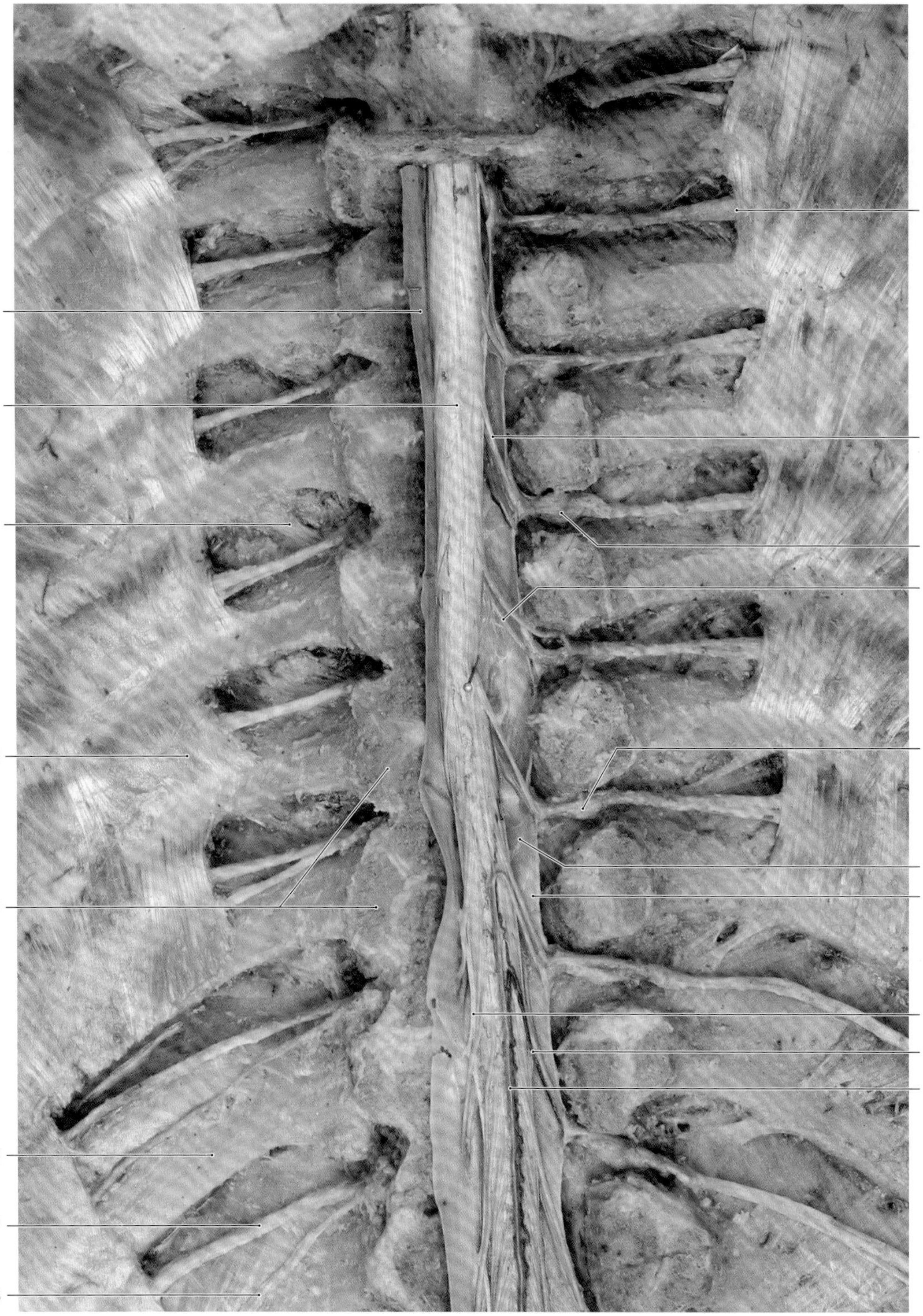

1
2
3
4
5
6
7
8
9
10
11
12
11
13
1
16
15
14

Fig. 2.107 **Spinal cord with intercostal nerves.** Inferior thoracic region (anterior aspect). Anterior portion of thoracic vertebrae removed, dural sheath opened, and spinal cord slightly reflected to the right to display the dorsal and ventral roots.

1 Dura mater
2 Spinal cord
3 Costotransverse ligament
4 Innermost intercostal muscle
5 Vertebral arches (cut surfaces)
6 Eleventh rib
7 Intercostal nerve
8 Collateral branch of intercostal nerve
9 Intercostal nerve (entering the intermuscular interval)
10 Anterior root filaments
11 Spinal (dorsal root) ganglion
12 Posterior root filaments
13 Arachnoid mater and denticulate ligament
14 Anterior spinal artery
15 Artery of Adamkiewicz
16 Denticulate ligament

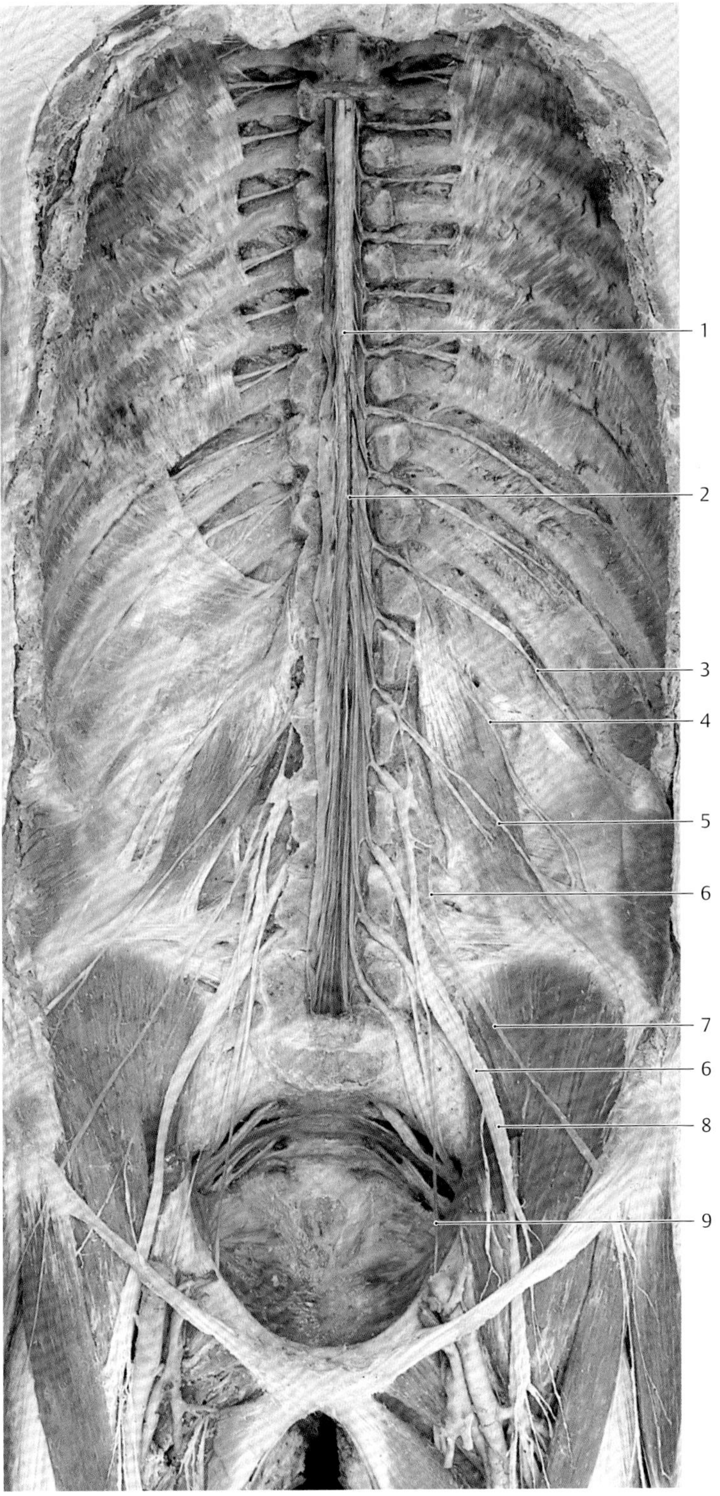


Fig. 2.108 **Spinal cord and lumbar plexus in situ** (anterior aspect). The spinal cord here ends at the level of T10 and fuses with the filum terminale. The femoral nerve arises from the lumbar plexus.

1 Conus medullaris
2 Filum terminale
3 Subcostal nerve
4 Iliohypogastric nerve
5 Ilio-inguinal nerve
6 Genitofemoral nerve
7 Lateral femoral cutaneous nerve
8 Femoral nerve
9 Obturator nerve

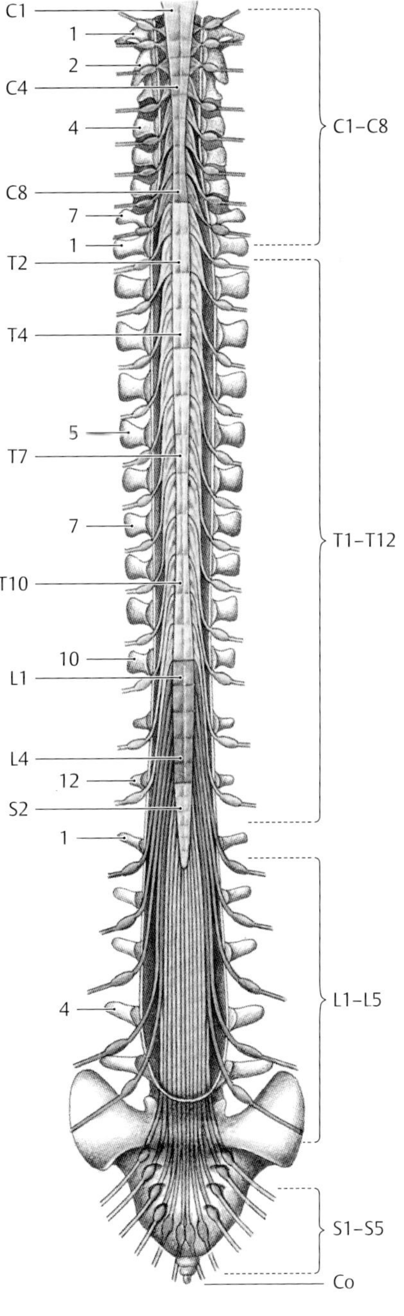


Fig. 2.109 **Organization of spinal cord segments in relation to the vertebral column** (anterior aspect).

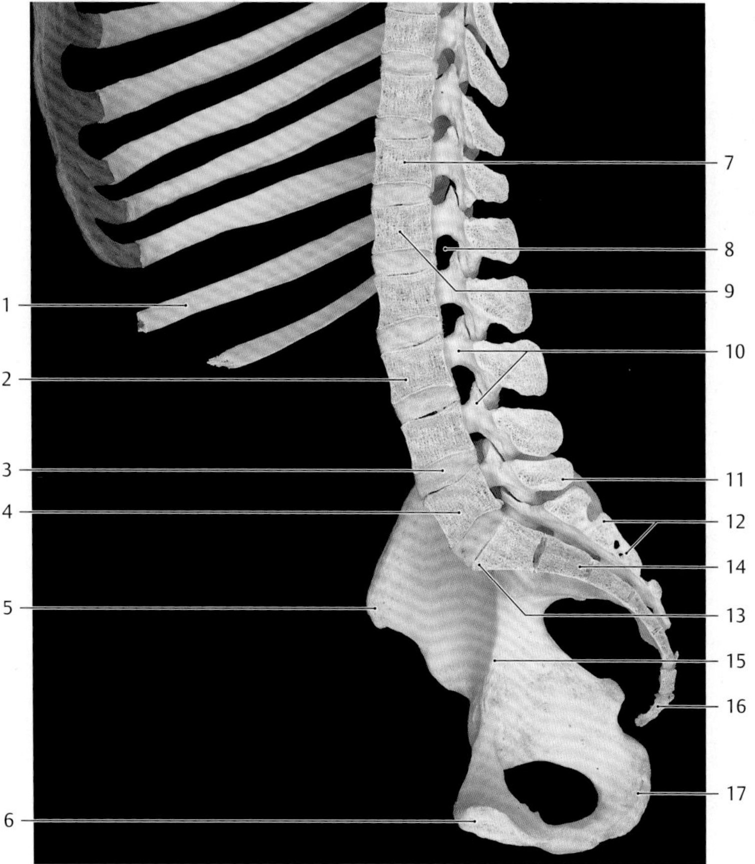


Fig. 2.110 **Lumbar part of vertebral column with pelvis and lower thoracic part** (sagittal section, medial aspect).

1 Eleventh rib
2 Body of third lumbar vertebra
3 Intervertebral disc
4 Body of fifth lumbar vertebra
5 Anterior superior iliac spine
6 Symphysial surface
7 Body of twelfth thoracic vertebra
8 Intervertebral foramen
9 Body of first lumbar vertebra
10 Vertebral canal
11 Spinous process of fifth lumbar vertebra
12 Sacrum (median sacral crest)
13 Promontory (promontorium)
14 Sacrum
15 Arcuate line
16 Coccyx
17 Ischial tuberosity
18 Sympathetic trunk with ganglia
19 Ureter
20 Iliohypogastric nerve (T12, L1)
21 Ilio-inguinal nerve (L1)
22 Femoral nerve (L1–L4)
23 Genitofemoral nerve (L1, L2)
24 Inferior hypogastric plexus
25 Ductus deferens
26 Urinary bladder
27 Medullary cone of spinal cord
28 Root filaments of spinal nerves
29 Subarachnoid space (filled with cerebrospinal fluid) (blue)
30 Terminal filament of spinal cord
31 Sacral plexus
32 Pelvic splanchnic nerves (nervi erigentes)
33 Rectum

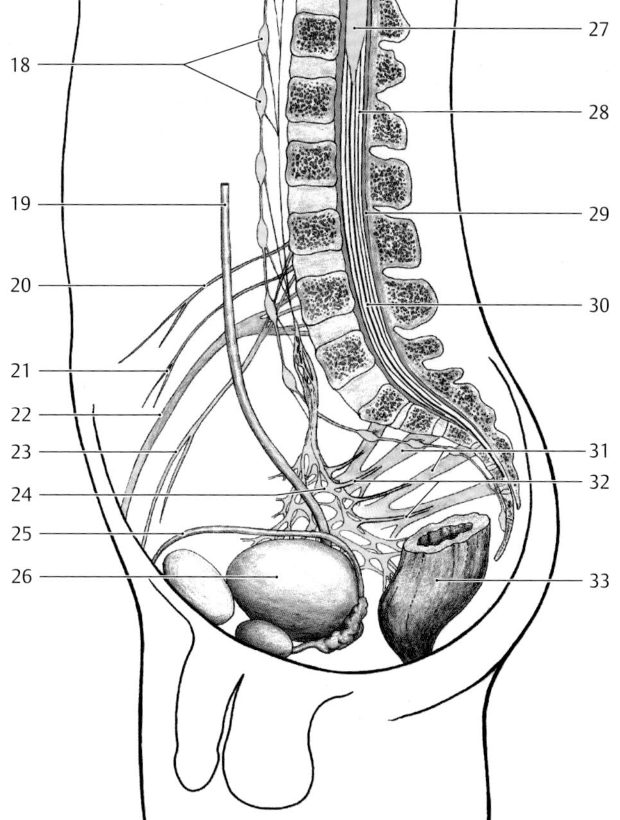


Fig. 2.111 **Lumbar part of vertebral column with spinal cord and root filaments** (sagittal section). Note the high location of the medullary cone. Sacral plexus and inferior hypogastric plexus are schematically shown.

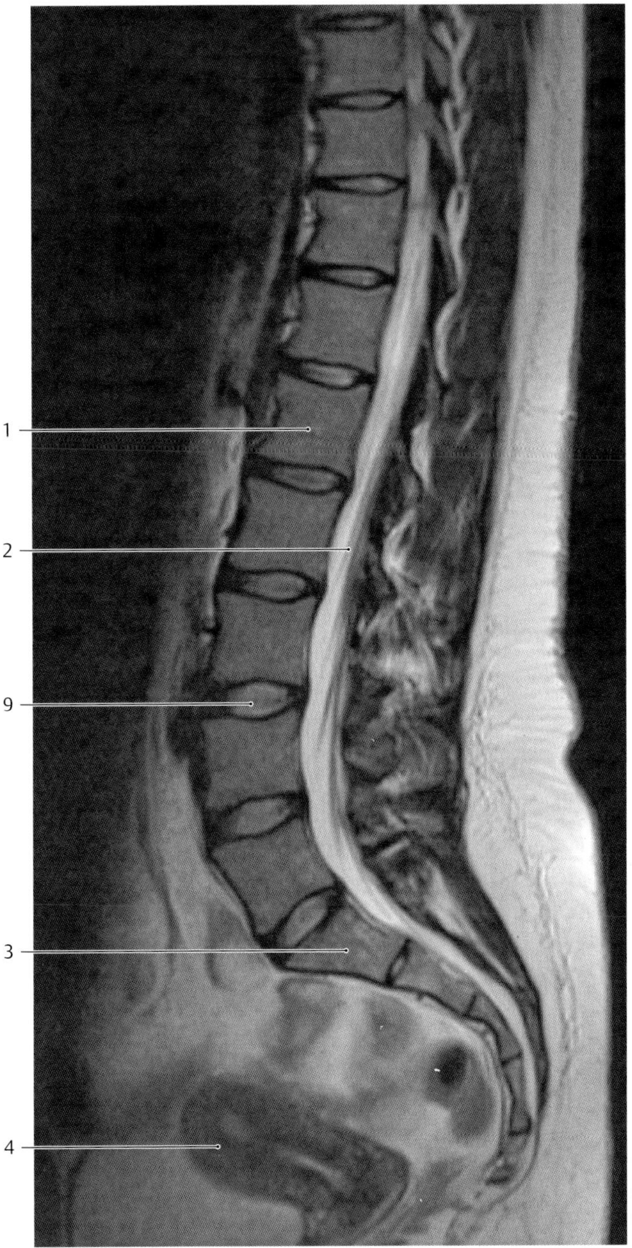


Fig. 2.112 **Paramedian section through the lumbar part of vertebral column with vertebral canal and spinal cord** (MRI scan; dashed line in the schematic drawing). (Courtesy of Prof. Uder, Institute of Radiology, University Hospital Erlangen, Germany.)

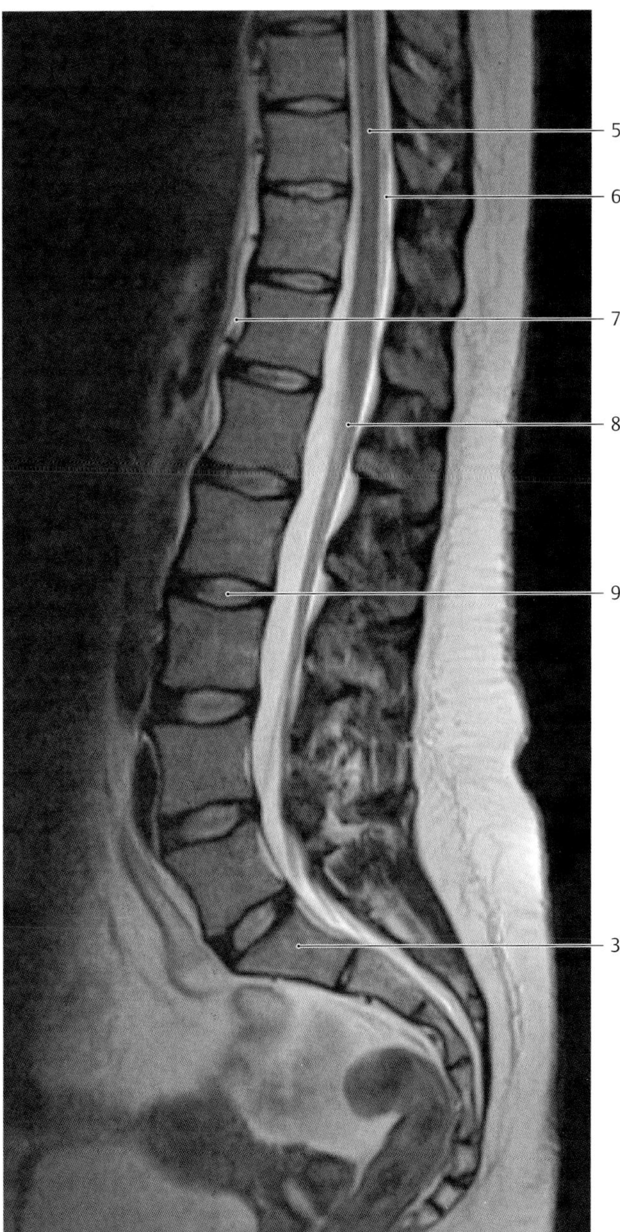


Fig. 2.113 **Median section through the lumbar part of vertebral column with vertebral canal and spinal cord** (MRI scan; continuous line in the schematic drawing). (Courtesy of Prof. Uder, Institute of Radiology, University Hospital Erlangen, Germany.)

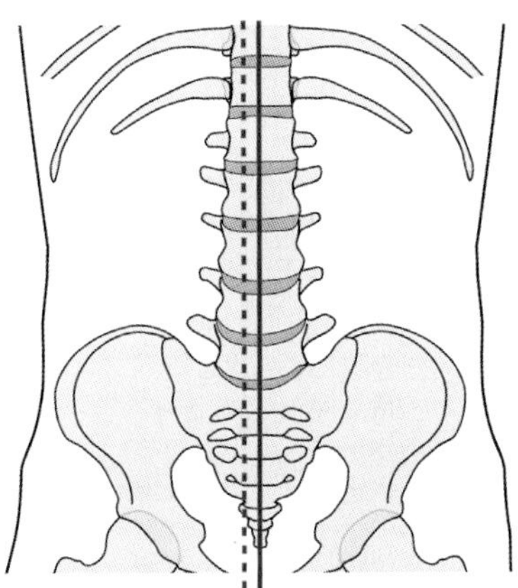

1 First lumbar vertebra (L1)
2 Root filaments of spinal nerves
3 Sacrum
4 Uterus
5 Spinal cord
6 Dura mater of spinal cord
7 Anterior longitudinal ligament
8 Medullary cone of spinal cord
9 Intervertebral disc of lumbar vertebra

Fig. 2.114 **Localization of the sections** (red lines; T10–T12, L1–L5, and sacrum).

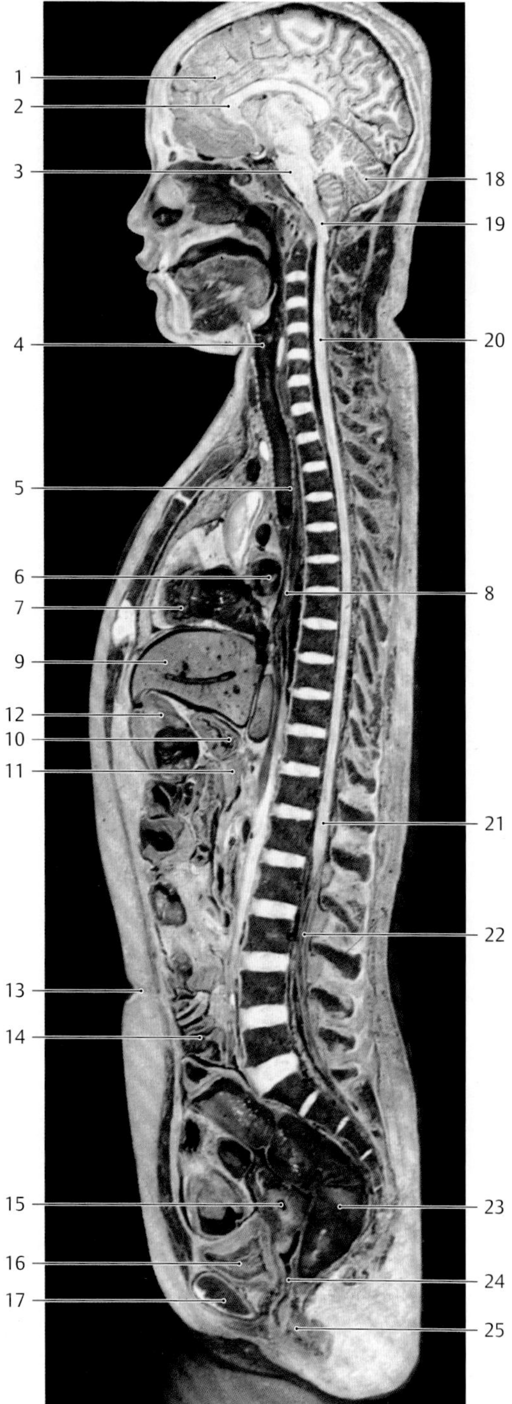


Fig. 2.115 **Median section through the head and trunk in the adult** (female). The conus medullaris of the spinal cord is located at the level of L1.

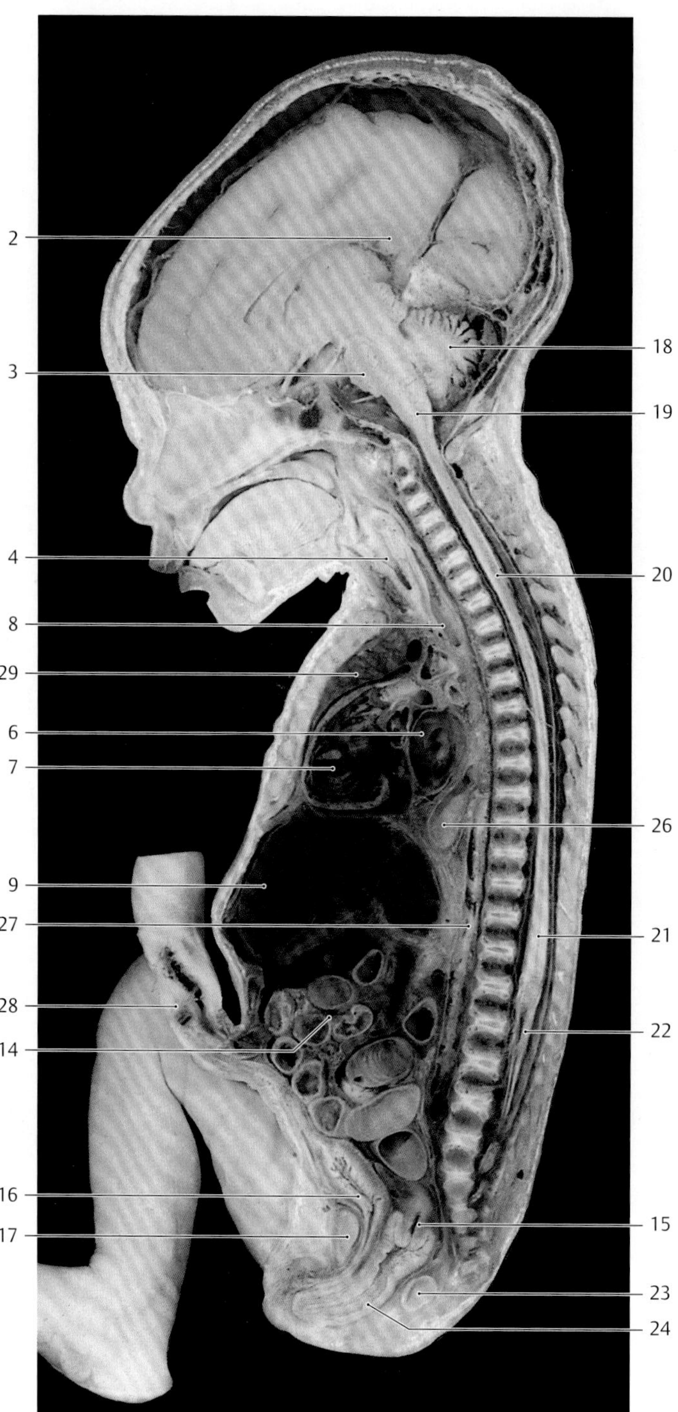


Fig. 2.116 **Median section through the head and trunk in the neonate.** Note that in the neonate the conus medullaris of the spinal cord extends far more caudally than in the adult.

1 Cerebrum
2 Corpus callosum
3 Pons
4 Larynx
5 Trachea
6 Left atrium
7 Right ventricle
8 Esophagus
9 Liver
10 Stomach
11 Pancreas
12 Transverse colon
13 Umbilicus
14 Small intestine
15 Uterus
16 Urinary bladder
17 Pubic symphysis
18 Cerebellum
19 Medulla oblongata
20 Spinal cord
21 Conus medullaris
22 Cauda equina
23 Rectum
24 Vagina
25 Anus
26 Inferior vena cava
27 Aorta
28 Umbilical cord
29 Thymus

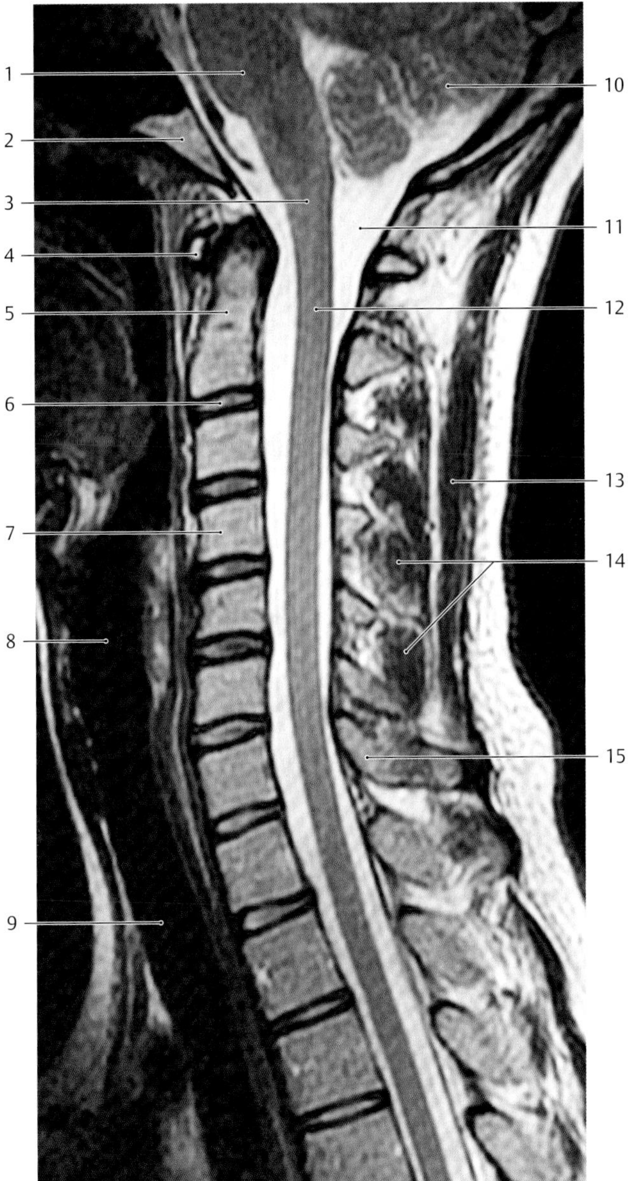


Fig. 2.117 **Midsagittal section through the cervical vertebral column** showing the spinal cord in connection with the medulla oblongata (MRI scan). (Heuck A, et al. MRT-Atlas des muskuloskelettalen Systems. Stuttgart, Germany: Schattauer, 2009.)

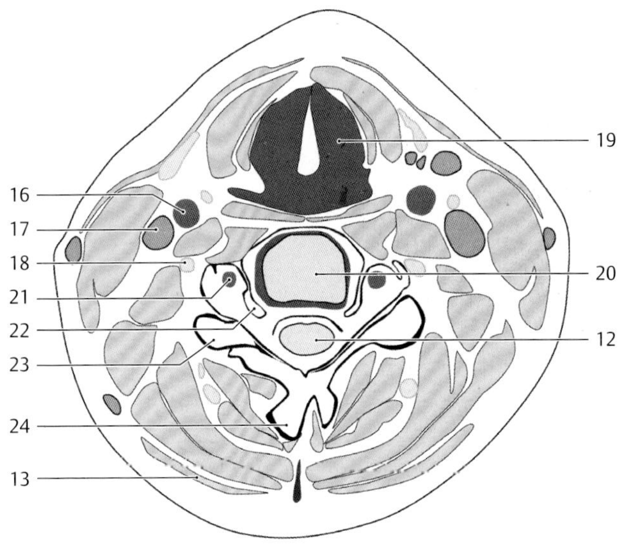


Fig. 2.118

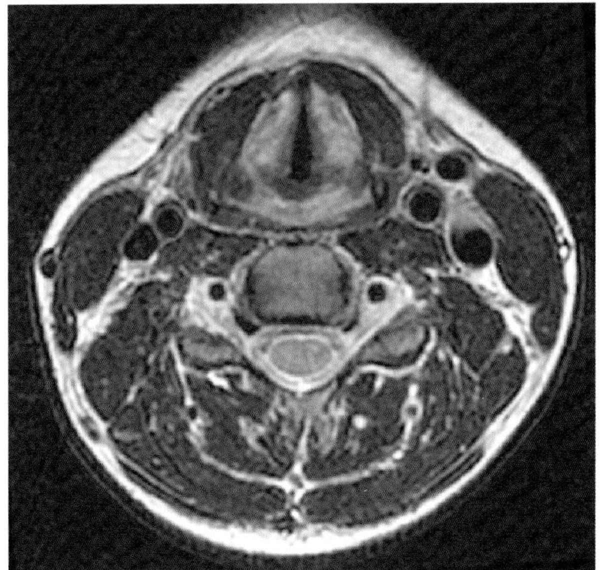

Fig. 2.119

Figs. 2.118 and 2.119 **Horizontal section through the neck** at the level of the larynx (schematic and MRI scan respectively). (Heuck A, et al. MRT-Atlas des muskuloskelettalen Systems. Stuttgart, Germany: Schattauer, 2009.)

1 Pons
2 Base of skull (clivus)
3 Medulla oblongata
4 Atlas (anterior arch)
5 Dens of axis
6 Intervertebral disc
7 Body of cervical vertebra (C4)
8 Site of larynx
9 Trachea
10 Cerebellum
11 Cerebellomedullary cistern
12 Spinal cord
13 Trapezius muscle
14 Muscles of the neck
15 Spinous process of cervical vertebra (C7)
16 Internal jugular vein
17 Common carotid artery
18 Vagus nerve (CN X)
19 Larynx
20 Body of cervical vertebra
21 Vertebral artery
22 Spinal nerve with spinal ganglion
23 Transverse process of cervical vertebra
24 Spinous process of cervical vertebra

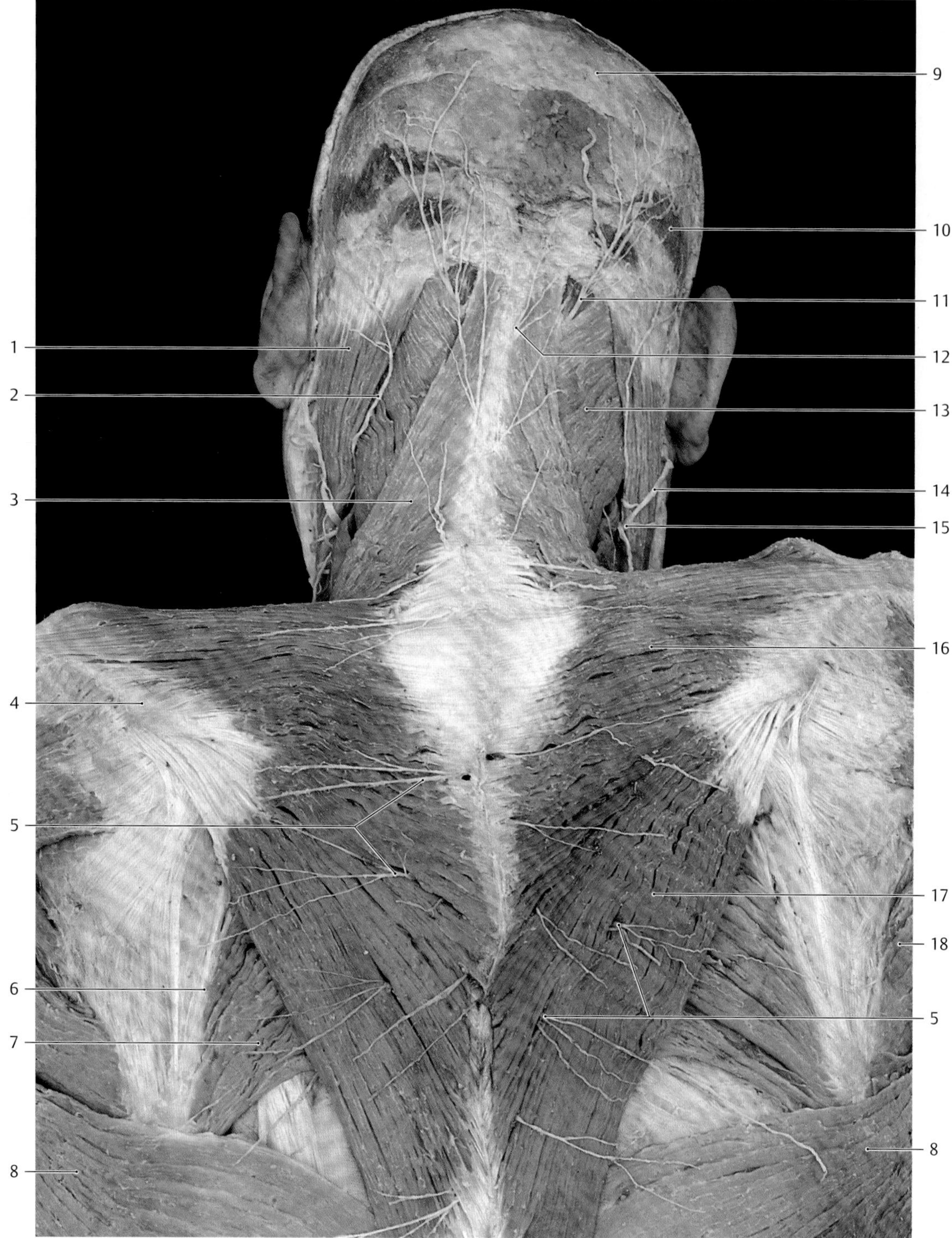


Fig. 2.120 **Posterior aspect of the neck** (superficial layer). Dissection of the trapezius muscle and the cutaneous branches of the dorsal branches of spinal nerves.

1 Sternocleidomastoid muscle
2 Lesser occipital nerve
3 Descending fibers of trapezius muscle
4 Spine of scapula
5 Medial cutaneous branches of dorsal rami of spinal nerves
6 Medial margin of scapula
7 Rhomboid major muscle
8 Latissimus dorsi muscle
9 Galea aponeurotica
10 Occipital belly of occipitofrontalis muscle
11 Greater occipital nerve
12 Third occipital nerve
13 Splenius capitis muscle
14 Great auricular nerve
15 Cutaneous nerves of cervical plexus
16 Transverse fibers of trapezius muscle
17 Ascending fibers of trapezius muscle
18 Teres major muscle

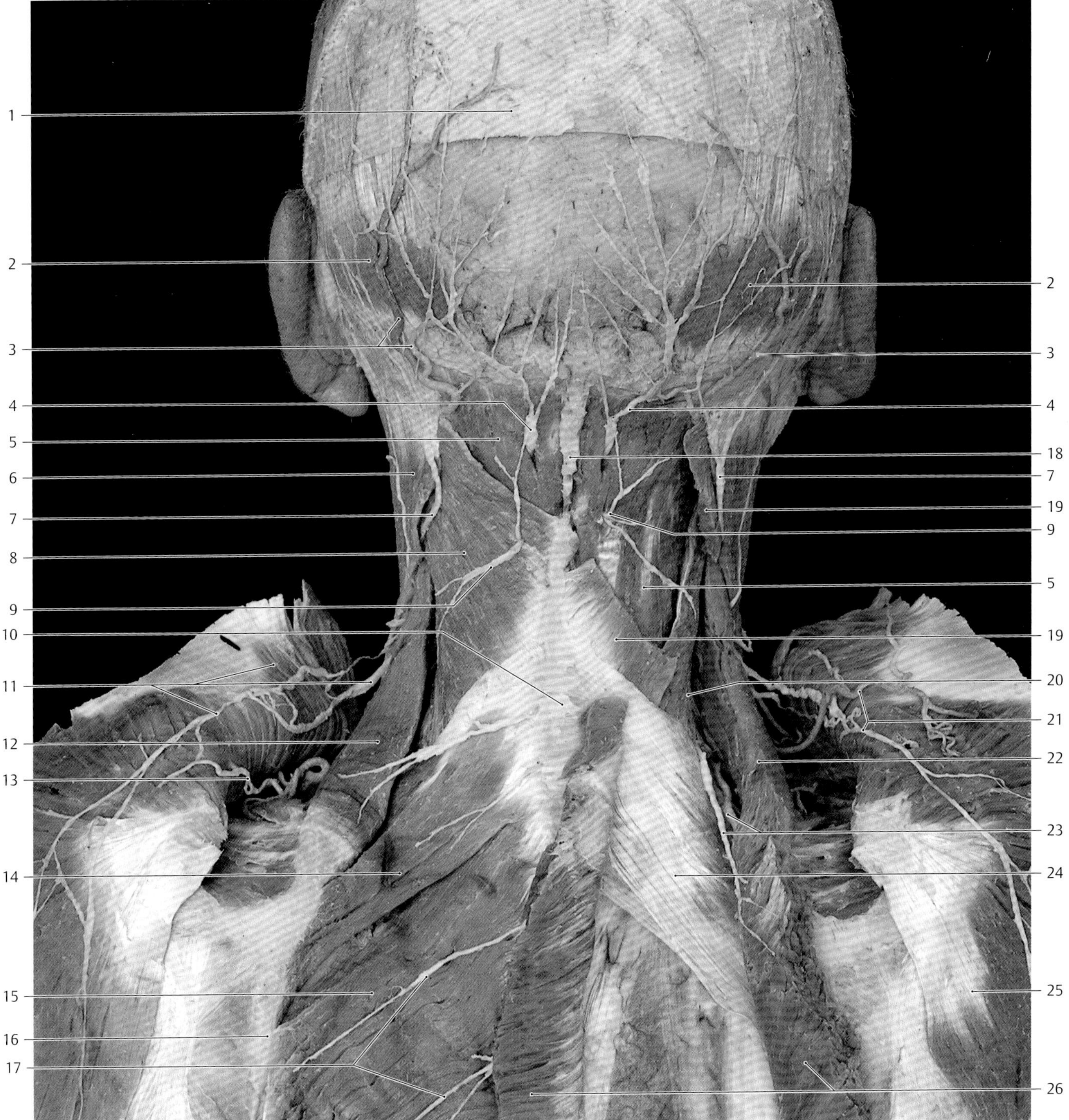


Fig. 2.121 **Posterior aspect of the neck** (deeper layer). The left trapezius muscle has been divided and reflected. On the right, the trapezius, rhomboid, and splenius muscles have been divided. The right levator scapulae muscle has been slightly reflected.

1 Galea aponeurotica
2 Occipital belly of occipitofrontalis muscle
3 Occipital artery
4 Greater occipital nerve (C2)
5 Semispinalis capitis muscle
6 Sternocleidomastoid muscle
7 Lesser occipital nerve
8 Left splenius capitis muscle
9 Third occipital nerve (C3)
10 Spinous process of vertebra prominens (C7)
11 Left trapezius muscle and accessory nerve
12 Levator scapulae muscle
13 Superficial branch of transverse cervical artery
14 Rhomboid minor muscle
15 Rhomboid major muscle
16 Medial margin of scapula
17 Medial branches of dorsal rami of spinal nerves
18 Ligamentum nuchae
19 Splenius capitis muscle (divided)
20 Splenius cervicis muscle
21 Right accessory nerve and superficial branch of transverse cervical artery
22 Right levator scapulae muscle
23 Dorsal scapular nerve and deep branch of transverse cervical artery
24 Serratus posterior superior muscle
25 Right trapezius muscle (divided and reflected)
26 Right rhomboid major muscle (divided and reflected)

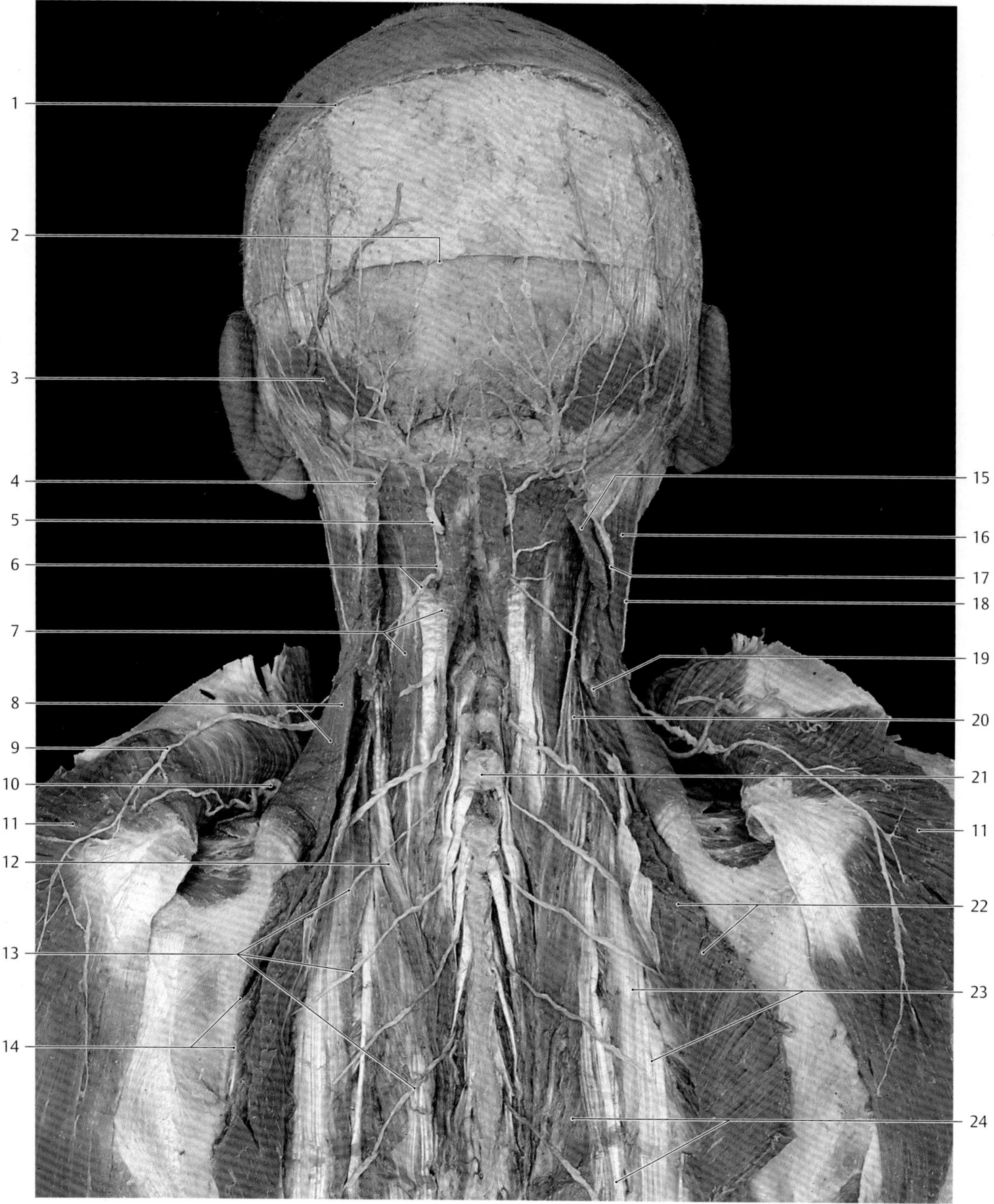


Fig. 2.122 **Posterior aspect of the neck** (deep layer). Trapezius, splenius capitis, and cervicis muscles have been divided and partly removed or reflected.

1 Skin of scalp
2 Galea aponeurotica
3 Occipital belly of occipitofrontalis muscle
4 Occipital artery
5 Greater occipital nerve
6 Third occipital nerve
7 Semispinalis capitis muscle
8 Levator scapulae muscle
9 Accessory nerve (CN XI)
10 Superficial cervical artery
11 Trapezius muscle (reflected)
12 Longissimus cervicis muscle
13 Medial cutaneous branches of dorsal rami of spinal nerves
14 Medial margin of scapula
15 Splenius capitis muscle (divided)
16 Sternocleidomastoid muscle
17 Lesser occipital nerve
18 Great auricular nerve
19 Splenius cervicis muscle
20 Longissimus cervicis muscle
21 Spinous process of vertebra prominens (C7)
22 Rhomboid muscles (divided)
23 Iliocostalis thoracis muscle
24 Longissimus thoracis muscle

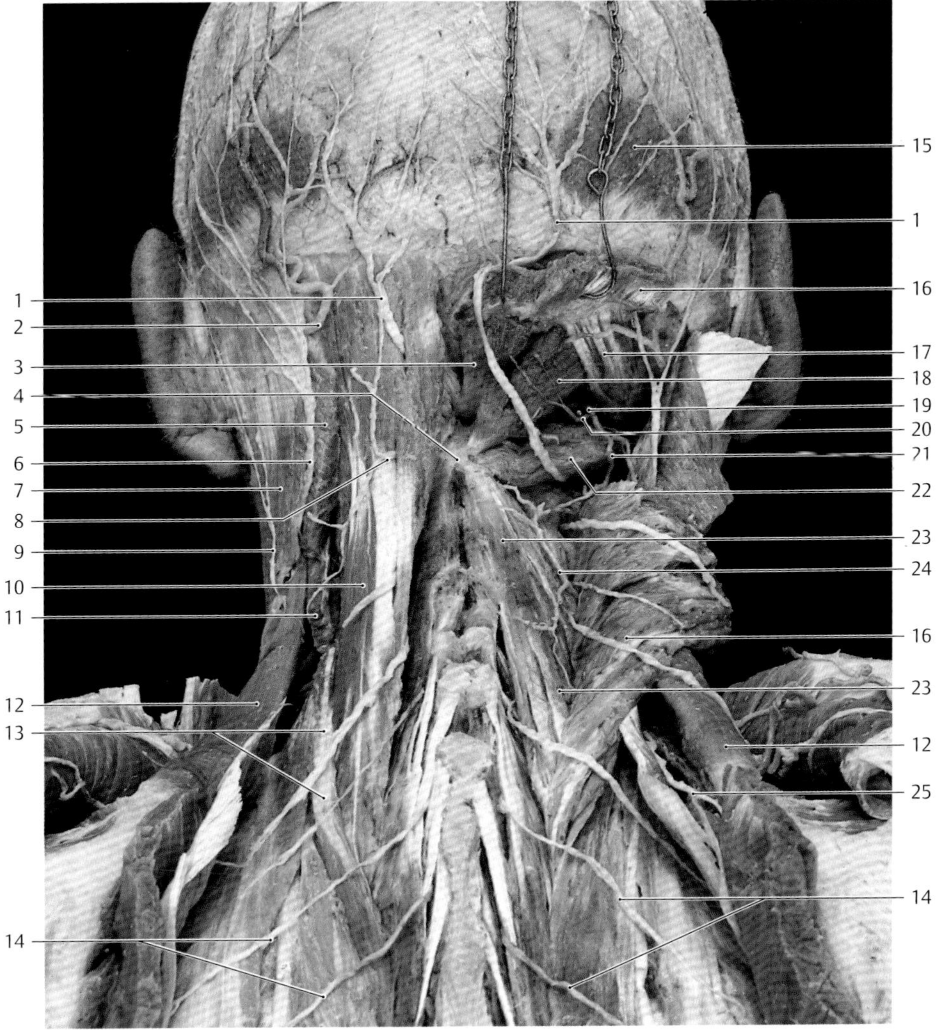


Fig. 2.123 **Posterior aspect of the neck** (deep layer). Dissection of suboccipital triangle. The right semispinalis capitis muscle has been divided and reflected.

1 Greater occipital nerve
2 Occipital artery
3 Rectus capitis posterior minor muscle
4 Spinous process of axis
5 Left splenius capitis muscle (cut)
6 Lesser occipital nerve
7 Left sternocleidomastoid muscle
8 Third occipital nerve (C3)
9 Great auricular nerve
10 Left semispinalis capitis muscle
11 Left semispinalis cervicis muscle (cut)
12 Levator scapulae muscle
13 Left longissimus cervicis muscle
14 Medial branches of dorsal rami of spinal nerves
15 Occipital belly of occipitofrontalis muscle
16 Semispinalis capitis muscle (cut)
17 Obliquus capitis superior muscle
18 Rectus capitis posterior major muscle
19 Vertebral artery
20 Suboccipital nerve (C1)
21 Muscular branch of vertebral artery
22 Obliquus capitis inferior muscle
23 Right semispinalis cervicis muscle
24 Deep cervical artery
25 Dorsal scapular nerve
26 External occipital protuberance
27 Trapezius muscle (cut)
28 Cervical vertebra (C3)
29 Mastoid process and splenius capitis muscle
30 Atlas
31 Axis
32 Spinous process of third cervical vertebra

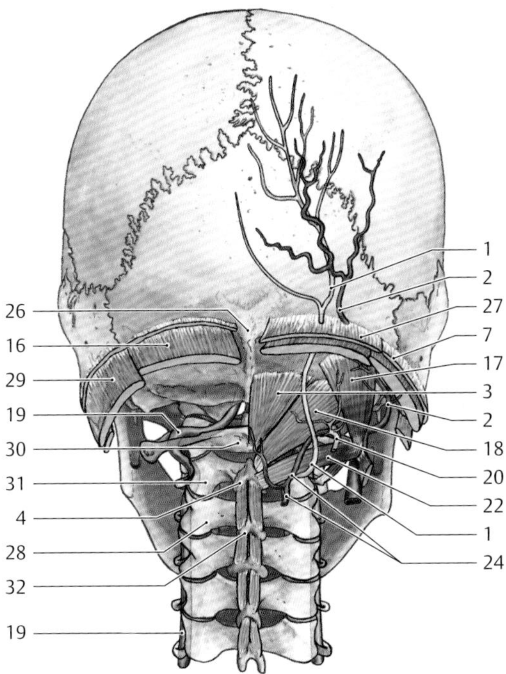


Fig. 2.124 **Suboccipital triangle and position of the greater occipital nerve** on the right and the vertebral artery on the left.

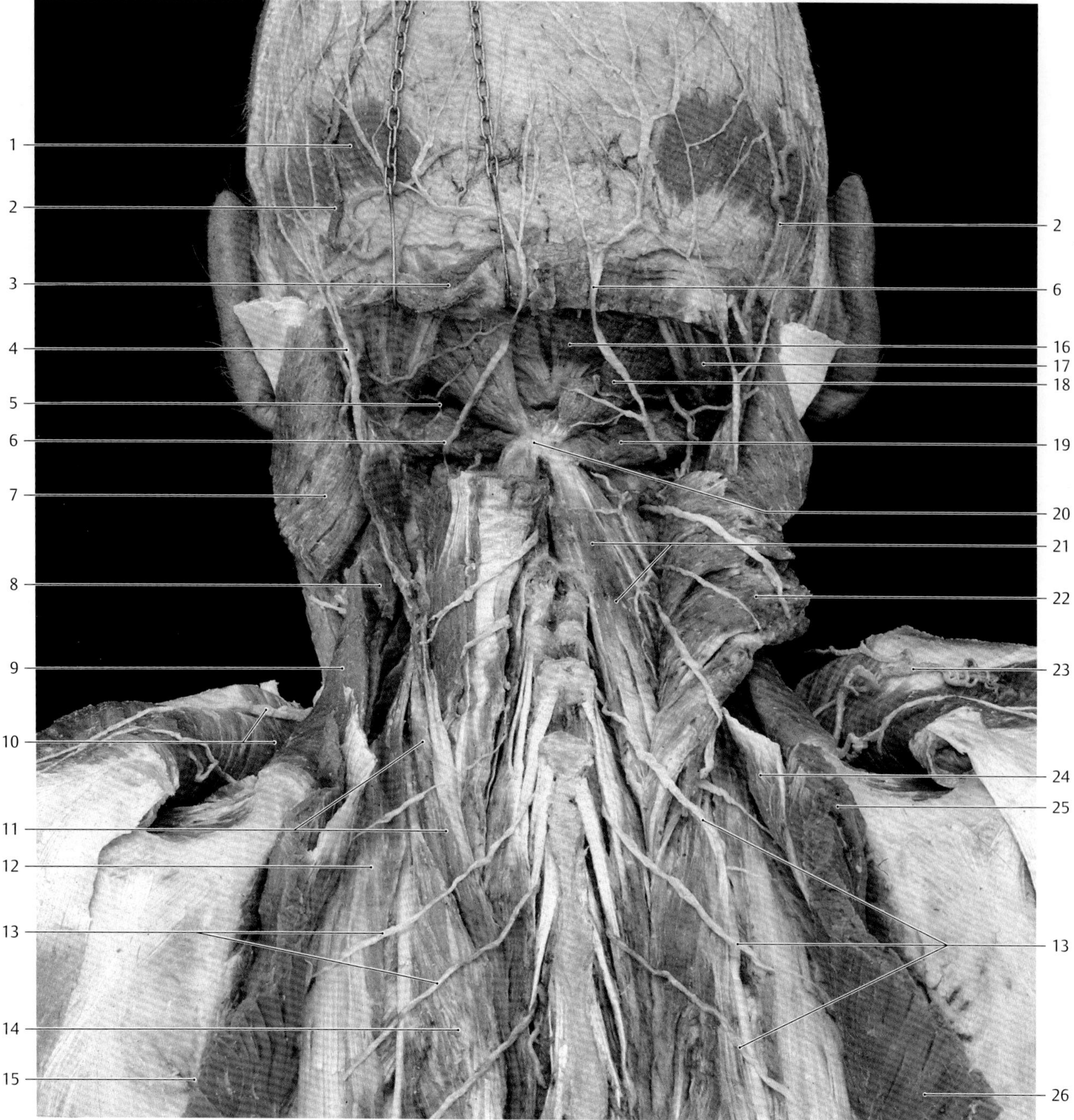


Fig. 2.125 **Posterior aspect of the neck** (deepest layer). Dissection of suboccipital triangle on both sides.

1 Occipital belly of occipitofrontalis muscle
2 Occipital artery
3 Insertion of semispinalis capitis muscle (divided)
4 Lesser occipital nerve (from cervical plexus)
5 Suboccipital nerve (C1)
6 Greater occipital nerve (C2)
7 Splenius capitis muscle (reflected)
8 Splenius cervicis muscle
9 Levator scapulae muscle
10 Accessory nerve (CN XI) and trapezius muscle
11 Longissimus cervicis muscle
12 Iliocostalis cervicis muscle
13 Medial cutaneus branches of dorsal rami of spinal nerves (C7, C8)
14 Longissimus thoracis muscle
15 Medial margin of scapula
16 Rectus capitis posterior minor muscle
17 Obliquus capitis superior muscle
18 Rectus capitis posterior major muscle
19 Obliquus capitis inferior muscle
20 Spinous process of axis
21 Semispinalis cervicis muscle
22 Semispinalis capitis muscle (divided and reflected)
23 Transverse cervical artery (superficial branch)
24 Serratus posterior superior muscle (divided and reflected)
25 Rhomboid minor muscle (divided and reflected)
26 Rhomboid major muscle (divided and reflected)

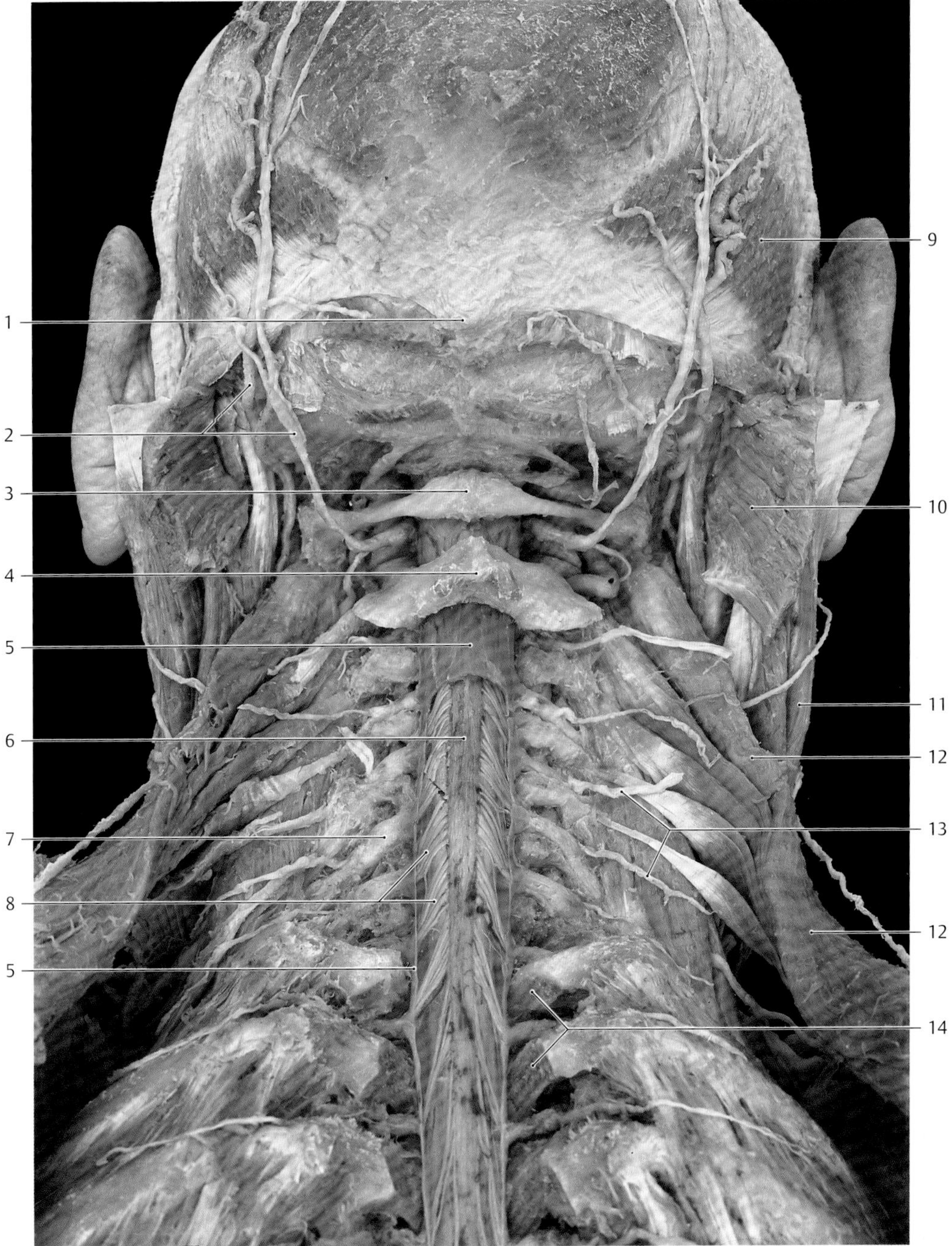


Fig. 2.126 **Posterior aspect of the neck** (deepest layer). The vertebral canal caudally of the atlas and axis has been opened to show the spinal cord. The dura mater has been partly removed.

1 External occipital protuberance
2 Greater occipital nerve (C2) and occipital artery
3 Atlas (posterior arch)
4 Axis (posterior arch)
5 Spinal dura mater
6 Spinal cord
7 Spinal ganglion
8 Posterior root filaments (fila radicularia posterior)
9 Occipital belly of occipitofrontalis muscle
10 Splenius capitis muscle (cut and reflected)
11 Sternocleidomastoid muscle
12 Levator scapulae muscle
13 Posterior branches of spinal nerves
14 Arches of cervical and upper thoracic vertebrae (cut)

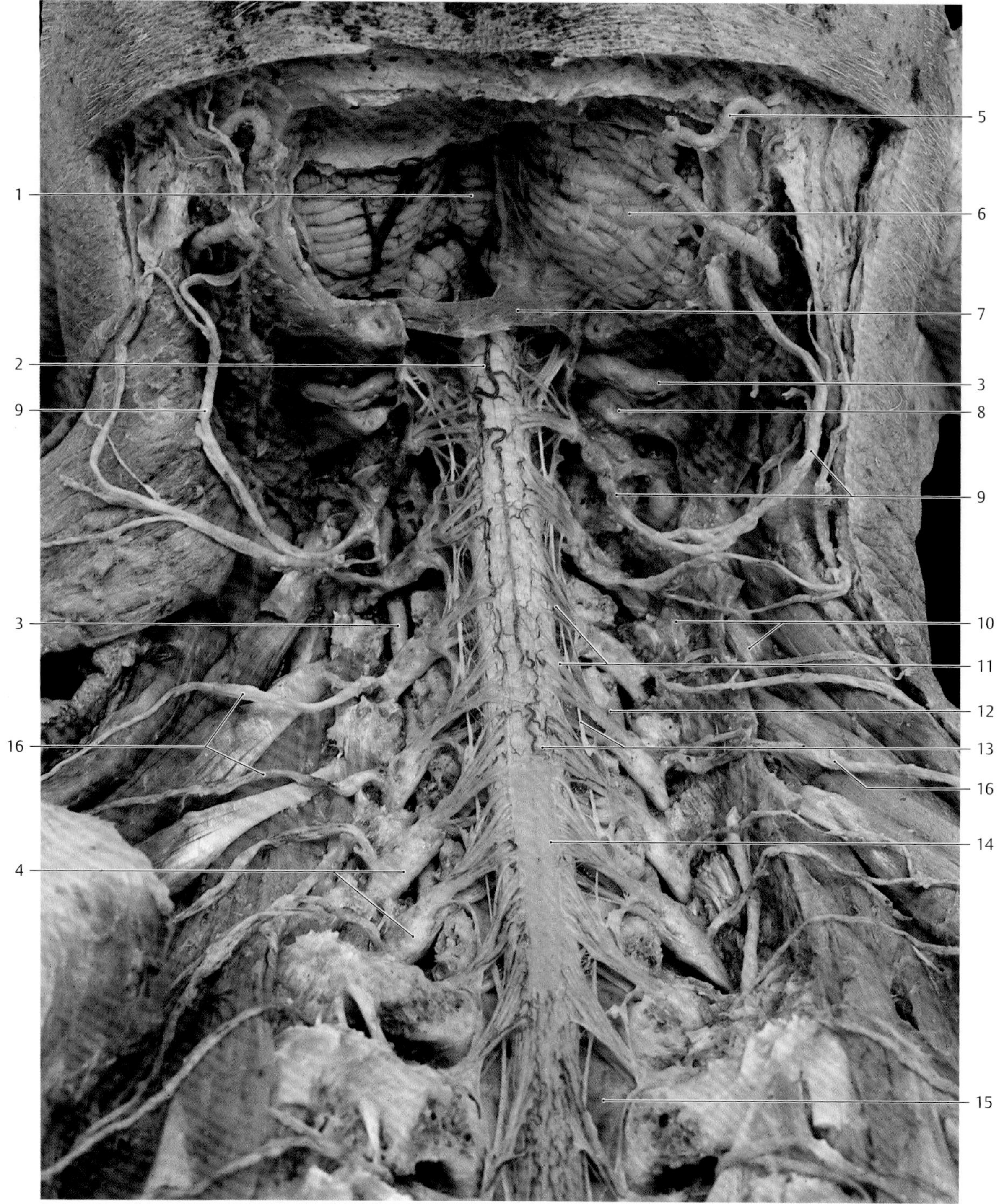


Fig. 2.127 **Posterior aspect of the neck** (deepest layer). Dissection of medulla oblongata and spinal cord. The cranial cavity has been opened.

1 Vermis of the cerebellum
2 Medulla oblongata and posterior spinal artery
3 Vertebral artery
4 Spinal ganglion
5 Occipital artery
6 Cerebellum
7 Cerebellomedullary cistern
8 Posterior arch of atlas
9 Greater occipital nerve (C2)
10 Levator scapulae muscle and intertransverse ligament
11 Dorsal roots of spinal nerves
12 Vertebral arch
13 Denticulate ligament and arachnoid mater
14 Area where pia mater has been removed
15 Spinal dura mater
16 Dorsal rami of spinal nerves

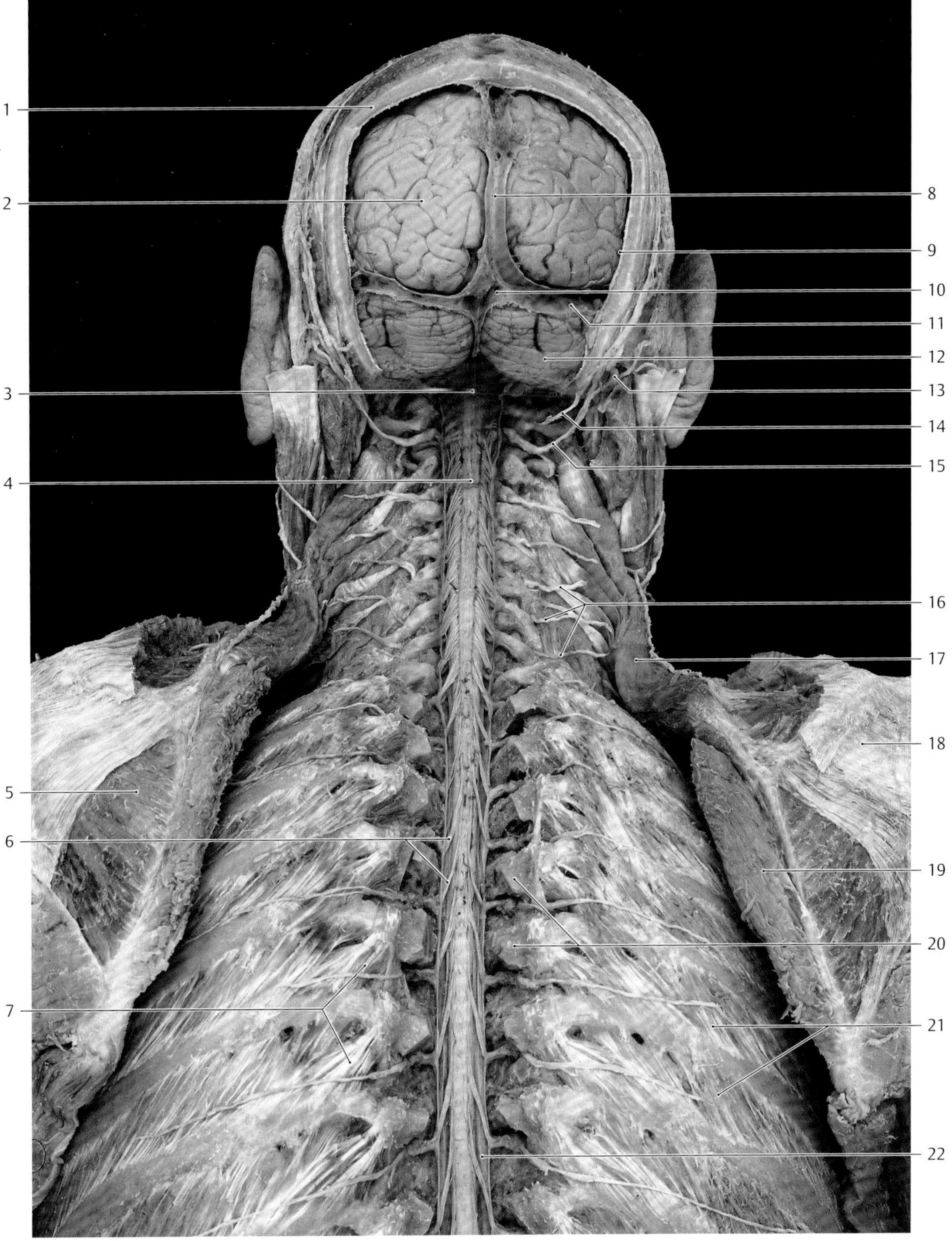


Fig. 2.128 **Posterior aspect of the neck** (deepest layer). Dissection of medulla oblongata and spinal cord in relation to the brain.

1 Calvaria
2 Left hemisphere of the brain
3 Cerebellomedullary cistern
4 Spinal cord
5 Scapula with infraspinous muscle
6 Posterior root filaments (fila radicularia posterior)
7 Levatores costarum muscles
8 Falx cerebri with sinus sagittalis superior
9 Subarachnoid space
10 Confluence of sinuses
11 Transverse sinus
12 Cerebellum
13 Occipital artery
14 Suboccipital nerve (C1)
15 Greater occipital nerve (C2)
16 Posterior branches of spinal nerves
17 Levator scapulae muscle
18 Deltoid muscle
19 Rhomboid muscles
20 Vertebral arches (cut)
21 External intercostal muscles
22 Spinal dura mater

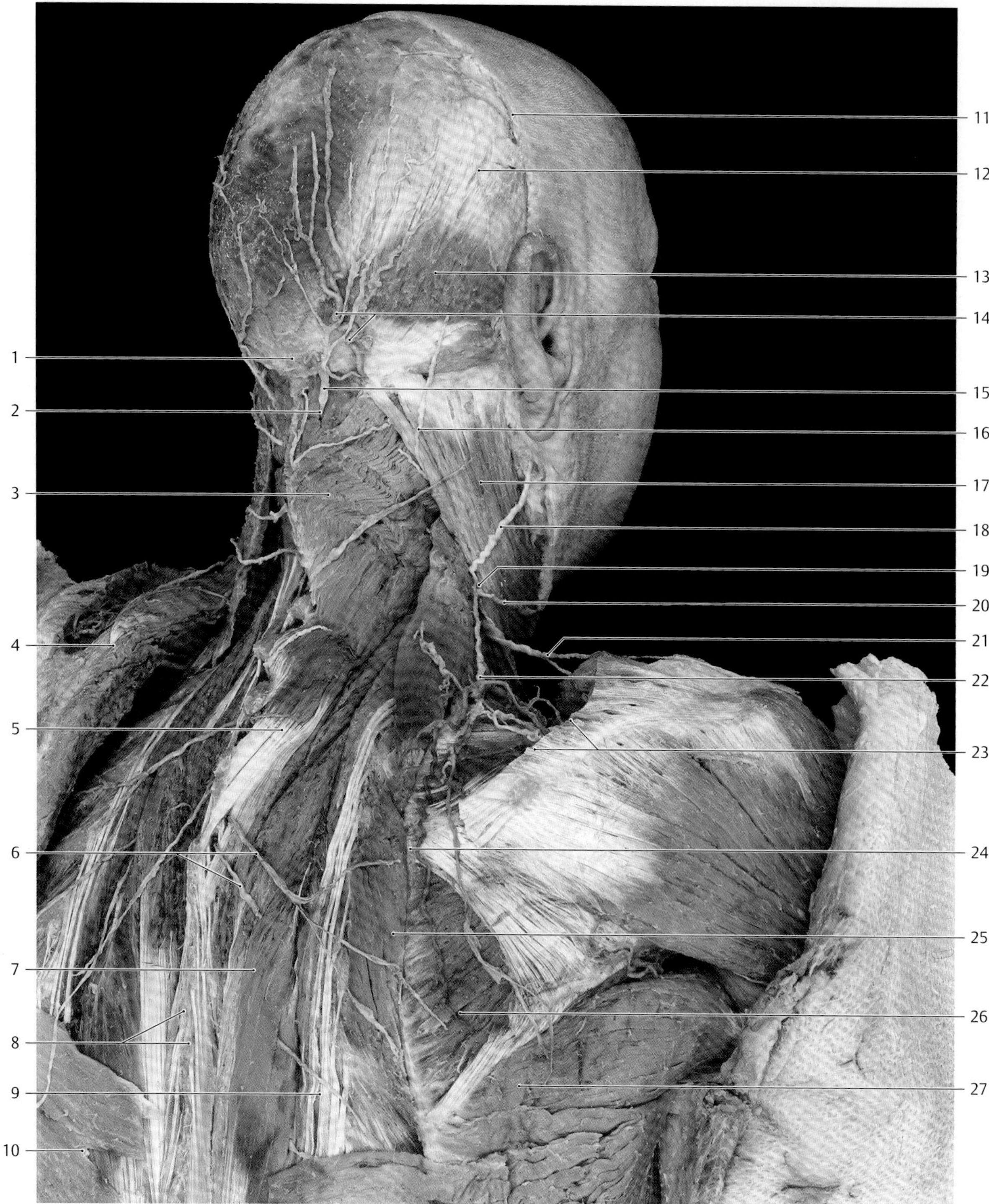


Fig. 2.129 **Oblique-lateral aspect of the neck** (deeper layer). The trapezius muscle has been removed.

1 External occipital protuberance
2 Semispinalis capitis muscle
3 Splenius capitis muscle
4 Scapula
5 Splenius cervicis muscle
6 Posterior branches of spinal nerves
7 Longissimus muscle
8 Spinous processes of thoracic vertebrae
9 Iliocostalis muscle
10 Latissimus dorsi muscle
11 Epidermis of the head (scalp)
12 Galea aponeurotica
13 Occipital belly of occipitofrontalis muscle
14 Occipital artery
15 Greater occipital nerve (C2)
16 Lesser occipital nerve
17 Sternocleidomastoid muscle
18 Great auricular nerve
19 Punctum nervosum
20 Transverse cervical nerve
21 Supraclavicular nerves
22 Accessory nerve (CN XI)
23 Trapezius muscle (cut edge)
24 Medial margin of scapula
25 Rhomboid major muscle
26 Infraspinous muscle
27 Teres major muscle

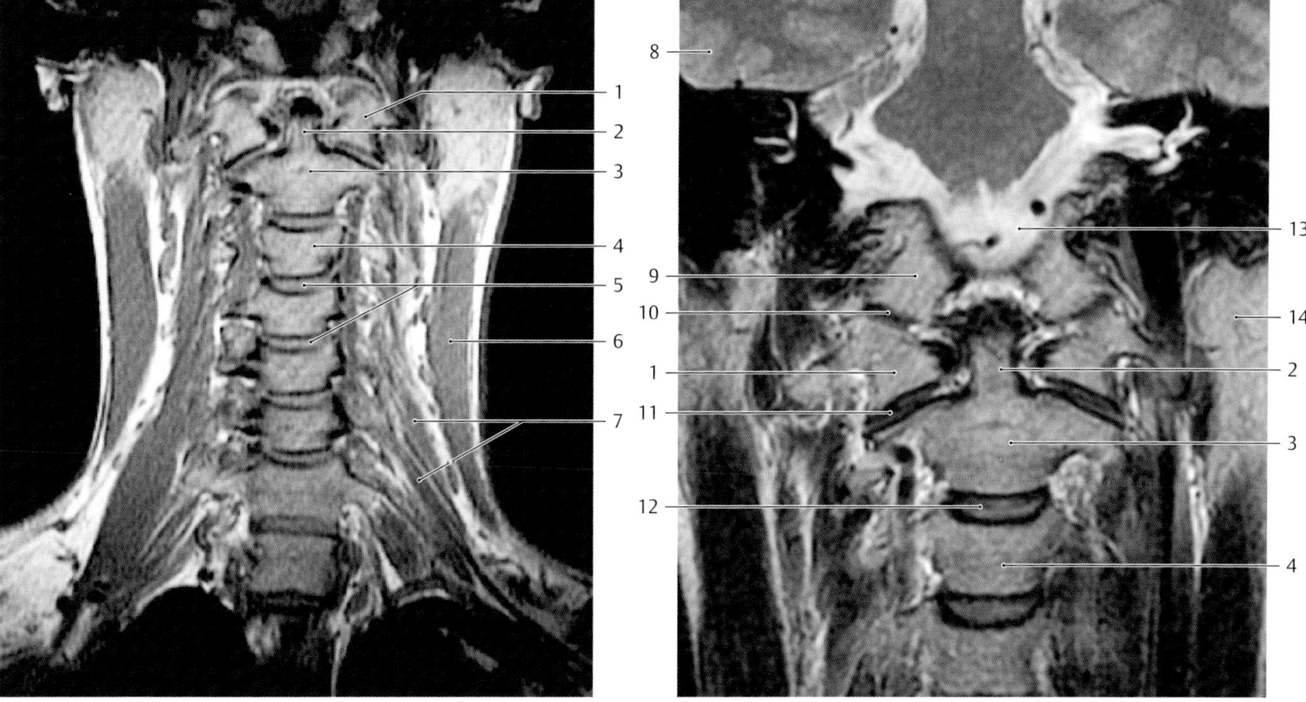


**Fig. 2.130 Coronal section through the cervical vertebral column** at the level of the vertical bodies (MRI scan). (Heuck A, et al. MRT-Atlas des muskuloskelettalen Systems. Stuttgart, Germany: Schattauer, 2009.)

**Fig. 2.131 Coronal section through the cervical vertebral column** at the level of the dens of axis (MRI scan). (Heuck A, et al. MRT-Atlas des muskuloskelettalen Systems. Stuttgart, Germany: Schattauer, 2009.)

1 Atlas
2 Dens of axis
3 Axis
4 Body of cervical vertebra (C3)
5 Intervertebral discs
6 Sternocleidomastoid muscle
7 Scalene muscles
8 Cerebellum
9 Occipital condyle
10 Atlanto-occipital joint
11 Lateral atlanto-axial joint
12 Intervertebral disc
13 Cistern of pons
14 Head of mandible

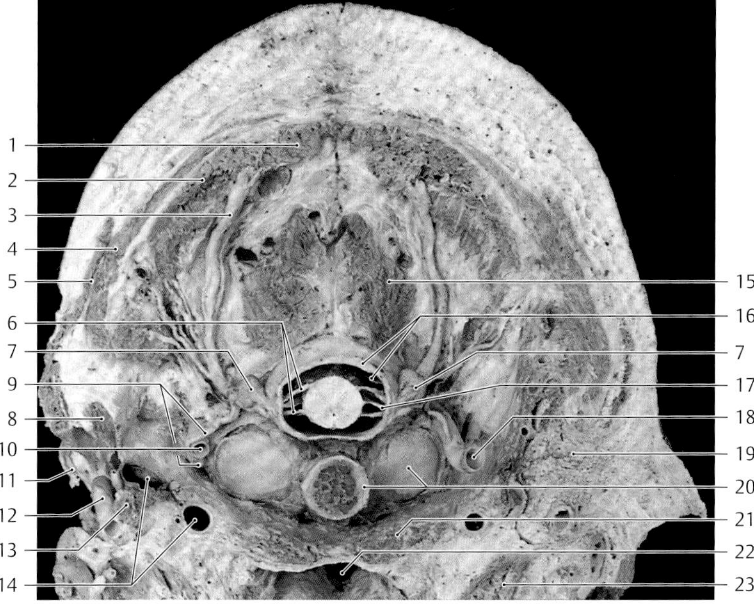


**Fig. 2.132 Horizontal section through the neck.** Dissection of the second cervical spinal nerve. Posterior surface at top of figure.

1 Trapezius muscle
2 Semispinalis capitis muscle
3 Dorsal ramus of spinal nerve
4 Sternocleidomastoid muscle
5 Platysma muscle
6 Dorsal and ventral roots of spinal nerves
7 Spinal ganglion
8 Posterior belly of digastric muscle
9 Ventral ramus of spinal nerve
10 Vertebral artery
11 Great auricular nerve
12 Superficial temporal artery
13 Styloid process
14 Internal jugular vein and internal carotid artery
15 Rectus capitis posterior major muscle
16 Dura mater and subarachnoid space
17 Denticulate ligament
18 Vertebral artery
19 Parotid gland
20 Dens of axis (divided) and inferior articular facet of atlas
21 Longus capitis muscle
22 Pharyngeal cavity
23 Medial pterygoid muscle

# 3 Upper Limb

## General Anatomy and Musculoskeletal System

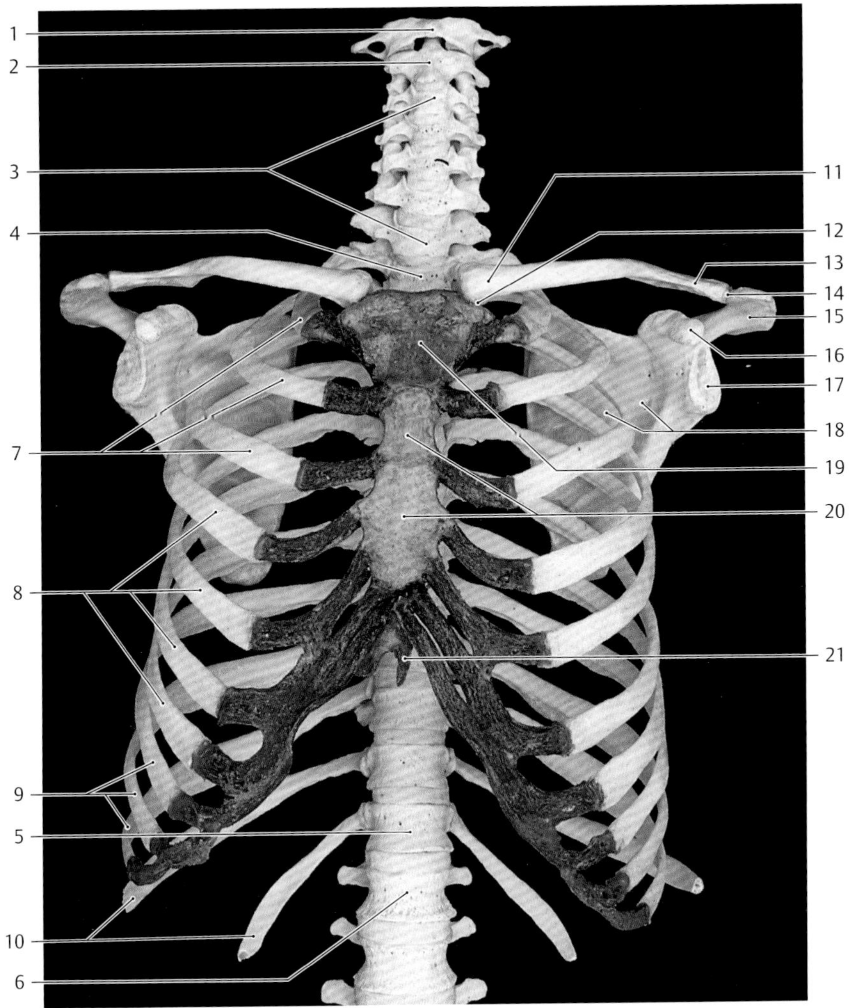


**Vertebral column**
1 Atlas (C1)
2 Axis (C2)
3 Third to seventh cervical vertebrae (C3–C7)
4 First thoracic vertebra (T1)
5 Twelfth thoracic vertebra (T12)
6 First lumbar vertebra (L1)

**Ribs**
7 First to third ribs } True ribs
8 Fourth to seventh ribs }
9 Eighth to tenth ribs } False ribs
10 Eleventh and twelfth ribs (floating ribs) }

**Clavicle (A)**
11 Sternal end
12 Sternoclavicular joint
13 Acromial end
14 Acromioclavicular joint

**Scapula (B)**
15 Acromion
16 Coracoid process
17 Glenoid cavity
18 Costal surface

**Sternum (C)**
19 Manubrium
20 Body
21 Xiphoid process

Fig. 3.1 **Skeleton of shoulder girdle and thorax** (anterior aspect). The cartilaginous parts of the ribs appear dark brown.

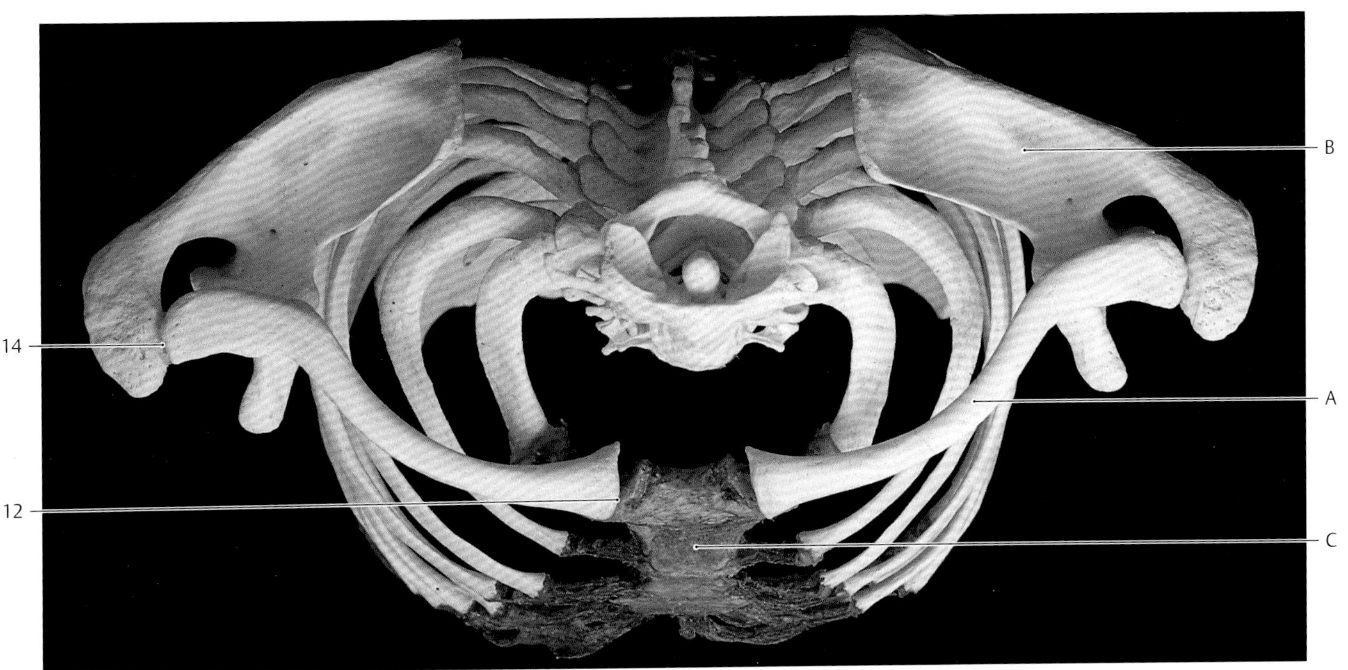


Fig. 3.2 **Skeleton of shoulder girdle and thorax** (superior aspect).

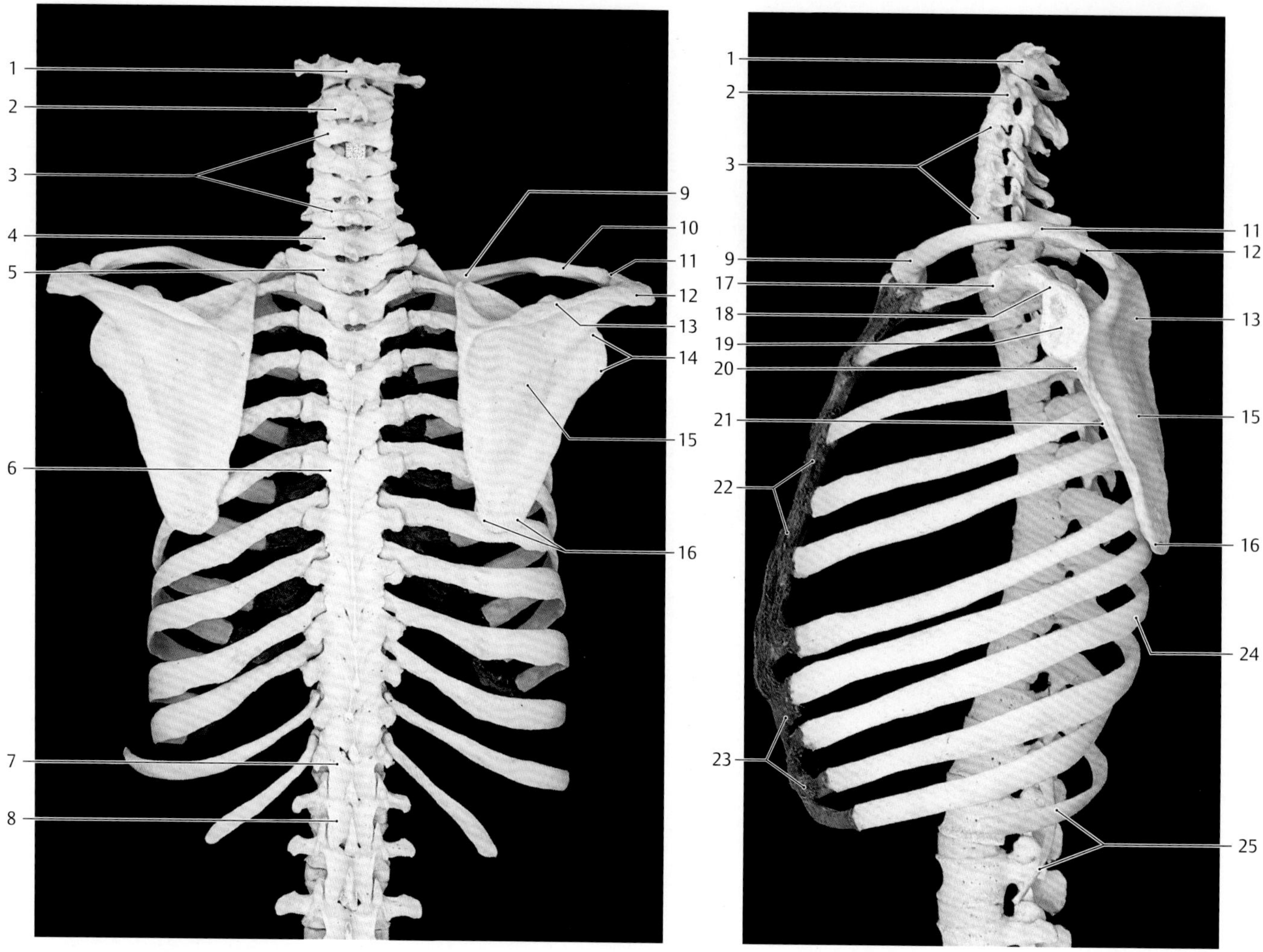


**Fig. 3.3 Skeleton of shoulder girdle and thorax** (posterior aspect).

**Fig. 3.4 Skeleton of shoulder girdle and thorax** (lateral aspect).

**Vertebral column**
1 Atlas (C1)
2 Axis (C2)
3 Third to sixth cervical vertebrae (C3–C6)
4 Seventh vertebra (vertebra prominens) (C7)
5 First thoracic vertebra (T1)
6 Sixth thoracic vertebra (T6)
7 Twelfth thoracic vertebra (T12)
8 First lumbar vertebra (L1)

**Clavicle**
9 Sternal end
10 Acromial end
11 Acromioclavicular joint

**Scapula**
12 Acromion
13 Spine of scapula
14 Lateral angle
15 Posterior surface
16 Inferior angle
17 Coracoid process
18 Supraglenoid tubercle
19 Glenoid cavity
20 Infraglenoid tubercle
21 Lateral margin

**Thorax**
22 Body of sternum
23 Subcostal angle
24 Angle of rib
25 Floating ribs

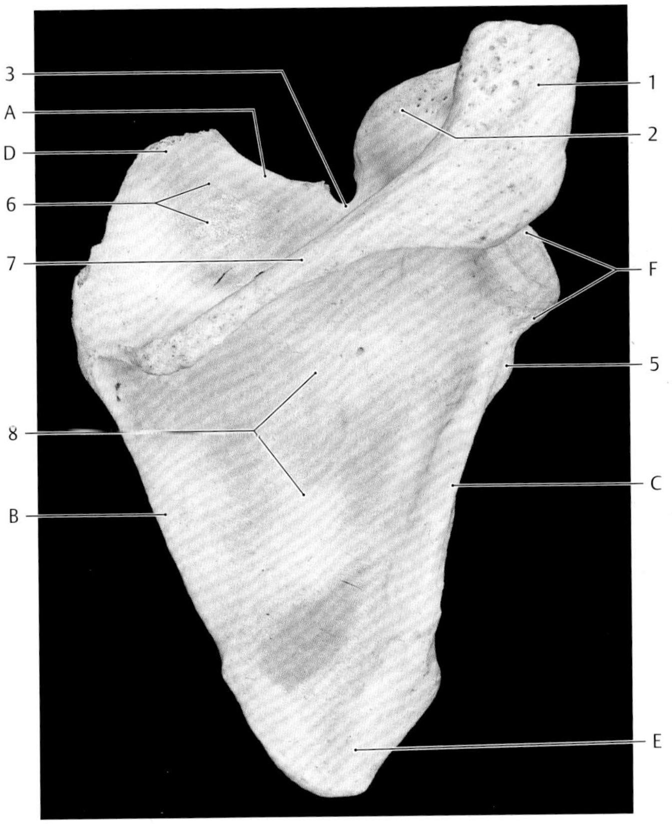

Fig. 3.5 **Right scapula** (posterior aspect).

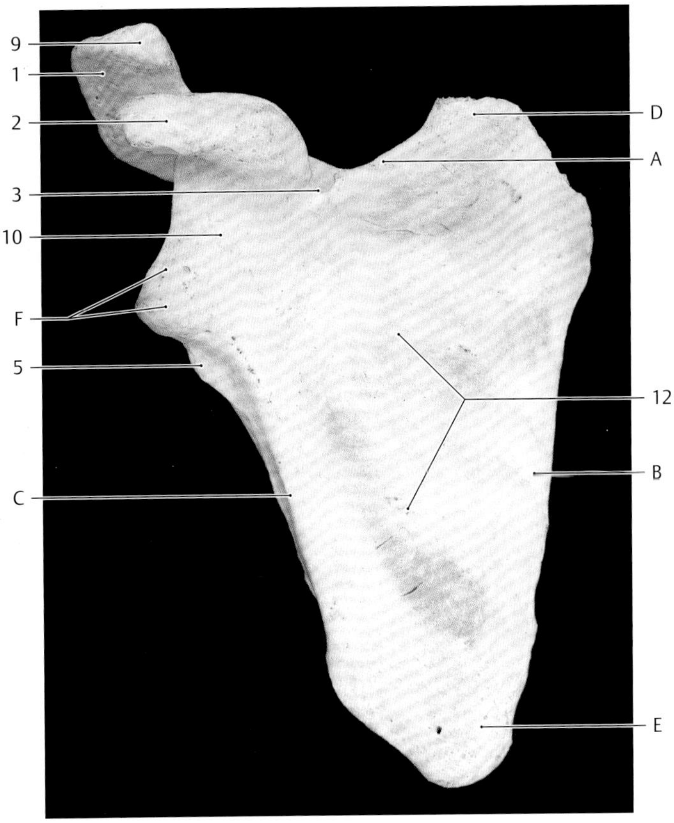

Fig. 3.6 **Right scapula** (anterior aspect, costal surface).

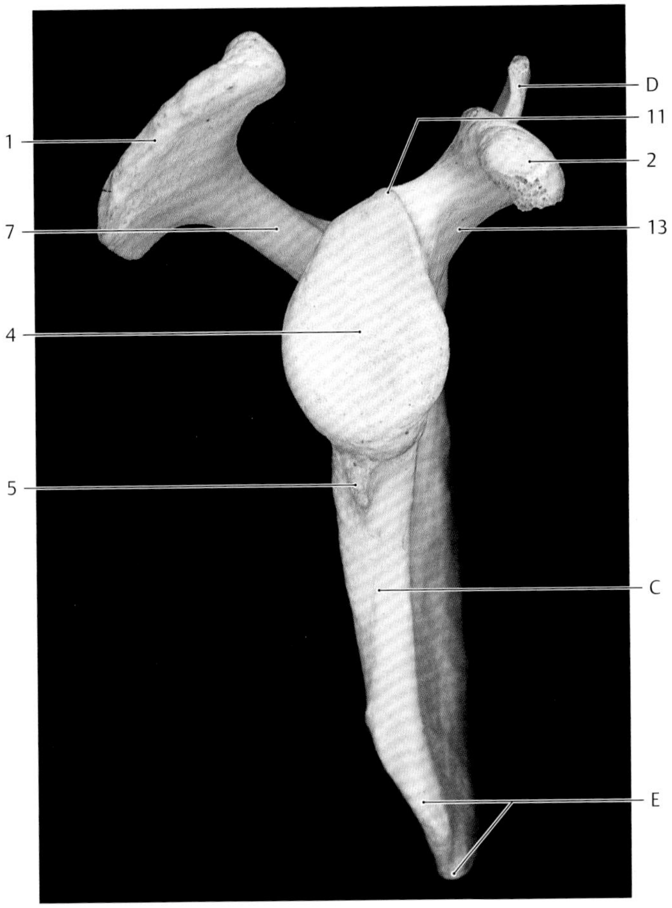

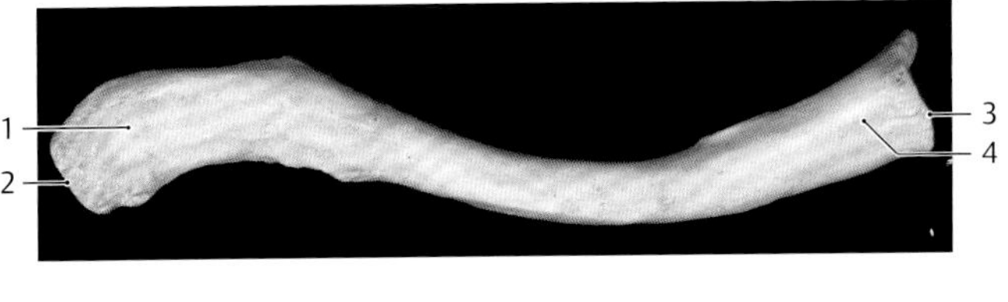


Fig. 3.8 **Right clavicle** (superior aspect).

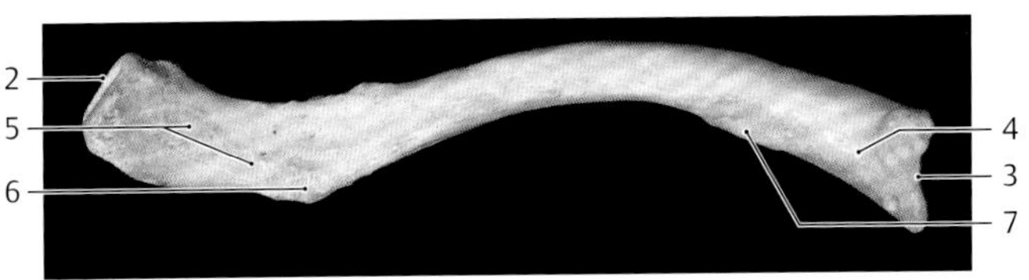


Fig. 3.9 **Right clavicle** (inferior aspect).

Fig. 3.7 **Right scapula** (lateral aspect).

**Scapula**

A = Superior border
B = Medial border
C = Lateral border
D = Superior angle
E = Inferior angle
F = Lateral angle

1 Acromion
2 Coracoid process
3 Scapular notch
4 Glenoid cavity
5 Infraglenoid tubercle
6 Supraspinous fossa
7 Spine
8 Infraspinous fossa
9 Articular facet for the acromion
10 Neck
11 Supraglenoid tubercle
12 Costal (anterior) surface
13 Base of coracoid process

**Clavicle**

1 Acromial end
2 Articular facet for the acromion
3 Articular facet for the sternum
4 Sternal end
5 Trapezoid line
6 Conoid tubercle
7 Impression of costoclavicular ligament

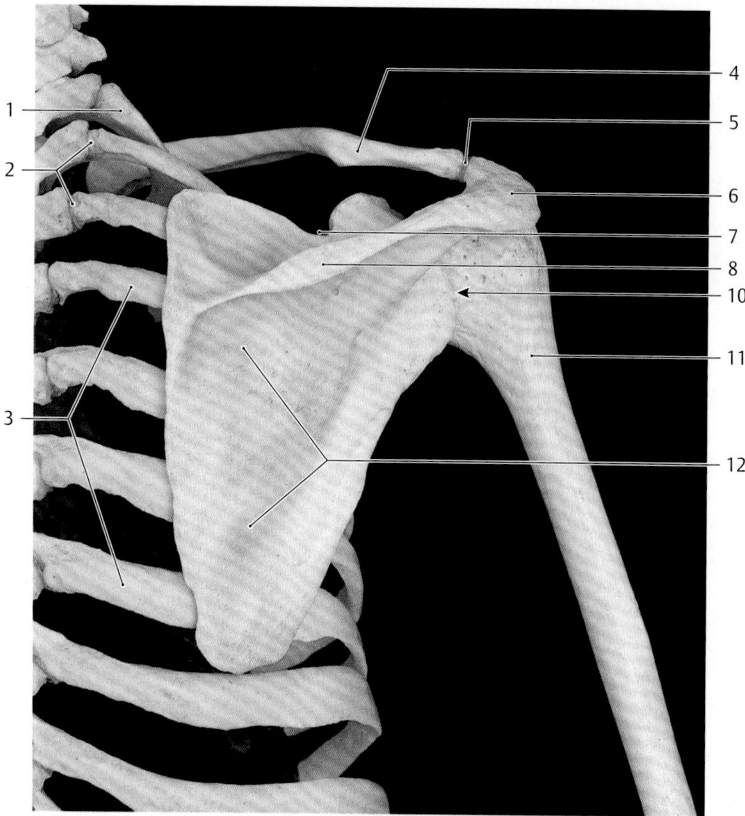


Fig. 3.10 **Bones of shoulder joint** (posterior aspect).

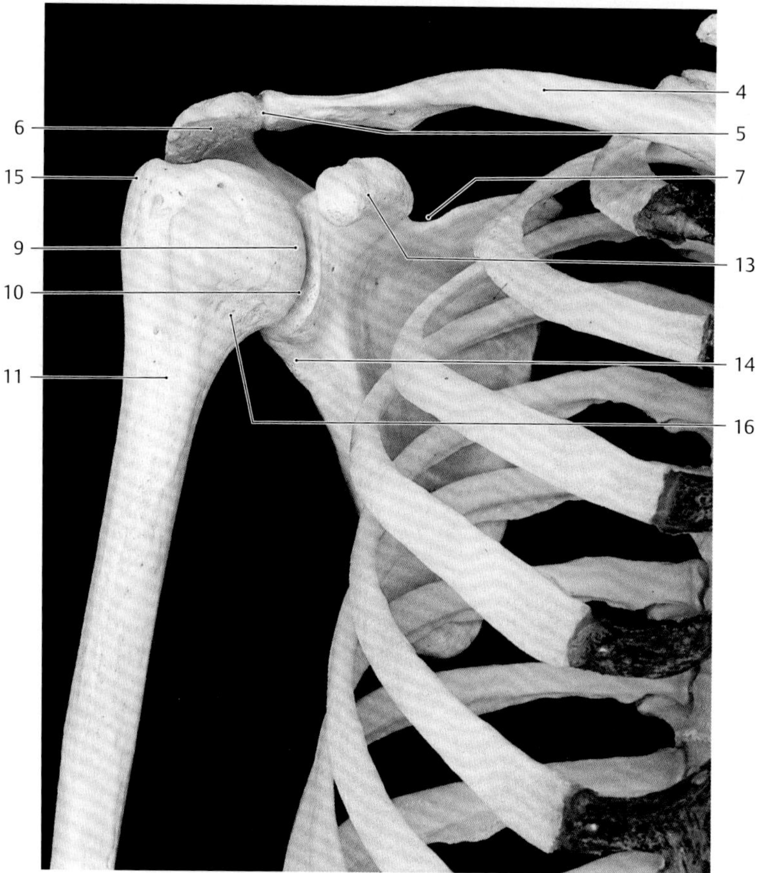


Fig. 3.11 **Bones of shoulder joint** (anterior aspect)

1 First rib
2 Position of costotransverse joints
3 Fourth to seventh ribs
4 Clavicle
5 Position of acromioclavicular joint
6 Acromion
7 Scapular notch
8 Spine of scapula
9 Head of humerus
10 Glenoid cavity
11 Surgical neck of humerus
12 Posterior surface of scapula
13 Coracoid process
14 Infraglenoid tubercle
15 Greater tubercle of humerus
16 Anatomical neck of humerus

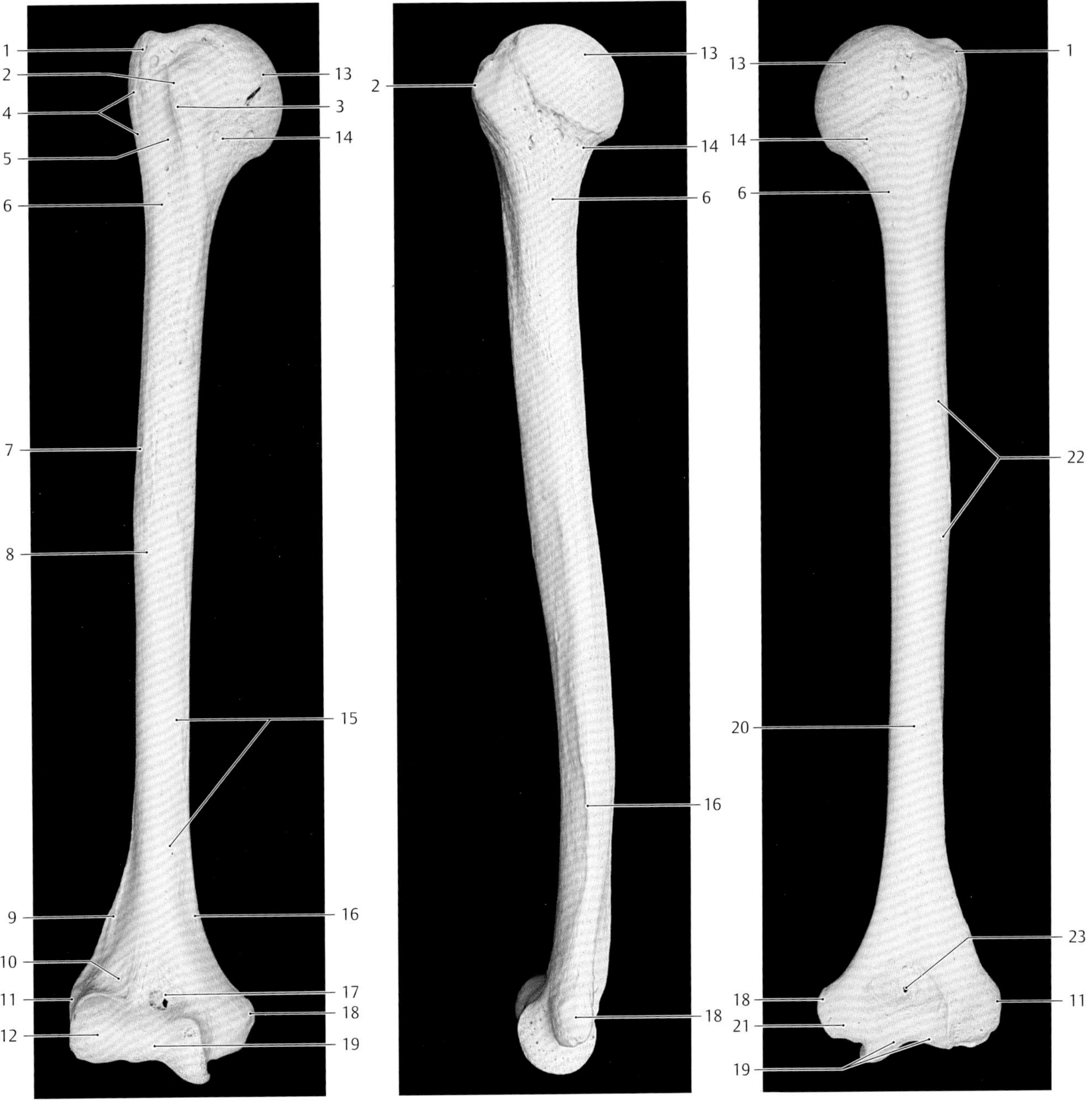


Fig. 3.12 **Right humerus** (anterior aspect).

Fig. 3.13 **Right humerus** (medial aspect).

Fig. 3.14 **Right humerus** (posterior aspect).

**Humerus**

1 Greater tubercle
2 Lesser tubercle
3 Crest of lesser tubercle
4 Crest of greater tubercle
5 Intertubercular sulcus
6 Surgical neck
7 Deltoid tuberosity
8 Antero-lateral surface
9 Lateral supracondylar ridge
10 Radial fossa
11 Lateral epicondyle
12 Capitulum
13 Head
14 Anatomical neck
15 Antero-medial surface
16 Medial supracondylar ridge
17 Coronoid fossa
18 Medial epicondyle
19 Trochlea
20 Posterior surface
21 Groove for ulnar nerve
22 Groove for radial nerve
23 Olecranon fossa

Fig. 3.15 **Bones of right forearm, radius, and ulna** (anterior aspect).

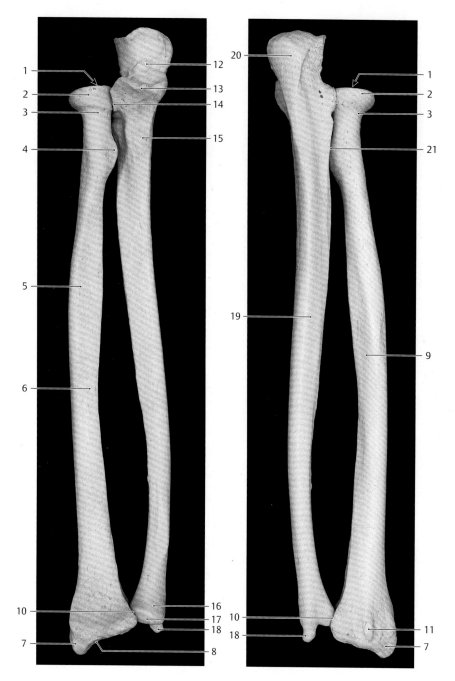

Fig. 3.16 **Bones of right forearm, radius, and ulna** (posterior aspect).

**Radius**

1 Head
2 Articular circumference
3 Neck
4 Radial tuberosity
5 Shaft
6 Anterior surface
7 Styloid process
8 Articular surface
9 Posterior surface
10 Ulnar notch
11 Dorsal tubercle

**Ulna**

12 Trochlear notch
13 Coronoid process
14 Radial notch
15 Ulnar tuberosity
16 Head
17 Articular circumference
18 Styloid process
19 Posterior surface
20 Olecranon
21 Supinator crest

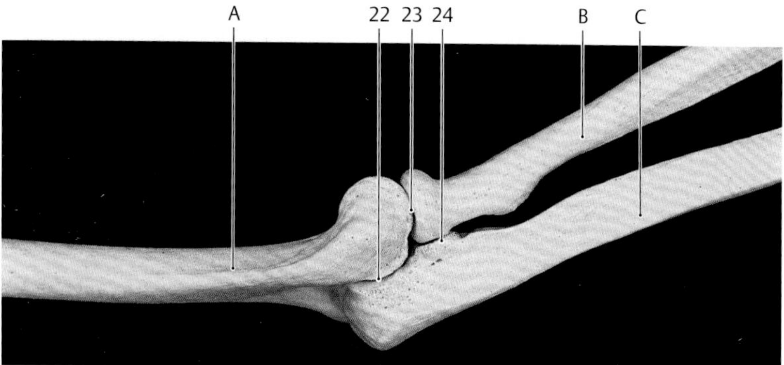


Fig. 3.17 **Bones of the right elbow joint** (lateral aspect).

**Articulations at the right elbow** (sites of joints).

22 Site of humero-ulnar joint
23 Site of humeroradial joint
24 Site of proximal radio-ulnar joint

A = Humerus
B = Radius
C = Ulna

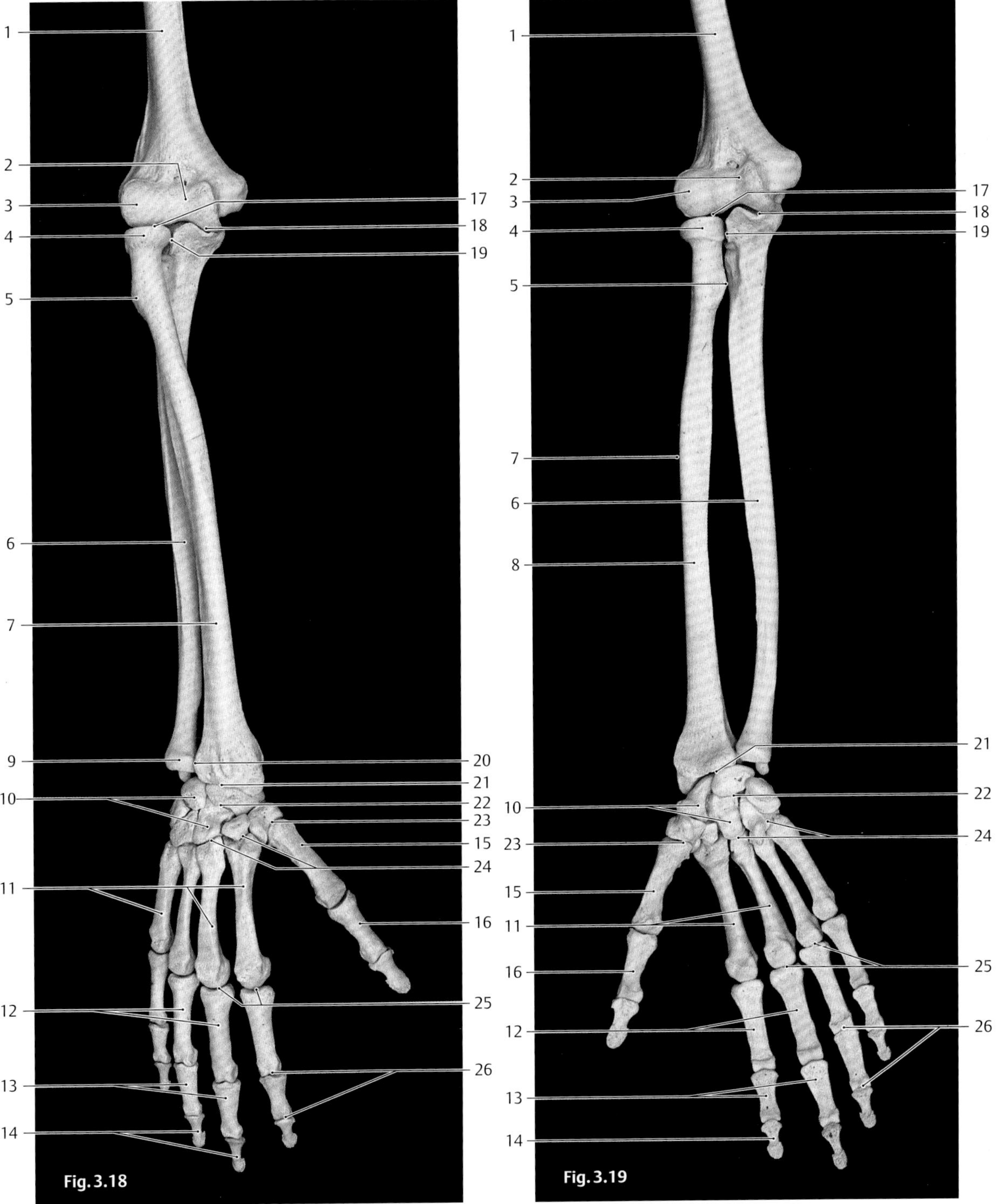


**Figs. 3.18 and 3.19 Skeleton of right forearm and hand in pronation** (left) **and supination** (right).

1 Humerus
2 Trochlea of humerus
3 Capitulum of humerus
4 Articular circumference of radius
5 Radial tuberosity
6 Anterior surface of ulna
7 Posterior surface of radius
8 Anterior surface of radius
9 Articular circumference of ulna
10 Carpal bones
11 Metacarpal bones
12 Proximal phalanges
13 Middle phalanges
14 Distal phalanges
15 Metacarpal bone of thumb
16 Proximal phalanx of thumb

**Sites of joints**

17 Humeroradial joint
18 Humero-ulnar joint
19 Proximal radio-ulnar joint
20 Distal radio-ulnar joint
21 Wrist joint
22 Midcarpal joint
23 Carpometacarpal joint of thumb
24 Carpometacarpal joints
25 Metacarpophalangeal joints
26 Interphalangeal joints of the hand

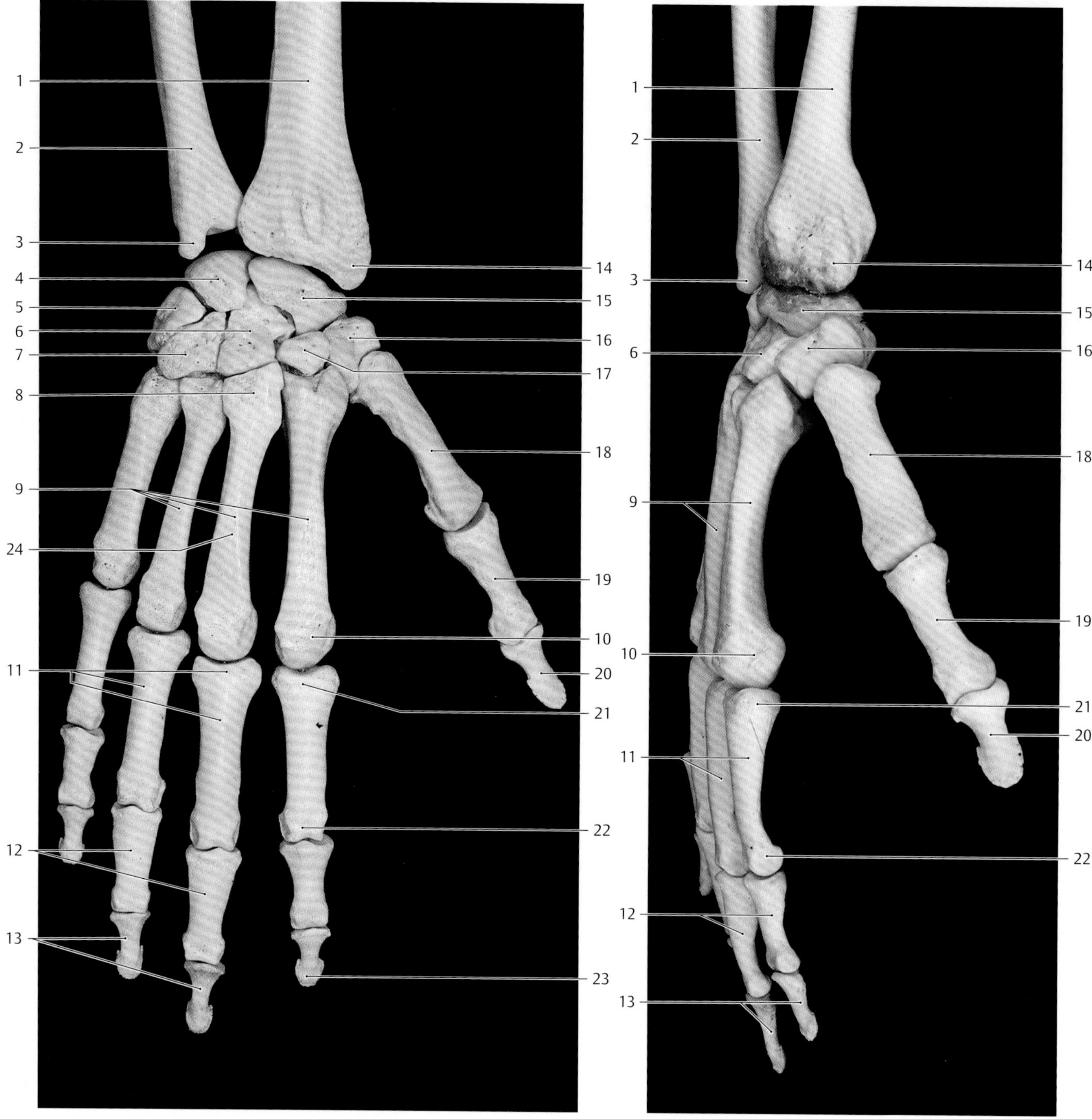


Fig. 3.20 **Skeleton of right wrist and hand** (dorsal aspect).

Fig. 3.21 **Skeleton of right wrist and hand** (medial aspect).

1 Radius
2 Ulna
3 Styloid process of ulna
4 Lunate bone } Carpal bones
5 Triquetral bone } Carpal bones
6 Capitate bone } Carpal bones
7 Hamate bone } Carpal bones
8 Base of third metacarpal bone
9 Metacarpal bones
10 Head of metacarpal bone
11 Proximal phalanges of the hand
12 Middle phalanges of the hand
13 Distal phalanges of the hand
14 Styloid process of radius
15 Scaphoid bone } Carpal bones
16 Trapezium bone } Carpal bones
17 Trapezoid bone } Carpal bones
18 Metacarpal bone of thumb
19 Proximal phalanx of thumb
20 Distal phalanx of thumb
21 Base of second proximal phalanx
22 Head of second proximal phalanx
23 Tuberosity of distal phalanx
24 Body of third metacarpal bone

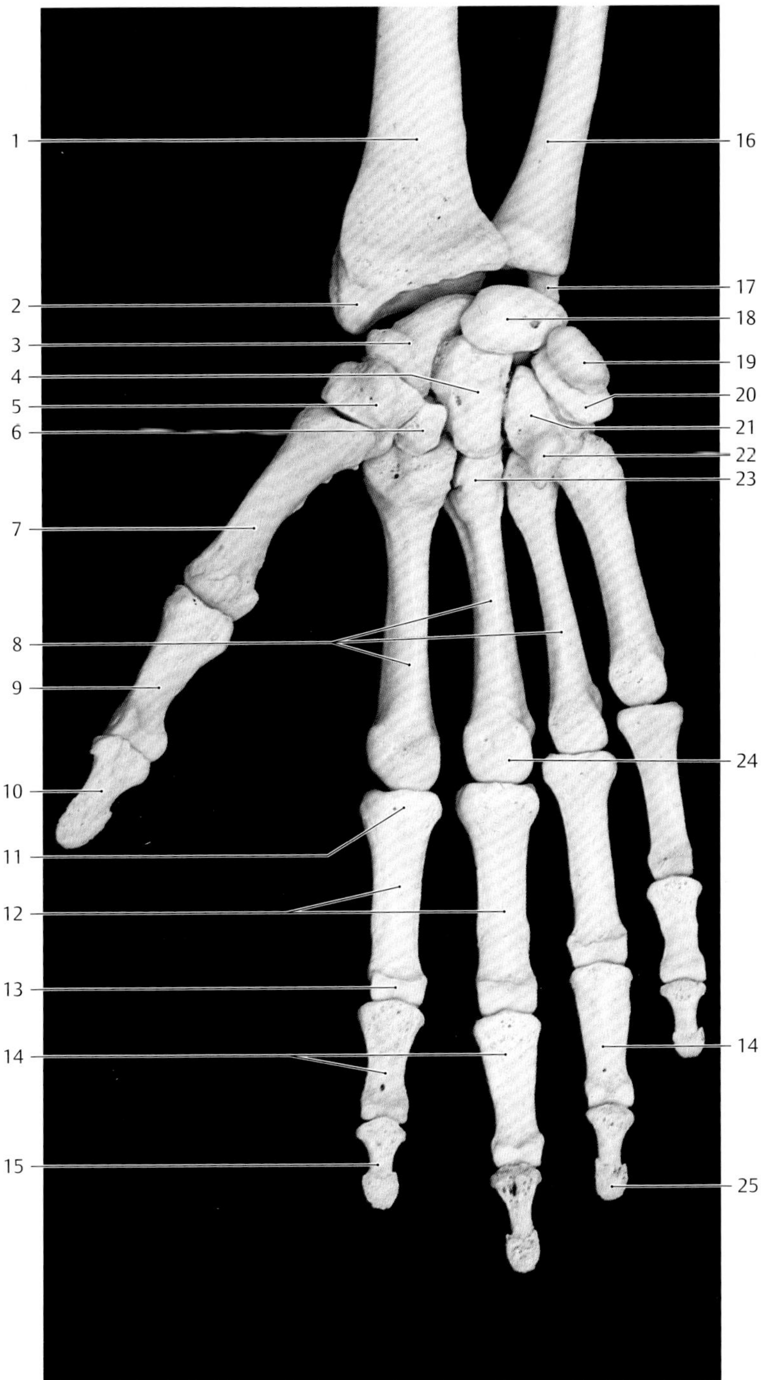

Fig. 3.22 **Skeleton of right wrist and hand** (palmar aspect).

1 Radius
2 Styloid process of radius
3 Scaphoid bone (Carpal bones)
4 Capitate bone (Carpal bones)
5 Trapezium (Carpal bones)
6 Trapezoid bone (Carpal bones)
7 First metacarpal bone
8 Second to fourth metacarpal bones
9 Proximal phalanx of thumb
10 Distal phalanx of thumb
11 Base of second proximal phalanx
12 Proximal phalanges
13 Head of second proximal phalanx
14 Middle phalanges
15 Distal phalanx
16 Ulna
17 Styloid process of ulna
18 Lunate bone (Carpal bones)
19 Pisiform bone (Carpal bones)
20 Triquetral bone (Carpal bones)
21 Hamate bone (Carpal bones)
22 Hamulus or hook of hamate bone
23 Base of third metacarpal bone
24 Head of metacarpal bone
25 Tuberosity of distal phalanx

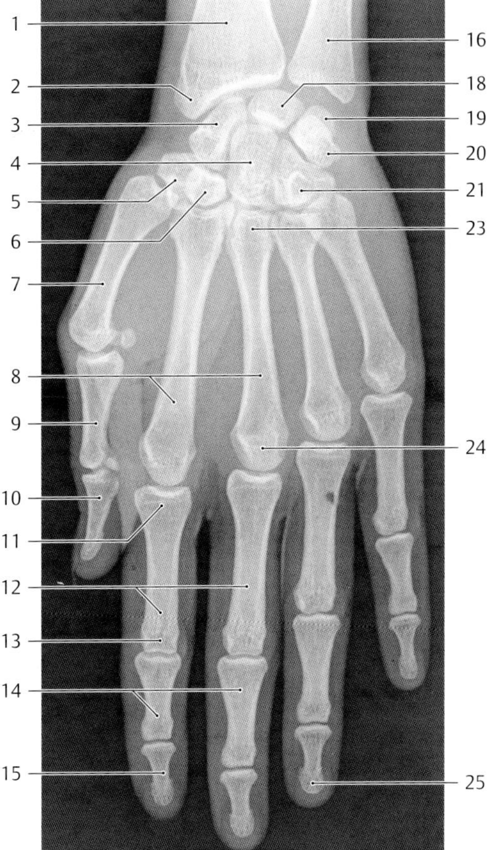

Fig. 3.23 **X-ray of wrist and hand** (palmar aspect). (Courtesy of Prof. Uder, Institute of Radiology, University Hospital Erlangen, Germany.)

The human hand is one of the most admirable structures of the human body. The carpometacarpal joint of the thumb, a saddle joint, enjoys wide mobility so that the thumb can come into contact with all other fingers, thus enabling the hand to become an instrument for grasping and psychologic expression. During evolution, these newly developed functions appeared after the erect posture of the human body was achieved. An inevitable prerequisite for the development of human cultures is not only the differentiation of the brain but also the development of an organ capable of realizing its ideas: the human hand.

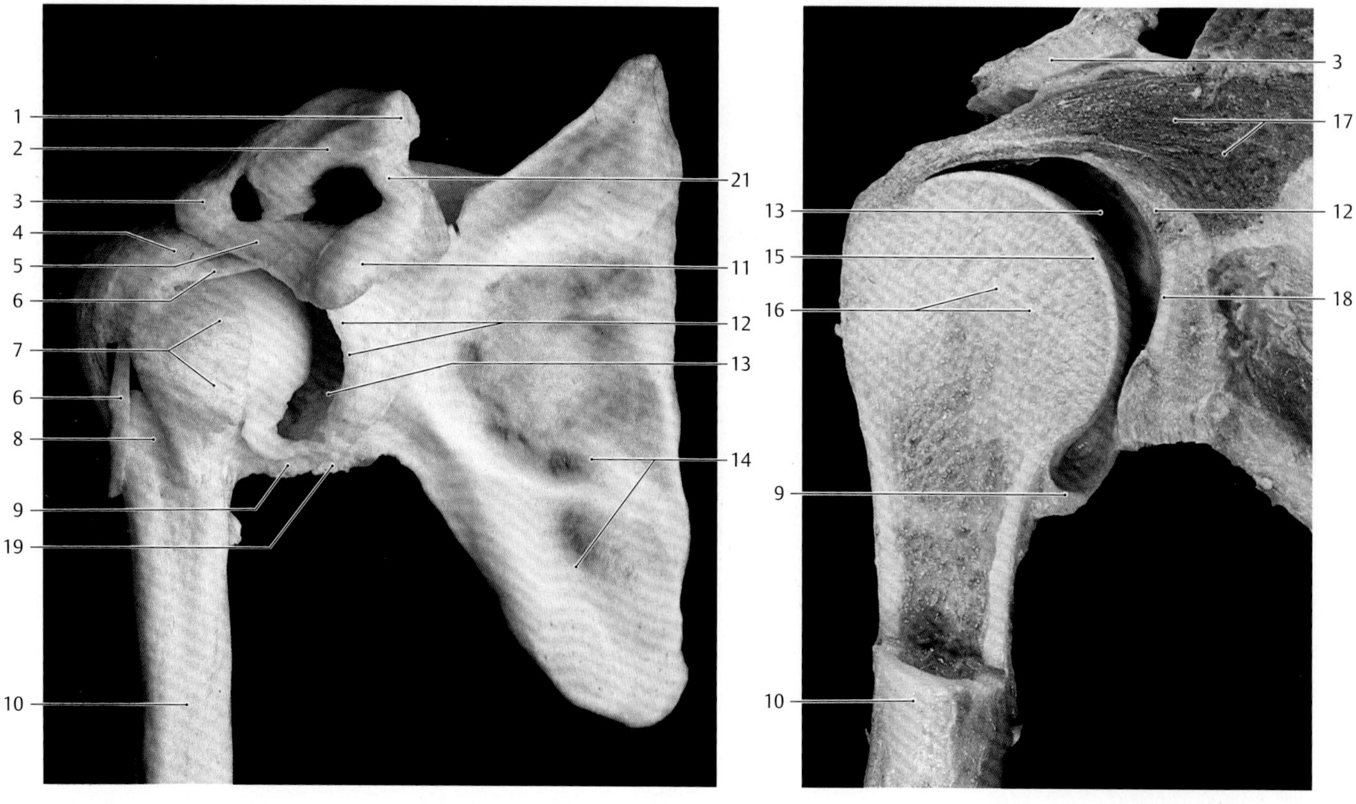


**Fig. 3.24 Right shoulder joint.** The anterior part of the articular capsule has been removed and the head of the humerus has been slightly rotated outward to show the cavity of the joint.

**Fig. 3.25 Coronal section through the right shoulder joint** (anterior aspect).

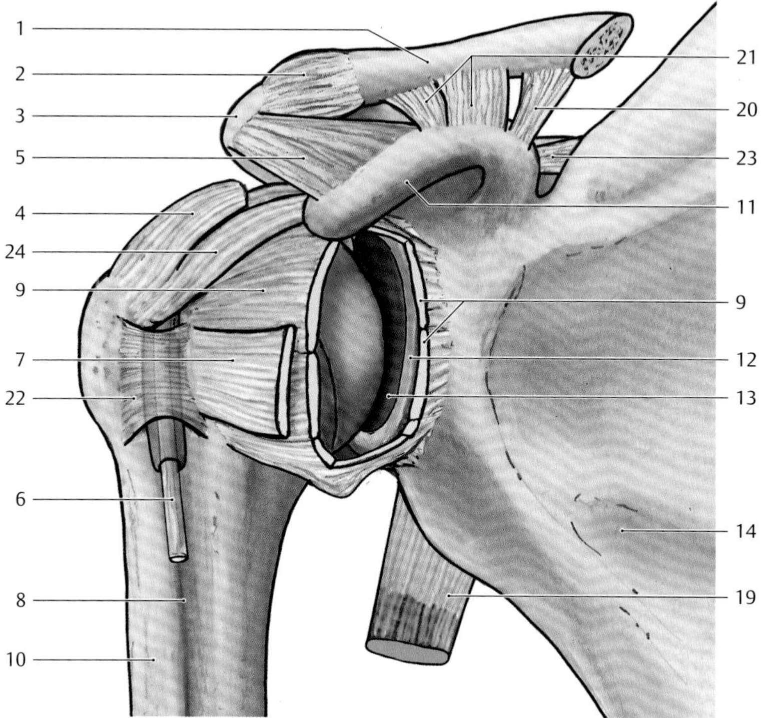


**Fig. 3.26 Shoulder joint with tendon of biceps brachii muscle, articular capsule, and ligaments** (anterior aspect).

1 Acromial end of clavicle
2 Acromioclavicular joint
3 Acromion
4 Tendon of supraspinatus muscle (attached to the articular capsule)
5 Coraco-acromial ligament
6 Tendon of long head of biceps brachii muscle
7 Tendon of subscapularis muscle (attached to the articular capsule)
8 Intertubercular sulcus
9 Articular capsule of shoulder joint
10 Humerus
11 Coracoid process
12 Glenoid labrum
13 Shoulder joint (joint cavity)
14 Scapula
15 Head of humerus
16 Epiphysial line
17 Supraspinatus muscle
18 Glenoid cavity
19 Tendon of long head of triceps brachii muscle
20 Conoid ligament (coracoclaviculare ligament)
21 Trapezoid ligament (coracoclaviculare ligament)
22 Transverse humeral ligament
23 Superior transverse ligament of the scapula
24 Coraco-humeral ligament

1 Humerus
2 Lateral epicondyle of humerus
3 Articular capsule
4 Anular ligament of proximal radio-ulnar joint
5 Radius
6 Tendon of biceps brachii muscle
7 Medial epicondyle of humerus
8 Ulnar collateral ligament
9 Oblique chord
10 Ulna
11 Interosseous membrane
12 Radial fossa
13 Capitulum of humerus
14 Head of radius
15 Radial collateral ligament
16 Coronoid fossa
17 Trochlea of humerus
18 Coronoid process of ulna
19 Olecranon
20 Radial tuberosity

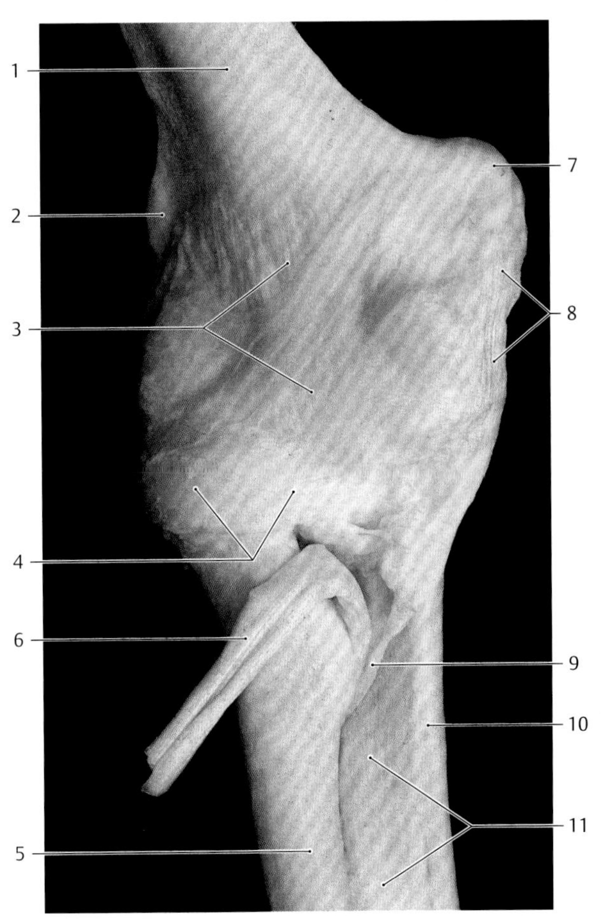


Fig. 3.27 **Ligaments of the elbow joint** (anterior aspect).

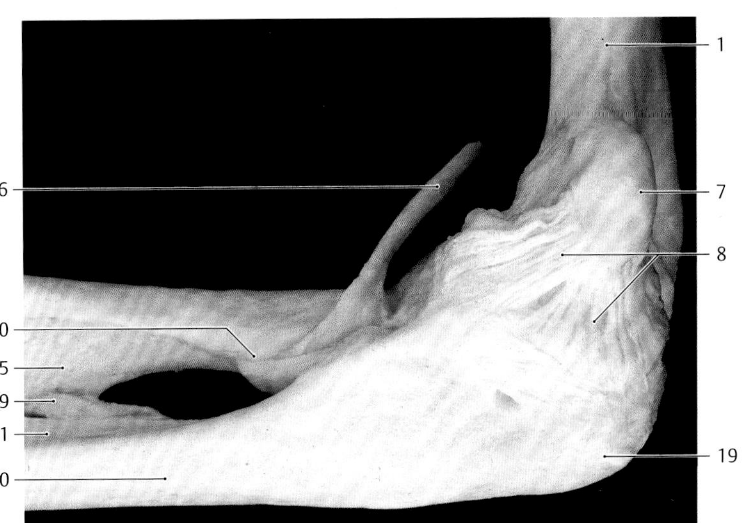


Fig. 3.28 **Ligaments of the elbow joint** (medial aspect).

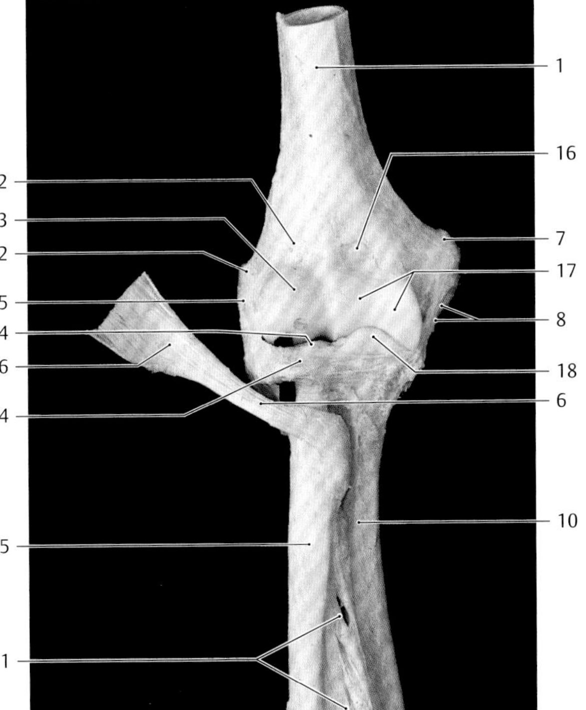


Fig. 3.29 **Elbow joint with ligaments** (anterior aspect). Articular capsule has been removed to show the anular ligament.

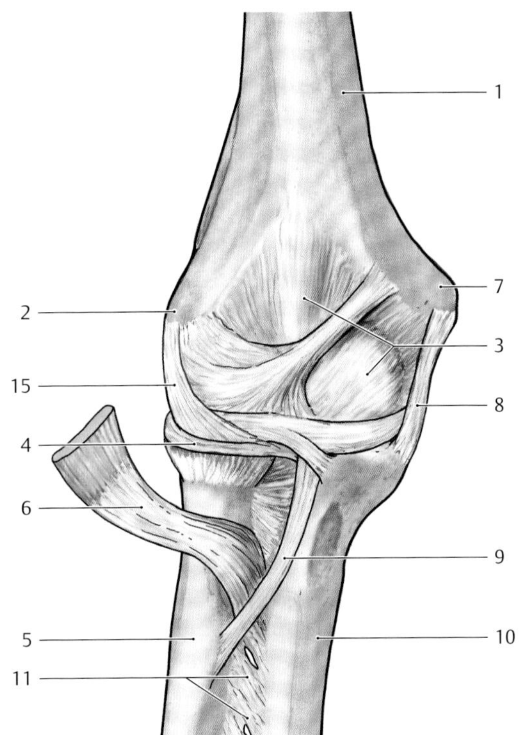


Fig. 3.30 **Elbow joint with ligaments, schematic** (anterior aspect). Articular capsule has been removed to show the anular ligament.

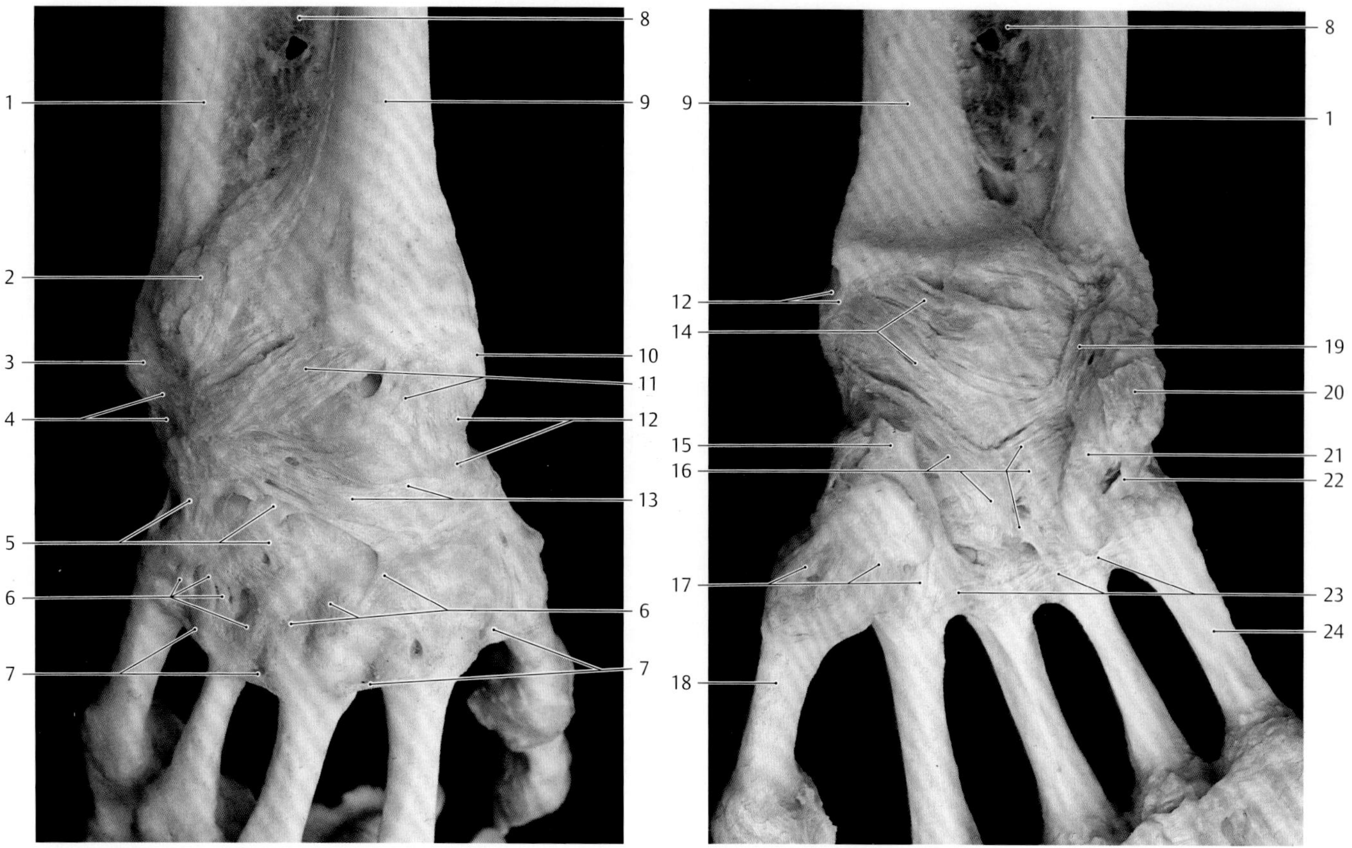

Fig. 3.31 **Ligaments of hand and wrist** (dorsal aspect).

Fig. 3.32 **Ligaments of hand and wrist** (palmar aspect).

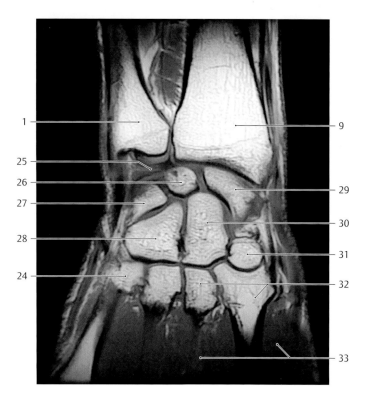

Fig. 3.33 **Coronal section through the hand and wrist** (MRI scan). Note the location of the wrist joint. (Heuck A, et al. MRT-Atlas des muskuloskelettalen Systems. Stuttgart, Germany: Schattauer, 2009.)

1 Ulna
2 Exostosis (pathological)
3 Head of ulna
4 Ulnar carpal collateral ligament
5 Deep intercarpal ligaments
6 Dorsal carpometacarpal ligaments
7 Dorsal metacarpal ligaments
8 Interosseous membrane
9 Radius
10 Styloid process of radius
11 Dorsal radiocarpal ligament
12 Radial collateral ligament
13 Articular capsule and dorsal intercarpal ligaments
14 Palmar radiocarpal ligament
15 Tendon of flexor carpi radialis muscle (cut)
16 Radiating carpal ligament
17 Palmar carpometacarpal ligaments
18 First metacarpal bone
19 Palmar ulnocarpal ligament
20 Tendon of flexor carpi ulnaris muscle (cut)
21 Pisohamate ligament
22 Pisometacarpal ligament
23 Palmar metacarpal ligaments
24 Fifth metacarpal bone
25 Articular disc (ulnocarpal)
26 Lunate bone
27 Triquetral bone
28 Hamate bone
29 Scaphoid (navicular) bone
30 Capitate bone
31 Trapezoid bone
32 Second and third metacarpal bones
33 Dorsal interossei muscles

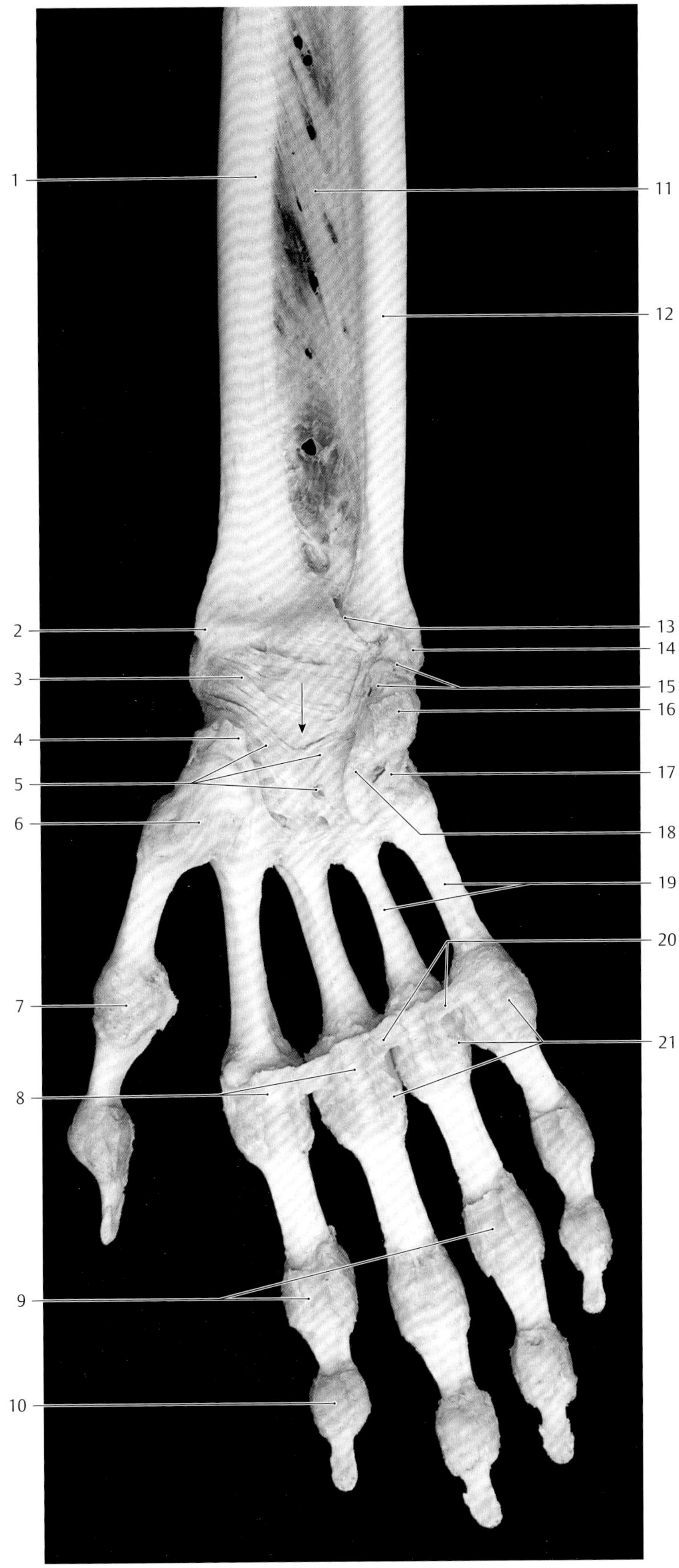

1 Radius
2 Styloid process of radius
3 Palmar radiocarpal ligament
4 Tendon of flexor carpi radialis muscle (cut)
5 Radiating carpal ligament
6 Articular capsule of carpometacarpal joint of thumb
7 Articular capsule of metacarpophalangeal joint of thumb
8 Palmar ligaments and articular capsule of metacarpophalangeal joints
9 Palmar ligaments and articular capsule of interphalangeal joints
10 Articular capsule
11 Interosseous membrane
12 Ulna
13 Distal radio-ulnar joint
14 Styloid process of ulna
15 Palmar ulnocarpal ligament
16 Pisiform bone with tendon of flexor carpi ulnaris muscle
17 Pisometacarpal ligament
18 Pisohamate ligament
19 Metacarpal bones
20 Deep transverse metacarpal ligaments
21 Collateral ligaments of metacarpophalangeal joints
22 Metacarpophalangeal joints

Fig. 3.34 **Ligaments of forearm, hand, and fingers** (palmar aspect). The arrow indicates the location of the carpal tunnel.

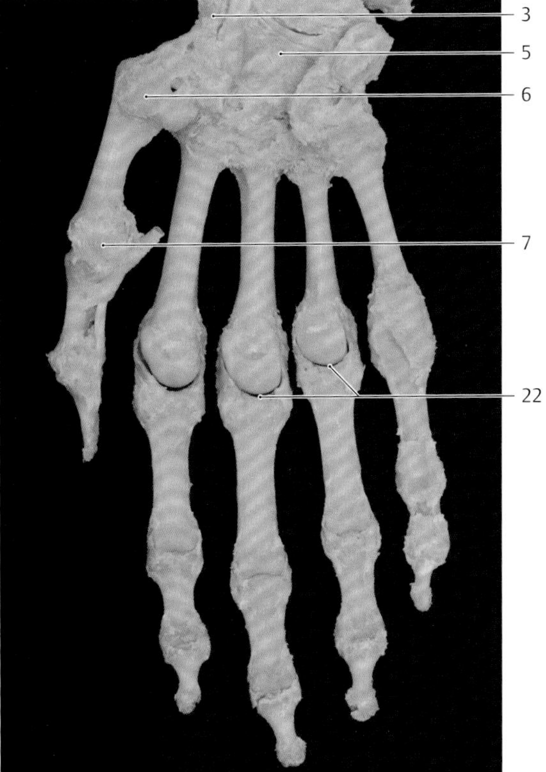


Fig. 3.35 **Second, fourth, and fifth metacarpophalangeal joints.** Articular capsules have been removed.

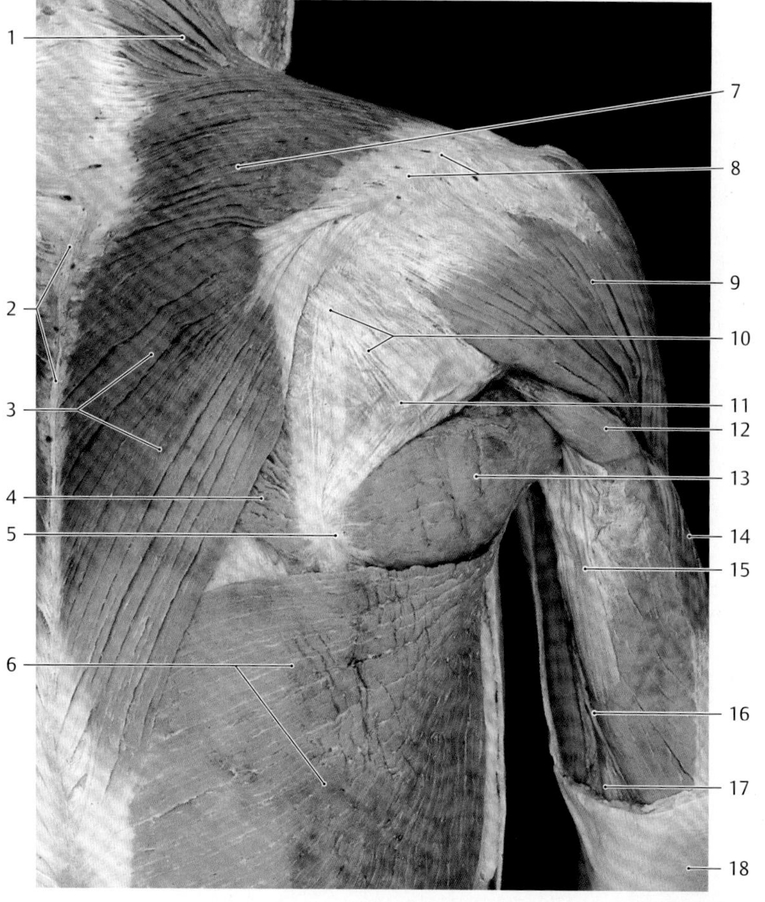


1 Descending fibers of trapezius muscle
2 Spinous processes of thoracic vertebrae
3 Ascending fibers of trapezius muscle
4 Rhomboid major muscle
5 Inferior angle of scapula
6 Latissimus dorsi muscle
7 Transverse fibers of trapezius muscle
8 Spine of scapula
9 Posterior fibers of deltoid muscle
10 Infraspinatus muscle and infraspinous fascia
11 Teres minor muscle and fascia
12 Long head of triceps brachii muscle
13 Teres major muscle
14 Lateral head of triceps brachii muscle
15 Tendon of triceps brachii muscle
16 Medial intermuscular septum
17 Ulnar nerve
18 Olecranon

Fig. 3.36 **Muscles of shoulder and arm,** superficial layer (right side, posterior aspect).

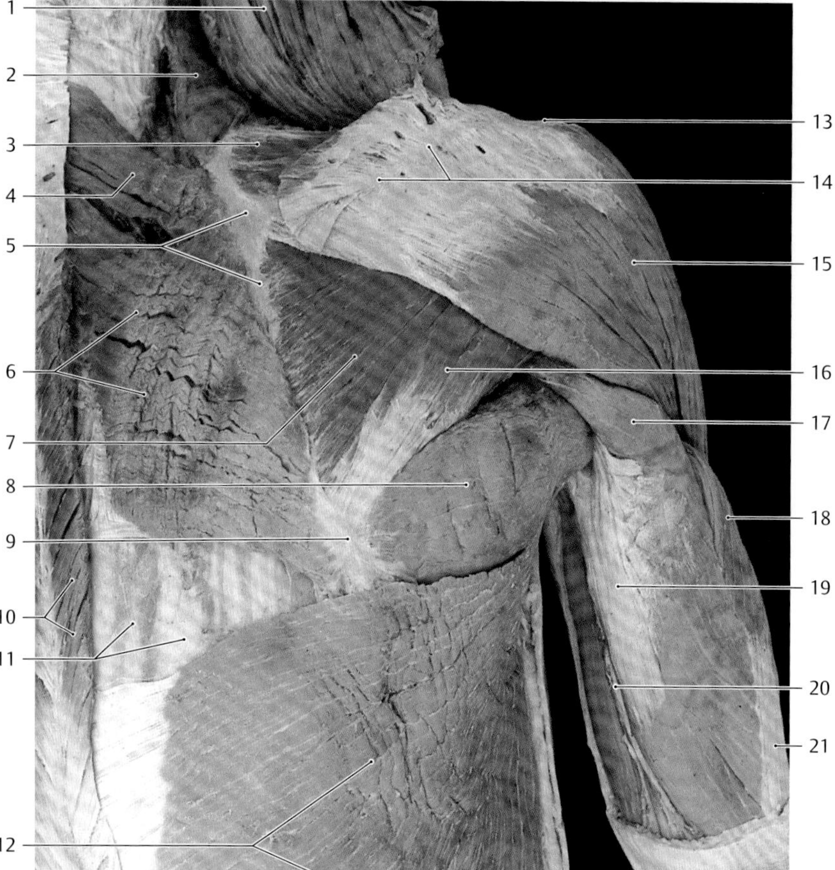


1 Trapezius muscle (reflected)
2 Levator scapulae muscle
3 Supraspinatus muscle
4 Rhomboid minor muscle
5 Medial border of scapula
6 Rhomboid major muscle
7 Infraspinatus muscle
8 Teres major muscle
9 Inferior angle of scapula
10 Cut edge of trapezius muscle
11 Intrinsic muscles of back with fascia
12 Latissimus dorsi muscle
13 Acromion
14 Spine of scapula
15 Deltoid muscle
16 Teres minor muscle
17 Long head of triceps brachii muscle
18 Lateral head of triceps brachii muscle
19 Medial head of triceps brachii muscle
20 Medial intermuscular septum
21 Tendon of triceps brachii muscle

Fig. 3.37 **Muscles of shoulder and arm,** deeper layer (right side, posterior aspect). The trapezius muscle has been cut near its origin at the vertebral column and reflected upward.

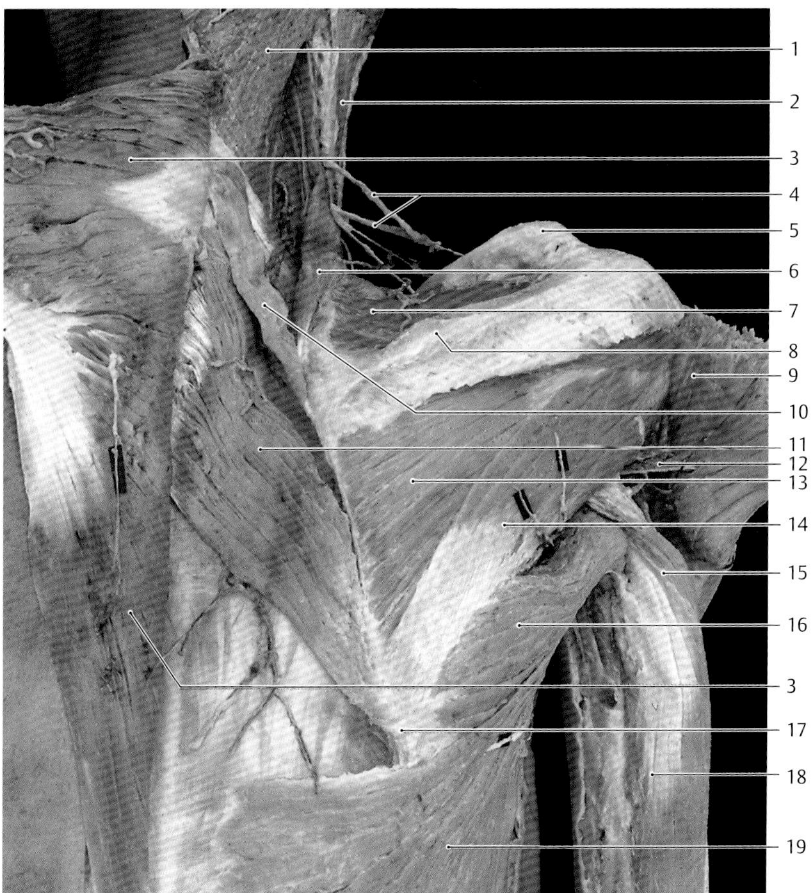

1 Splenius capitis muscle
2 Sternocleidomastoid muscle
3 Trapezius muscle (reflected)
4 Lateral supraclavicular nerves
5 Clavicle
6 Levator scapulae muscle
7 Supraspinatus muscle
8 Spine of scapula
9 Deltoid muscle (reflected)
10 Rhomboid minor muscle
11 Rhomboid major muscle
12 Axillary nerve and posterior circumflex humeral artery
13 Infraspinatus muscle
14 Teres minor muscle
15 Long head of triceps brachii muscle
16 Teres major muscle
17 Inferior angle of scapula
18 Triceps brachii muscle
19 Latissimus dorsi muscle

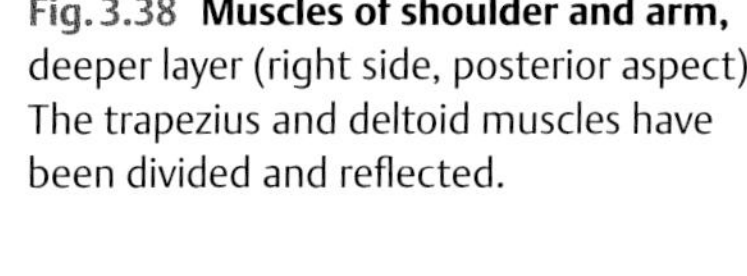

**Fig. 3.38 Muscles of shoulder and arm,** deeper layer (right side, posterior aspect). The trapezius and deltoid muscles have been divided and reflected.

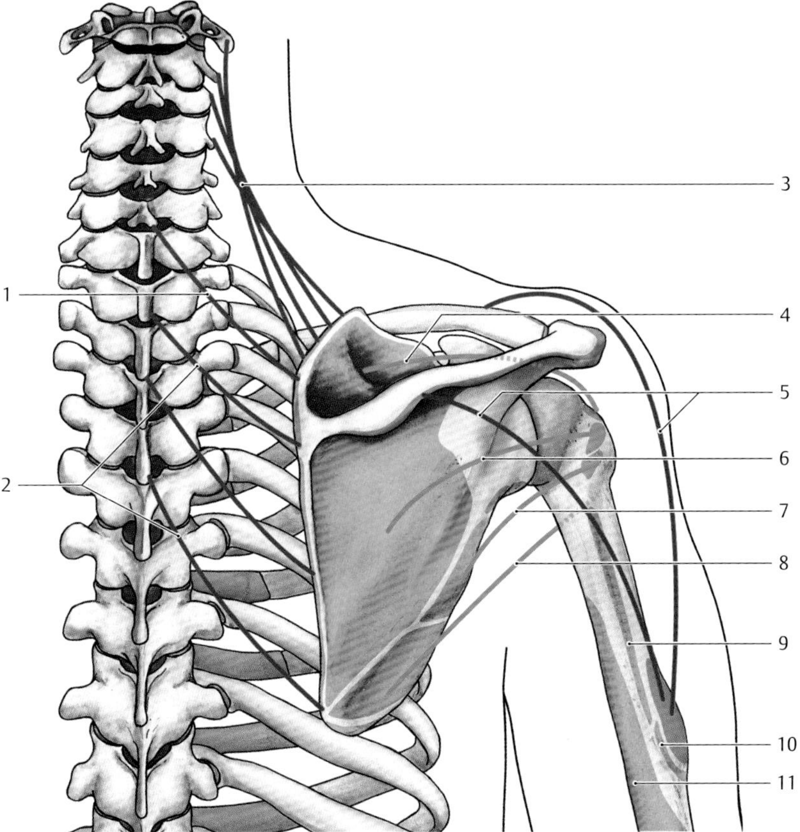

1 Rhomboid minor muscle
2 Rhomboid major muscle
3 Levator scapulae muscle
4 Supraspinatus muscle
5 Deltoid muscle
6 Infraspinatus muscle
7 Teres minor muscle
8 Teres major muscle
9 Origin of triceps brachii muscle, lateral head
10 Origin of brachialis muscle
11 Origin of triceps brachii muscle, medial head

**Fig. 3.39 Position and course of the main shoulder muscles** (posterior aspect). Blue = deeper muscles; red = superficial muscles.

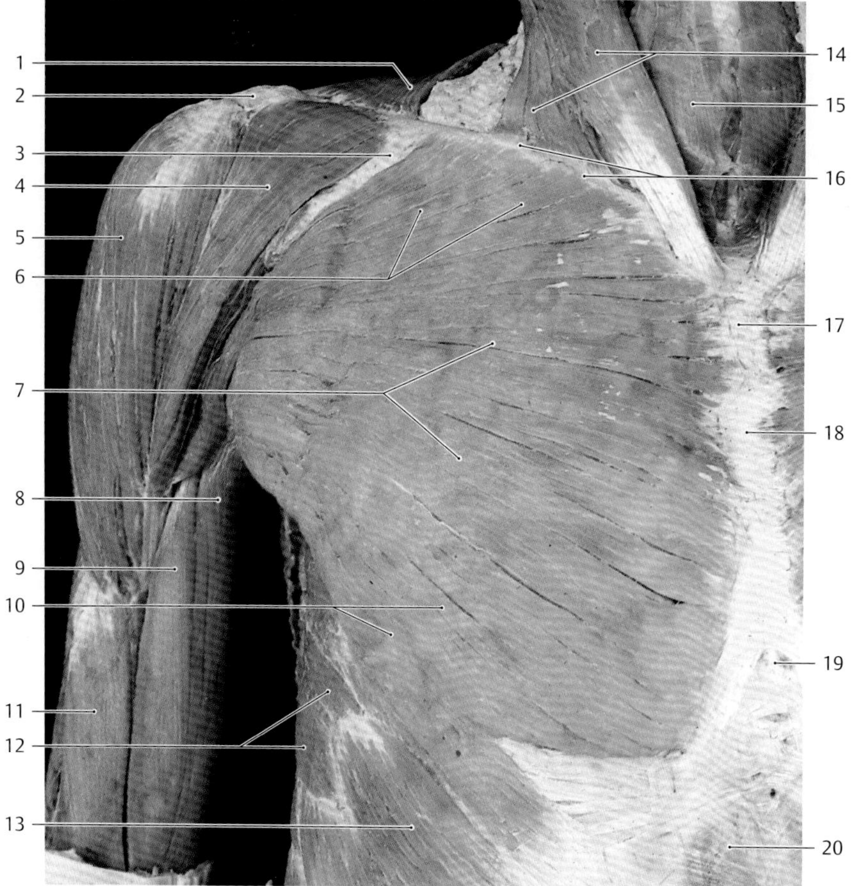


1 Trapezius muscle
2 Acromion
3 Deltopectoral triangle
4 Clavicular part of deltoid muscle (anterior fibers)
5 Acromial part of deltoid muscle (central fibers)
6 Clavicular part of pectoralis major muscle
7 Sternocostal part of pectoralis major muscle
8 Short head of biceps brachii muscle
9 Long head of biceps brachii muscle
10 Abdominal part of pectoralis major muscle
11 Brachialis muscle
12 Serratus anterior muscle
13 External abdominal oblique muscle
14 Sternocleidomastoid muscle
15 Infrahyoid muscles
16 Clavicle
17 Manubrium sterni
18 Body of sternum
19 Xiphoid process
20 Anterior layer of sheath of rectus abdominis muscle

Fig. 3.40 **Shoulder, arm, and pectoral muscles,** superficial layer (right side, anterior aspect).

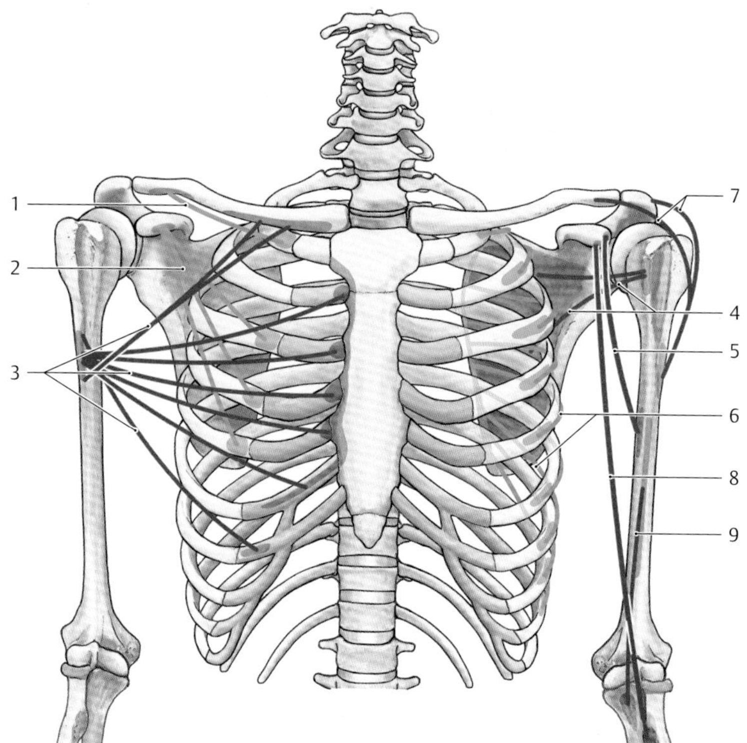


1 Subclavius muscle
2 Pectoralis minor muscle
3 Pectoralis major muscle
4 Subscapularis muscle
5 Coracobrachialis muscle
6 Serratus anterior muscle
7 Clavicular and acromial part of deltoid muscle
8 Short head of biceps brachii muscle
9 Brachialis muscle

Fig. 3.41 **Position and course of pectoral and shoulder muscles** (anterior aspect). Blue = deeper muscles; red = superficial muscles; green = serratus anterior muscle.

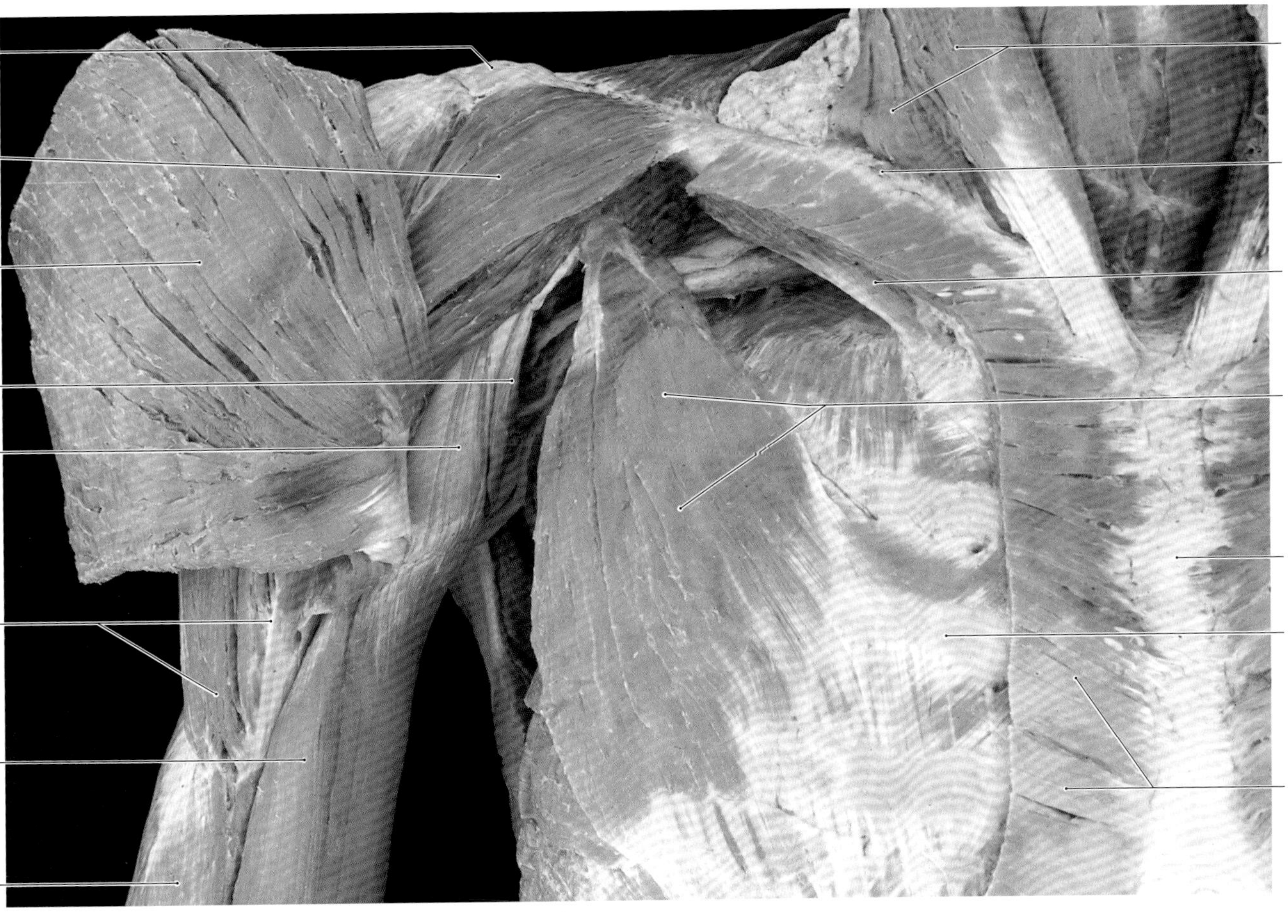

Fig. 3.42 **Shoulder, arm, and pectoral muscles,** deep layer (right side, anterior aspect).

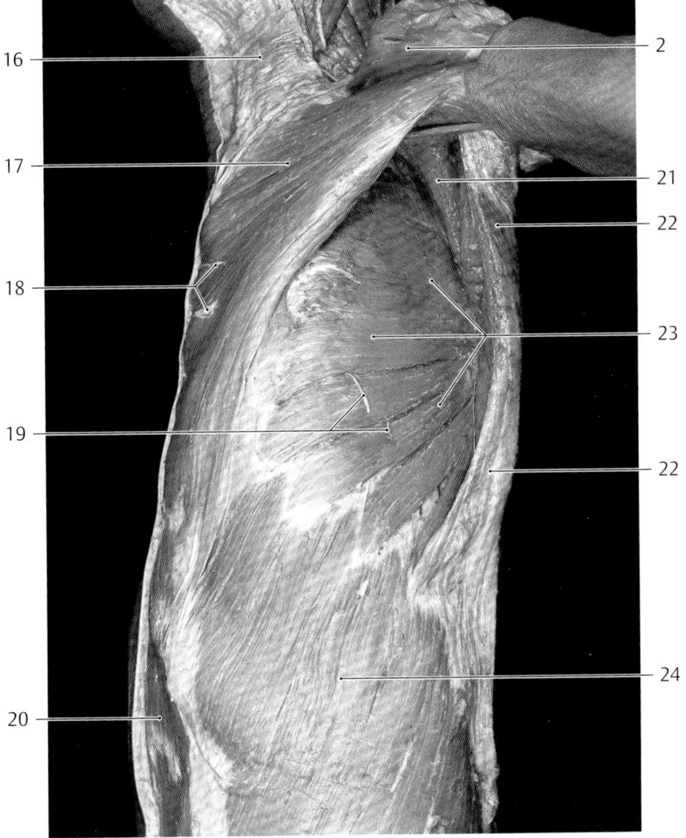


1 Acromion
2 Clavicular part of deltoid muscle
3 Pectoralis major muscle (reflected)
4 Coracobrachialis muscle
5 Short head of biceps brachii muscle
6 Deltoid muscle (insertion on humerus)
7 Long head of biceps brachii muscle
8 Brachialis muscle
9 Sternocleidomastoid muscle
10 Clavicle
11 Subclavius muscle
12 Pectoralis minor muscle
13 Sternum
14 Third rib
15 Pectoralis major muscle (cut)
16 Platysma muscle
17 Pectoralis major muscle forming the anterior axillary fold
18 Anterior cutaneous branches of intercostal nerves
19 Lateral cutaneous branches of intercostal nerves
20 Rectus abdominis muscle
21 Subscapularis muscle
22 Latissimus dorsi muscle forming the posterior axillary fold
23 Serratus anterior muscle forming the medial wall of the axilla
24 External abdominal oblique muscle

Fig. 3.43 **Axillary fossa and serratus anterior muscle** (left side, lateral aspect).

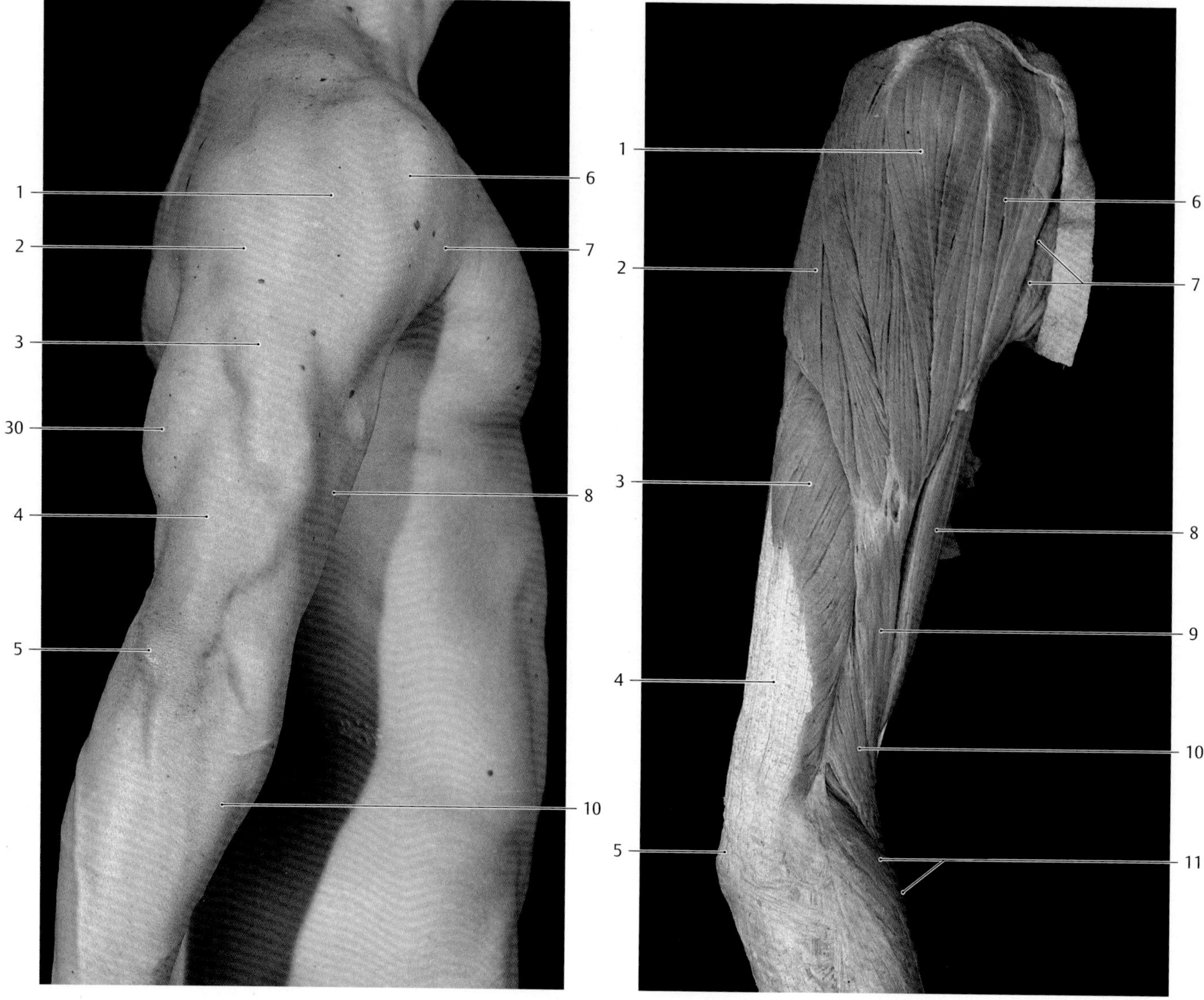


**Fig. 3.44 Muscles of the upper arm** (right side, lateral aspect). Triceps brachii muscle strongly contracted.

**Fig. 3.45 Muscles of the upper arm** (right side, lateral aspect).

1 Acromial part of deltoid muscle (central fibers)
2 Scapular part of deltoid muscle (posterior fibers)
3 Triceps brachii muscle
4 Tendon of triceps brachii muscle
5 Olecranon
6 Clavicular part of deltoid muscle (anterior fibers)
7 Deltopectoral groove
8 Biceps brachii muscle
9 Brachialis muscle
10 Brachioradialis muscle
11 Extensor carpi radialis longus muscle
12 Clavicle (divided)
13 Pectoralis major muscle
14 Medial intermuscular septum with vessels and nerves
15 Lateral intermuscular septum
16 Tendon of biceps brachii muscle
17 Bicipital aponeurosis
18 Axillary artery
19 Rhomboid major muscle
20 Subscapularis muscle
21 Latissimus dorsi muscle (divided)
22 Medial intermuscular septum
23 Medial epicondyle of humerus
24 Brachial artery and median nerve
25 Pronator teres muscle
26 Tendon of short head of biceps brachii muscle
27 Coracobrachialis muscle
28 Distal part of biceps brachii muscle
29 Teres major muscle
30 Long head of triceps brachii muscle
31 Medial head of triceps brachii muscle
32 Radius
33 Head of humerus
34 Coracoid process
35 Humerus
36 Trochlea
37 Ulna
38 Coraco-acromial ligament
39 Articular capsule of shoulder joint
40 Tendon of long head of biceps brachii muscle

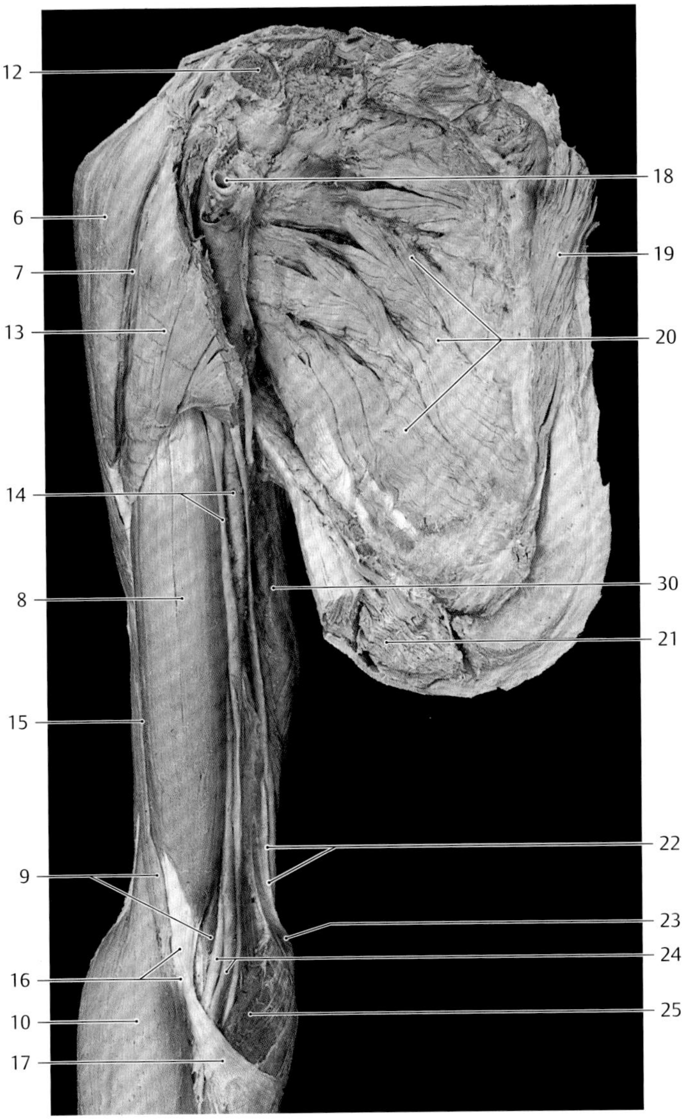

12
6
7
13
14
8
15
9
16
10
17
18
19
20
30
21
22
23
24
25

Fig. 3.46 **Muscles of the arm** (right side, anterior aspect). The arm with the scapula and attached muscles has been removed from the trunk.

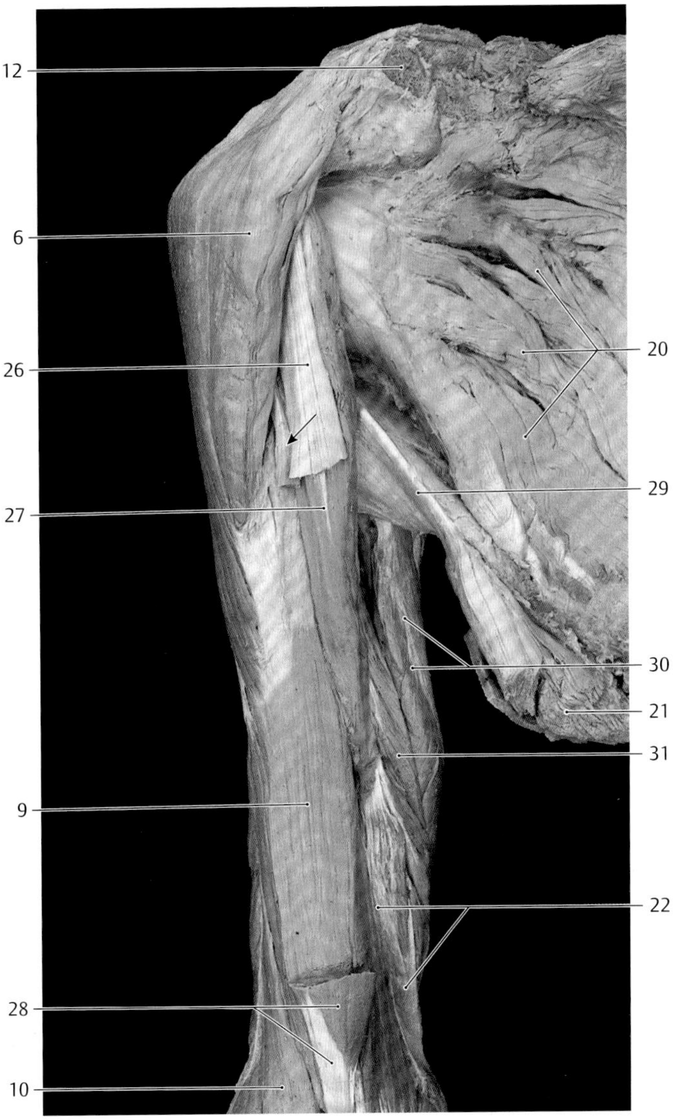

12
6
26
27
9
28
10
20
29
30
21
31
22

Fig. 3.47 **Muscles of the arm** (right side, anterior aspect). Part of the biceps brachii muscle has been removed. Arrow = tendon of long head of biceps brachii muscle.

34
33
35
A
B
C
D
36
32
37

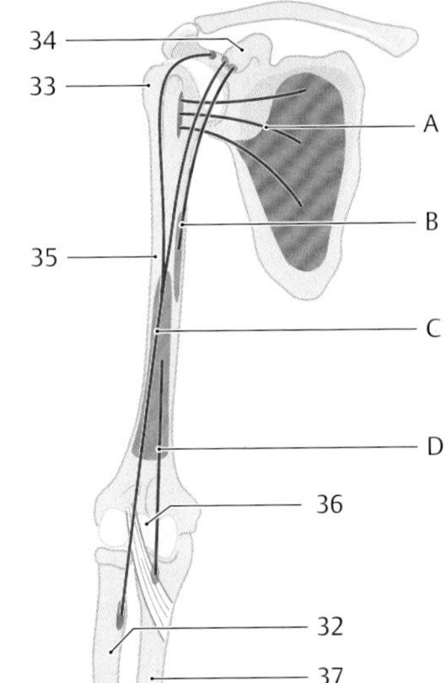

Fig. 3.48 **Position and course of flexors of the arm** (anterior aspect).

A = Subscapularis muscle (red)
B = Coracobrachialis muscle (blue)
C = Biceps brachii muscle (red)
D = Brachialis muscle (blue)

38
39
40
26

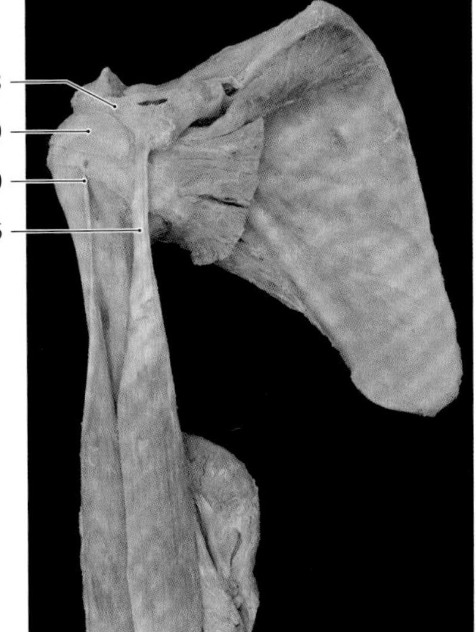

Fig. 3.49 **Position and course of tendons of long and short head of biceps brachii muscle** (right side, anterior aspect).

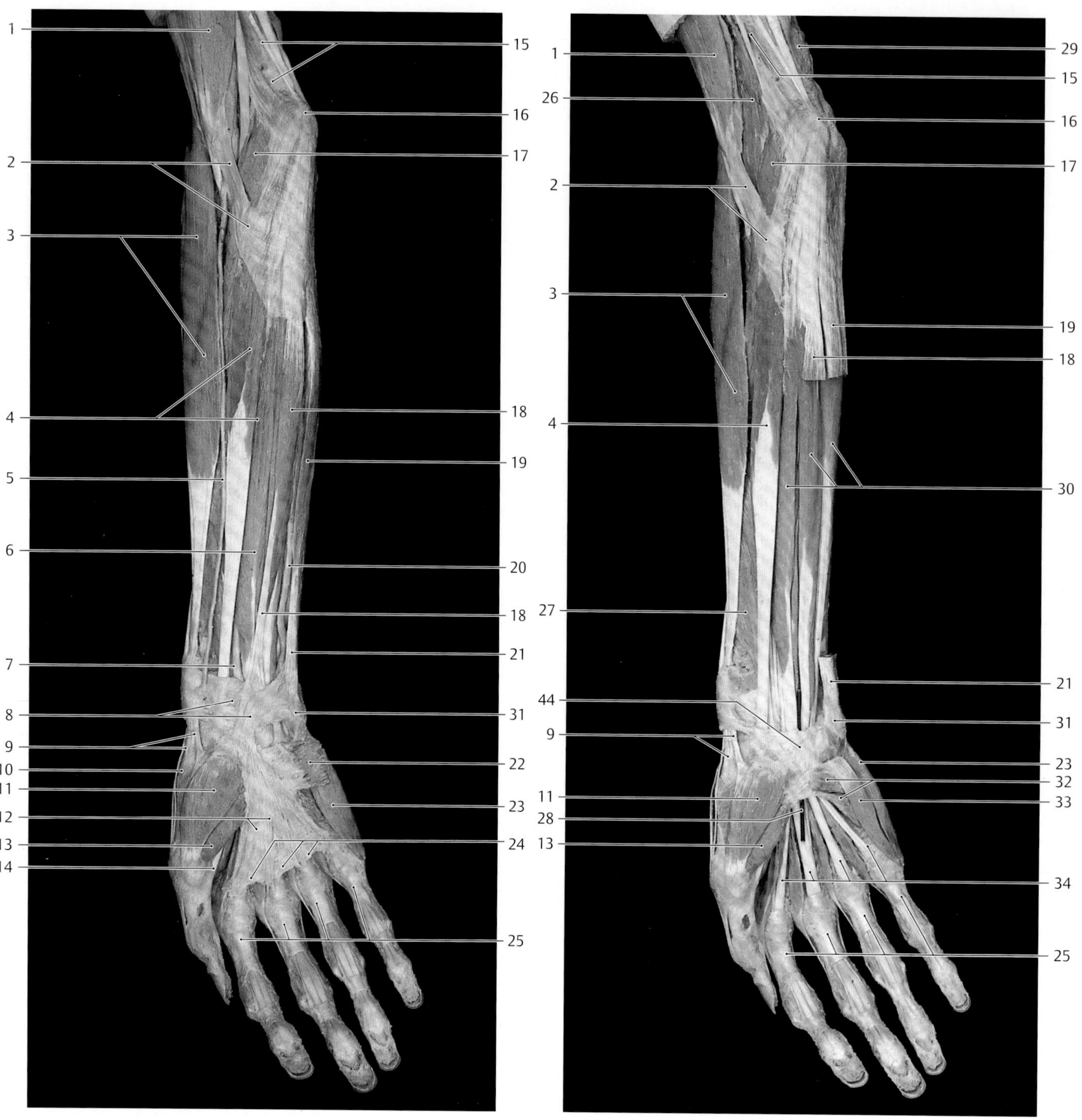


Fig. 3.50 **Flexor muscles of forearm and hand,** superficial layer (right side, anterior aspect).

Fig. 3.51 **Flexor muscles of forearm and hand,** superficial layer (right side, anterior aspect). The palmaris longus and flexor carpi ulnaris muscles have been removed.

1 Biceps brachii muscle
2 Bicipital aponeurosis
3 Brachioradialis muscle
4 Flexor carpi radialis muscle
5 Radial artery
6 Flexor digitorum superficialis muscle
7 Median nerve
8 Antebrachial fascia and tendon of palmaris longus muscle
9 Tendon of abductor pollicis longus muscle
10 Tendon of extensor pollicis brevis muscle
11 Abductor pollicis brevis muscle
12 Palmar aponeurosis
13 Superficial head of flexor pollicis brevis muscle
14 Tendon of flexor pollicis longus muscle
15 Medial intermuscular septum
16 Medial epicondyle of humerus
17 Humeral head of pronator teres muscle
18 Palmaris longus muscle
19 Flexor carpi ulnaris muscle
20 Ulnar artery
21 Tendon of flexor carpi ulnaris muscle
22 Palmaris brevis muscle
23 Abductor digiti minimi muscle
24 Transverse fasciculi of palmar aponeurosis
25 Digital fibrous sheaths of tendons of flexor digitorum muscle
26 Brachialis muscle

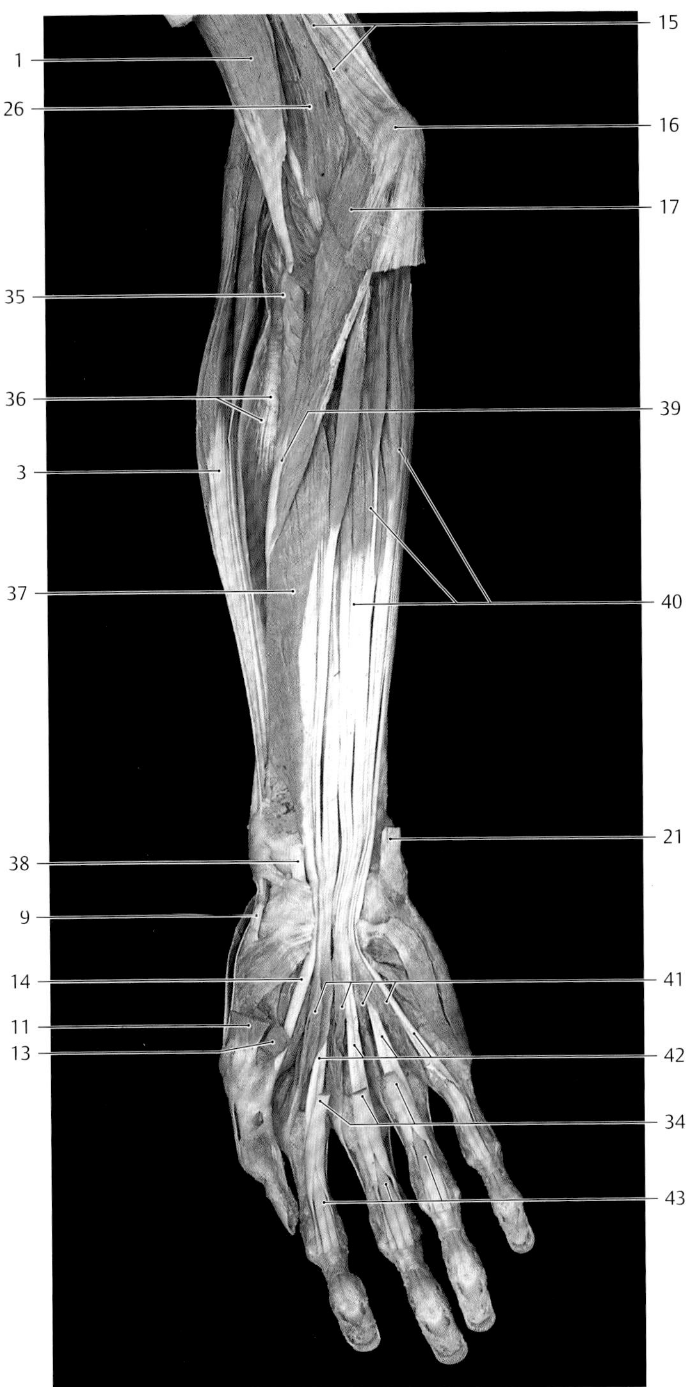


Fig. 3.52 **Flexor muscles of forearm and hand,** middle layer (right side, anterior aspect). The palmaris longus, flexor carpi radialis, and ulnaris muscles have been removed. The flexor retinaculum has been divided.

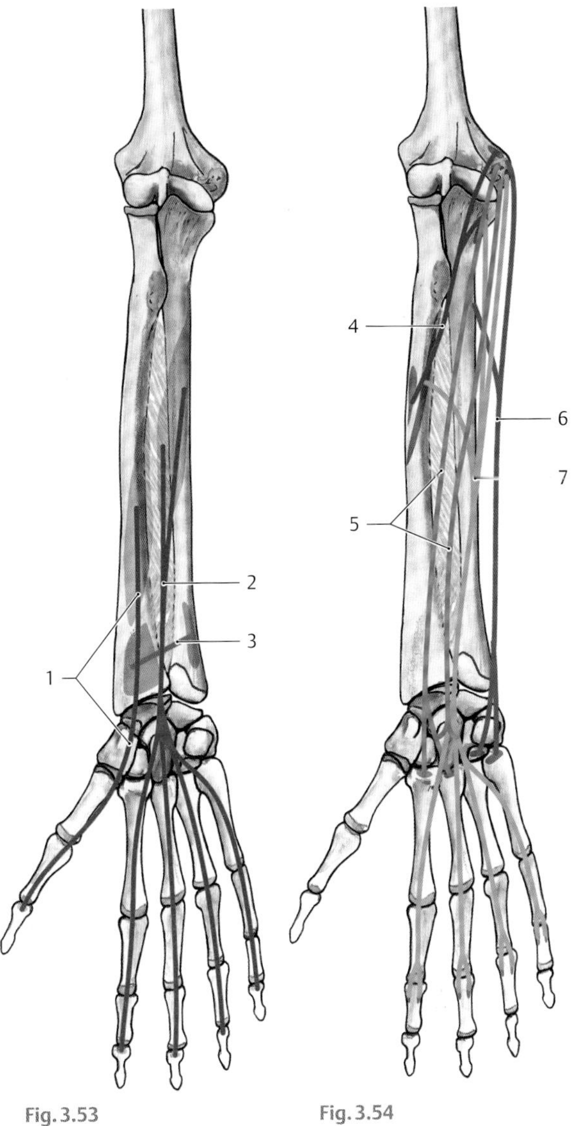


Fig. 3.53 Fig. 3.54

Figs. 3.53 and 3.54 **Position and course of flexors of forearm and hand** (anterior aspect).

**Deep flexors**
1 Flexor pollicis longus muscle (red)
2 Flexor digitorum profundus muscle (red)
3 Pronator quadratus muscle (blue)

**Superficial flexors**
4 Pronator teres muscle (red)
5 Flexor carpi radialis muscle (orange)
6 Flexor carpi ulnaris muscle (deep blue)
7 Flexor digitorum superficialis muscle (light blue)

27 Flexor pollicis longus muscle
28 Carpal tunnel (canalis carpi, probe)
29 Triceps brachii muscle
30 Flexor digitorum superficialis muscle
31 Pisiform bone and palmar carpal ligament
32 Opponens digiti minimi muscle
33 Flexor digiti minimi brevis muscle
34 Tendons of flexor digitorum superficialis muscle
35 Supinator muscle
36 Radius and extensor carpi radialis brevis muscle
37 Flexor pollicis longus muscle
38 Tendon of flexor carpi radialis muscle
39 Pronator teres muscle (insertion of radius)
40 Flexor digitorum profundus muscle
41 Lumbrical muscles
42 Tendons of flexor digitorum profundus muscle
43 Tendons of flexor digitorum profundus muscle having passed through the divided tendons of the flexor digitorum superficialis muscle
44 Flexor retinaculum

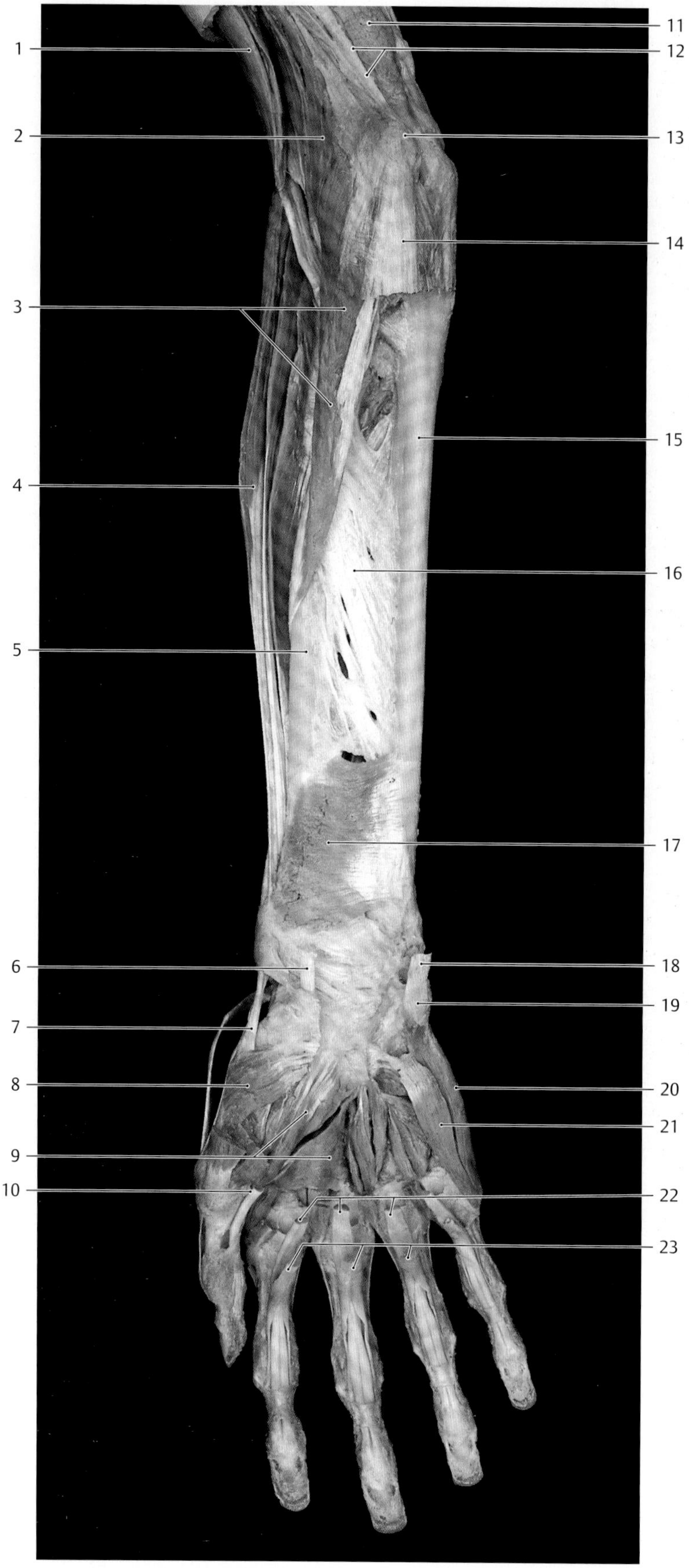

1 Biceps brachii muscle
2 Brachialis muscle
3 Pronator teres muscle
4 Brachioradialis muscle
5 Radius
6 Tendon of flexor carpi radialis muscle
7 Tendon of abductor pollicis longus muscle
8 Opponens pollicis muscle
9 Adductor pollicis muscle
10 Tendon of flexor pollicis longus muscle
11 Triceps brachii muscle
12 Medial intermuscular septum
13 Medial epicondyle of humerus
14 Common flexor mass (divided)
15 Ulna
16 Interosseous membrane
17 Pronator quadratus muscle
18 Tendon of flexor carpi ulnaris muscle
19 Pisiform bone
20 Abductor digiti minimi muscle
21 Flexor digiti minimi brevis muscle
22 Tendons of flexor digitorum profundus muscle
23 Tendons of flexor digitorum superficialis muscle
24 Flexor retinaculum
25 Hypothenar muscles
26 Thenar muscles
27 Common synovial sheath of flexor tendons
28 Synovial sheath of tendon of flexor pollicis longus muscle
29 Digital synovial sheaths of flexor tendons

**Fig. 3.55 Flexor muscles of forearm and hand,** deep layer (right side, anterior aspect). All flexors have been removed to display the pronator quadratus and pronator teres muscles together with the interosseous membrane. Forearm in supination.

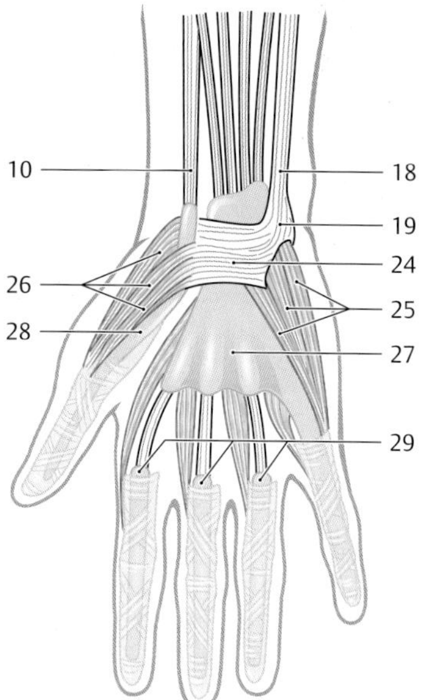


**Fig. 3.56 Synovial sheaths of flexor tendons,** indicated in blue (palmar aspect of right hand).

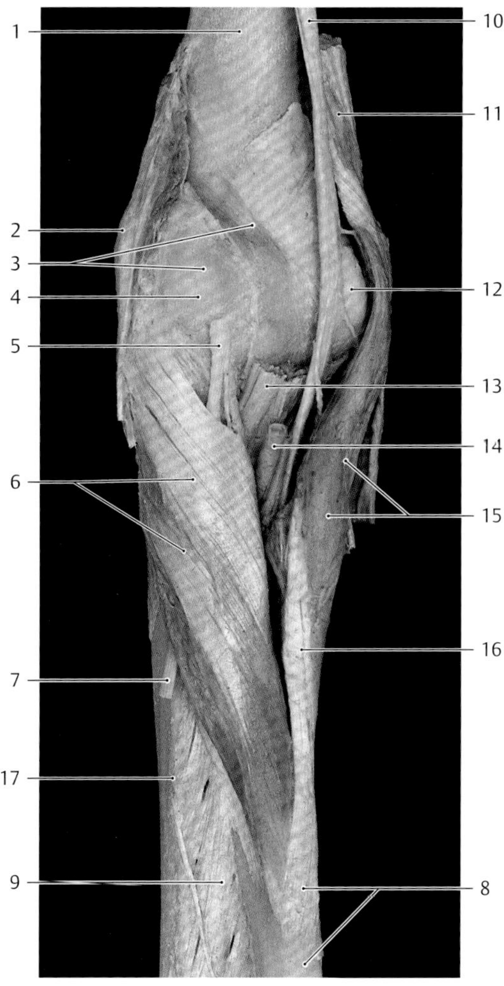


Fig. 3.57 **Right supinator muscle and elbow joint** (anterior aspect). Forearm in pronation.

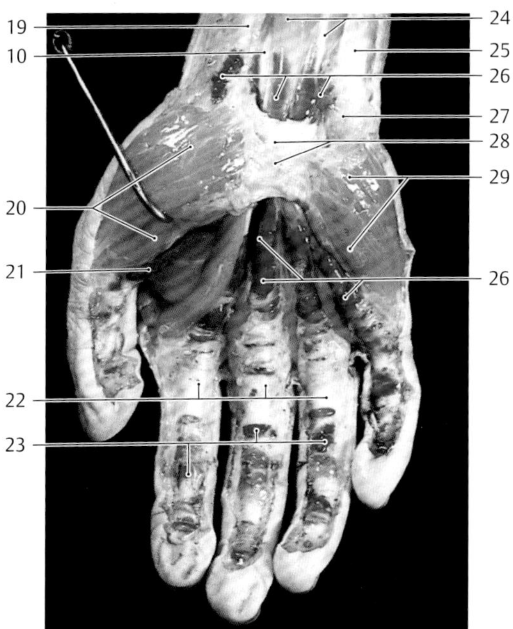


Fig. 3.58 **Synovial sheaths of flexor tendons** (palmar aspect of right hand). The sheaths have been injected with blue gelatin.

1 Humerus
2 Lateral epicondyle of humerus
3 Articular capsule
4 Position of capitulum of humerus
5 Deep branch of radial nerve
6 Supinator muscle
7 Entrance of deep branch of radial nerve to extensor muscles
8 Radius and insertion of pronator teres muscle
9 Interosseous membrane
10 Median nerve
11 Triceps brachii muscle
12 Trochlea of humerus
13 Tendon of biceps brachii muscle
14 Brachial artery
15 Pronator teres muscle
16 Tendon of pronator teres muscle
17 Ulna
18 Pronator quadratus muscle
19 Tendon of flexor carpi radialis muscle
20 Thenar muscles
21 Synovial sheath of tendon of flexor pollicis longus muscle
22 Fibrous sheath of flexor tendons
23 Digital synovial sheath of flexor tendons
24 Flexor digitorum superficialis muscle
25 Tendon of flexor carpi ulnaris muscle
26 Common synovial sheath of flexor tendons
27 Position of pisiform bone
28 Flexor retinaculum
29 Hypothenar muscles

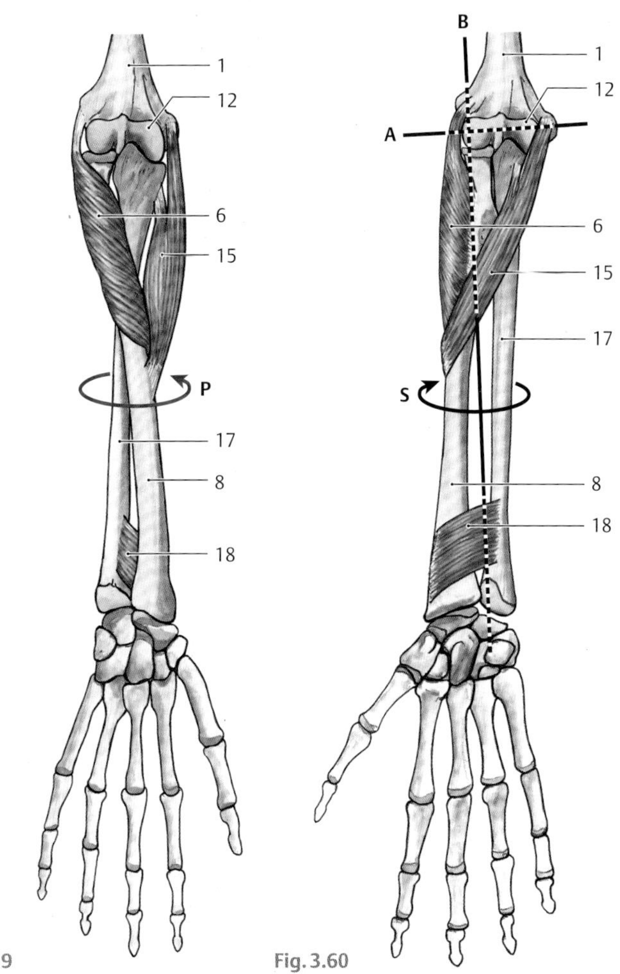


Fig. 3.59

Fig. 3.60

A = Axis of flexion and extension
B = Axis of rotation

Arrows: S = Supination, P = Pronation

Figs. 3.59 and 3.60 **Diagram illustrating the two axes of the elbow joint.**

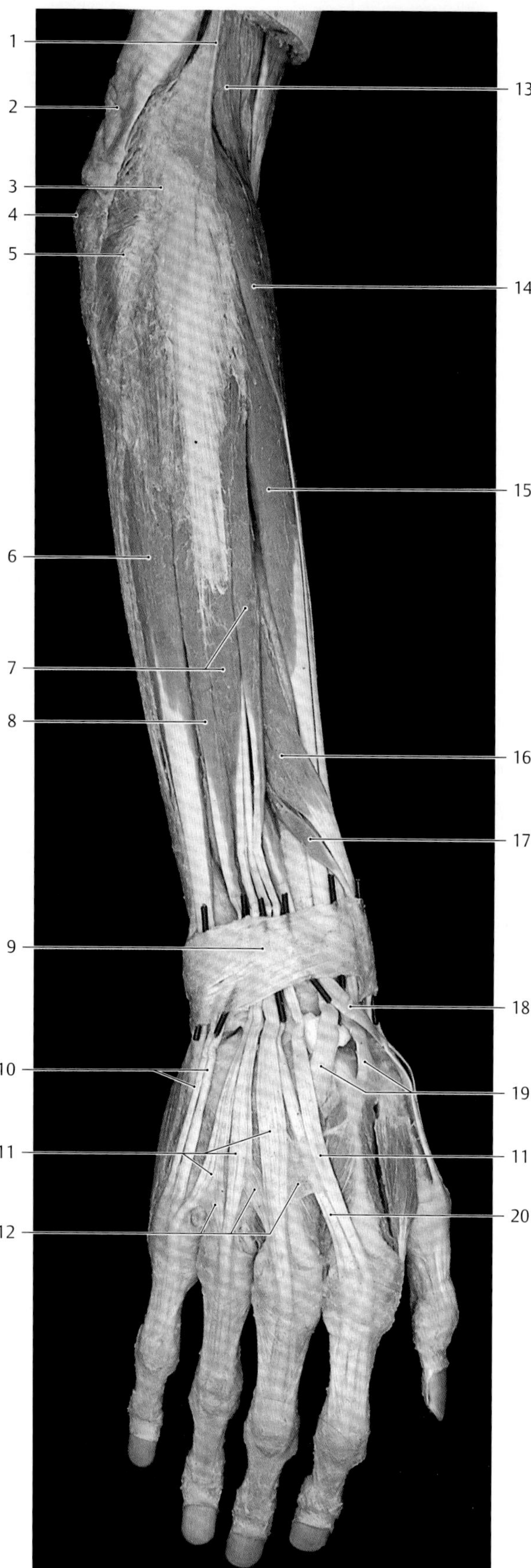


Fig. 3.61 **Extensor muscles of forearm and hand,** superficial layer (right side, posterior aspect). Tunnels for extensor tendons indicated by probes.

1 Lateral intermuscular septum
2 Tendon of triceps brachii muscle
3 Lateral epicondyle of humerus
4 Olecranon
5 Anconeus muscle
6 Extensor carpi ulnaris muscle
7 Extensor digitorum muscle
8 Extensor digiti minimi muscle
9 Extensor retinaculum
10 Tendons of extensor digiti minimi muscle
11 Tendons of extensor digitorum muscle
12 Intertendinous connections
13 Brachioradialis muscle
14 Extensor carpi radialis longus muscle
15 Extensor carpi radialis brevis muscle
16 Abductor pollicis longus muscle
17 Extensor pollicis brevis muscle
18 Tendon of extensor pollicis longus muscle
19 Tendons of both extensor carpi radialis longus and extensor carpi radialis brevis muscles
20 Tendon of extensor indicis muscle
21 First tunnel:
Abductor pollicis longus muscle, extensor pollicis brevis muscle
22 Second tunnel:
Extensor carpi radialis longus and brevis muscles
23 Third tunnel:
Extensor pollicis longus muscle
24 Fourth tunnel:
Extensor digitorum muscle, extensor indicis muscle
25 Fifth tunnel:
Extensor digiti minimi muscle
26 Sixth tunnel:
Extensor carpi ulnaris muscle

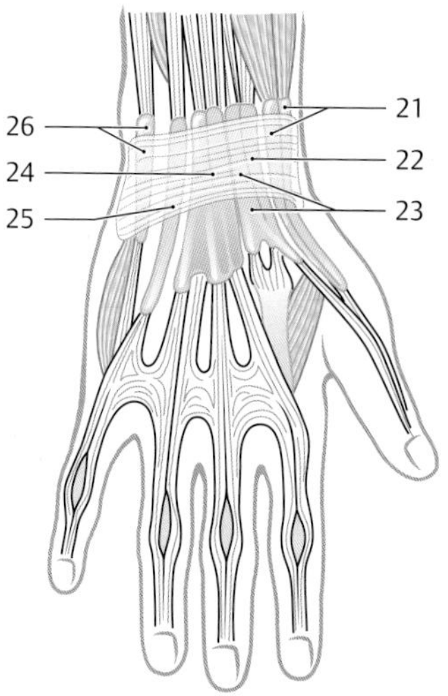


Fig. 3.62 **Synovial sheaths of extensor tendons,** indicated in blue (dorsal aspect of right hand). Notice the six tunnels for the passage of the extensor tendons beneath the extensor retinaculum.

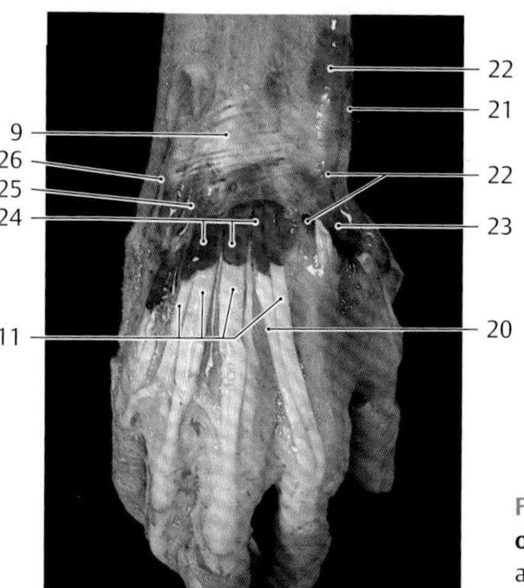


Fig. 3.63 **Synovial sheaths of extensor tendons** (dorsal aspect of right hand). The sheaths have been injected with blue gelatin.

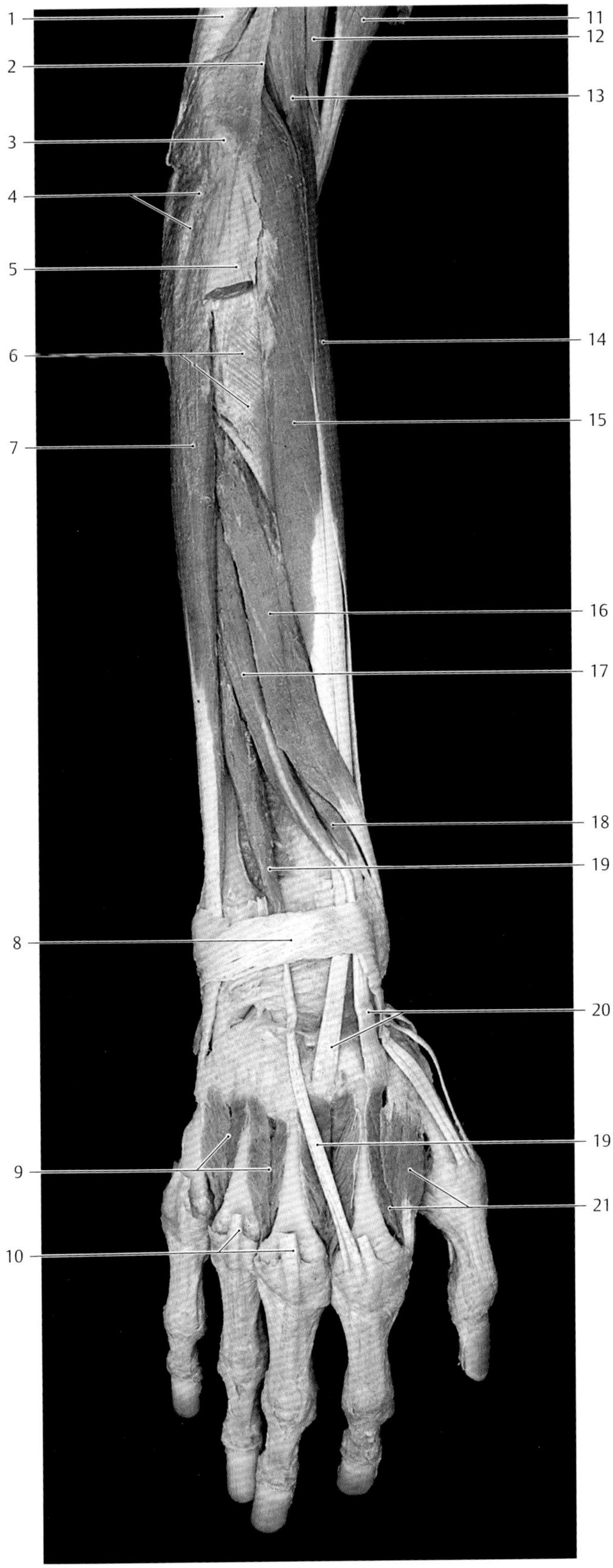

1 Triceps brachii muscle
2 Lateral intermuscular septum
3 Lateral epicondyle of humerus
4 Anconeus muscle
5 Extensor digitorum and extensor digiti minimi muscles (cut)
6 Supinator muscle
7 Extensor carpi ulnaris muscle
8 Extensor retinaculum
9 Third and fourth dorsal interossei muscles
10 Tendons of extensor digitorum muscle (cut)
11 Biceps brachii muscle
12 Brachialis muscle
13 Brachioradialis muscle
14 Extensor carpi radialis longus muscle
15 Extensor carpi radialis brevis muscle
16 Abductor pollicis longus muscle
17 Extensor pollicis longus muscle
18 Extensor pollicis brevis muscle
19 Extensor indicis muscle
20 Tendons of extensor carpi radialis longus and extensor carpi radialis brevis muscles
21 First dorsal interosseous muscle

Fig. 3.64 **Extensor muscles of forearm and hand,** deep layer (right side, posterior aspect).

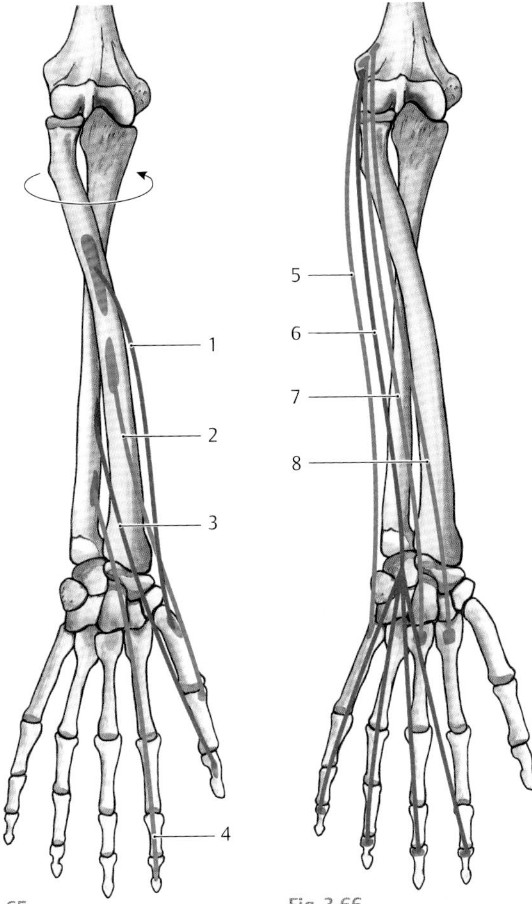


Figs. 3.65 and 3.66 **Position and course of extensors of forearm and hand** (posterior aspect).

**Extensors of thumb**
1 Abductor pollicis longus muscle (red)
2 Extensor pollicis brevis muscle (blue)
3 Extensor pollicis longus muscle (red)
4 Extensor indicis muscle (blue)

**Extensors of fingers and hand**
5 Extensor carpi ulnaris muscle (blue)
6 Extensor digitorum muscle (red)
7 Extensor carpi radialis brevis muscle (blue)
8 Extensor carpi radialis longus muscle (blue)

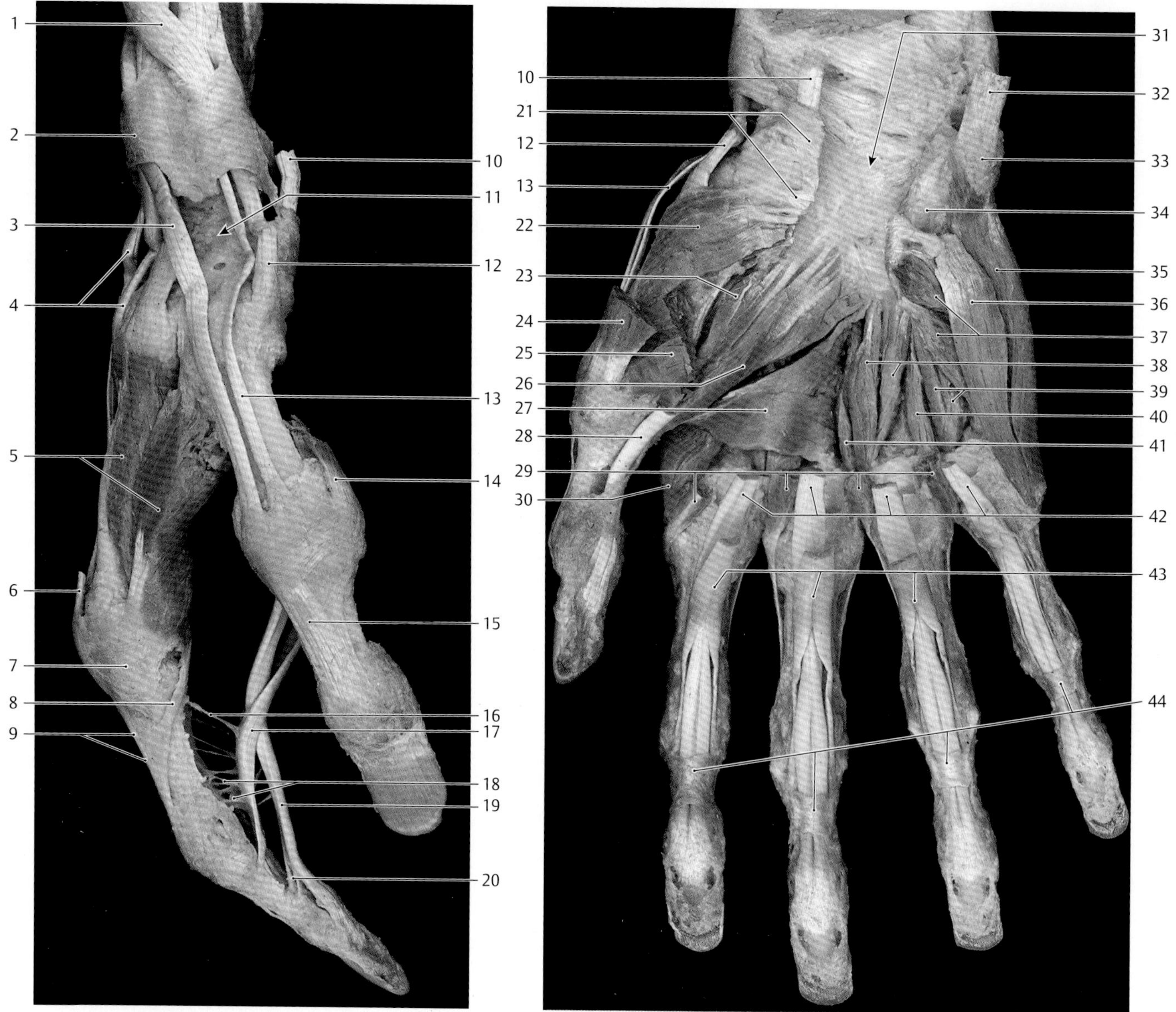


**Fig. 3.67 Muscles of thumb and index finger** (medial aspect). The tendons of the extensor muscles of the thumb and the insertion of the flexor tendons of the index finger are displayed.

**Fig. 3.68 Muscles of the hand** (right side, palmar aspect). The tendons of the flexor muscles and parts of the thumb muscles have been removed. The carpal tunnel has been opened.

1 Tendons of extensor pollicis brevis and abductor pollicis longus muscles
2 Extensor retinaculum
3 Tendon of extensor pollicis longus muscle
4 Tendons of extensor carpi radialis longus and brevis muscles
5 First dorsal interosseous muscle
6 Tendon of extensor digitorum muscle for index finger
7 Location of metacarpophalangeal joint
8 Tendon of lumbrical muscle
9 Extensor expansion of index finger
10 Tendon of flexor carpi radialis muscle (cut)
11 Anatomical snuffbox
12 Tendon of abductor pollicis longus muscle
13 Tendon of extensor pollicis brevis muscle
14 Tendon of abductor pollicis brevis muscle
15 Extensor expansion of extensor of thumb
16 Vinculum longum
17 Tendons of flexor digitorum superficialis muscle dividing to allow passage of deep tendons
18 Vincula of flexor tendons
19 Tendon of flexor digitorum profundus muscle
20 Vinculum breve
21 Radial carpal eminence (cut edge of flexor retinaculum)
22 Opponens pollicis muscle
23 Deep head of flexor pollicis brevis muscle
24 Abductor pollicis brevis muscle (cut)
25 Superficial head of flexor pollicis brevis muscle (cut)
26 Oblique head of adductor pollicis muscle
27 Transverse head of adductor pollicis muscle
28 Tendon of flexor pollicis longus muscle (cut)
29 Lumbrical muscles (cut)
30 First dorsal interosseous muscle
31 Position of carpal tunnel
32 Tendon of flexor carpi ulnaris muscle
33 Location of pisiform bone
34 Hook of hamate bone
35 Abductor digiti minimi muscle
36 Flexor digiti minimi brevis muscle
37 Opponens digiti minimi muscle
38 Second palmar interosseous muscle
39 Third palmar interosseous muscle
40 Fourth dorsal interosseous muscle
41 Third dorsal interosseous muscle
42 Tendon of flexor digitorum profundus muscle (cut)
43 Tendons of flexor digitorum superficialis muscle (cut)
44 Fibrous flexor sheaths

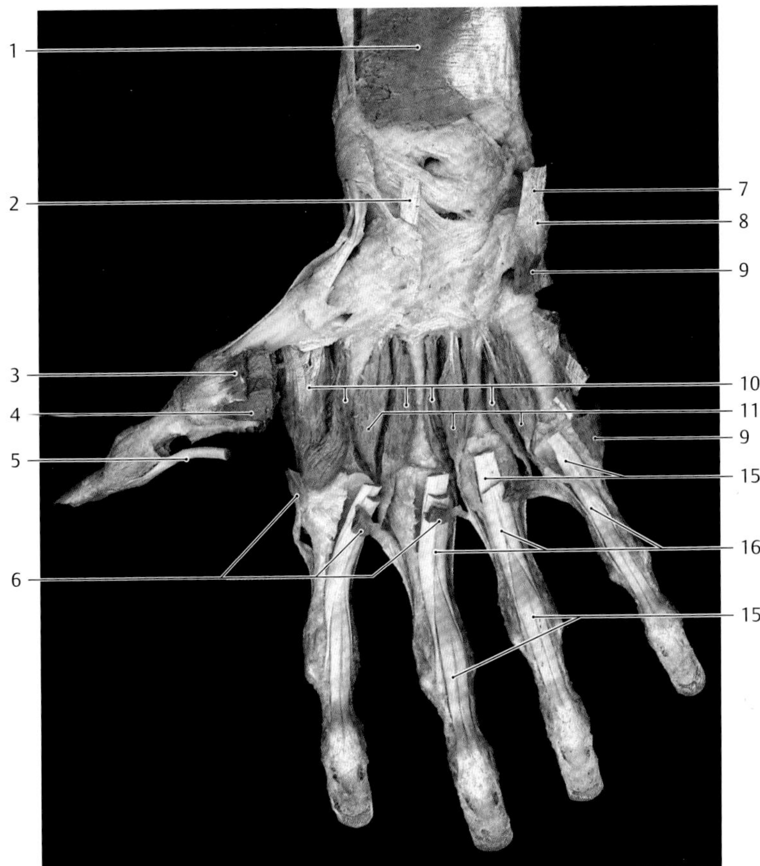


Fig. 3.69 **Muscles of the hand,** deep layer (right side, palmar aspect). The thenar and hypothenar muscles have been removed to display the interossei muscles.

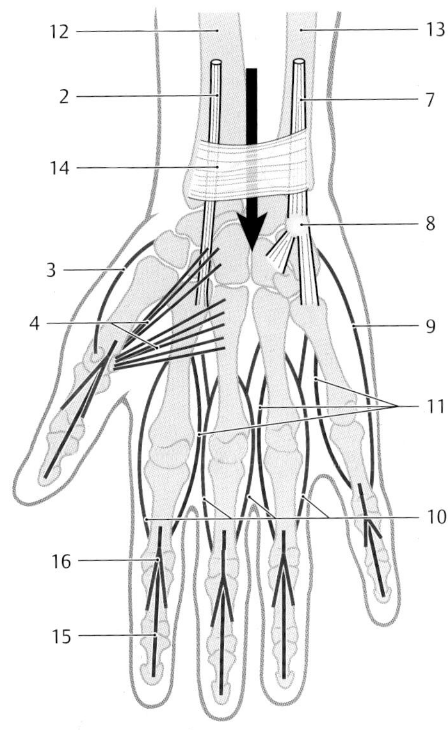


Fig. 3.70 **Actions of interossei muscles** in abduction and adduction of fingers (palmar aspect of right hand).
Arrow = carpal tunnel.
Red = abduction (dorsal interossei, abductor digiti minimi, and abductor pollicis brevis muscles)
Blue = adduction (palmar interossei muscles, adductor pollicis muscle)

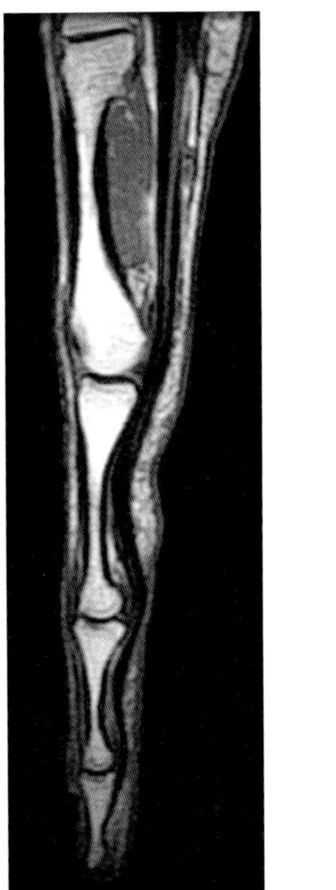

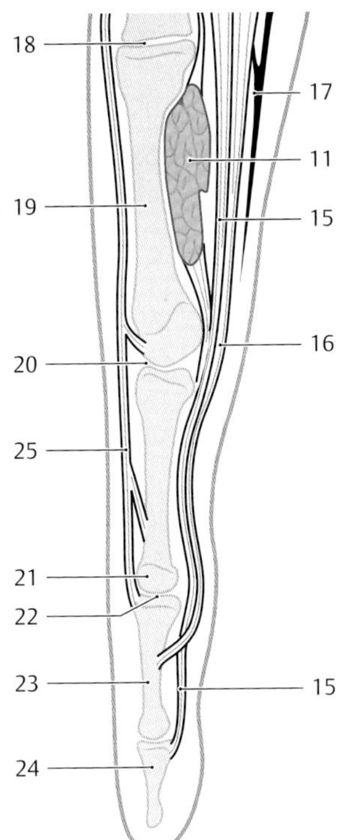


Figs. 3.71 and 3.72 **Longitudinal section through the third finger** (MRI scan and schematic respectively). (Heuck A, et al. MRT-Atlas des muskuloskelettalen Systems. Stuttgart, Germany: Schattauer, 2009.)

1 Pronator quadratus muscle
2 Tendon of flexor carpi radialis muscle
3 Abductor pollicis brevis muscle (divided)
4 Adductor pollicis muscle (divided)
5 Tendon of flexor pollicis longus muscle
6 Lumbrical muscles (cut)
7 Tendon of flexor carpi ulnaris muscle
8 Pisiform bone
9 Abductor digiti minimi muscle (divided)
10 Dorsal interossei muscles
11 Palmar interossei muscles
12 Radius
13 Ulna
14 Flexor retinaculum
15 Tendons of flexor digitorum profundus muscle
16 Tendons of flexor digitorum superficialis muscle
17 Palmar aponeurosis
18 Carpometacarpal joint
19 Third metacarpal bone
20 Metacarpophalangeal joint
21 Head of third proximal phalanx
22 Proximal interphalangeal joint
23 Middle phalanx
24 Distal phalanx
25 Aponeurosis of extensors

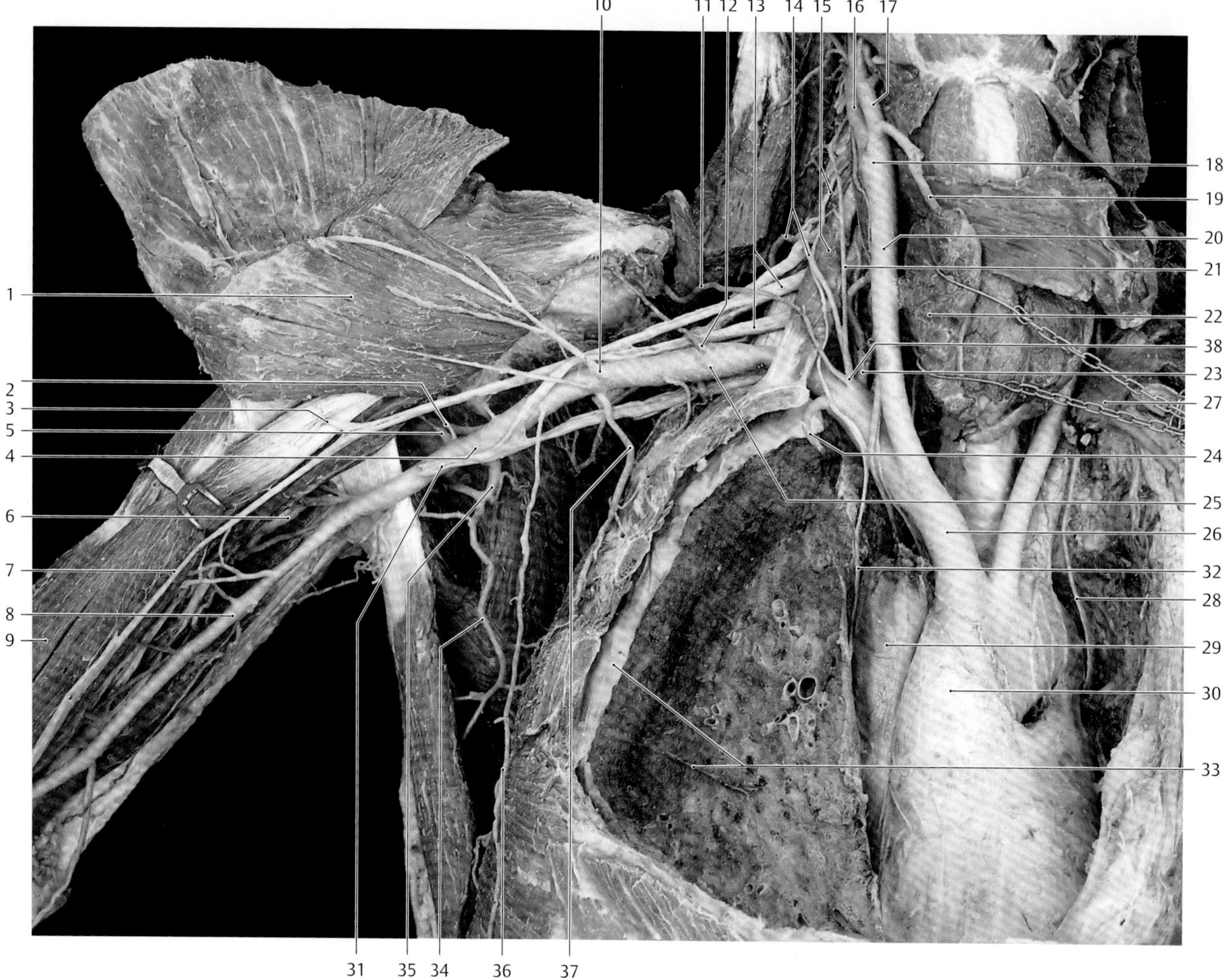


Fig. 3.73 **Main branches of subclavian and axillary arteries** (right side, anterior aspect). Pectoralis muscles have been reflected, the clavicle and anterior wall of the thorax removed, and the right lung divided. Left lung with pleura and thyroid gland have been reflected laterally to display the aortic arch and common carotid artery with their branches.

1 Pectoralis minor muscle (reflected)
2 Anterior circumflex humeral artery
3 Musculocutaneous nerve (divided)
4 Axillary artery
5 Posterior circumflex humeral artery
6 Profunda brachii artery
7 Median nerve (var.)
8 Brachial artery
9 Biceps brachii muscle
10 Thoraco-acromial artery
11 Suprascapular artery
12 Descending scapular artery
13 Brachial plexus (middle trunk)
14 Transverse cervical artery
15 Anterior scalene muscle and phrenic nerve
16 Right internal carotid artery
17 Right external carotid artery
18 Carotid sinus
19 Superior thyroid artery
20 Right common carotid artery
21 Ascending cervical artery
22 Thyroid gland
23 Inferior thyroid artery
24 Internal thoracic artery
25 Right subclavian artery
26 Brachiocephalic trunk
27 Left brachiocephalic vein (divided)
28 Left vagus nerve
29 Superior vena cava (divided)
30 Ascending aorta
31 Median nerve (divided)
32 Phrenic nerve
33 Right lung (divided) and pulmonary pleura
34 Thoracodorsal artery
35 Subscapular artery
36 Lateral mammary branches (var.)
37 Lateral thoracic artery
38 Thyrocervical trunk
39 Supreme intercostal artery
40 Superior ulnar collateral artery
41 Inferior ulnar collateral artery
42 Middle collateral artery
43 Radial collateral artery
44 Radial recurrent artery
45 Radial artery
46 Anterior and posterior interosseous arteries
47 Princeps pollicis artery
48 Deep palmar arch
49 Common palmar digital arteries
50 Ulnar recurrent artery
51 Recurrent interosseous artery
52 Common interosseous artery
53 Ulnar artery
54 Superficial palmar arch
55 Median nerve and brachial artery
56 Biceps brachii muscle
57 Ulnar nerve
58 Flexor pollicis longus muscle
59 Proper palmar digital arteries
60 Anterior interosseous artery
61 Flexor carpi ulnaris muscle
62 Superficial palmar branch of radial artery

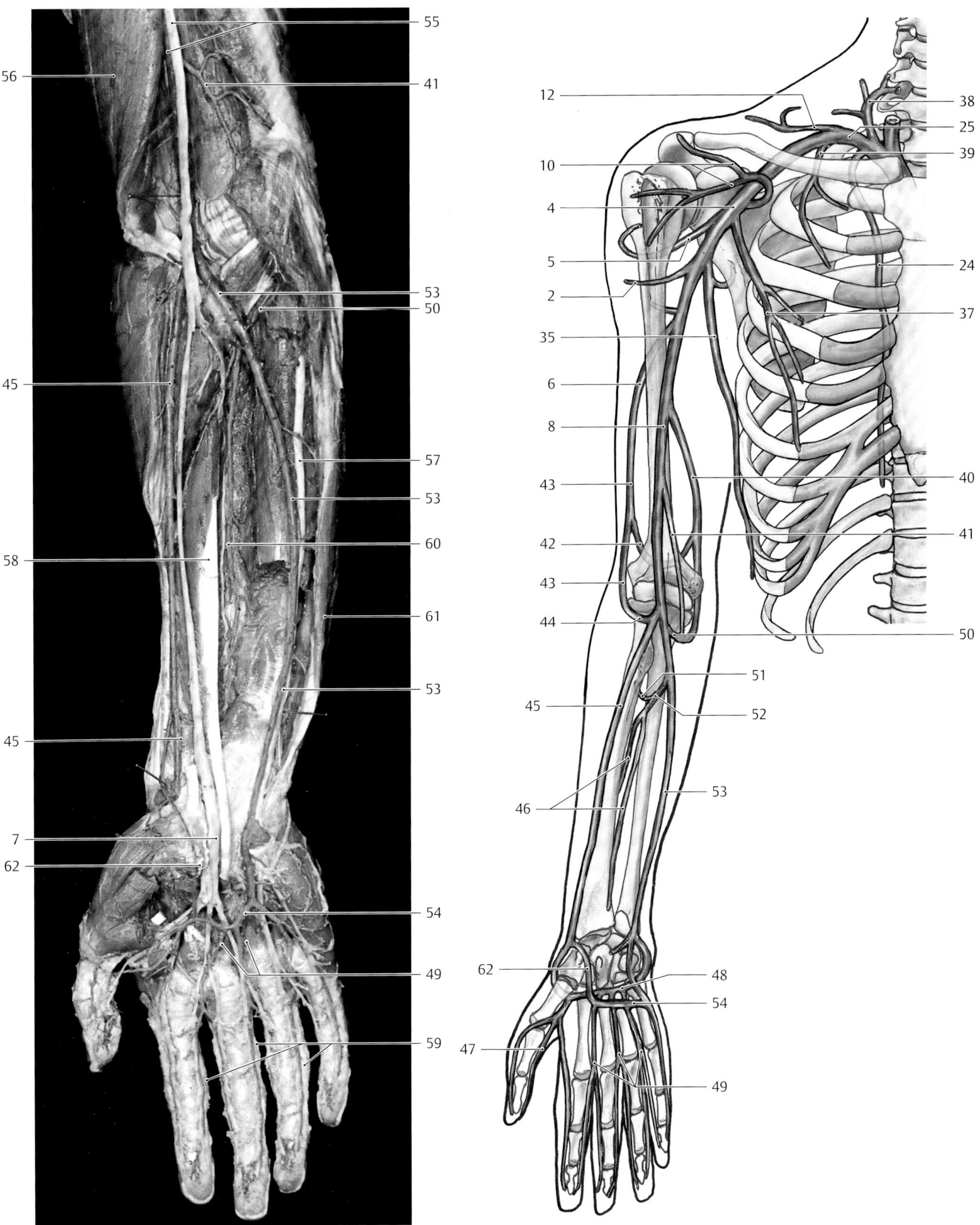


Fig. 3.74 **Main arteries of forearm and hand** (right side, anterior aspect). The superficial flexor muscles have been removed, the carpal tunnel opened, and the flexor retinaculum cut. The arteries have been filled with colored resin.

Fig. 3.75 **Main arteries of the upper limb** (right side). Branches of the right subclavian artery, the axillary artery, and the brachial artery are shown.

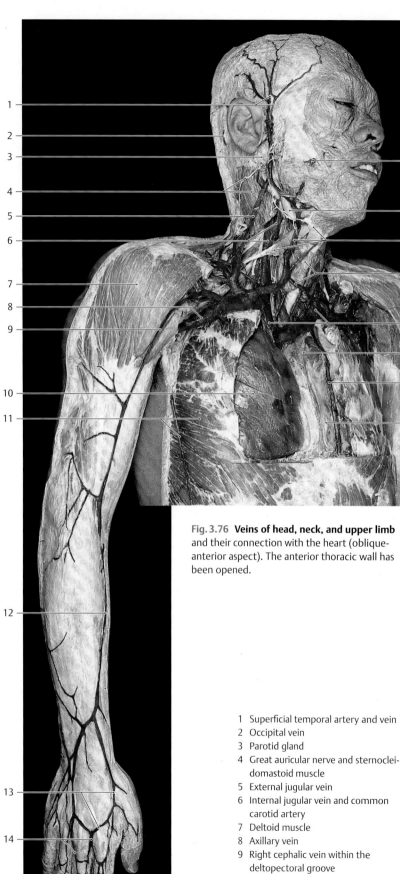

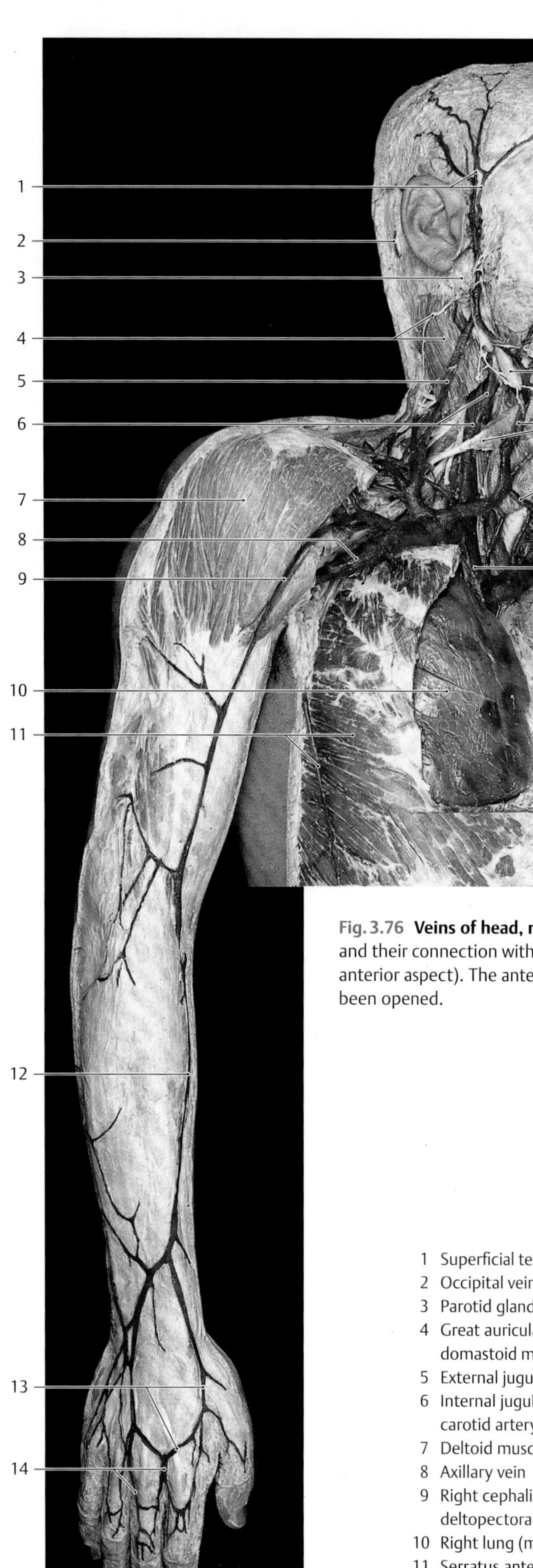


**Fig. 3.76 Veins of head, neck, and upper limb** and their connection with the heart (oblique-anterior aspect). The anterior thoracic wall has been opened.

**Fig. 3.77 Main truncal veins of the upper limb** (right side).

1 Superficial temporal artery and vein
2 Occipital vein
3 Parotid gland
4 Great auricular nerve and sternocleidomastoid muscle
5 External jugular vein
6 Internal jugular vein and common carotid artery
7 Deltoid muscle
8 Axillary vein
9 Right cephalic vein within the deltopectoral groove
10 Right lung (middle lobe)
11 Serratus anterior muscle and lateral thoracic vein
12 Cephalic vein on forearm
13 Venous network on dorsum of hand
14 Dorsal metacarpal veins
15 Facial artery and vein
16 Submandibular gland
17 Anterior jugular vein, hyoid bone, and omohyoid muscle
18 Jugular venous arch and thyroid gland
19 Right and left brachiocephalic veins
20 Retrosternal body (remnant of thymus gland)
21 Internal thoracic artery and vein
22 Heart with pericardium
23 Right venous angle
24 Brachial vein
25 Basilic vein
26 Median cubital vein
27 Digital veins

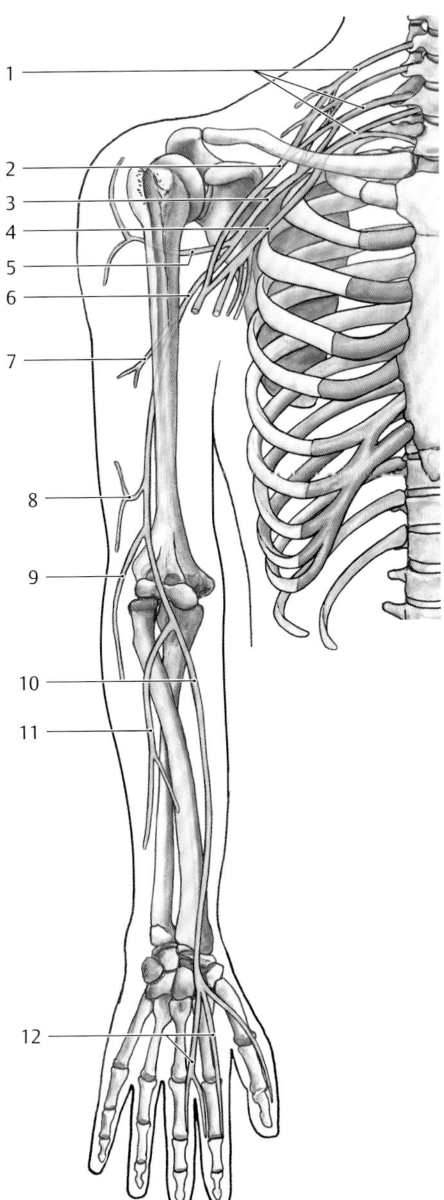


**Fig. 3.78 Main branches of radial and axillary nerves** (right side).

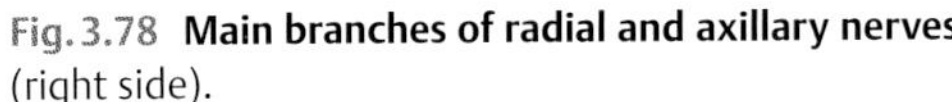

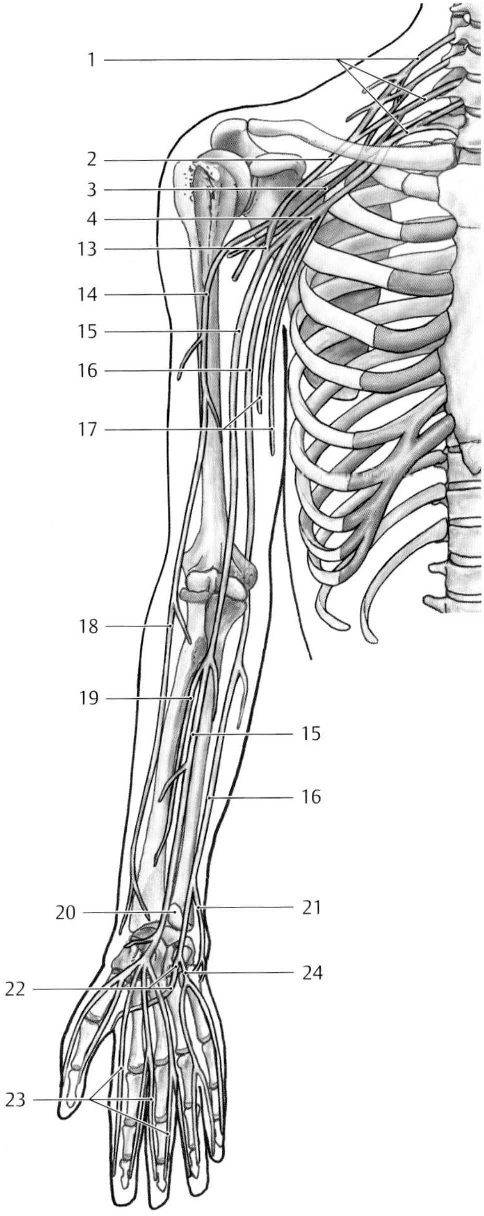


**Fig. 3.79 Main branches of musculocutaneous, median, and ulnar nerves** (right side). The posterior trunk of brachial plexus is indicated in orange.

1 Brachial plexus
2 Lateral cord of brachial plexus
3 Posterior cord of brachial plexus
4 Medial cord of brachial plexus
5 Axillary nerve
6 Radial nerve
7 Posterior cutaneous nerve of arm
8 Lower lateral cutaneous nerve of arm
9 Posterior cutaneous nerve of forearm
10 Superficial branch of radial nerve
11 Deep branch of radial nerve
12 Dorsal digital nerves
13 Roots of median nerve
14 Musculocutaneous nerve
15 Median nerve
16 Ulnar nerve
17 Medial cutaneous nerves of arm and forearm
18 Lateral cutaneous nerve of forearm
19 Anterior interosseous nerve
20 Palmar branch of median nerve
21 Dorsal branch of ulnar nerve
22 Deep branch of ulnar nerve
23 Common palmar digital nerves of median nerve
24 Superficial branch of ulnar nerve

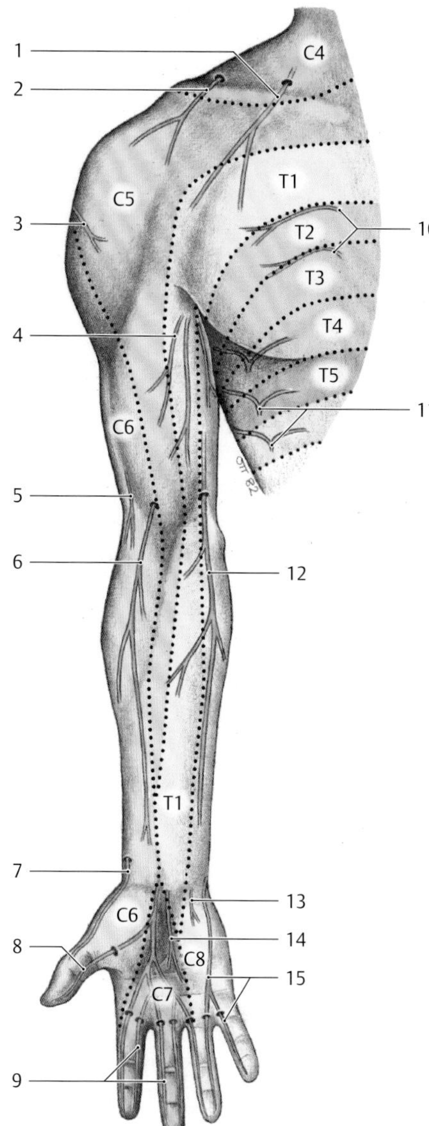


**Fig. 3.80 Cutaneous nerves of the upper limb** (right side, anterior aspect).

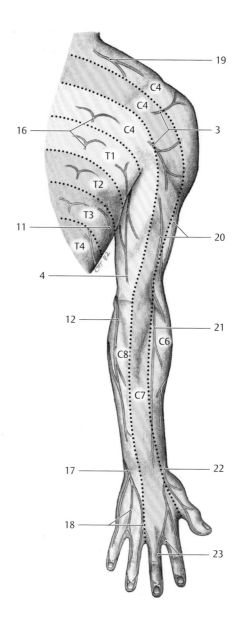

**Fig. 3.81 Cutaneous nerves of the upper limb** (right side, posterior aspect).

1 Medial supraclavicular nerve
2 Intermediate supraclavicular nerve
3 Upper lateral cutaneous nerve of arm
4 Terminal branches of intercostobrachial nerves
5 Lower lateral cutaneous nerve of arm
6 Lateral cutaneous nerve of forearm
7 Terminal branch of superficial branch of radial nerve
8 Palmar digital nerve of thumb (branch of median nerve)
9 Palmar digital branches of median nerve
10 Anterior cutaneous branches of intercostal nerves
11 Lateral cutaneous branches of intercostal nerves
12 Medial cutaneous nerve of forearm
13 Palmar cutaneous branch of ulnar nerve
14 Palmar branch of median nerve
15 Palmar digital branches of ulnar nerve
16 Cutaneous branches of dorsal rami of spinal nerves
17 Dorsal branch of ulnar nerve
18 Dorsal digital nerves
19 Posterior supraclavicular nerve
20 Posterior cutaneous nerve of arm (from radial nerve)
21 Posterior cutaneous nerve of forearm (from radial nerve)
22 Superficial branch (from radial nerve)
23 Dorsal digital branches (from radial nerve)

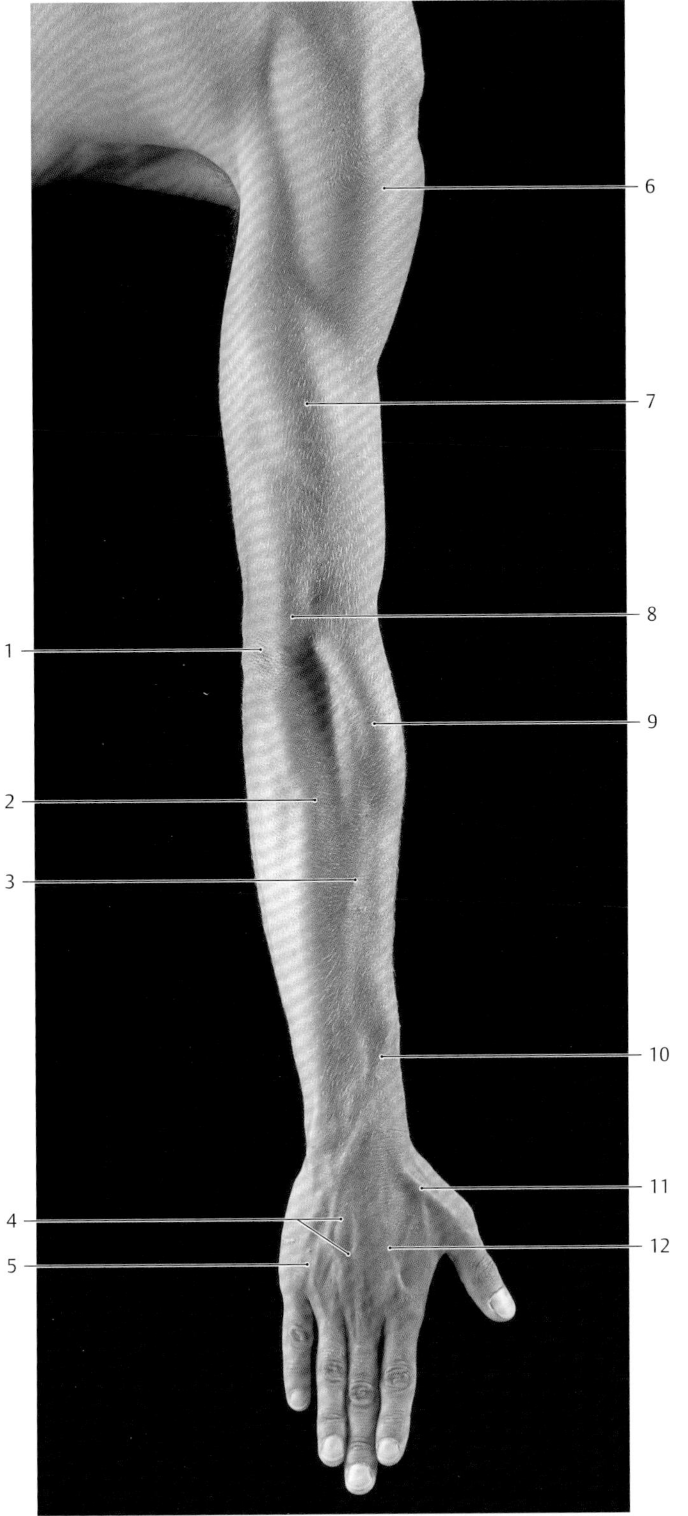


Fig. 3.82 **Surface anatomy of the upper limb** (right side, posterior aspect).

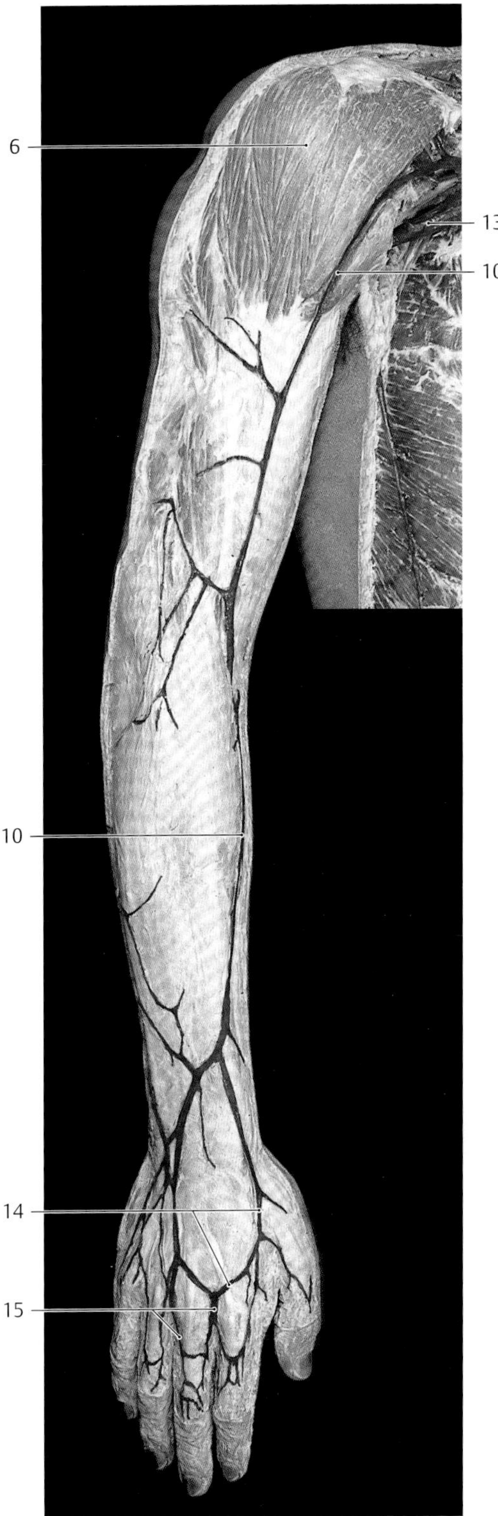


Fig. 3.83 **Superficial veins of the arm** (right side, posterior aspect). The veins have been injected with blue gelatin.

1 Olecranon
2 Extensor muscles of forearm
3 Accessory cephalic vein
4 Tendons of extensor digitorum muscle
5 Dorsal venous network of hand (ulnar)
6 Deltoid muscle
7 Triceps brachii muscle
8 Lateral epicondyle of humerus
9 Brachioradialis muscle
10 Cephalic vein
11 Tendon of abductor pollicis longus muscle
12 Tendon of extensor indicis muscle
13 Axillary vein
14 Dorsal venous network of hand (radial)
15 Dorsal metacarpal veins

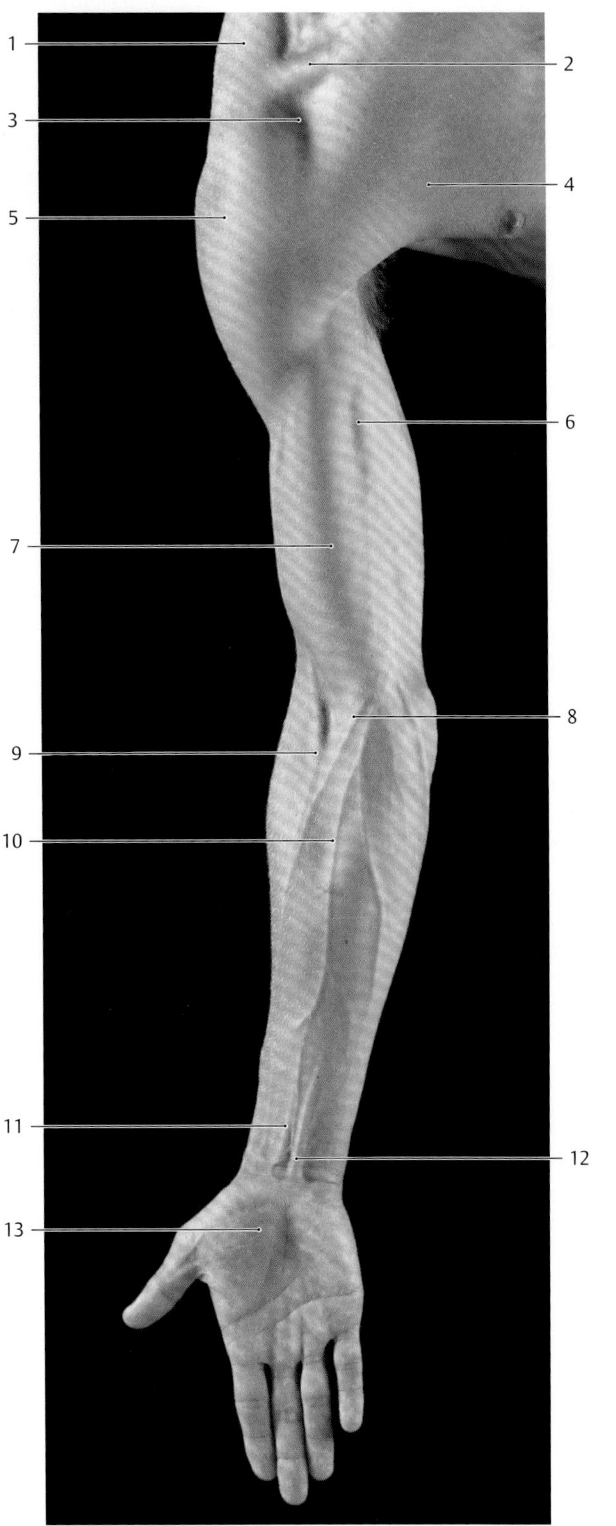


Fig. 3.84 **Surface anatomy of the upper limb** (right side, anterior aspect).

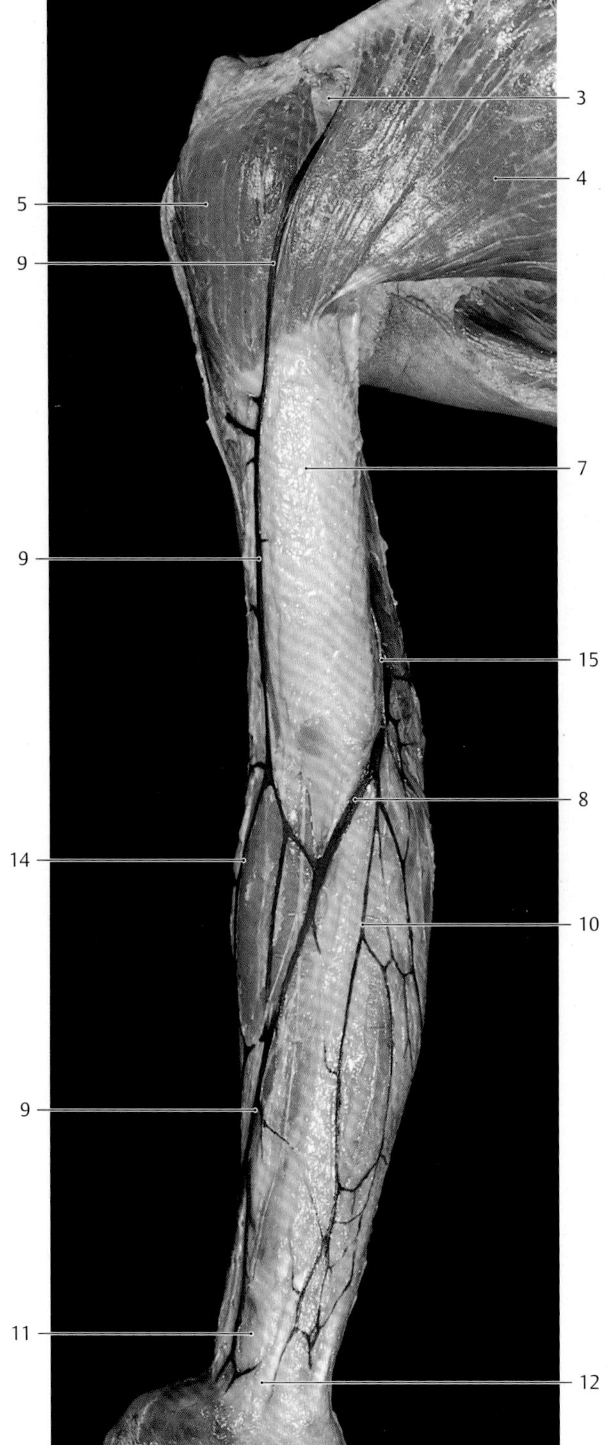


Fig. 3.85 **Superficial veins of the arm** (right side, anterior aspect). The veins have been injected with blue gelatin.

1 Trapezius muscle
2 Clavicle
3 Deltopectoral triangle
4 Pectoralis major muscle
5 Deltoid muscle
6 Brachial vein
7 Biceps brachii muscle
8 Median cubital vein
9 Cephalic vein
10 Median vein of forearm
11 Tendon of flexor carpi radialis
12 Tendon of palmaris longus muscle
13 Location of adductor pollicis muscle
14 Accessory cephalic vein
15 Basilic vein

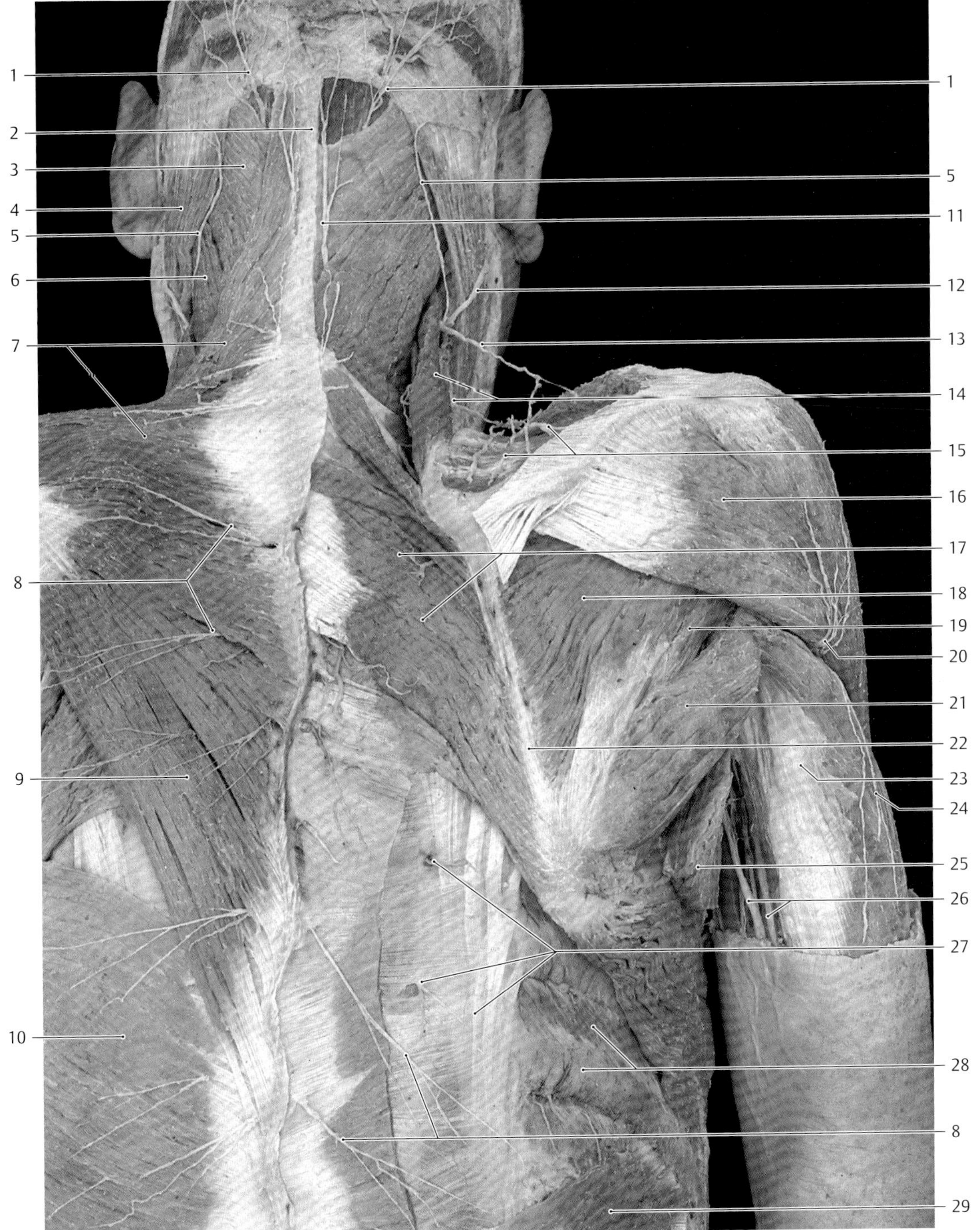


**Fig. 3.86 Posterior regions of neck and shoulder** (superficial layer [left side]; trapezius and latissimus dorsi muscles removed [right side]). Dissection of dorsal branches of spinal nerves.

1 Greater occipital nerve
2 Ligamentum nuchae
3 Splenius capitis muscle
4 Sternocleidomastoid muscle
5 Lesser occipital nerve
6 Splenius cervicis muscle
7 Descending and transverse fibers of trapezius muscle
8 Medial cutaneous branches of dorsal rami of spinal nerves
9 Ascending fibers of trapezius muscle
10 Latissimus dorsi muscle
11 Cutaneous branch of third occipital nerve
12 Great auricular nerve
13 Accessory nerve (CN XI)
14 Posterior supraclavicular nerve and levator scapulae muscle
15 Branches of suprascapular artery
16 Deltoid muscle
17 Rhomboid major muscle
18 Infraspinatus muscle
19 Teres minor muscle
20 Upper lateral cutaneous nerve of arm (branch of axillary nerve)
21 Teres major muscle
22 Medial margin of scapula
23 Long head of triceps muscle
24 Posterior cutaneous nerve of arm (branch of radial nerve)
25 Latissimus dorsi muscle (divided)
26 Ulnar nerve and brachial artery
27 Lateral cutaneous branches of dorsal rami of spinal nerves and iliocostalis thoracis muscle
28 External intercostal muscle and seventh rib
29 Serratus posterior inferior muscle

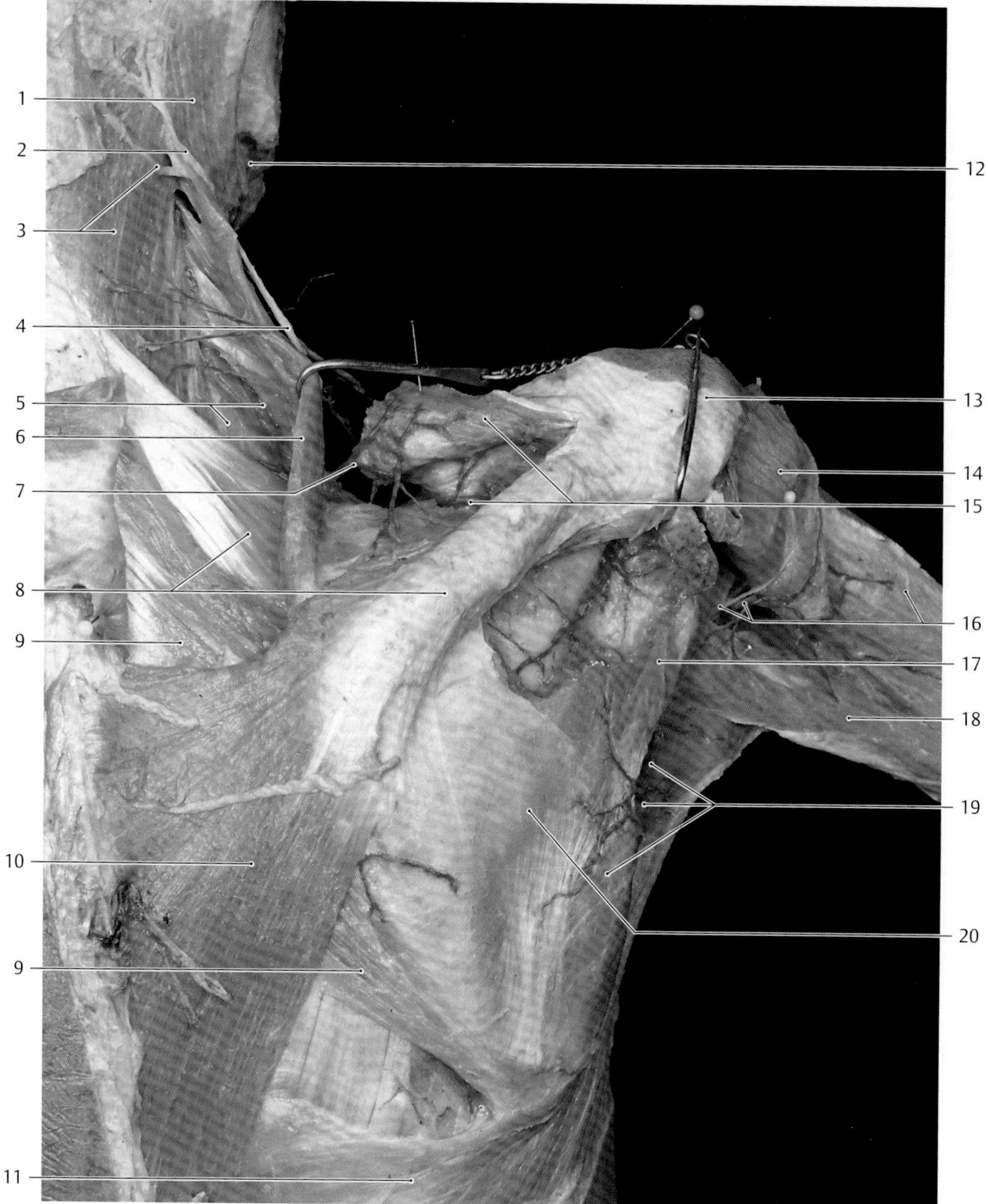


Fig. 3.87 **Posterior region of the shoulder,** deep layer. The arteries of the scapular region have been injected with red gelatin. Trapezius, deltoid, and infraspinatus muscles have been partially removed or reflected.

1 Sternocleidomastoid muscle
2 Lesser occipital nerve
3 Splenius capitis muscle and third occipital nerve
4 Accessory nerve (CN XI)
5 Splenius cervicis muscle and transverse cervical artery (deep branch)
6 Levator scapulae muscle
7 Transverse cervical artery (superficial branch)
8 Spine of scapula and serratus posterior superior muscle
9 Rhomboid major muscle
10 Trapezius muscle
11 Latissimus dorsi muscle
12 Facial artery
13 Acromion
14 Deltoid muscle
15 Suprascapular artery and supraspinatus muscle (reflected)
16 Axillary nerve, posterior circumflex humeral artery, and lateral head of triceps brachii muscle
17 Teres minor muscle
18 Long head of triceps brachii muscle
19 Circumflex scapular artery and teres major muscle
20 Infraspinatus muscle with fascia

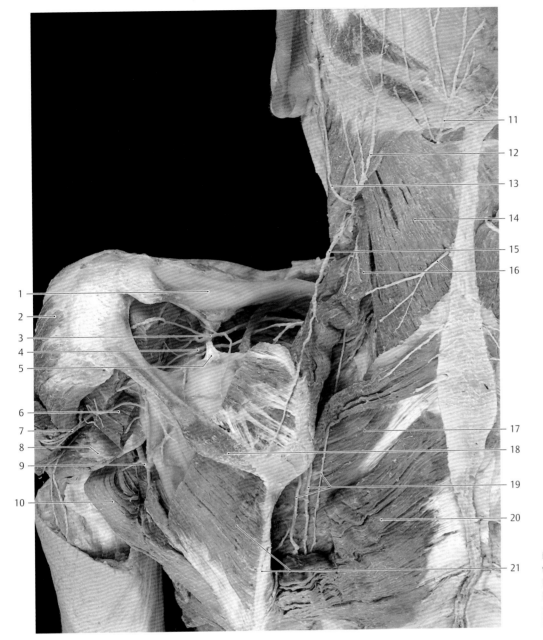

1 Clavicle
2 Deltoid muscle
3 Suprascapular artery
4 Suprascapular nerve
5 Superior transverse scapular ligament
6 Teres minor muscle
7 Axillary nerve and posterior circumflex humeral artery
8 Long head of triceps muscle
9 Circumflex scapular artery
10 Teres major muscle
11 Greater occipital nerve
12 Lesser occipital nerve
13 Great auricular nerve
14 Splenius capitis muscle
15 Accessory nerve (CN XI)
16 Third occipital nerve and levator scapulae muscle
17 Serratus posterior superior muscle
18 Spine of scapula
19 Descending scapular artery and dorsal scapular nerve
20 Rhomboid major muscle
21 Infraspinatus muscle and medial margin of scapula
22 Axillary artery
23 Radial nerve and brachial artery
24 Thoracodorsal artery
25 Thyrocervical trunk
26 Brachial plexus

Fig. 3.88 **Posterior region of the shoulder,** deepest layer. Rhomboid and scapular muscles have been fenestrated; the posterior part of deltoid muscle has been reflected.

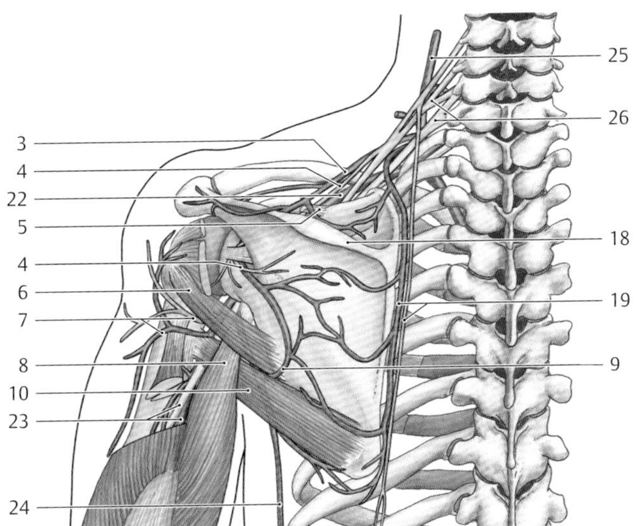


Fig. 3.89 **Collateral circulation of the shoulder** (posterior aspect). Anastomosis of suprascapular and circumflex scapular arteries.

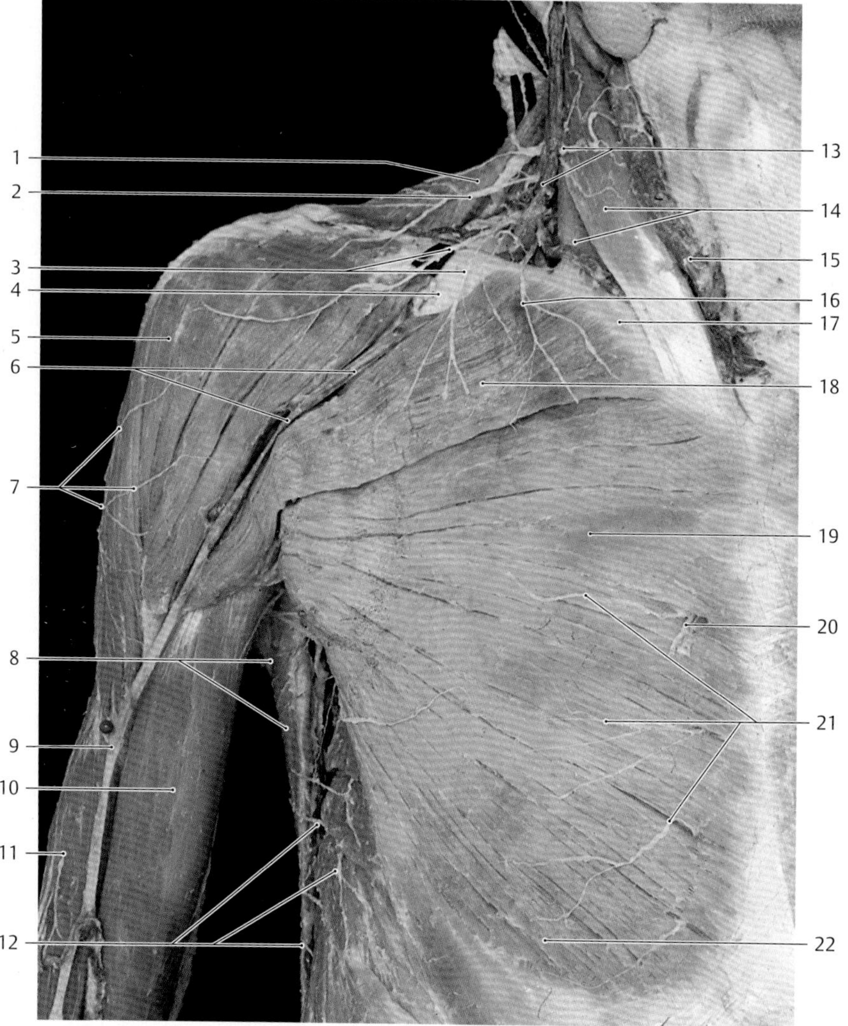


Fig. 3.90 **Anterior regions of shoulder and thoracic wall,** superficial layer. Dissection of the cutaneous nerves and veins.

1 Trapezius muscle
2 Posterior supraclavicular nerve
3 Middle supraclavicular nerve
4 Deltopectoral triangle
5 Deltoid muscle
6 Cephalic vein within the deltopectoral groove
7 Upper lateral cutaneous nerve of arm (branch of axillary nerve)
8 Latissimus dorsi muscle
9 Cephalic vein
10 Biceps brachii muscle
11 Triceps brachii muscle
12 Lateral cutaneous branches of intercostal nerves
13 Transverse cervical nerve and external jugular vein
14 Sternocleidomastoid muscle
15 Anterior jugular vein
16 Anterior supraclavicular nerve
17 Clavicle
18 Clavicular part of pectoralis major muscle
19 Sternocostal part of pectoralis major muscle
20 Perforating branch of internal thoracic artery
21 Anterior cutaneous branches of intercostal nerves
22 Abdominal part of pectoralis major muscle
23 Sternocleidomastoid muscle, cervical branch of facial nerve, and anterior jugular vein
24 External jugular vein and transverse cervical nerve (inferior branch)
25 Sternoclavicular joint (opened) with articular disc
26 Pectoralis major muscle
27 Omohyoid muscle and external jugular vein
28 Jugular venous arch and sternohyoid muscle
29 Sternoclavicular joint (not opened)

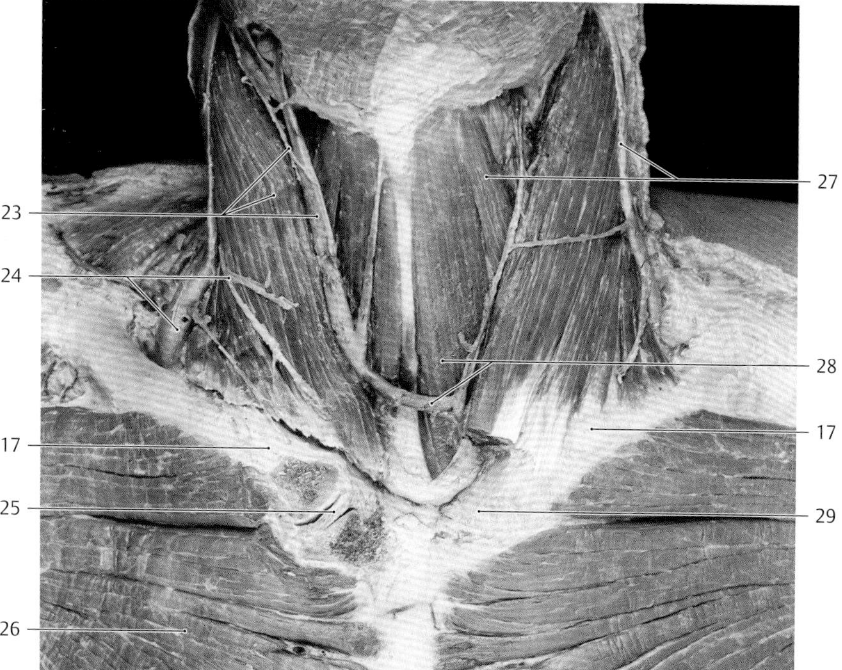


Fig. 3.91 **Anterior regions of thoracic wall and neck.** The sternoclavicular joint is depicted. On the right side the joint has been opened by a coronal section. Note the articular disc.

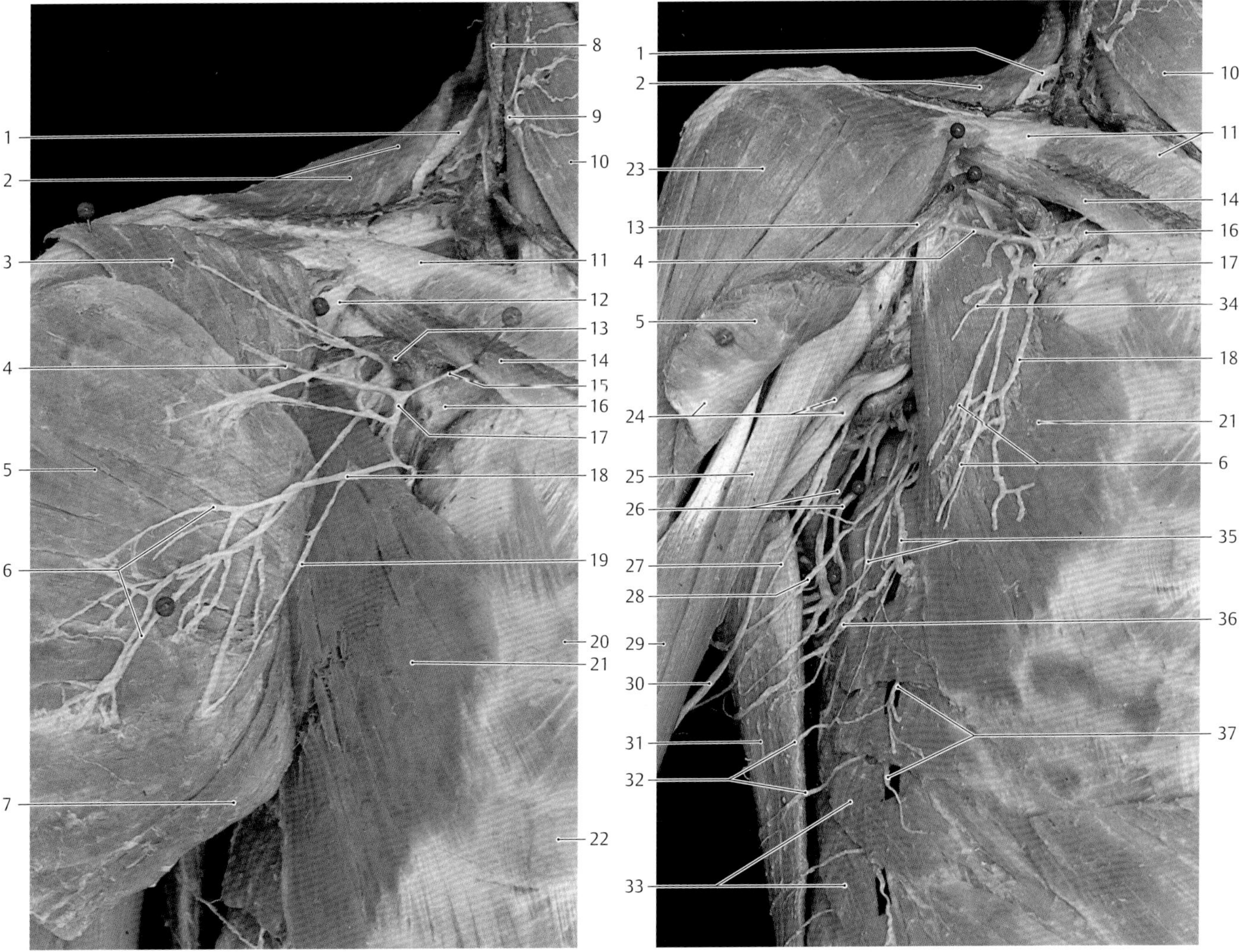


Fig. 3.92 **Deltopectoral triangle and infraclavicular region** (anterior aspect). The pectoralis major muscle has been cut and reflected.

Fig. 3.93 **Anterior regions of shoulder and thoracic wall** with axillary region, deep layer. The pectoralis major muscle has been cut and partly removed.

1 Accessory nerve
2 Trapezius muscle
3 Pectoralis major muscle (clavicular part)
4 Acromial branch of thoraco-acromial artery
5 Pectoralis major muscle
6 Lateral pectoral nerves
7 Abdominal part of pectoralis major muscle
8 External jugular vein
9 Cutaneous branches of cervical plexus
10 Sternocleidomastoid muscle
11 Clavicle
12 Clavipectoral fascia
13 Cephalic vein
14 Subclavius muscle
15 Clavicular branch of thoraco-acromial artery
16 Subclavian vein
17 Thoraco-acromial artery
18 Pectoral branch of thoraco-acromial artery
19 Medial pectoral nerve
20 Second rib
21 Pectoralis minor muscle
22 Third rib
23 Deltoid muscle
24 Pectoralis major muscle (reflected), brachial artery, and median nerve
25 Short head of biceps brachii muscle
26 Thoracodorsal artery and nerve
27 Medial cutaneous nerve of arm
28 Intercostobrachial nerve (T2)
29 Long head of biceps brachii muscle
30 Medial cutaneous nerve of forearm
31 Latissimus dorsi muscle
32 Lateral cutaneous branches of intercostal nerves (posterior branches)
33 Serratus anterior muscle
34 Medial pectoral nerve
35 Long thoracic nerve and lateral thoracic artery
36 Intercostobrachial nerve (T3)
37 Lateral cutaneous branches of intercostal nerves (anterior branches)

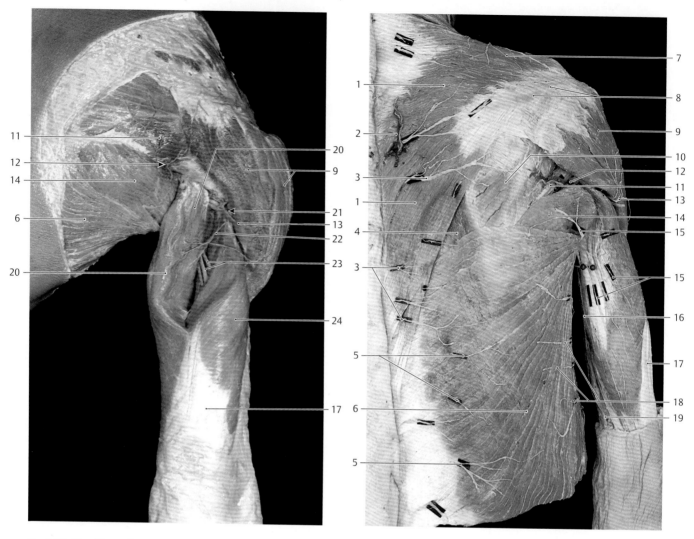

Fig. 3.94 **Shoulder and arm** (posterior aspect). Dissection of the quadrangular and triangular spaces of the axillary region.

Fig. 3.95 **Shoulder region and arm,** superficial layer (posterior aspect). Note the segmental arrangement of the cutaneous nerves of the back.

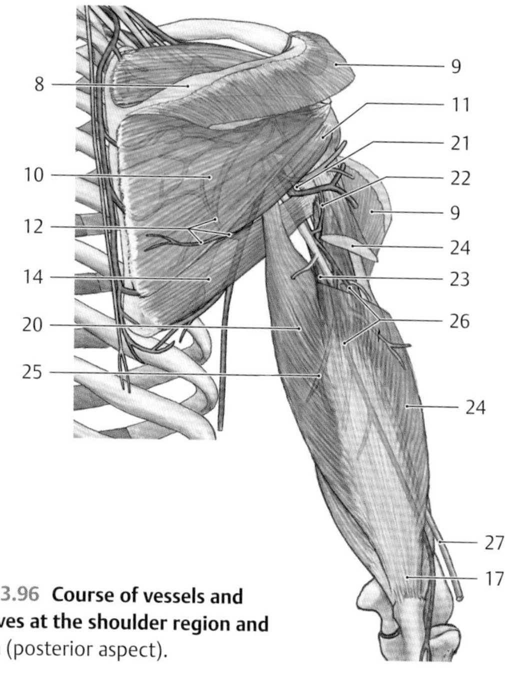


Fig. 3.96 **Course of vessels and nerves at the shoulder region and arm** (posterior aspect).

1 Trapezius muscle
2 Dorsal branches of posterior intercostal artery and vein (medial cutaneous branches)
3 Medial branches of dorsal rami of spinal nerves
4 Rhomboid major muscle
5 Lateral branches of dorsal rami of spinal nerves
6 Latissimus dorsi muscle
7 Posterior supraclavicular nerves
8 Spine of scapula
9 Deltoid muscle
10 Infraspinatus muscle
11 Teres minor muscle
12 Triangular space with circumflex scapular artery and vein
13 Upper lateral cutaneous nerve of arm with artery
14 Teres major muscle
15 Terminal branches of intercostobrachial nerve
16 Medial cutaneous nerve of arm
17 Tendon of triceps brachii muscle
18 Lateral cutaneous branches of intercostal nerves
19 Medial cutaneous nerve of forearm
20 Long head of triceps brachii muscle
21 Quadrangular space with axillary nerve and posterior humeral circumflex artery
22 Anastomosis between profunda brachii artery and posterior humeral circumflex artery
23 Course of radial nerve and profunda brachii artery
24 Lateral head of triceps brachii muscle
25 Medial collateral artery
26 Radial collateral artery
27 Radial nerve

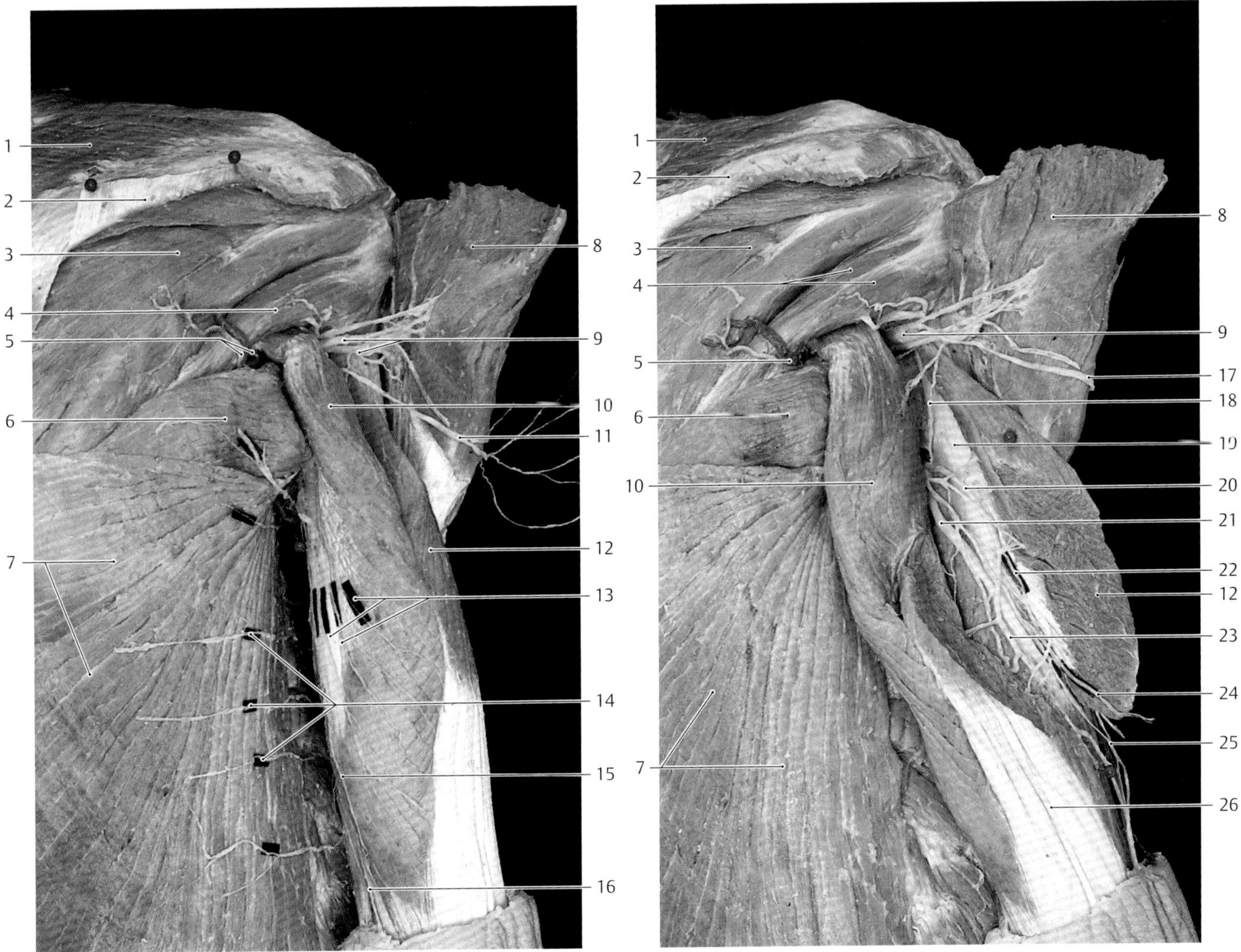


**Fig. 3.97 Shoulder region and arm,** deep layer (posterior aspect). Part of deltoid muscle has been cut and reflected to display the quadrangular and triangular spaces of the axillary region.

**Fig. 3.98 Shoulder region and arm,** deep layer (posterior aspect). The lateral head of the triceps brachii muscle has been cut to display the radial nerve and accompanying vessels.

1 Trapezius muscle
2 Spine of scapula
3 Infraspinatus muscle
4 Teres minor muscle
5 Triangular space containing circumflex scapular artery and vein
6 Teres major muscle
7 Latissimus dorsi muscle
8 Deltoid muscle (cut and reflected)
9 Quadrangular space containing axillary nerve and posterior circumflex humeral artery and vein
10 Long head of triceps brachii muscle
11 Cutaneous branch of axillary nerve
12 Lateral head of triceps brachii muscle
13 Terminal branches of intercostobrachial nerve
14 Lateral cutaneous branches of intercostal nerves
15 Medial cutaneous nerve of arm
16 Medial cutaneous nerve of forearm
17 Upper lateral cutaneous nerve of arm
18 Anastomosis between profunda brachii artery and posterior humeral circumflex artery
19 Humerus
20 Profunda brachii artery
21 Radial nerve
22 Radial collateral artery
23 Middle collateral artery
24 Lower lateral cutaneous nerve of arm
25 Posterior cutaneous nerve of forearm
26 Tendon of triceps brachii muscle

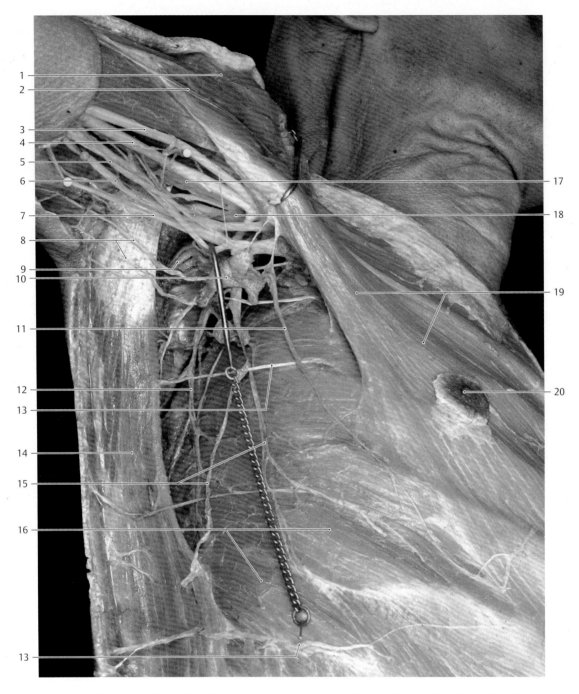


**Fig. 3.99 Axillary region** (right side, inferior aspect). Dissection of superficial axillary lymph nodes and lymphatic vessels. The pectoralis major muscle has been slightly elevated.

1 Deltoid muscle
2 Cephalic vein
3 Median nerve
4 Brachial artery
5 Medial cutaneous nerves of arm and forearm
6 Ulnar nerve
7 Basilic vein
8 Intercostobrachial nerves
9 Circumflex scapular artery
10 Superficial axillary lymph nodes
11 Lateral thoracic artery
12 Thoracodorsal artery
13 Lateral cutaneous branch of intercostal nerve
14 Latissimus dorsi muscle
15 Thoraco-epigastric vein
16 Serratus anterior muscle
17 Musculocutaneous nerve
18 Radial nerve
19 Pectoralis major muscle
20 Nipple

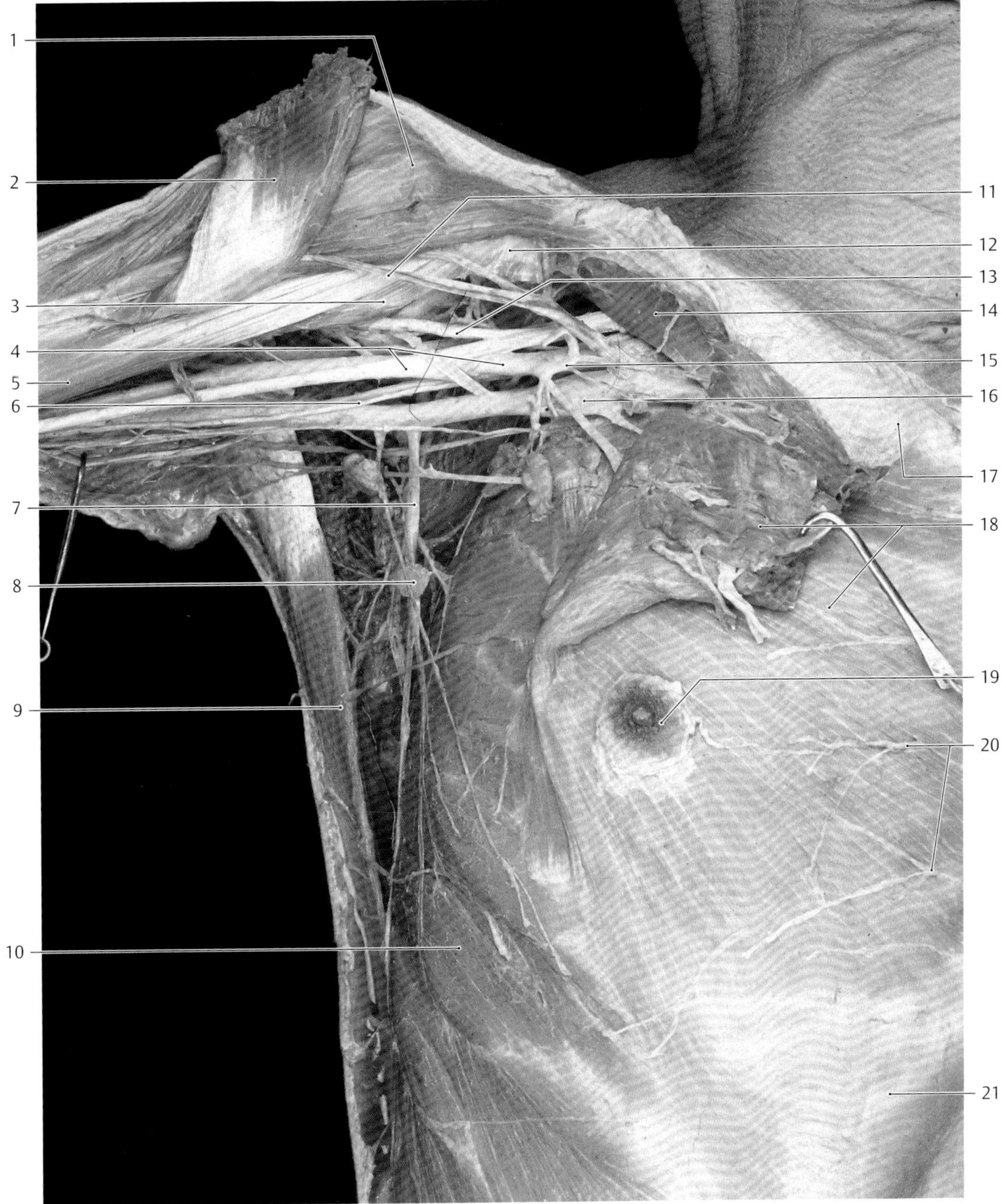


Fig. 3.100 **Axillary region** (right side, anterior aspect). Dissection of deep axillary lymph nodes. Pectoralis major and minor muscles have been divided and reflected. Shoulder girdle and arm have been elevated and reflected.

1 Deltoid muscle
2 Insertion of pectoralis major muscle
3 Coracobrachialis muscle
4 Roots of median nerve and axillary artery
5 Short head of biceps brachii muscle
6 Ulnar nerve and medial cutaneous nerve of forearm
7 Thoraco-epigastric vein
8 Deep axillary lymph nodes
9 Latissimus dorsi muscle
10 Serratus anterior muscle
11 Cephalic vein
12 Insertion of pectoralis minor muscle (coracoid process)
13 Musculocutaneous nerve
14 Subclavius muscle
15 Thoraco-acromial artery
16 Axillary vein
17 Clavicle
18 Pectoralis major and minor muscles (reflected)
19 Nipple
20 Anterior cutaneous branches of intercostal nerves
21 Anterior layer of rectus sheath

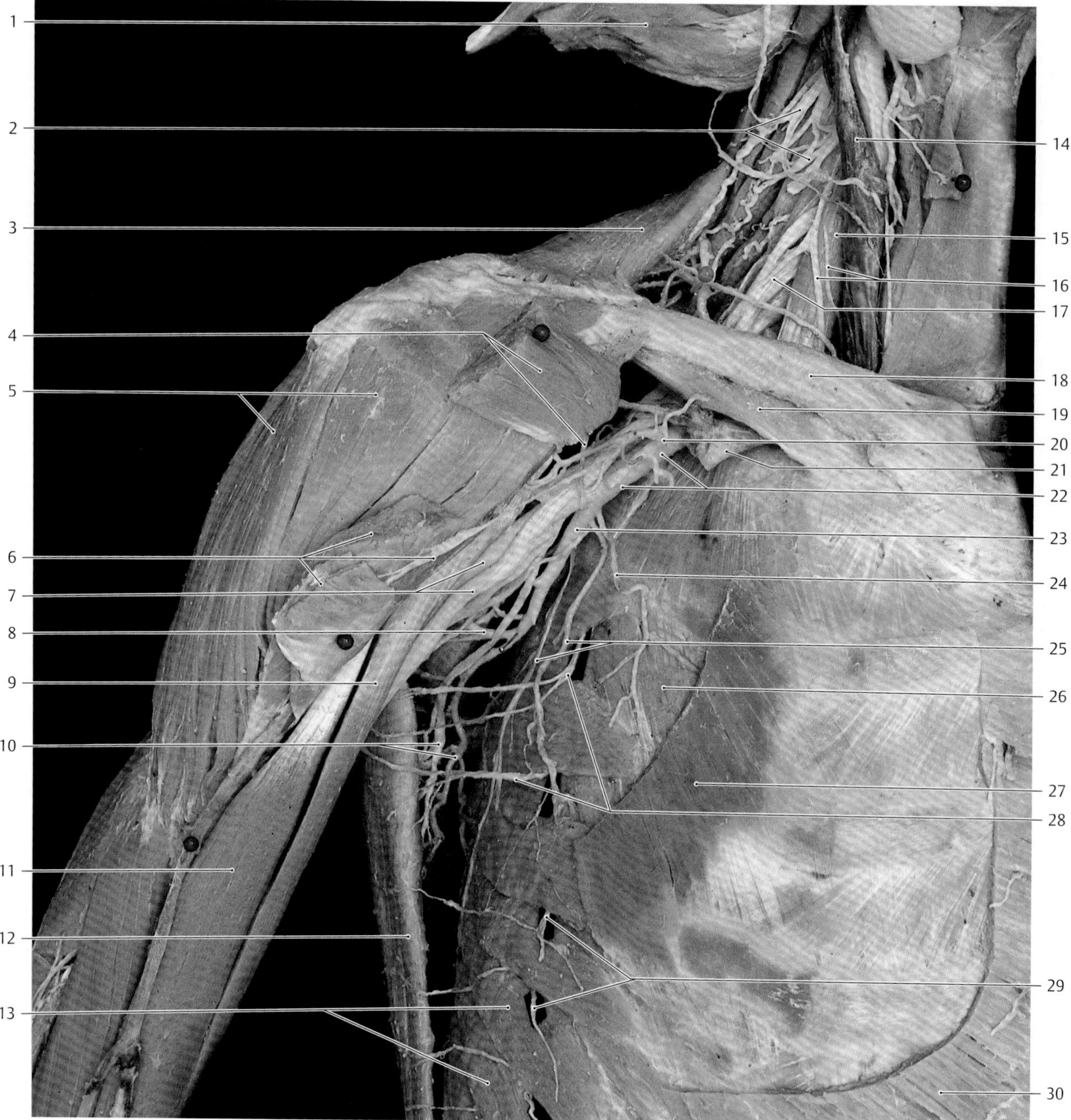


**Fig. 3.101 Axillary region** (right side, anterior aspect). Pectoralis major and minor muscles have been cut and reflected to display the vessels and nerves of the axilla.

1 Sternocleidomastoid muscle (cut and reflected)
2 Cervical plexus
3 Trapezius muscle
4 Pectoralis minor muscle and medial pectoral nerve
5 Deltoid muscle
6 Pectoralis major muscle and lateral pectoral nerve
7 Median nerve and brachial artery
8 Circumflex scapular artery
9 Short head of biceps brachii muscle
10 Thoracodorsal artery and nerve
11 Long head of biceps brachii muscle
12 Latissimus dorsi muscle
13 Serratus anterior muscle
14 Internal jugular vein
15 Anterior scalene muscle
16 Phrenic nerve and ascending cervical artery
17 Brachial plexus (at the levels of the trunks)
18 Clavicle
19 Subclavius muscle
20 Thoraco-acromial artery
21 Subclavian vein (cut)
22 Axillary artery
23 Subscapular artery
24 Superior thoracic artery
25 Lateral thoracic artery and long thoracic nerve
26 External intercostal muscle
27 Insertion of pectoralis minor muscle
28 Intercostobrachial nerves
29 Lateral cutaneous branches of intercostal nerves
30 Insertion of pectoralis major muscle

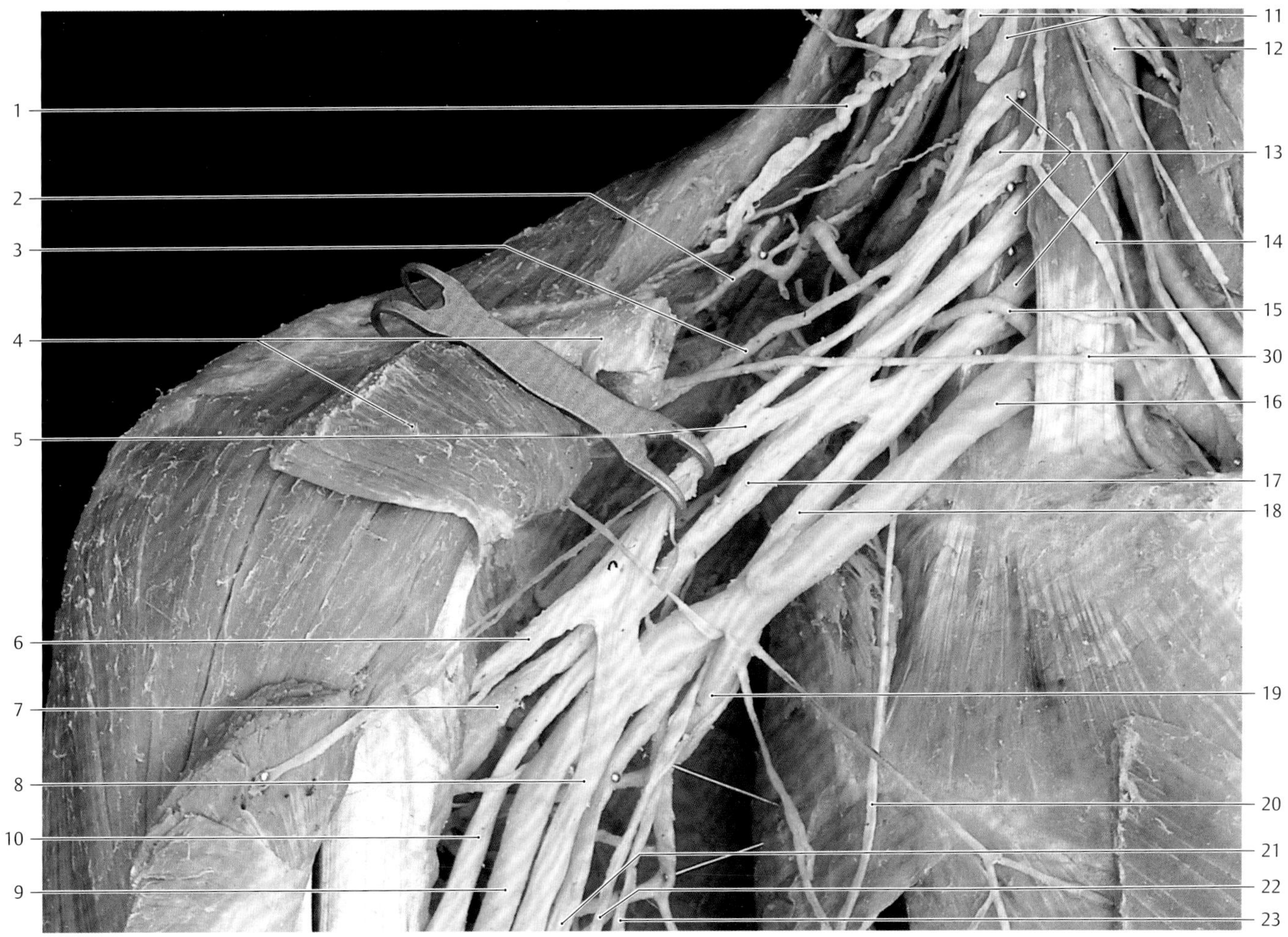

Fig. 3.102 **Brachial plexus** (anterior aspect). The clavicle and the two pectoralis muscles have been partly removed.

1 Accessory nerve
2 Dorsal scapular artery
3 Suprascapular nerve
4 Clavicle and pectoralis minor muscle
5 Lateral cord of brachial plexus
6 Musculocutaneous nerve
7 Axillary nerve
8 Median nerve
9 Brachial artery
10 Radial nerve
11 Cervical plexus
12 Common carotid artery
13 Roots of brachial plexus (C5–T1)
14 Phrenic nerve
15 Transverse cervical artery
16 Subclavian artery
17 Posterior cord of brachial plexus
18 Medial cord of brachial plexus
19 Subscapular artery
20 Long thoracic nerve
21 Ulnar nerve
22 Medial cutaneous nerve of forearm
23 Thoracodorsal nerve
24 Intercostobrachial nerves
25 Medial cutaneous nerves of arm and forearm
26 Anterior scalene muscle
27 Middle scalene muscle
28 Intercostal nerve (T3)
29 Axillary artery
30 Suprascapular artery

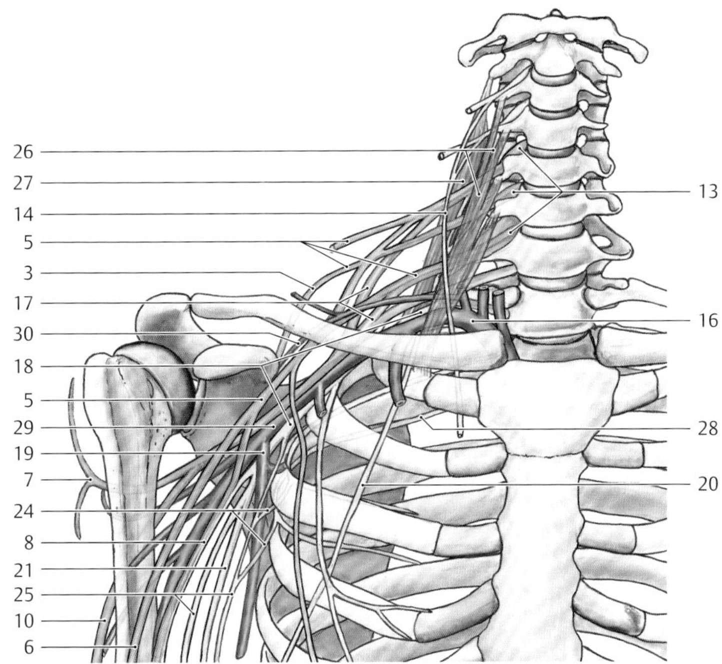


Fig. 3.103 **Main branches of brachial plexus.** Posterior cord in orange, lateral cord in ocher, and medial cord in light yellow.

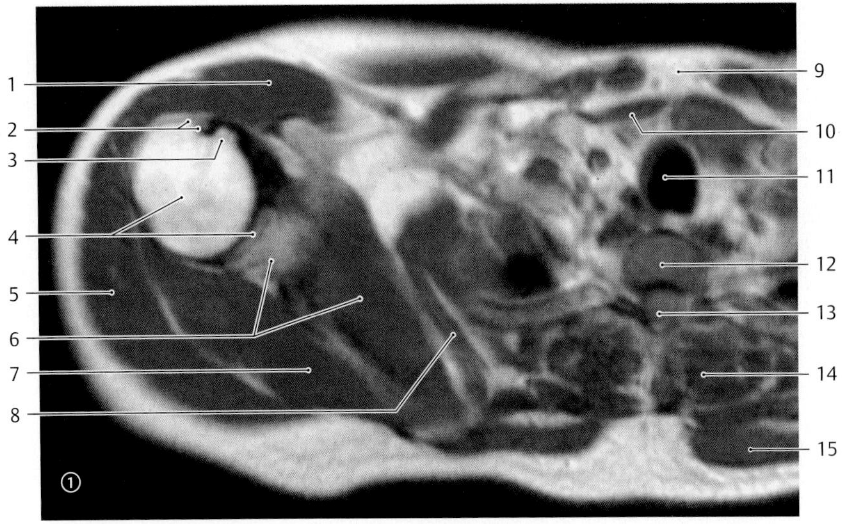


**Fig. 3.104 Horizontal section through the right shoulder joint.** Section 1 (inferior aspect, MRI scan). (Heuck A, et al. MRT-Atlas des muskuloskelettalen Systems. Stuttgart, Germany: Schattauer, 2009.)

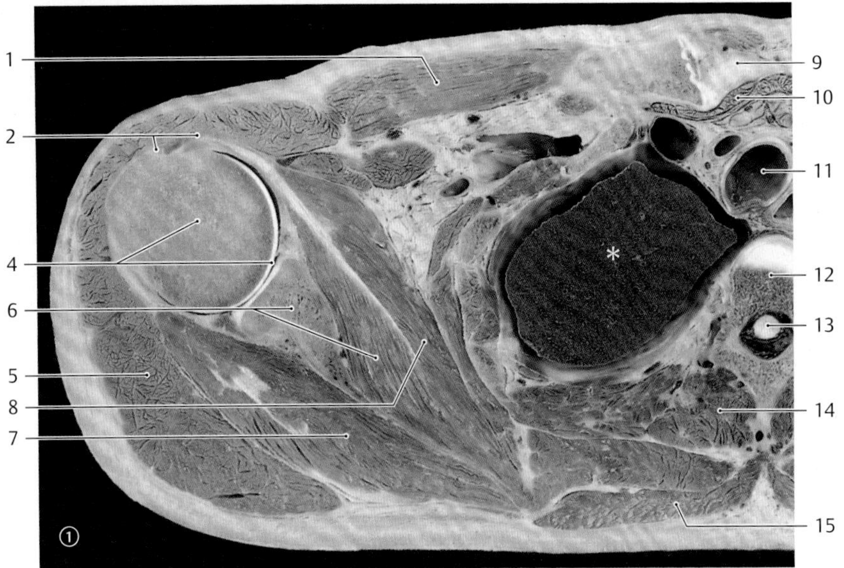


**Fig. 3.105 Horizontal section through the right shoulder joint.** Section 1 (inferior aspect). * = Upper lobe of lung.

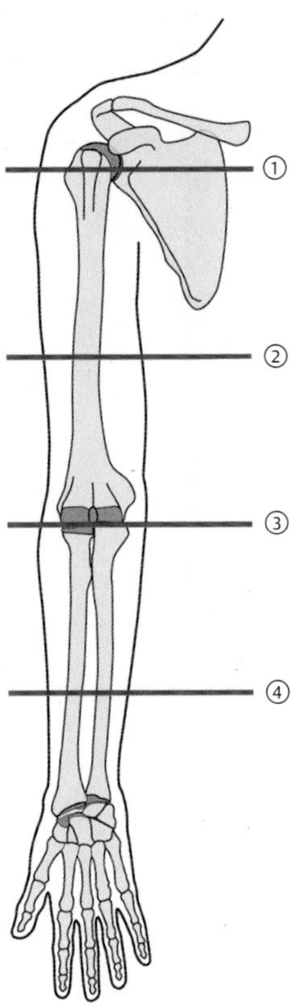


**Fig. 3.106 Location of the sections through the upper limb.**

1 Pectoralis major muscle
2 Greater tubercle and tendon of biceps muscle
3 Lesser tubercle
4 Head of humerus and articular cavity of shoulder joint
5 Deltoid muscle
6 Scapula
7 Infraspinatus muscle
8 Serratus anterior muscle
9 Sternum
10 Infrahyoid muscles
11 Trachea
12 Body of thoracic vertebra
13 Vertebral canal and spinal cord
14 Deep muscles of the back
15 Trapezius muscle
16 Brachialis muscle
17 Radial nerve and profunda brachii artery
18 Triceps brachii muscle
19 Cephalic vein
20 Biceps brachii muscle
21 Musculocutaneous nerve
22 Ulnar nerve
23 Median nerve
24 Brachial artery and vein
25 Shaft of humerus
26 Brachioradialis muscle
27 Radial nerve
28 Olecranon and articular cavity of elbow joint
29 Basilic vein
30 Humerus
31 Pronator teres muscle
32 Extensor muscles of forearm
33 Deep branch of radial nerve
34 Anterior interosseus artery and nerve
35 Interosseous membrane
36 Ulna
37 Radius
38 Superficial branch of radial artery
39 Flexor pollicis longus muscle
40 Flexor digitorum superficialis and profundus muscles
41 Ulnar nerve, artery, and vein
42 Flexor carpi ulnaris muscle
43 Radial artery

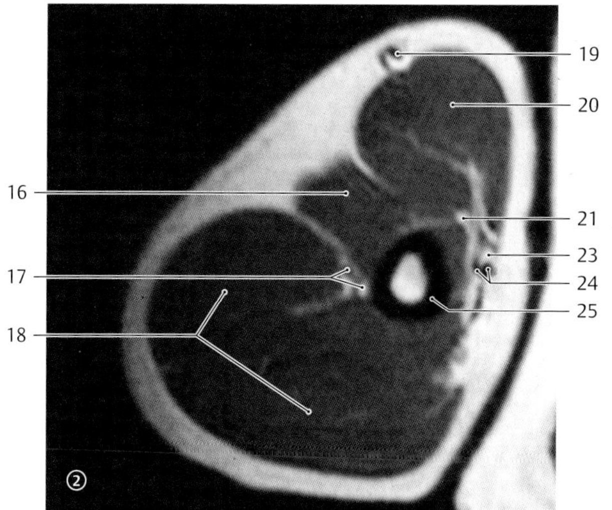


Fig. 3.107 **Axial section through the middle of the right arm.** Section 2 (inferior aspect, MRI scan). (Courtesy of Prof. Uder, Institute of Radiology, University Hospital Erlangen, Germany.)

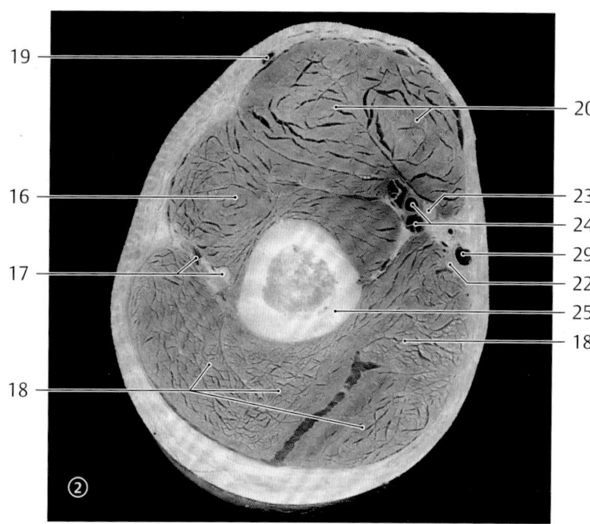


Fig. 3.108 **Axial section through the middle of the right arm.** Section 2 (inferior aspect).

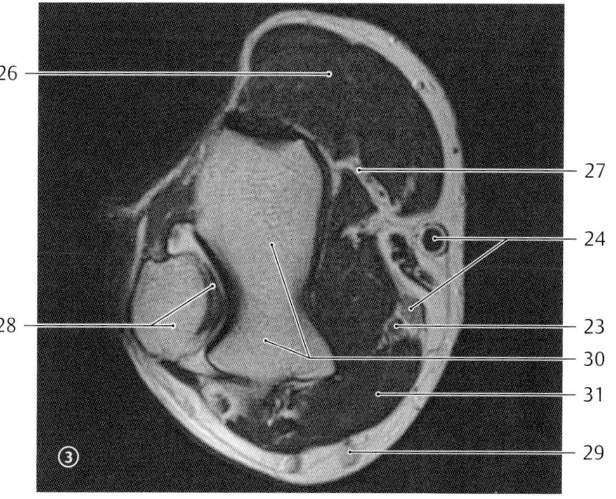


Fig. 3.109 **Axial section through the right elbow joint.** Section 3 (inferior aspect, MRI scan). (Courtesy of Prof. Uder, Institute of Radiology, University Hospital Erlangen, Germany.)

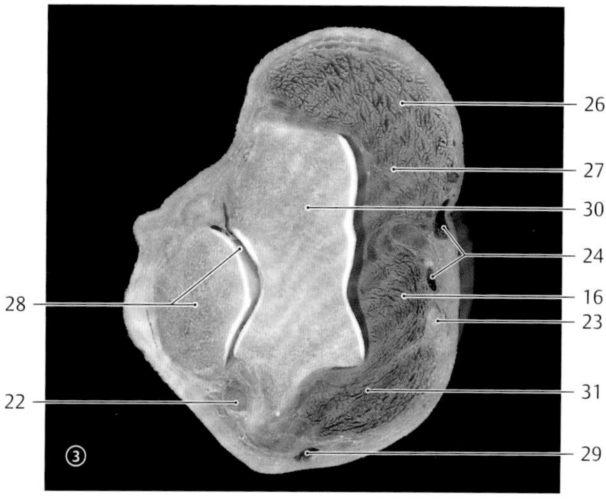


Fig. 3.110 **Axial section through the right elbow joint.** Section 3 (inferior aspect).

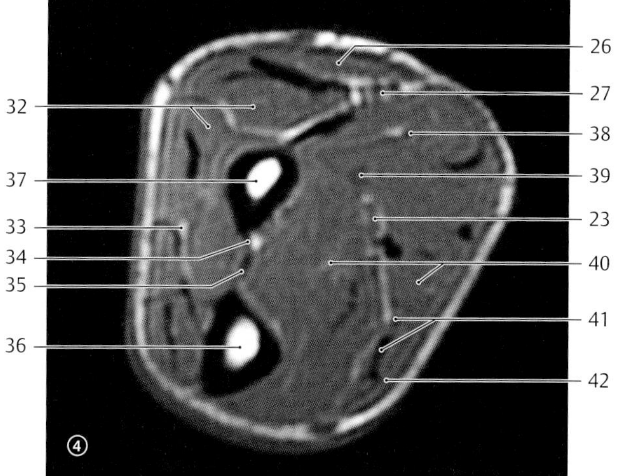


Fig. 3.111 **Axial section through the middle of the right forearm.** Section 4 (inferior aspect, MRI scan). (Courtesy of Prof. Uder, Institute of Radiology, University Hospital Erlangen, Germany.)

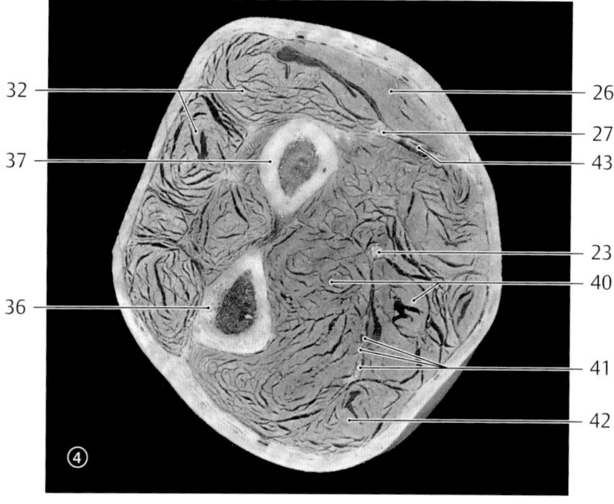


Fig. 3.112 **Axial section through the middle of the right forearm.** Section 4 (inferior aspect).

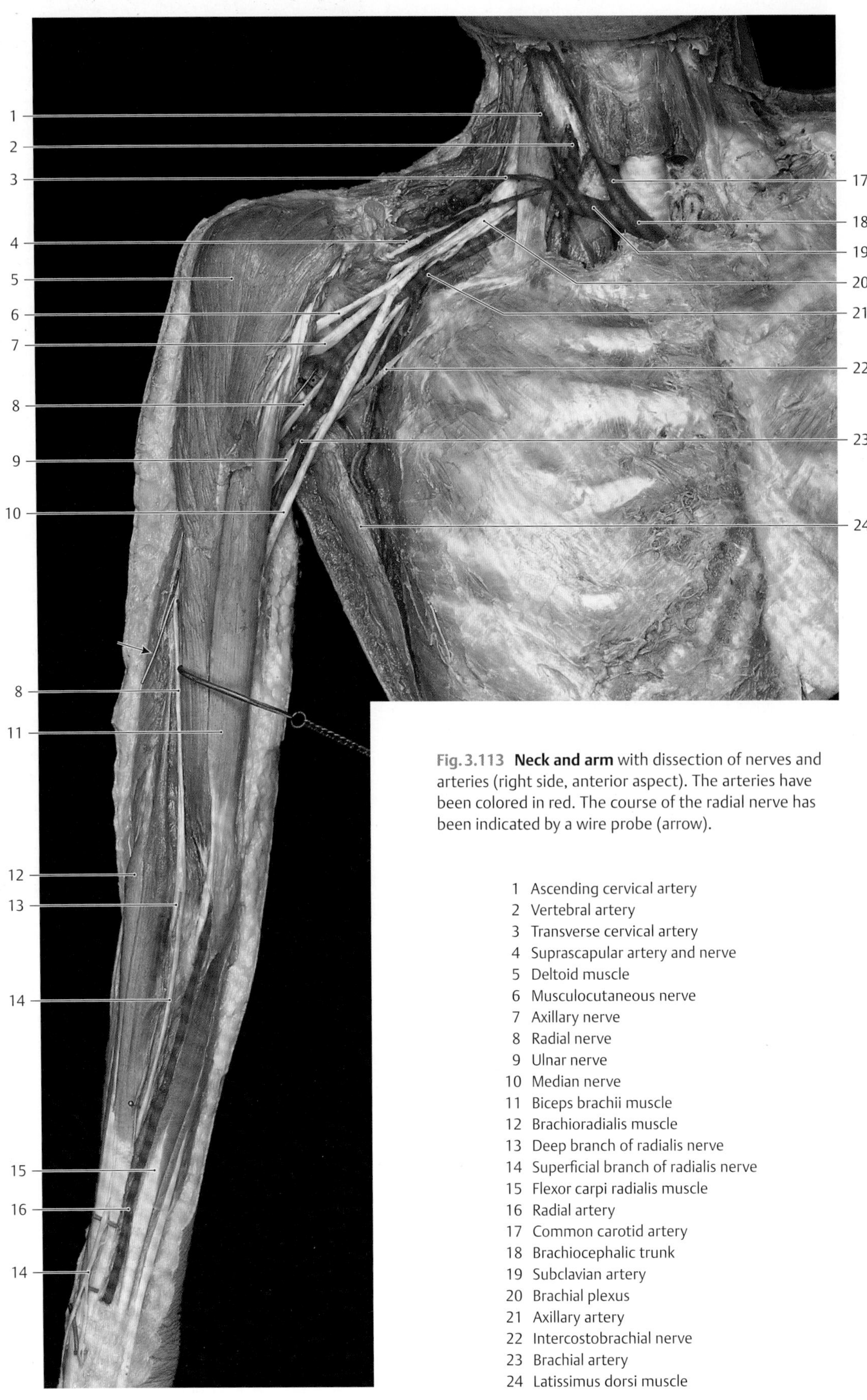


Fig. 3.113 **Neck and arm** with dissection of nerves and arteries (right side, anterior aspect). The arteries have been colored in red. The course of the radial nerve has been indicated by a wire probe (arrow).

1 Ascending cervical artery
2 Vertebral artery
3 Transverse cervical artery
4 Suprascapular artery and nerve
5 Deltoid muscle
6 Musculocutaneous nerve
7 Axillary nerve
8 Radial nerve
9 Ulnar nerve
10 Median nerve
11 Biceps brachii muscle
12 Brachioradialis muscle
13 Deep branch of radialis nerve
14 Superficial branch of radialis nerve
15 Flexor carpi radialis muscle
16 Radial artery
17 Common carotid artery
18 Brachiocephalic trunk
19 Subclavian artery
20 Brachial plexus
21 Axillary artery
22 Intercostobrachial nerve
23 Brachial artery
24 Latissimus dorsi muscle

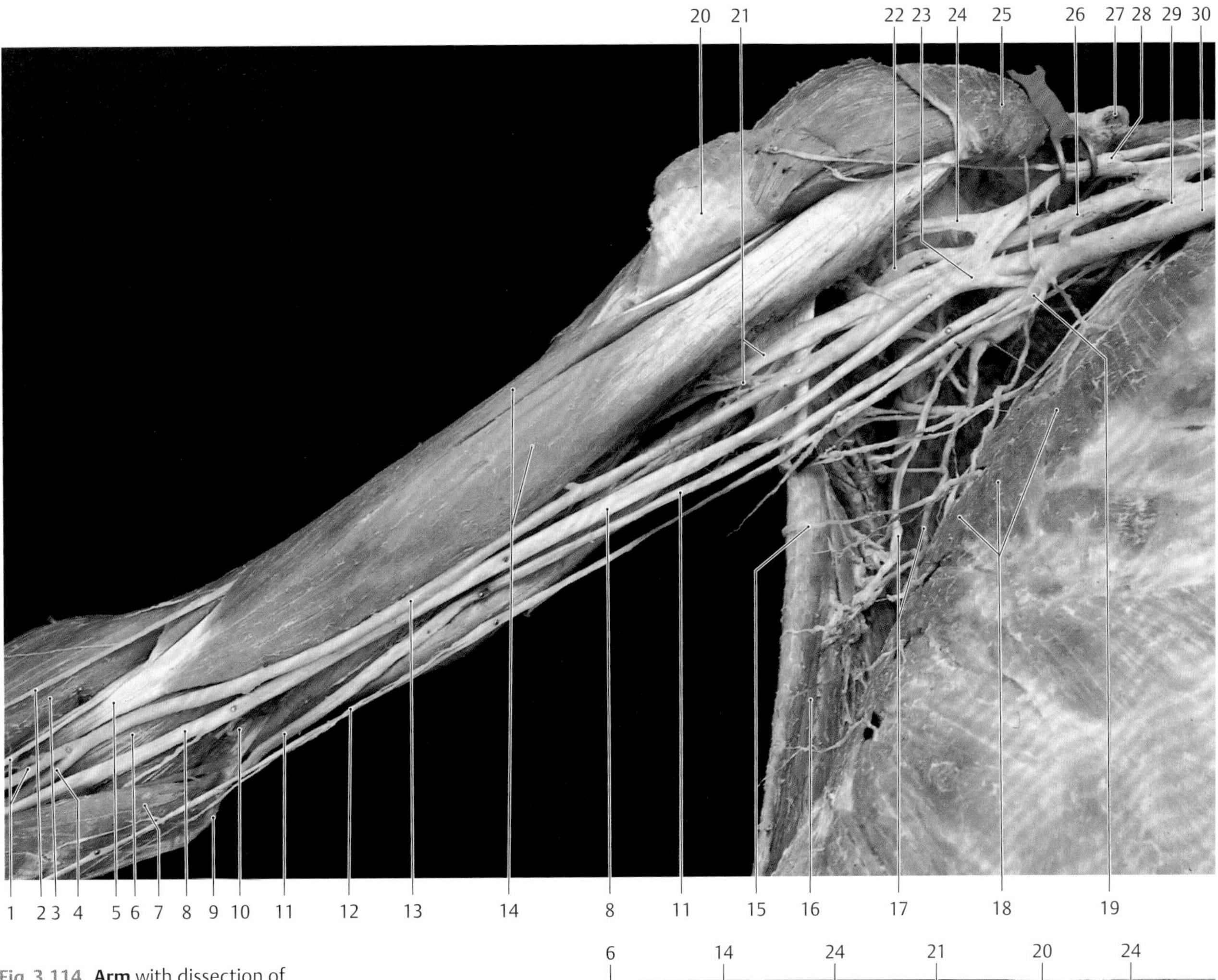


**Fig. 3.114** **Arm** with dissection of nerves and vessels (right side, anterior aspect).The shoulder girdle has been reflected slightly.

6 14 24 21 20 24
8 31 11 13 16

**Fig. 3.115** **Arm** with dissection of nerves and vessels, deeper layer (right side, antero-inferior aspect). The biceps brachii muscle has been reflected.

1 Radial artery and superficial branch of radial nerve
2 Lateral cutaneous nerve of forearm
3 Brachioradialis muscle
4 Ulnar artery
5 Tendon of biceps brachii muscle
6 Brachialis muscle
7 Pronator teres muscle
8 Median nerve
9 Medial epicondyle of humerus
10 Inferior ulnar collateral artery
11 Ulnar nerve
12 Medial cutaneous nerve of forearm
13 Brachial artery
14 Biceps brachii muscle
15 Intercostobrachial nerve (T3)
16 Latissimus dorsi muscle
17 Thoracodorsal nerve and artery
18 Serratus anterior muscle
19 Subscapular artery
20 Pectoralis major muscle (reflected) and lateral pectoral nerve
21 Radial nerve and profunda brachii artery
22 Axillary nerve
23 Roots of the median nerve with axillary artery
24 Musculocutaneous nerve
25 Pectoralis minor muscle (reflected) and medial pectoral nerve
26 Posterior cord of brachial plexus
27 Clavicle (cut)
28 Lateral cord of brachial plexus
29 Medial cord of brachial plexus
30 Subclavian artery
31 Brachial vein

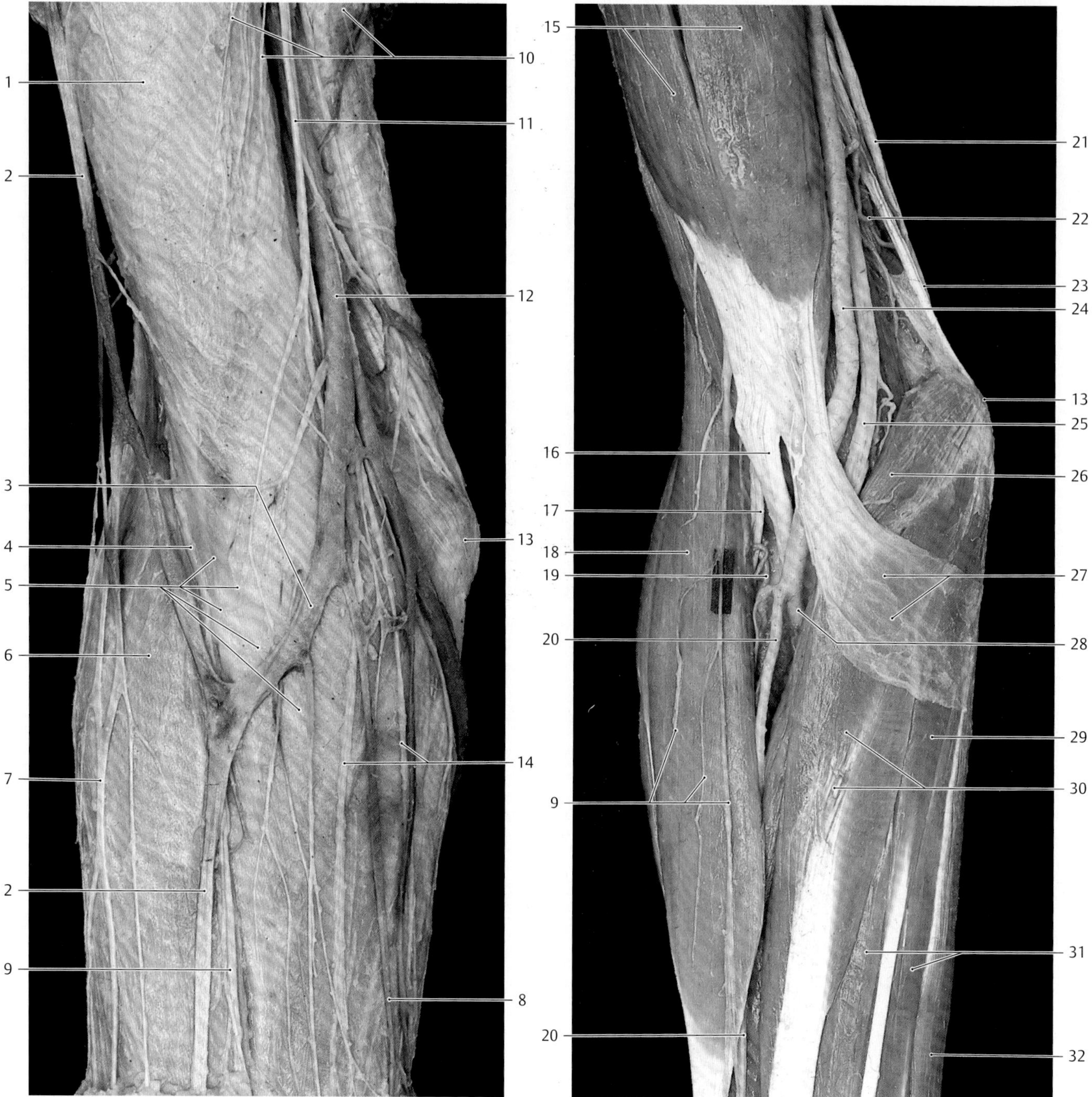


**Fig. 3.116 Cubital region** (anterior aspect). Dissection of cutaneous nerves and veins.

**Fig. 3.117 Cubital region,** superficial layer (anterior aspect). The fasciae of the muscles have been removed.

1 Biceps brachii muscle with fascia
2 Cephalic vein
3 Median cubital vein
4 Lateral cutaneous nerve of forearm
5 Tendon and aponeurosis of biceps brachii muscle (covered by the antebrachial fascia)
6 Brachioradialis muscle with fascia
7 Accessory cephalic vein
8 Median vein of forearm
9 Branches of lateral cutaneous nerve of forearm
10 Terminal branches of medial cutaneous nerve of arm
11 Medial cutaneous nerve of forearm
12 Basilic vein
13 Medial epicondyle of humerus
14 Terminal branches of medial cutaneous nerve of forearm
15 Biceps brachii muscle
16 Tendon of biceps brachii muscle
17 Radial nerve
18 Brachioradialis muscle
19 Radial recurrent artery
20 Radial artery
21 Ulnar nerve
22 Superior ulnar collateral artery
23 Medial intermuscular septum
24 Brachial artery
25 Median nerve
26 Pronator teres muscle
27 Bicipital aponeurosis
28 Ulnar artery
29 Palmaris longus muscle
30 Flexor carpi radialis muscle
31 Flexor digitorum superficialis muscle
32 Flexor carpi ulnaris muscle

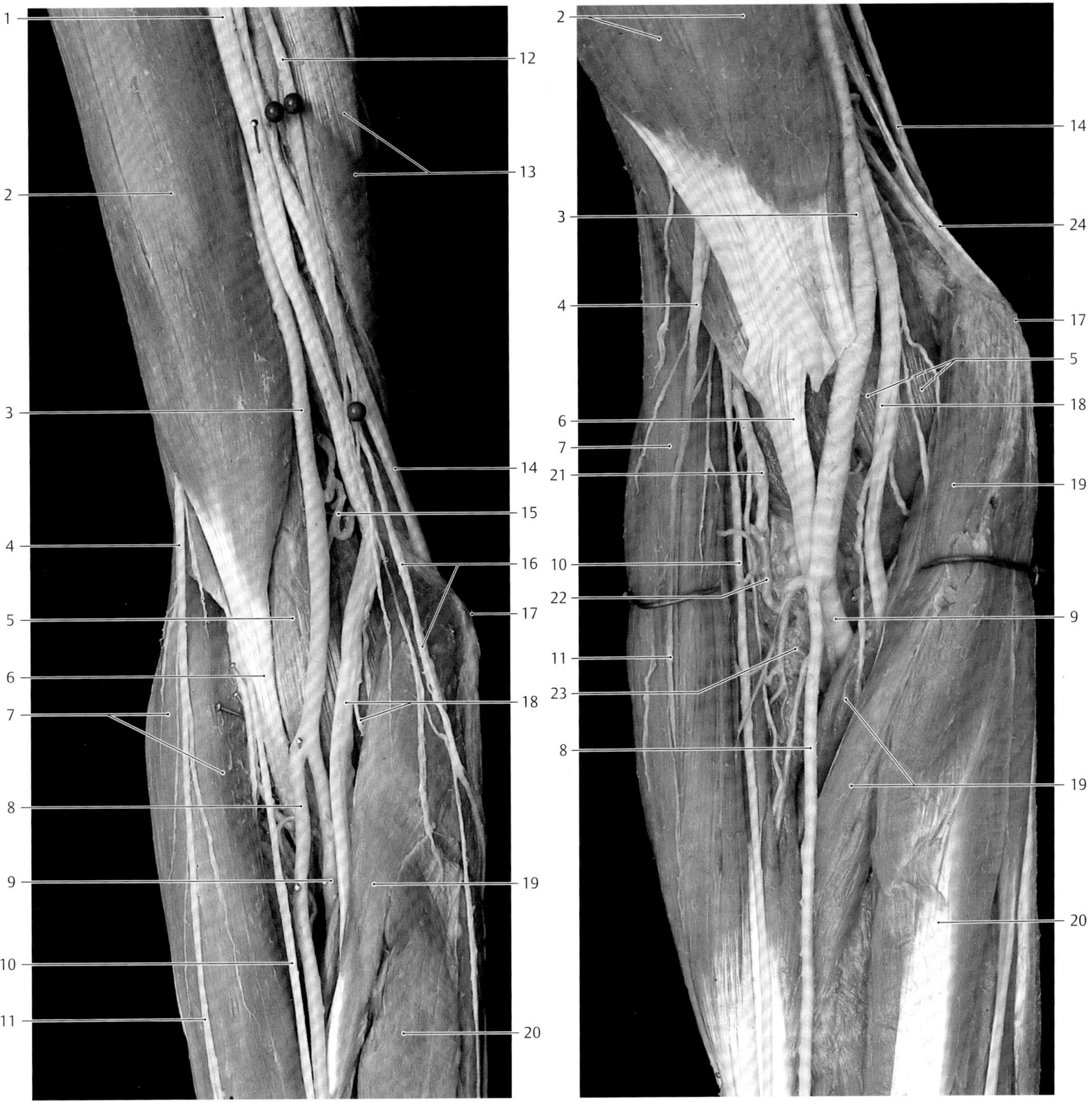


**Fig. 3.118 Cubital region,** middle layer (anterior aspect). The bicipital aponeurosis has been removed.

**Fig. 3.119 Cubital region,** middle layer (anterior aspect). Pronator teres and brachioradialis muscles have been slightly reflected.

1 Median nerve
2 Biceps brachii muscle
3 Brachial artery
4 Lateral cutaneous nerve of forearm (terminal branch of musculocutaneous nerve)
5 Brachialis muscle
6 Tendon of biceps brachii muscle
7 Brachioradialis muscle
8 Radial artery
9 Ulnar artery
10 Superficial branch of radial nerve
11 Lateral cutaneous nerve of forearm
12 Medial cutaneous nerve of forearm
13 Triceps brachii muscle
14 Ulnar nerve
15 Inferior ulnar collateral artery
16 Anterior branch of medial cutaneous nerve of forearm
17 Medial epicondyle of humerus
18 Median nerve with branches to pronator teres muscle
19 Pronator teres muscle
20 Flexor carpi radialis muscle
21 Deep branch of radial nerve
22 Radial recurrent artery
23 Supinator muscle
24 Medial intermuscular septum of arm

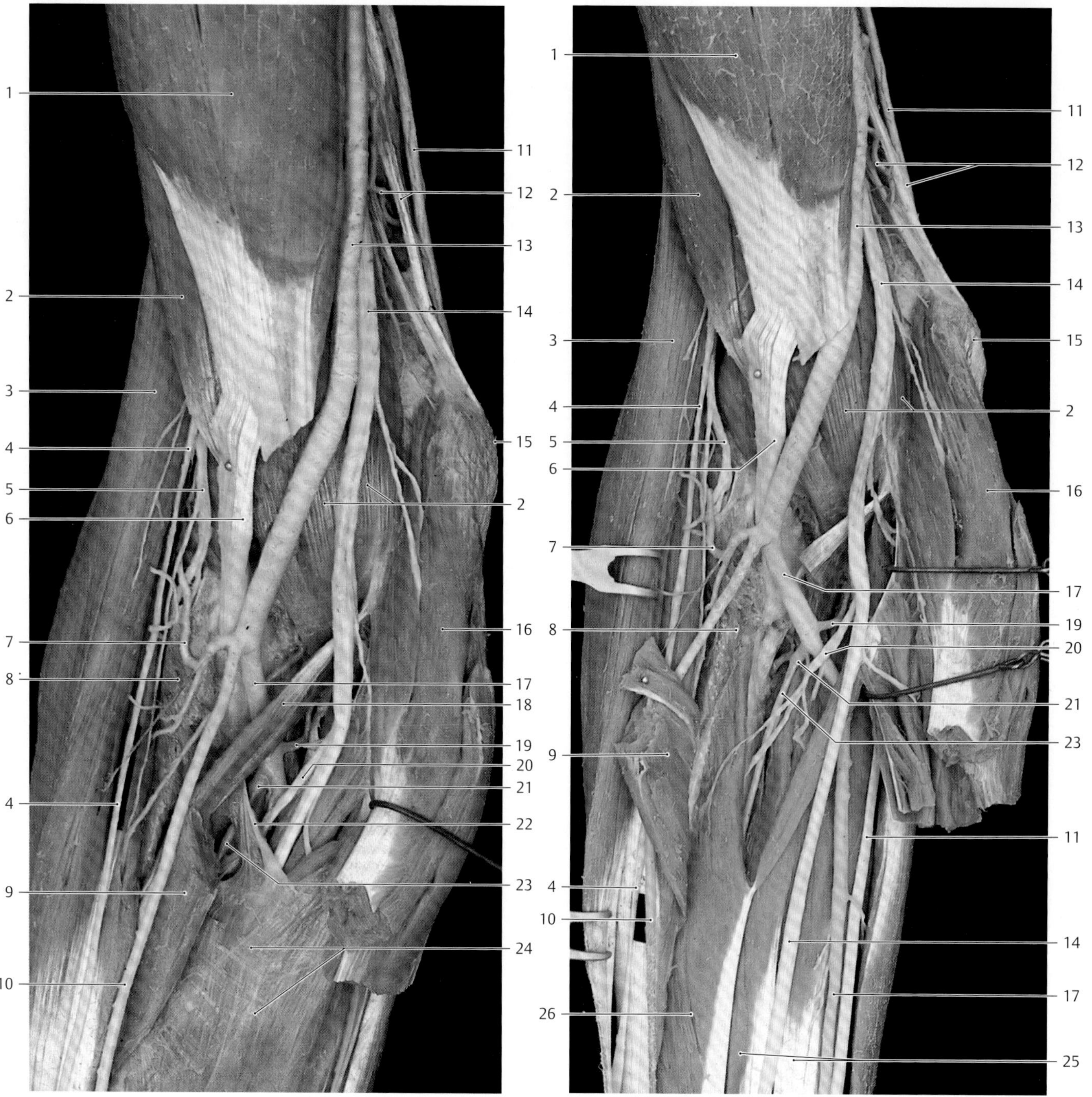


Fig. 3.120 **Cubital region,** deep layer (anterior aspect). Pronator teres and flexor carpi ulnaris muscles have been cut and reflected.

Fig. 3.121 **Cubital region,** deepest layer (anterior aspect). Flexor digitorum superficialis muscle and the ulnar head of the pronator teres muscle have been cut and reflected.

1 Biceps brachii muscle
2 Brachialis muscle
3 Brachioradialis muscle
4 Superficial branch of radial nerve
5 Deep branch of radial nerve
6 Tendon of biceps brachii muscle
7 Radial recurrent artery
8 Supinator muscle
9 Insertion of pronator teres muscle
10 Radial artery
11 Ulnar nerve
12 Medial intermuscular septum of arm and superior ulnar collateral artery
13 Brachial artery
14 Median nerve
15 Medial epicondyle of humerus
16 Humeral head of pronator teres muscle
17 Ulnar artery
18 Ulnar head of pronator teres muscle
19 Ulnar recurrent artery
20 Anterior interosseous nerve
21 Common interosseous artery
22 Tendinous arch of flexor digitorum superficialis muscle (radial head)
23 Anterior interosseous artery
24 Flexor digitorum superficialis muscle
25 Flexor digitorum profundus muscle
26 Flexor pollicis longus muscle

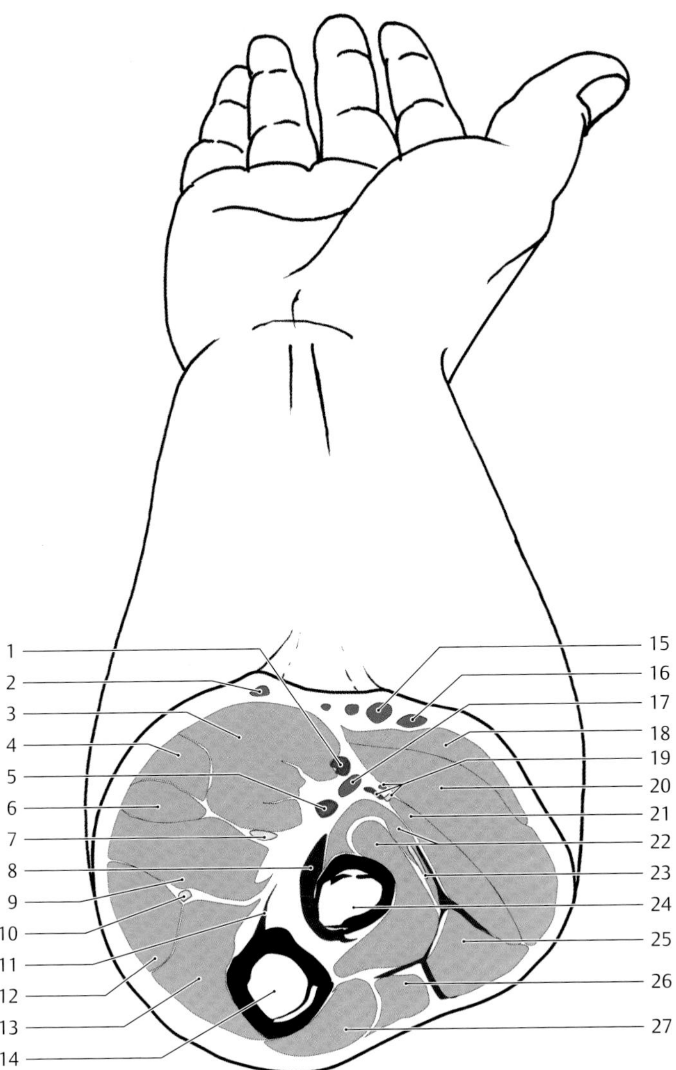


1 Radial artery
2 Basilic vein
3 Pronator teres muscle
4 Flexor carpi radialis muscle
5 Ulnar artery
6 Palmaris longus muscle
7 Median nerve
8 Tendon of biceps brachii muscle
9 Flexor digitorum superficialis muscle
10 Ulnar nerve
11 Tendon of brachialis muscle
12 Flexor carpi ulnaris muscle
13 Flexor digitorum profundus muscle
14 Ulna
15 Median cubital vein
16 Cephalic antebrachii vein
17 Radial vein
18 Brachioradialis muscle
19 Superficial branch of radial nerve, radial artery and vein
20 Extensor carpi radialis longus muscle
21 Extensor carpi radialis brevis muscle
22 Supinator muscle
23 Deep branch of radial nerve
24 Radius
25 Extensor digitorum muscle
26 Extensor carpi ulnaris muscle
27 Anconeus muscle

Fig. 3.122 **Axial section through the forearm** distally of the elbow joint revealing the arrangement of muscles, nerves, and vessels (compare with the MRI scan below).

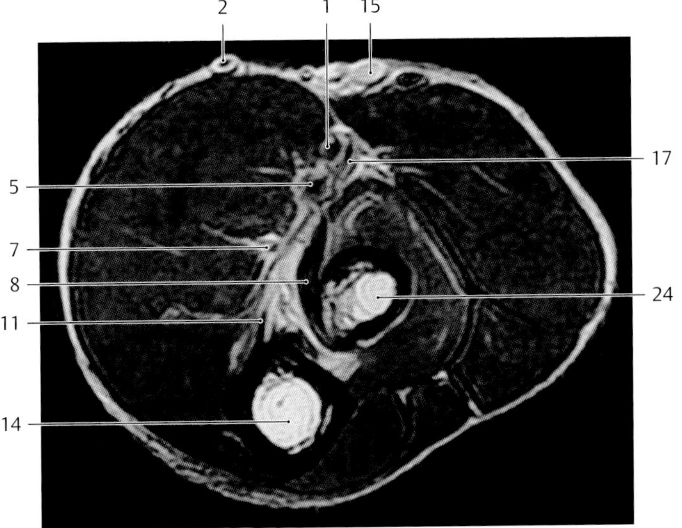


Fig. 3.123 **Axial section through the forearm** distally of the elbow joint (MRI scan; for details see schematic drawing above). (Heuck A, et al. MRT-Atlas des muskuloskelettalen Systems. Stuttgart, Germany: Schattauer, 2009.)

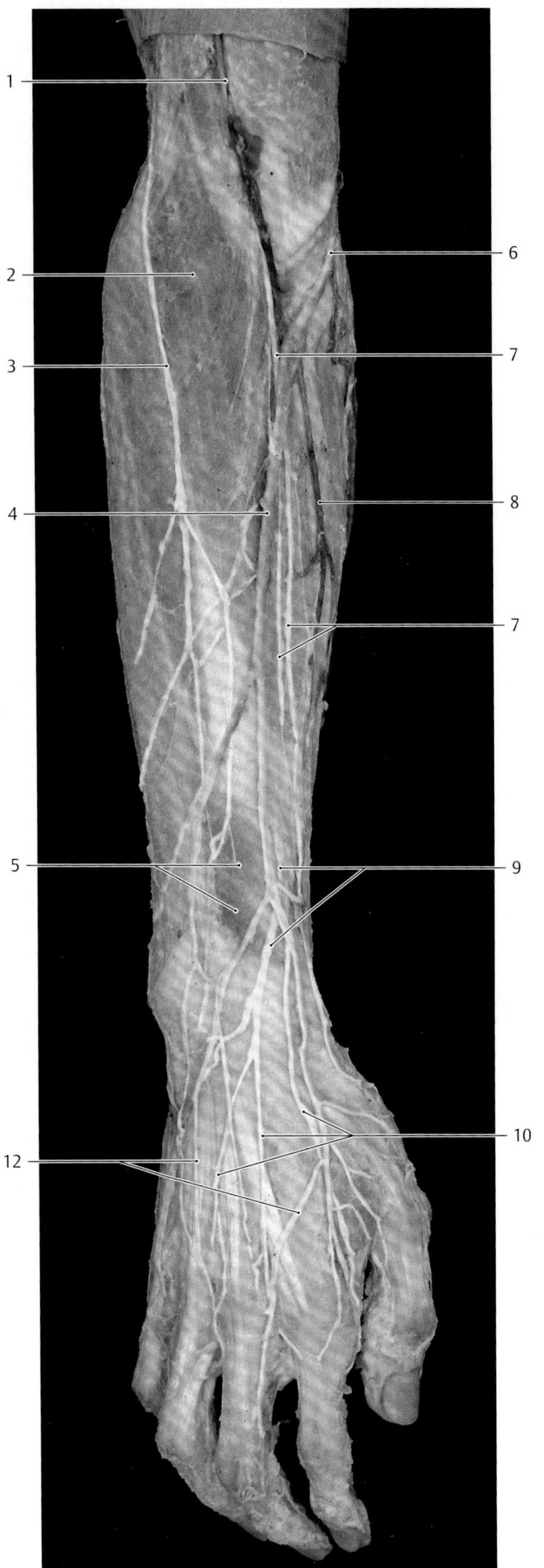


Fig. 3.124 **Posterior regions of forearm and hand** with superficial veins and cutaneous nerves (right side).

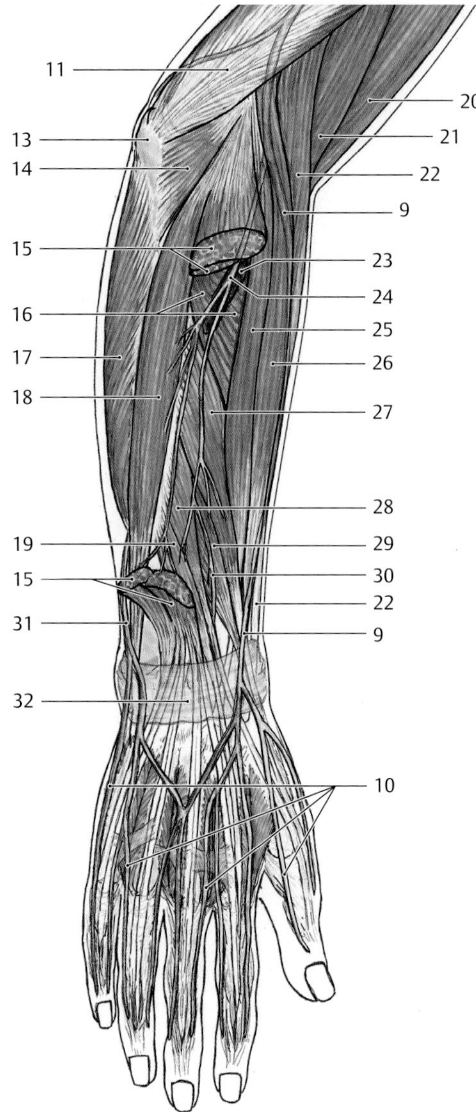


Fig. 3.125 **Course of the nerves to forearm and hand** (posterior aspect). Yellow = radial and ulnar nerves.

1 Cephalic vein
2 Brachioradialis muscle covered by its fascia
3 Posterior cutaneous nerve of forearm (branch of radial nerve)
4 Cephalic vein of forearm
5 Extensor pollicis longus and brevis muscles covered by their fascia
6 Median cubital vein
7 Lateral cutaneous nerves of forearm (branch of musculo-cutaneous nerve)
8 Intermedian vein of forearm
9 Superficial branch of radial nerve
10 Dorsal digital branches of radial nerve
11 Triceps brachii muscle
12 Dorsal venous network of hand
13 Olecranon
14 Anconeus muscle
15 Extensor digitorum and extensor digiti minimi muscles
16 Supinator muscle
17 Flexor carpi ulnaris muscle
18 Extensor carpi ulnaris muscle
19 Extensor indicis muscle
20 Biceps brachii muscle
21 Brachialis muscle
22 Brachioradialis muscle
23 Supinator channel
24 Deep branch of radial nerve
25 Extensor carpi radialis brevis muscle
26 Extensor carpi radialis longus muscle
27 Abductor pollicis longus muscle
28 Extensor pollicis longus muscle
29 Extensor pollicis brevis muscle
30 Posterior interosseus nerve
31 Ulnar nerve
32 Extensor retinaculum

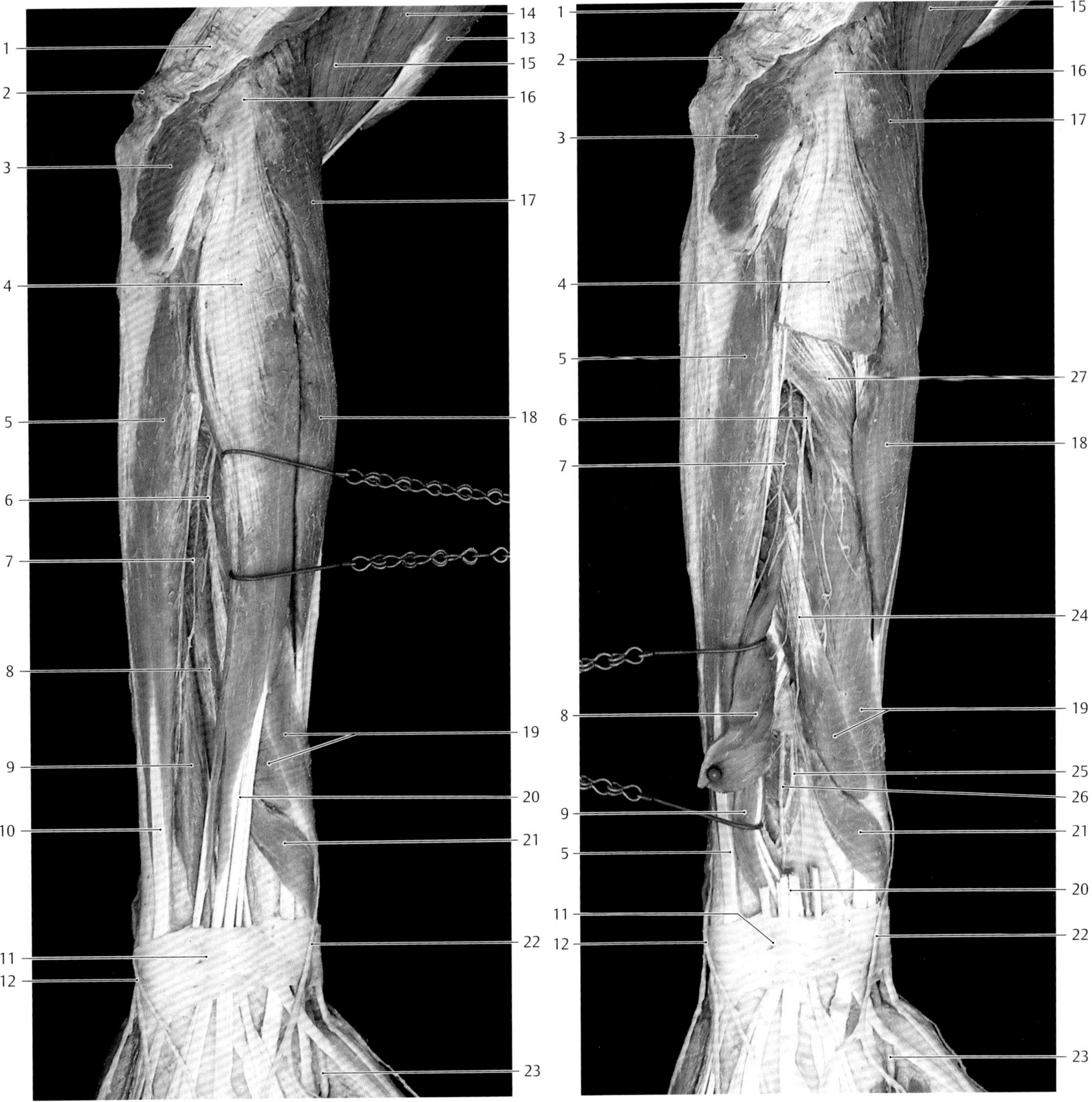


**Fig. 3.126 Posterior region of the forearm** with vessels and nerves, superficial layer (right side).

**Fig. 3.127 Posterior region of the forearm** with vessels and nerves, deep layer (right side).

1 Tendon of triceps brachii muscle
2 Olecranon
3 Anconeus muscle
4 Extensor digitorum muscle
5 Extensor carpi ulnaris muscle
6 Deep branch of radial nerve
7 Posterior interosseous artery
8 Extensor pollicis longus muscle
9 Extensor indicis muscle
10 Tendon of extensor carpi ulnaris muscle
11 Extensor retinaculum
12 Dorsal branch of ulnar nerve
13 Biceps brachii muscle
14 Brachialis muscle
15 Brachioradialis muscle
16 Lateral epicondyle of humerus
17 Extensor carpi radialis longus muscle
18 Extensor carpi radialis brevis muscle
19 Abductor pollicis longus muscle
20 Tendons of extensor digitorum muscle
21 Extensor pollicis brevis muscle
22 Superficial branch of radial nerve
23 Radial artery
24 Posterior interosseous nerve
25 Posterior interosseous branch of radial nerve
26 Posterior branch of anterior interosseous artery
27 Supinator muscle

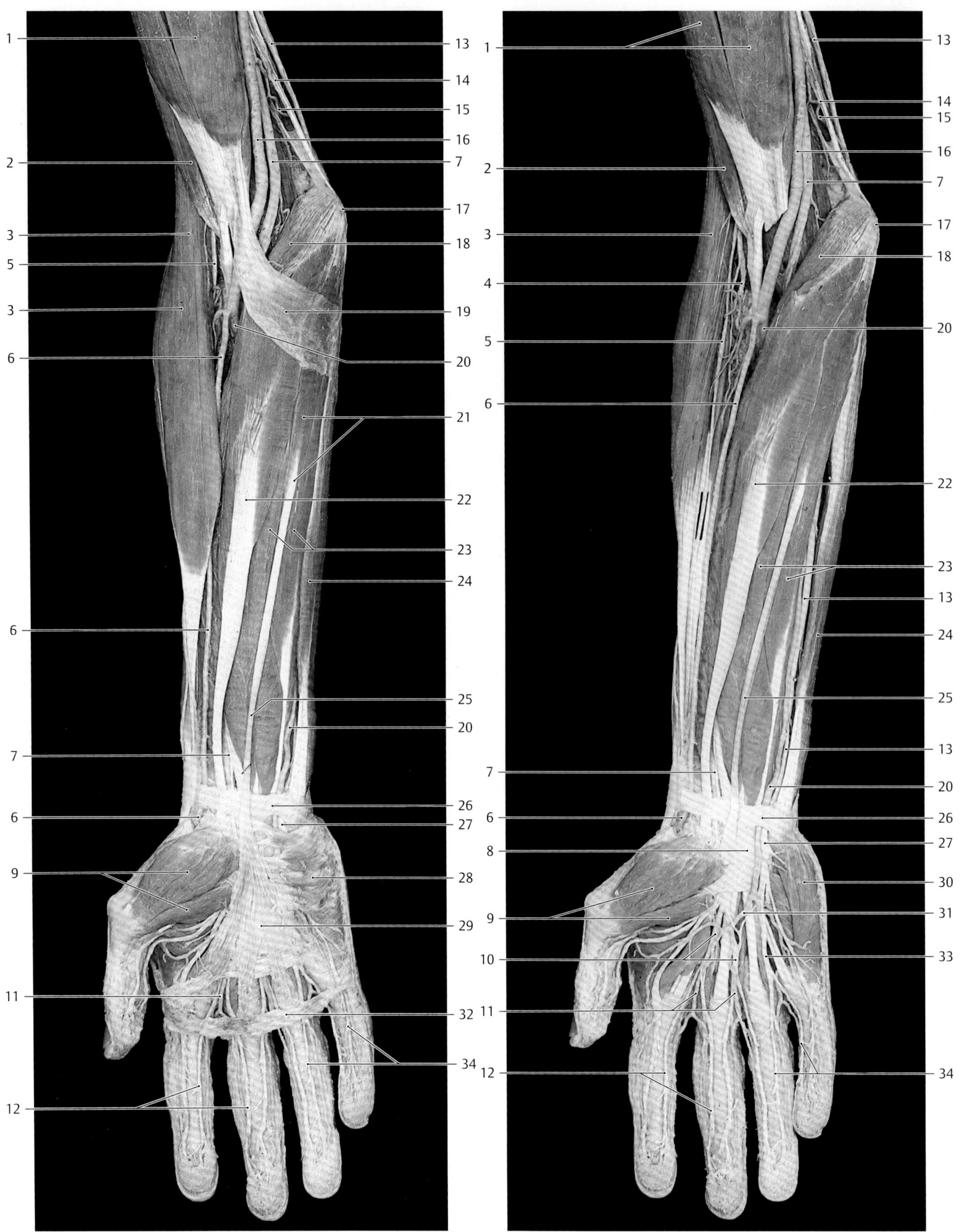


Fig. 3.128 **Anterior regions of forearm and hand** with vessels and nerves, superficial layer (right side).

Fig. 3.129 **Anterior regions of forearm and hand** with vessels and nerves, superficial layer (right side). The palmar aponeurosis of the hand and the bicipital aponeurosis have been removed.

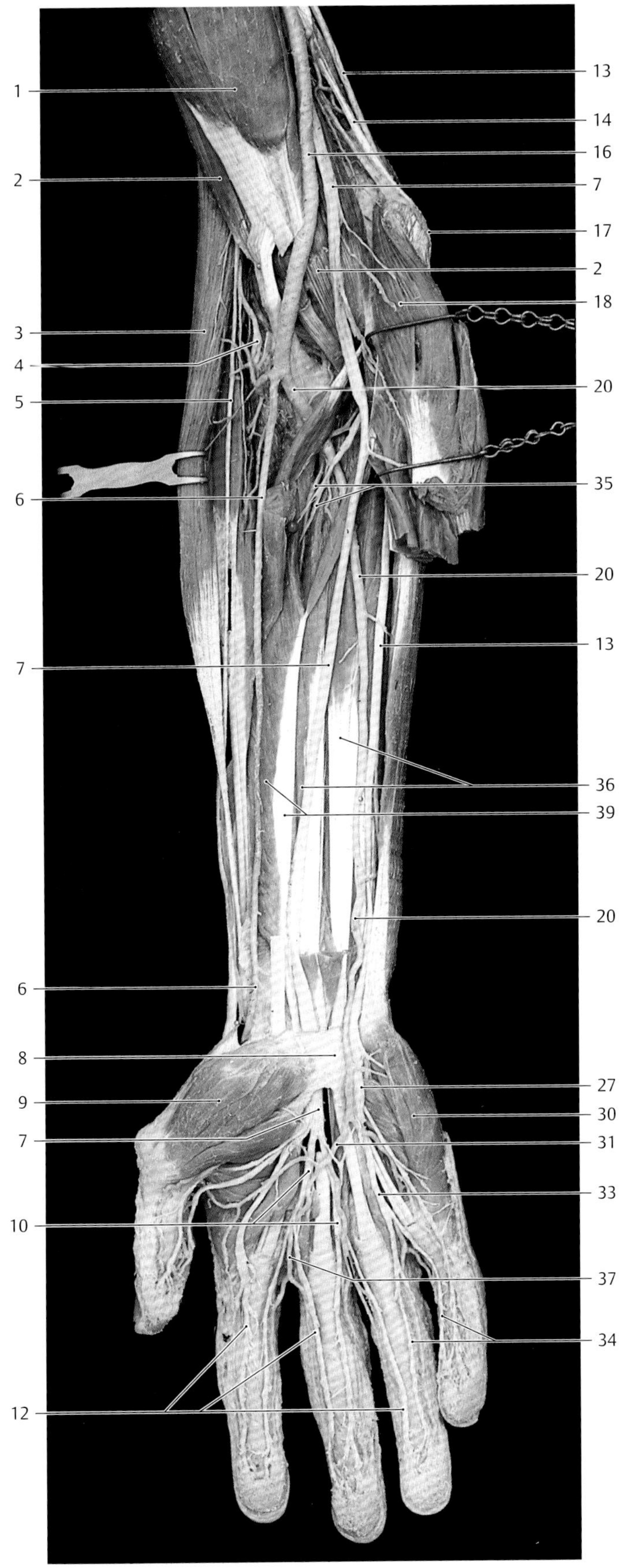

1 Biceps brachii muscle
2 Brachialis muscle
3 Brachioradialis muscle
4 Deep branch of radial nerve
5 Superficial branch of radial nerve
6 Radial artery
7 Median nerve
8 Flexor retinaculum
9 Thenar muscles
10 Common palmar digital nerves of median nerve
11 Common palmar digital arteries
12 Proper palmar digital nerves of median nerve
13 Ulnar nerve
14 Medial intermuscular septum of arm
15 Superior ulnar collateral artery
16 Brachial artery
17 Medial epicondyle of humerus
18 Pronator teres muscle
19 Bicipital aponeurosis
20 Ulnar artery
21 Palmaris longus muscle
22 Flexor carpi radialis muscle
23 Flexor digitorum superficialis muscle
24 Flexor carpi ulnaris muscle
25 Tendon of palmaris longus muscle
26 Remnant of antebrachial fascia (palmar ligament)
27 Superficial branch of ulnar nerve
28 Palmaris brevis muscle
29 Palmar aponeurosis
30 Hypothenar muscles
31 Superficial palmar arch
32 Superficial transverse metacarpal ligament
33 Common palmar digital branch of ulnar nerve
34 Proper palmar digital branches of ulnar nerve
35 Anterior interosseous artery and nerve
36 Flexor digitorum profundus muscle
37 Common palmar digital arteries
38 Palmar branch of median nerve
39 Flexor pollicis longus muscle
40 Palmar cutaneous branch of ulnar nerve

**Fig. 3.130 Anterior regions of forearm and hand** with vessels and nerves, deep layer (right side). The superficial layer of the flexor muscles has been removed.

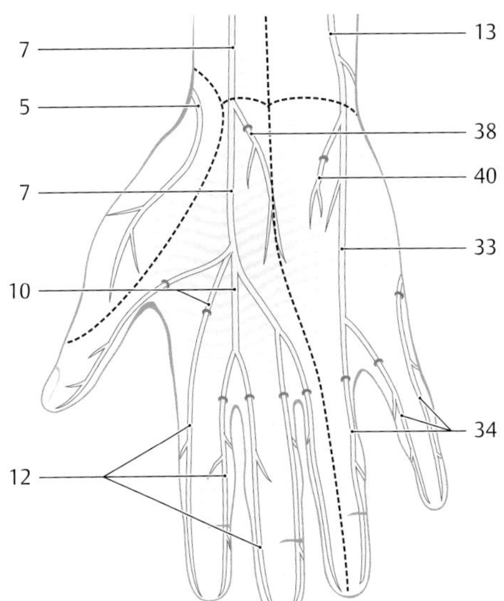


**Fig. 3.131 Innervation pattern of the hand** (palmar aspect). 3½ digits by median nerve; 1½ digits by ulnar nerve.

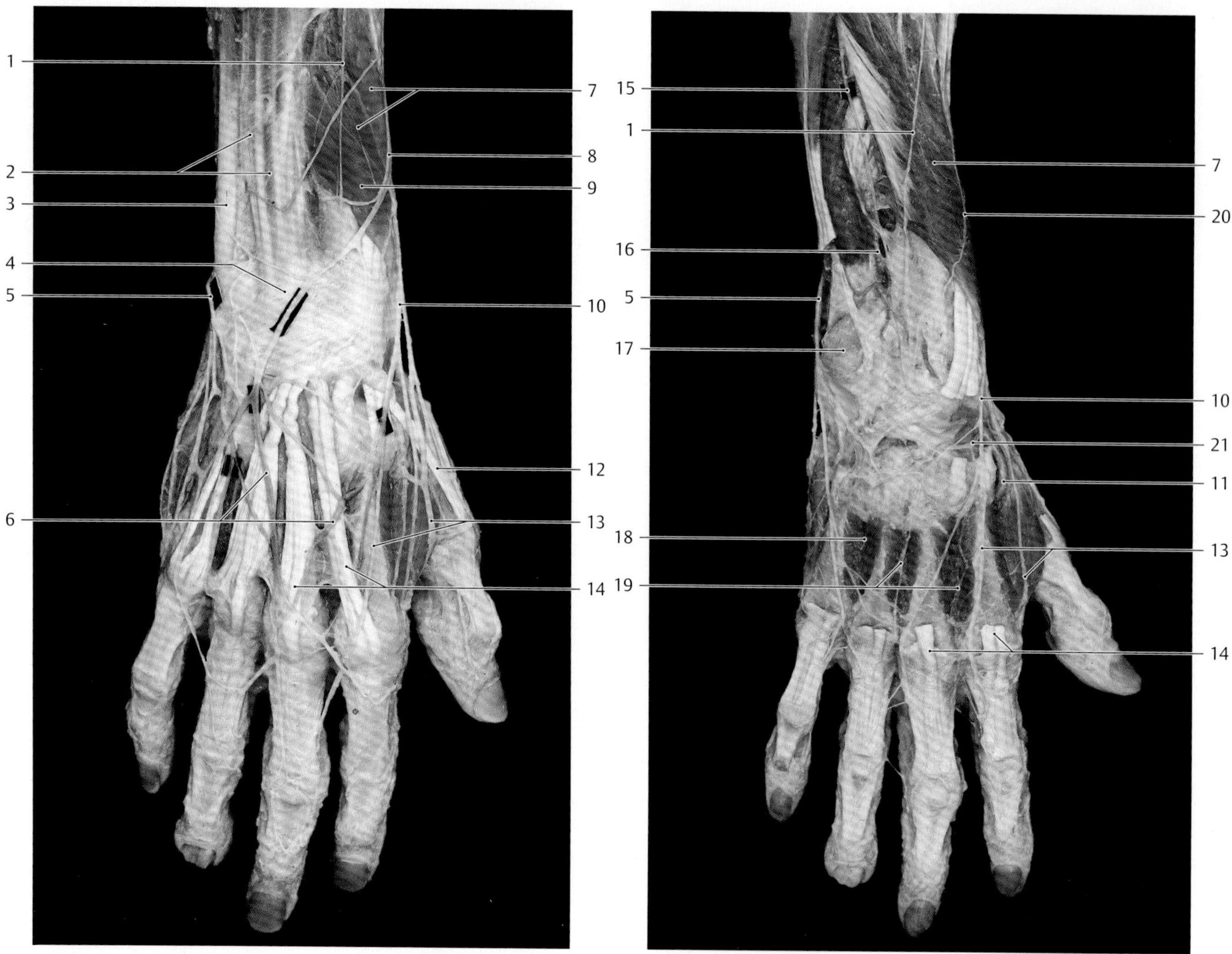


Fig. 3.132 **Dorsum of the right hand,** superficial layer. Cutaneous nerves and veins are depicted.

Fig. 3.133 **Dorsum of the right hand,** deeper layer. Extensor digitorum muscle has been partly removed.

Fig. 3.134 **Innervation pattern of the hand** (dorsal aspect). 2½ digits by radial nerve; 2½ digits by ulnar nerve. Note that the terminal branches to the dorsal surfaces of the distal phalanges are derived from the palmar digital nerves. The cutaneous distribution varies; often 3½ digits are innervated by the radial and 1½ digits by the ulnar nerve.

1 Posterior cutaneous nerve of forearm (branch of radial nerve)
2 Extensor digitorum muscle
3 Tendon of extensor carpi ulnaris muscle
4 Extensor retinaculum
5 Ulnar nerve
6 Dorsal venous network of hand
7 Abductor pollicis brevis muscle
8 Cephalic vein
9 Extensor pollicis brevis muscle
10 Superficial branch of radial nerve
11 Radial artery
12 Tendon of extensor pollicis longus muscle
13 Dorsal digital branches of radial nerve
14 Tendons of extensor digitorum muscle with intertendinous connections
15 Posterior interosseus nerve (branch of the deep radial nerve)
16 Posterior interosseous artery
17 Styloid process of ulna
18 Dorsal interosseus muscle
19 Dorsal carpal branch of radial artery
20 Lateral cutaneous nerve of forearm (branch of musculocutaneous nerve)
21 Dorsal metacarpal artery
22 Dorsal digital branches of ulnar nerve
23 Regions supplied by palmar digital nerves (ulnar nerve)
24 Regions supplied by palmar digital nerves (median nerve)
25 Communicating branch with ulnar nerve

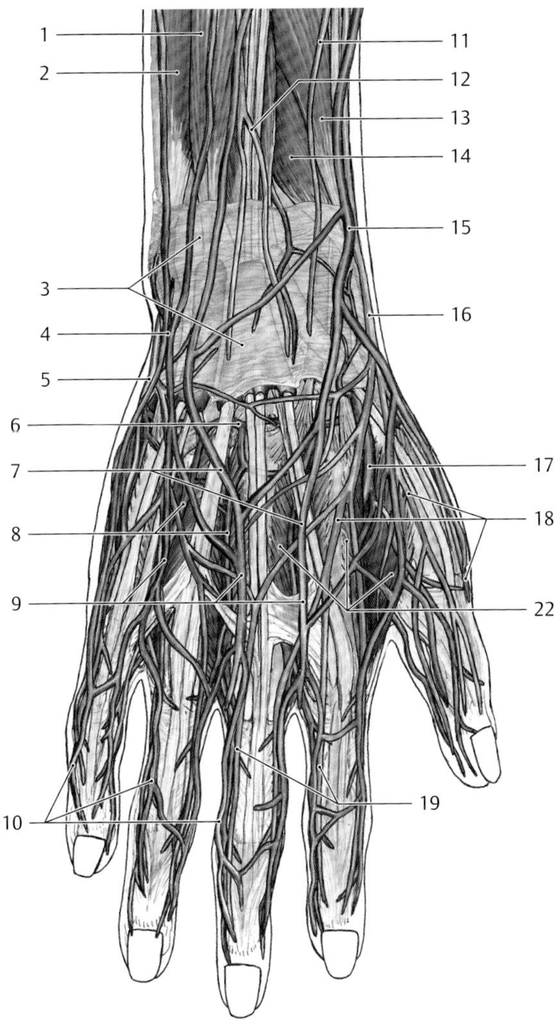


Fig. 3.135 **Dorsum of the right hand,** superficial layer. Cutaneous veins, nerves, and arteries are depicted. The dorsal fascia of the hand has been removed.

1 Extensor digiti minimi muscle
2 Extensor carpi ulnaris muscle
3 Extensor retinaculum
4 Basilic vein
5 Dorsal branch of ulnar nerve
6 Dorsal carpal branch of ulnar artery
7 Dorsal venous network of hand
8 Dorsal metacarpal arteries
9 Dorsal metacarpal veins
10 Dorsal digital veins
11 Lateral cutaneous nerve of forearm
12 Posterior cutaneous nerve of forearm
13 Abductor pollicis longus muscle
14 Abductor pollicis brevis muscle
15 Cephalic vein
16 Superficial branch of radial nerve
17 Radial artery
18 Dorsal digital branches of radial nerve
19 Dorsal digital nerves for the fingers
20 Hamate bone
21 Capitate bone
22 Dorsal interossei muscles
23 Collateral ligament
24 Proximal phalanges II–V
25 Middle phalanges II–V
26 Distal phalanges IV and V
27 Os trapezoideum
28 Metacarpal bones II–IV
29 Opponens pollicis muscle
30 Second metacarpophalangeal joint
31 Proper palmar digital artery

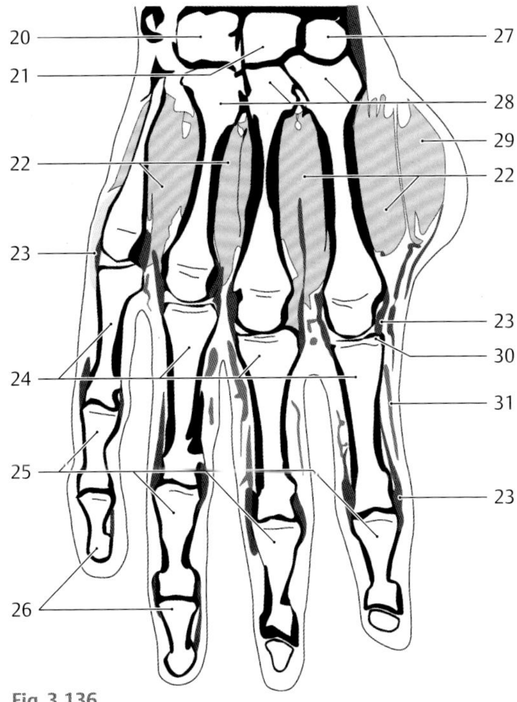


Fig. 3.136

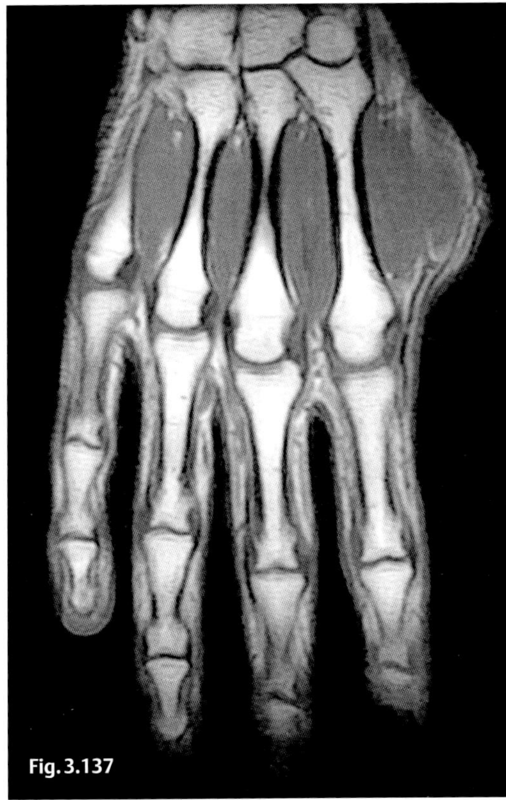


Figs. 3.136 and 3.137 **Coronal section through the right hand** (dorsal aspect; schematic and MRI scan respectively). (Heuck A, et al. MRT-Atlas des muskuloskelettalen Systems. Stuttgart, Germany: Schattauer, 2009.)

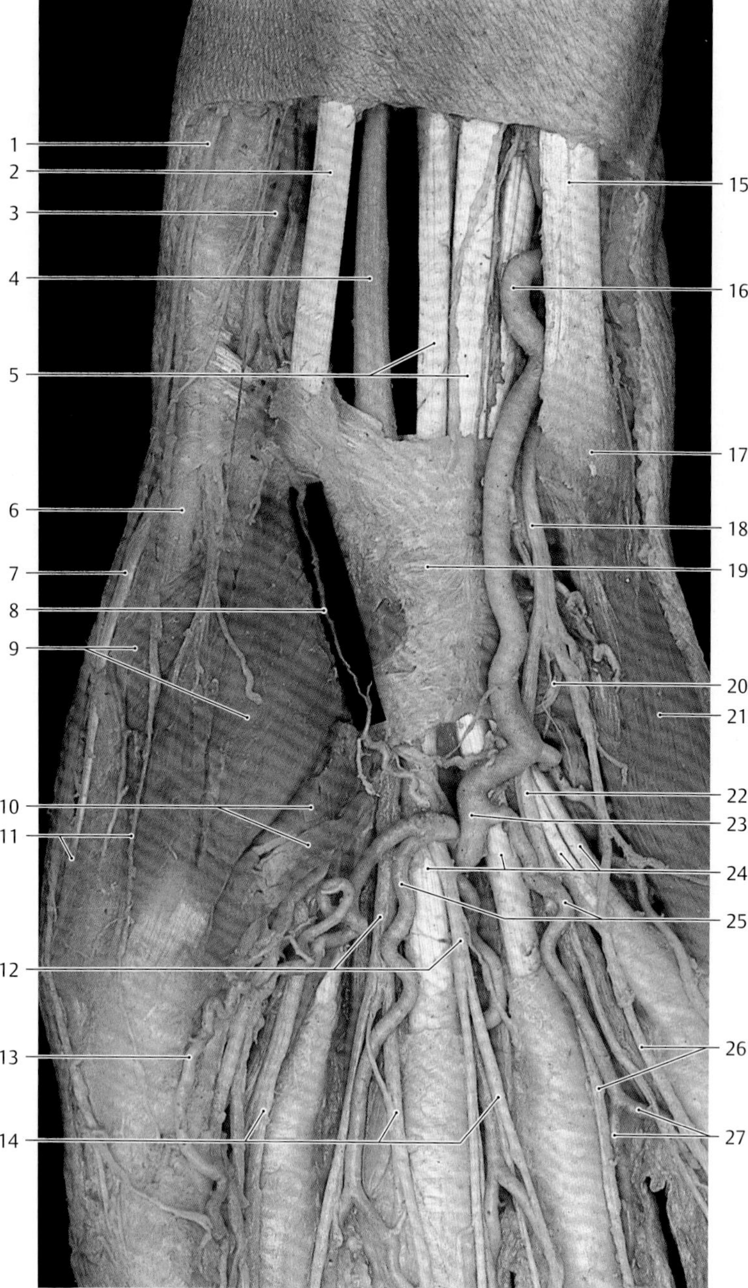


Fig. 3.138 **Anterior region of wrist and palm of the right hand,** superficial layer. Dissection of the superficial palmar arch.

1 Superficial branch of radial nerve
2 Tendon of flexor carpi radialis muscle
3 Radial artery
4 Median nerve
5 Tendon of flexor digitorum superficialis muscle
6 Tendon of abductor pollicis longus muscle
7 Tendon of extensor pollicis brevis muscle
8 Superficial palmar branch of radial artery
9 Abductor pollicis brevis muscle
10 Superficial head of flexor pollicis brevis muscle
11 Terminal branches of superficial branch of radial nerve
12 Common palmar digital nerves (median nerve)
13 Proper palmar digital arteries of thumb
14 Proper palmar digital nerves (median nerve)
15 Tendon of flexor carpi ulnaris muscle
16 Ulnar artery
17 Position of pisiform bone
18 Superficial branch of ulnar nerve
19 Flexor retinaculum
20 Deep branch of ulnar nerve
21 Abductor digiti minimi muscle
22 Common palmar digital nerve (ulnar nerve)
23 Superficial palmar arch
24 Tendons of flexor digitorum muscles
25 Common palmar digital arteries
26 Palmar digital nerves (ulnar nerve)
27 Proper palmar digital arteries
28 Carpal tunnel
29 Fibrous sheaths for the tendons of flexor digitorum muscles
30 Deep palmar arch
31 Princeps pollicis artery
32 Palmar branch of median nerve
33 Common digital palmar artery
34 Ulnar nerve
35 Capillary network of fingers
36 Dorsal branch of ulnar nerve

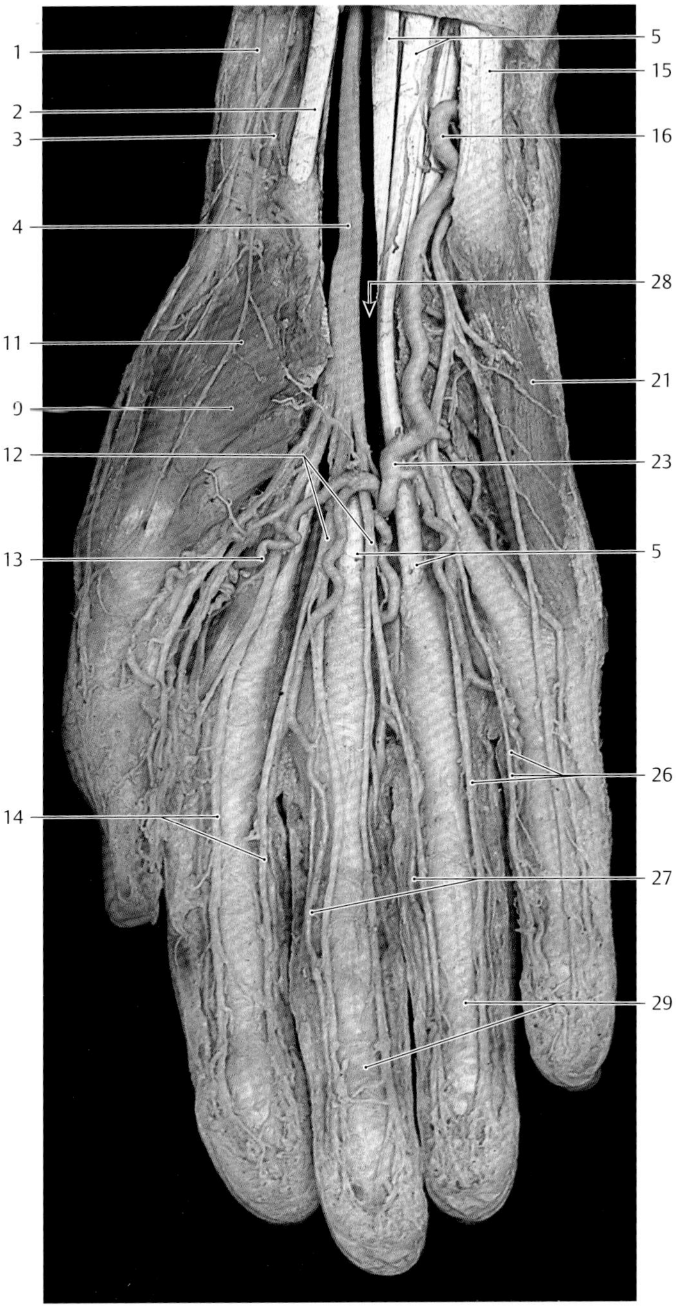

Fig. 3.139 **Palm of the right hand,** deeper layer. The flexor retinaculum has been removed.

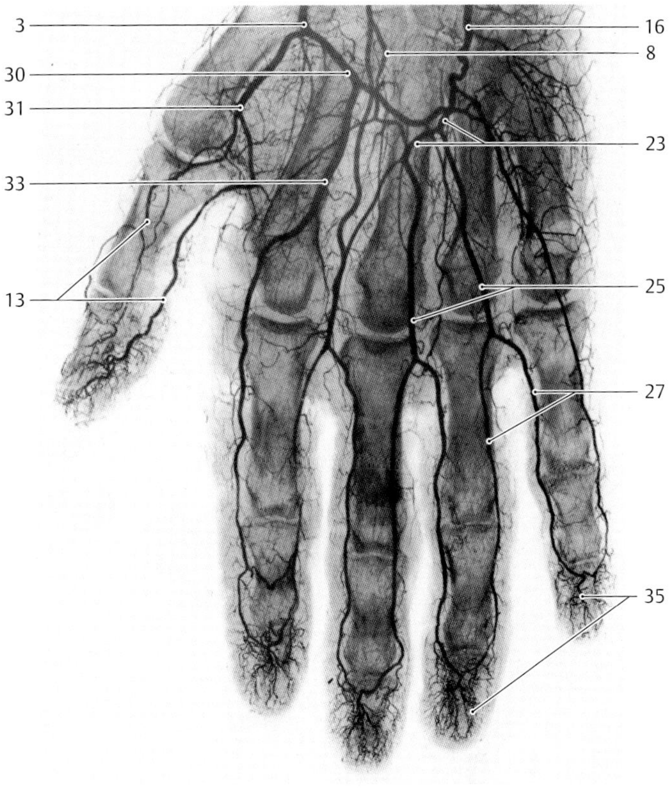

Fig. 3.140 **Arteriogram of the right hand** (palmar aspect).

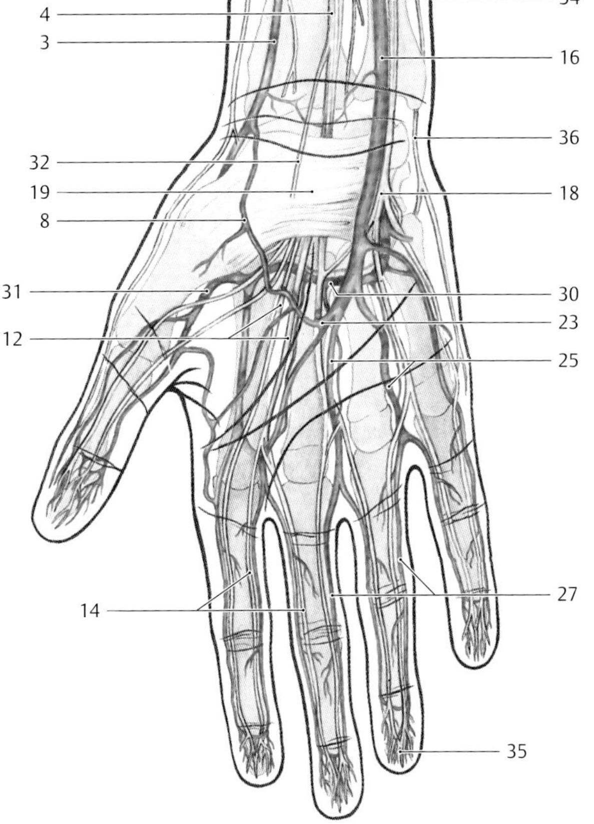


Fig. 3.141 **Palm of the right hand** with arteries and nerves.

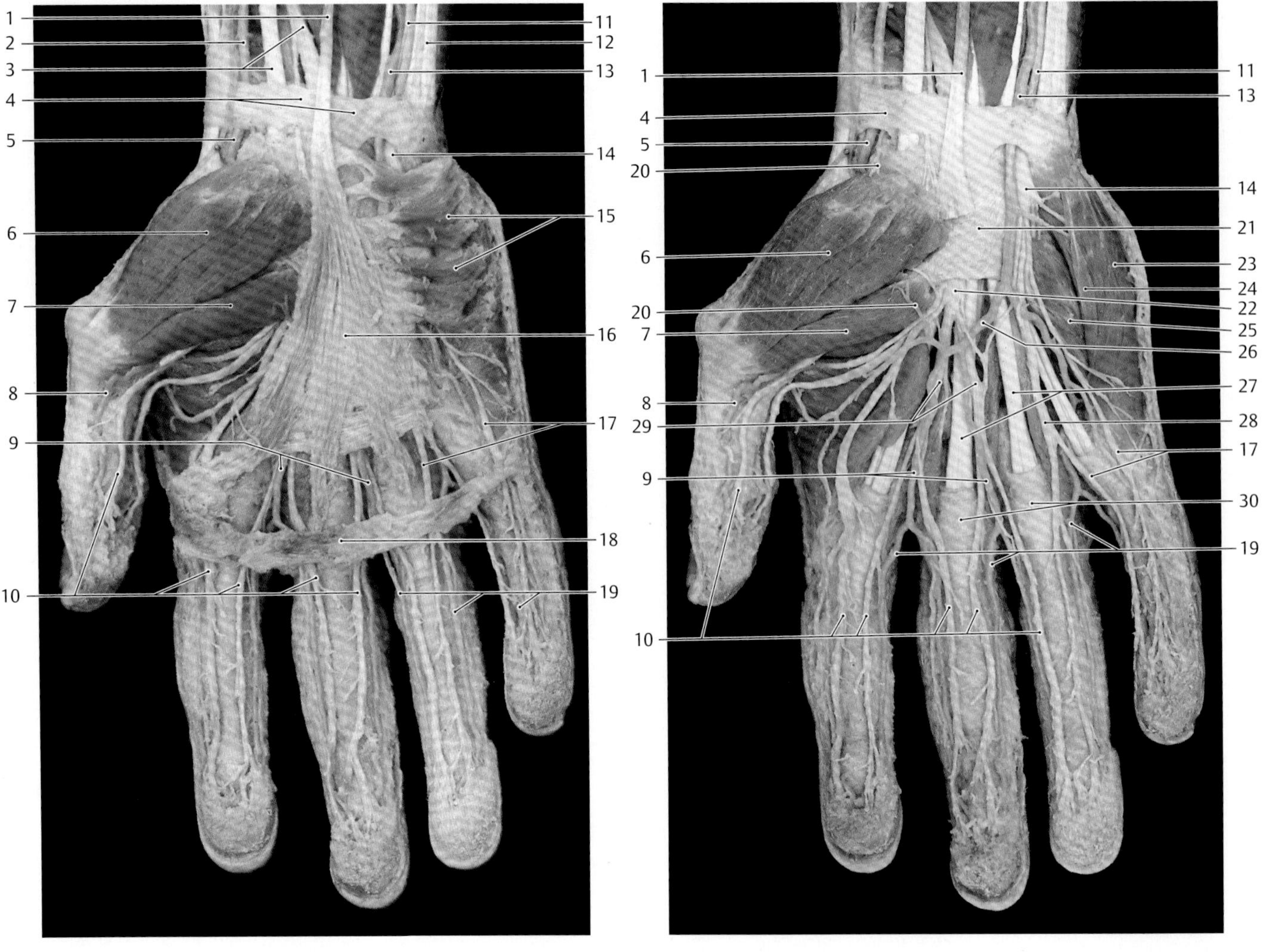


**Fig. 3.142 Palm of the right hand,** superficial layer. Dissection of vessels and nerves.

**Fig. 3.143 Palm of the right hand,** superficial layer. Dissection of vessels and nerves. The palmar aponeurosis has been removed to display the superficial palmar arch.

1 Tendon of palmaris longus muscle
2 Radial artery
3 Tendon of flexor carpi radialis muscle and median nerve
4 Distal part of antebrachial fascia
5 Radial artery passing into the anatomical snuffbox
6 Abductor pollicis brevis muscle
7 Superficial head of flexor pollicis brevis muscle
8 Palmar digital artery of thumb
9 Common palmar digital arteries
10 Proper palmar digital nerves (median nerve)
11 Ulnar nerve
12 Tendon of flexor carpi ulnaris muscle
13 Ulnar artery
14 Superficial branch of ulnar nerve
15 Palmaris brevis muscle
16 Palmar aponeurosis
17 Palmar digital nerves (ulnar nerve)
18 Superficial transverse metacarpal ligament
19 Proper palmar digital arteries
20 Superficial palmar branch of radial artery (contributing to the superficial palmar arch)
21 Flexor retinaculum
22 Median nerve
23 Abductor digiti minimi muscle
24 Flexor digiti minimi brevis muscle
25 Opponens digiti minimi muscle
26 Superficial palmar arch
27 Tendons of flexor digitorum superficialis muscle
28 Common palmar digital branch of ulnar nerve
29 Common palmar digital branches of median nerve
30 Fibrous sheaths of tendons of flexor muscles

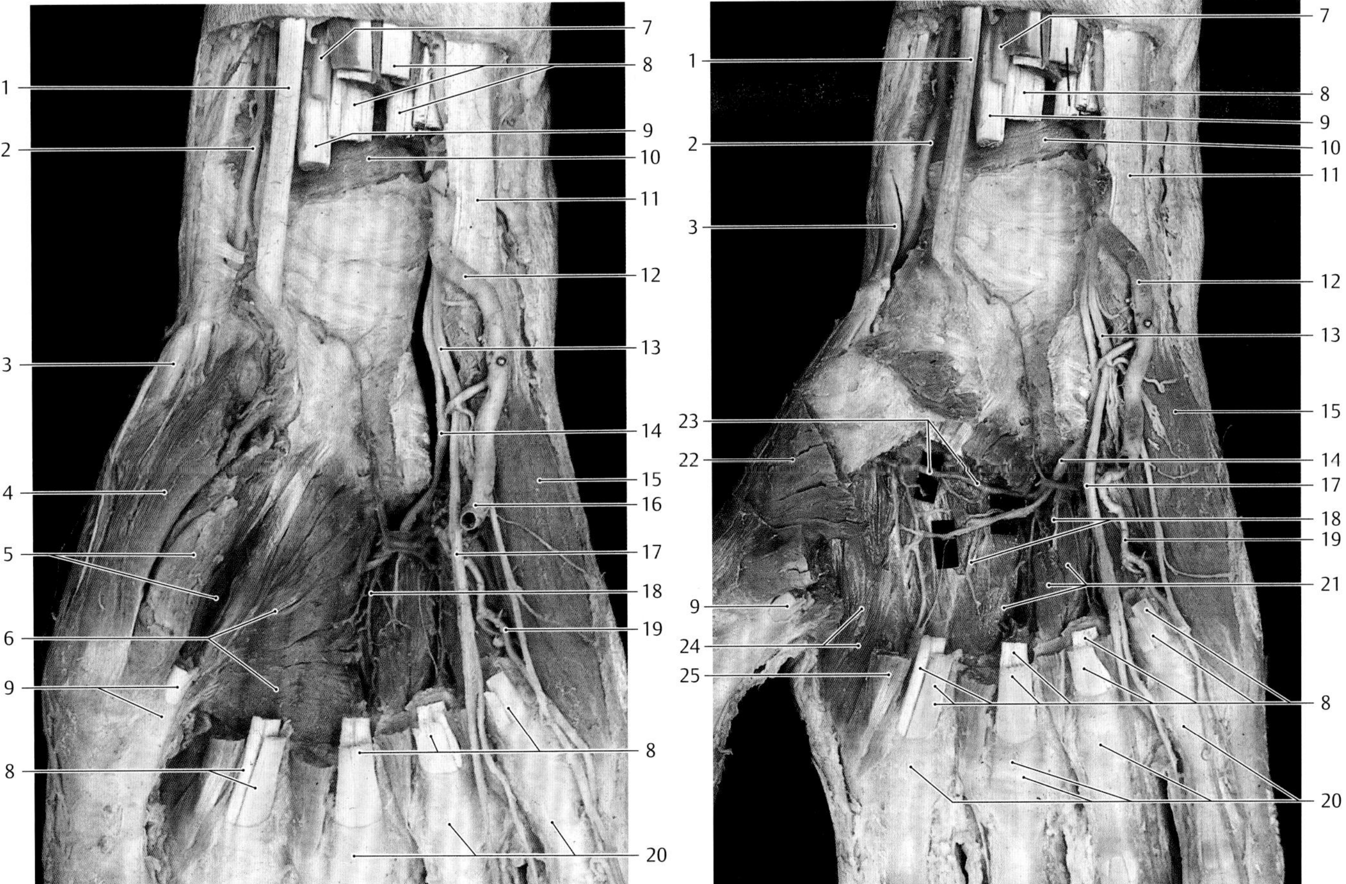


**Fig. 3.144 Anterior region of wrist and palm of the right hand,** deep layer. The carpal tunnel has been opened, the tendons of the flexor muscles have been removed, and the superficial palmar arch has been cut.

**Fig. 3.145 Anterior region of wrist and palm of the right hand,** deep layer. Dissection of the deep palmar arch.

1 Tendon of flexor carpi radialis muscle
2 Radial artery
3 Tendon of abductor pollicis longus muscle
4 Abductor pollicis brevis muscle
5 Superficial and deep heads of flexor pollicis brevis muscle
6 Oblique and transverse heads of adductor pollicis muscle
7 Median nerve
8 Tendons of flexor digitorum superficialis and profundus muscles
9 Tendon of flexor pollicis longus muscle
10 Pronator quadratus muscle
11 Tendon of flexor carpi ulnaris muscle
12 Ulnar artery
13 Superficial branch of ulnar nerve
14 Deep branch of ulnar nerve
15 Abductor digiti minimi muscle
16 Superficial palmar arch (cut end)
17 Common palmar digital nerve (ulnar nerve)
18 Palmar metacarpal arteries of deep palmar arch
19 Palmar digital artery of the fifth finger
20 Fibrous sheaths of tendons of flexor muscles
21 Palmar interossei muscles
22 Opponens pollicis muscle (cut)
23 Deep palmar arch
24 First dorsal interosseous muscle
25 First lumbrical muscle

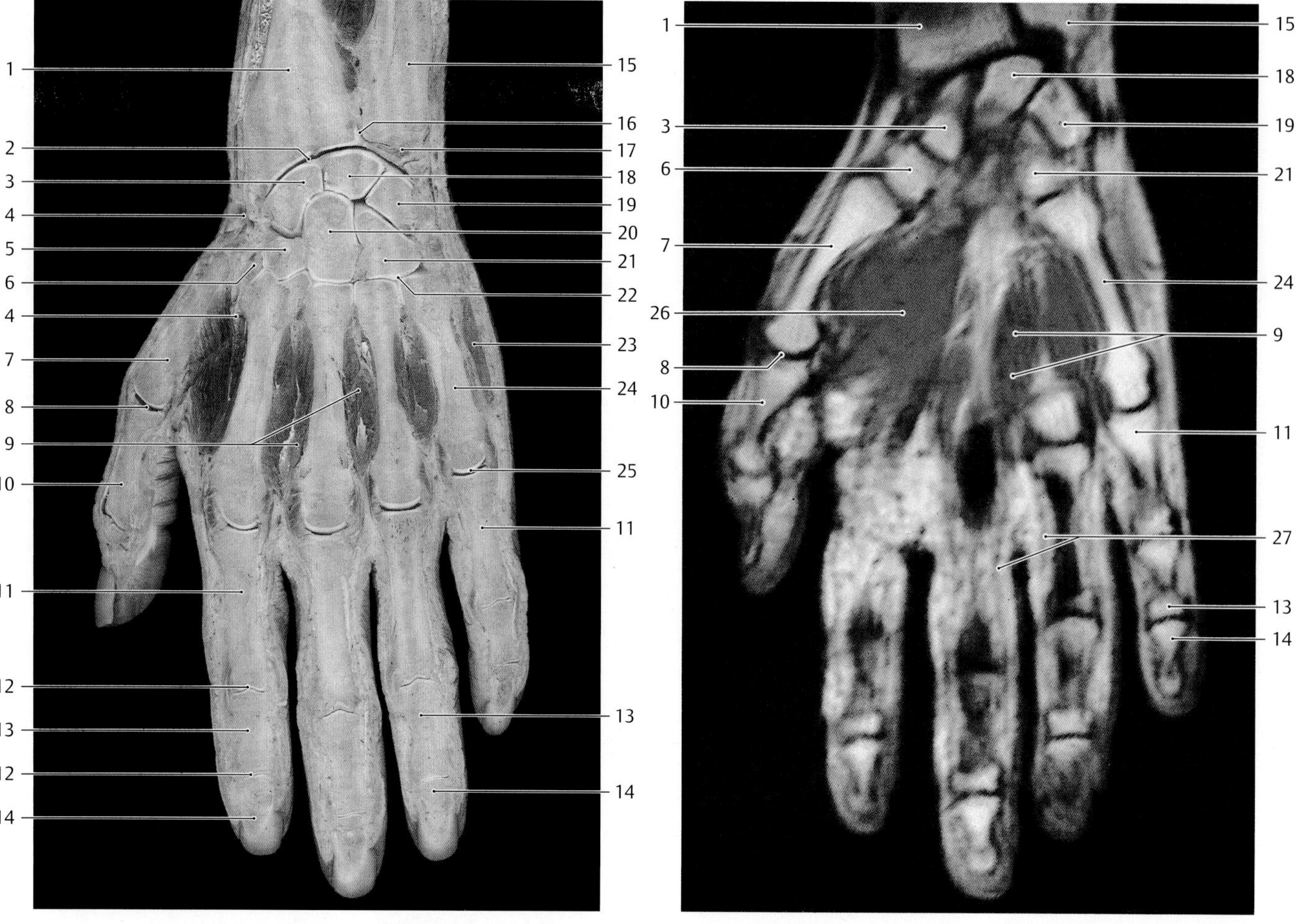

**Fig. 3.146 Coronal section through the left hand** at the level of the interossei muscles (dorsal aspect).

**Fig. 3.147 Coronal section through the left hand** at the level of the interossei muscles (dorsal aspect, MRI scan). (Heuck A, et al. MRT-Atlas des muskuloskelettalen Systems. Stuttgart, Germany: Schattauer, 2009.)

**Fig. 3.148 Coronal section through the left hand** at the level of the interossei muscles (dorsal aspect).

1 Radius
2 Radiocarpal joint
3 Scaphoid (navicular) bone
4 Radial artery
5 Trapezoid bone
6 Trapezium bone
7 First metacarpal bone
8 Metacarpophalangeal joint of thumb
9 Interossei muscles
10 Proximal phalanx of thumb
11 Proximal phalanx of fingers
12 Interphalangeal joints
13 Middle phalanx
14 Distal phalanx
15 Ulna
16 Distal radio-ulnar joint
17 Articular disc
18 Lunate bone
19 Triquetral bone
20 Capitate bone
21 Hamate bone
22 Carpometacarpal joints
23 Abductor digiti minimi muscle
24 Fifth metacarpal bone
25 Metacarpophalangeal joint
26 Adductor pollicis muscle
27 Proper palmar digital arteries
28 Metacarpal joint
29 Opponens pollicis muscle
30 Ulnar collateral ligament
31 Pisiform bone

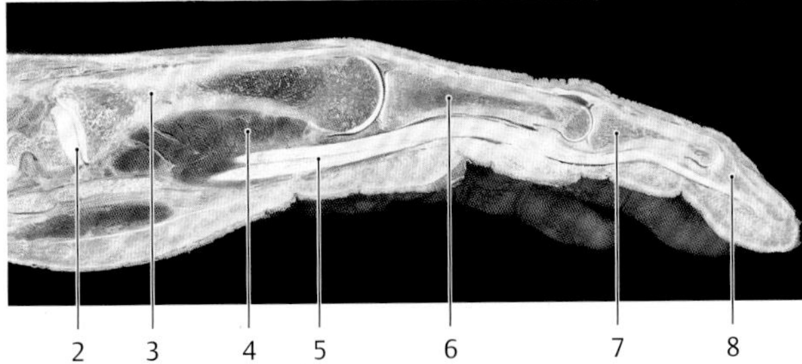


Fig. 3.149 **Longitudinal section through the hand** at the level of the third finger.

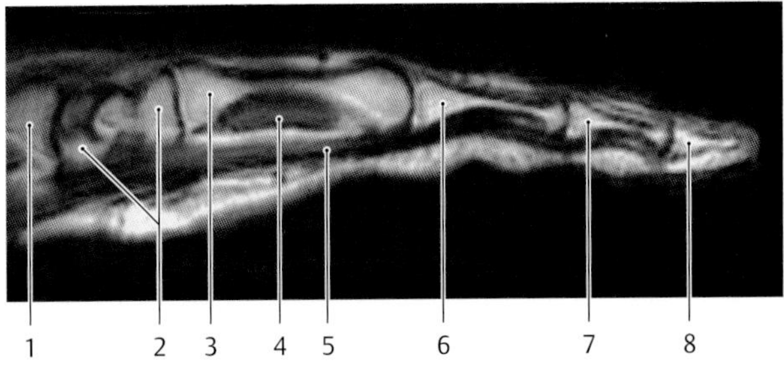


Fig. 3.150 **Longitudinal section through the hand at the level of the third finger** (MRI scan). (Heuck A, et al. MRT-Atlas des muskuloskelettalen Systems. Stuttgart, Germany: Schattauer, 2009.)

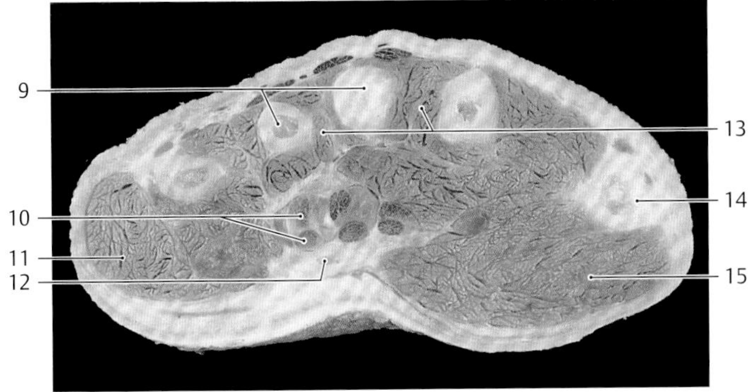


Fig. 3.151 **Axial section through the right hand** at the level of the metacarpus (inferior aspect).

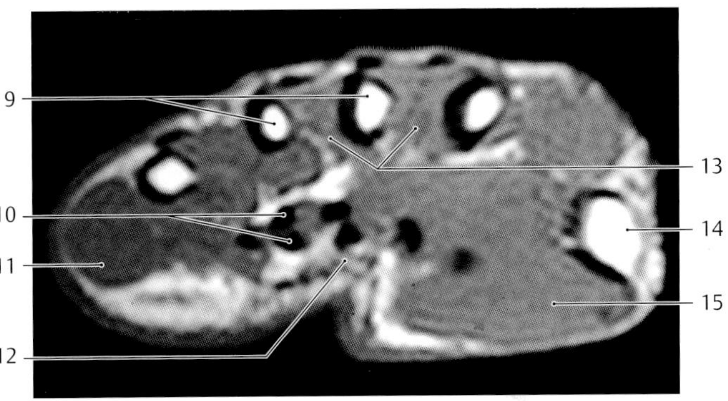


Fig. 3.152 **Axial section through the right hand** at the level of the metacarpus (inferior aspect, MRI scan). (Courtesy of Prof. Uder, Institute of Radiology, University Hospital Erlangen, Germany.)

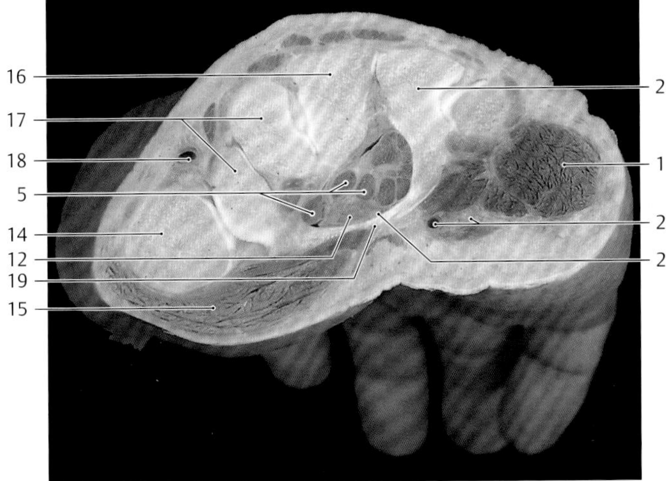


Fig. 3.153 **Axial section through the right hand** at the level of the carpal tunnel (proximal aspect).

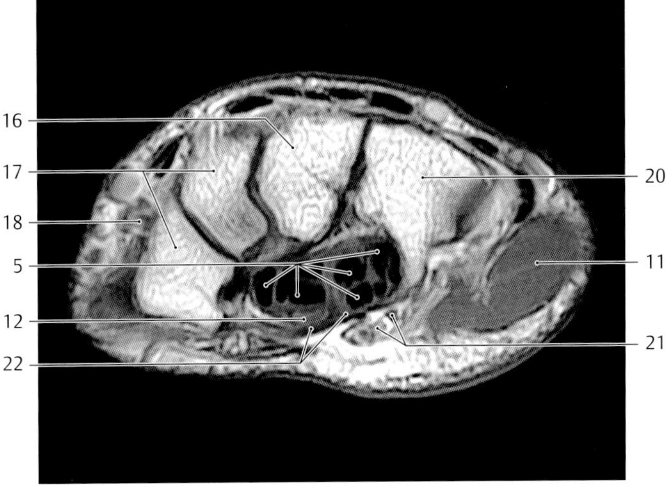


Fig. 3.154 **Axial section through the right hand** at the level of the carpal tunnel (proximal aspect, MRI scan). (Heuck A, et al. MRT-Atlas des muskuloskelettalen Systems. Stuttgart, Germany: Schattauer, 2009.)

1 Radius
2 Carpal bones
3 Metacarpal bone
4 Interossei muscles
5 Tendons of flexor digitorum profundus (upper) and superficialis (lower) muscles
6 Proximal phalanx
7 Middle phalanx
8 Distal phalanx
9 Third and fourth metacarpal bones
10 Carpal tunnel with tendons of flexor digitorum muscles
11 Hypothenar muscles
12 Median nerve
13 Interossei muscles
14 First metacarpal bone
15 Thenar muscles
16 Capitate bone
17 Trapezium and trapezoid bones
18 Radial artery
19 Flexor retinaculum
20 Hamate bone
21 Ulnar artery and nerve
22 Carpal tunnel

# 4 Lower Limb

## General Anatomy and Musculoskeletal System

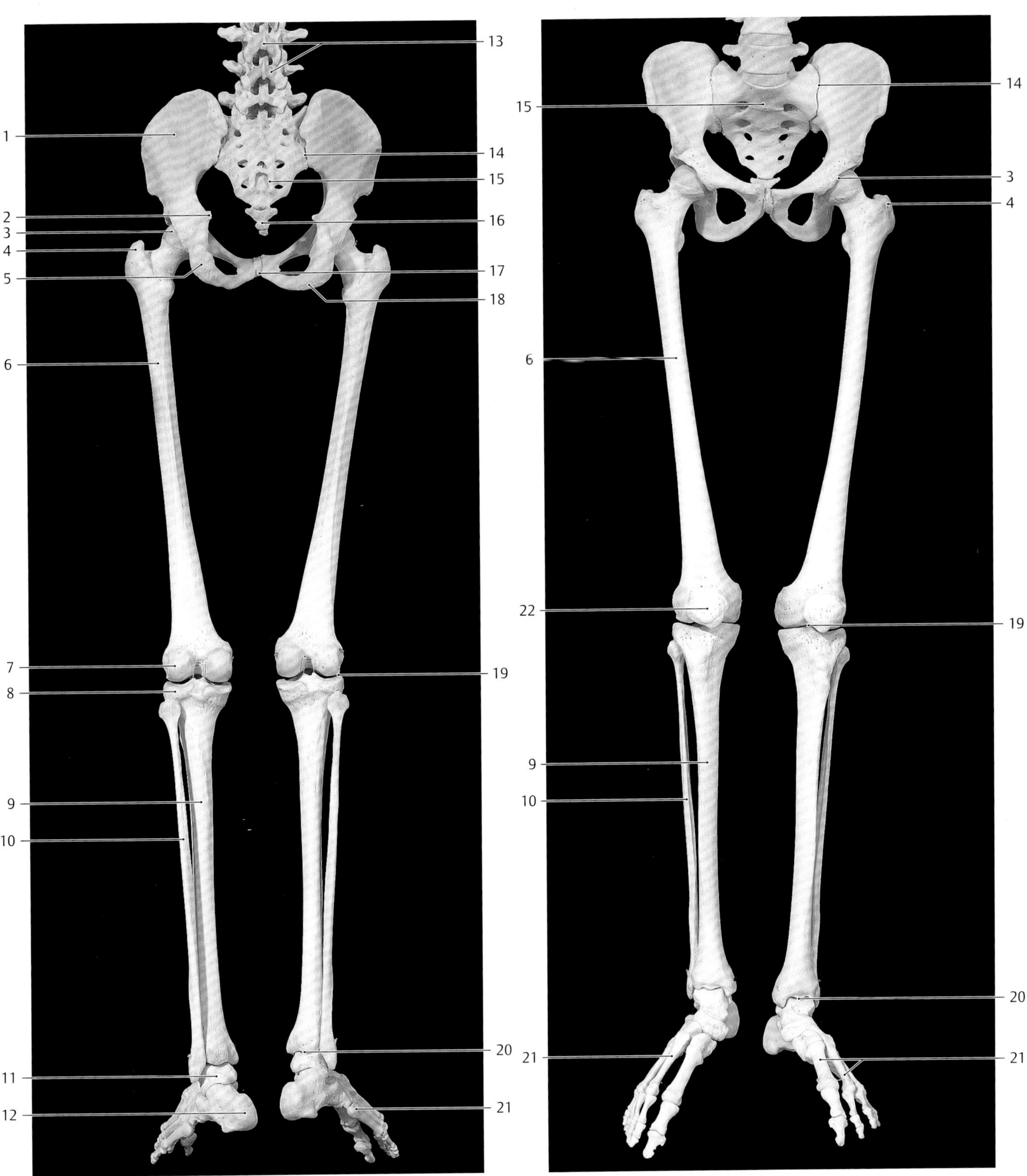


Fig. 4.1 **Skeleton of pelvic girdle and lower limb** (posterior aspect).

Fig. 4.2 **Skeleton of pelvic girdle and lower limb** (anterior aspect).

1 Ilium
2 Ischial spine
3 Hip joint
4 Greater trochanter
5 Ischial tuberosity
6 Femur
7 Lateral condyle of femur
8 Lateral condyle of tibia
9 Tibia
10 Fibula
11 Talus
12 Calcaneus
13 Lumbar vertebrae
14 Sacro-iliac joint
15 Sacrum
16 Coccyx
17 Pubic symphysis
18 Ischial tuberosity
19 Knee joint
20 Ankle joint
21 Metatarsal bones
22 Patella

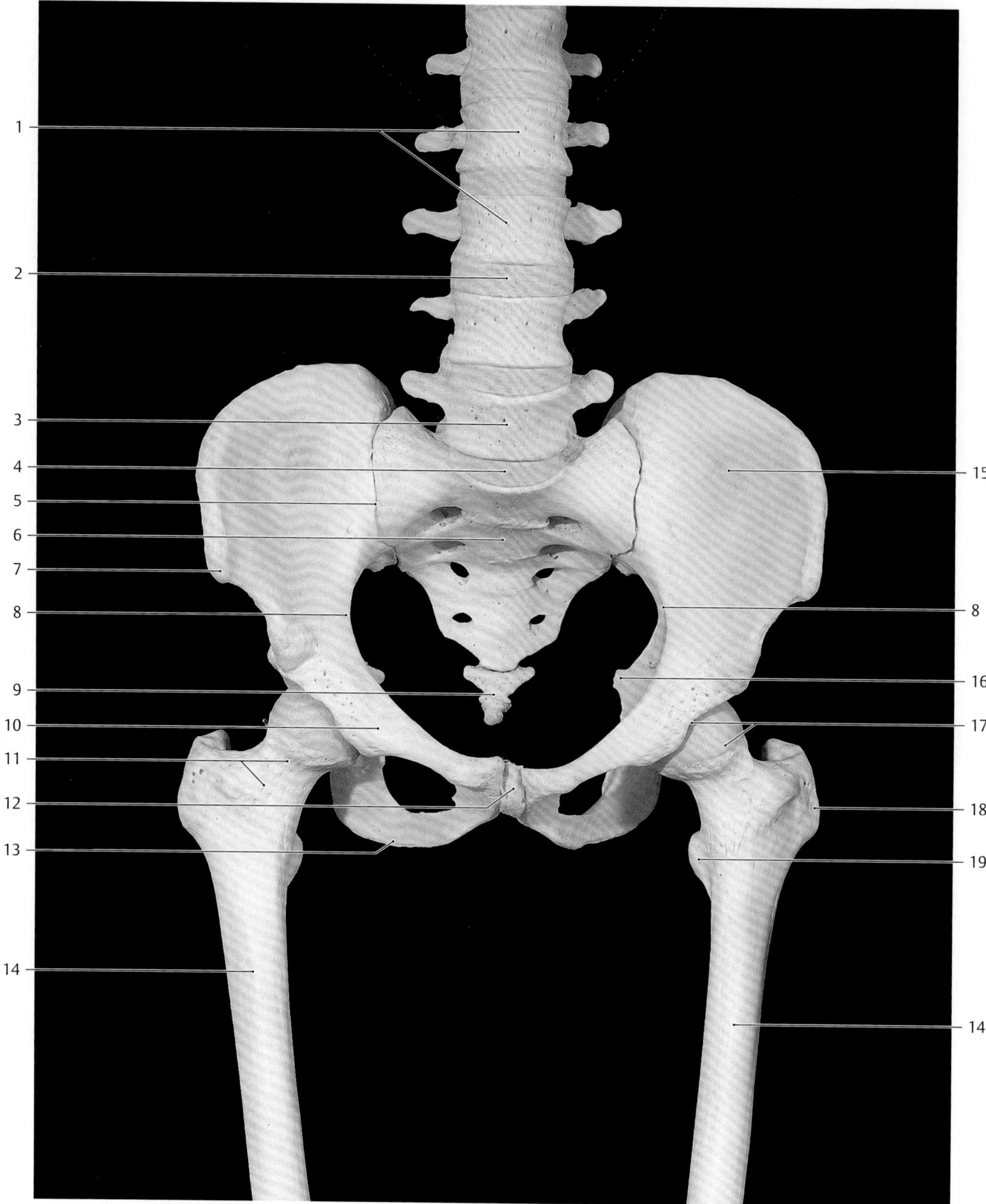


Fig. 4.3 **Lumbar vertebrae and skeleton of pelvic girdle with both femurs** (anterior aspect).

1 Second and third lumbar vertebrae
2 Intervertebral disc
3 Fifth lumbar vertebra
4 Intervertebral disc between fifth lumbar vertebra and sacrum
5 Sacro-iliac joint
6 Sacrum
7 Anterior superior iliac spine
8 Linea terminalis
9 Coccyx
10 Pubis
11 Neck of femur
12 Pubic symphysis
13 Ischial tuberosity
14 Femur
15 Iliac fossa
16 Ischial spine
17 Head of femur (and localization of hip joint)
18 Greater trochanter
19 Lesser trochanter

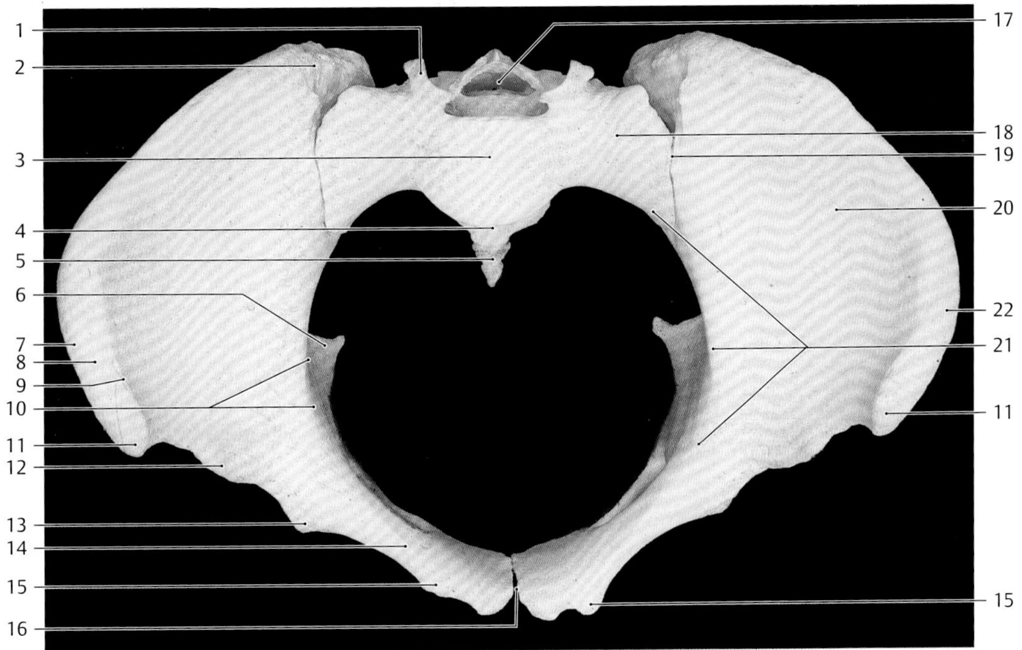


Fig. 4.4 **Female pelvis** (superior aspect). Note the differences between the male and female pelvis, predominantly in the form and dimensions of the sacrum, the superior and inferior apertures, and the alae of the ilium.

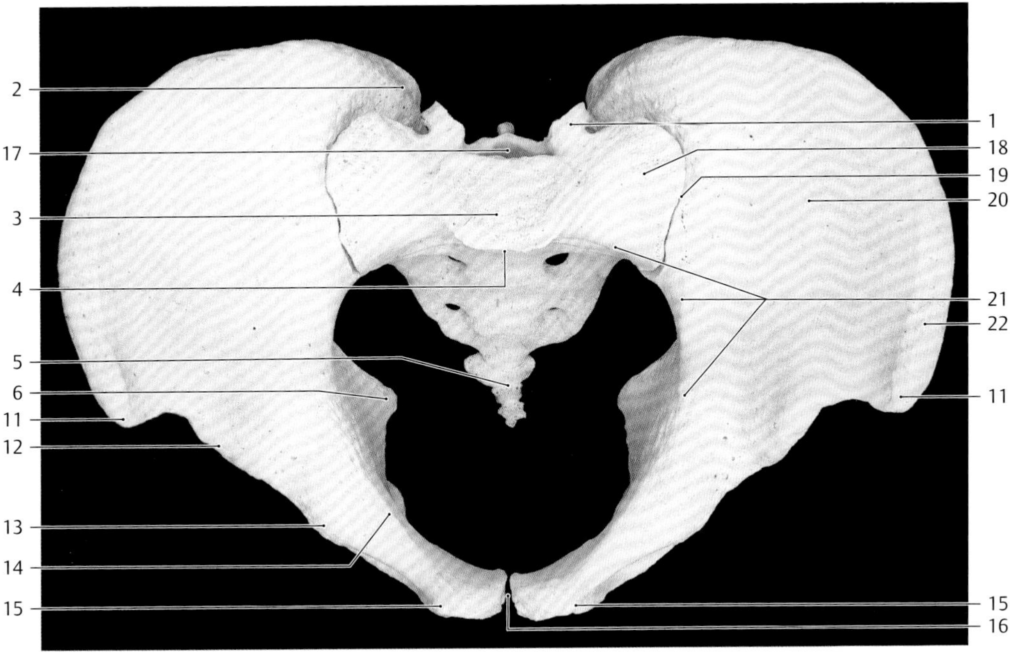


Fig. 4.5 **Male pelvis** (superior aspect). Compare with the female pelvis (depicted in Fig. 4.4 above).

1 Superior articular process of sacrum
2 Posterior superior iliac spine
3 Base of sacrum
4 Sacral promontory
5 Coccyx
6 Ischial spine
7 External lip } of iliac crest
8 Intermediate line } of iliac crest
9 Internal lip } of iliac crest
10 Arcuate line
11 Anterior superior iliac spine
12 Anterior inferior iliac spine
13 Iliopubic eminence
14 Pecten pubis
15 Pubic tubercle
16 Pubic symphysis
17 Sacral canal
18 Ala of sacrum
19 Position of sacro-iliac joint
20 Iliac fossa
21 Linea terminalis
22 Iliac crest

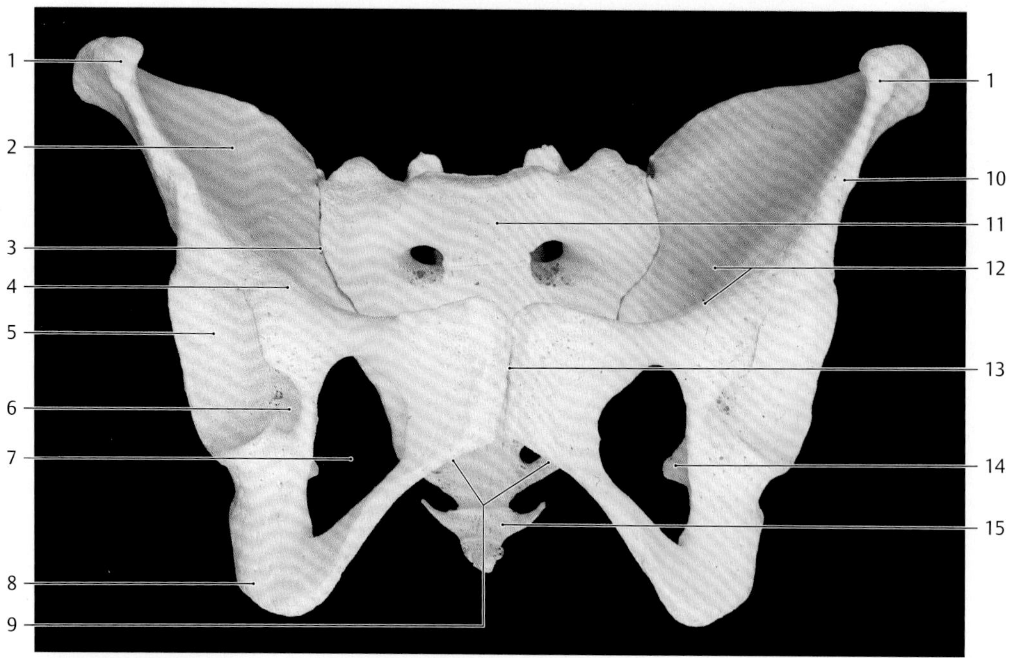


**Fig. 4.6 Female pelvis** (anterior aspect). Note the differences between the form and dimensions of the male and female pelvis. The female pubic arch is wider than the male. The obturator foramen in the female pelvis is triangular, while that in the male pelvis is ovoid.

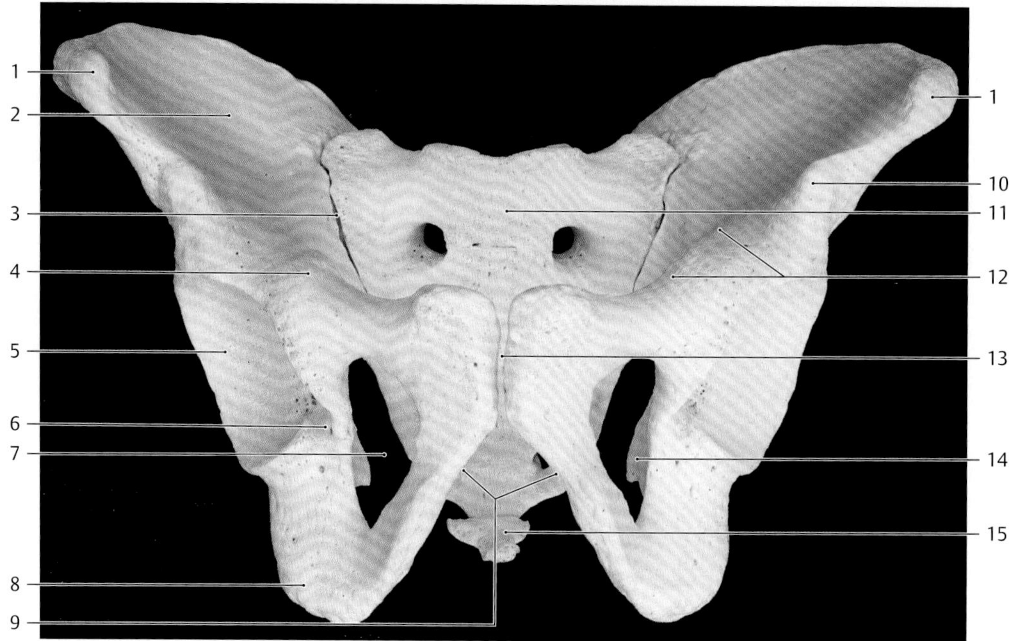


**Fig. 4.7 Male pelvis** (anterior aspect). Compare with the female pelvis (depicted in Fig. 4.6 above).

1 Anterior superior iliac spine
2 Iliac fossa
3 Position of sacro-iliac joint
4 Iliopubic eminence
5 Lunate surface of acetabulum
6 Acetabular notch
7 Obturator foramen
8 Ischial tuberosity
9 Pubic arch
10 Anterior inferior iliac spine
11 Sacrum
12 Linea terminalis (at margin of superior aperture)
13 Pubic symphysis
14 Ischial spine
15 Coccyx

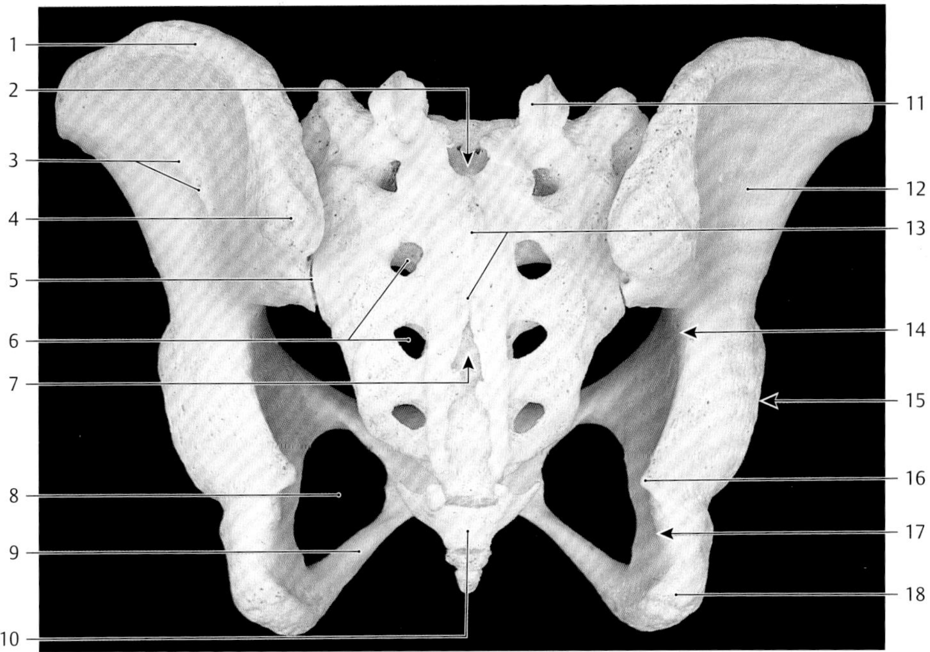


Fig. 4.8 **Female pelvis** (posterior aspect). Note the differences between the female and male pelvis, especially with respect to the inferior aperture, the shape of the sacrum, the two sciatic notches, and the pubic arch.

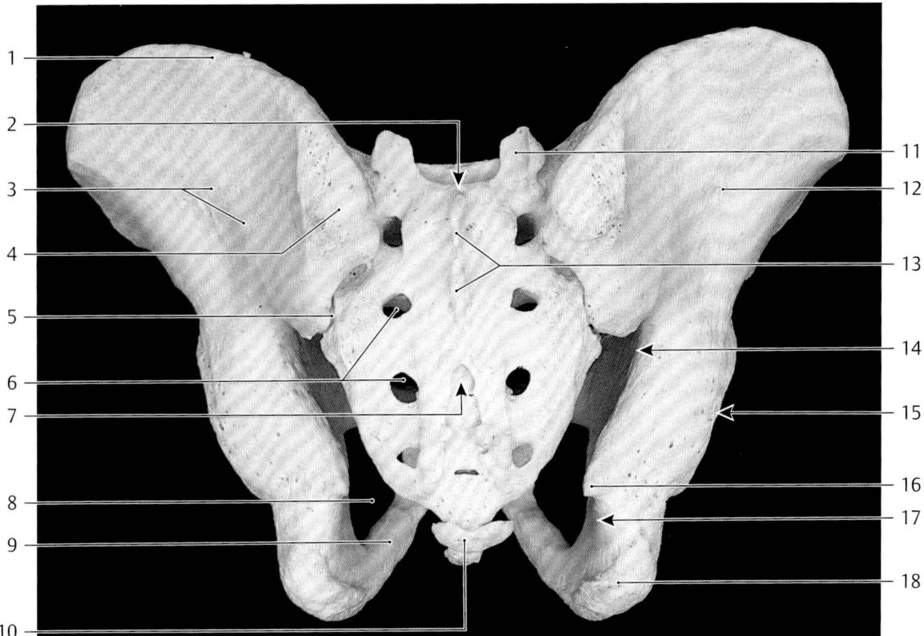


Fig. 4.9 **Male pelvis** (posterior aspect). Compare with the female pelvis (depicted in Fig. 4.8 above).

1 Iliac crest
2 Sacral canal
3 Posterior gluteal line
4 Posterior superior iliac spine
5 Position of sacro-iliac joint
6 Dorsal sacral foramina
7 Sacral hiatus
8 Obturator foramen
9 Ramus of ischium
10 Coccyx
11 Superior articular process of sacrum
12 Gluteal surface of ilium
13 Median sacral crest
14 Greater sciatic notch
15 Position of acetabulum
16 Ischial spine
17 Lesser sciatic notch
18 Ischial tuberosity

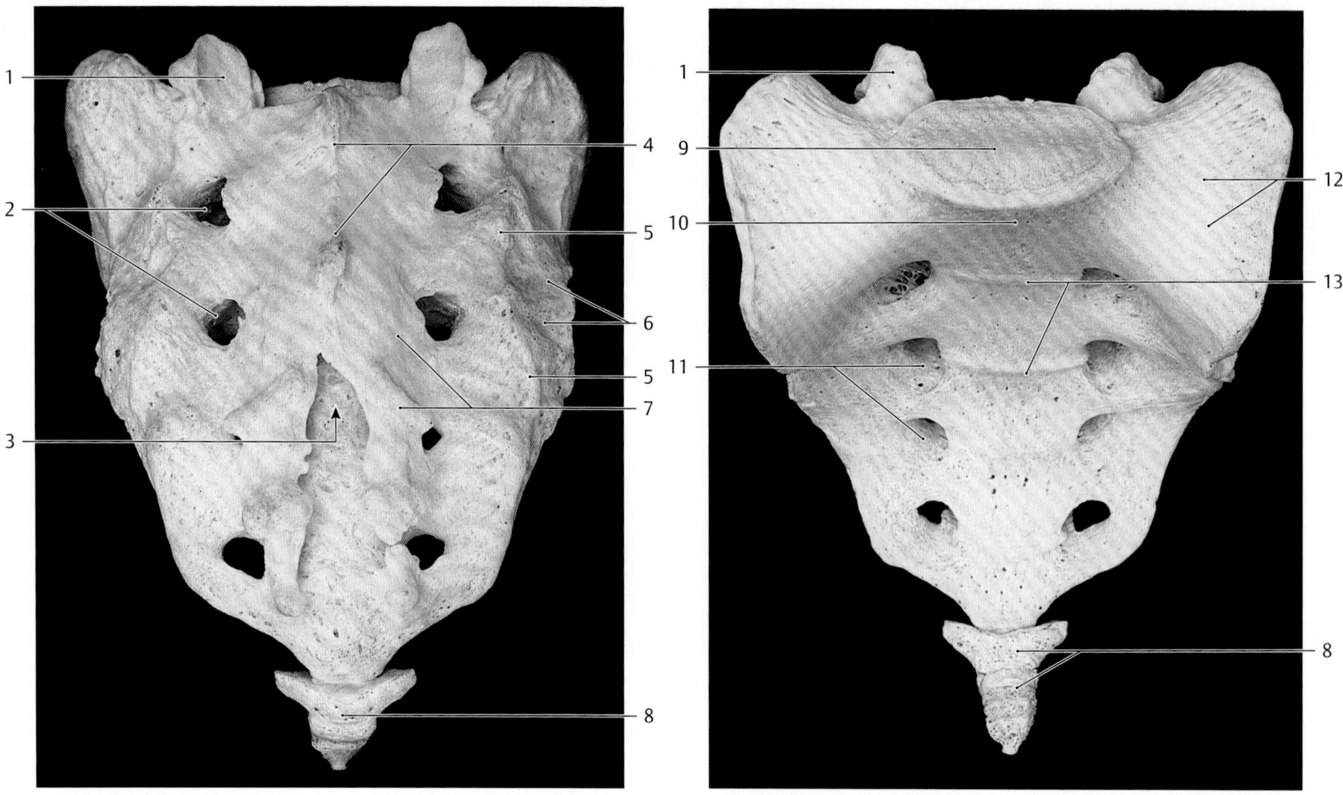


Fig. 4.10 **Sacrum** (posterior aspect).

Fig. 4.11 **Sacrum** (anterior aspect).

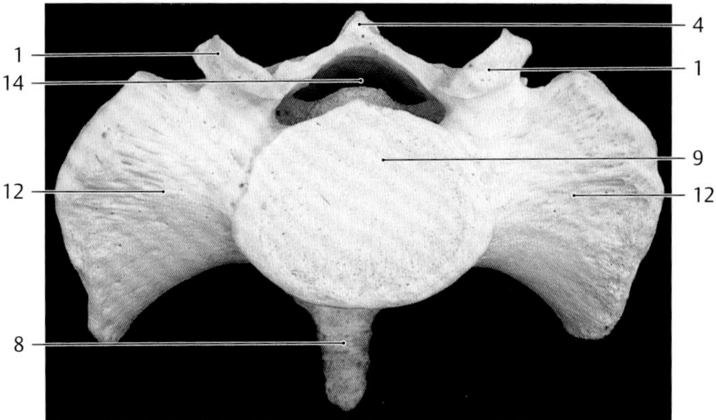


Fig. 4.12 **Sacrum** (superior aspect).

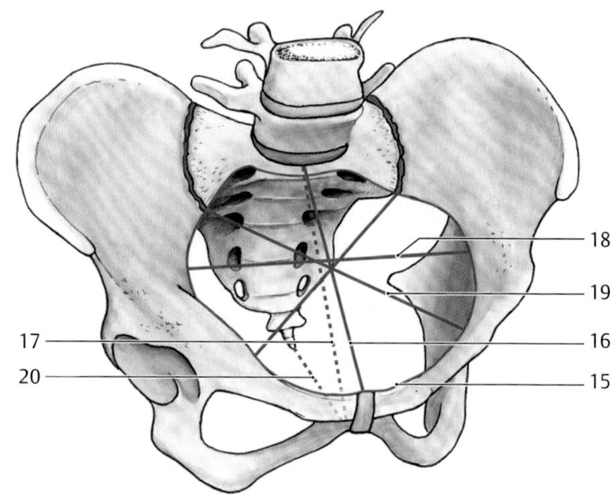


Fig. 4.13 **Diameters of pelvis** (oblique-superior aspect).

1 Superior articular process of sacrum
2 Posterior sacral foramina
3 Sacral hiatus
4 Median sacral crest
5 Lateral sacral crest
6 Sacral tuberosity
7 Intermediate sacral crest
8 Coccyx
9 Base of sacrum
10 Sacral promontory
11 Anterior sacral foramina
12 Lateral part of sacrum (ala)
13 Transverse line of sacrum
14 Sacral canal
15 Linea terminalis
16 True conjugate
17 Diagonal conjugate
18 Transverse diameter
19 Oblique diameter
20 Inferior pelvic aperture or outlet

The pelvic girdle is firmly connected to the vertebral column at the sacro-iliac joint. Therefore, the body can be kept upright more easily even if only one limb is used for support (as in walking). The mobility of the lower limb is more limited than that of the upper limb.

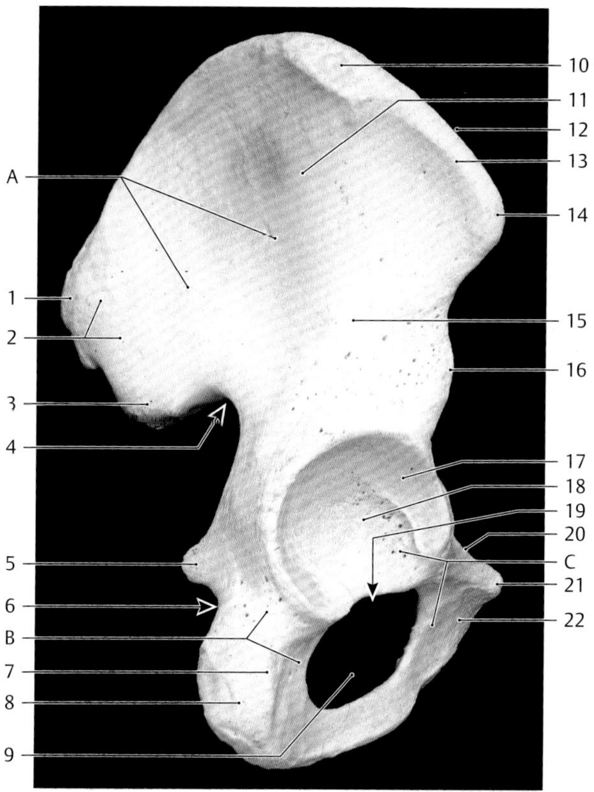


Fig. 4.14 **Right hip bone** (lateral aspect).

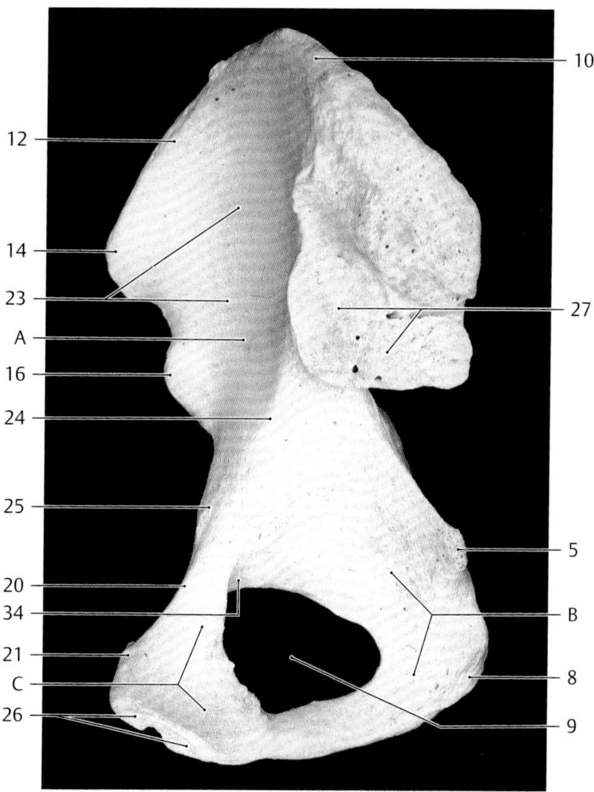


Fig. 4.15 **Right hip bone** (medial aspect).

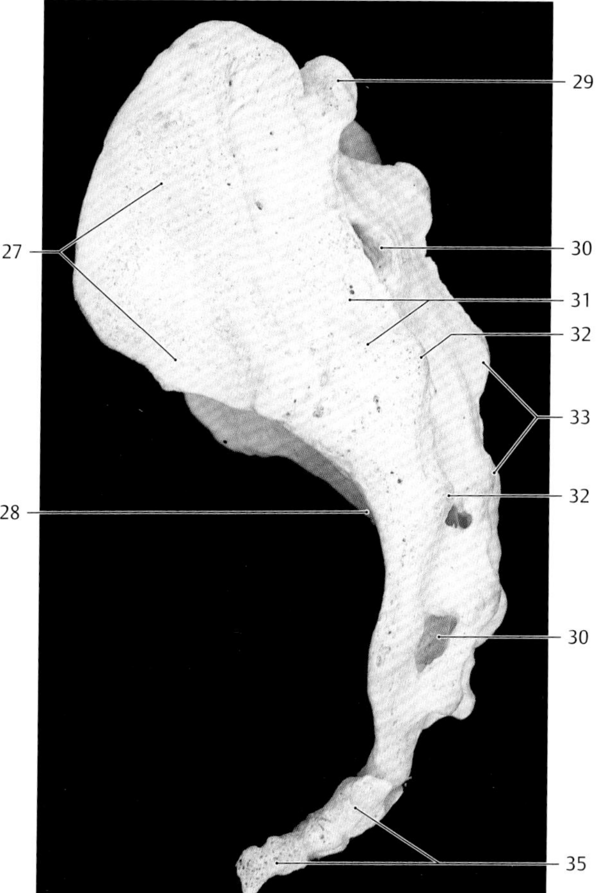


Fig. 4.16 **Sacrum and coccyx** (lateral aspect).

A = Ilium
B = Ischium
C = Pubis

1 Posterior superior iliac spine
2 Posterior gluteal line
3 Posterior inferior iliac spine
4 Greater sciatic notch
5 Ischial spine
6 Lesser sciatic notch
7 Body of ischium
8 Ischial tuberosity
9 Obturator foramen
10 Iliac crest
11 Anterior gluteal line
12 Internal lip of iliac crest
13 External lip of iliac crest
14 Anterior superior iliac spine
15 Inferior gluteal line
16 Anterior inferior iliac spine
17 Lunate surface of acetabulum
18 Acetabular fossa
19 Acetabular notch
20 Pecten pubis
21 Pubic tubercle
22 Body of pubis
23 Iliac fossa
24 Arcuate line
25 Iliopubic eminence
26 Symphysial surface of pubis
27 Auricular surface
28 Pelvic surface of sacrum
29 Superior articular process of sacrum
30 Dorsal sacral foramina
31 Sacral tuberosity
32 Lateral sacral crest
33 Median sacral crest
34 Obturator groove
35 Coccyx

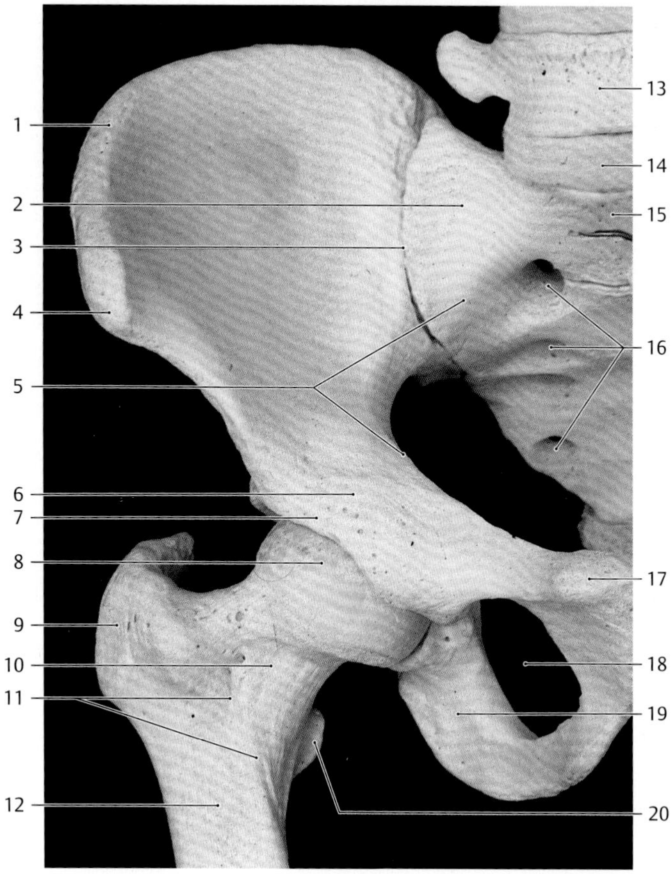

**Fig. 4.17 Bones of the right hip joint** (anterior aspect).

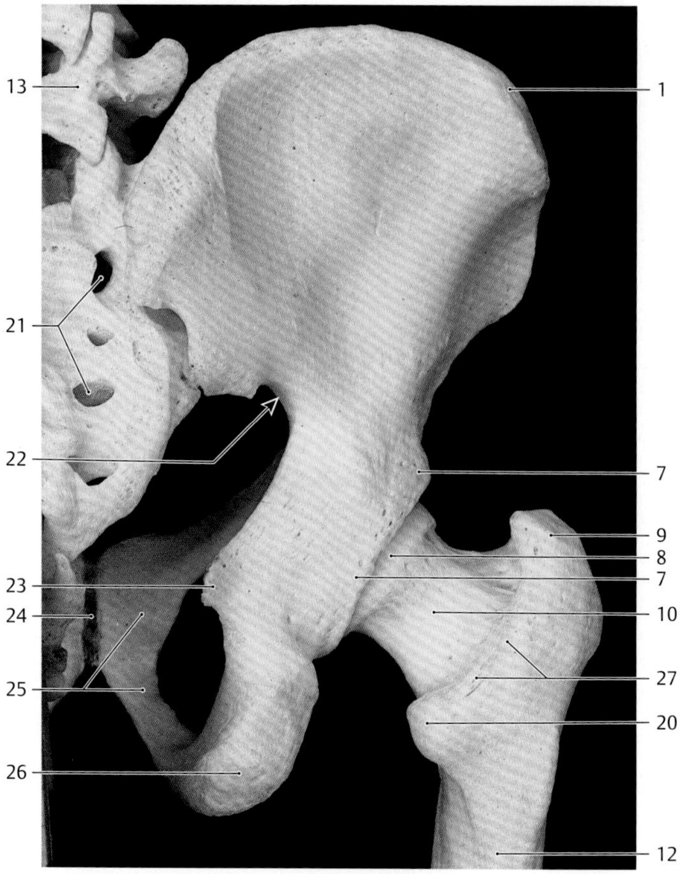

**Fig. 4.18 Bones of the right hip joint** (posterior aspect).

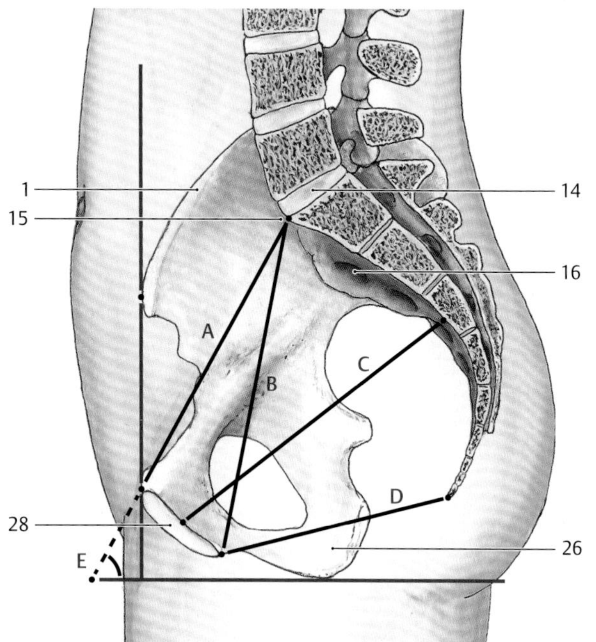


**Fig. 4.19 Inclination and diameters of the female pelvis,** right half (medial aspect).

1 Iliac crest
2 Lateral part of sacrum (ala)
3 Position of sacro-iliac joint
4 Anterior superior iliac spine
5 Linea terminalis
6 Iliopubic eminence
7 Bony margin of acetabulum
8 Head of femur
9 Greater trochanter
10 Neck of femur
11 Intertrochanteric line
12 Shaft of femur
13 Fifth lumbar vertebra
14 Intervertebral disc between fifth lumbar vertebra and sacrum (imitation)
15 Sacral promontory
16 Anterior sacral foramina
17 Pubic tubercle
18 Obturator foramen
19 Ramus of ischium
20 Lesser trochanter
21 Posterior sacral foramina
22 Greater sciatic notch
23 Ischial spine
24 Pubic symphysis
25 Pubis
26 Ischial tuberosity
27 Intertrochanteric crest
28 Symphysial surface

**Diameters of the pelvis**

A = True conjugate (11–11.5 cm) (conjugata vera)
B = Diagonal conjugate (12.5–13 cm)
C = Largest diameter of pelvis
D = Inferior pelvic aperture
E = Pelvic inclination (60°)

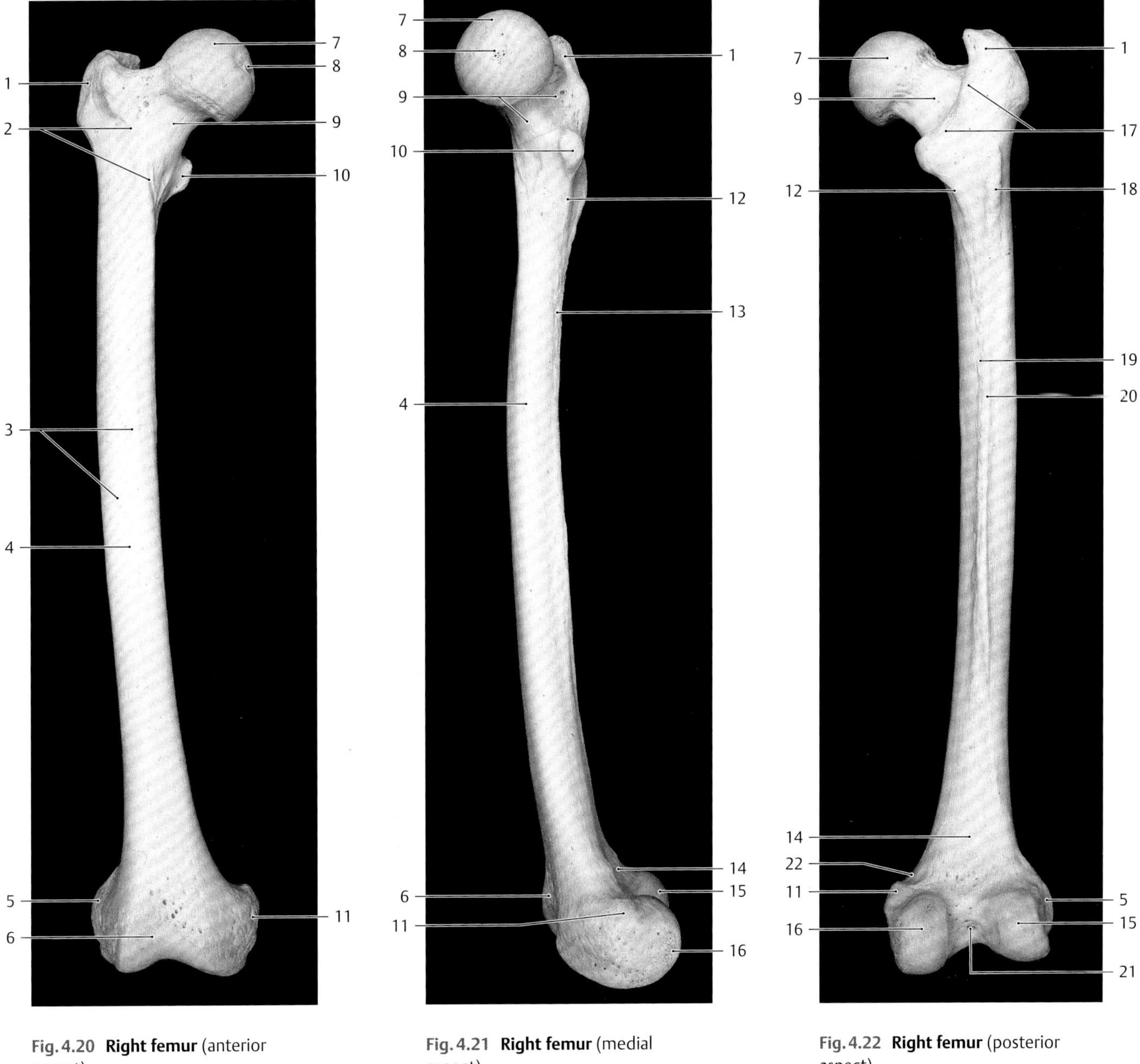


**Fig. 4.20 Right femur** (anterior aspect).

**Fig. 4.21 Right femur** (medial aspect).

**Fig. 4.22 Right femur** (posterior aspect).

1 Greater trochanter
2 Intertrochanteric line
3 Nutrient foramina
4 Shaft of femur (diaphysis)
5 Lateral epicondyle
6 Patellar surface
7 Head
8 Fovea of head
9 Neck
10 Lesser trochanter
11 Medial epicondyle
12 Pectineal line
13 Linea aspera
14 Popliteal surface
15 Lateral condyle
16 Medial condyle
17 Intertrochanteric crest
18 Third trochanter
19 Medial lip } of linea aspera
20 Lateral lip } of linea aspera
21 Intercondylar fossa
22 Adductor tubercle

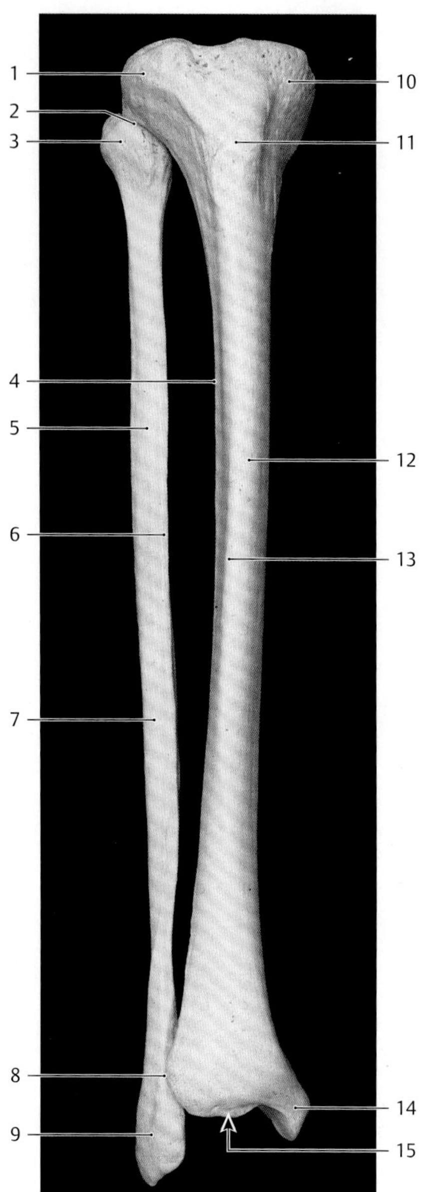


Fig. 4.23 **Bones of the leg. Right tibia and fibula** (anterior aspect).

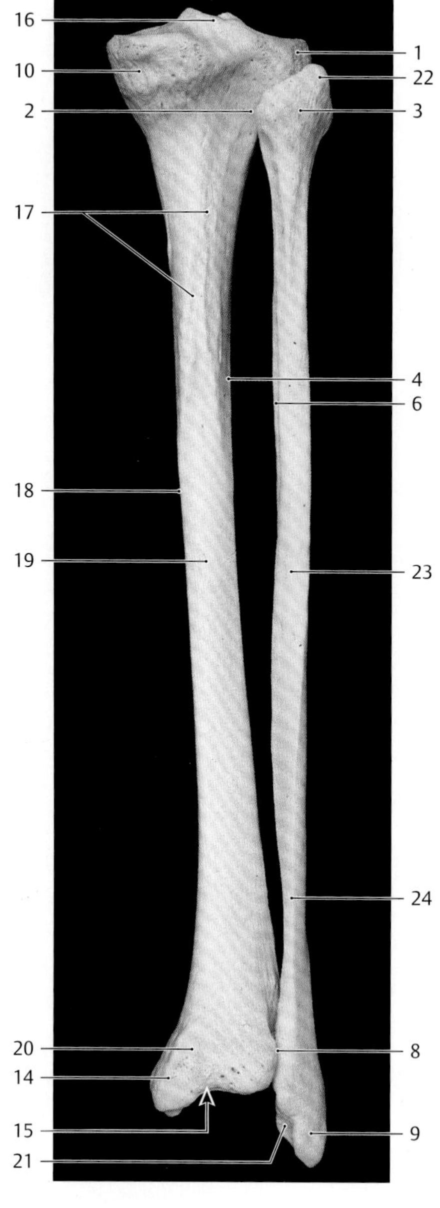


Fig. 4.24 **Bones of the leg. Right tibia and fibula** (posterior aspect).

1 Lateral condyle of tibia
2 Position of tibiofibular joint
3 Head of fibula
4 Interosseous border of tibia
5 Shaft of fibula
6 Interosseous border of fibula
7 Lateral surface of fibula
8 Position of tibiofibular syndesmosis
9 Lateral malleolus
10 Medial condyle of tibia
11 Tuberosity of tibia
12 Shaft of tibia (diaphysis)
13 Anterior margin of tibia
14 Medial malleolus
15 Inferior articular surface of tibia
16 Intercondylar eminence
17 Soleal line
18 Medial border of tibia
19 Posterior surface of tibia
20 Malleolar sulcus of tibia
21 Malleolar articular surface of fibula
22 Apex of head of fibula
23 Posterior surface of fibula
24 Posterior border of fibula
25 Medial intercondylar tubercle
26 Posterior intercondylar area
27 Anterior intercondylar area
28 Lateral intercondylar tubercle

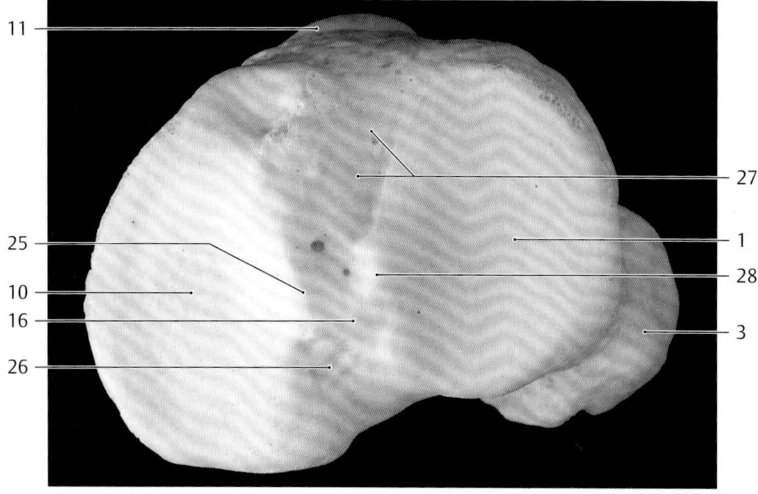


Fig. 4.25 **Upper end of the right tibia with fibula** (from above), anterior margin of tibia above. Superior articular surface of tibia.

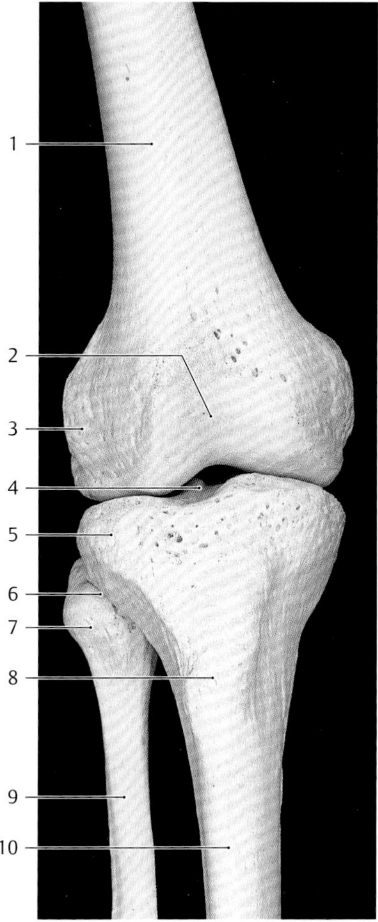


Fig. 4.26 **Bones of the right knee joint** (anterior aspect).

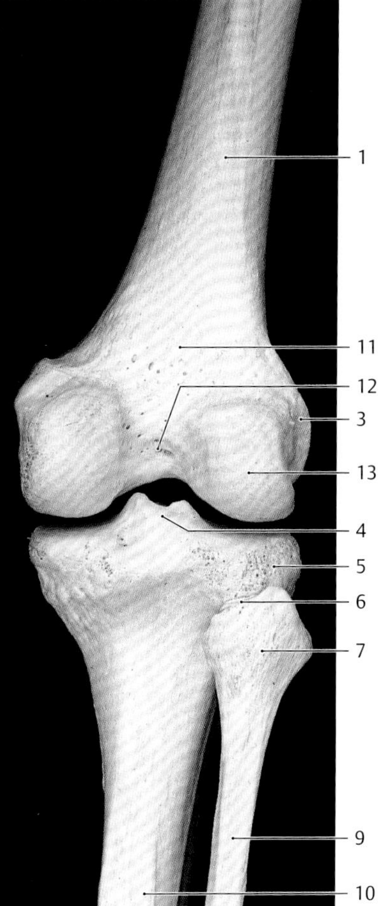


Fig. 4.27 **Bones of the right knee joint** (posterior aspect).

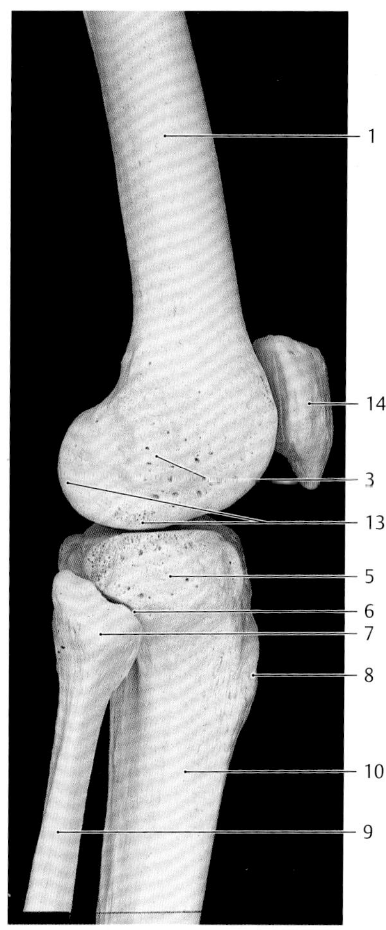


Fig. 4.28 **Bones of the right knee joint** (lateral aspect).

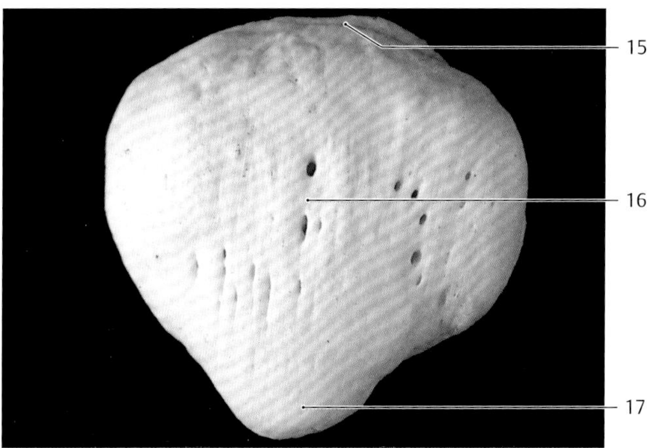


Fig. 4.29 **Right patella** (anterior aspect).

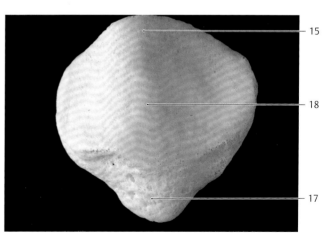


Fig. 4.30 **Right patella** (posterior aspect).

1 Femur
2 Patellar surface of femur
3 Lateral epicondyle of femur
4 Intercondylar eminence of tibia
5 Lateral condyle of tibia
6 Position of tibiofibular joint
7 Head of fibula
8 Tuberosity of tibia
9 Fibula
10 Shaft of tibia
11 Popliteal surface of femur
12 Intercondylar fossa of femur
13 Lateral condyle of femur
14 Patella
15 Base of patella
16 Anterior surface of patella
17 Apex of patella
18 Articular surface of patella

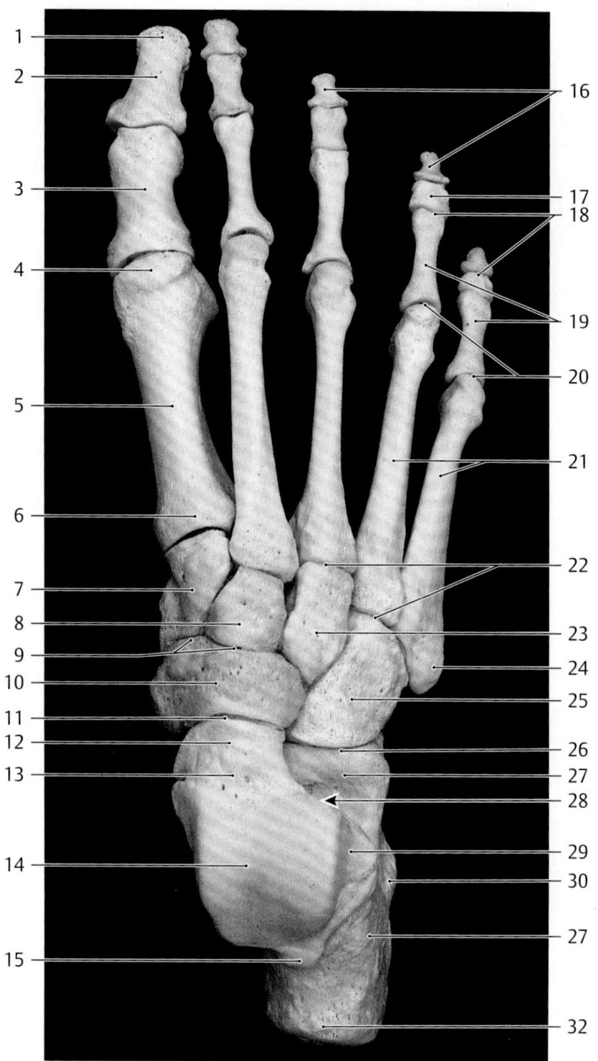


Fig. 4.31 **Bones of the right foot** (dorsal aspect).

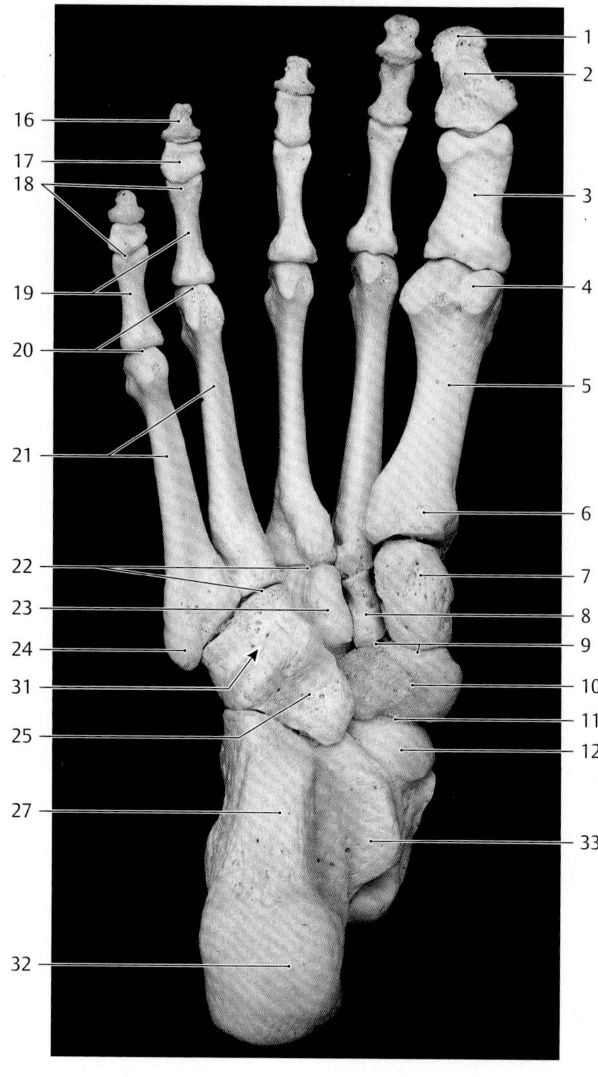


Fig. 4.32 **Bones of the right foot** (plantar aspect).

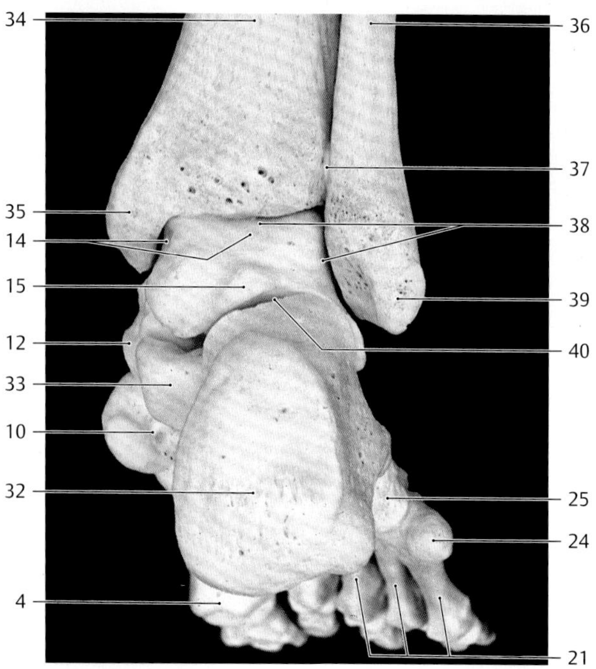


Fig. 4.33 **Bones of the right foot** together with tibia and fibula (posterior aspect).

1 Tuberosity of distal phalanx of great toe
2 Distal phalanx of great toe
3 Proximal phalanx of great toe
4 Head of first metatarsal bone
5 First metatarsal bone
6 Base of first metatarsal bone
7 Medial cuneiform bone
8 Intermediate cuneiform bone
9 Position of cuneonavicular joint
10 Navicular bone
11 Position of talocalcaneonavicular joint
12 Head of talus
13 Neck of talus
14 Trochlea of talus
15 Posterior talar process
16 Distal phalanges
17 Middle phalanx
18 Position of interphalangeal joints
19 Proximal phalanges
20 Position of metatarsophalangeal joints
21 Metatarsal bones

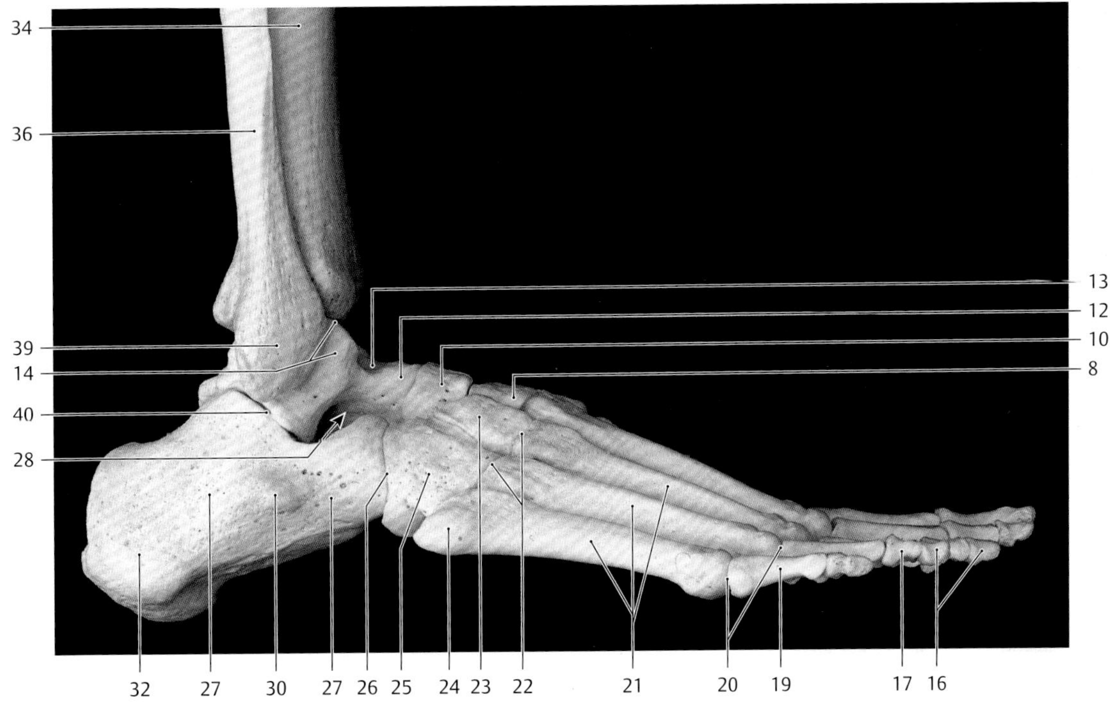


Fig. 4.34 **Bones of the right foot, tibia, and fibula** (lateral aspect).

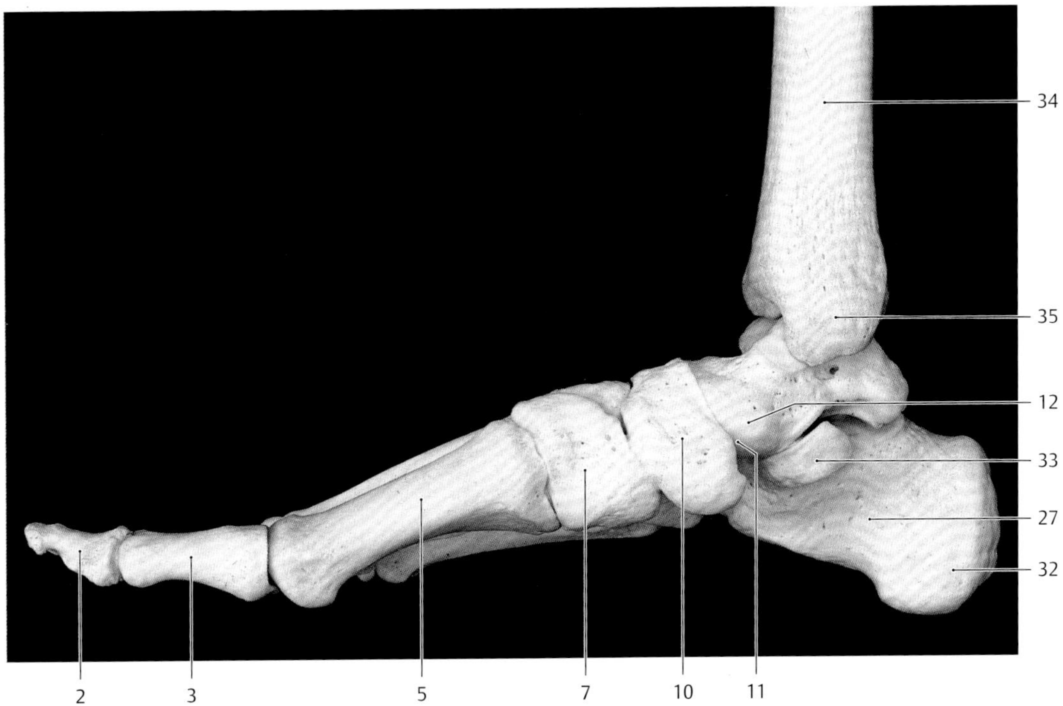


Fig. 4.35 **Bones of the right foot, tibia, and fibula** (medial aspect).

22 Position of tarsometatarsal joints
23 Lateral cuneiform bone
24 Tuberosity of fifth metatarsal bone
25 Cuboid bone
26 Position of calcaneocuboid joint
27 Calcaneus
28 Tarsal sinus
29 Lateral malleolar surface of talus
30 Peroneal trochlea of calcaneus
31 Groove for the tendon of peroneus longus muscle
32 Calcaneal tuberosity
33 Sustentaculum tali
34 Tibia
35 Medial malleolus
36 Fibula
37 Position of tibiofibular syndesmosis
38 Position of ankle joint
39 Lateral malleolus
40 Position of subtalar joint

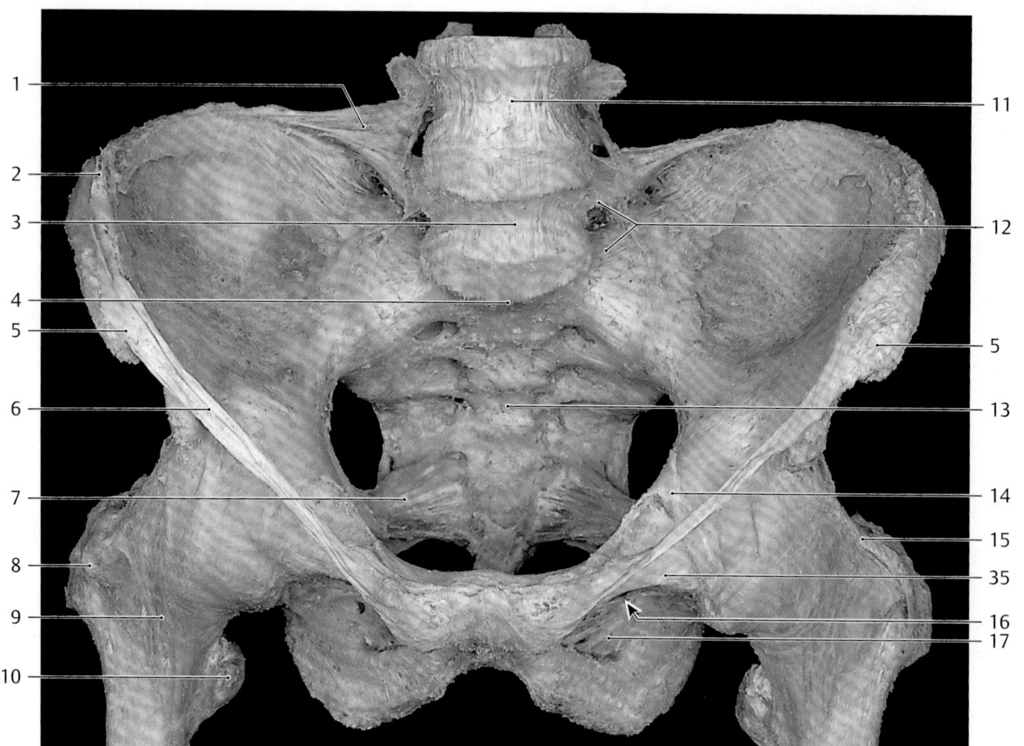


**Fig. 4.36 Ligaments of pelvis and hip joint** (anterior aspect).

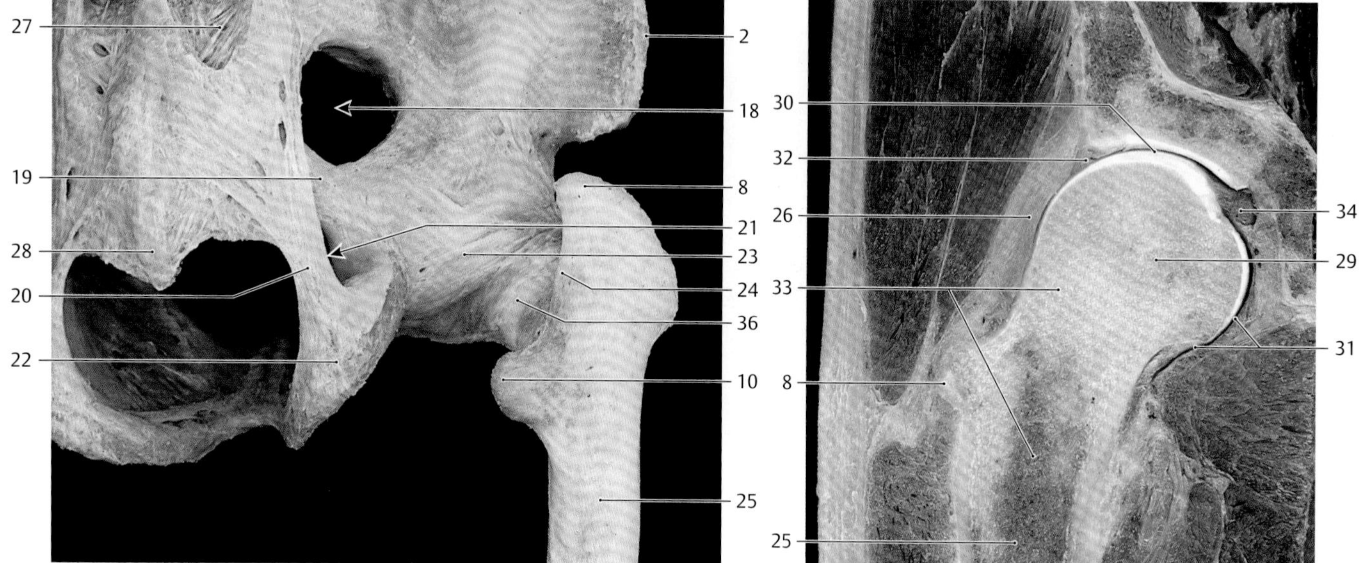


**Fig. 4.37 Ligaments of pelvis and hip joint** (right posterior aspect).

**Fig. 4.38 Coronal section through the right hip joint** (anterior aspect).

1 Iliolumbar ligament
2 Iliac crest
3 Fifth lumbar vertebra
4 Sacral promontory
5 Anterior superior iliac spine
6 Inguinal ligament
7 Sacrospinous ligament
8 Greater trochanter
9 Iliofemoral ligament (vertical band)
10 Lesser trochanter
11 Fourth lumbar vertebra
12 Iliolumbar and ventral sacro-iliac ligaments
13 Sacrum
14 Iliopectineal arch
15 Iliofemoral ligament (horizontal band)
16 Obturator canal
17 Obturator membrane
18 Greater sciatic foramen
19 Sacrospinous ligament
20 Sacrotuberous ligament
21 Lesser sciatic foramen
22 Ischial tuberosity
23 Ischiofemoral ligament
24 Intertrochanteric crest
25 Femur
26 Articular capsule of hip joint
27 Dorsal sacro-iliac ligaments
28 Coccyx with superficial dorsal sacrococcygeal ligament
29 Head of femur
30 Articular cartilage of head of femur
31 Articular cavity of hip joint
32 Acetabular lip
33 Spongy bone
34 Ligament of head of femur
35 Pubofemoral ligament
36 Zona orbicularis

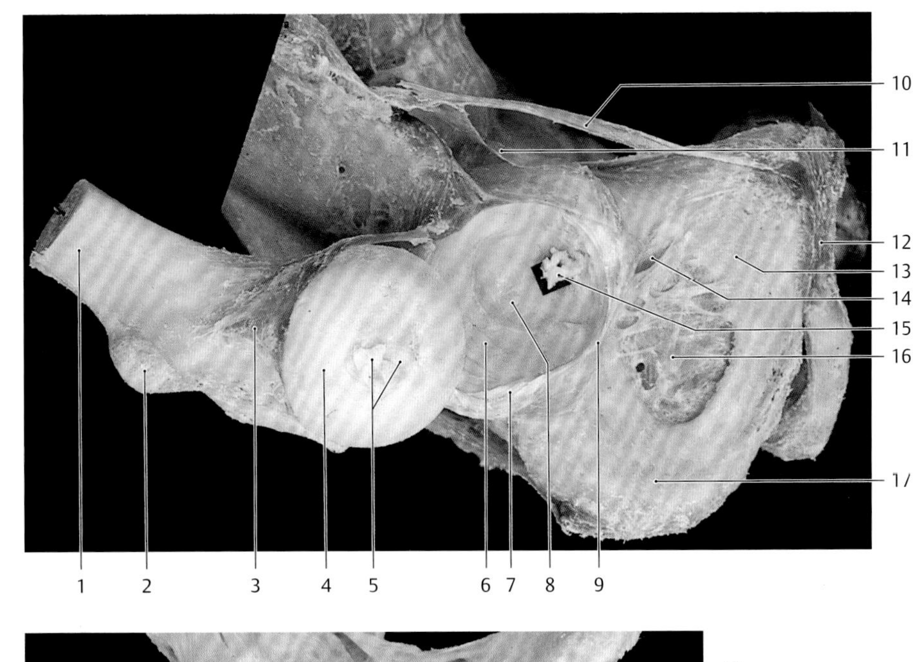


Fig. 4.39 **Right hip joint,** opened (latero-anterior aspect). The ligament of the head of the femur has been divided, and the femur has been posteriorly reflected.

1 Femur
2 Lesser trochanter
3 Neck of femur
4 Head of femur
5 Fovea of head with cut edge of ligament of head
6 Lunate surface of acetabulum
7 Acetabular lip
8 Acetabular fossa
9 Transverse acetabular ligament
10 Inguinal ligament
11 Iliopectineal arch
12 Pubic symphysis
13 Pubis
14 Obturator canal
15 Ligament of head of femur
16 Obturator membrane
17 Ischium
18 Anterior longitudinal ligament (level of fifth lumbar vertebra)
19 Sacral promontory
20 Iliolumbar ligament
21 Iliac crest
22 Anterior superior iliac spine
23 Iliofemoral ligament (horizontal band)
24 Iliofemoral ligament (vertical band)
25 Greater trochanter
26 Pubofemoral ligament
27 Anterior inferior iliac spine
28 Ventral sacro-iliac ligaments
29 Sacrospinous ligament
30 Sacrotuberous ligament
31 Intertrochanteric line
32 Ischiofemoral ligament
33 Zona orbicularis

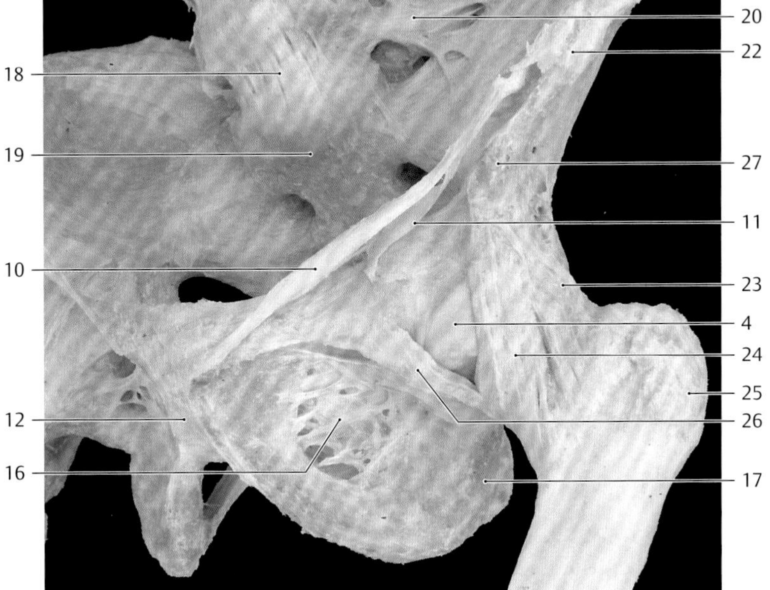


Fig. 4.40 **Ligaments of pelvis and hip joint** (antero-lateral aspect).

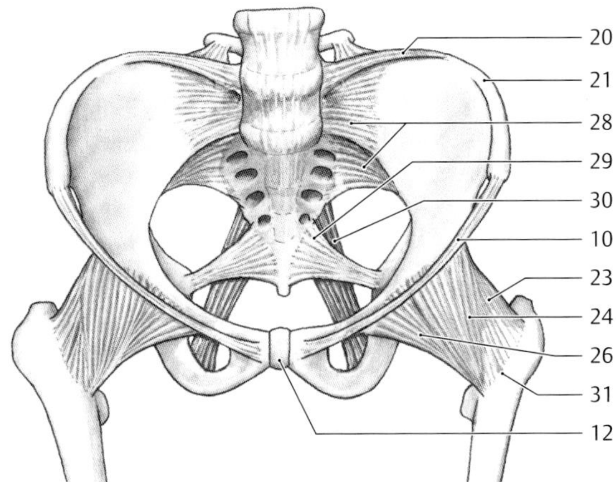


Fig. 4.41 **Ligaments of pelvis and hip joint** (anterior aspect).

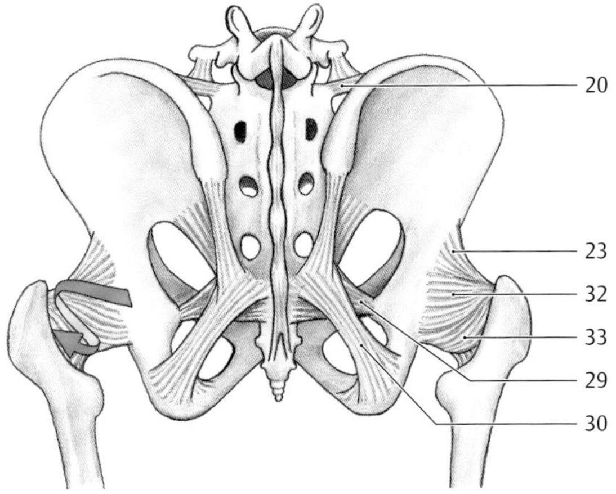


Fig. 4.42 **Ligaments of pelvis and hip joint** (posterior aspect).

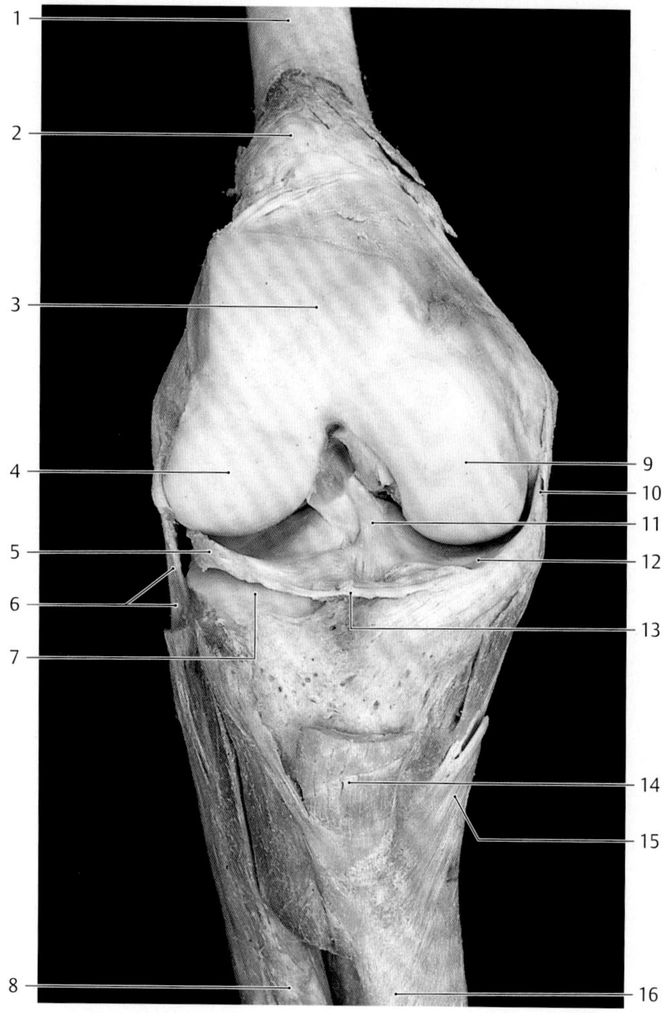

**Fig. 4.43 Right knee joint with ligaments** (anterior aspect). The patella and articular capsule have been removed and the femur slightly flexed.

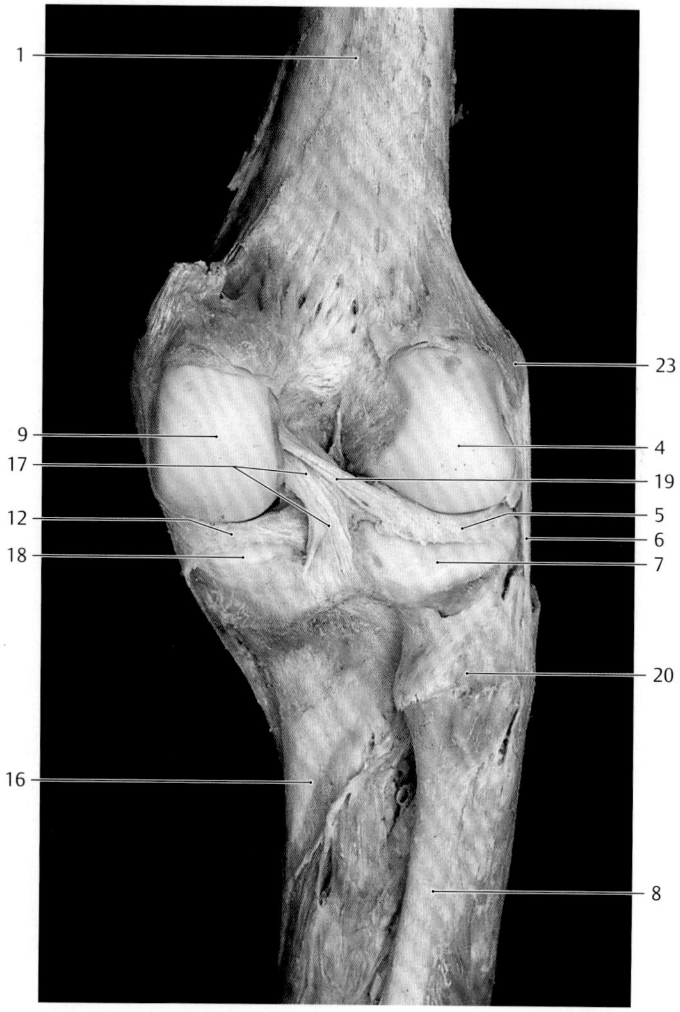

**Fig. 4.44 Right knee joint with ligaments** (posterior aspect). The joint is extended and the articular capsule has been removed.

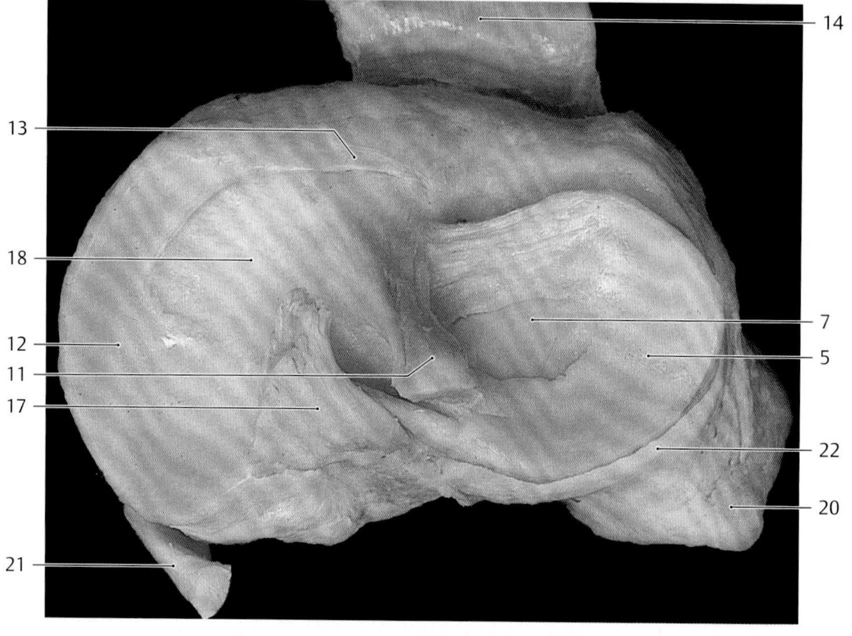


**Fig. 4.45 Articular surface of right tibia, menisci, and cruciate ligaments** (superior aspect). Anterior margin of tibia above.

1 Femur
2 Articular capsule with suprapatellar bursa
3 Patellar surface
4 Lateral condyle of femur
5 Lateral meniscus of knee joint
6 Fibular collateral ligament
7 Lateral condyle of tibia (superior articular surface)
8 Fibula
9 Medial condyle of femur
10 Tibial collateral ligament
11 Anterior cruciate ligament
12 Medial meniscus of knee joint
13 Transverse ligament of knee
14 Patellar ligament
15 Common tendon of sartorius, semitendinosus, and gracilis muscles
16 Tibia
17 Posterior cruciate ligament
18 Medial condyle of tibia (superior articular surface)
19 Posterior meniscofemoral ligament
20 Head of fibula
21 Tendon of semimembranosus muscle
22 Posterior attachment of articular capsule of knee joint
23 Lateral epicondyle of femur

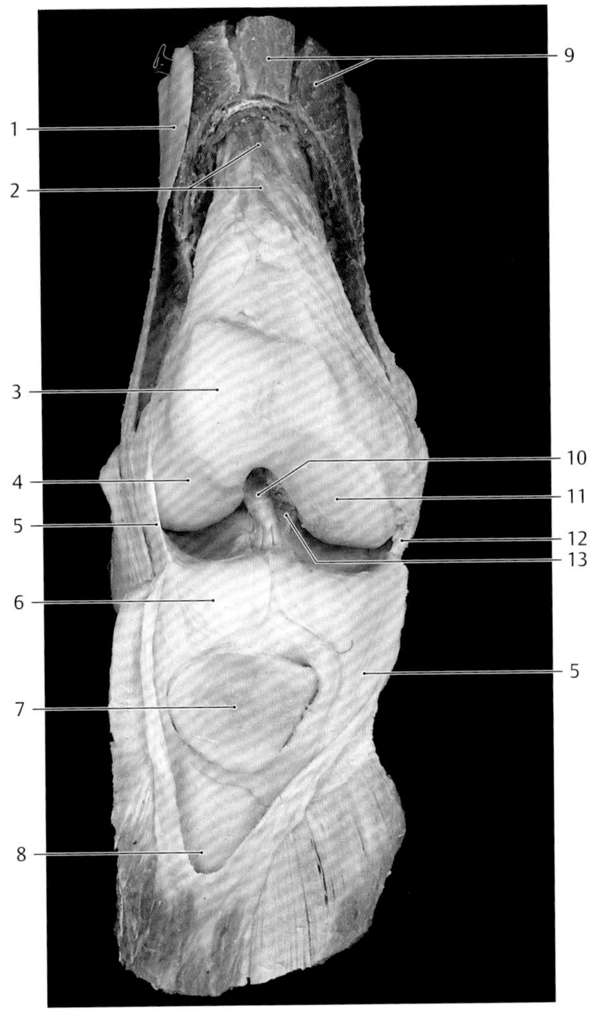

**Fig. 4.46 Right knee joint,** opened (anterior aspect). The patellar ligament with the patella has been reflected.

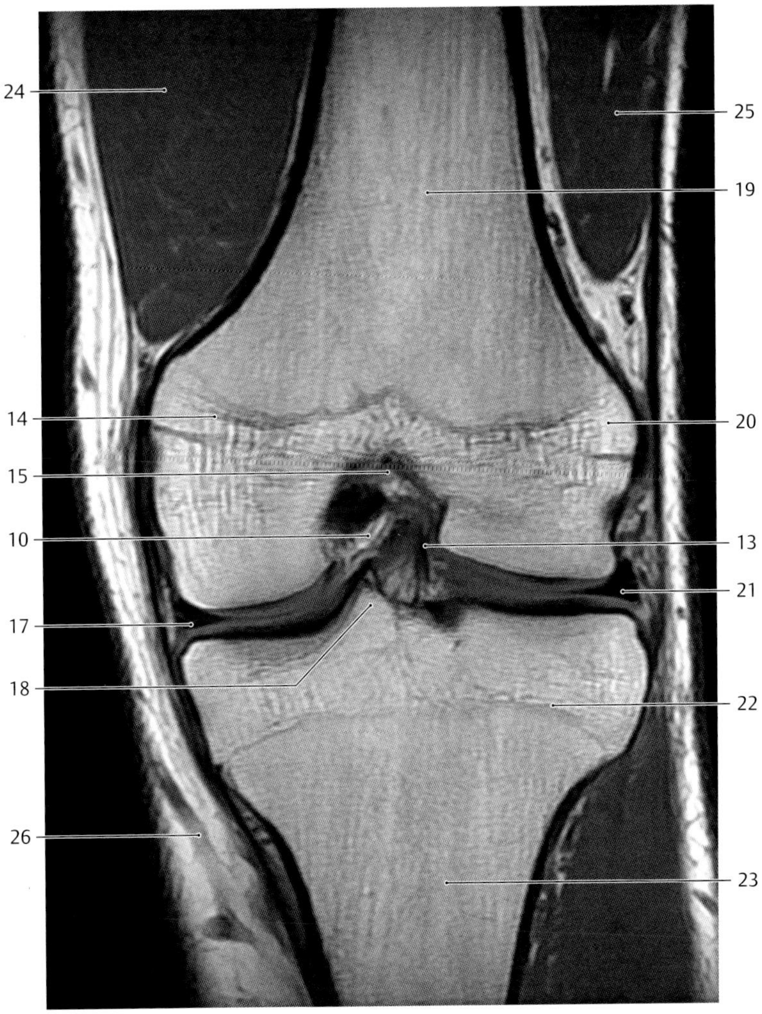

**Fig. 4.47 Coronal section through the knee joint** (MRI scan). (Heuck A, et al. MRT-Atlas des muskuloskelettalen Systems. Stuttgart, Germany: Schattauer, 2009.)

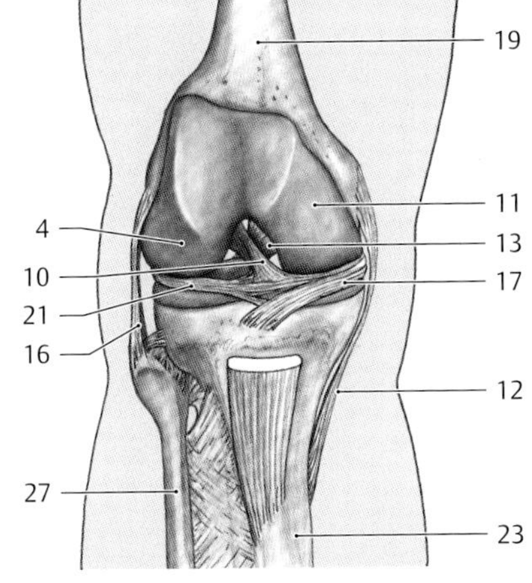


**Fig. 4.48 Ligaments of the right knee joint** (anterior aspect).

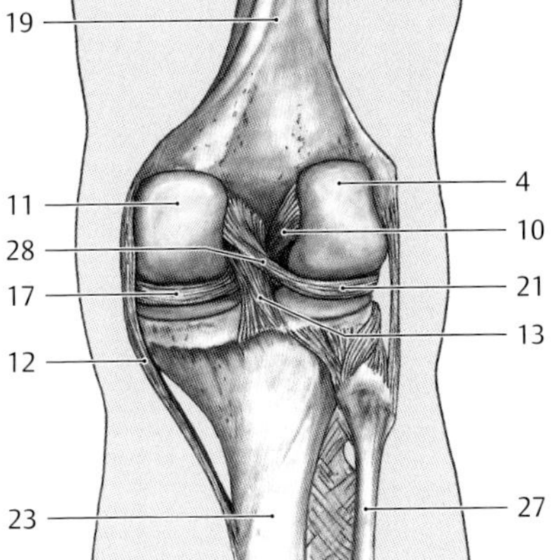


**Fig. 4.49 Ligaments of the right knee joint** (posterior aspect).

1 Iliotibial tract
2 Articular muscle of knee
3 Patellar surface
4 Lateral condyle of femur
5 Articular capsule
6 Infrapatellar fat pad
7 Patella (articular surface)
8 Suprapatellar bursa
9 Quadriceps femoris muscle
10 Anterior cruciate ligament
11 Medial condyle of femur
12 Tibial collateral ligament
13 Posterior cruciate ligament
14 Medial epicondyle of femur
15 Intercondylar fossa of femur
16 Fibular collateral ligament
17 Medial meniscus
18 Medial intercondylar tubercle
19 Femur
20 Lateral epicondyle of femur
21 Lateral meniscus
22 Epiphysial line of tibia
23 Tibia
24 Vastus medialis muscle
25 Vastus lateralis muscle
26 Great saphenous vein
27 Fibula
28 Posterior meniscofemoral ligament

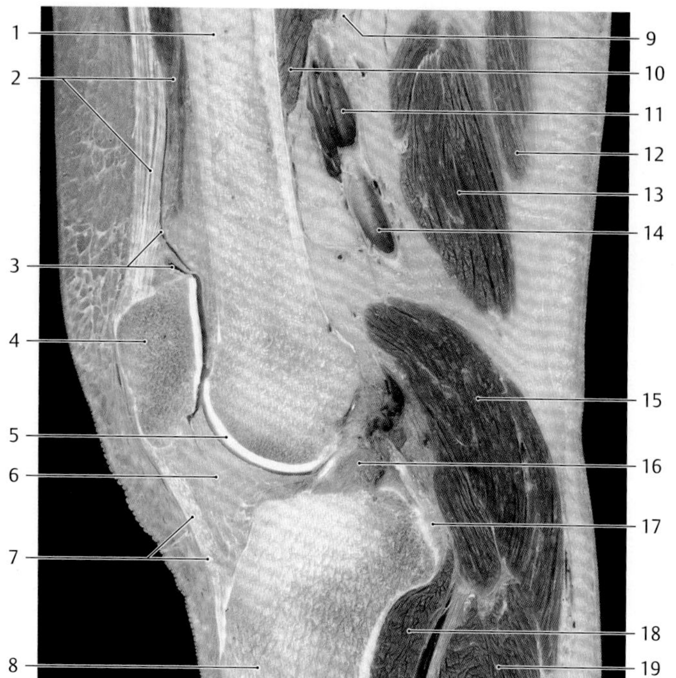


**Fig. 4.50 Sagittal section through the knee joint** (lateral aspect). Anterior surface to the left.

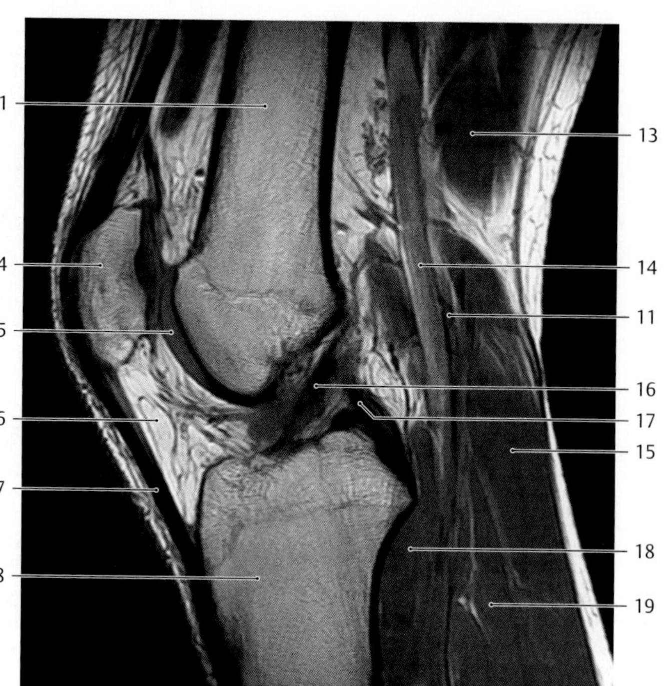


**Fig. 4.51 Sagittal section through the knee joint** (MRI scan). (Heuck A, et al. MRT-Atlas des muskuloskelettalen Systems. Stuttgart, Germany: Schattauer, 2009.)

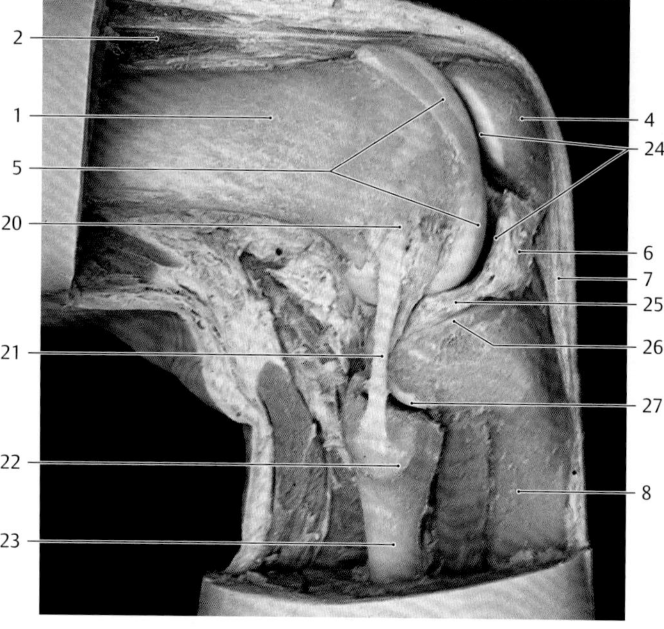


**Fig. 4.52 Right knee joint** and tibiofibular joint with ligaments (lateral aspect). Note the position of the lateral meniscus.

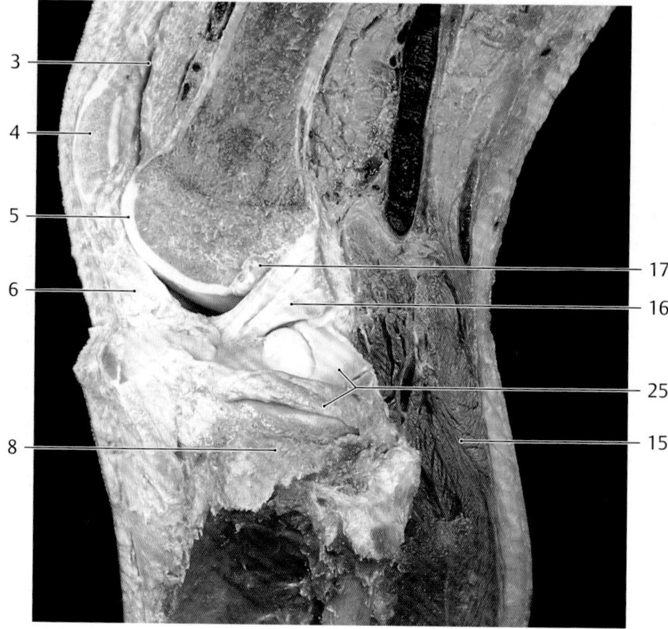


**Fig. 4.53 Left knee joint** with anterior cruciate ligament (lateral aspect).

1 Femur
2 Quadriceps femoris muscle
3 Suprapatellar bursa and articular cavity
4 Patella
5 Articular cartilage of femur
6 Infrapatellar fat pad
7 Patellar ligament
8 Tibia
9 Tibial nerve
10 Adductor magnus muscle
11 Popliteal vein
12 Semitendinosus muscle
13 Semimembranosus muscle
14 Popliteal artery
15 Gastrocnemius muscle
16 Anterior cruciate ligament
17 Posterior cruciate ligament
18 Popliteus muscle
19 Soleus muscle
20 Lateral epicondyle of femur
21 Fibular collateral ligament
22 Head of fibula
23 Fibula
24 Articular cavity of knee joint
25 Lateral meniscus of knee joint
26 Lateral condyle of tibia
27 Tibiofibular joint

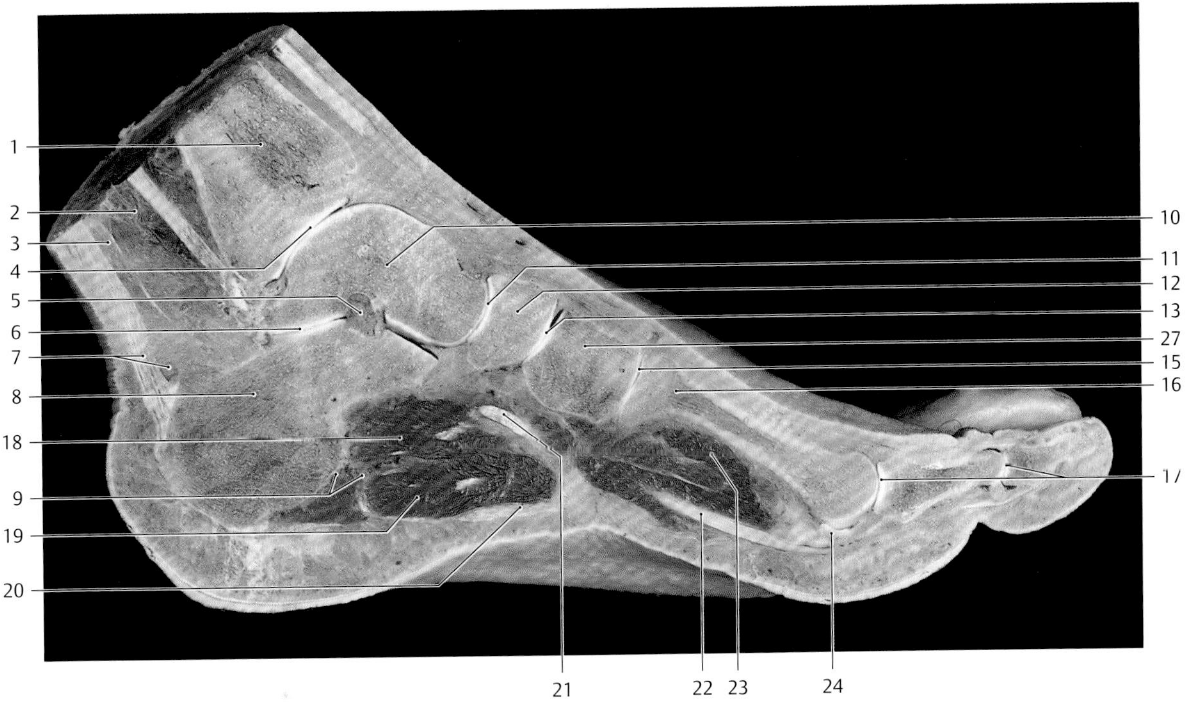


Fig. 4.54 **Sagittal section through the foot** at the level of the first phalanx.

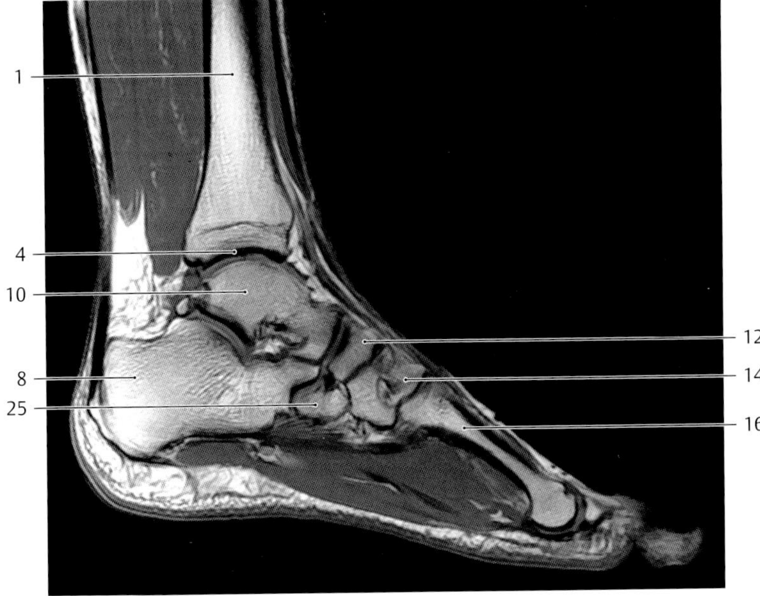


Fig. 4.55 **Sagittal section through the foot and leg** (MRI scan). (Heuck A, et al. MRT-Atlas des muskuloskelettalen Systems. Stuttgart, Germany: Schattauer, 2009.)

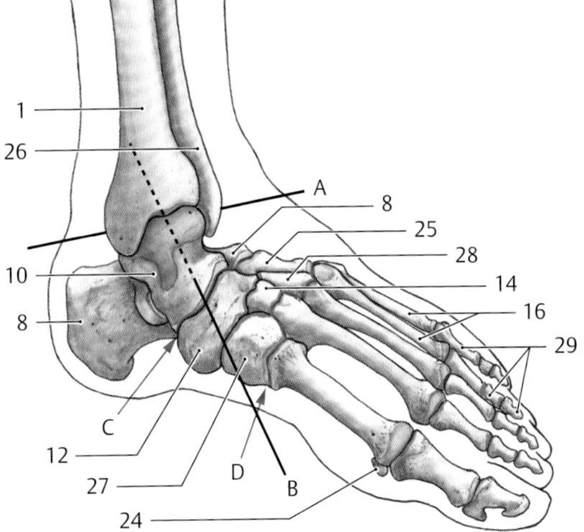


Fig. 4.56 **Skeleton of the left foot.** Joints are indicated in blue. Red lines = axis of joints.

A = Talocrural joint
B = Talocalcaneonaviwcular joint
C = Transverse tarsal joint (Chopart joint line)
D = Tarsometatarsal joints (Lisfranc joint line)

1 Tibia
2 Deep flexor muscles of leg
3 Superficial flexor muscles of leg
4 Ankle joint
5 Interosseous talocalcaneal ligament
6 Subtalar joint
7 Calcaneal or Achilles tendon and bursa
8 Calcaneus
9 Vessels and nerves of foot
10 Talus
11 Talocalcaneonavicular joint
12 Navicular bone
13 Cuneonavicular joint
14 Intermediate cuneiform bone
15 First tarsometatarsal joint
16 Metatarsal bones
17 Metatarsophalangeal and interphalangeal joints
18 Quadratus plantae muscle with flexor tendons
19 Flexor digitorum brevis muscle
20 Plantar aponeurosis
21 Tendon of tibialis posterior muscle
22 Tendon of flexor hallucis longus muscle
23 Flexor hallucis brevis muscle
24 Sesamoid bone
25 Cuboid bone
26 Fibula
27 Medial cuneiform bone
28 Lateral cuneiform bone
29 Phalanges

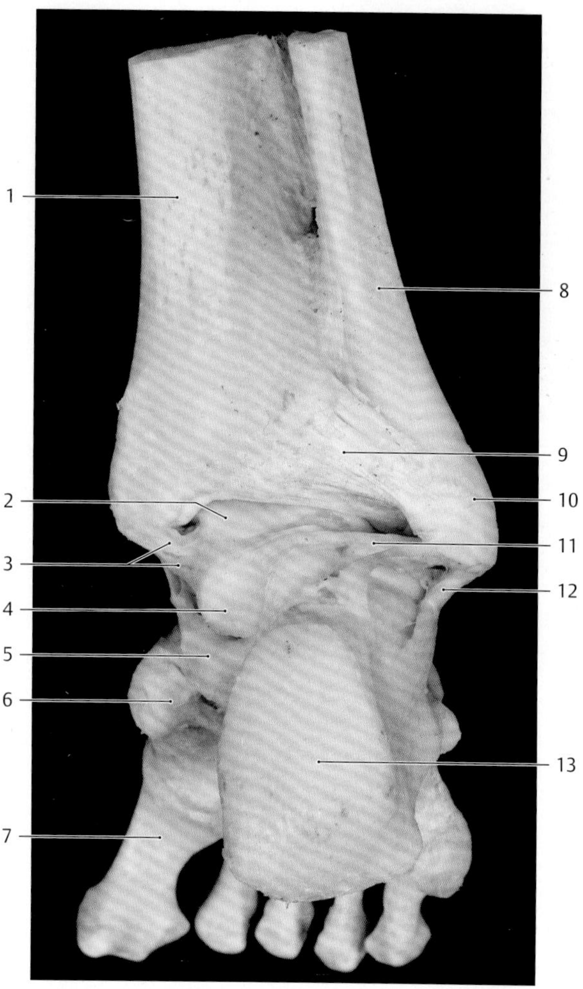


Fig. 4.57 **Ligaments of the ankle joint of the right foot** (dorsal aspect).

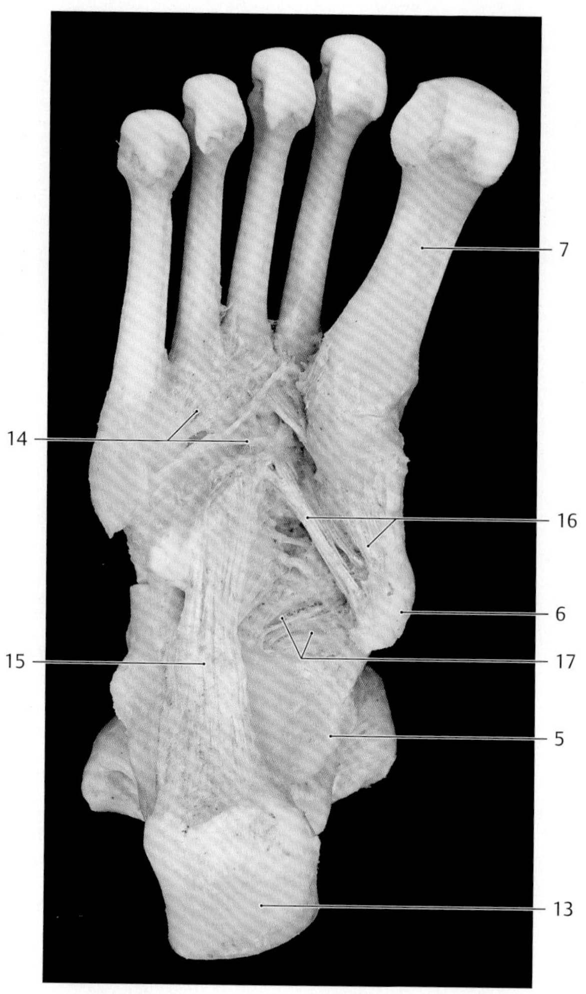


Fig. 4.58 **Deep ligaments of the right foot** (plantar aspect). The toes have been removed.

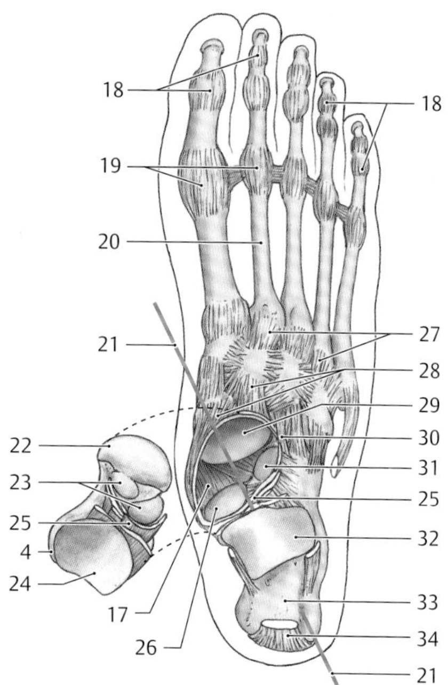


Fig. 4.59 **Ligaments of the foot.** Top view of the talocalcaneonavicular joint. The talus has been rotated to show the articular surfaces of the joint.

1 Tibia
2 Trochlea of talus
3 Medial or deltoid ligament of ankle (posterior tibiotalar part)
4 Talus
5 Sustentaculum tali
6 Navicular bone
7 First metatarsal bone
8 Fibula
9 Posterior tibiofibular ligament
10 Lateral malleolus
11 Posterior talofibular ligament
12 Calcaneofibular ligament
13 Calcaneal tuberosity
14 Plantar tarsometatarsal ligaments
15 Long plantar ligament
16 Plantar cuneonavicular ligaments
17 Plantar calcaneonavicular ligament
18 Articular capsules of interphalangeal joints
19 Articular capsules of metatarsophalangeal joints
20 Second metatarsal bone
21 Axis for inversion and eversion of foot
22 Navicular articular surface } of talus
23 Anterior and middle calcaneal surfaces } of talus
24 Posterior calcaneal surface } of talus
25 Talocalcaneal interosseous ligament
26 Middle talar articular surface of calcaneus
27 Dorsal tarsometatarsal ligaments
28 Talonavicular ligament
29 Articular surface of navicular bone
30 Bifurcate ligament
31 Anterior talar articular surface } of calcaneus
32 Posterior talar articular surface } of calcaneus
33 Calcaneus
34 Calcaneal or Achilles tendon and bursa

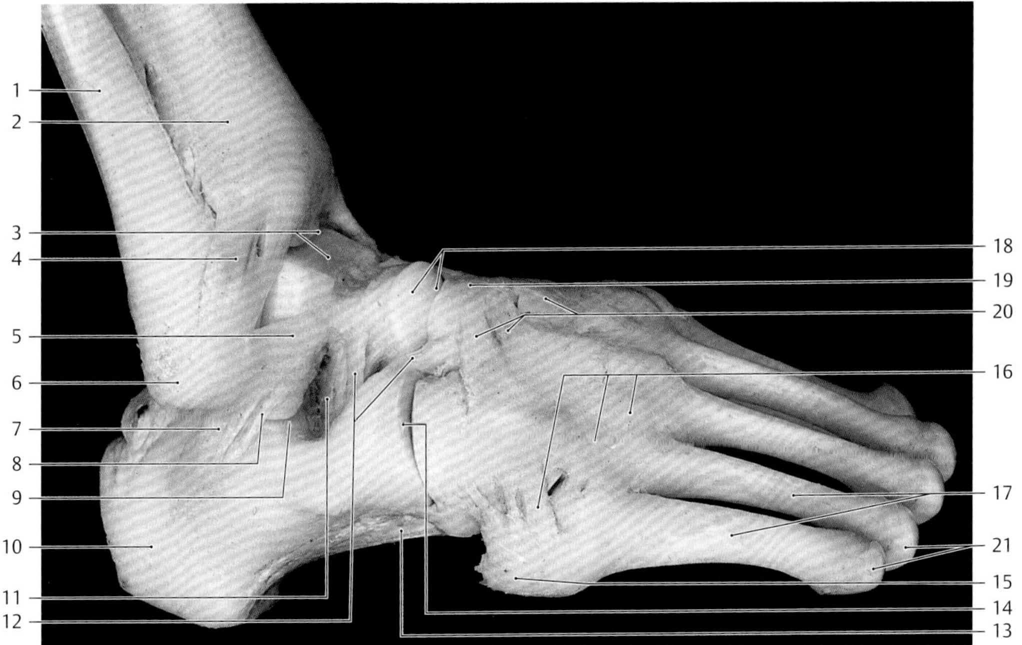


Fig. 4.60 **Ligaments of the right foot** (lateral aspect).

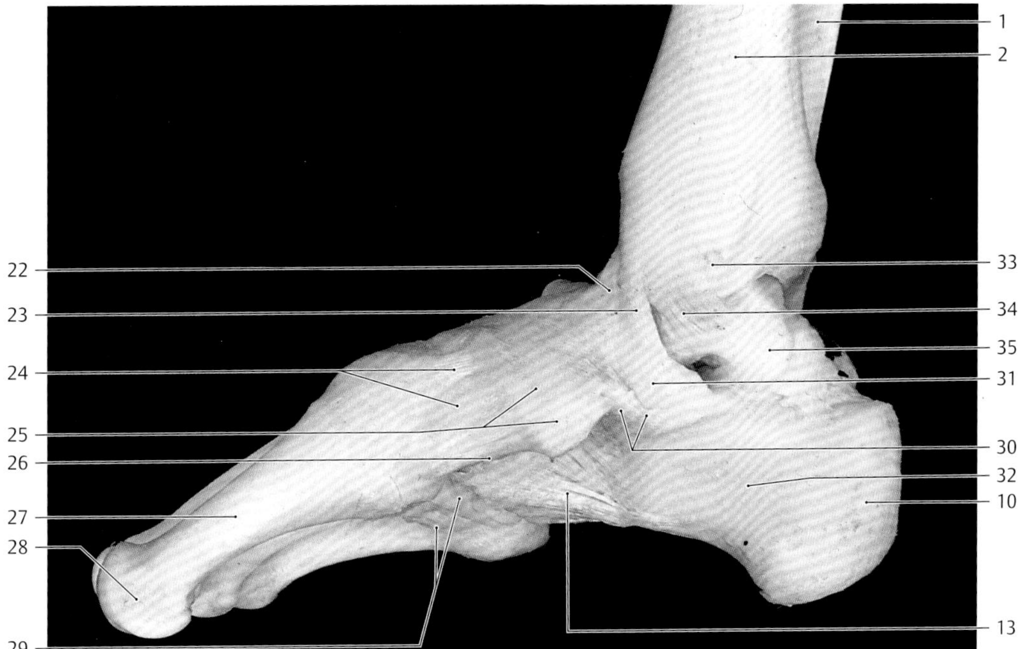


Fig. 4.61 **Ligaments of the right foot** (medial aspect).

1 Fibula
2 Tibia
3 Trochlea of talus and ankle joint
4 Anterior tibiofibular ligament
5 Anterior talofibular ligament
6 Lateral malleolus
7 Calcaneofibular ligament
8 Lateral talocalcaneal ligament
9 Subtalar joint
10 Calcaneal tuberosity
11 Interosseous talocalcaneal ligament
12 Bifurcate ligament
13 Long plantar ligament
14 Calcaneocuboid joint
15 Tuberosity of fifth metatarsal bone
16 Dorsal tarsometatarsal ligaments
17 Metatarsal bones
18 Head of talus and talocalcaneonavicular joint
19 Navicular bone
20 Dorsal cuneonavicular ligaments
21 Heads of metatarsal bones
22 Medial or deltoid ligament of ankle (tibionavicular part)
23 Medial or deltoid ligament of ankle (tibiocalcaneal part)
24 Dorsal cuneonavicular ligaments
25 Navicular bone
26 Plantar cuneonavicular ligament
27 First metatarsal bone
28 Head of first metatarsal bone
29 Plantar tarsometatarsal ligaments
30 Plantar calcaneonavicular ligament
31 Sustentaculum tali
32 Calcaneus
33 Medial malleolus
34 Medial or deltoid ligament of ankle (posterior tibiotalar part)
35 Talus

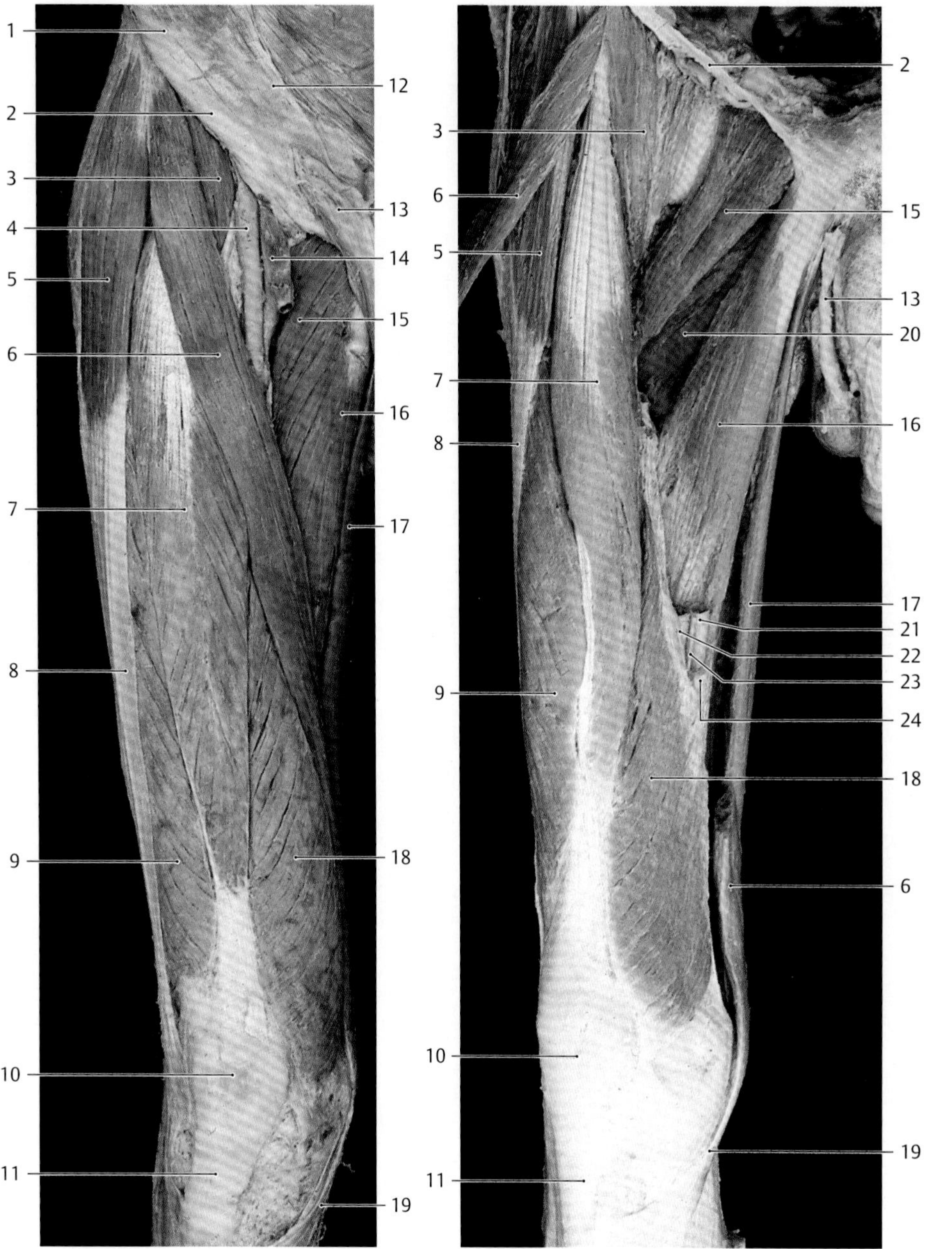


**Fig. 4.62 Extensor and adductor muscles of the thigh** (right side, anterior aspect).

**Fig. 4.63 Quadriceps muscle and superficial layer of adductor muscles of the thigh** (right side, anterior aspect). The sartorius muscle has been divided.

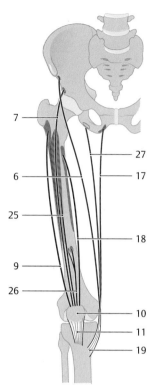

**Fig. 4.64 Course of the extensor muscles of the thigh** and muscles inserting with common tendon on the tibia (anterior aspect).

1 Anterior superior iliac spine
2 Inguinal ligament
3 Iliopsoas muscle
4 Femoral artery
5 Tensor fasciae latae muscle
6 Sartorius muscle
7 Rectus femoris muscle
8 Iliotibial tract
9 Vastus lateralis muscle
10 Patella
11 Patellar ligament
12 Aponeurosis of external abdominal oblique muscle
13 Spermatic cord
14 Femoral vein
15 Pectineus muscle
16 Adductor longus muscle
17 Gracilis muscle
18 Vastus medialis muscle
19 Common tendon of sartorius, gracilis, and semitendinosus muscles (pes anserinus)
20 Adductor brevis muscle
21 Femoral artery } entering the adductor canal
22 Femoral vein } entering the adductor canal
23 Saphenous nerve } entering the adductor canal
24 Vasto-adductor membrane
25 Vastus intermedius muscle
26 Articularis genus muscle
27 Semitendinosus muscle

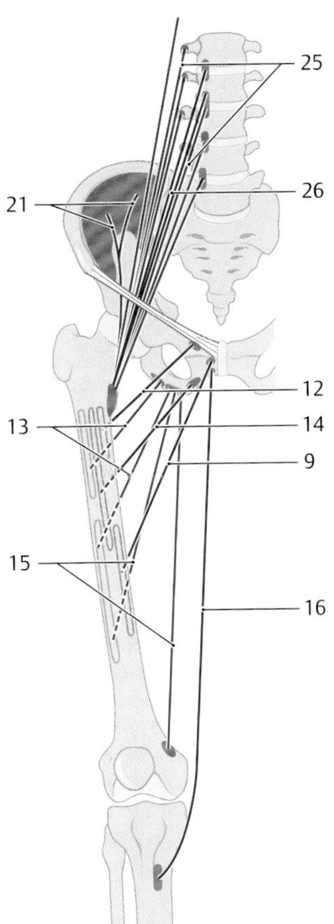


**Fig. 4.65 Course of the adductor muscles of the thigh** (anterior aspect).

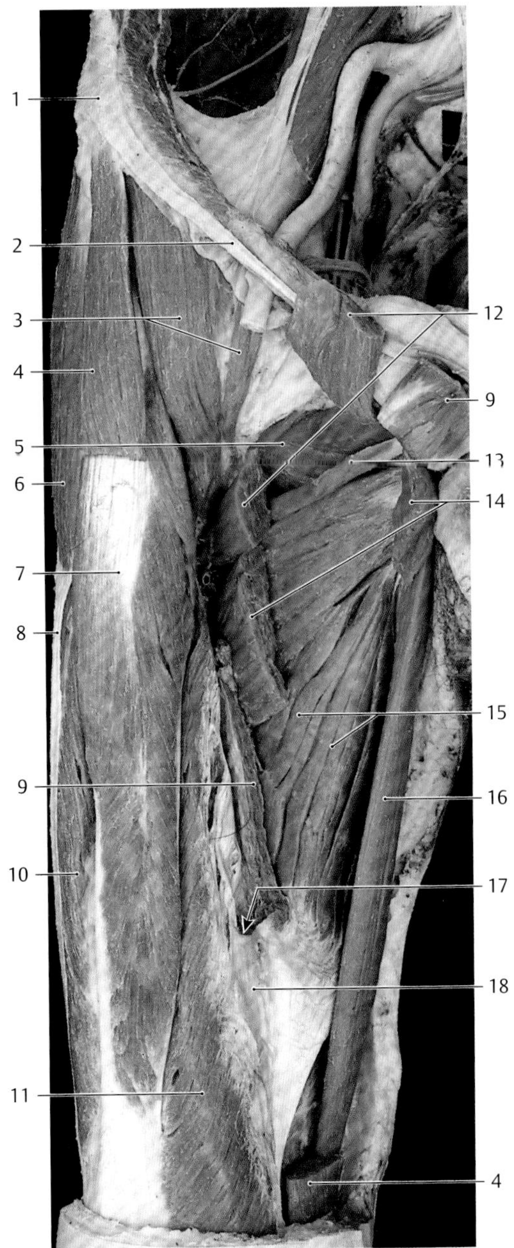


**Fig. 4.66 Adductor magnus muscle and deep layer of adductor muscles of the thigh** (right side, anterior aspect). Pectineus, adductor longus, and brevis muscles have been divided.

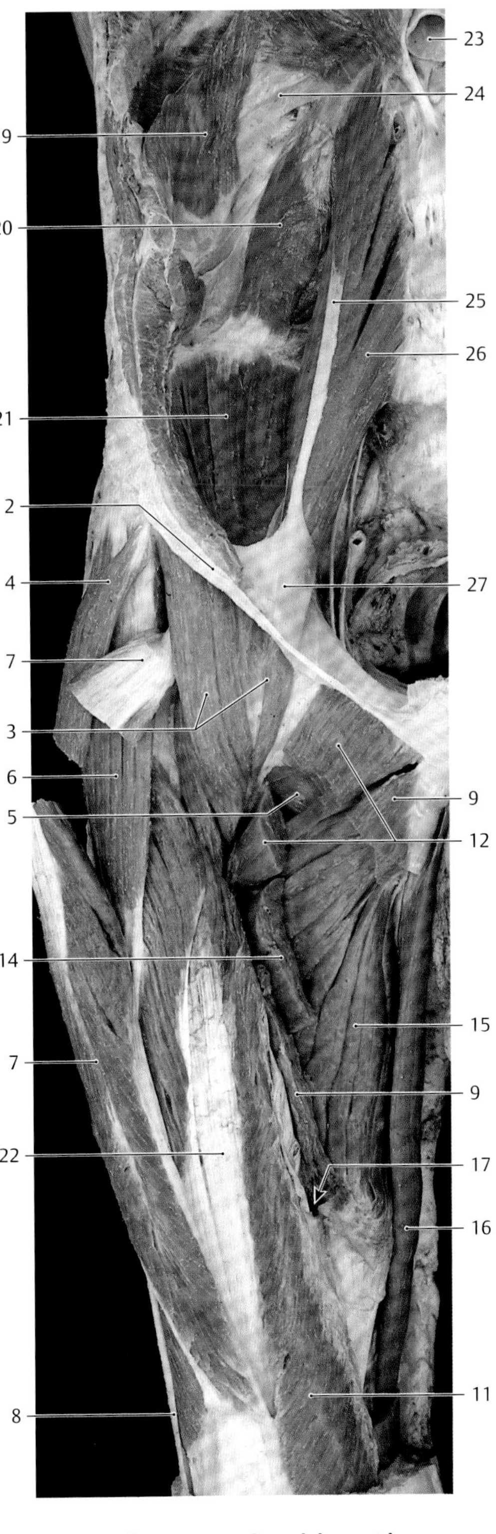


**Fig. 4.67 Iliopsoas muscle and deepest layer of adductor muscles of the thigh** (right side, anterior aspect). Pectineus, adductor longus, and brevis muscles have been divided. Note: The iliac, psoas minor, and psoas major muscles collectively form the iliopsoas muscle.

1 Anterior superior iliac spine
2 Inguinal ligament
3 Iliopsoas muscle
4 Sartorius muscle
5 Obturator externus muscle
6 Tensor fasciae latae muscle
7 Rectus femoris muscle
8 Iliotibial tract
9 Adductor longus muscle (divided)
10 Vastus lateralis muscle
11 Vastus medialis muscle
12 Pectineus muscle (divided)
13 Adductor minimus muscle
14 Adductor brevis muscle (cut)
15 Adductor magnus muscle
16 Gracilis muscle
17 Adductor canal
18 Vasto-adductor membrane
19 Diaphragm
20 Quadratus lumborum muscle
21 Iliacus muscle
22 Vastus intermedius muscle
23 Aortic hiatus
24 Twelfth rib
25 Psoas minor muscle
26 Psoas major muscle
27 Iliopectineal arch

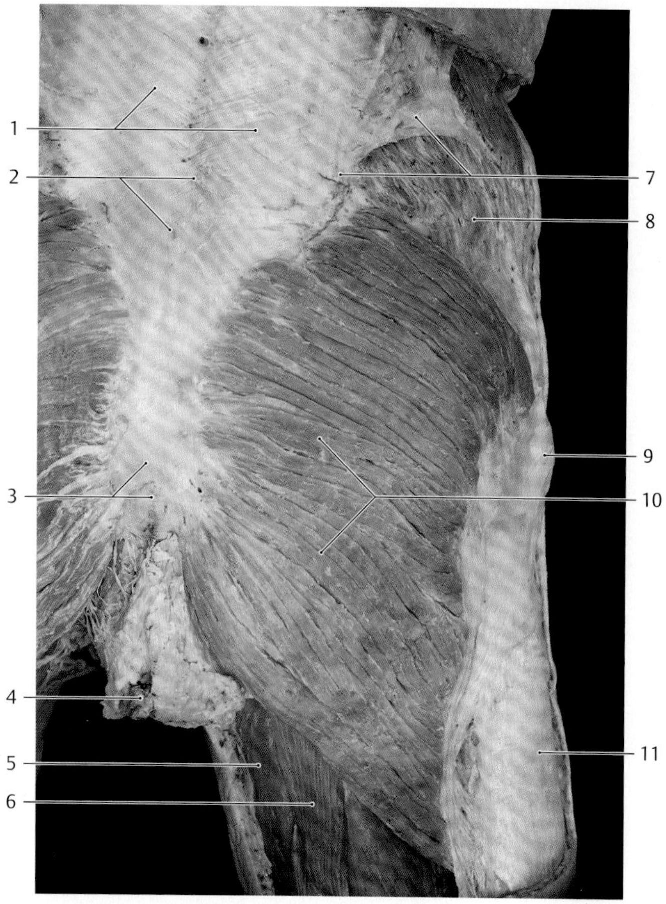

Fig. 4.68 **Gluteal muscles,** superficial layer (right side, posterior aspect).

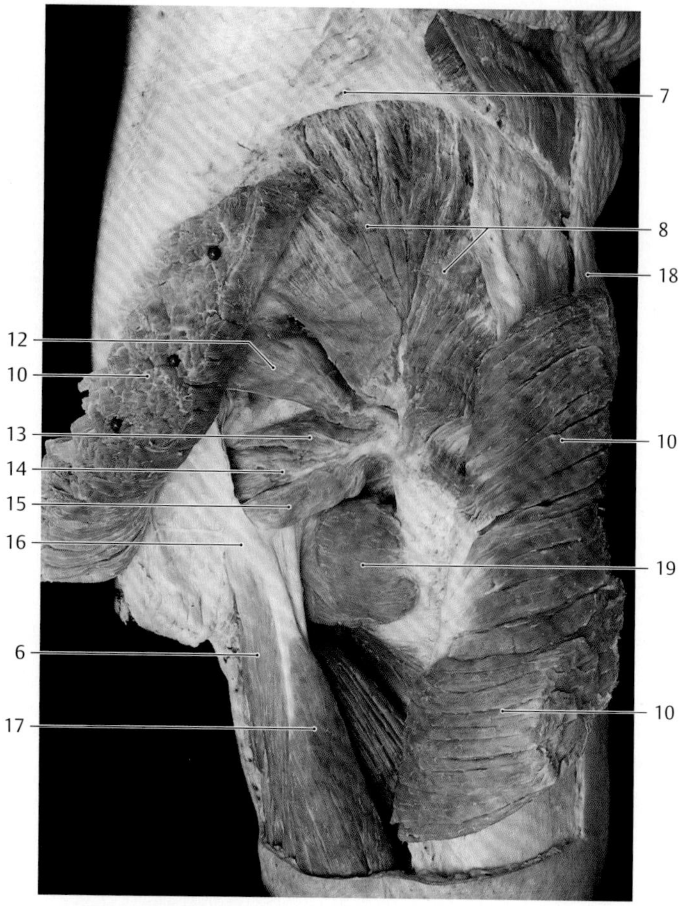

Fig. 4.69 **Gluteal muscles,** deeper layer (right side, posterior aspect).

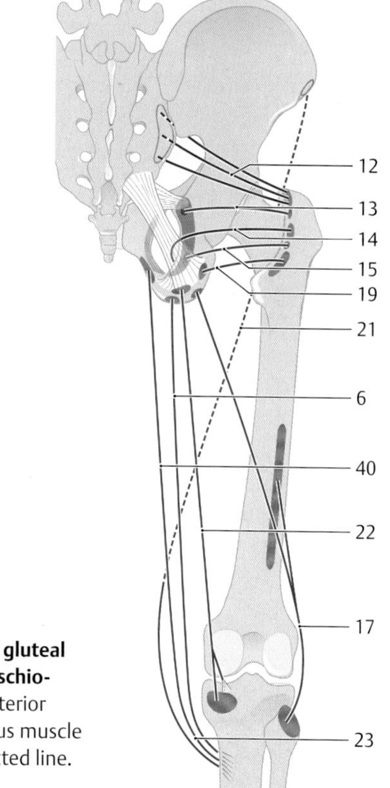


Fig. 4.70 **Course of gluteal** (deeper layer) **and ischio-crural muscles** (posterior aspect). The sartorius muscle is indicated by a dotted line.

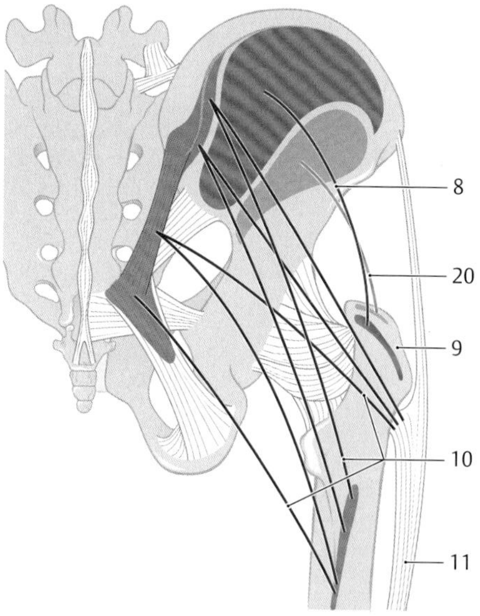

Fig. 4.71 **Course of the gluteal muscles** (posterior aspect).

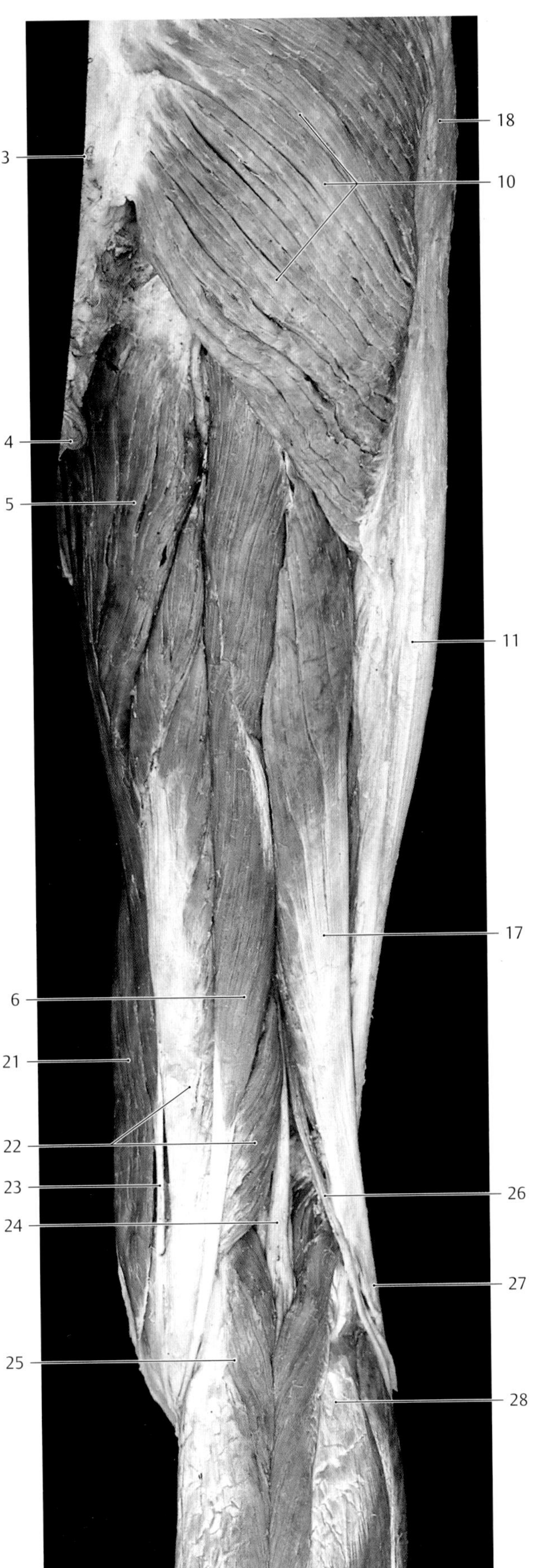


Fig. 4.72 **Flexor muscles of the thigh,** superficial layer (right side, posterior aspect).

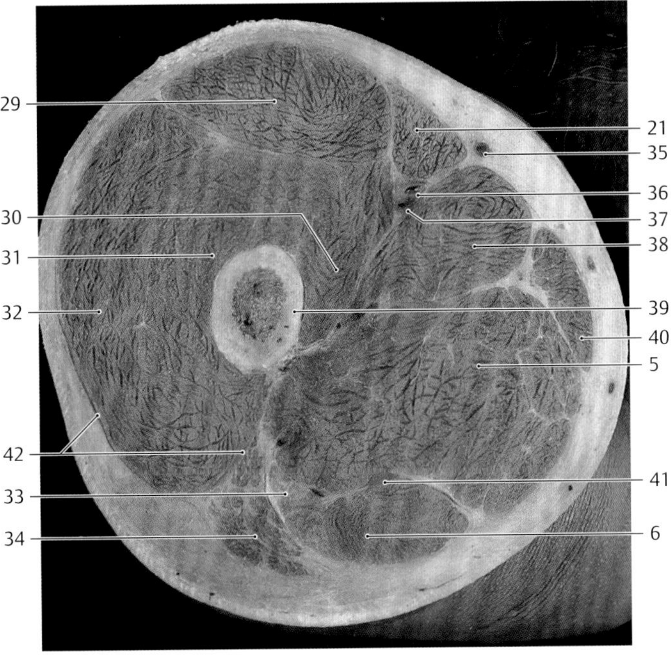


Fig. 4.73 **Cross section through the right thigh** (inferior aspect). Anterior side on top.

1 Thoracolumbar fascia
2 Spinous processes of lumbar vertebrae
3 Coccyx
4 Anus
5 Adductor magnus muscle
6 Semitendinosus muscle
7 Iliac crest
8 Gluteus medius muscle
9 Greater trochanter
10 Gluteus maximus muscle
11 Iliotibial tract
12 Piriformis muscle
13 Superior gemellus muscle
14 Obturator internus muscle
15 Inferior gemellus muscle
16 Ischial tuberosity
17 Biceps femoris muscle
18 Tensor fasciae latae muscle
19 Quadratus femoris muscle
20 Gluteus minimus muscle
21 Sartorius muscle
22 Semimembranosus muscle
23 Tendon of gracilis muscle
24 Tibial nerve
25 Medial head of gastrocnemius muscle
26 Common fibular nerve
27 Tendon of biceps femoris muscle
28 Lateral head of gastrocnemius muscle
29 Rectus femoris muscle
30 Vastus medialis muscle
31 Vastus intermedius muscle
32 Vastus lateralis muscle
33 Sciatic nerve
34 Gluteus maximus muscle (insertion)
35 Great saphenous vein
36 Femoral artery
37 Femoral vein
38 Adductor longus muscle
39 Femur
40 Gracilis muscle
41 Septum between semitendinosus and semimembranosus muscles
42 Lateral intermuscular septum

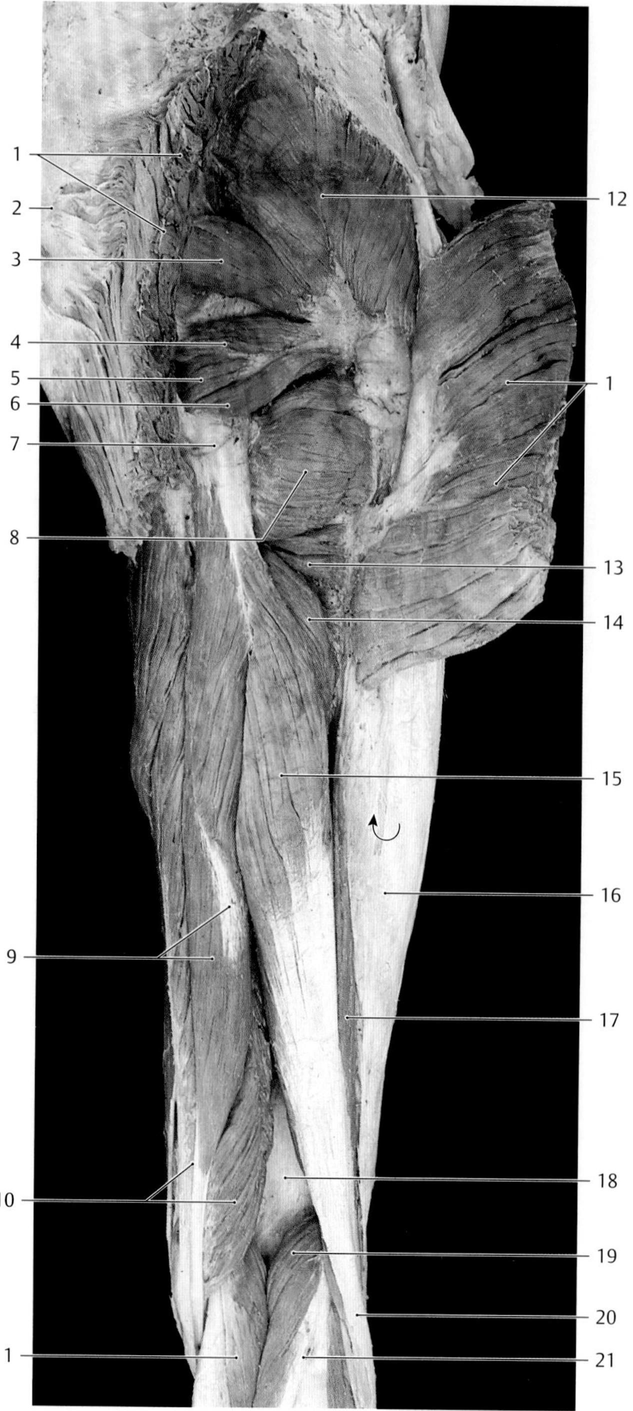


Fig. 4.74 **Flexor muscles of the thigh** (right side, posterior aspect). The gluteus maximus muscle has been cut and reflected. Arrow = entrance to muscular septum.

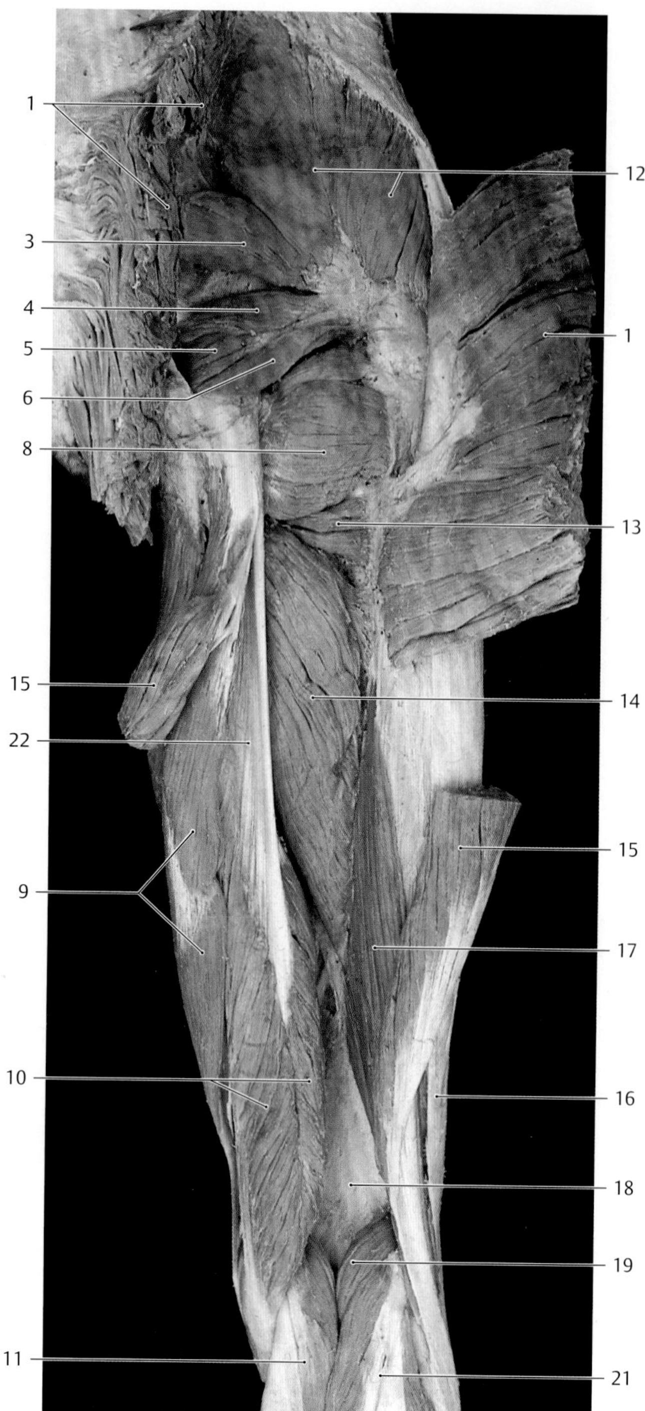


Fig. 4.75 **Flexor muscles of the thigh** (right side, posterior aspect). The gluteus maximus muscle and the long head of the biceps femoris muscle have been divided and displaced.

1 Gluteus maximus muscle (divided)
2 Position of coccyx
3 Piriformis muscle
4 Superior gemellus muscle
5 Obturator internus muscle
6 Inferior gemellus muscle
7 Ischial tuberosity
8 Quadratus femoris muscle
9 Semitendinosus muscle with intermediate tendon
10 Semimembranosus muscle
11 Medial head of gastrocnemius muscle
12 Gluteus medius muscle
13 Adductor minimus muscle
14 Adductor magnus muscle
15 Long head of biceps femoris muscle
16 Iliotibial tract
17 Short head of biceps femoris muscle
18 Popliteal surface of femur
19 Plantaris muscle
20 Tendon of biceps femoris muscle
21 Lateral head of gastrocnemius muscle
22 Tendon of semimembranosus muscle

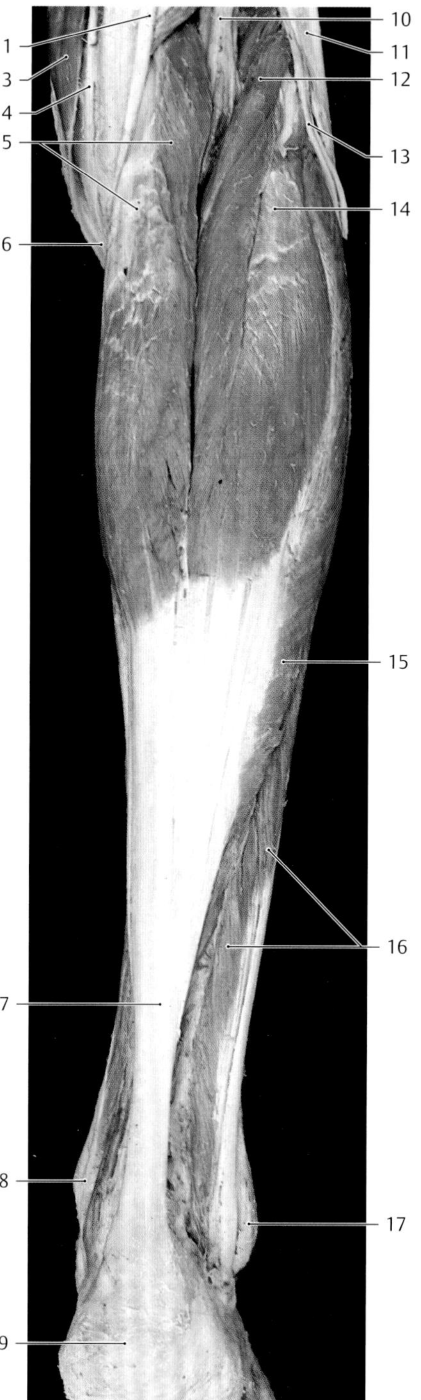


Fig. 4.76 **Flexor muscles of the leg** (right side, posterior aspect).

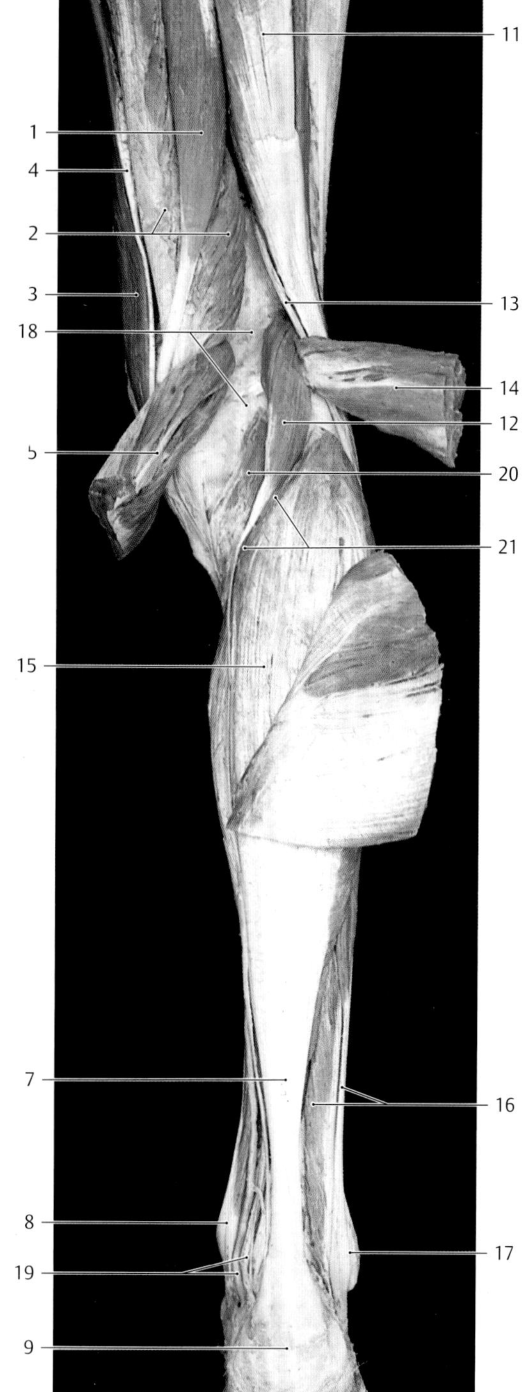


Fig. 4.77 **Flexor muscles of the leg** (right side, posterior aspect). Both heads of the gastrocnemius muscle have been cut and reflected.

Fig. 4.78 **Course of the flexor muscles of the leg** (posterior aspect).

1 Semitendinosus muscle
2 Semimembranosus muscle
3 Sartorius muscle
4 Tendon of gracilis muscle
5 Medial head of gastrocnemius muscle
6 Common tendon of gracilis, sartorius, and semitendinosus muscles (pes anserinus)
7 Calcaneal or Achilles tendon
8 Medial malleolus
9 Calcaneal tuberosity
10 Tibial nerve
11 Biceps femoris muscle
12 Plantaris muscle
13 Common fibular nerve
14 Lateral head of gastrocnemius muscle
15 Soleus muscle
16 Peroneus longus and brevis muscles
17 Lateral malleolus
18 Popliteal fossa
19 Tibial nerve and posterior tibial artery
20 Popliteus muscle
21 Tendinous arch of soleus muscle
22 Femur
23 Fibula
24 Tibia

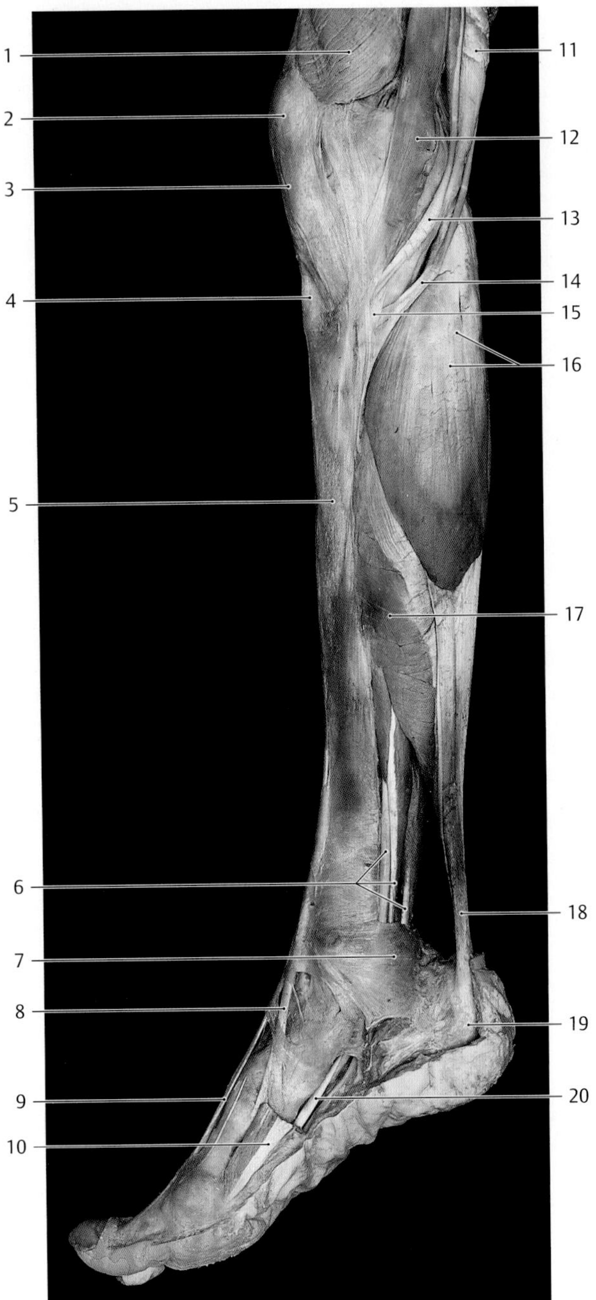


Fig. 4.79 **Muscles of leg and foot** (right side, medial aspect).

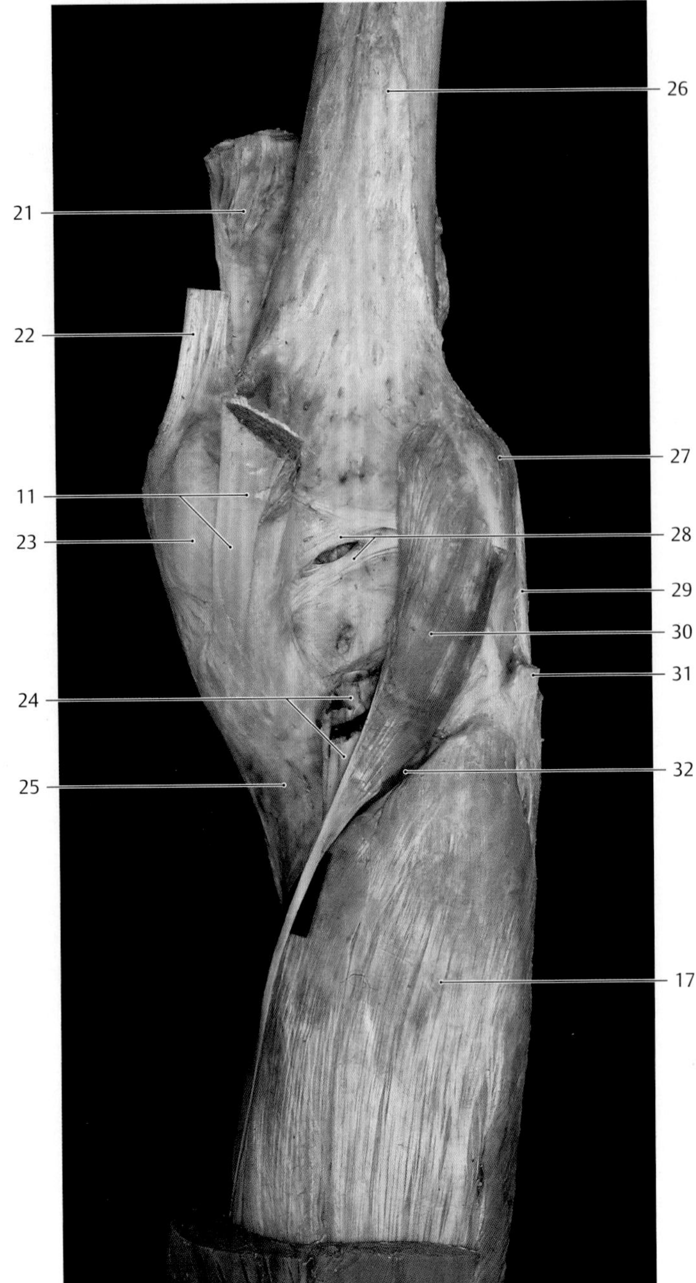


Fig. 4.80 **Popliteal region with plantaris and soleus muscles** (right side, posterior aspect). Notice the insertion of the tendon of the semimembranosus muscle.

1 Vastus medialis muscle
2 Patella
3 Patellar ligament
4 Tibial tuberosity
5 Tibia
6 Tendons of deep flexor muscles (from anterior to posterior: [1] tibialis posterior; [2] flexor digitorum longus; [3] flexor hallucis longus muscles)
7 Flexor retinaculum
8 Tendon of tibialis anterior muscle
9 Tendon of extensor hallucis longus muscle
10 Abductor hallucis muscle
11 Tendon of semimembranosus muscle
12 Sartorius muscle
13 Tendon of gracilis muscle
14 Tendon of semitendinosus muscle
15 Common tendon of gracilis, semitendinosus, and sartorius muscles (pes anserinus)
16 Medial head of gastrocnemius muscle
17 Soleus muscle
18 Calcaneal or Achilles tendon
19 Calcaneus muscle
20 Tendon of flexor hallucis longus muscle
21 Quadriceps femoris muscle (divided)
22 Tendon of adductor magnus muscle (divided)
23 Medial condyle of femur
24 Popliteal artery and vein, and tibial nerve
25 Tibia
26 Femur
27 Lateral epicondyle of femur
28 Oblique popliteal ligament
29 Lateral (fibular) collateral ligament
30 Plantaris muscle
31 Tendon of biceps femoris muscle (divided)
32 Tendinous arch of soleus muscle

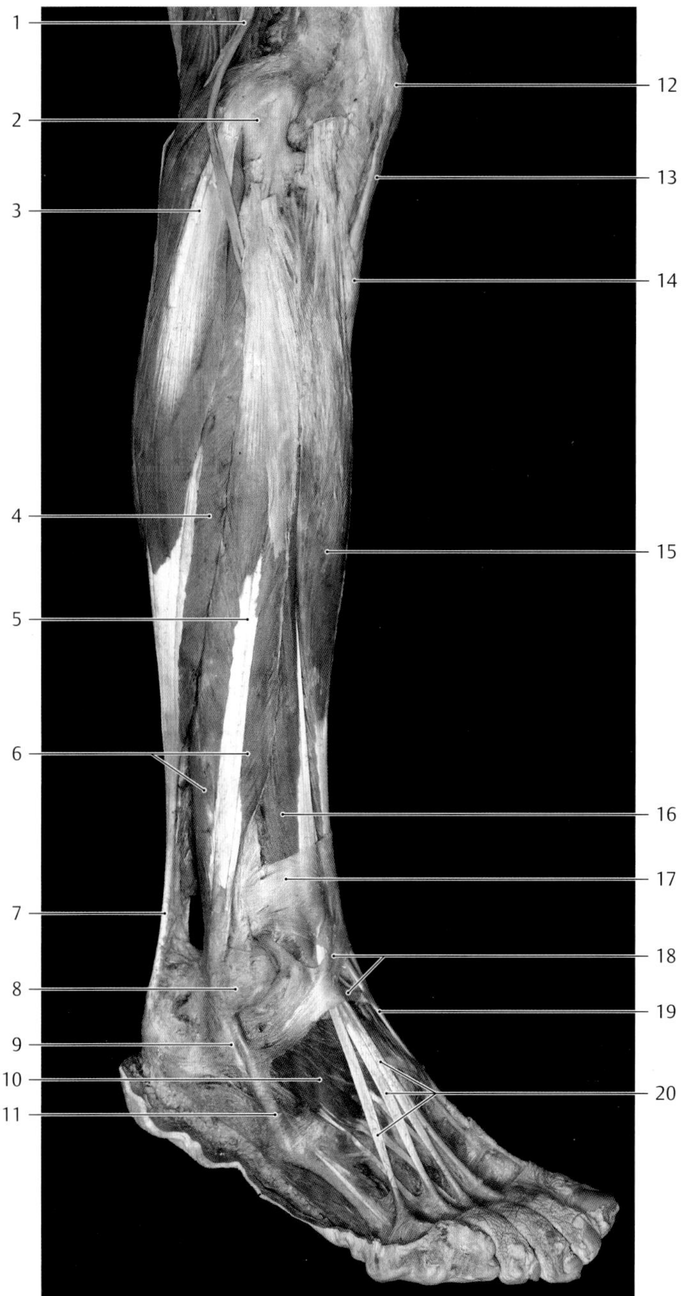


Fig. 4.81 **Muscles of leg and foot** (right side, lateral aspect).

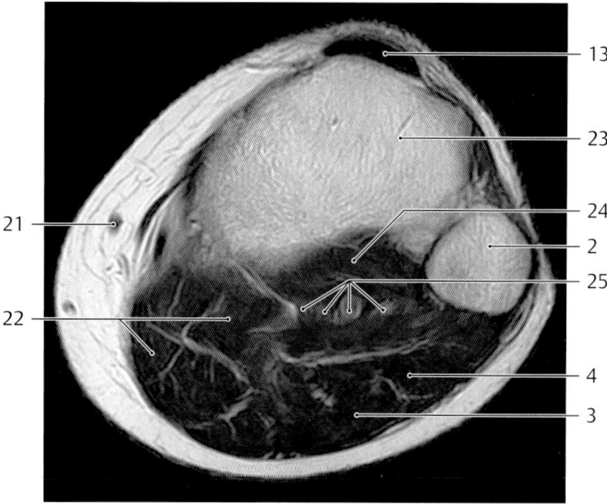


Fig. 4.82 **Axial section through the right leg** distally of the knee joint (MRI scan; see corresponding Fig. 4.83). (Heuck A, et al. MRT-Atlas des muskuloskelettalen Systems. Stuttgart, Germany: Schattauer, 2009.)

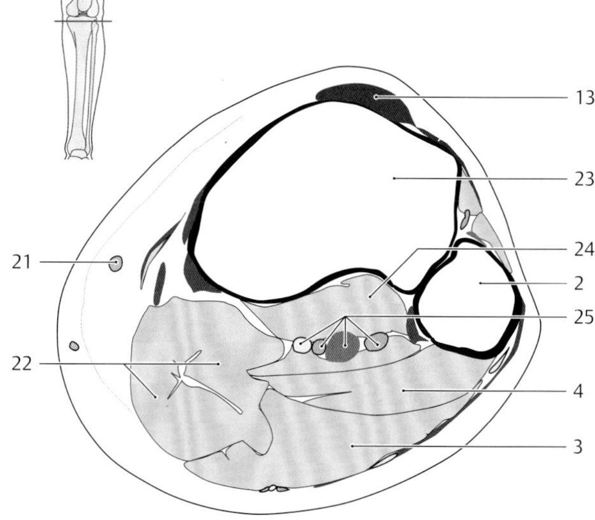


Fig. 4.83 **Axial section through the right leg** distally of the knee joint (schematic of Fig. 4.82 above). (Heuck A, et al. MRT-Atlas des muskuloskelettalen Systems. Stuttgart, Germany: Schattauer, 2009.)

1 Common fibular nerve
2 Head of fibula
3 Lateral head of gastrocnemius muscle
4 Soleus muscle
5 Peroneus longus muscle
6 Peroneus brevis muscle
7 Calcaneal or Achilles tendon
8 Lateral malleolus muscle
9 Tendon of peroneus longus muscle
10 Extensor digitorum brevis muscle
11 Tendon of peroneus brevis muscle
12 Patella
13 Patellar ligament
14 Tuberosity of tibia
15 Tibialis anterior muscle
16 Extensor digitorum longus muscle
17 Superior extensor retinaculum
18 Inferior extensor retinaculum
19 Tendon of extensor hallucis longus muscle
20 Tendons of extensor digitorum longus muscle
21 Great saphenous vein
22 Medial head of gastrocnemius muscle
23 Tibia
24 Popliteus muscle
25 Tibial nerve, popliteal artery, and veins

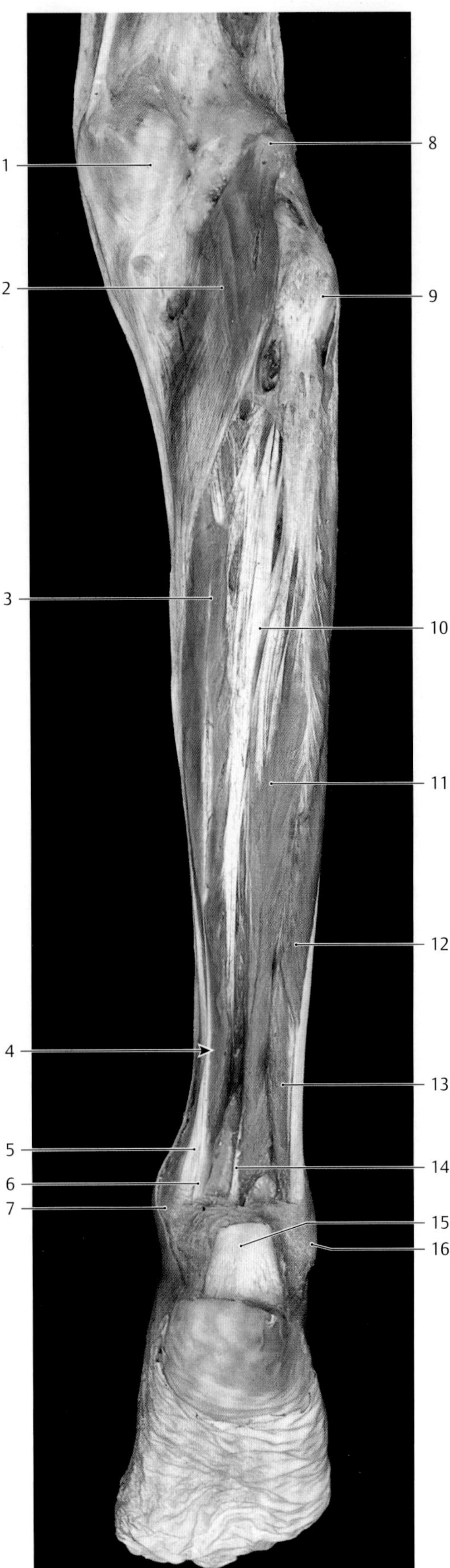


1 Medial condyle of femur
2 Popliteus muscle
3 Flexor digitorum longus muscle
4 Crossing of tendons in the leg
5 Tendon of tibialis posterior muscle
6 Tendon of flexor digitorum longus muscle
7 Medial malleolus
8 Lateral condyle of femur
9 Head of fibula
10 Tibialis posterior muscle
11 Flexor hallucis longus muscle
12 Peroneus longus muscle
13 Peroneus brevis muscle
14 Tendon of flexor hallucis longus muscle
15 Calcaneal or Achilles tendon (divided)
16 Lateral malleolus

**Fig. 4.84 Deep flexor muscles of leg and foot** (right side, posterior aspect).

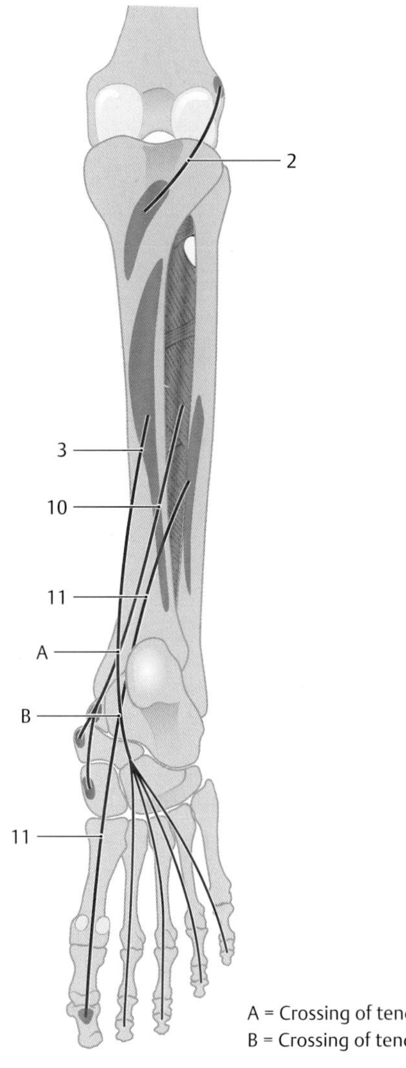


**Fig. 4.85 Course of the deep flexor muscles of the leg** (posterior aspect).

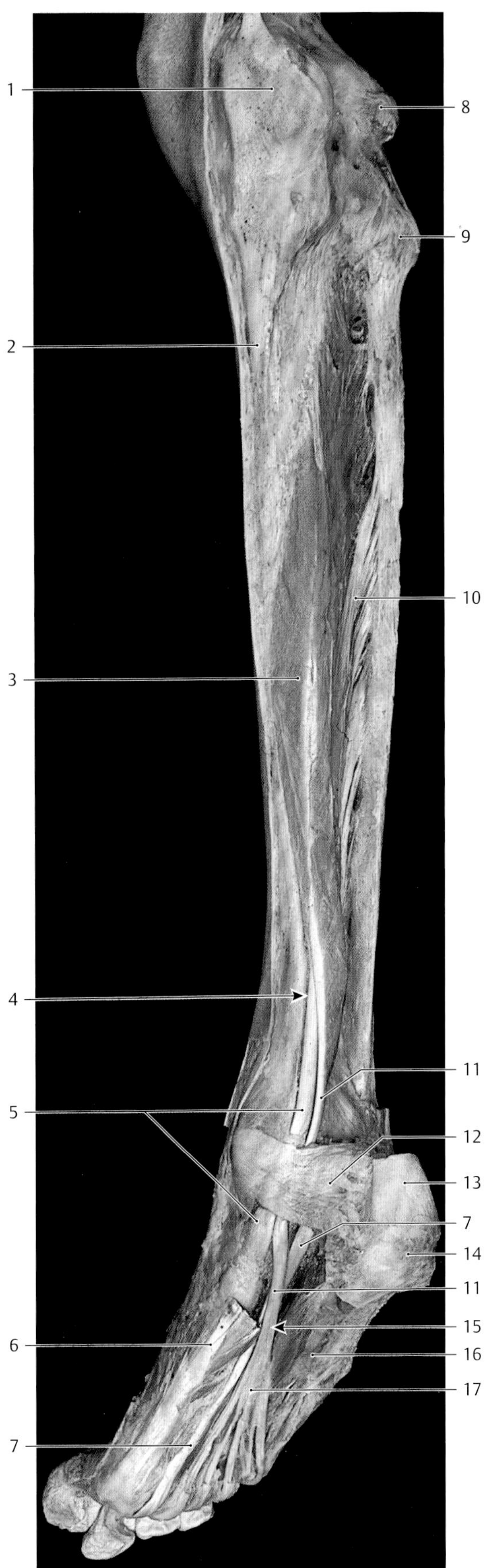


Fig. 4.86 **Deep flexor muscles of leg and foot** (right side, posterior oblique-medial aspect). Flexor digitorum brevis and flexor hallucis longus muscles have been removed.

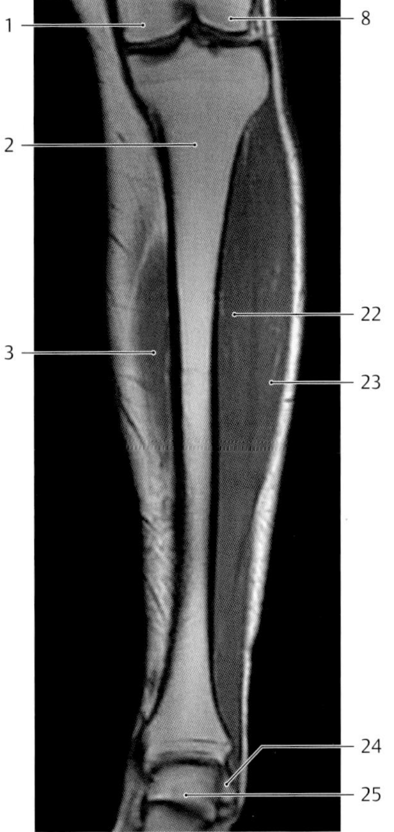


Fig. 4.87 **Coronal section through the leg** (MRI scan). (Heuck A, et al. MRT-Atlas des muskuloskelettalen Systems. Stuttgart, Germany: Schattauer, 2009.)

1 Medial condyle of femur
2 Tibia
3 Flexor digitorum longus muscle
4 Crossing of tendons in the leg
5 Tendon of tibialis posterior muscle
6 Abductor hallucis muscle
7 Tendon of flexor hallucis longus muscle
8 Lateral condyle of femur
9 Head of fibula
10 Tibialis posterior muscle
11 Tendon of flexor digitorum longus muscle
12 Flexor retinaculum
13 Calcaneal or Achilles tendon
14 Calcaneal tuberosity
15 Crossing of tendons in the sole
16 Quadratus plantae muscle
17 Tendons of flexor digitorum longus muscle
18 Tendon of tibialis anterior muscle
19 Area of insertion of tibialis posterior muscle
20 Lumbrical muscles
21 Flexor hallucis longus muscle
22 Tibialis anterior muscle
23 Extensor hallucis longus muscle
24 Lateral malleolus of fibula
25 Trochlea of talus

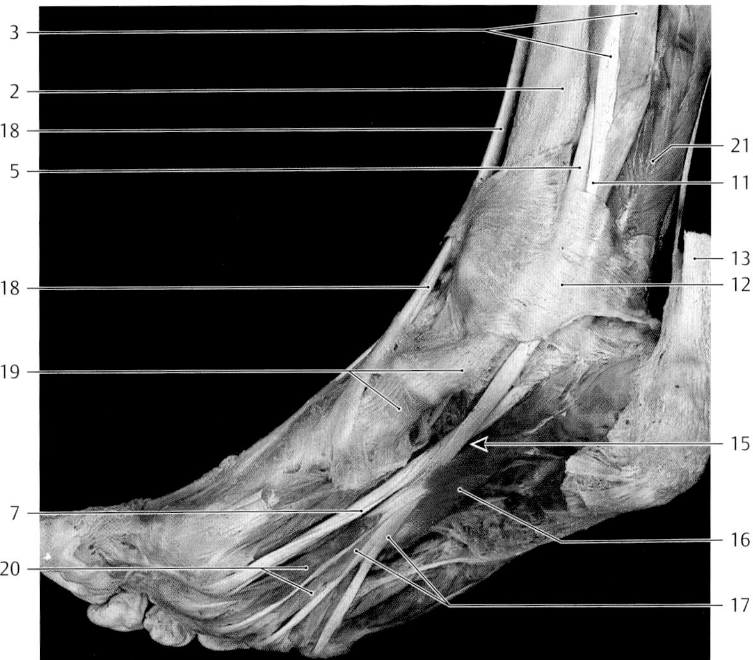


Fig. 4.88 **Sole of the right foot with tendons of long flexor muscles** (oblique-medial and inferior aspect).

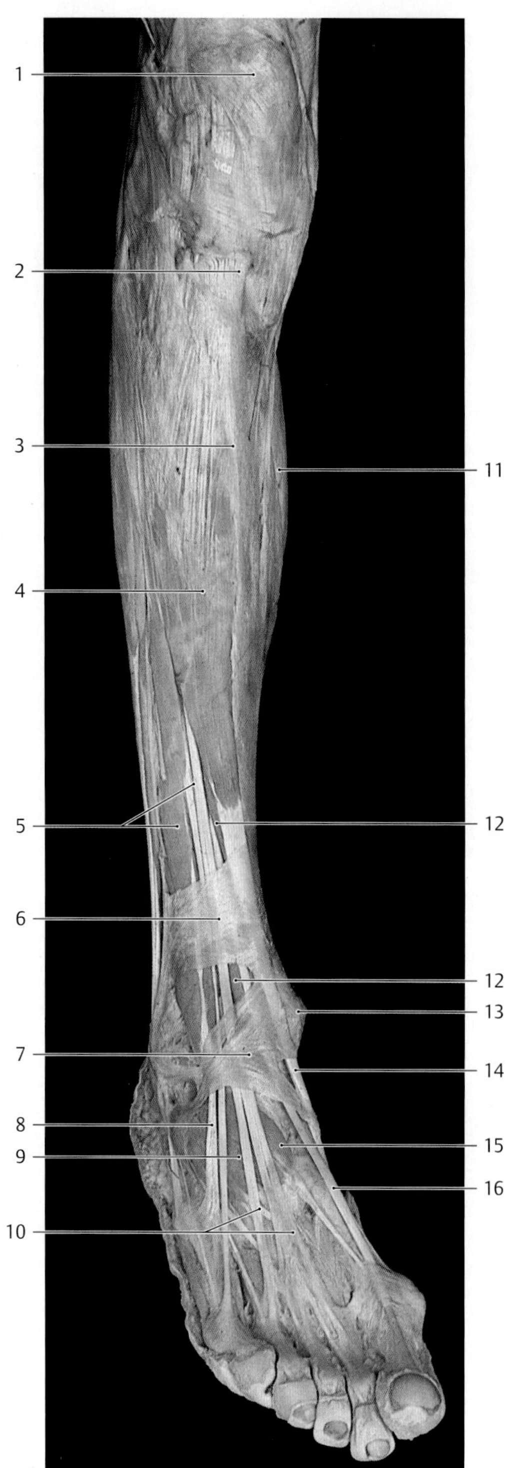


Fig. 4.89 **Extensor muscles of leg and foot** (right side, oblique antero-lateral aspect).

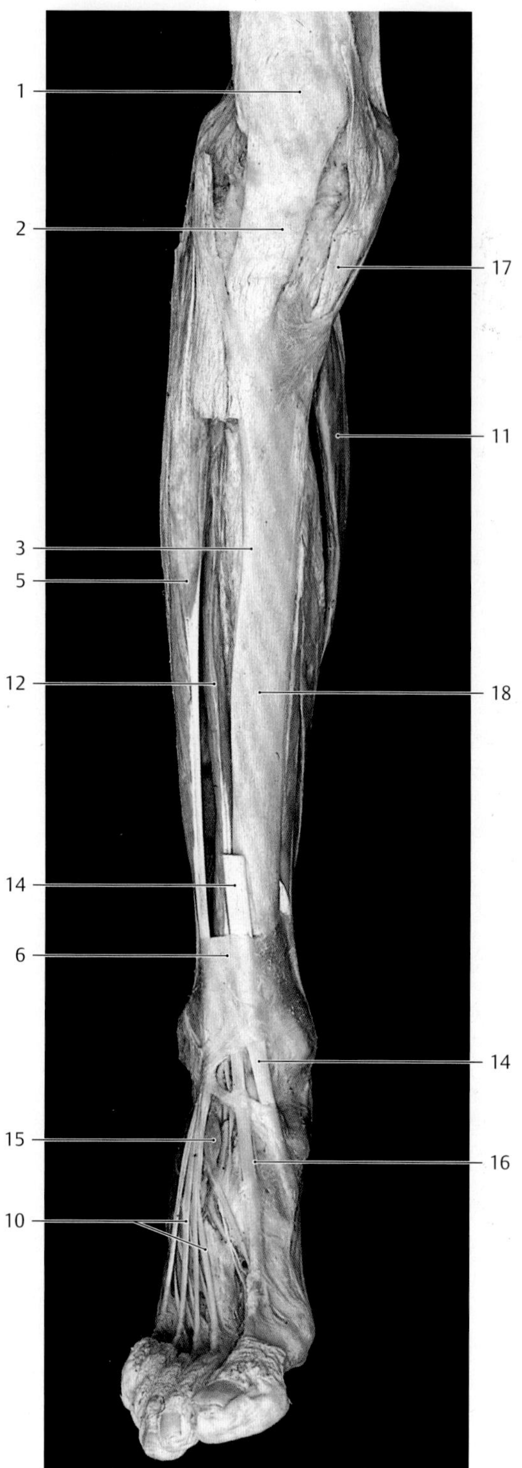


Fig. 4.90 **Extensor muscles of leg and foot** (right side, anterior aspect). Part of the tibialis anterior muscle has been removed.

1 Patella
2 Patellar ligament
3 Anterior margin of tibia
4 Tibialis anterior muscle
5 Extensor digitorum longus muscle
6 Superior extensor retinaculum
7 Inferior extensor retinaculum
8 Tendon of peroneus tertius muscle
9 Extensor digitorum brevis muscle
10 Tendons of extensor digitorum longus muscle
11 Soleus muscle
12 Extensor hallucis longus muscle
13 Medial malleolus
14 Tendon of tibialis anterior muscle
15 Extensor hallucis brevis muscle
16 Tendon of extensor hallucis longus muscle
17 Common tendon of gracilis, semitendinosus, and sartorius muscles (pes anserinus)
18 Tibia

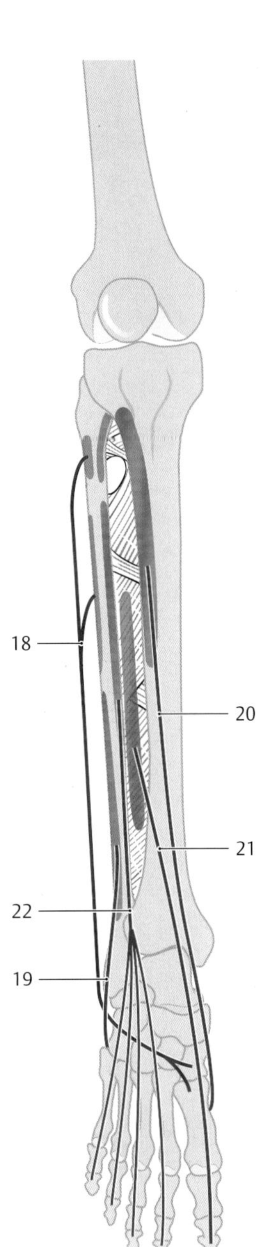


Fig. 4.91 **Course of the extensor muscles of the leg** (anterior aspect).

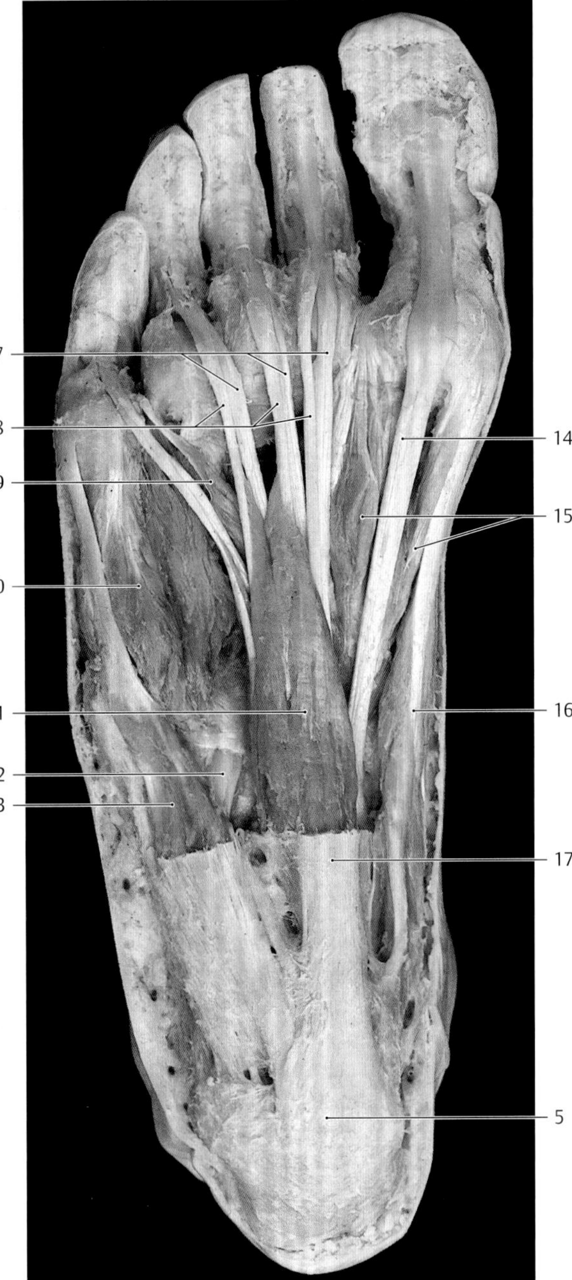


Fig. 4.92 **Muscles of the sole of foot,** superficial layer. The plantar aponeurosis and the fasciae of the superficial muscles have been removed.

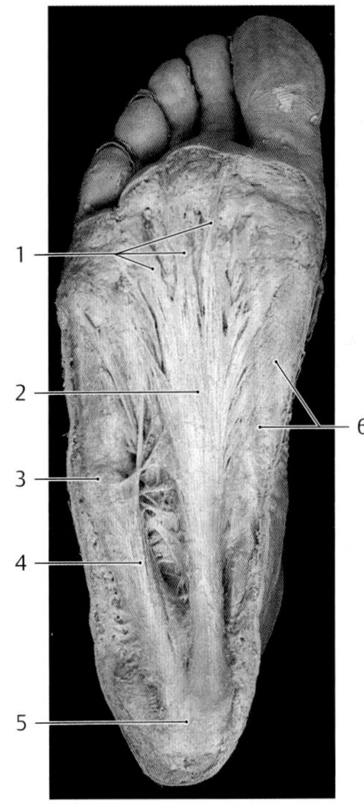


Fig. 4.93 **Sole of the foot with the plantar aponeurosis.**

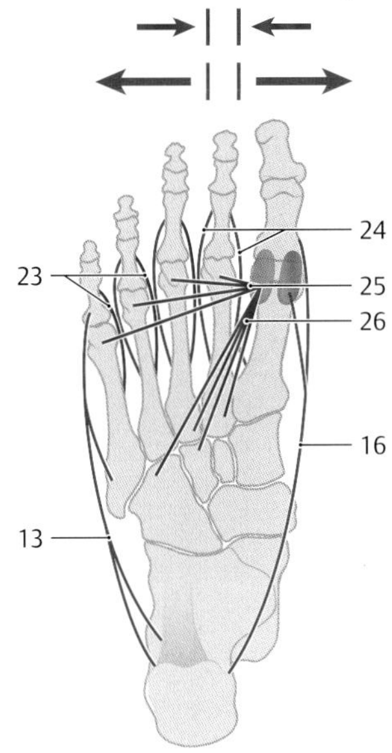


Fig. 4.94 **Course of abductor and adductor muscles of the foot** (plantar aspect). Red arrows = abduction; blue arrows = adduction.

1 Longitudinal bands of plantar aponeurosis
2 Plantar aponeurosis
3 Position of tuberosity of fifth metatarsal bone
4 Muscles of fifth toe with fascia
5 Calcaneal tuberosity
6 Muscles of great toe with fascia
7 Tendons of flexor digitorum longus muscle
8 Tendons of flexor digitorum brevis muscle
9 Lumbrical muscle
10 Flexor digiti minimi brevis muscle
11 Flexor digitorum brevis muscle
12 Tendon of peroneus longus muscle
13 Abductor digiti minimi muscle
14 Tendon of flexor hallucis longus muscle
15 Flexor hallucis brevis muscle
16 Abductor hallucis muscle
17 Plantar aponeurosis (cut)
18 Peroneus longus muscle
19 Peroneus brevis muscle
20 Tibialis anterior muscle
21 Extensor hallucis longus muscle
22 Extensor digitorum longus muscle
23 Plantar interossei muscles (blue)
24 Dorsal interossei muscles (red)
25 Transverse head of adductor hallucis muscle (blue)
26 Oblique head of adductor hallucis muscle (blue)

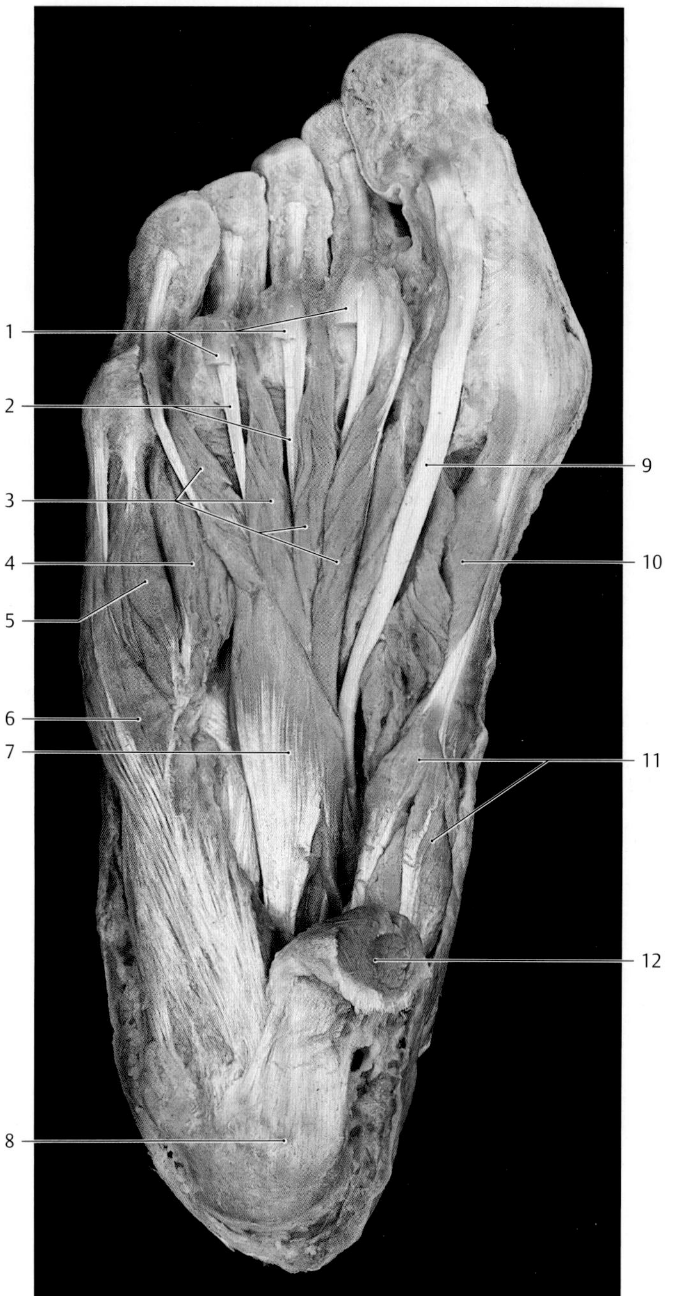


Fig. 4.95 **Muscles of the sole of foot,** middle layer. The flexor digitorum brevis muscle has been divided.

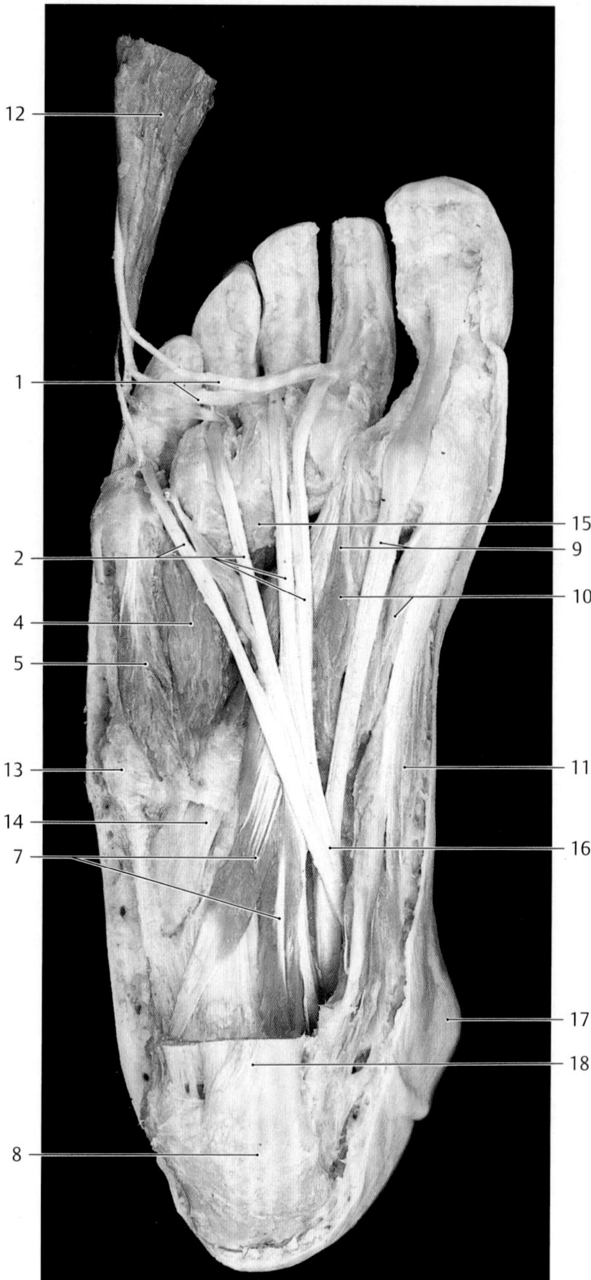


Fig. 4.96 **Muscles of the sole of foot,** middle layer. The tendons of the flexor muscles and the crossing of tendons are displayed. The flexor digitorum brevis muscle has been divided and reflected.

1 Tendons of flexor digitorum brevis muscle
2 Tendons of flexor digitorum longus muscle
3 Lumbrical muscles
4 Interossei muscles
5 Flexor digiti minimi brevis muscle
6 Abductor digiti minimi muscle
7 Quadratus plantae muscle
8 Calcaneal tuberosity
9 Tendon of flexor hallucis longus muscle
10 Flexor hallucis brevis muscle
11 Abductor hallucis muscle
12 Flexor digitorum brevis muscle (divided)
13 Tuberosity of fifth metatarsal bone
14 Tendon of peroneus longus muscle
15 Transverse head of adductor hallucis muscle
16 Crossing of tendons in the sole of foot
17 Medial malleolus
18 Plantar aponeurosis (divided)

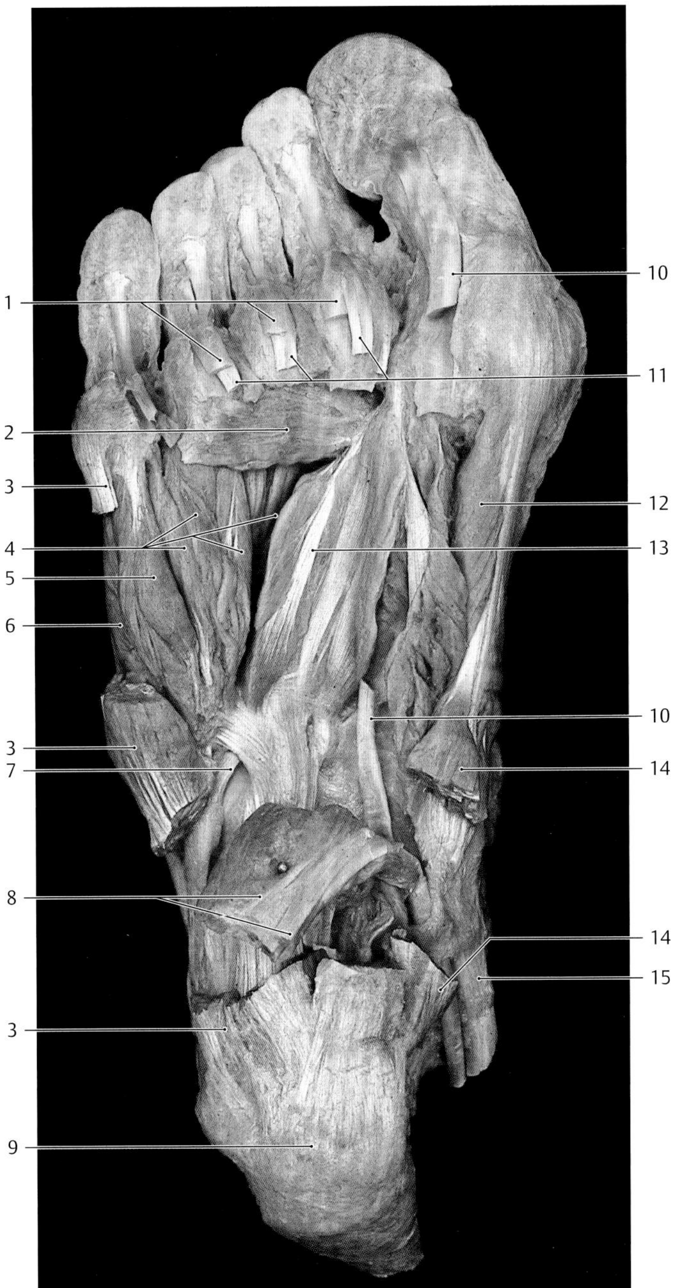


Fig. 4.97 **Muscles of the sole of foot,** deep layer. The flexor digitorum brevis muscle has been removed, and the quadratus plantae, abductor hallucis, and digiti minimi muscles have been divided.

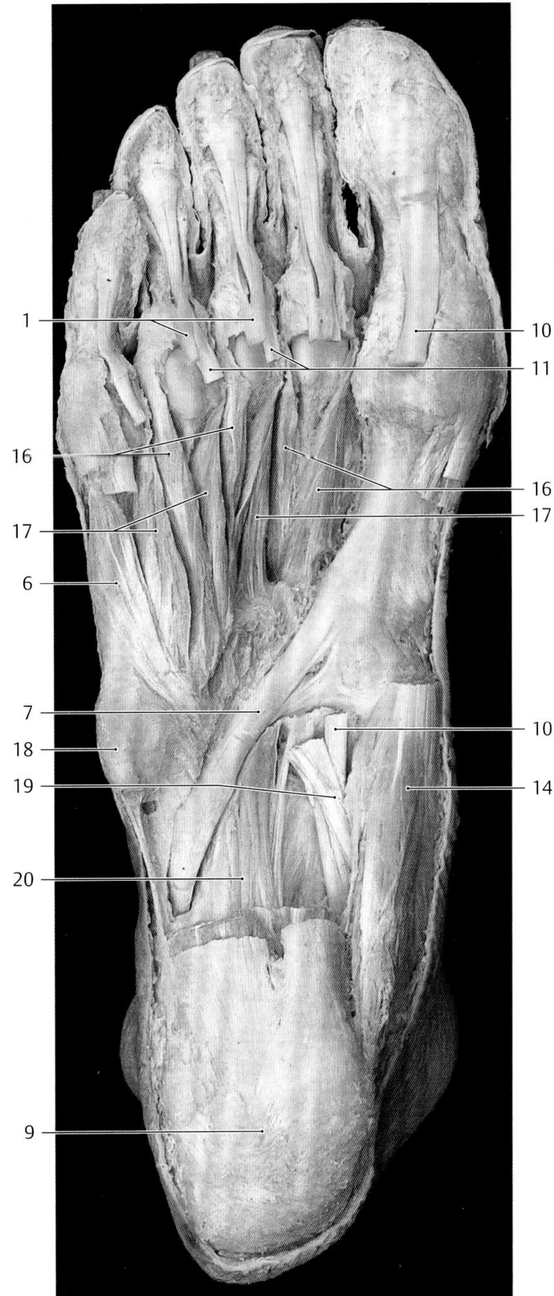


Fig. 4.98 **Muscles of the sole of foot,** deepest layer. The interossei muscles and the canal for the tendon of peroneus longus muscle are shown.

1 Tendons of flexor digitorum brevis muscle
2 Transverse head of adductor hallucis muscle
3 Abductor digiti minimi muscle
4 Interossei muscles
5 Flexor digiti minimi brevis muscle
6 Opponens digiti minimi muscle
7 Tendon of peroneus longus muscle
8 Quadratus plantae muscle with tendon of flexor digitorum longus muscle
9 Calcaneal tuberosity
10 Tendon of flexor hallucis longus muscle (divided)
11 Tendons of flexor digitorum longus muscle
12 Flexor hallucis brevis muscle
13 Oblique head of adductor hallucis muscle
14 Abductor hallucis muscle (cut)
15 Tendon of tibialis posterior muscle
16 Dorsal interossei muscles
17 Plantar interossei muscles
18 Tuberosity of fifth metatarsal bone
19 Tendon of flexor digitorum longus muscle (crossing of plantar tendons)
20 Long plantar ligament

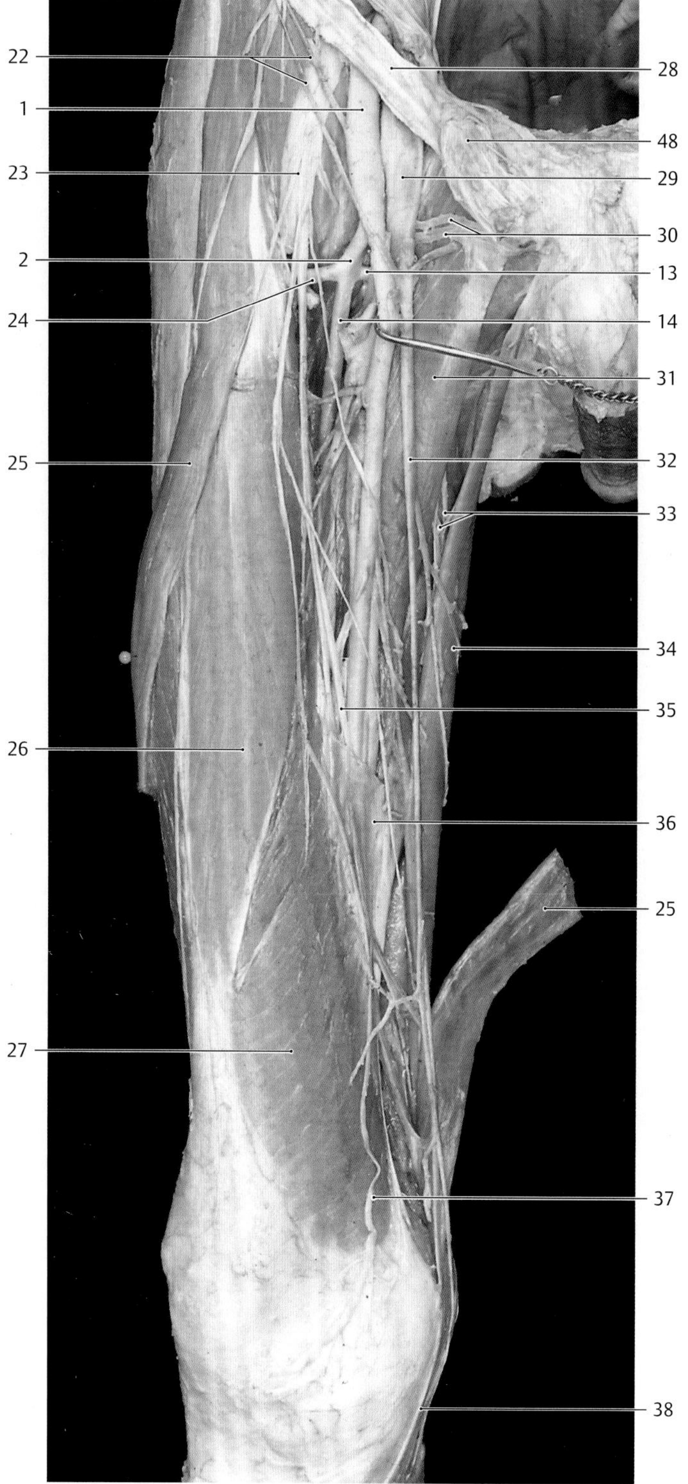


**Fig. 4.99 Main arteries and nerves of the thigh** (right side, anterior aspect). The sartorius muscle has been divided and reflected. The femoral vein has been partly removed to show the deep femoral artery. Note that the vessels enter the adductor canal to reach the popliteal fossa.

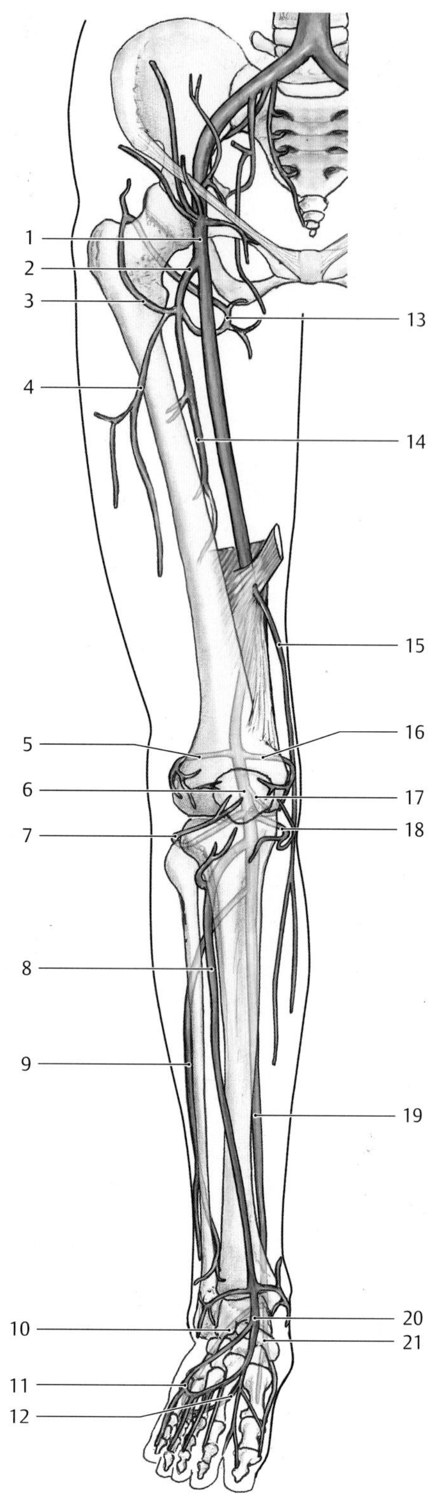


**Fig. 4.100 Main arteries of the lower limb** (anterior aspect).

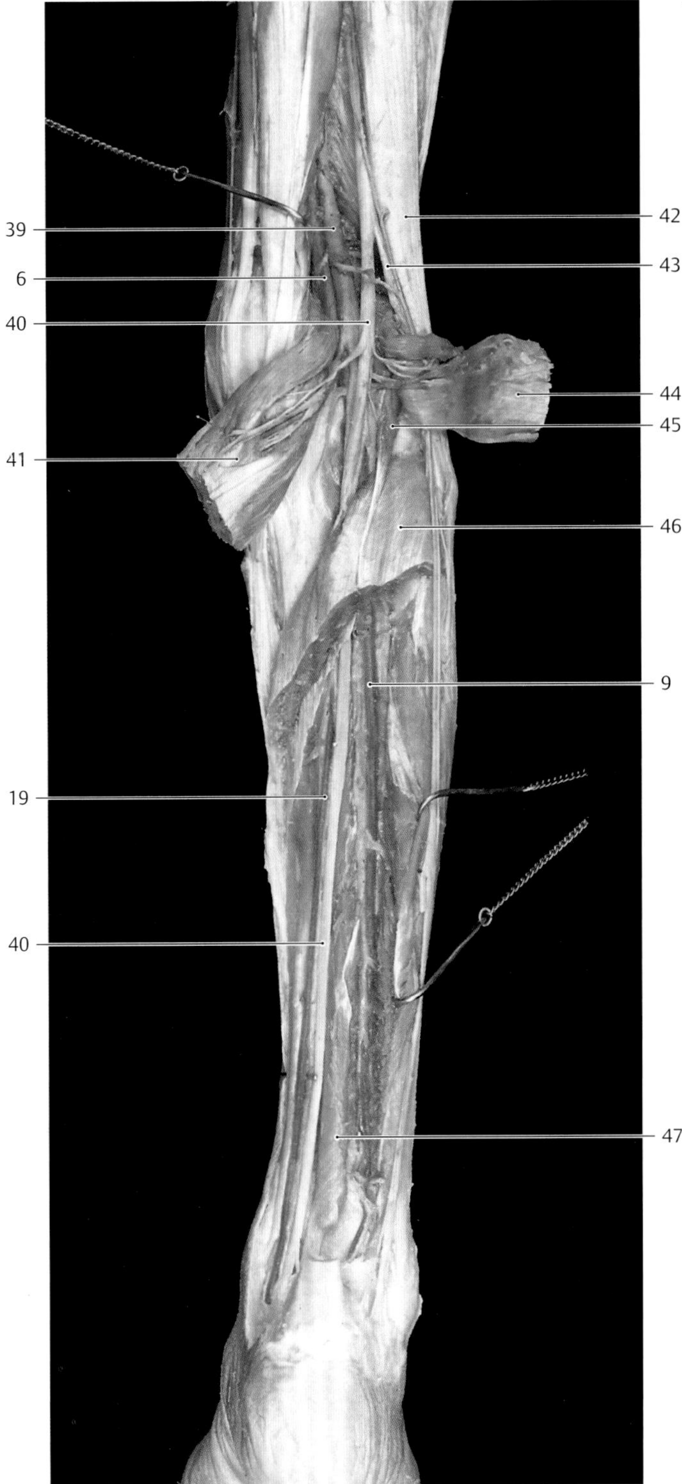


1 Femoral artery
2 Deep artery of thigh
3 Ascending branch of lateral circumflex femoral artery
4 Descending branch of lateral circumflex femoral artery
5 Lateral superior genicular artery
6 Popliteal artery
7 Lateral inferior genicular artery
8 Anterior tibial artery
9 Peroneal artery
10 Lateral plantar artery
11 Arcuate artery with dorsal metatarsal arteries
12 Plantar arch with plantar metatarsal arteries
13 Medial circumflex femoral artery
14 Deep artery of thigh with perforating arteries
15 Descending genicular artery
16 Medial superior genicular artery
17 Middle genicular artery
18 Medial inferior genicular artery
19 Posterior tibial artery
20 Dorsalis pedis artery
21 Medial plantar artery
22 Superficial and deep circumflex iliac arteries
23 Femoral nerve
24 Lateral circumflex femoral artery
25 Sartorius muscle (cut and reflected)
26 Rectus femoris muscle
27 Vastus medialis muscle
28 Inguinal ligament
29 Femoral vein
30 External pudendal artery and vein
31 Adductor longus muscle
32 Great saphenous vein
33 Obturator artery and nerve
34 Gracilis muscle
35 Saphenous nerve
36 Vasto-adductor membrane
37 Anterior cutaneous branch of femoral nerve
38 Infrapatellar branch of saphenous nerve
39 Popliteal vein
40 Tibial nerve
41 Medial head of gastrocnemius muscle
42 Biceps femoris muscle
43 Common fibular nerve
44 Lateral head of gastrocnemius muscle
45 Plantaris muscle
46 Soleus muscle
47 Flexor hallucis longus muscle
48 Spermatic cord

Fig. 4.101 **Arteries of the leg** (right side, posterior aspect).

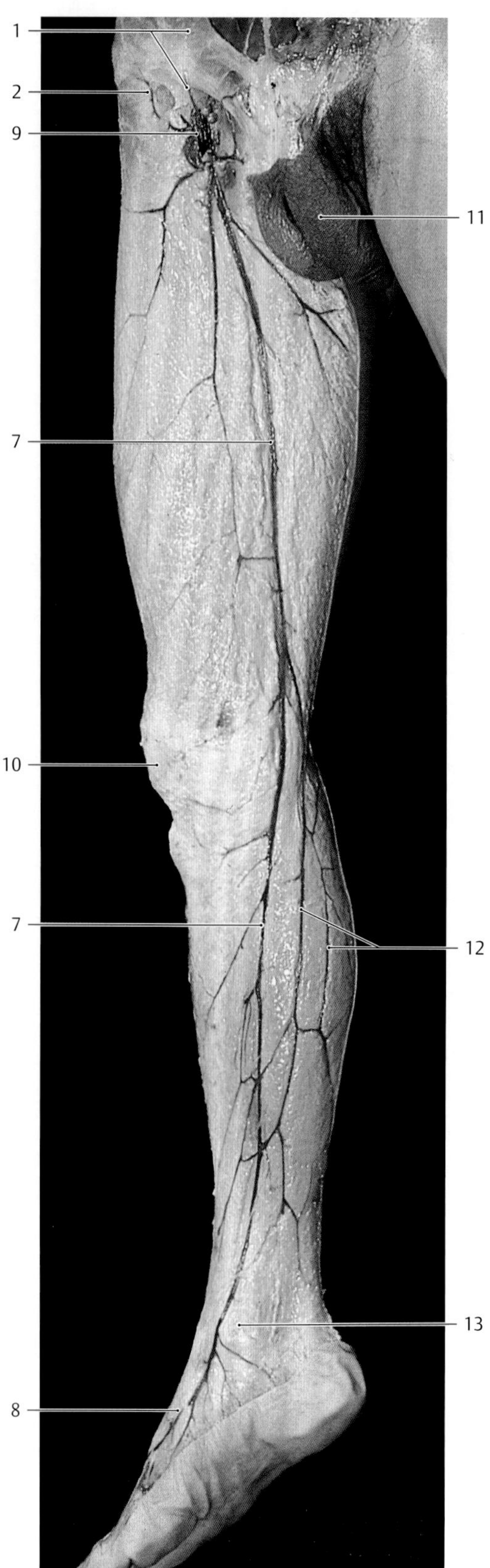


Fig. 4.102 **Superficial veins of the lower limb** (right side, medio-anterior aspect). The veins have been injected with red solution.

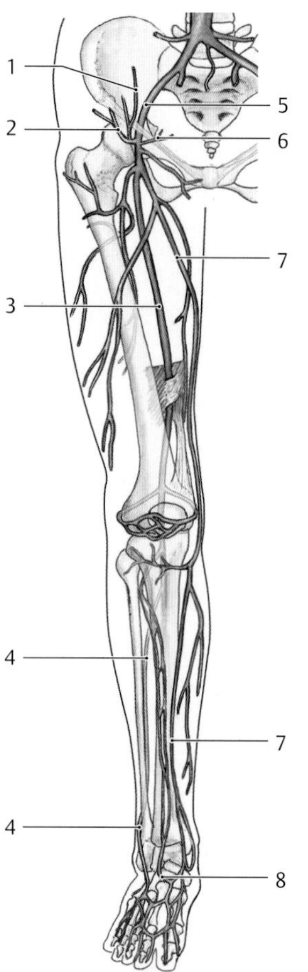


Fig. 4.103 **Main veins of the lower limb** (anterior aspect).

1 Superficial epigastric vein
2 Superficial circumflex iliac vein
3 Femoral vein
4 Small saphenous vein
5 External iliac vein
6 External pudendal vein
7 Great saphenous vein
8 Dorsal venous arch of foot
9 Saphenous opening with femoral vein
10 Patella
11 Penis
12 Anastomoses between great and small saphenous veins
13 Medial malleolus
14 Saphenous nerve
15 Posterior tibial artery and veins
16 Tibial nerve
17 Medial dorsal cutaneous nerve
18 Posterior tibial vein
19 Popliteal fossa
20 Perforating veins
21 Lateral malleolus
22 Superficial layer of crural fascia
23 Perforating veins I–III (of Cockett)
24 Tibia
25 Dorsal digital veins of foot
26 Dorsal venous arch of foot
27 Dorsal metatarsal veins
28 Anterior tibial artery and vein
29 Fibula
30 Peroneal artery and vein
31 Deep layer of crural fascia

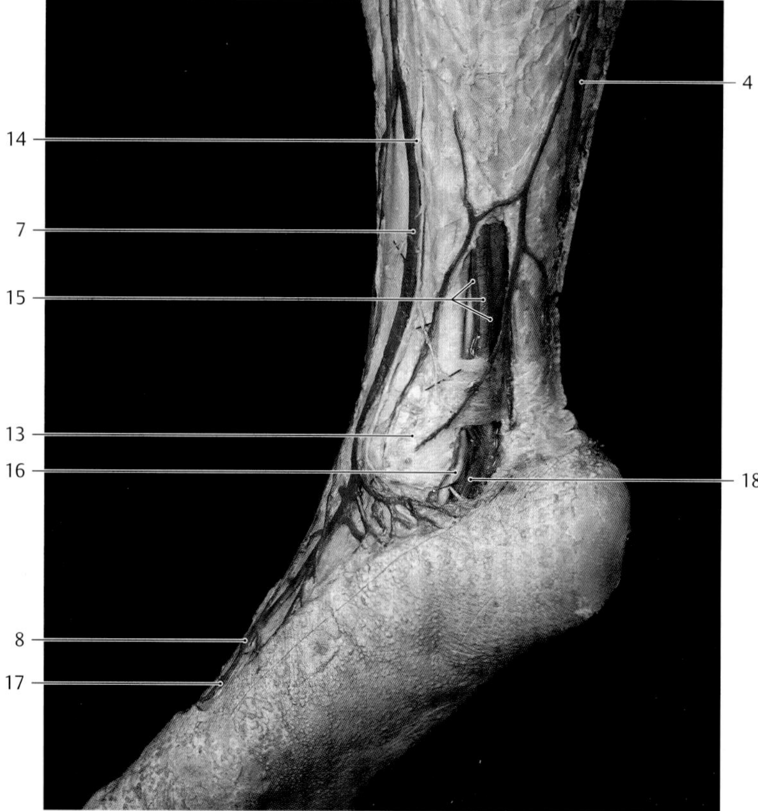


Fig. 4.104 **Medial malleolar region of the right foot.** Dissection of tibial nerve, posterior tibial vessels, and great saphenous vein. The veins have been injected with blue resin.

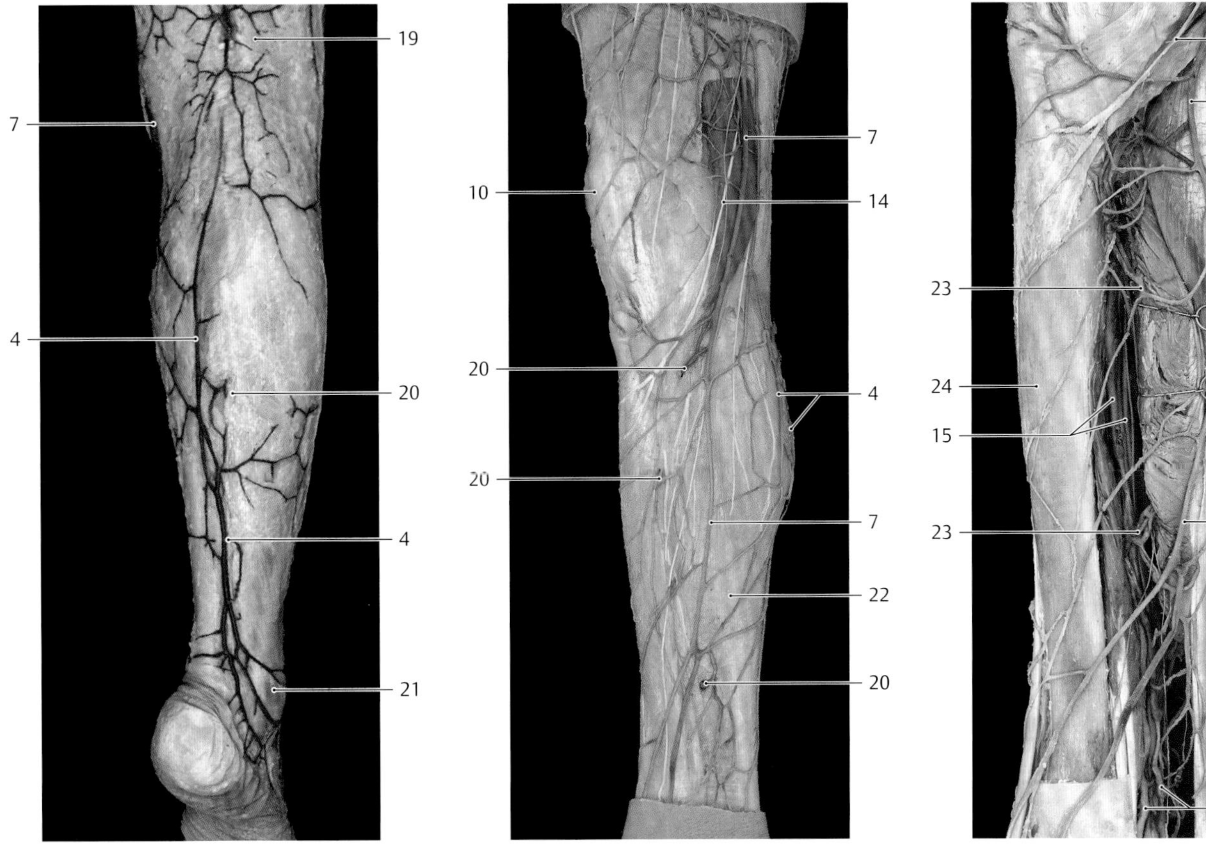


**Fig. 4.105 Superficial veins of the leg** (right side, posterior aspect). The veins have been injected with blue resin.

**Fig. 4.106 Superficial veins of the leg** (left side, medial aspect). The perforating veins of Cockett have been dissected.

**Fig. 4.107 Veins of the leg** (left side, medial aspect). The anastomoses between the superficial and deeper veins have been dissected.

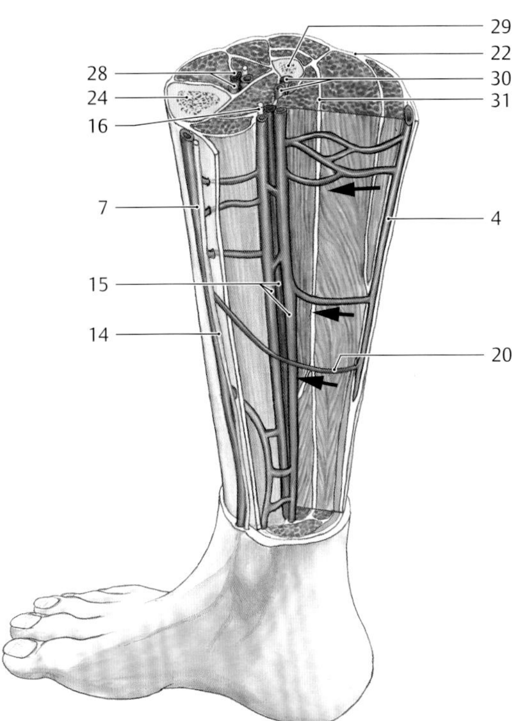


**Fig. 4.108 Anastomoses between the superficial and deeper veins of the leg.** Arrows = directions of blood flow.

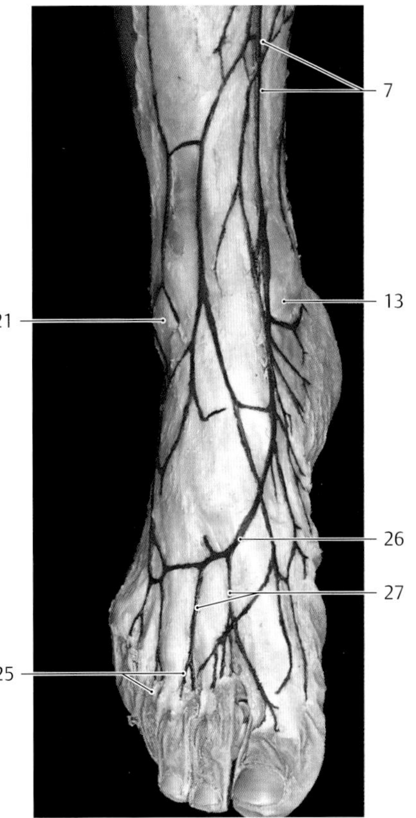


**Fig. 4.109 Superficial veins of the dorsum of the right foot.** The veins have been injected with blue resin.

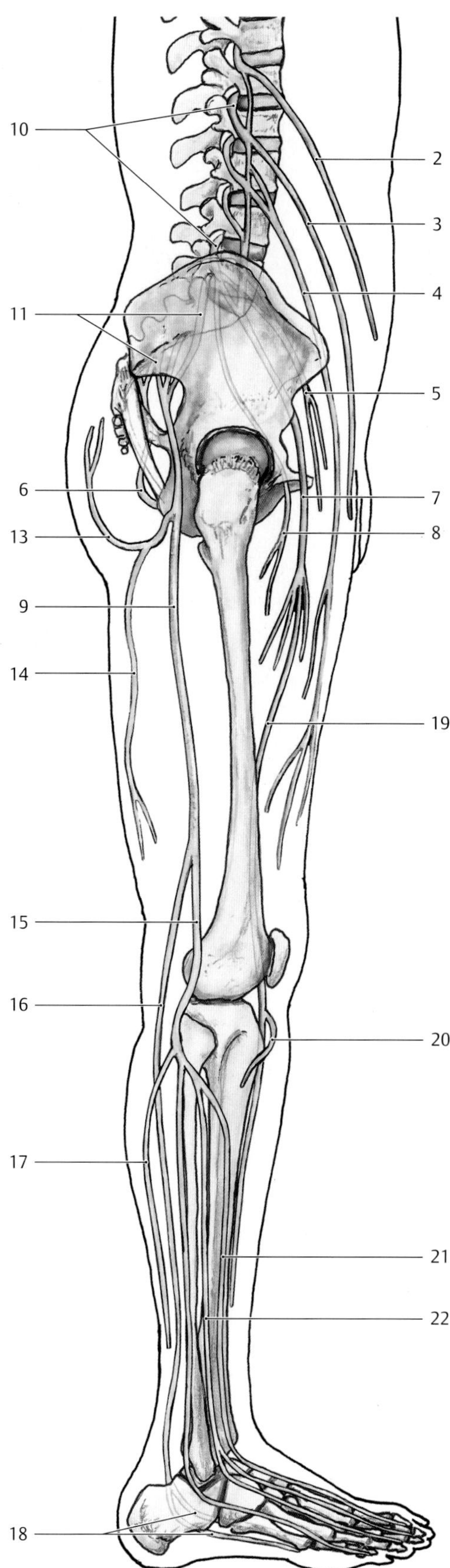


Fig. 4.110 **Nerves of the lower limb** (lateral aspect).

1 Subcostal nerve
2 Iliohypogastric nerve
3 Ilio-inguinal nerve
4 Lateral femoral cutaneous nerve
5 Genitofemoral nerve
6 Pudendal nerve
7 Femoral nerve
8 Obturator nerve
9 Sciatic nerve
10 Lumbar plexus (L1–L4)
11 Sacral plexus (L4–S4)
12 “Pudendal” plexus (S2–S4)
(10–12: lumbosacral plexus)
13 Inferior cluneal nerves
14 Posterior femoral cutaneous nerve
15 Common fibular nerve
16 Tibial nerve
17 Lateral sural cutaneous nerve
18 Medial and lateral plantar nerves
19 Saphenous nerve
20 Infrapatellar branch of saphenous nerve
21 Deep fibular nerve
22 Superficial fibular nerve
23 Anterior cutaneous branch of iliohypogastric nerve
24 Lateral cutaneous branch of iliohypogastric nerve
25 Femoral branch of genitofemoral nerve
26 Lateral cutaneous branches of intercostal nerves
27 Anterior cutaneous branches of intercostal nerves
28 Genital branch of genitofemoral nerve
29 Anterior scrotal nerves

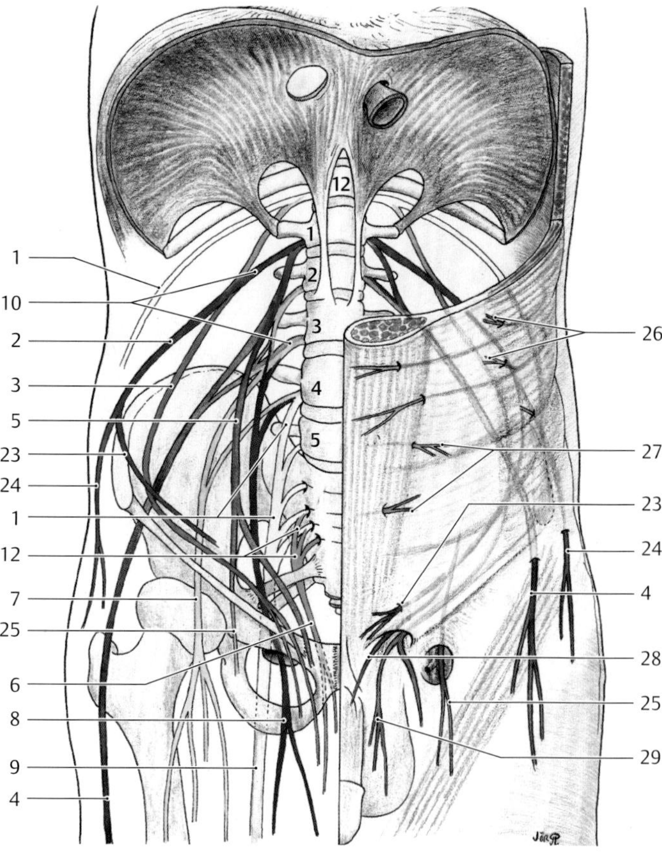


Fig. 4.111 **Main branches of the lumbosacral plexus** (anterior aspect).

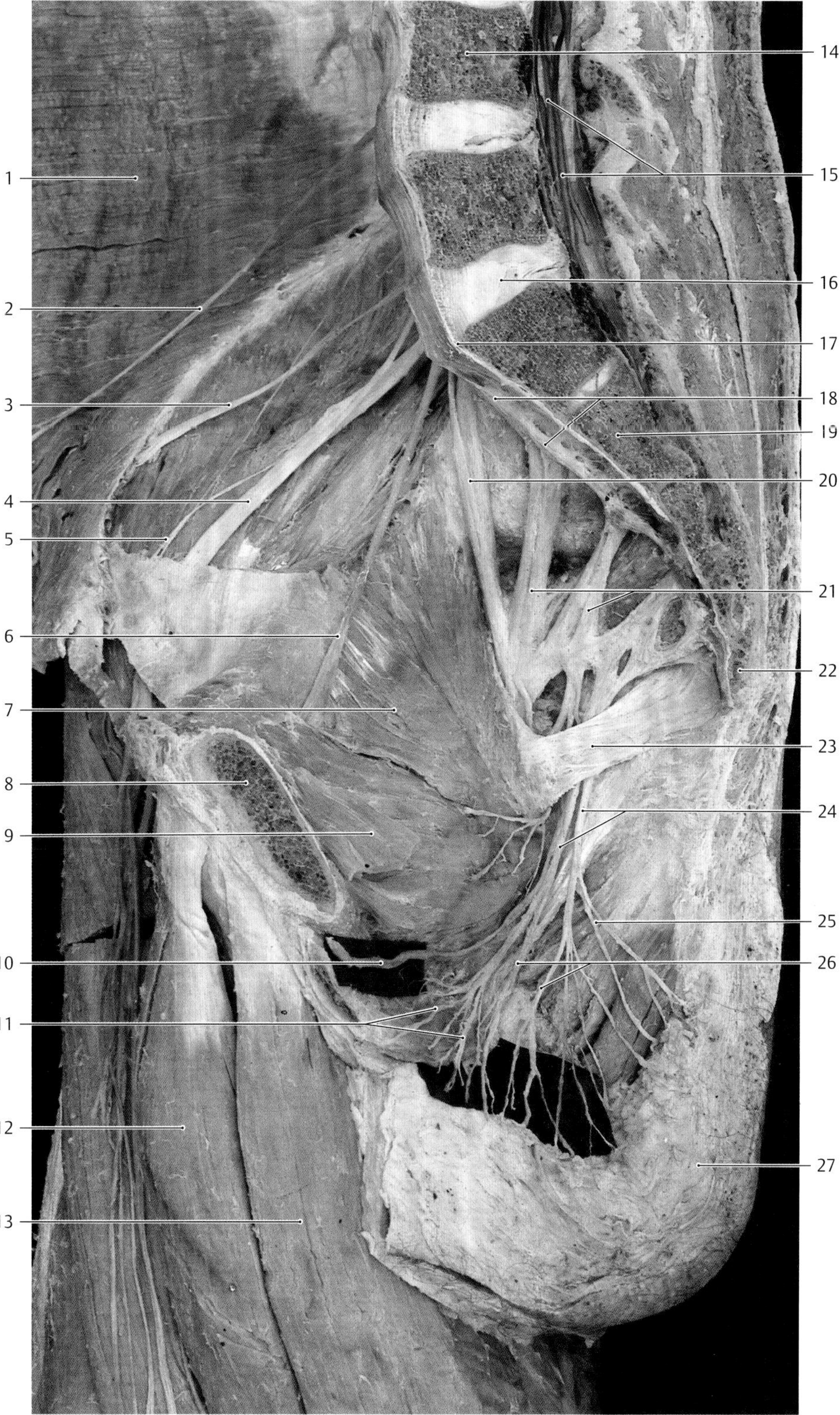


1 Transverse abdominal muscle
2 Iliohypogastric nerve
3 Ilio-inguinal nerve
4 Femoral nerve
5 Lateral femoral cutaneous nerve
6 Obturator nerve
7 Obturator internus muscle
8 Pubis (cut edge)
9 Levator ani muscle (remnant)
10 Dorsal nerve of penis
11 Posterior scrotal nerves of pudendal nerve
12 Adductor longus muscle
13 Gracilis muscle
14 Body of fourth lumbar vertebra
15 Cauda equina
16 Intervertebral disc
17 Sacral promontory
18 Sympathetic trunk
19 Sacrum
20 Lumbosacral trunk
21 Sacral plexus
22 Coccyx
23 Sacrospinous ligament
24 Pudendal nerve
25 Inferior rectal nerves
26 Perineal nerves of pudendal nerve
27 Subcutaneous fat tissue of gluteal region

Fig. 4.112 **Lumbosacral plexus in situ** (right side, medial aspect). The pelvic organs with the peritoneum and part of the levator ani muscle have been removed.

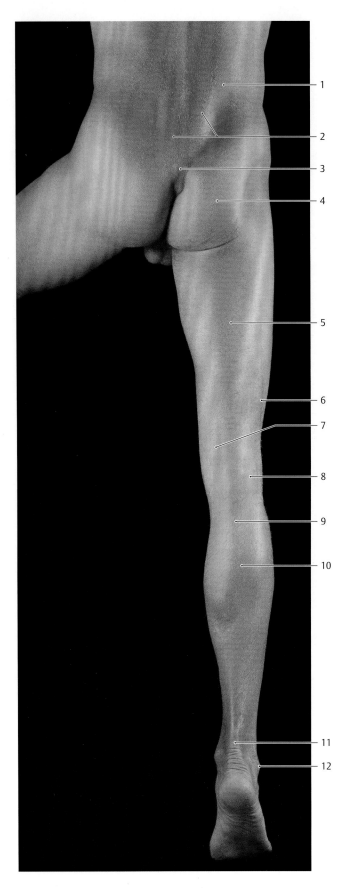

**Fig. 4.113 Surface anatomy of the lower limb** (right side, posterior aspect). The gluteal muscles are contracted.

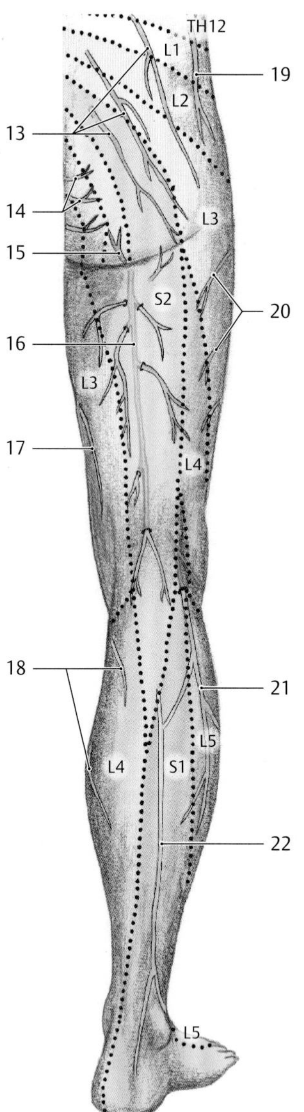


**Fig. 4.114 Cutaneous nerves of the lower limb** (posterior aspect). Dotted lines = border of segments.

1 Iliac crest
2 Sacrum
3 Coccyx
4 Gluteus maximus muscle
5 Ischiocrural muscles
6 Iliotibial tract
7 Tendon of semimembranosus muscle
8 Tendon of biceps femoris muscle
9 Popliteal fossa
10 Triceps surae muscle
11 Calcaneal or Achilles tendon
12 Lateral malleolus
13 Superior cluneal nerves
14 Middle cluneal nerves
15 Inferior cluneal nerves
16 Posterior femoral cutaneous nerve
17 Obturator nerve
18 Saphenous nerve
19 Iliohypogastric nerve
20 Lateral femoral cutaneous nerves
21 Common fibular nerve
22 Sural nerve

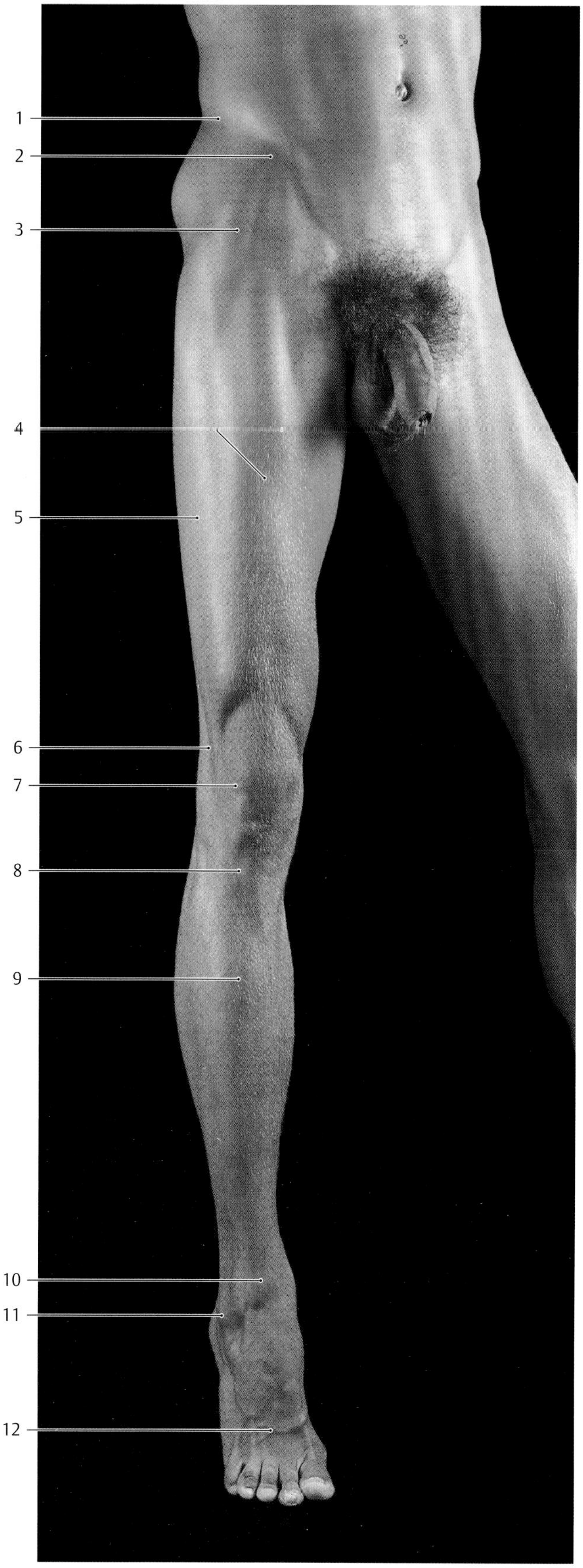

**Fig. 4.115 Surface anatomy of the lower limb** (right side, anterior aspect).

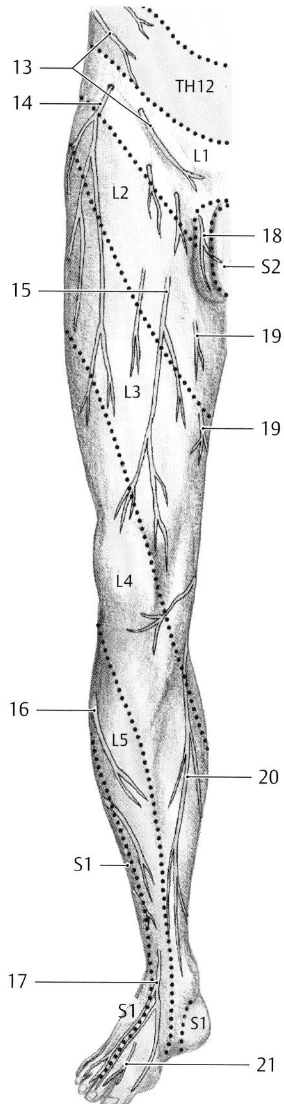


**Fig. 4.116 Cutaneous nerves of the lower limb** (anterior aspect). Dotted lines = border of segments.

1 Iliac crest
2 Anterior superior iliac spine
3 Tensor fasciae latae muscle
4 Quadriceps femoris muscle
5 Iliotibial tract
6 Tendon of biceps femoris muscle
7 Patella
8 Patellar ligament
9 Tibia
10 Tendon of tibialis anterior muscle
11 Lateral malleolus
12 Dorsal venous arch of foot
13 Iliohypogastric nerve
14 Lateral femoral cutaneous nerve
15 Femoral nerve
16 Common fibular nerve
17 Superficial fibular nerve
18 Ilio-inguinal nerve
19 Obturator nerve
20 Saphenous nerve
21 Deep fibular nerve

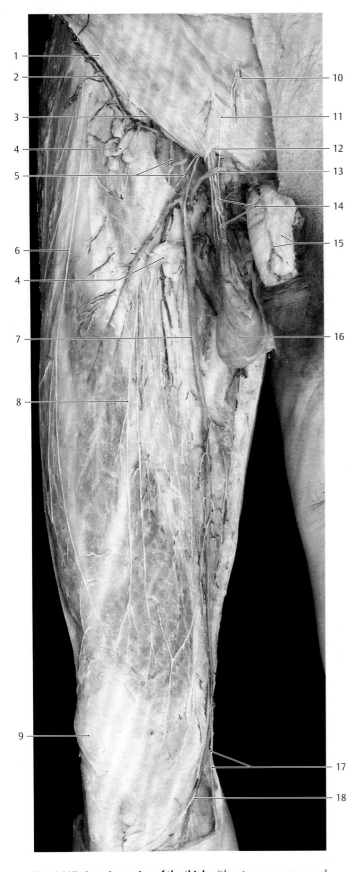

**Fig. 4.117 Anterior region of the thigh** with cutaneous nerves and veins (right side).

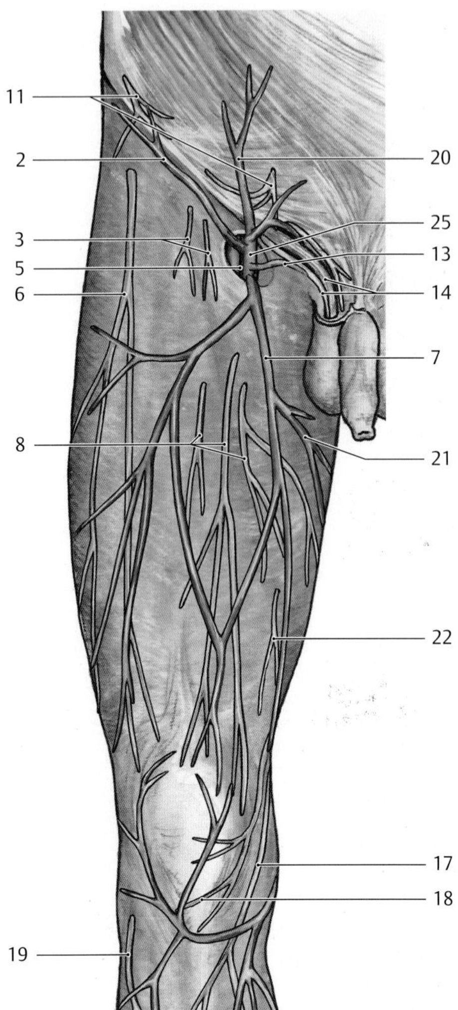


**Fig. 4.118 Anterior region of the thigh** with cutaneous nerves and veins (right side; see corresponding dissection in Fig. 4.117).

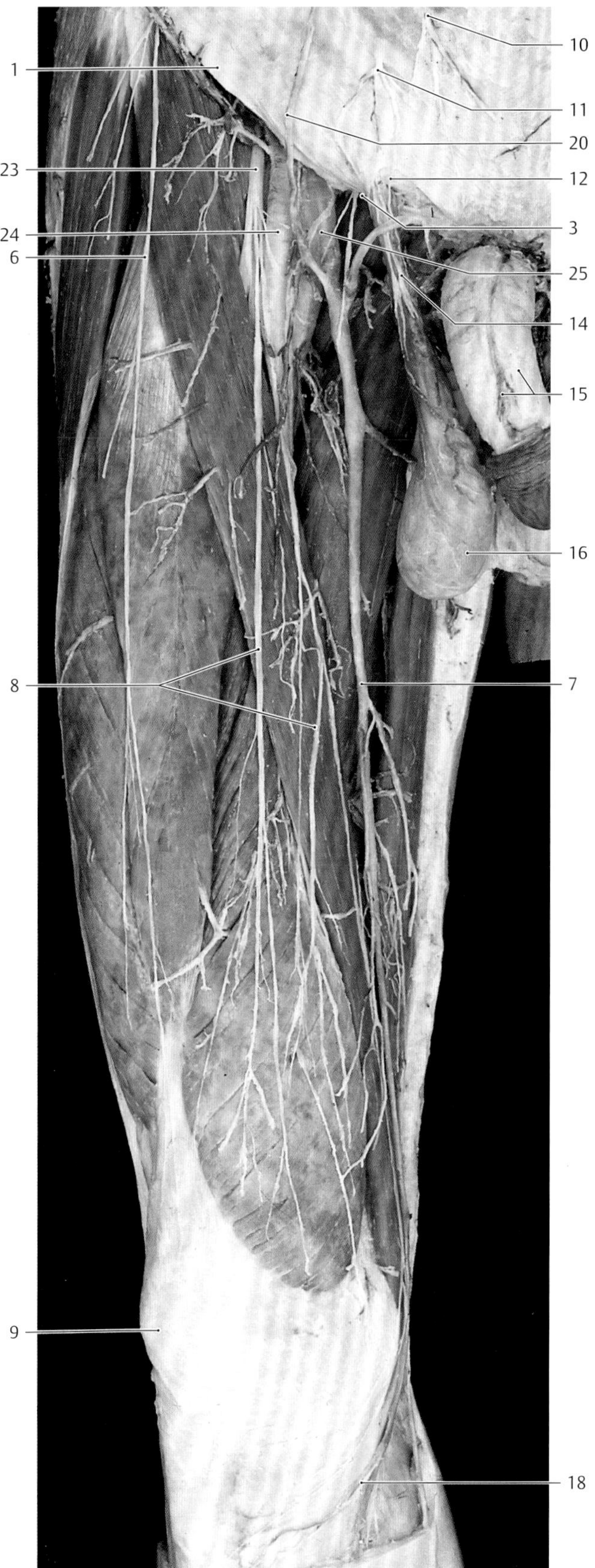


Fig. 4.119 **Anterior region of the thigh** with cutaneous nerves and veins (right side). The fascia lata and the fasciae of the thigh muscles have been removed.

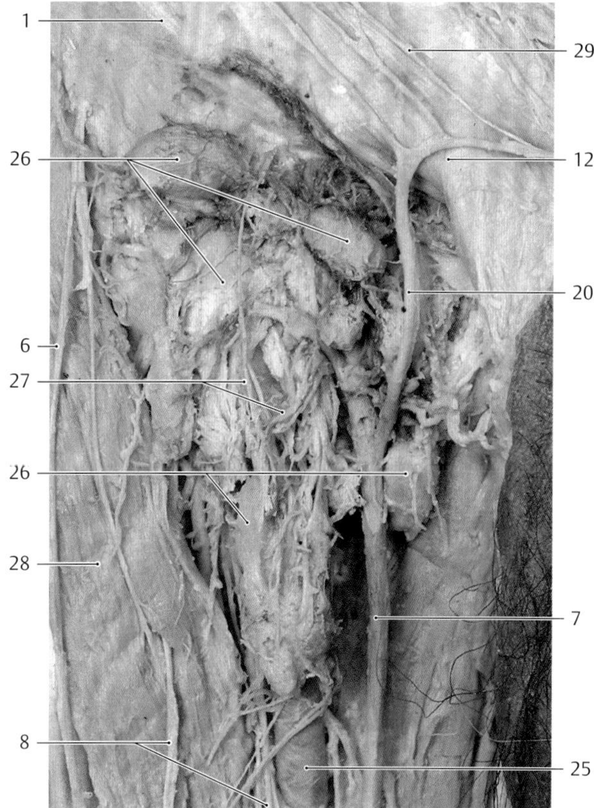


Fig. 4.120 **Inguinal nodes with lymphatic vessels** (anterior aspect).

1 Inguinal ligament
2 Superficial circumflex iliac vein
3 Femoral branch of genitofemoral nerve
4 Superficial inguinal lymph nodes
5 Saphenous opening with femoral artery and vein
6 Lateral femoral cutaneous nerve
7 Great saphenous vein
8 Anterior cutaneous branches of femoral nerve
9 Patella
10 Terminal branches of subcostal nerve
11 Terminal branches of iliohypogastric nerve
12 Superficial inguinal ring
13 External pudendal vein
14 Spermatic cord with genital branch of genitofemoral nerve
15 Penis with superficial dorsal vein of penis
16 Testis and its coverings
17 Saphenous nerve
18 Infrapatellar branch of saphenous nerve
19 Lateral sural cutaneous nerve
20 Superficial epigastric vein
21 Accessory saphenous vein
22 Cutaneous branch of obturator nerve
23 Femoral nerve
24 Femoral artery
25 Femoral vein
26 Superficial and inferior inguinal lymph nodes (enlarged)
27 Lymphatic vessels
28 Sartorius muscle
29 Iliohypogastric nerve

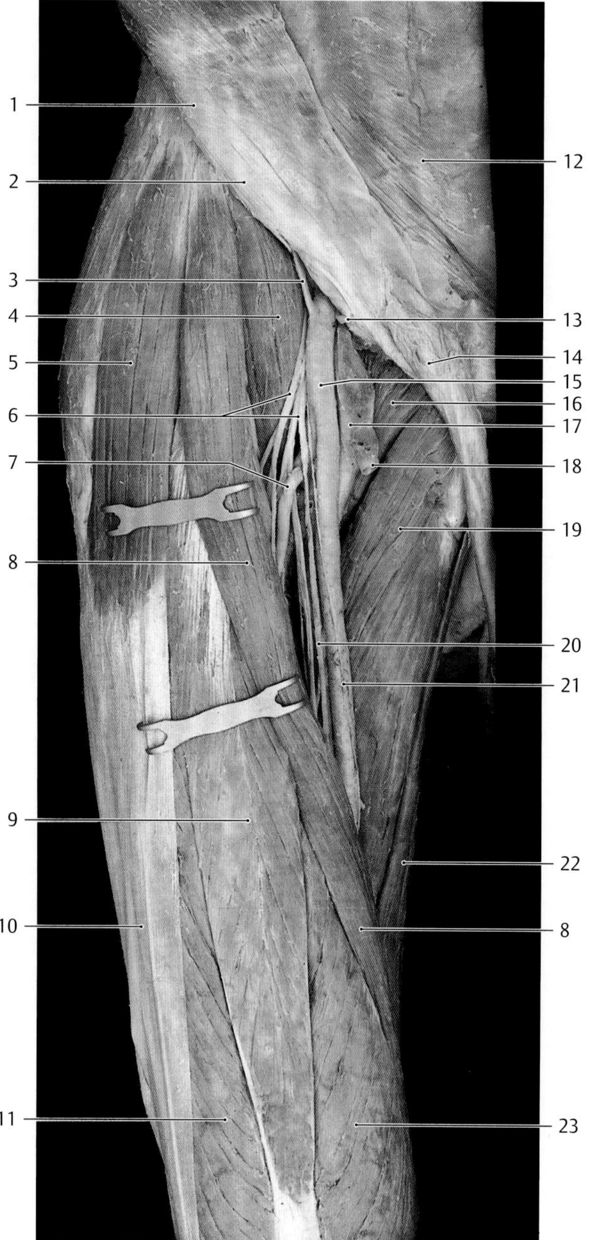


Fig. 4.121 **Anterior region of the thigh** (right side, anterior aspect). The fascia lata has been removed and the sartorius muscle has been slightly reflected.

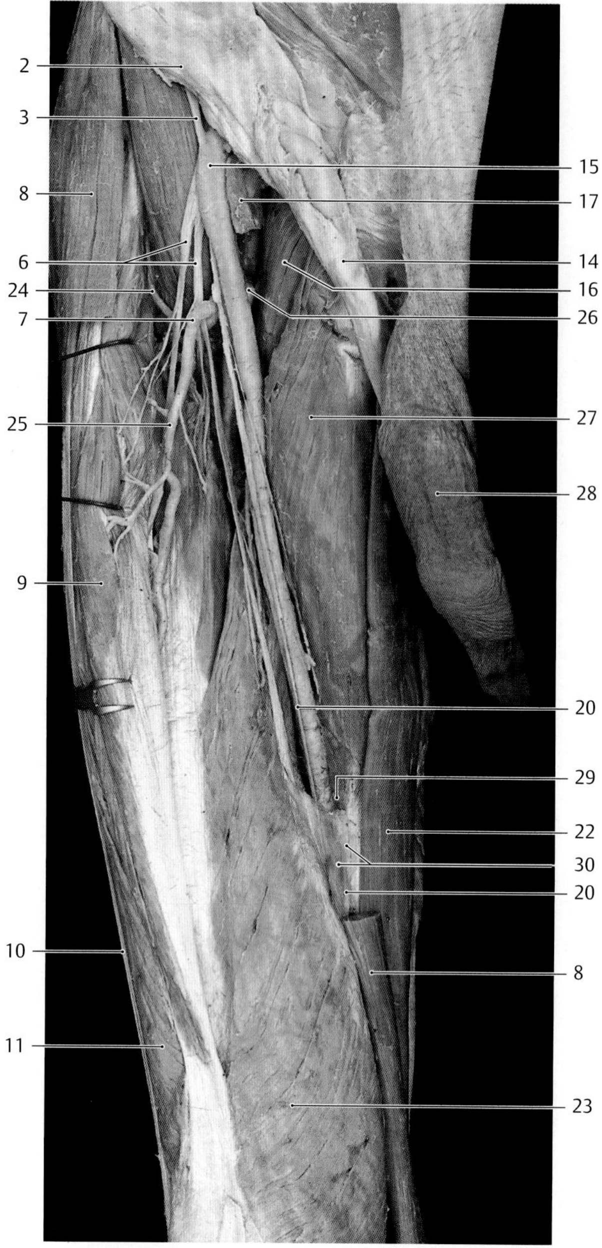


Fig. 4.122 **Anterior region of the thigh** (right side, anterior aspect). The fascia lata has been removed and the sartorius muscle has been divided.

1 Anterior superior iliac spine
2 Inguinal ligament
3 Deep circumflex iliac artery
4 Iliopsoas muscle
5 Tensor fasciae latae muscle
6 Femoral nerve
7 Lateral circumflex femoral artery
8 Sartorius muscle
9 Rectus femoris muscle
10 Iliotibial tract
11 Vastus lateralis muscle
12 Anterior sheath of rectus abdominis muscle
13 Inferior epigastric artery
14 Spermatic cord
15 Femoral artery
16 Pectineus muscle
17 Femoral vein
18 Great saphenous vein (divided)
19 Adductor longus muscle
20 Saphenous nerve
21 Muscular branch of femoral nerve
22 Gracilis muscle
23 Vastus medialis muscle
24 Ascending branch of lateral circumflex femoral artery
25 Descending branch of lateral circumflex femoral artery
26 Medial circumflex femoral artery
27 Adductor longus muscle
28 Penis
29 Entrance to adductor canal
30 Vasto-adductor membrane of fascia beneath sartorius muscle

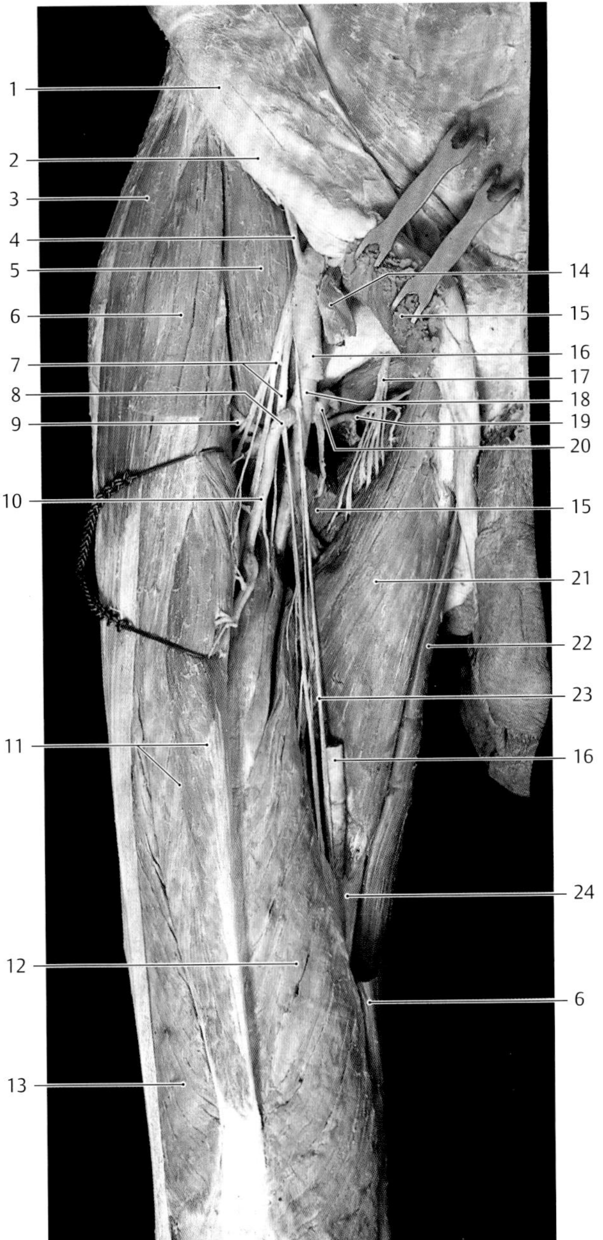


Fig. 4.123 **Anterior region of the thigh** (right side, anterior aspect). The fascia lata has been removed. Sartorius and pectineus muscles, and the femoral artery have been cut to display the deep femoral artery with its branches. The rectus femoris muscle has been slightly reflected.

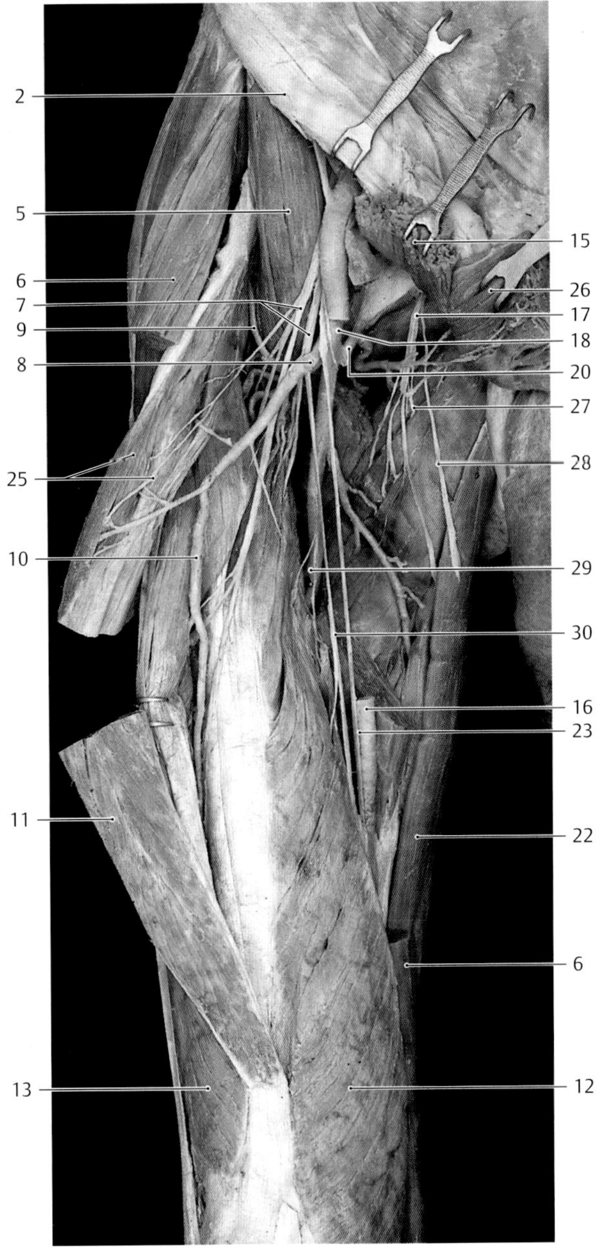


Fig. 4.124 **Anterior region of the thigh** (right side, anterior aspect). The sartorius, pectineus, adductor longus, and rectus femoris muscles have been divided and reflected. The greater part of the femoral artery has been removed.

1 Anterior superior iliac spine
2 Inguinal ligament
3 Tensor fasciae latae muscle
4 Deep circumflex iliac artery
5 Iliopsoas muscle
6 Sartorius muscle (cut)
7 Femoral nerve
8 Lateral circumflex femoral artery
9 Ascending branch of lateral circumflex femoral artery
10 Descending branch of lateral circumflex femoral artery
11 Rectus femoris muscle
12 Vastus medialis muscle
13 Vastus lateralis muscle
14 Femoral vein
15 Pectineus muscle (cut)
16 Femoral artery (cut)
17 Obturator nerve
18 Deep artery of thigh
19 Ascending branch of medial circumflex femoral artery
20 Medial circumflex femoral artery
21 Adductor longus muscle
22 Gracilis muscle
23 Saphenous nerve
24 Distal part of vasto-adductor membrane
25 Rectus femoris muscle with muscular branches of femoral nerve
26 Adductor longus muscle (divided)
27 Posterior branch of obturator nerve
28 Anterior branch of obturator nerve
29 Point at which perforating artery branches off from deep artery of thigh
30 Muscular branch of femoral nerve to vastus medialis muscle

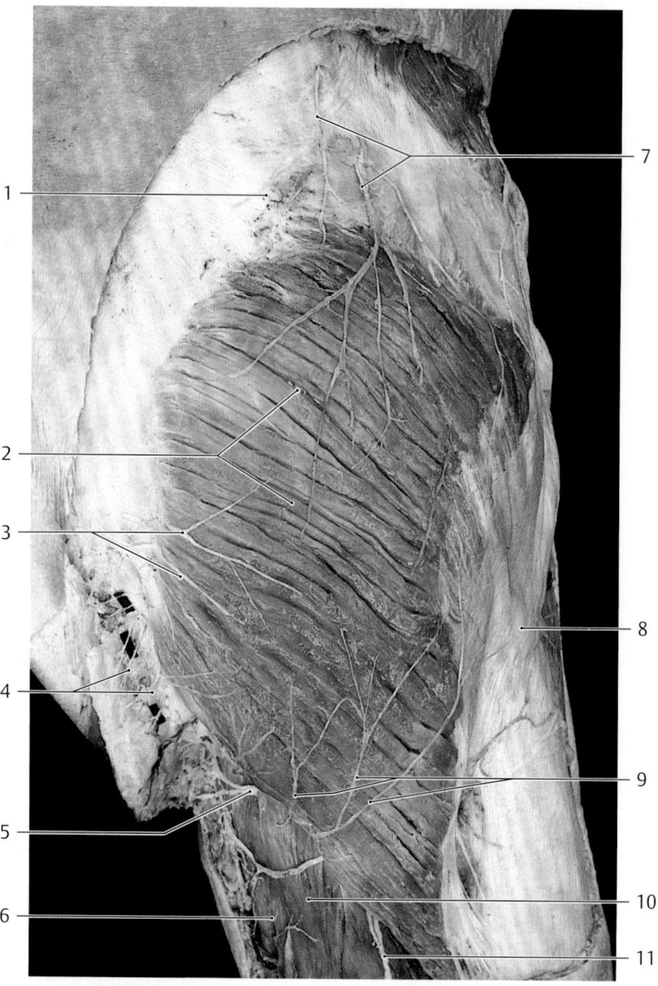


Fig. 4.125 **Gluteal region** (right side). Dissection of the cutaneous nerves.

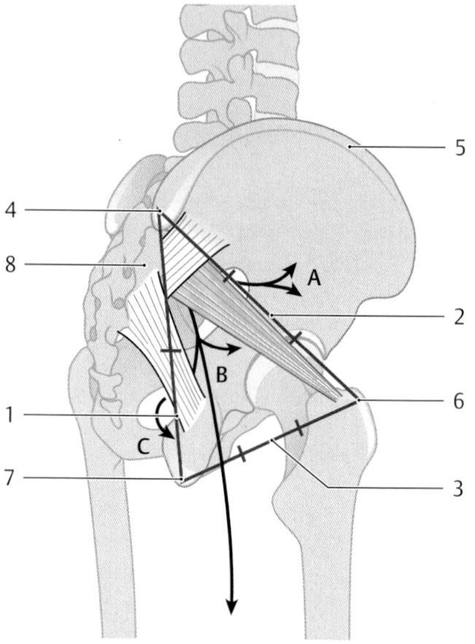

1 Iliac crest
2 Gluteus maximus muscle
3 Middle cluneal nerves
4 Anococcygeal nerves
5 Perineal branch of posterior femoral cutaneous nerve
6 Adductor magnus muscle
7 Superior cluneal nerves
8 Position of greater trochanter
9 Inferior cluneal nerves
10 Semitendinosus muscle
11 Posterior femoral cutaneous nerve
12 Long head of biceps femoris muscle

Fig. 4.126 **Location of the sciatic foramina** (A, B, C) **in relation to the bones at the gluteal region** (postero-lateral aspect).

**Red lines**

1 **Spine-tuber line**
(the infrapiriform foramen is situated in the middle of this line)
2 **Spine-trochanter line**
(the suprapiriform foramen is located in the upper third)
3 **Tuber-trochanter line**
(the ischiadic nerve can be found between the middle and posterior third)

**Other structures**

4 Posterior superior iliac spine
5 Iliac crest
6 Greater trochanter
7 Ischial tuberosity
8 Sacrum

**A Suprapiriform foramen (of greater sciatic foramen)**
Superior gluteal artery, vein, and nerve

**B Infrapiriform foramen (of greater sciatic foramen)**
- Sciatic nerve
- Inferior gluteal artery, vein, and nerve
- Posterior femoral cutaneous nerve
- Internal pudendal artery and vein
- Pudendal nerve
- Internal obturator nerve
- Nerve to quadratus femoris muscle

**C Lesser sciatic foramen**
- Pudendal nerve
- Internal pudendal artery and vein
- Internal obturator nerve

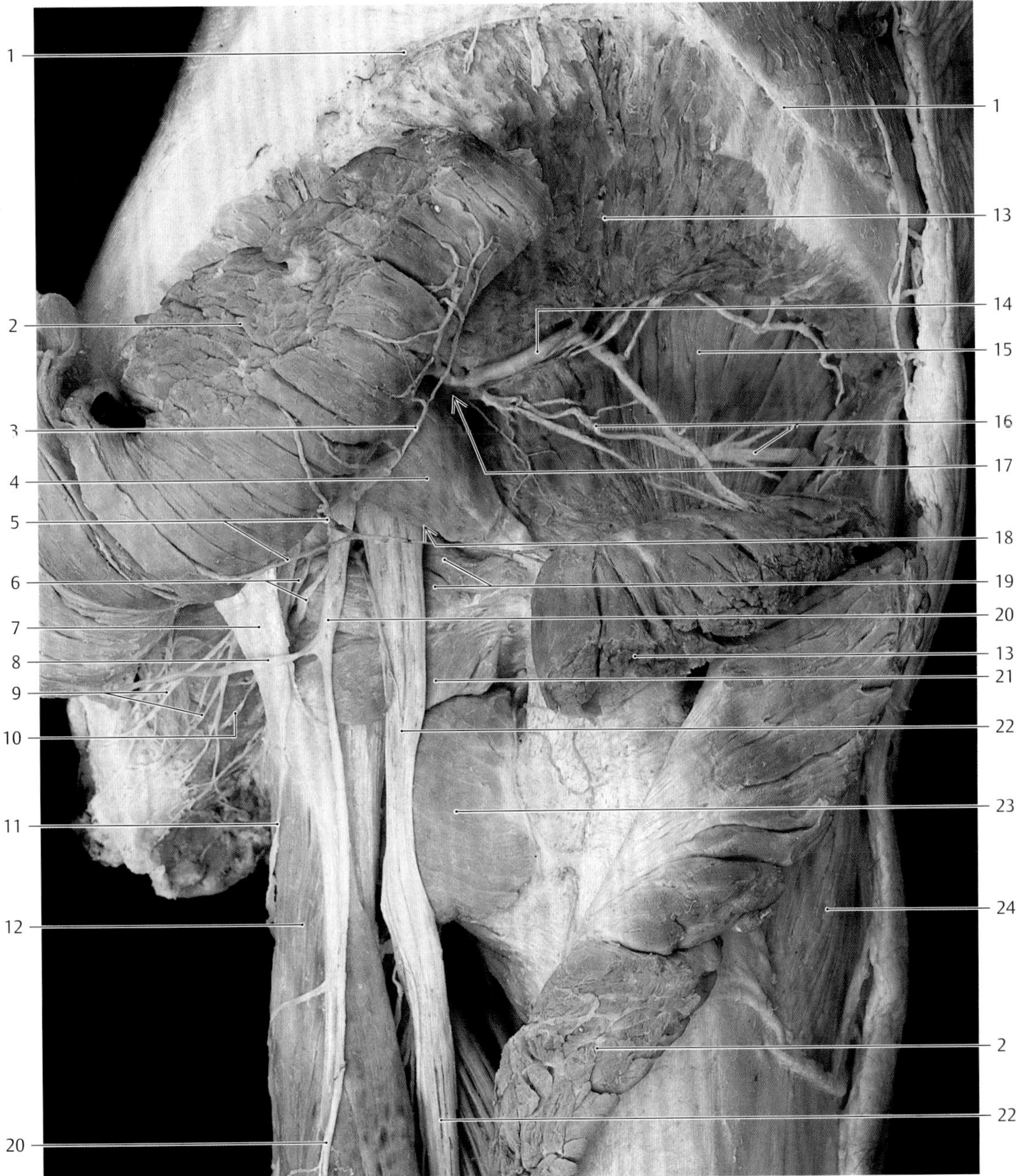


**Fig. 4.127 Gluteal region** (right side). Gluteus maximus and gluteus medius muscles have been divided and reflected. Notice the position of the foramina above and below the piriformis muscle and the lesser sciatic foramen.

1 Iliac crest
2 Gluteus maximus muscle (cut)
3 Inferior gluteal nerve
4 Piriformis muscle
5 Muscular branches of inferior gluteal artery
6 Pudendal nerve and internal pudendal artery within the lesser sciatic foramen (entrance to the pudendal canal)
7 Sacrotuberous ligament
8 Inferior cluneal nerve
9 Inferior rectal nerves
10 Inferior rectal arteries
11 Perforating cutaneous nerve of posterior femoral cutaneous nerve
12 Long head of biceps femoris muscle
13 Gluteus medius muscle (cut)
14 Deep branch of superior gluteal artery
15 Gluteus minimus muscle
16 Superior gluteal nerve
17 Suprapiriform foramen } greater sciatic foramen
18 Infrapiriform foramen } greater sciatic foramen
19 Obturator internus and superior gemellus muscles
20 Posterior femoral cutaneous nerve
21 Inferior gemellus muscle
22 Sciatic nerve
23 Quadratus femoris muscle
24 Tensor fasciae latae muscle

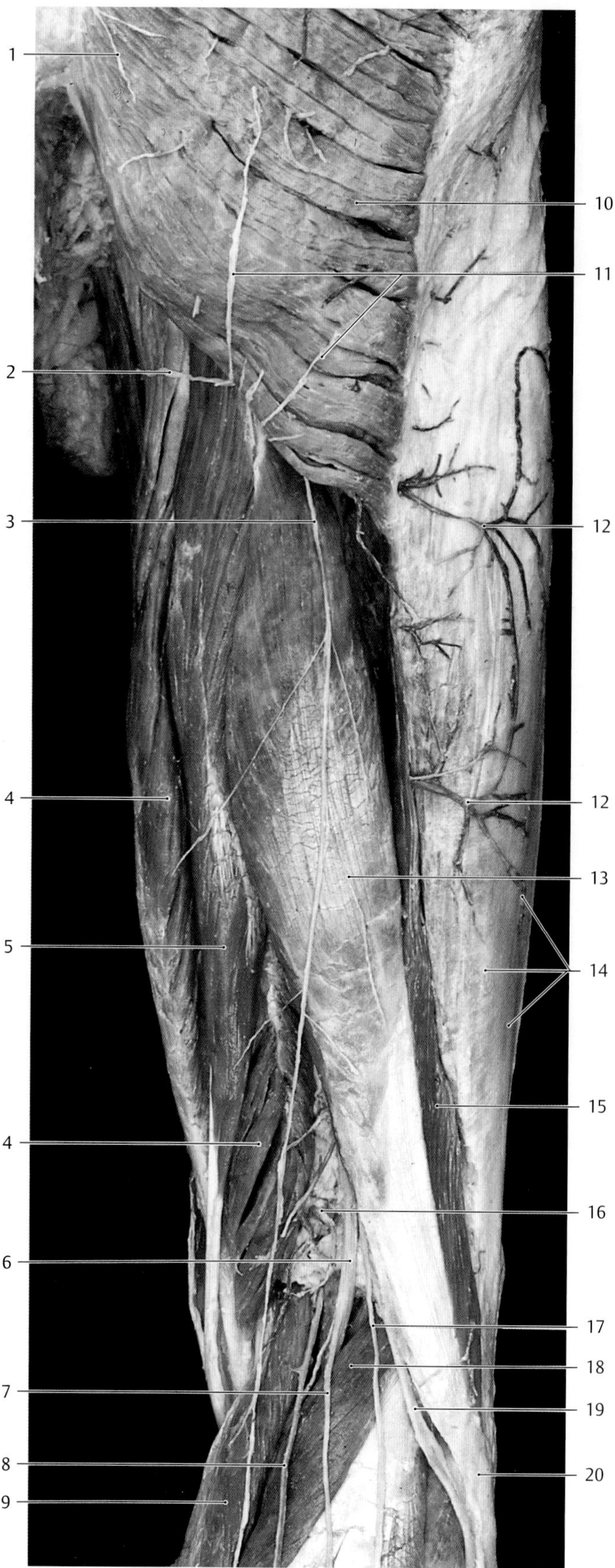


Fig. 4.128 **Gluteal and posterior regions of the thigh** with cutaneous nerves (right side). The fascia lata and the fasciae of the muscles have been removed.

1 Middle cluneal nerves
2 Perineal branch of posterior femoral cutaneous nerve
3 Posterior femoral cutaneous nerve
4 Semimembranosus muscle
5 Semitendinosus muscle
6 Tibial nerve
7 Medial sural cutaneous nerve
8 Small saphenous vein
9 Medial head of gastrocnemius muscle
10 Gluteus maximus muscle
11 Inferior cluneal nerves
12 Cutaneous veins
13 Long head of biceps femoris muscle
14 Iliotibial tract
15 Short head of biceps femoris muscle
16 Popliteal fossa
17 Lateral sural cutaneous nerve
18 Lateral head of gastrocnemius muscle
19 Common fibular nerve
20 Tendon of biceps femoris muscle
21 Inferior gluteal nerve
22 Sacrotuberous ligament
23 Inferior rectal branches of pudendal nerve
24 Anus
25 Gluteus medius muscle
26 Piriformis muscle
27 Sciatic nerve
28 Inferior gluteal artery
29 Gluteus maximus muscle (cut)
30 Quadratus femoris muscle
31 Sciatic nerve dividing into its two branches (the common fibular nerve and the tibial nerve)
32 Muscular branches of sciatic nerve to the ischiocrural muscles
33 Popliteal artery
34 Popliteal vein
35 Small saphenous vein (cut)
36 Long head of biceps femoris muscle (cut)
37 Superficial fibular nerve

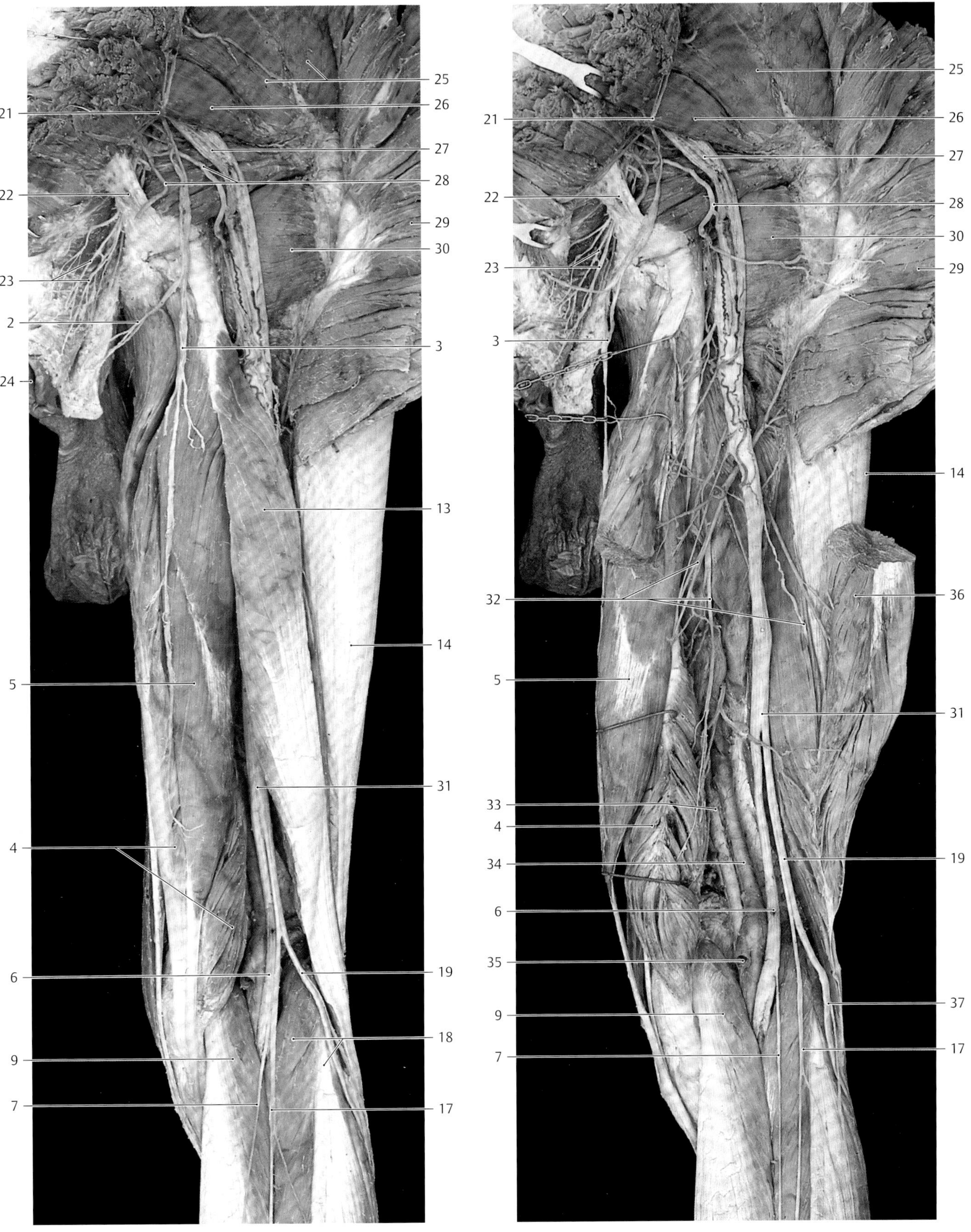


Fig. 4.129 **Gluteal and posterior regions of the thigh** (right side). The gluteus maximus muscle has been divided and reflected.

Fig. 4.130 **Gluteal and posterior regions of the thigh** (right side). The gluteus maximus muscle and the long head of the biceps femoris muscle have been divided and reflected.

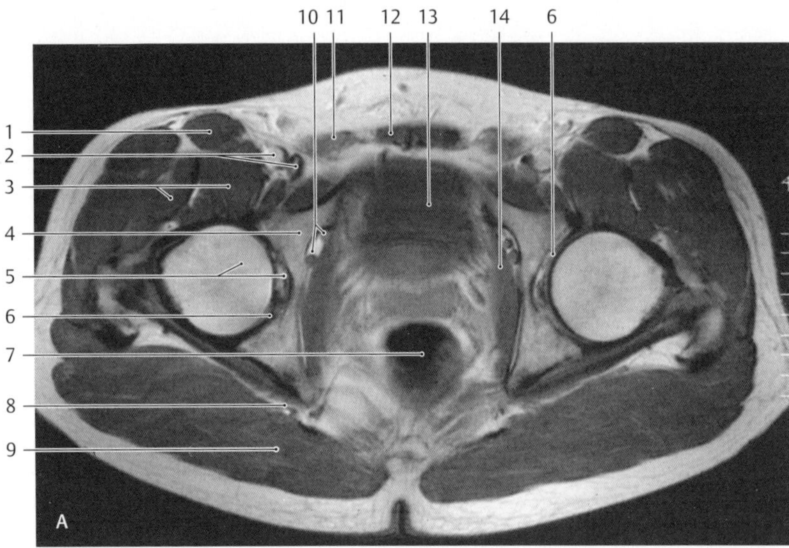


Fig. 4.131 **Axial section through the pelvis** at the level of the hip joints. Section A (inferior aspect, MRI scan). (Courtesy of Prof. Uder, Institute of Radiology, University Hospital Erlangen, Germany.)

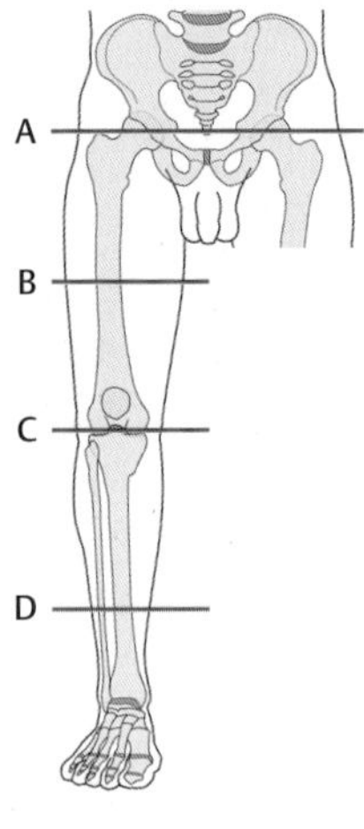


Fig. 4.133 **Lower limb, location of sections.**

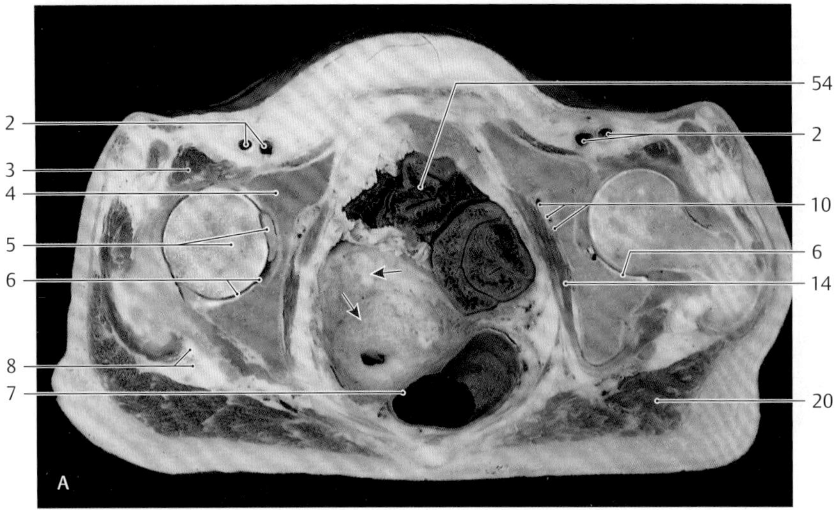


Fig. 4.132 **Axial section through the pelvis** at the level of the hip joints in a female. Section A (inferior aspect). Arrows = uterus (myometrium with myoma).

1 Sartorius muscle
2 Femoral artery and vein
3 Iliopsoas muscle
4 Pubis
5 Head of femur with ligament of head of femur
6 Articular cavity
7 Rectum
8 Sciatic nerve and accompanying artery
9 Gluteus maximus muscle
10 Obturator artery, vein, and nerve
11 Rectus abdominis muscle
12 Pyramidalis muscle
13 Urinary bladder
14 Obturator internus muscle
15 Rectus femoris muscle
16 Vastus intermedius and vastus lateralis muscles of quadriceps femoris muscle
17 Femur
18 Perforating artery
19 Sciatic nerve
20 Gluteus maximus muscle (insertion)
21 Vastus medialis muscle
22 Sartorius muscle
23 Femoral artery and vein
24 Great saphenous vein
25 Gracilis muscle
26 Adductor muscles
27 Biceps femoris muscle
28 Patellar ligament
29 Lateral condyle of femur
30 Posterior cruciate ligament
31 Tibial nerve
32 Popliteal artery and vein
33 Lateral head of gastrocnemius muscle
34 Medial condyle of femur
35 Medial head of gastrocnemius muscle
36 Tibialis anterior muscle
37 Tibia
38 Deep fibular nerve, anterior tibial artery, and vein
39 Patellar surface
40 Peroneus longus and brevis muscles
41 Fibula
42 Soleus muscle
43 Flexor digitorum longus muscle
44 Tibialis posterior muscle
45 Posterior tibial artery and vein, and tibial nerve
46 Peroneal artery
47 Small saphenous vein and sural nerve
48 Extensor hallucis longus muscle
49 Extensor digitorum longus muscle
50 Semimembranosus muscle
51 Semitendinosus muscle
52 Anterior cruciate ligament
53 Plantaris muscle
54 Small intestine

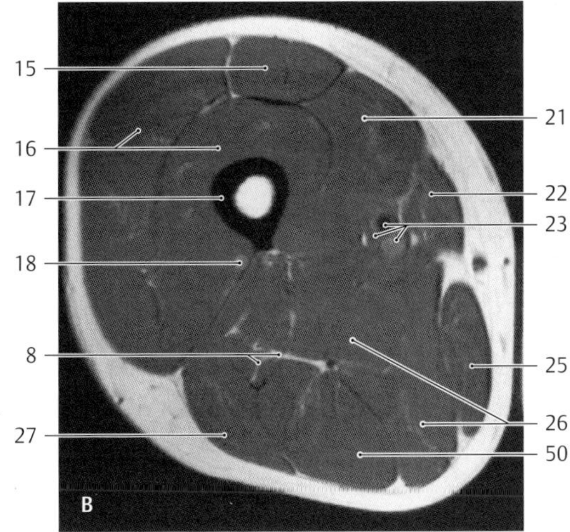


Fig. 4.134 **Axial section through the middle of the right thigh.** Section B (inferior aspect, MRI scan). (Courtesy of Prof. Uder, Institute of Radiology, University Hospital Erlangen, Germany.)

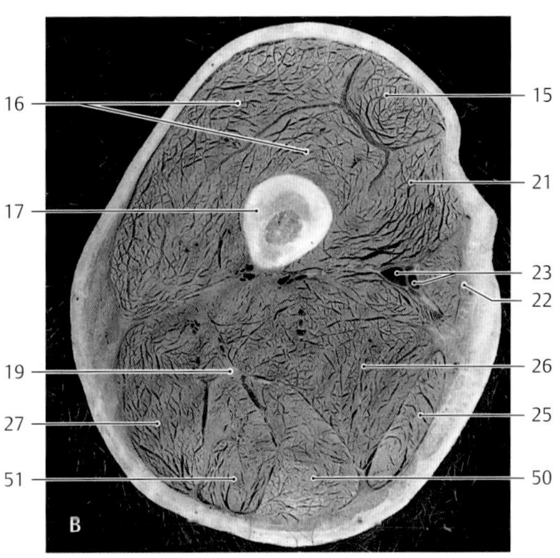


Fig. 4.135 **Axial section through the middle of the right thigh.** Section B (inferior aspect).

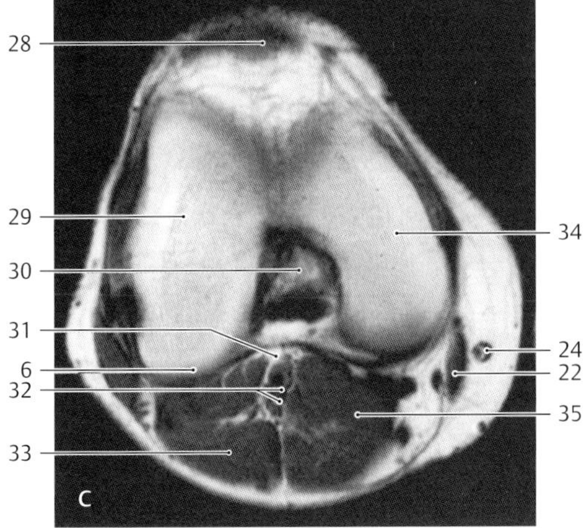


Fig. 4.136 **Axial section through the right knee joint.** Section C (inferior aspect, MRI scan). (Courtesy of Prof. Uder, Institute of Radiology, University Hospital Erlangen, Germany.)

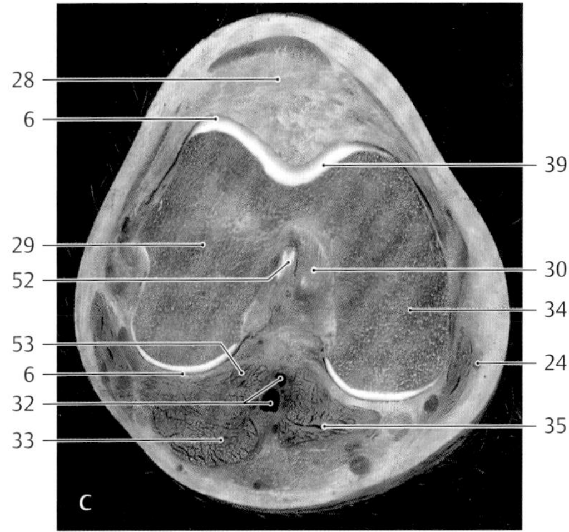


Fig. 4.137 **Axial section through the right knee joint.** Section C (inferior aspect).

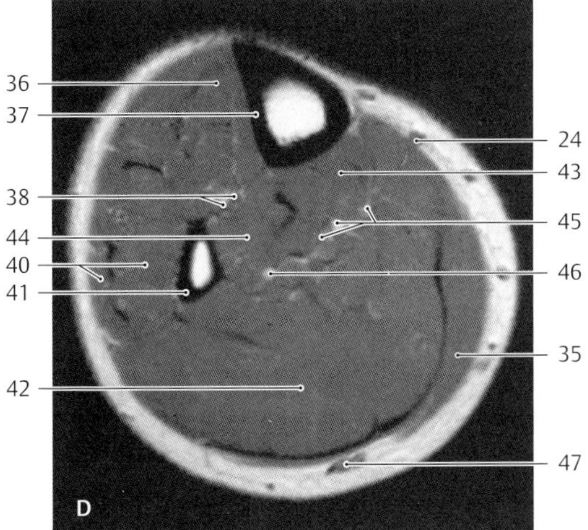


Fig. 4.138 **Axial section through the middle of the right leg.** Section D (inferior aspect, MRI scan). (Courtesy of Prof. Uder, Institute of Radiology, University Hospital Erlangen, Germany.)

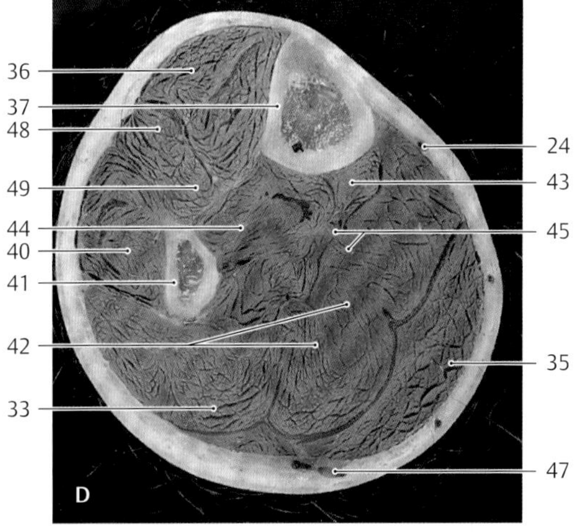


Fig. 4.139 **Axial section through the middle of the right leg.** Section D (inferior aspect).

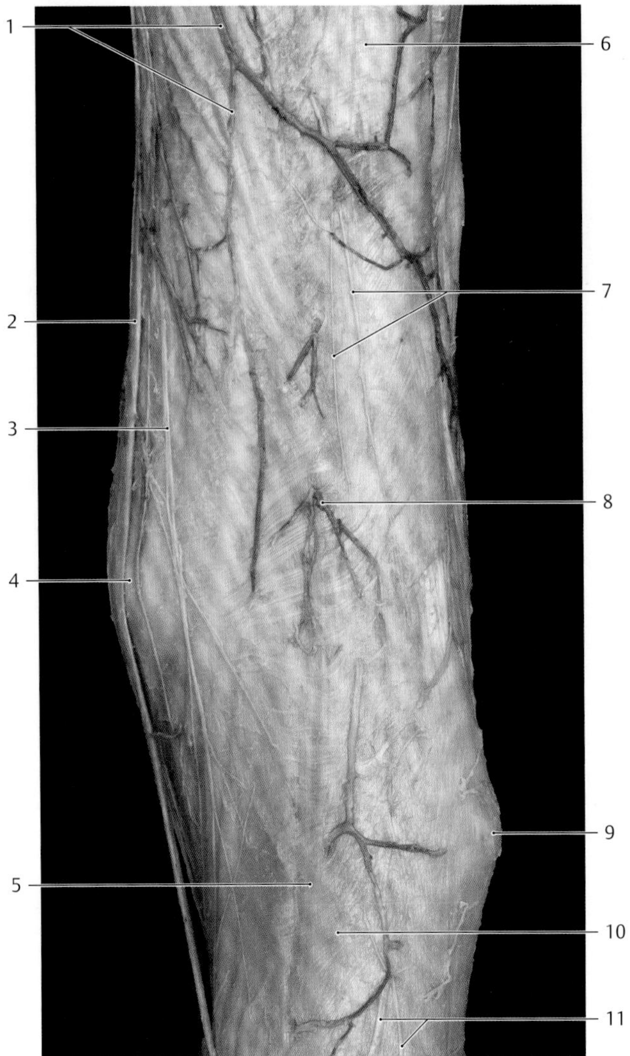


Fig. 4.140 **Posterior region of the knee** with cutaneous nerves and veins (right side).

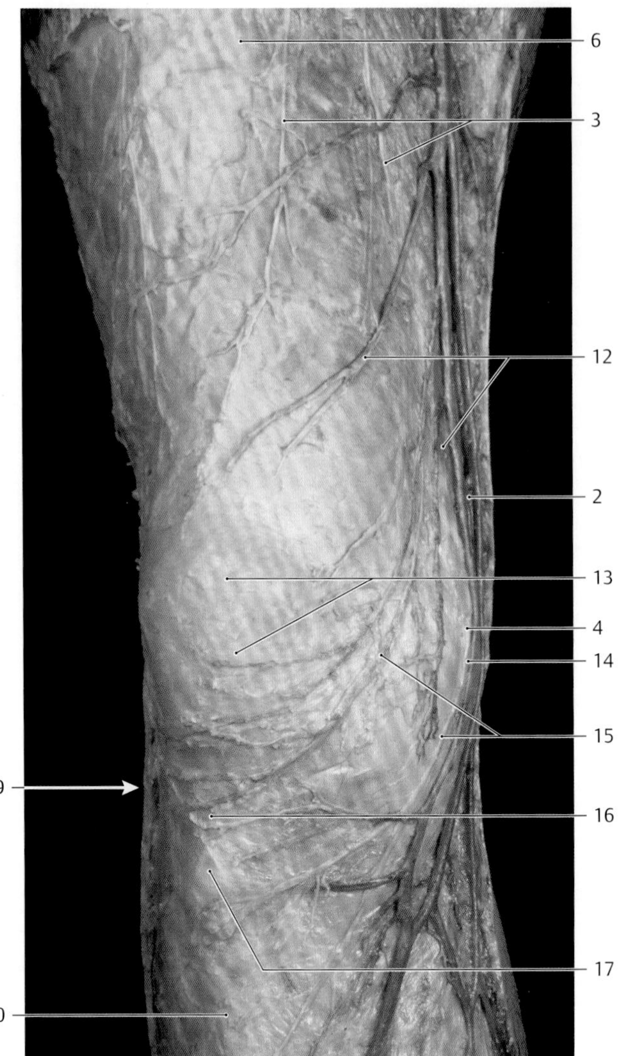


Fig. 4.141 **Anterior region of the knee** with cutaneous nerves and veins (right side).

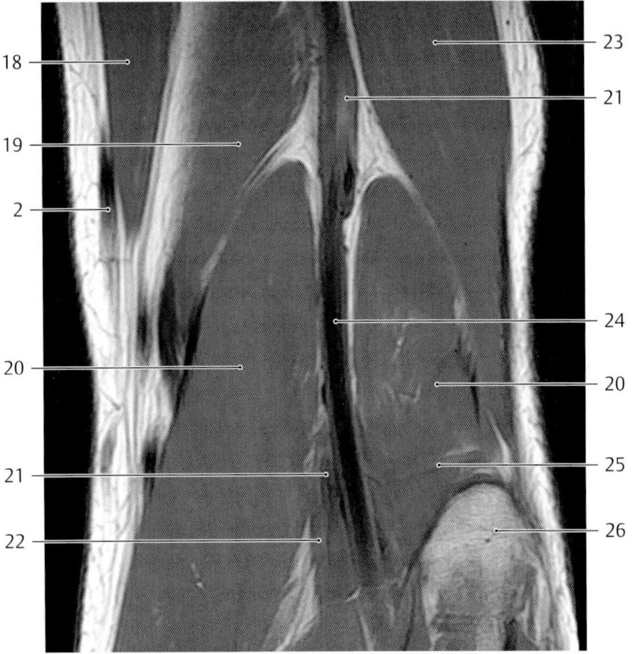


1 Cutaneous veins (tributaries of great saphenous vein)
2 Great saphenous vein
3 Cutaneous branches of femoral nerve
4 Position of medial condyle of femur
5 Position of small saphenous vein
6 Fascia lata
7 Terminal branches of posterior femoral cutaneous nerve
8 Cutaneous veins of popliteal fossa
9 Position of head of fibula
10 Superficial layer of crural fascia
11 Lateral sural cutaneous nerve
12 Venous network around knee
13 Patella
14 Saphenous nerve
15 Infrapatellar branch of saphenous nerve
16 Patellar ligament
17 Position of tibial tuberosity
18 Sartorius muscle
19 Semimembranosus muscle
20 Gastrocnemius muscle
21 Popliteal vein
22 Tibial nerve
23 Biceps femoris muscle
24 Popliteal artery
25 Lateral inferior genicular artery
26 Fibula

Fig. 4.142 **Coronal section through the popliteal fossa** (MRI scan). (Heuck A, et al. MRT-Atlas des muskuloskelettalen Systems. Stuttgart, Germany: Schattauer, 2009.)

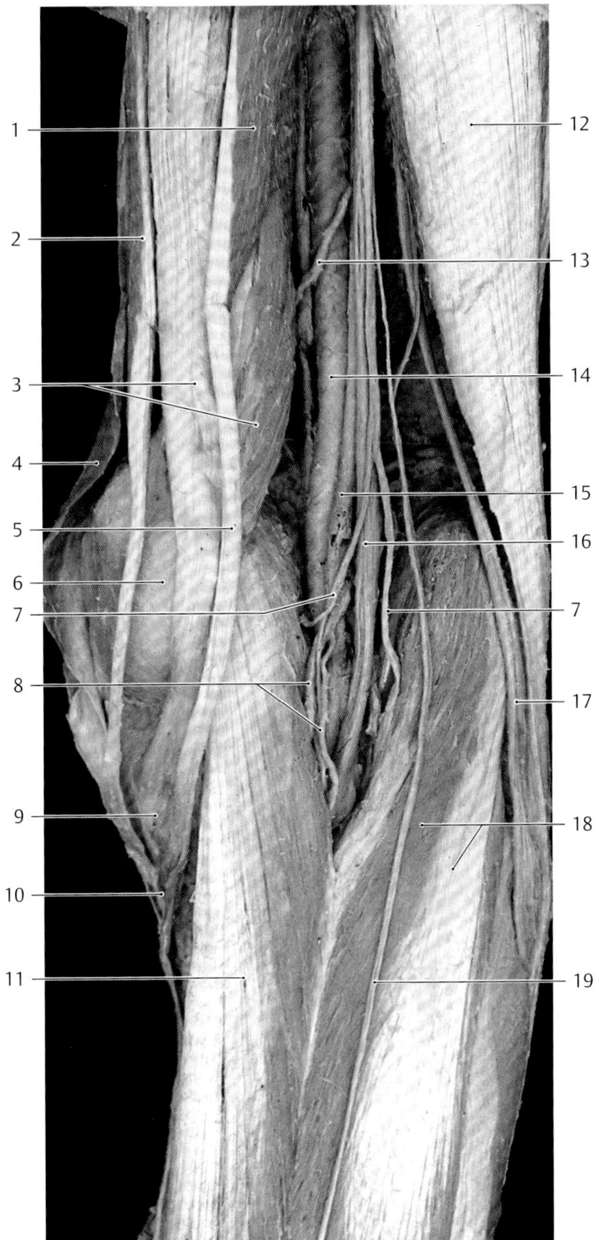


Fig. 4.143 **Popliteal fossa,** middle layer (right side). The gastrocnemius muscle has been divided and reflected.

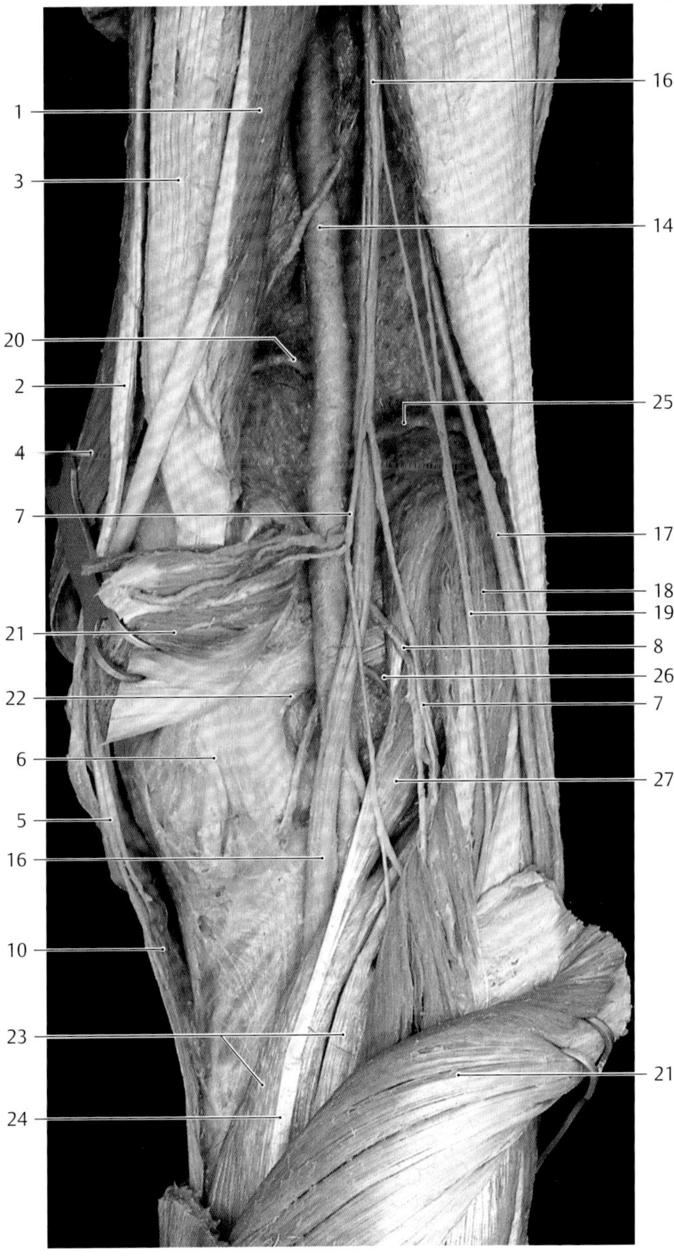


Fig. 4.144 **Popliteal fossa,** deep layer (right side). The gastrocnemius and soleus muscles have been divided and reflected.

1 Semitendinosus muscle
2 Gracilis muscle
3 Semimembranosus muscle
4 Sartorius muscle
5 Tendon of semitendinosus muscle
6 Position of medial condyle of femur
7 Muscular branches of tibial nerve
8 Sural arteries and veins
9 Tendon of semimembranosus muscle
10 Common tendon of gracilis, semitendinosus, and sartorius muscles (pes anserinus)
11 Medial head of gastrocnemius muscle
12 Biceps femoris muscle
13 Muscular branch of popliteal artery
14 Popliteal artery
15 Popliteal vein
16 Tibial nerve
17 Common fibular nerve
18 Lateral head of gastrocnemius muscle
19 Medial sural cutaneous nerve
20 Medial superior genicular artery
21 Medial head of gastrocnemius muscle (cut and reflected)
22 Medial inferior genicular artery
23 Soleus muscle
24 Tendon of plantaris muscle
25 Lateral superior genicular artery
26 Lateral inferior genicular artery
27 Plantaris muscle

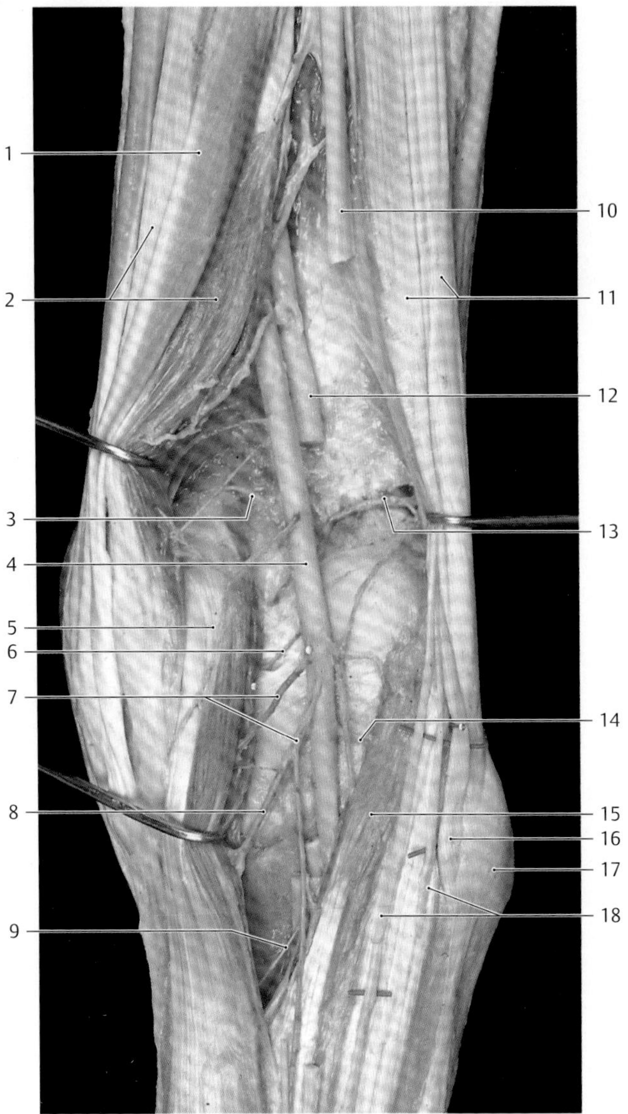


Fig. 4.145 **Popliteal fossa,** deep layer (right side). The muscles have been reflected to display the genicular arteries.

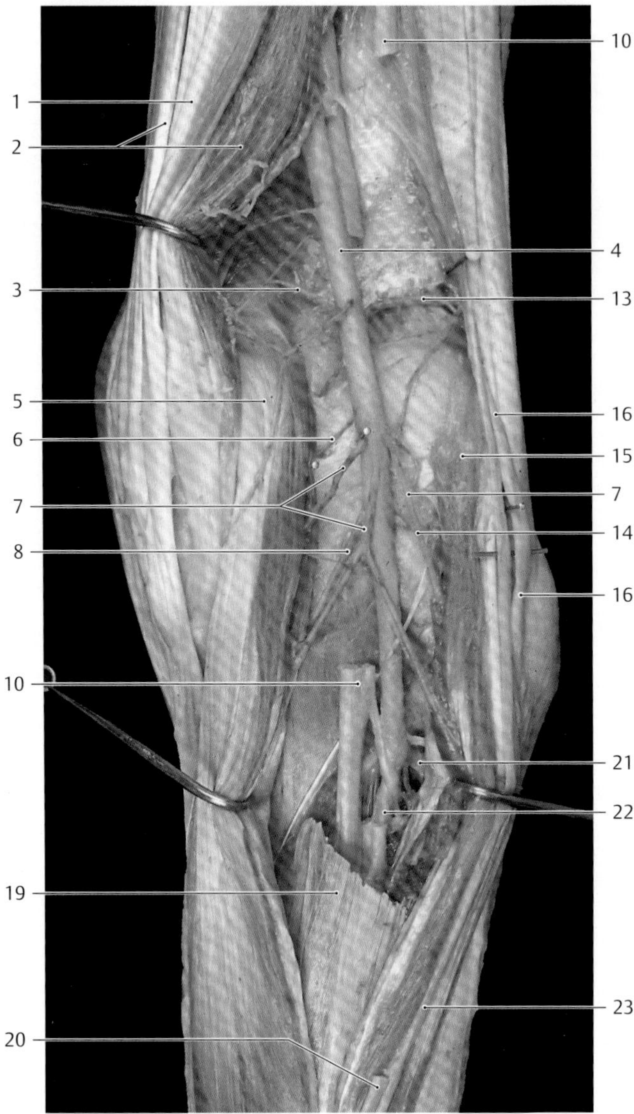


Fig. 4.146 **Popliteal fossa,** deepest layer (right side). Tibial nerve and popliteal vein have been partly removed and a portion of the soleus muscle was cut away to display the anterior tibial artery.

1 Semitendinosus muscle
2 Semimembranosus muscle
3 Medial superior genicular artery
4 Popliteal artery
5 Medial head of gastrocnemius muscle
6 Middle genicular artery
7 Muscular branches of popliteal artery
8 Medial inferior genicular artery
9 Tendon of plantaris muscle
10 Tibial nerve (cut)
11 Biceps femoris muscle
12 Popliteal vein (cut)
13 Lateral superior genicular artery
14 Lateral inferior genicular artery
15 Lateral head of gastrocnemius muscle
16 Common fibular nerve
17 Head of fibula
18 Lateral sural cutaneous nerves
19 Soleus muscle
20 Medial sural cutaneous nerve
21 Anterior tibial artery
22 Posterior tibial artery
23 Lateral sural cutaneous nerve

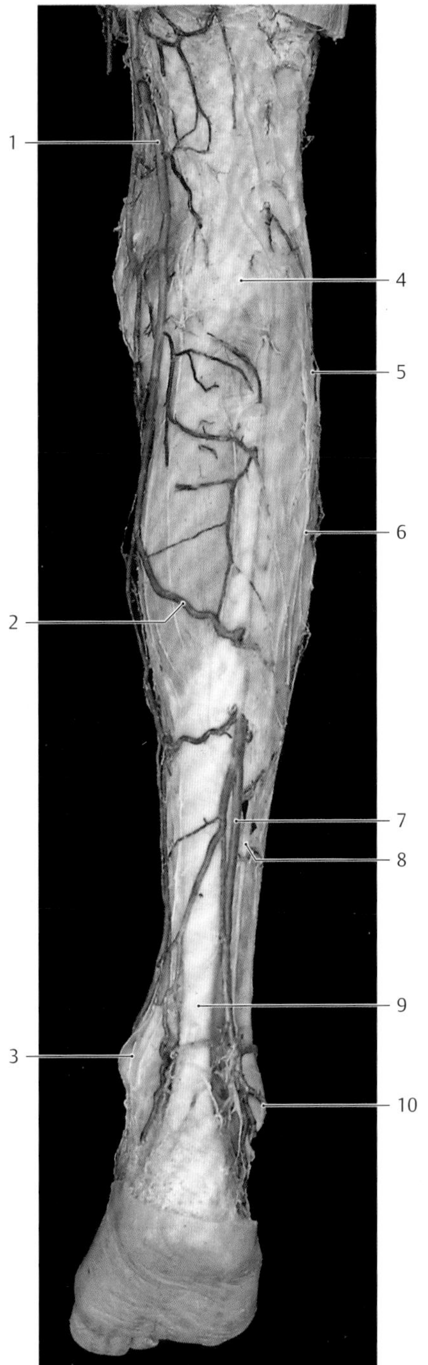


Fig. 4.147 **Posterior crural region and popliteal fossa** with cutaneous veins and nerves (right side).

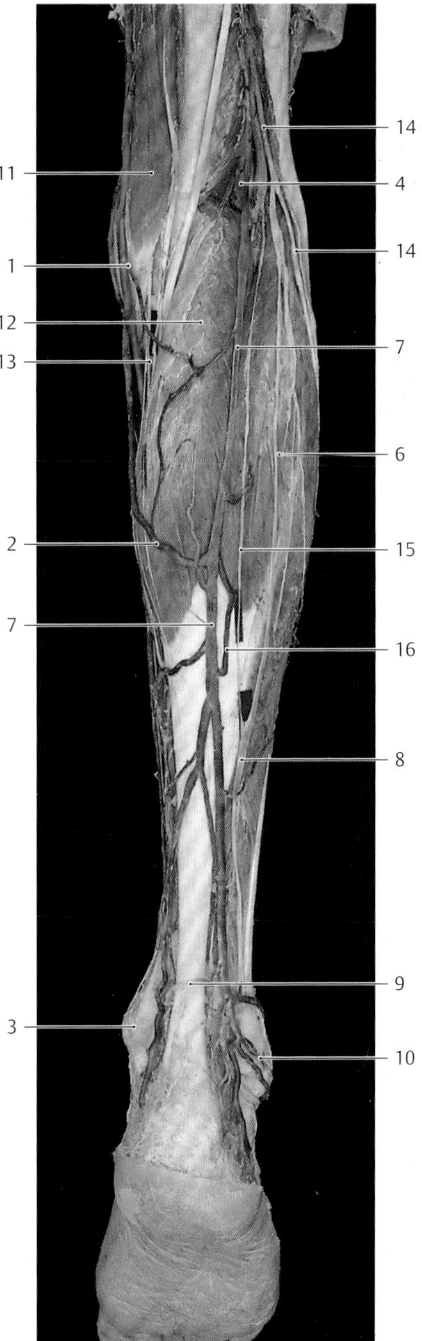


Fig. 4.148 **Posterior crural region and popliteal fossa** with cutaneous veins and nerves (right side). The superficial layer of the crural fascia has been removed.

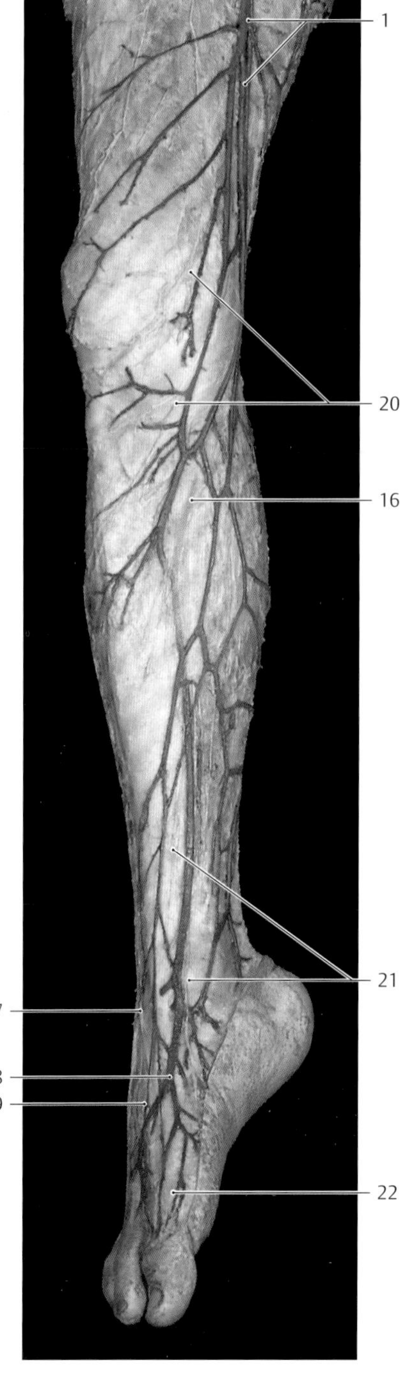


Fig. 4.149 **Antero-medial crural region** with cutaneous veins and nerves (right side).

1 Great saphenous vein
2 Anastomosis between small and great saphenous veins
3 Medial malleolus
4 Popliteal fossa
5 Position of head of fibula
6 Lateral sural cutaneous nerve
7 Small saphenous vein
8 Sural nerve
9 Calcaneal or Achilles tendon
10 Lateral malleolus
11 Semitendinosus muscle
12 Medial head of gastrocnemius muscle
13 Saphenous nerve
14 Common fibular nerve
15 Medial sural cutaneous nerve
16 Perforating veins
17 Superficial fibular nerve
18 Dorsal venous arch of foot
19 Intermediate dorsal cutaneous nerve
20 Infrapatellar branches of saphenous nerve
21 Terminal branches of saphenous nerve
22 Medial dorsal cutaneous nerve

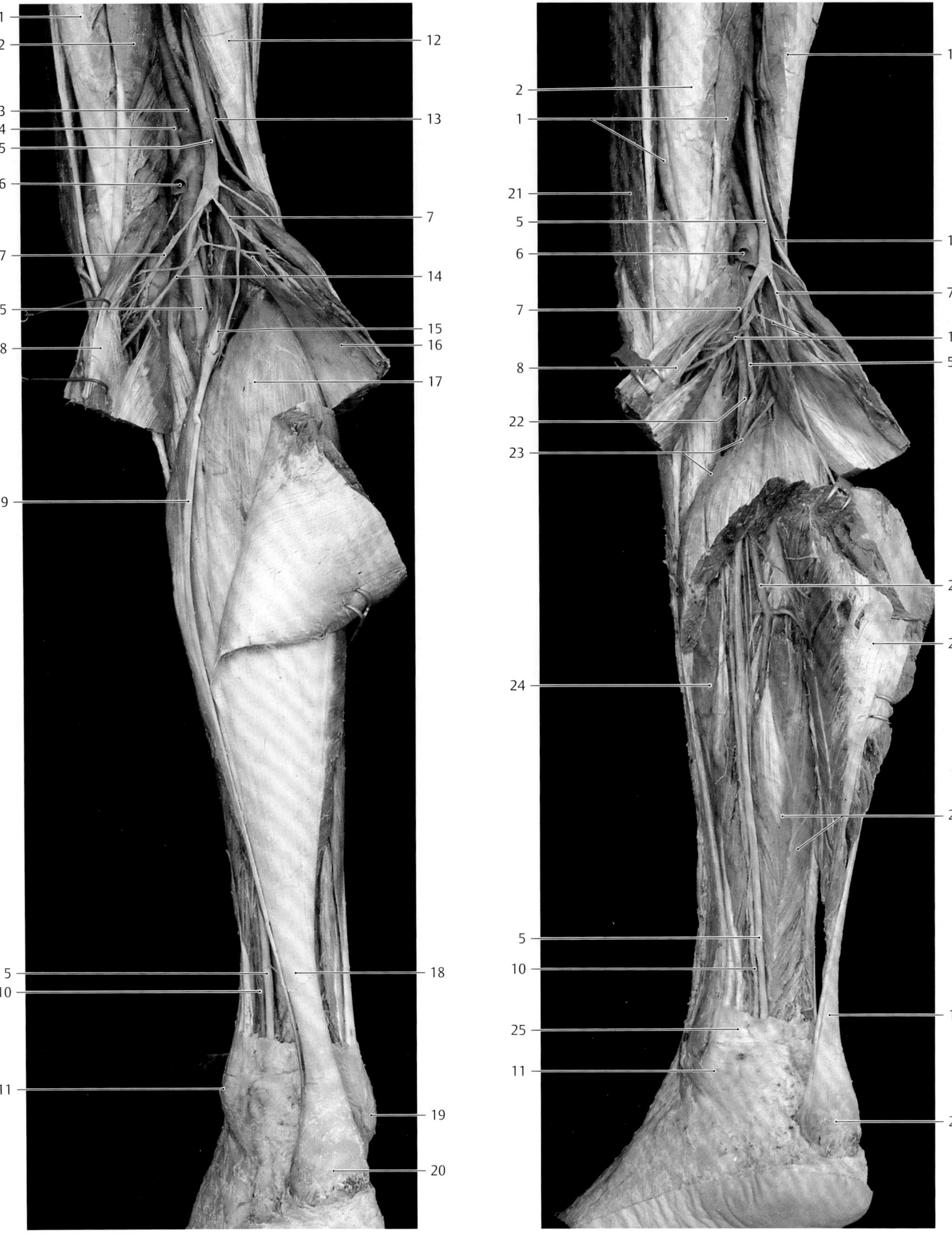


Fig. 4.150 **Posterior crural region and popliteal fossa,** superficial layer (right side). The cutaneous veins and nerves have been removed.

Fig. 4.151 **Posterior crural region and popliteal fossa,** middle layer (right side). The medial head of the gastrocnemius muscle has been divided and reflected.

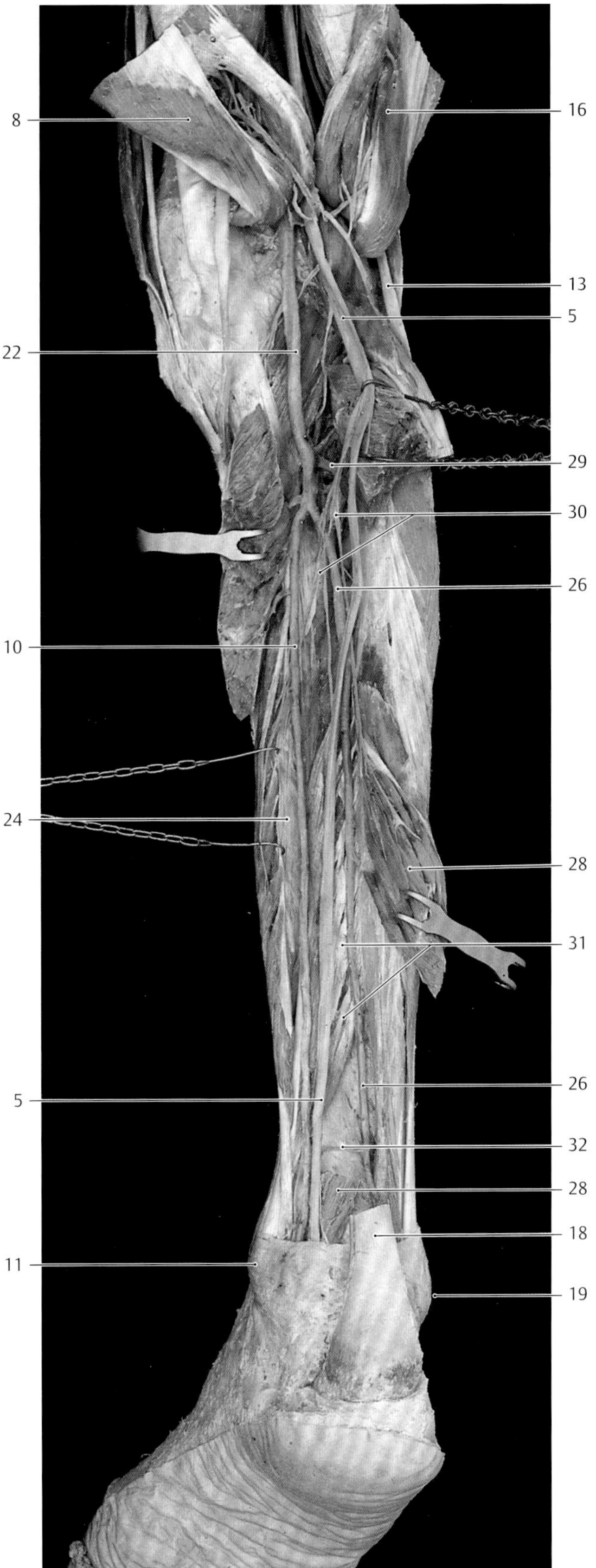


Fig. 4.152 **Posterior crural region and popliteal fossa,** deep layer (right side). Triceps surae (gastrocnemius and soleus) and flexor hallucis longus muscles have been cut and reflected.

1 Semimembranosus muscle
2 Semitendinosus muscle
3 Popliteal vein
4 Popliteal artery
5 Tibial nerve
6 Small saphenous vein (cut)
7 Muscular branch of tibial nerve
8 Medial head of gastrocnemius muscle
9 Tendon of plantaris muscle
10 Posterior tibial artery
11 Medial malleolus
12 Biceps femoris muscle
13 Common fibular nerve
14 Sural arteries
15 Plantaris muscle
16 Lateral head of gastrocnemius muscle
17 Soleus muscle
18 Calcaneal or Achilles tendon
19 Lateral malleolus
20 Calcaneal tuberosity
21 Sartorius muscle
22 Popliteal artery
23 Tendinous arch of soleus muscle
24 Flexor digitorum longus muscle
25 Flexor retinaculum
26 Peroneal artery
27 Triceps surae muscle (cut)
28 Flexor hallucis longus muscle
29 Anterior tibial artery
30 Muscular branches of tibial nerve
31 Tibialis posterior muscle
32 Communicating branch of peroneal artery
33 Tendon of tibialis anterior muscle
34 Tibia
35 Tendon of extensor hallucis longus muscle
36 Tendons of extensor digitorum longus muscle
37 Anterior tibial artery
38 Fibula
39 Tendons of peroneus longus and brevis muscles

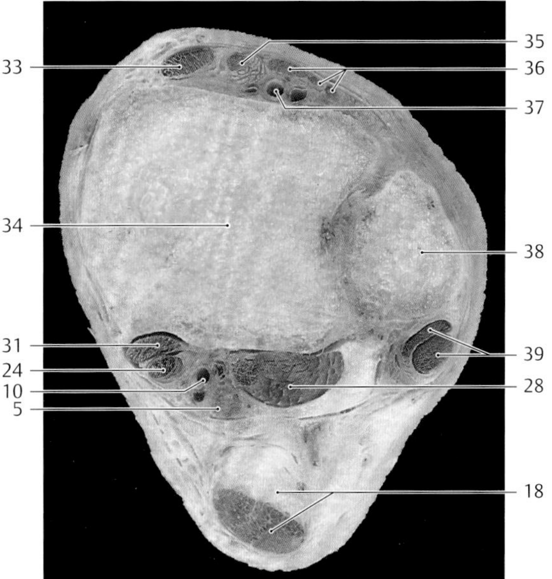


Fig. 4.153 **Cross section through the leg,** superior to the malleoli (inferior aspect).

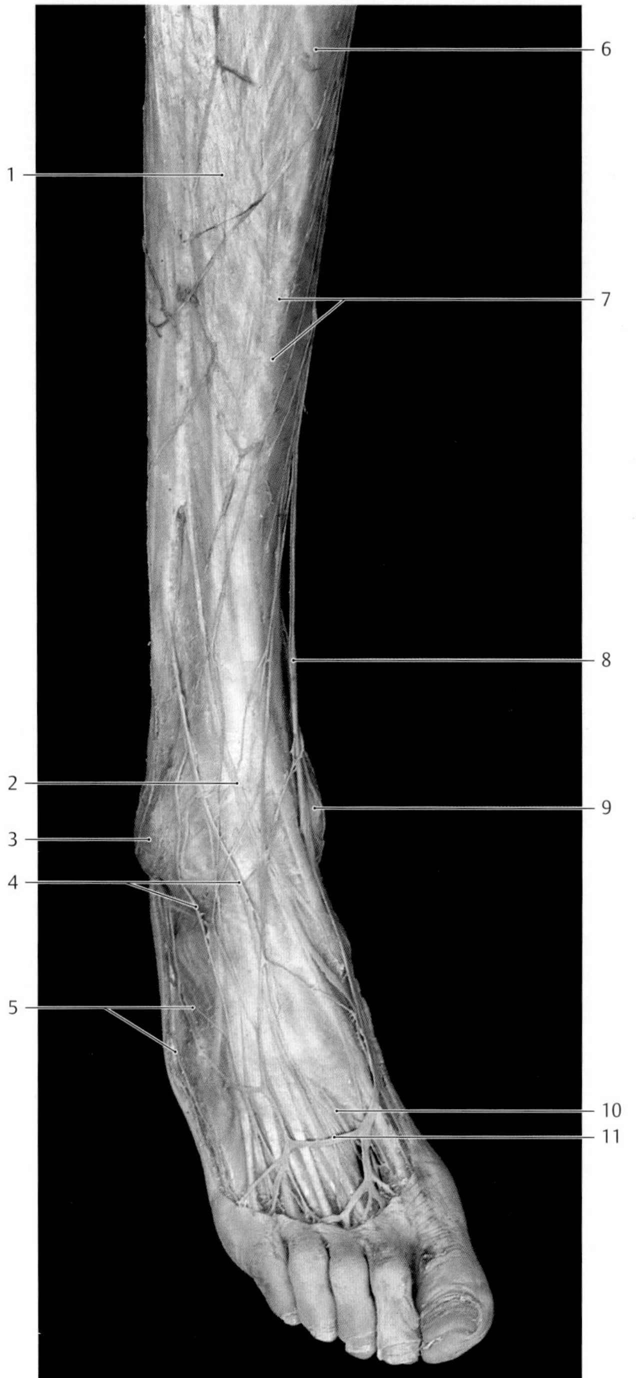


**Fig. 4.154 Anterior crural region and dorsum of the foot** with cutaneous nerves and veins (right side).

**Fig. 4.155 Medial crural region and foot** with cutaneous nerves and veins (right side).

1 Superficial crural fascia
2 Medial dorsal cutaneous branch of superficial fibular nerve
3 Lateral malleolus
4 Intermediate dorsal cutaneous branch of superficial fibular nerve
5 Lateral dorsal cutaneous branch of sural nerve
6 Position of tibial tuberosity
7 Anterior margin of tibia
8 Great saphenous vein
9 Medial malleolus
10 Deep fibular nerve
11 Dorsal venous arch of foot
12 Position of patella
13 Infrapatellar branches of saphenous nerve
14 Saphenous nerve
15 Small saphenous vein
16 Perforating vein
17 Calcaneal or Achilles tendon

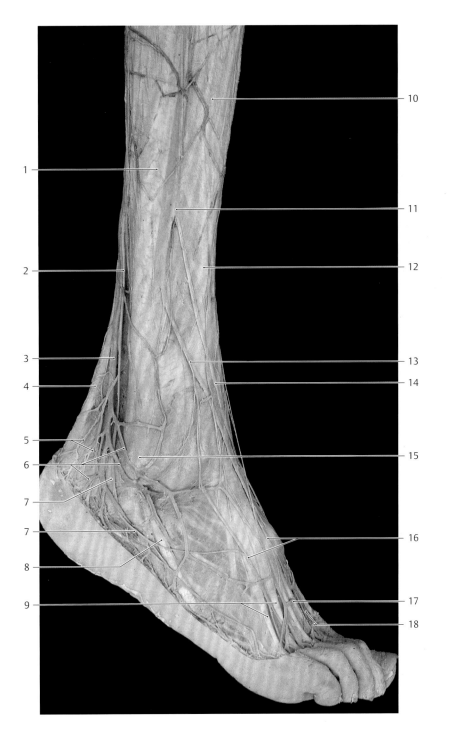

Fig. 4.156 **Lateral crural region and foot** with cutaneous nerves and veins (right side).

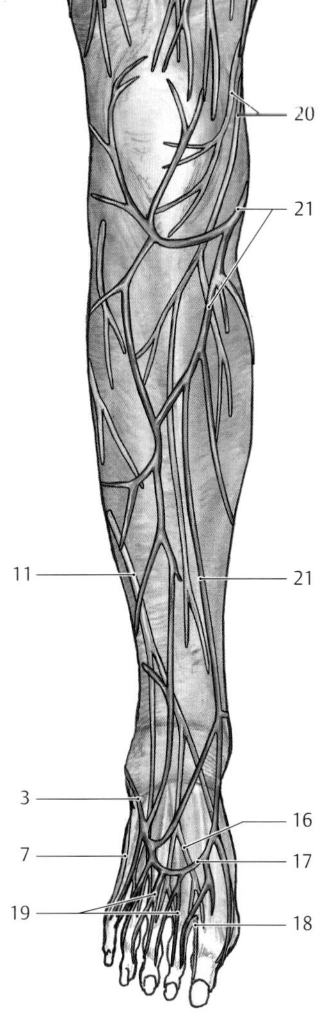


Fig. 4.157 **Anterior crural region and dorsum of the foot** with cutaneous nerves and veins.

1 Position of fibula
2 Sural nerve
3 Small saphenous vein
4 Calcaneal or Achilles tendon
5 Lateral calcaneal branches of sural nerve
6 Venous plexus of lateral malleolus
7 Lateral dorsal cutaneous branch of sural nerve
8 Tendon of peroneus brevis muscle
9 Tendons of extensor digitorum longus muscle
10 Crural fascia
11 Superficial fibular nerve
12 Position of tibia
13 Intermediate dorsal cutaneous branch of superficial fibular nerve
14 Medial dorsal cutaneous branch of superficial fibular nerve
15 Lateral malleolus
16 Dorsal digital nerves
17 Dorsal venous arch of foot
18 Deep fibular nerve
19 Dorsal metatarsal veins
20 Saphenous nerve
21 Great saphenous vein

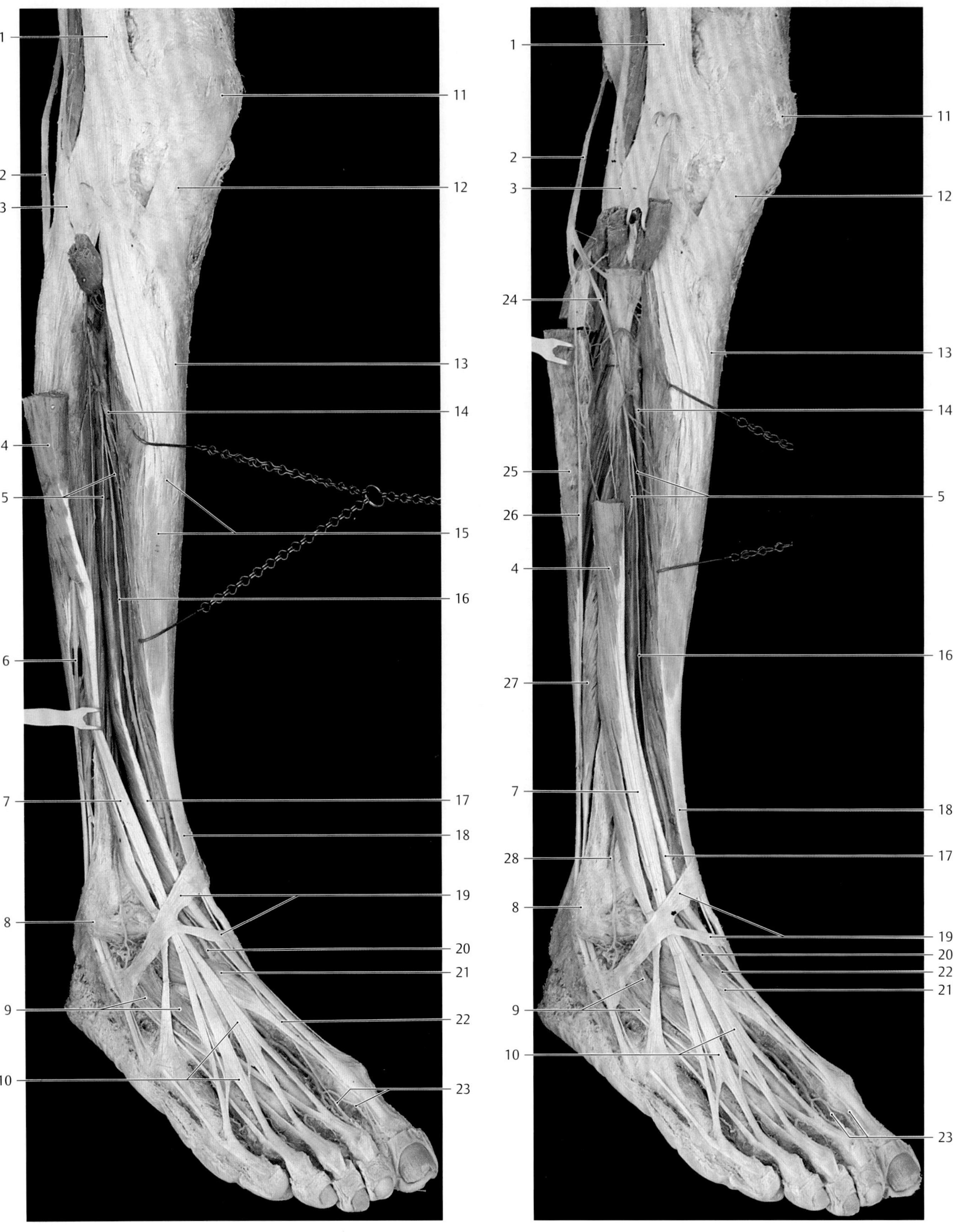


**Fig. 4.158 Lateral crural region and dorsum of the foot,** middle layer (right side, antero-lateral aspect). The extensor digitorum longus muscle has been divided and reflected laterally.

**Fig. 4.159 Lateral crural region and dorsum of the foot,** deep layer (right side, antero-lateral aspect). Extensor digitorum longus and peroneus longus muscles have been divided or removed. The common fibular nerve has been elevated to show its course around the head of the fibula.

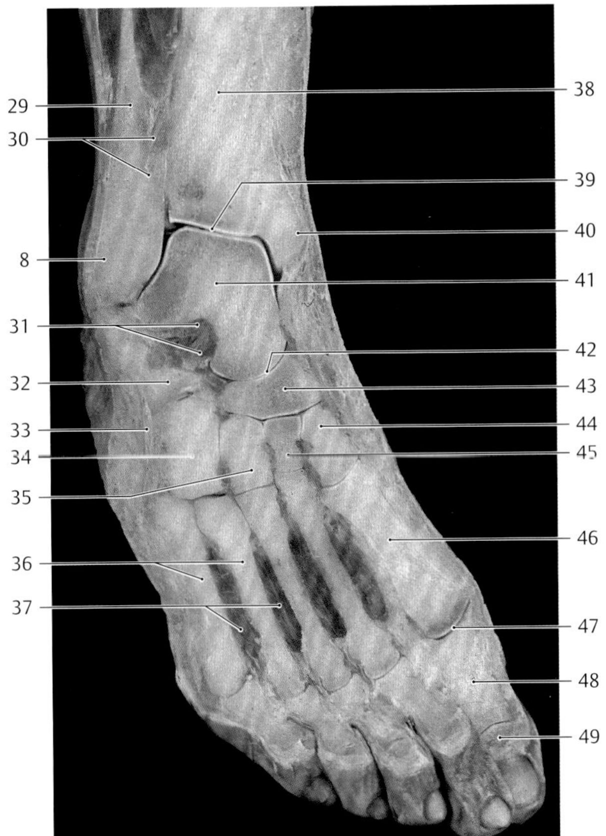


Fig. 4.160 **Coronal section through the right foot and ankle joint** (dorsal aspect).

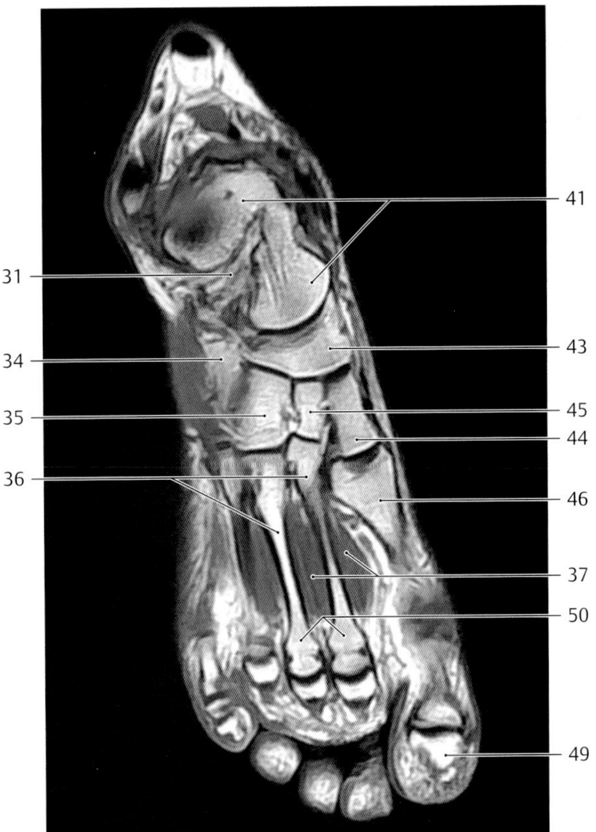


Fig. 4.161 **Coronal section through the right foot and ankle joint** (MRI scan). (Heuck A, et al. MRT-Atlas des muskuloskelettalen Systems. Stuttgart, Germany: Schattauer, 2009.)

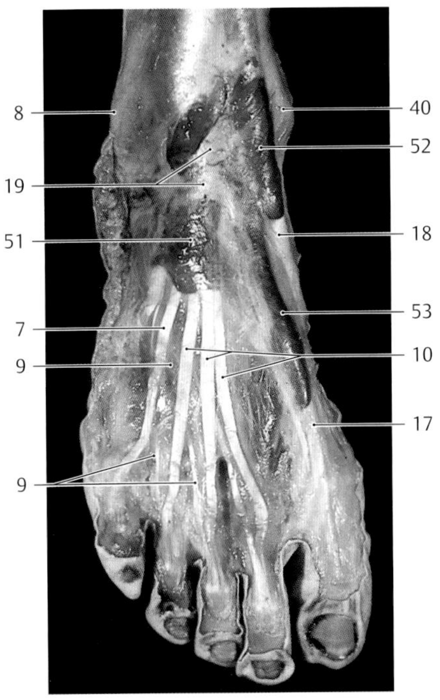


Fig. 4.162 **Synovial sheaths of extensor tendons** (dorsal aspect). The sheaths have been injected with blue gelatin.

1 Iliotibial tract
2 Common fibular nerve
3 Position of head of fibula
4 Extensor digitorum longus muscle
5 Muscular branches of deep fibular nerve
6 Superficial fibular nerve
7 Tendon of extensor digitorum longus muscle
8 Lateral malleolus
9 Extensor digitorum brevis muscle with tendons
10 Tendons of extensor digitorum longus muscle
11 Patella
12 Patellar ligament
13 Anterior margin of tibia
14 Anterior tibial artery
15 Tibialis anterior muscle
16 Deep fibular nerve
17 Extensor hallucis longus muscle
18 Tendon of tibialis anterior muscle
19 Inferior extensor retinaculum
20 Dorsalis pedis artery
21 Extensor hallucis brevis muscle
22 Deep fibular nerve (on dorsum of foot)
23 Terminal branches of deep fibular nerve
24 Deep fibular nerve
25 Peroneus longus muscle (cut)
26 Superficial fibular nerve (with peroneal muscles laterally reflected)
27 Peroneus brevis muscle
28 Lateral anterior malleolar artery
29 Fibula
30 Distal tibiofibular joint (syndesmosis)
31 Talocalcaneal interosseous ligament
32 Calcaneus
33 Tendon of peroneus brevis muscle
34 Cuboid bone
35 Lateral cuneiform bone
36 Metatarsal bones
37 Dorsal interossei muscles
38 Tibia
39 Ankle joint
40 Medial malleolus
41 Talus
42 Talocalcaneonavicular joint
43 Navicular bone
44 Medial cuneiform bone
45 Intermediate cuneiform bone
46 First metatarsal bone
47 Metatarsophalangeal joint of great toe
48 Proximal phalanx of great toe
49 Distal phalanx of great toe
50 Heads of the second and third metatarsal bones
51 Synovial sheath of tendons of extensor digitorum longus muscle
52 Synovial sheath of tendon of tibialis anterior muscle
53 Synovial sheath of tendon of extensor hallucis longus muscle

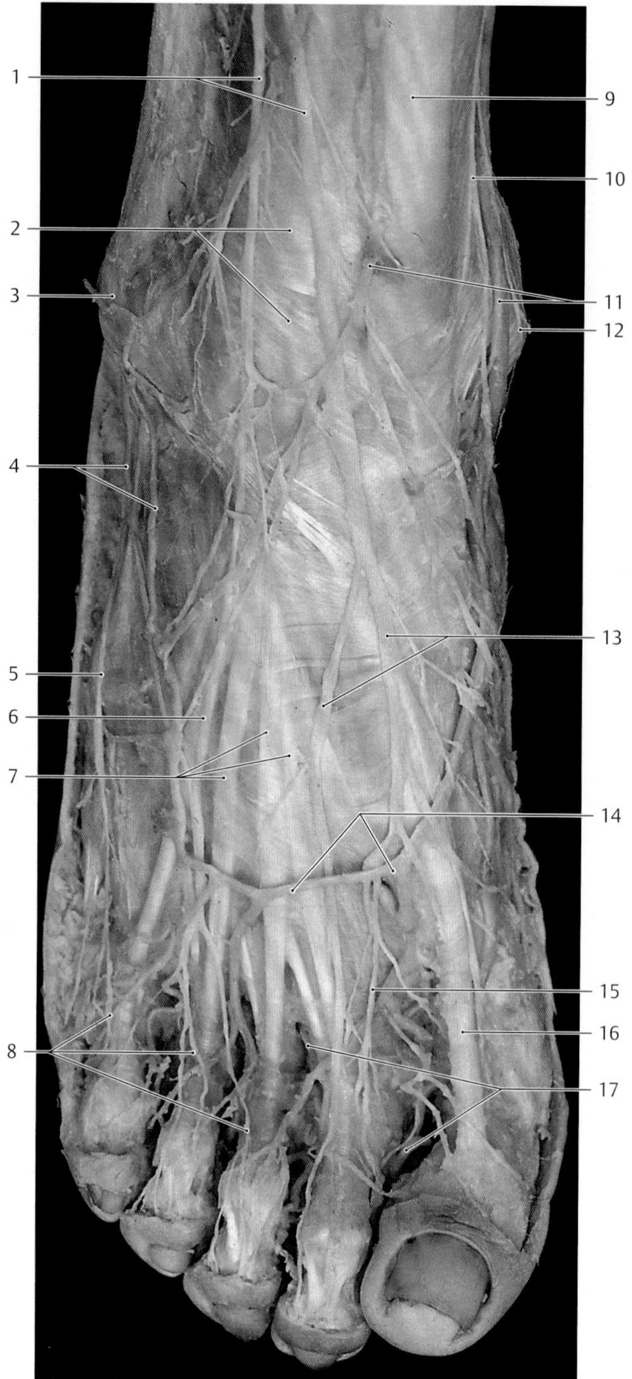


Fig. 4.163 **Dorsum of the right foot,** superficial layer.

Fig. 4.164 **Dorsum of the right foot,** superficial layer. The fascia of the dorsum has been removed.

1 Superficial fibular nerve
2 Superior extensor retinaculum
3 Lateral malleolus
4 Venous network of lateral malleolus and tributaries of small saphenous vein
5 Lateral dorsal cutaneous branch of sural nerve
6 Intermediate dorsal cutaneous nerve
7 Tendons of extensor digitorum longus muscle
8 Dorsal digital nerves
9 Tendon of tibialis anterior muscle
10 Saphenous nerve
11 Venous network of medial malleolus and tributaries of great saphenous vein
12 Medial malleolus
13 Medial dorsal cutaneous nerves
14 Dorsal venous arch of foot
15 Dorsal digital nerve (of deep fibular nerve)
16 Tendon of extensor hallucis longus muscle
17 Dorsal digital arteries
18 Peroneal muscles
19 Deep plantar branch of dorsalis pedis artery anastomosing with plantar arch
20 Extensor digitorum longus muscle
21 Extensor hallucis longus muscle
22 Inferior extensor retinaculum
23 Extensor hallucis brevis muscle

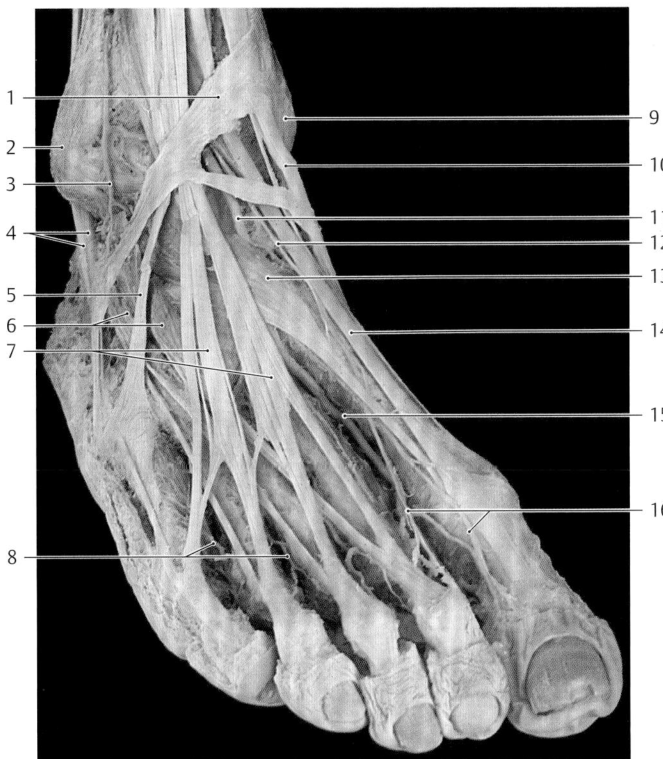


Fig. 4.165 **Dorsum of the right foot,** middle layer. The cutaneous nerves have been removed.

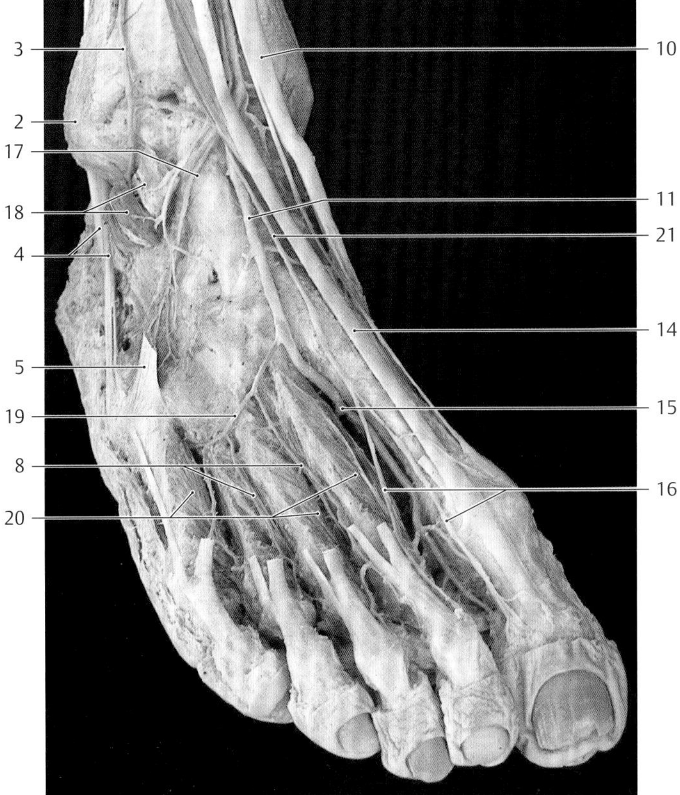


Fig. 4.166 **Dorsum of the right foot,** deep layer. Extensor digitorum and hallucis brevis muscles have been removed.

1 Inferior extensor retinaculum
2 Lateral malleolus
3 Lateral anterior malleolar artery
4 Tendons of peroneal muscles
5 Tendon of peroneus tertius muscle
6 Extensor digitorum brevis muscle
7 Tendons of extensor digitorum longus muscle
8 Dorsal metatarsal arteries
9 Medial malleolus
10 Tendon of tibialis anterior muscle
11 Dorsalis pedis artery
12 Deep fibular nerve (on dorsum of foot)
13 Extensor hallucis brevis muscle
14 Tendon of extensor hallucis longus muscle
15 Dorsalis pedis artery with deep plantar branch to the plantar arch
16 Terminal branches of deep fibular nerve
17 Lateral tarsal artery
18 Extensor digitorum brevis muscle (divided)
19 Arcuate artery
20 Dorsal interossei muscles
21 Deep fibular nerve

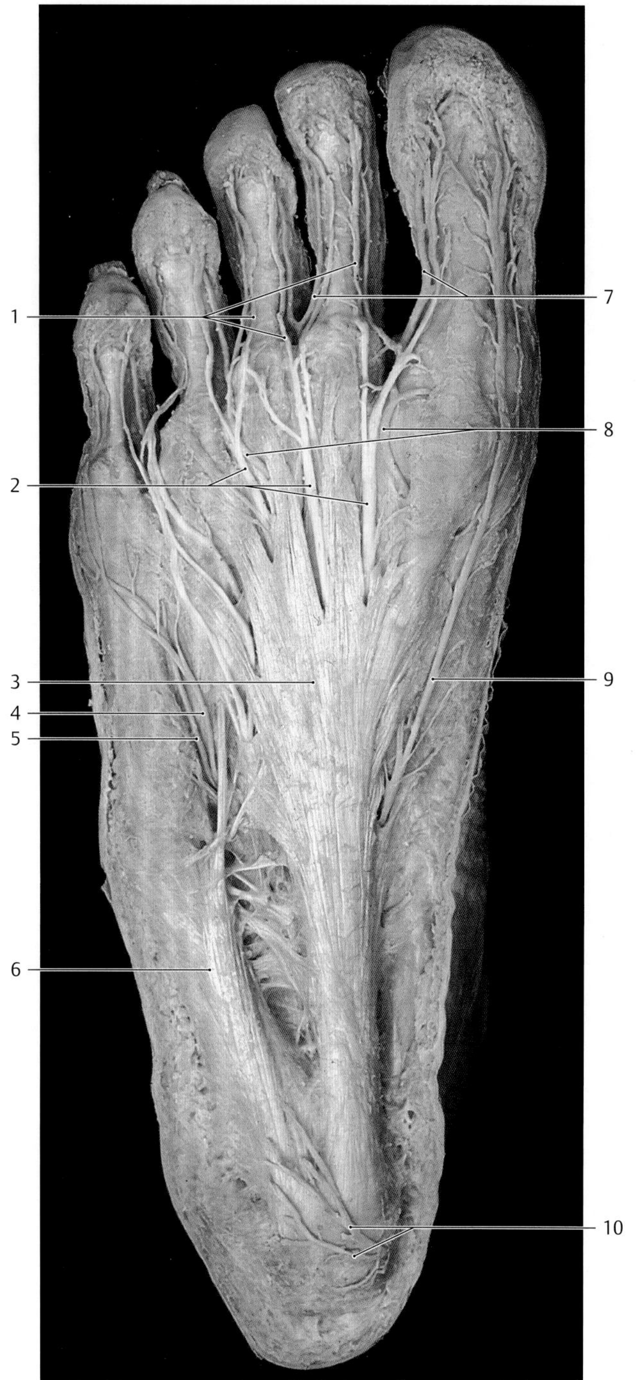


Fig. 4.167 **Sole of the right foot,** superficial layer. Dissection of cutaneous nerves and vessels.

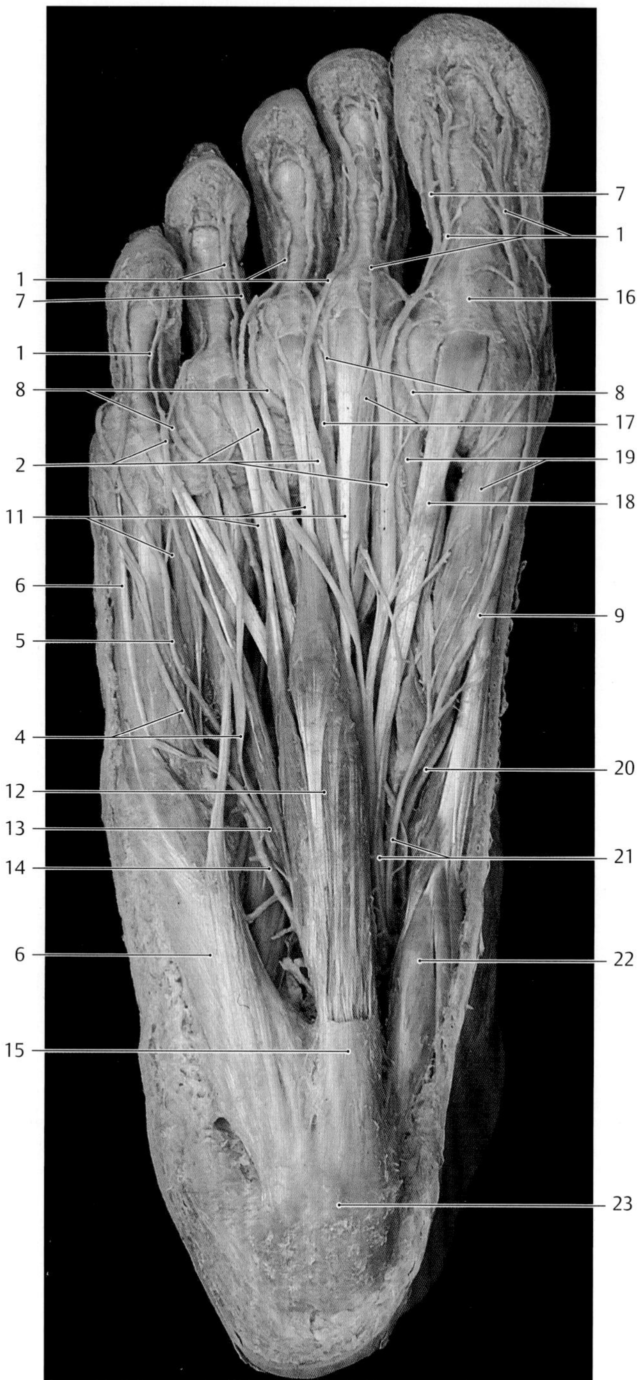


Fig. 4.168 **Sole of the right foot,** middle layer. The plantar aponeurosis has been removed.

1 Proper plantar digital nerves
2 Common plantar digital nerves
3 Plantar aponeurosis
4 Superficial branch of lateral plantar nerve
5 Superficial branch of lateral plantar artery
6 Abductor digiti minimi muscle
7 Proper plantar digital arteries
8 Common plantar digital arteries
9 Digital branch of medial plantar nerve to great toe
10 Medial calcaneal branches
11 Tendons of flexor digitorum brevis muscle
12 Flexor digitorum brevis muscle
13 Superficial branch of lateral plantar nerve
14 Lateral plantar artery
15 Plantar aponeurosis (remnant)
16 Fibrous sheath of toe
17 Lumbrical muscles
18 Tendon of flexor hallucis longus muscle
19 Flexor hallucis brevis muscle
20 Medial plantar artery
21 Medial plantar nerve
22 Abductor hallucis muscle
23 Calcaneal tuberosity

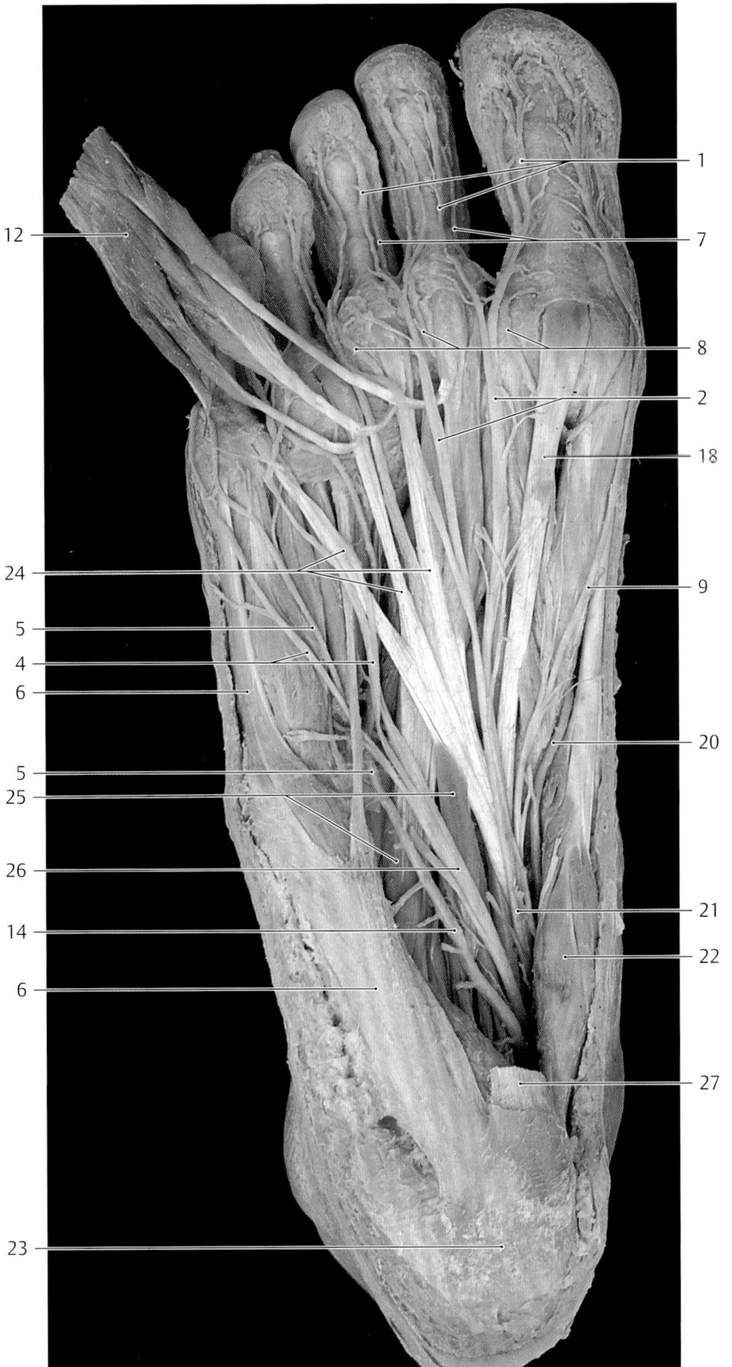


Fig. 4.169 **Sole of the right foot,** middle layer. Dissection of vessels and nerves. The flexor digitorum brevis muscle has been divided and anteriorly reflected.

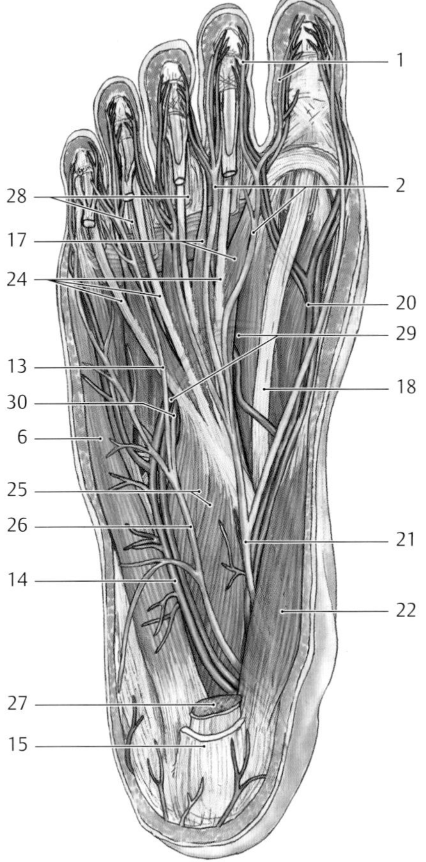


Fig. 4.170 **Sole of the right foot** with vessels and nerves. The flexor digitorum brevis muscle has been removed. Light blue = synovial sheaths of flexor tendons (28).

24 Tendons of flexor digitorum longus muscle
25 Quadratus plantae muscle
26 Lateral plantar nerve
27 Flexor digitorum brevis muscle (cut)
28 Synovial sheaths of tendons of flexor digitorum longus and brevis muscles
29 Plantar arch
30 Deep branch of lateral plantar nerve

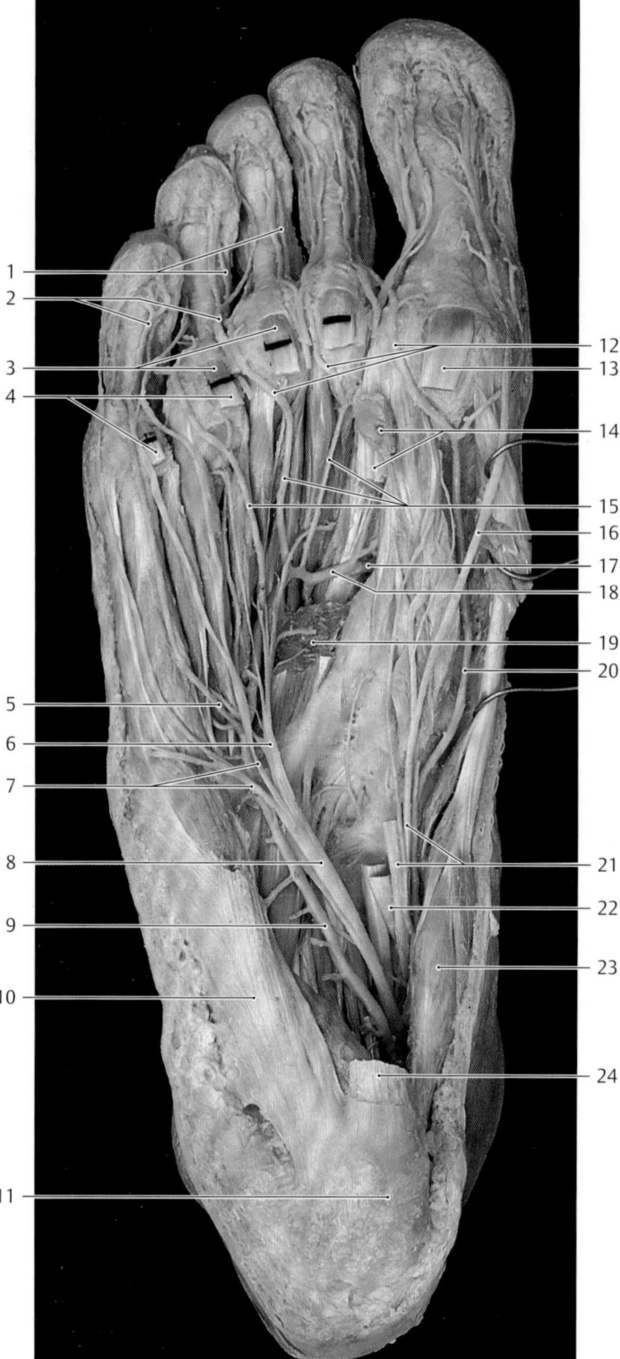


Fig. 4.171 **Sole of the right foot,** deep layer. Dissection of vessels and nerves. The flexor digitorum brevis muscle, the quadratus plantae muscle with the tendons of the flexor digitorum longus muscle, and some branches of the medial plantar nerve have been removed. The flexor hallucis brevis and adductor hallucis muscles have been cut and portions removed to show the somewhat atypical course of the medial plantar artery and deep muscles of the foot.

1 Proper plantar digital arteries
2 Proper plantar digital nerves
3 Tendons of flexor digitorum brevis muscle
4 Tendons of flexor digitorum longus muscle
5 Superficial branch of lateral plantar artery
6 Deep branch of lateral plantar nerve
7 Superficial branch of lateral plantar nerve
8 Lateral plantar nerve
9 Lateral plantar artery
10 Abductor digiti minimi muscle
11 Calcaneal tuberosity
12 Common plantar digital arteries
13 Tendon of flexor hallucis longus muscle
14 Insertion of both heads of adductor hallucis muscle
15 Plantar metatarsal arteries
16 Medial proper plantar digital nerve
17 Deep plantar branch of dorsal metatarsal artery (perforating branch)
18 Plantar arch
19 Oblique head of adductor hallucis muscle (cut)
20 Medial plantar artery
21 Medial plantar nerve
22 Crossing of tendons in the sole of foot (flexor hallucis longus and flexor digitorum longus muscles)
23 Abductor hallucis muscle
24 Origin of flexor hallucis brevis muscle
25 Medial cuneiform and first metatarsal bones
26 Tendon of peroneus longus muscle
27 Abductor hallucis and flexor hallucis brevis muscles
28 Medial plantar artery, vein, and nerve
29 Fourth and fifth metatarsal bones
30 Lateral plantar artery, vein, and nerve
31 Flexor digitorum brevis muscle
32 Plantar aponeurosis

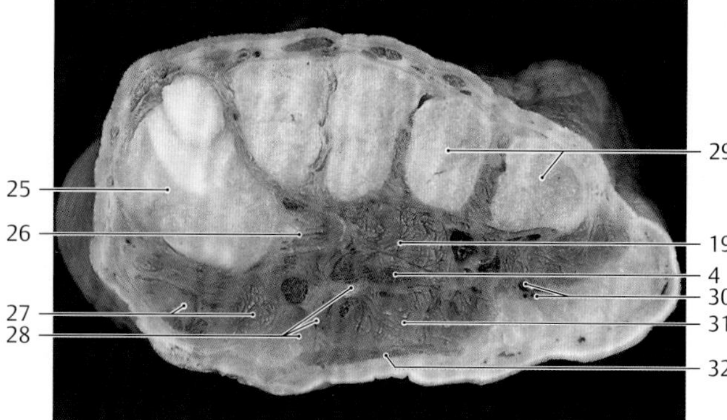


Fig. 4.172 **Cross section through the right foot** at the level of the metatarsal bones (posterior aspect; see corresponding sections in Fig. 4.175).

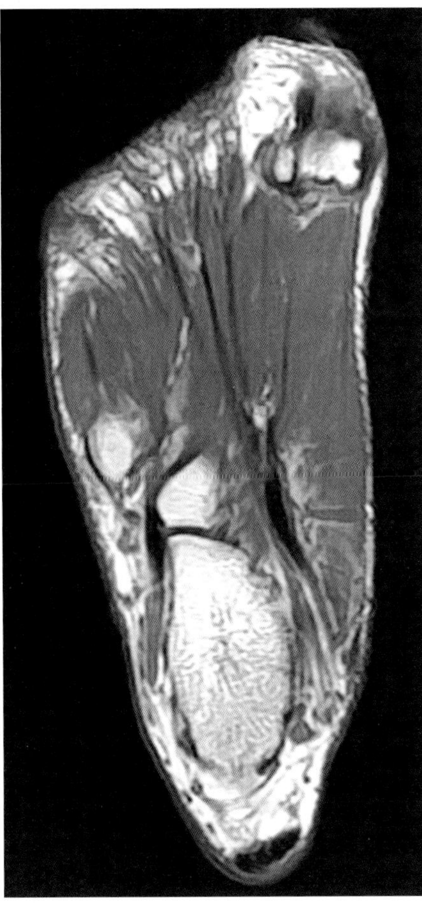

Fig. 4.173 **Sole of the right foot** (MRI scan; see corresponding schematic Fig. 4.174). (Heuck A, et al. MRT-Atlas des muskuloskelettalen Systems. Stuttgart, Germany: Schattauer, 2009.)

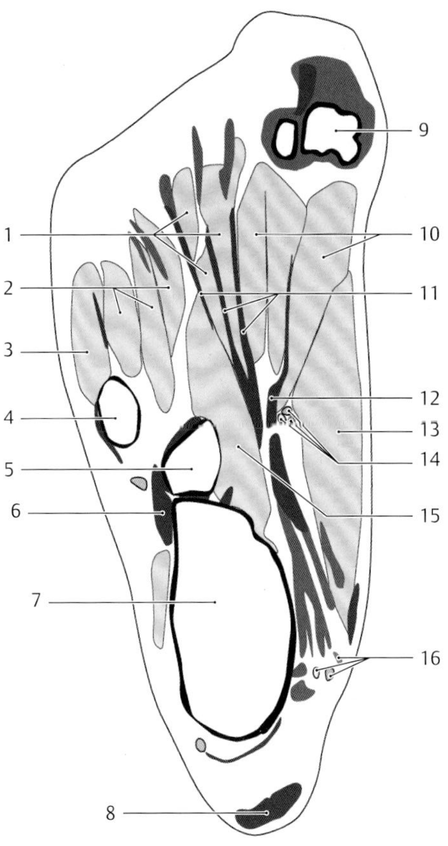


Fig. 4.174 **Sole of the right foot.** (Heuck A, et al. MRT-Atlas des muskuloskelettalen Systems. Stuttgart, Germany: Schattauer, 2009.)

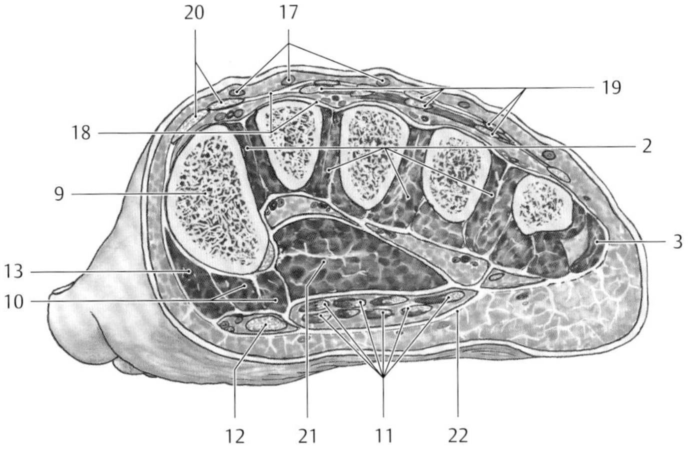


Fig. 4.175 **Cross section through the right foot** at the level of the metatarsal bones (posterior aspect; see corresponding Fig. 4.172).

1 Lumbrical muscles
2 Plantar interossei muscles
3 Abductor digiti minimi muscle
4 Tuberosity of fifth metatarsal bone
5 Cuboid bone
6 Tendon of peroneus longus muscle
7 Calcaneus
8 Calcaneal or Achilles tendon
9 First metatarsal bone
10 Flexor hallucis brevis muscle
11 Tendons of flexor digitorum longus and brevis muscles
12 Tendon of flexor hallucis longus muscle
13 Abductor hallucis muscle
14 Medial plantar artery, vein, and nerve
15 Quadratus plantae muscle
16 Lateral plantar artery, vein, and nerve
17 Dorsal venous network of foot
18 Superficial and deep dorsal fascia of foot
19 Tendons of extensor digitorum longus and brevis muscles
20 Tendons of extensor hallucis longus and brevis muscles
21 Adductor hallucis muscle
22 Plantar aponeurosis

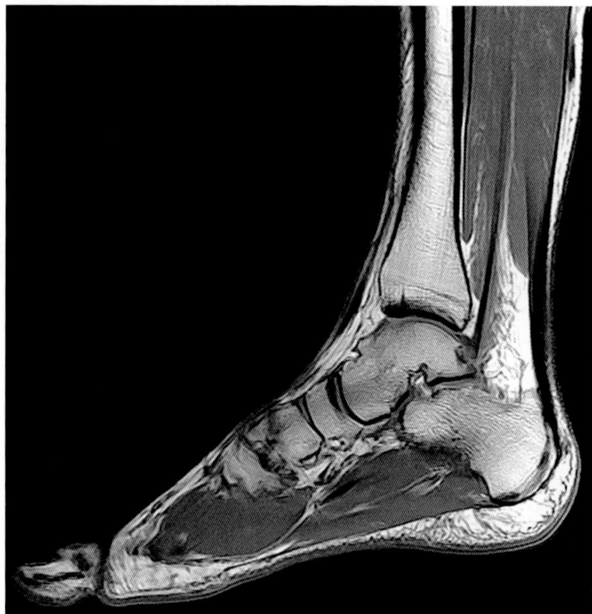

Fig. 4.176 **Sagittal section through the ankle joint and foot** at the level of the first toe (MRI scan; see corresponding schematic Fig. 4.177). (Heuck A, et al. MRT-Atlas des muskuloskelettalen Systems. Stuttgart, Germany: Schattauer, 2009.)

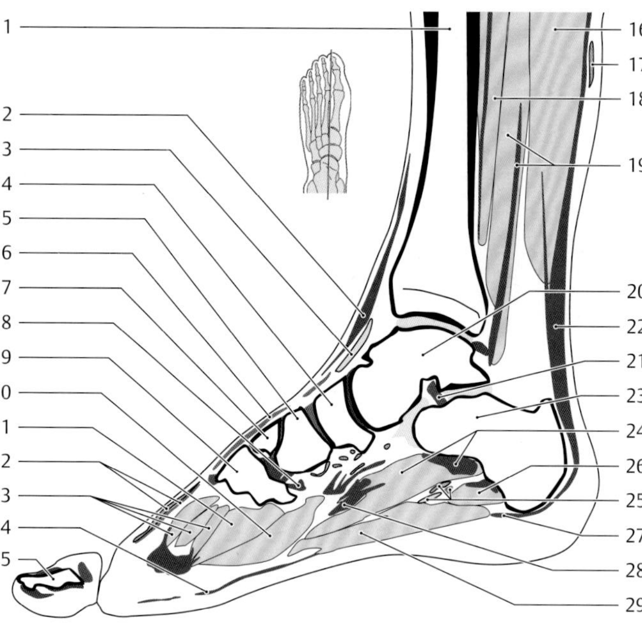


Fig. 4.177 **Sagittal section through the ankle joint and foot** at the level of the first toe. (Heuck A, et al. MRT-Atlas des muskuloskelettalen Systems. Stuttgart, Germany: Schattauer, 2009.)

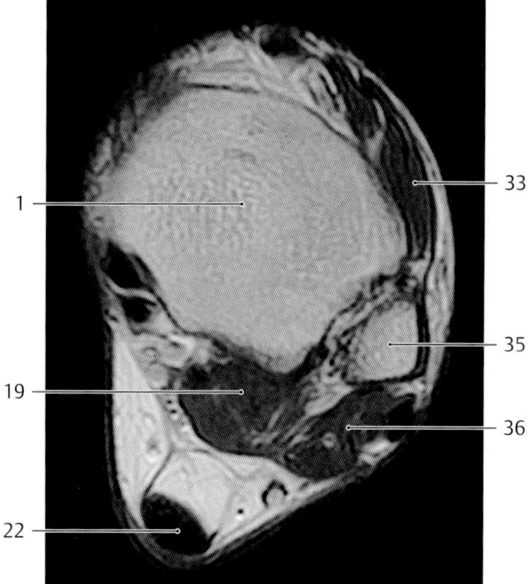


Fig. 4.178 **Cross section through the right leg,** superior to the malleoli (MRI scan). (Heuck A, et al. MRT-Atlas des muskuloskelettalen Systems. Stuttgart, Germany: Schattauer, 2009.)

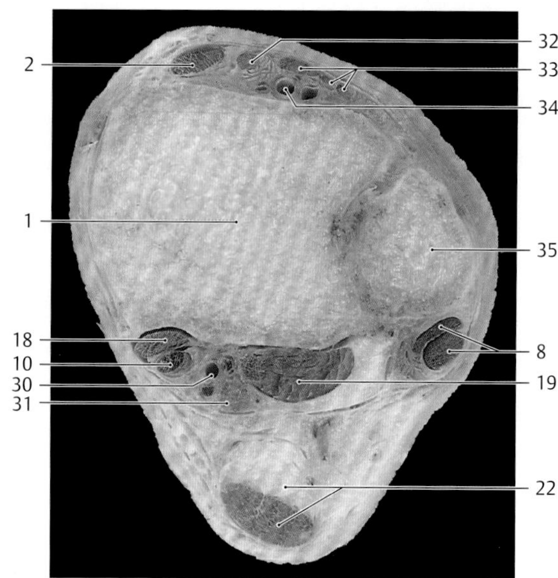


Fig. 4.179 **Cross section through the leg,** superior to the malleoli (inferior aspect).

1 Tibia
2 Tendon of tibialis anterior muscle
3 Deep peroneal nerve
4 Navicular bone
5 Intermediate cuneiform bone
6 Dorsal artery of the foot
7 Medial cuneiform bone
8 Tendon of peroneus longus muscle
9 Base of the first metatarsal bone
10 Flexor digitorum longus muscle
11 Adductor hallucis muscle
12 Dorsal metatarsal artery and vein
13 Interossei muscles
14 Plantar aponeurosis
15 Distal phalanx
16 Sole muscle
17 Small saphenous vein
18 Tibialis posterior muscle
19 Flexor hallucis longus muscle
20 Talus
21 Talocalcaneal interosseous ligament
22 Calcaneal or Achilles tendon
23 Calcaneus
24 Quadratus plantae muscle
25 Lateral plantar artery, vein, and nerve
26 Abductor digiti minimi muscle
27 Plantar aponeurosis
28 Tendon of flexor digitorum longus muscle
29 Flexor digitorum brevis muscle
30 Posterior tibial artery
31 Tibial nerve
32 Tendon of extensor hallucis longus muscle
33 Tendons of extensor digitorum longus muscle
34 Anterior tibial artery
35 Fibula
36 Peroneus brevis muscle

# 5 Thoracic Organs

Internal Organs

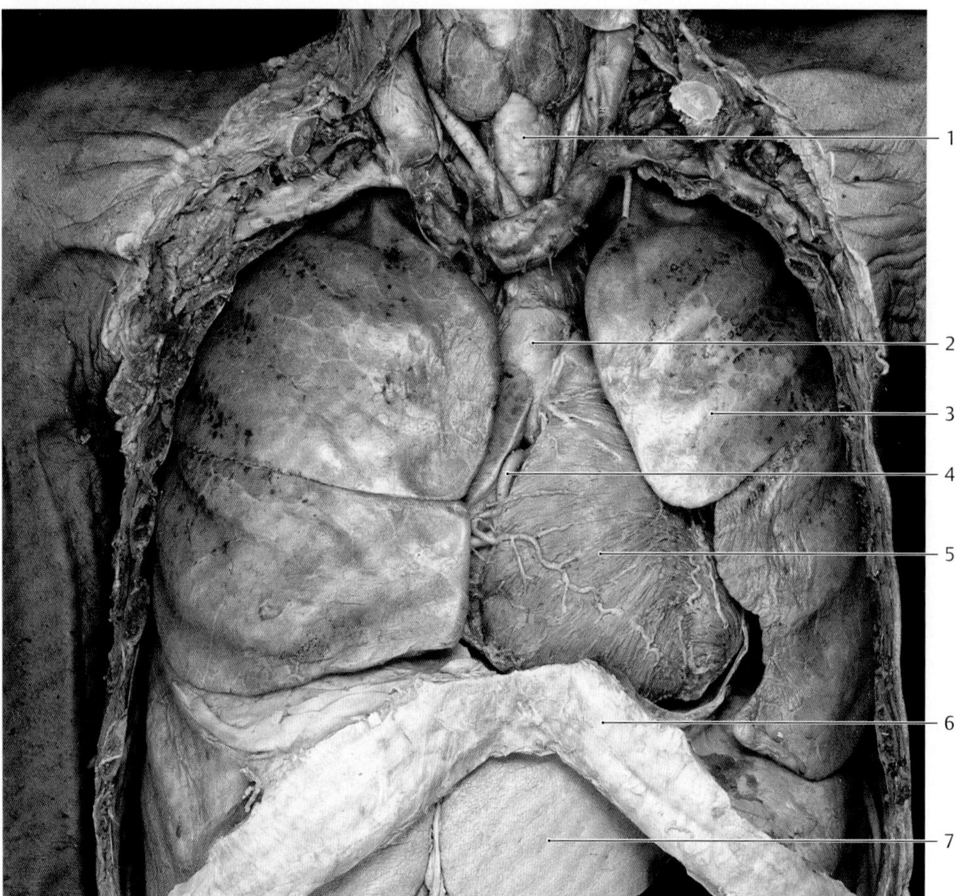


1 Trachea
2 Ascending aorta
3 Upper lobe of left lung
4 Right coronary artery
5 Right ventricle of the heart
6 Costal margin
7 Liver
8 Sternum
9 Right auricle of the heart
10 Middle lobe of right lung
11 Right atrium of the heart
12 Main bronchus
13 Azygos vein
14 Left ventricle of the heart and bulb of aorta
15 Esophagus
16 Descending aorta
17 Spinal cord

Fig. 5.1 **Thoracic organs in situ** (anterior aspect). The anterior thoracic wall has been removed.

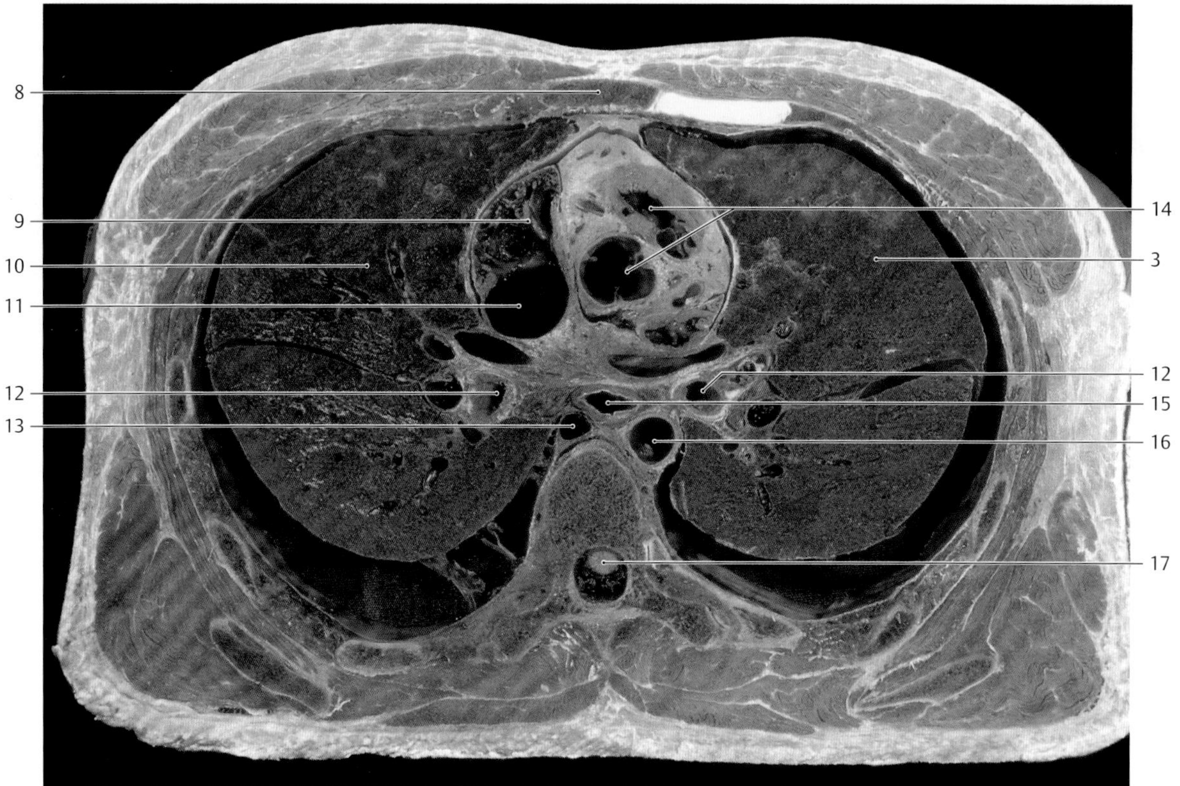


Fig. 5.2 **Horizontal section through the thorax** at the level of the seventh thoracic vertebra (from below).

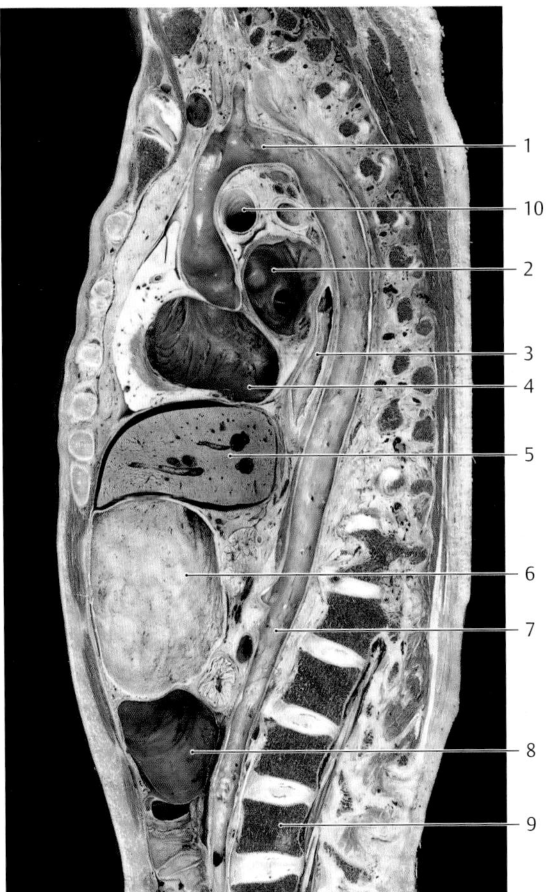


Fig. 5.3 **Sagittal section through the thoracic and abdominal cavities** (parasternal).

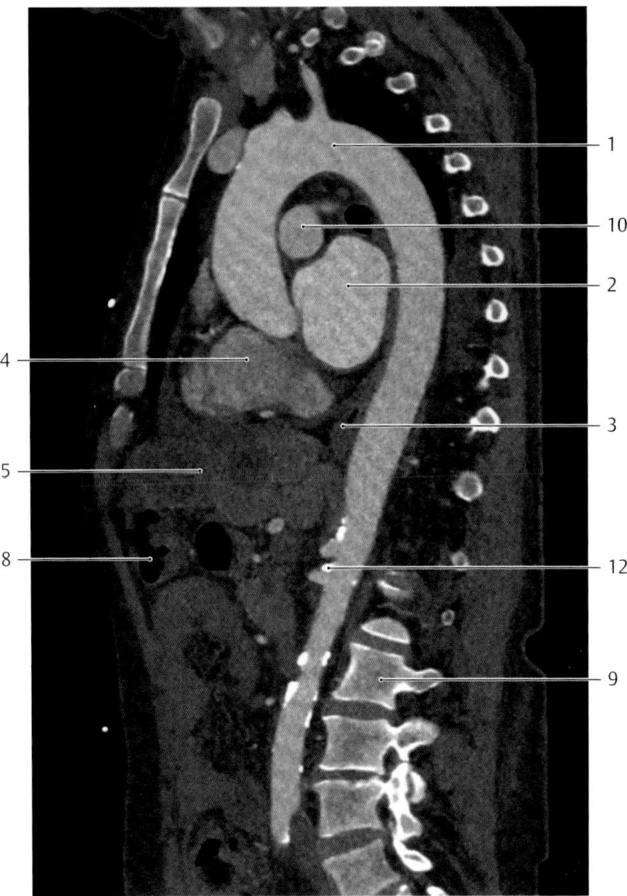


Fig. 5.4 **Sagittal section through the thoracic and abdominal cavities** (parasternal, CT scan). (Courtesy of Prof. Uder, Institute of Radiology, University Hospital Erlangen, Germany.)

1 Aortic arch
2 Left atrium of the heart
3 Esophagus
4 Right atrium of the heart
5 Liver
6 Stomach
7 Abdominal aorta
8 Transverse colon (dilated)
9 Body of lumbar vertebra
10 Pulmonary trunk
11 Right ventricle of the heart
12 Superior mesenteric artery
13 Trachea
14 Remaining parts of thymus gland
15 Ascending aorta
16 Pericardium

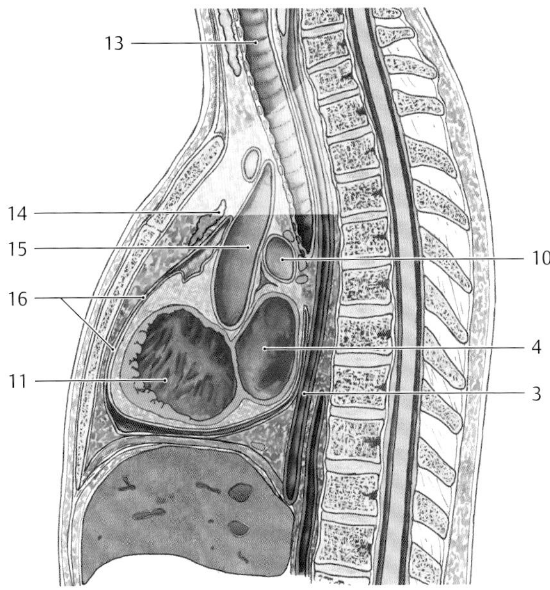


Fig. 5.5 **Sagittal section through the thoracic cavity.** The parts of the mediastinum are indicated by colors (see corresponding table to the right).

| Parts of mediastinum | Content |
|---|---|
| Superior mediastinum (yellow) | Trachea, brachiocephalic veins, thymus, aortic arch, esophagus, thoracic duct |
| Middle mediastinum (blue) | Heart, ascending aorta, pulmonary trunk, pulmonary veins, phrenic nerves |
| Posterior mediastinum (orange) | Esophagus with vagus nerves, descending aorta, thoracic duct, sympathetic trunks |
| Anterior mediastinum (pink) | Smaller vessels and nerves, fat and connective tissue, thymus (only in the child) |

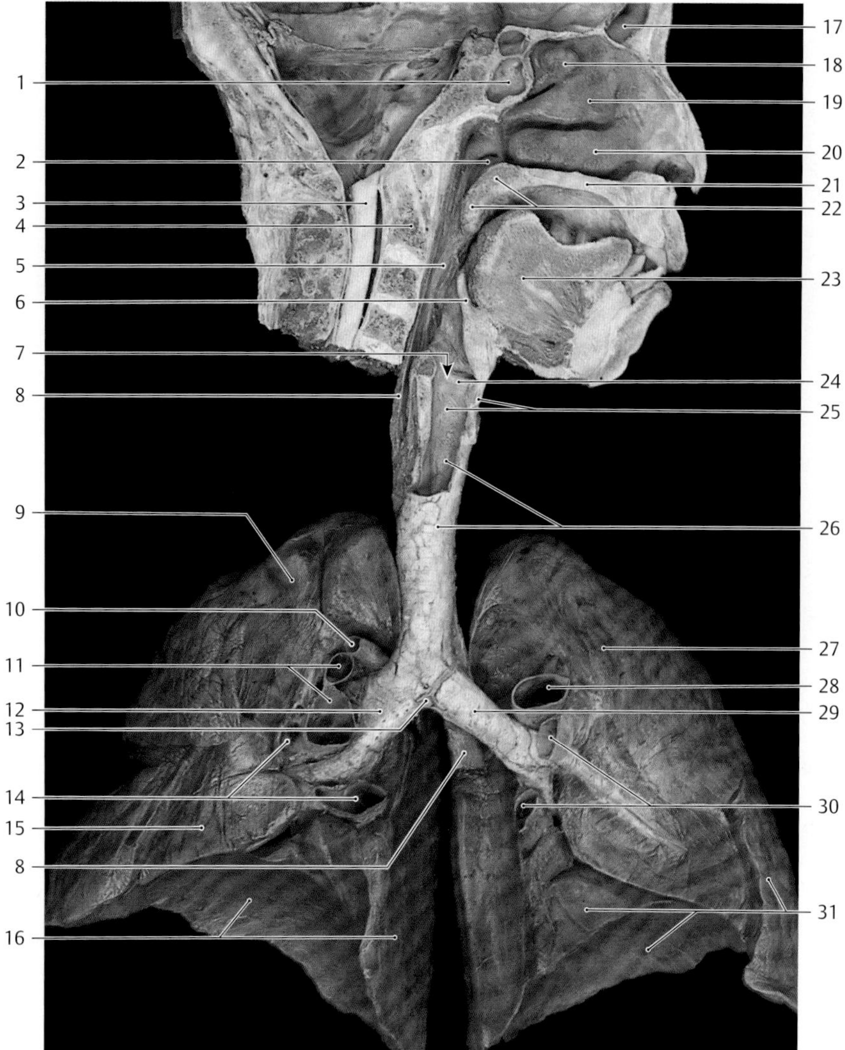


Fig. 5.6 **Respiratory system.** The lungs have been fixed in expiration and turned laterally. The head has been bisected and turned laterally.

1 Sphenoid sinus
2 Pharyngeal opening of auditory tube
3 Spinal cord
4 Dens of axis
5 Oropharynx (oropharyngeal isthmus)
6 Epiglottis
7 Entrance of larynx
8 Esophagus
9 Upper lobe of right lung
10 Azygos vein
11 Branches of pulmonary artery
12 Right main bronchus
13 Bifurcation of trachea
14 Tributaries of right pulmonary veins
15 Middle lobe of right lung
16 Lower lobe of right lung
17 Frontal sinus
18 Superior nasal concha
19 Middle nasal concha
20 Inferior nasal concha
21 Hard palate
22 Soft palate with uvula
23 Tongue
24 Vocal fold
25 Larynx
26 Trachea
27 Upper lobe of left lung
28 Left pulmonary artery
29 Left main bronchus
30 Left pulmonary veins
31 Lower lobe of left lung

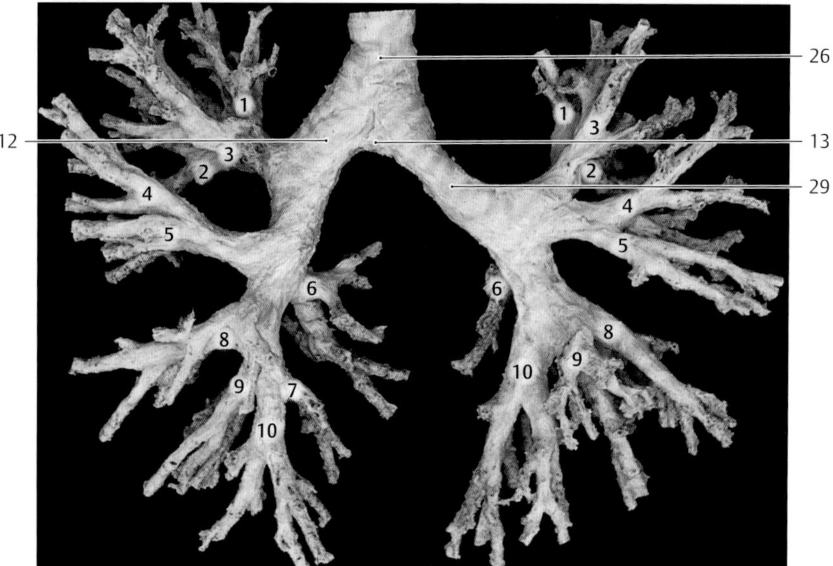


Fig. 5.7 **Bronchial tree** (anterior aspect). The lung tissue has been removed. The bronchopulmonary segments are numbered 1–10.

► **Labels correspond to the figures on page 223:**

1 Nasal cavity
2 Pharynx
3 Larynx (thyroid cartilage)
4 Trachea
5 Upper lobe of right lung
6 Bifurcation of trachea
7 Right main bronchus
8 Horizontal fissure of right lung
9 Middle lobe of right lung
10 Oblique fissures of lungs
11 Lower lobe of right lung
12 Clavicle
13 Upper lobe of left lung
14 Left main bronchus
15 Bronchi supplying broncho-pulmonary segments
16 Lower lobe of left lung
17 Costal margin
18 Hyoid bone
19 Right superior lobar bronchus
20 Right middle lobar bronchus
21 Right inferior lobar bronchus
22 Left superior lobar bronchus
23 Left inferior lobar bronchus
24 Segmental bronchi
25 Branches of pulmonary arteries
26 Branches of pulmonary veins

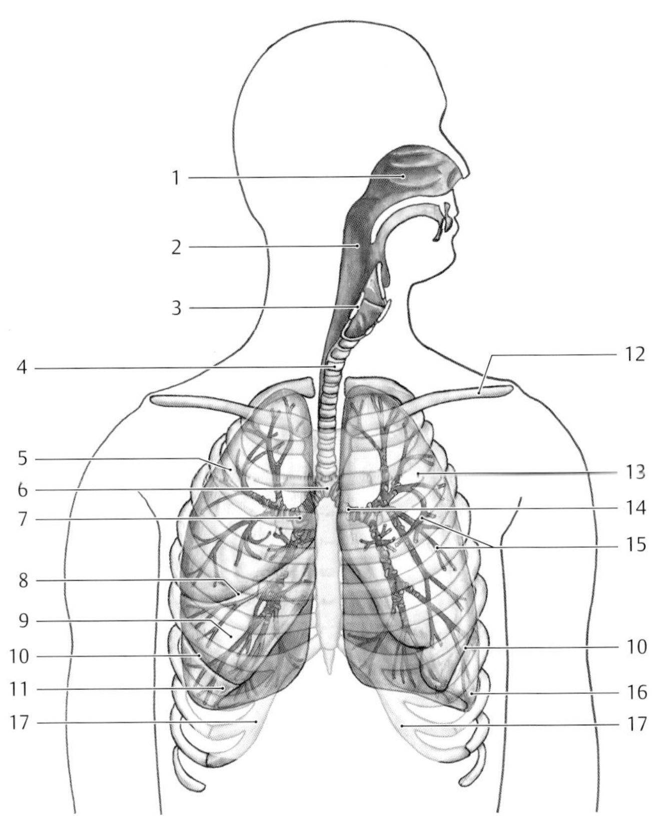


Fig. 5.8 **Organization and positions of the respiratory organs** (anterior aspect).

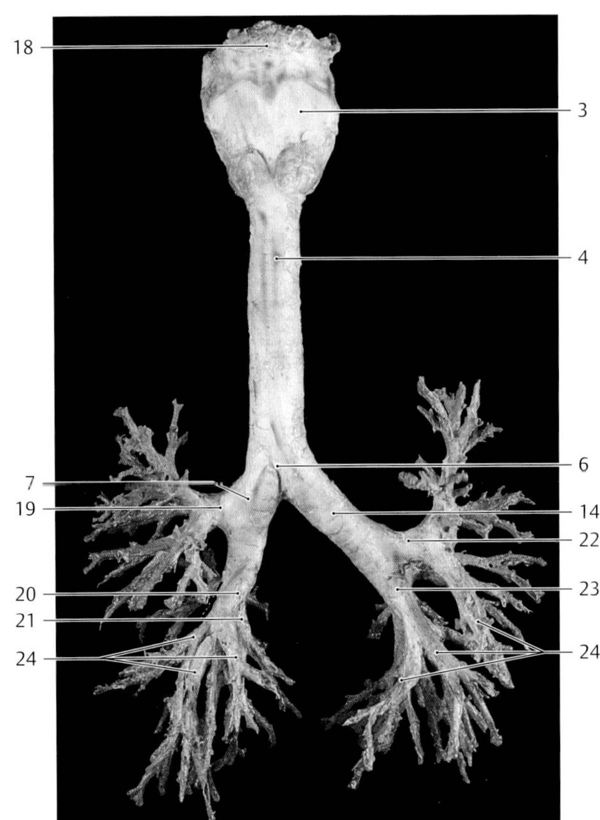


Fig. 5.9 **Larynx, trachea, and bronchial tree** (anterior aspect).

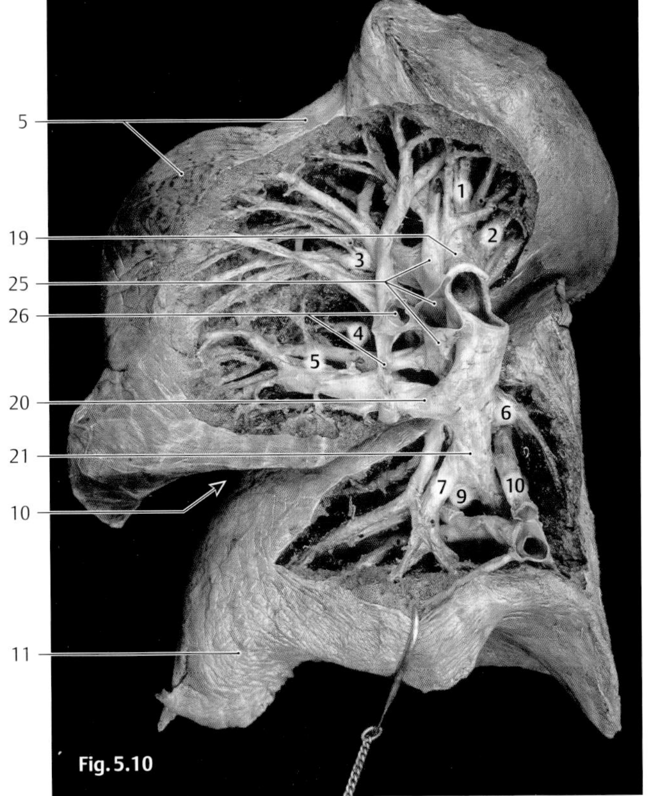


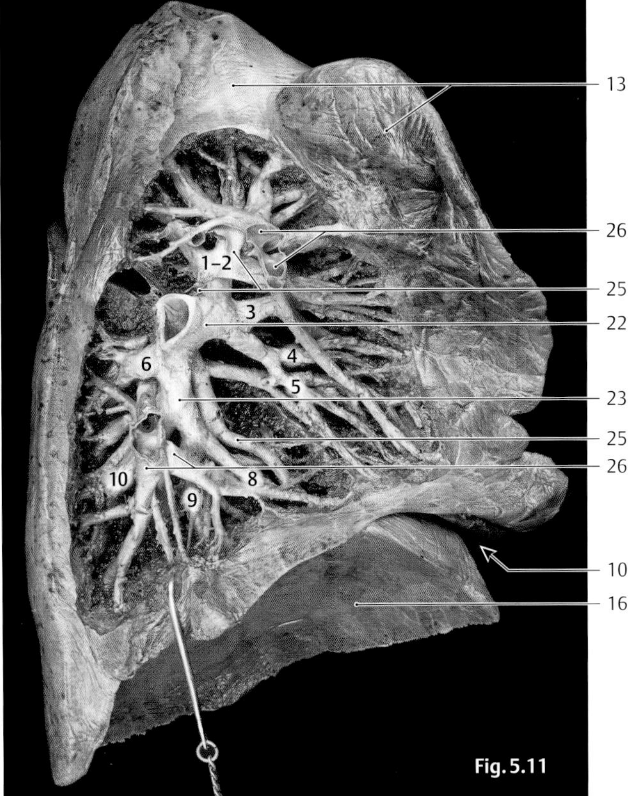


Figs. 5.10 and 5.11 **Mediastinal dissection of the bronchial tree, pulmonary veins, and pulmonary arteries** of right lung (Fig. 5.10) and left lung (Fig. 5.11) (medial aspect). The bronchopulmonary segments are numbered 1–10.

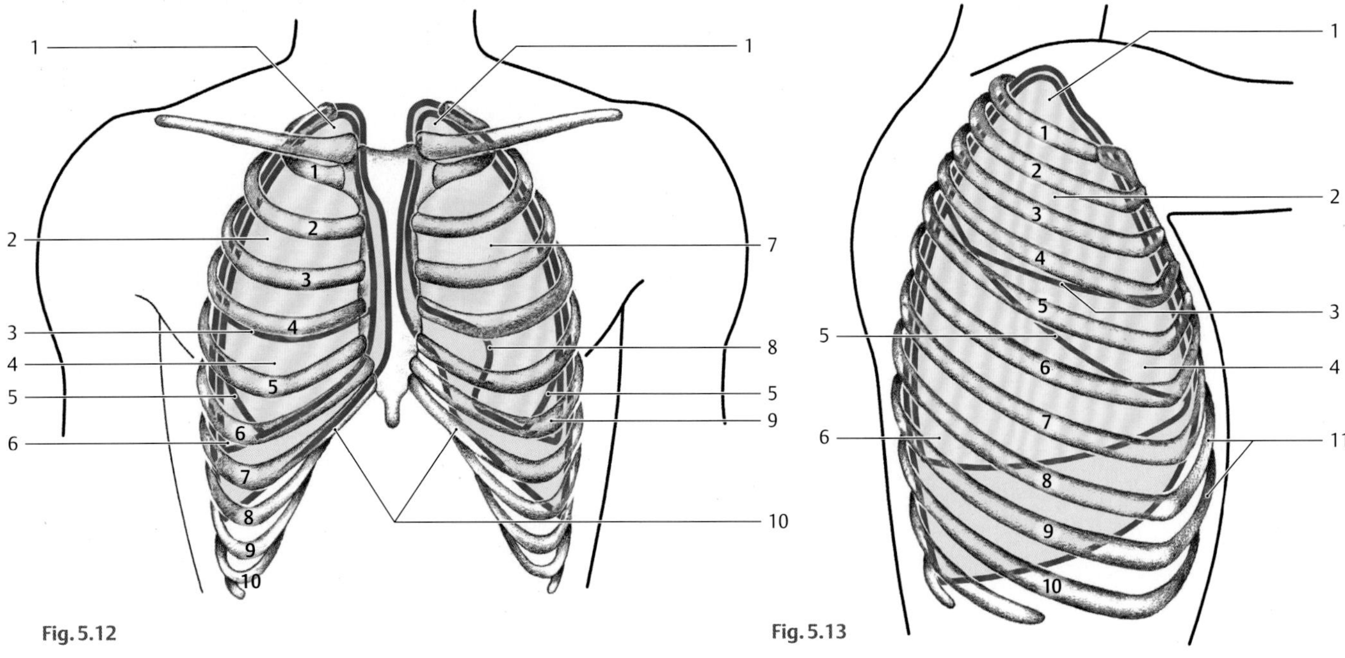


Fig. 5.12

Fig. 5.13

**Figs. 5.12 and 5.13 Surface projections of lungs and pleura on the thoracic wall** (anterior aspect [Fig. 5.12] and right-lateral aspect [Fig. 5.13]). Red = margins of the lung; blue = margins of pleura. The numbers indicate the ribs.

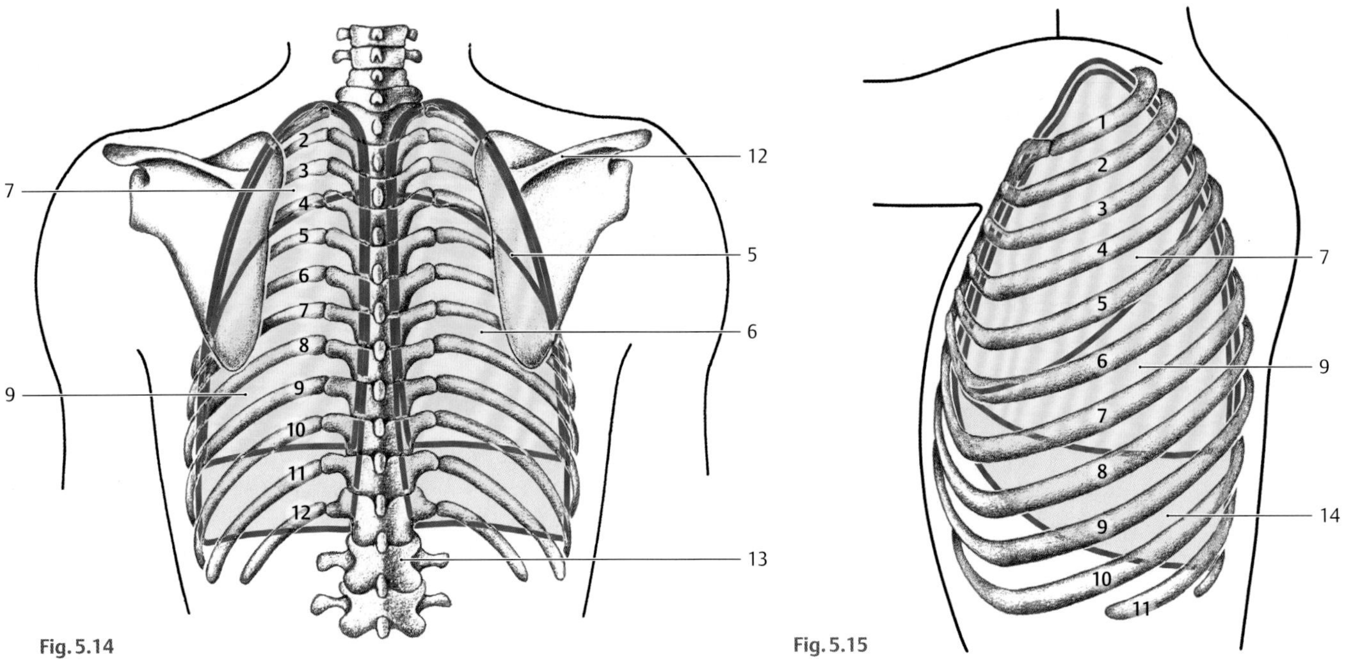


Fig. 5.14

Fig. 5.15

**Figs. 5.14 and 5.15 Surface projections of lungs and pleura on the thoracic wall** (posterior aspect [Fig. 5.14] and left-lateral aspect [Fig. 5.15]). Red = margins of lung; blue = margins of pleura. The numbers indicate the ribs.

1 Apex of lung
2 Upper lobe of right lung
3 Horizontal fissure of right lung
4 Middle lobe of right lung
5 Oblique fissures of lungs
6 Lower lobe of right lung
7 Upper lobe of left lung
8 Cardiac notch of left lung
9 Lower lobe of left lung
10 Infrasternal angle
11 Costal margin
12 Spine of scapula
13 First lumbar vertebra
14 Space between border of lung and pleura (costodiaphragmatic recess)

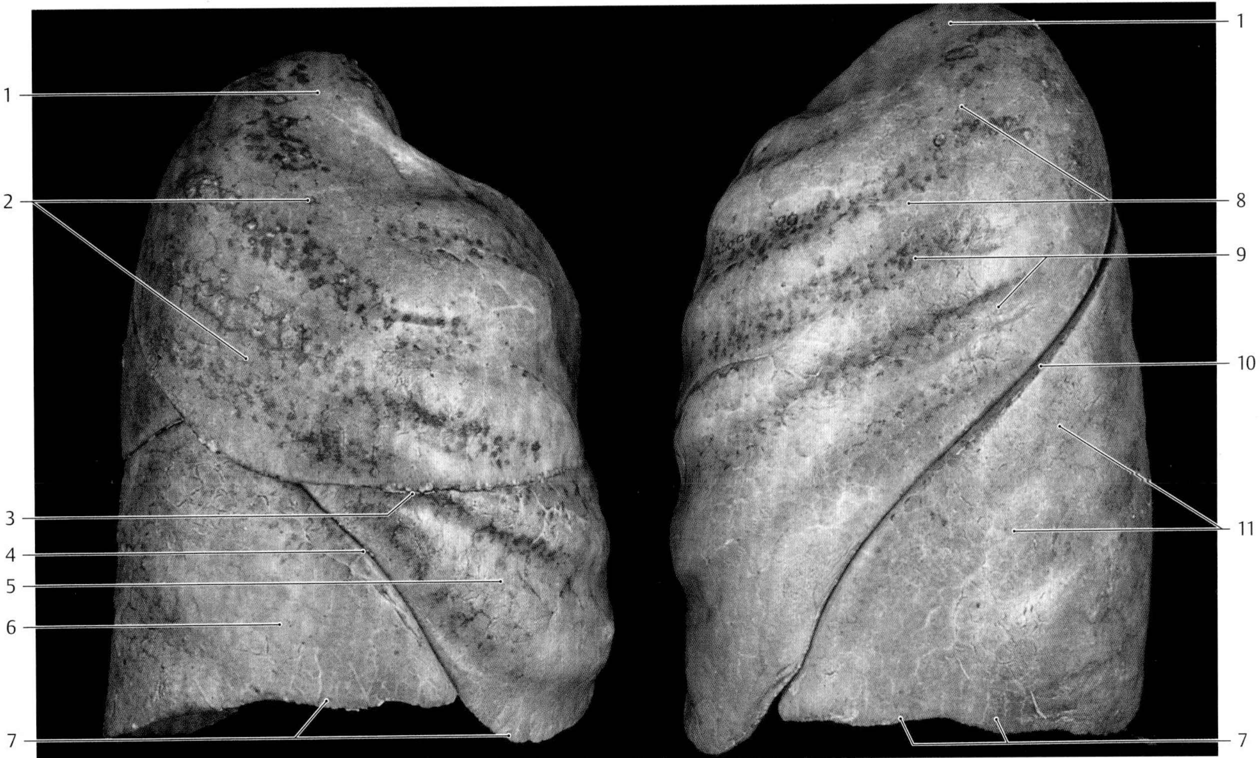


Fig. 5.16 **Right lung** (lateral aspect).

**Left lung** (lateral aspect).

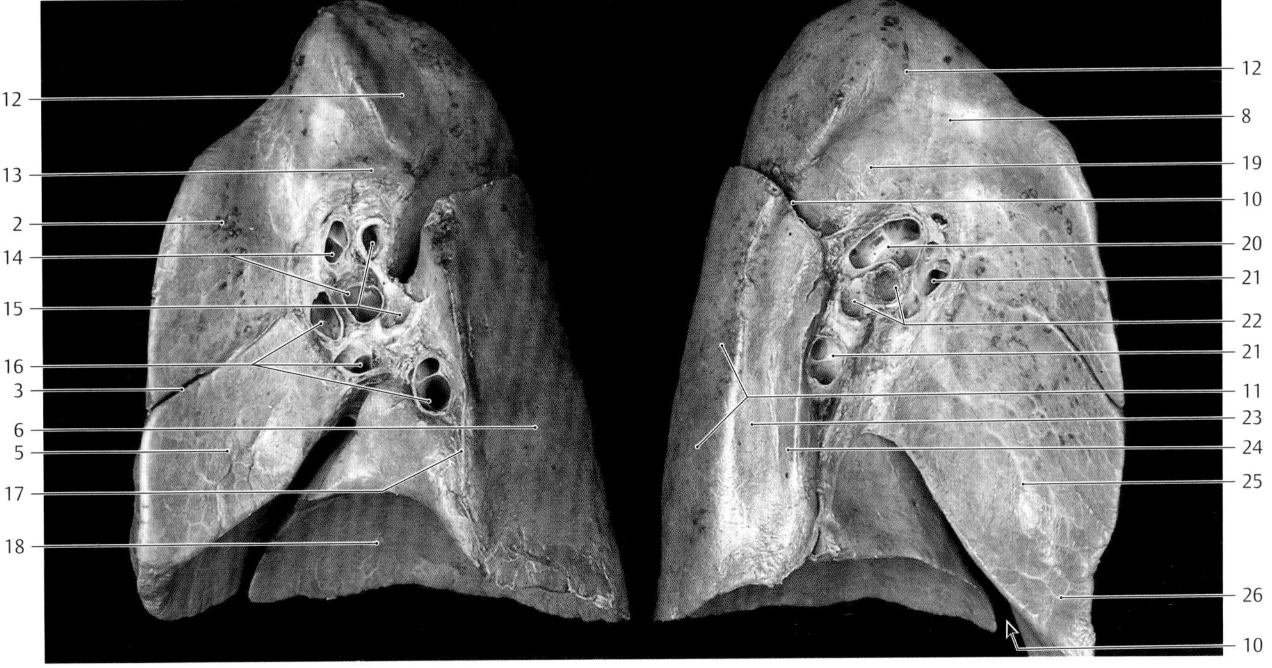


Fig. 5.17 **Right lung** (medial aspect).

**Left lung** (medial aspect).

1 Apex of lung
2 Upper lobe of right lung
3 Horizontal fissure of right lung
4 Oblique fissure of right lung
5 Middle lobe } of right lung
6 Lower lobe } of right lung
7 Inferior border
8 Upper lobe of left lung
9 Impressions of ribs
10 Oblique fissure of left lung
11 Lower lobe of left lung
12 Groove of subclavian artery
13 Groove of azygos arch
14 Branches of right pulmonary artery
15 Bronchi
16 Right pulmonary veins
17 Pulmonary ligament
18 Diaphragmatic surface
19 Groove of aortic arch
20 Left pulmonary artery
21 Branches of left pulmonary veins
22 Left secondary bronchi
23 Groove of thoracic aorta
24 Groove of esophagus
25 Cardiac impression
26 Lingula

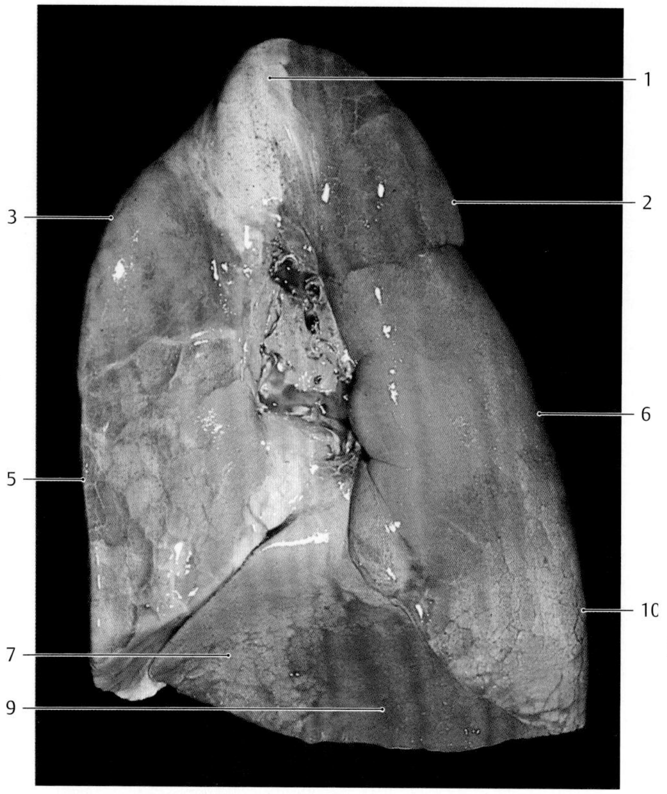

Fig. 5.18 **Right lung** (medial aspect).

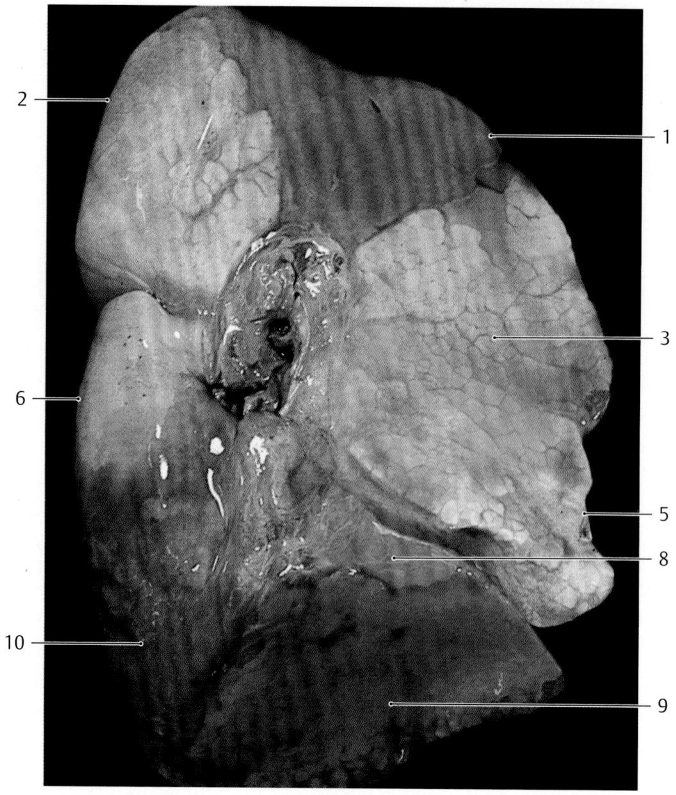

Fig. 5.19 **Left lung** (medial aspect).

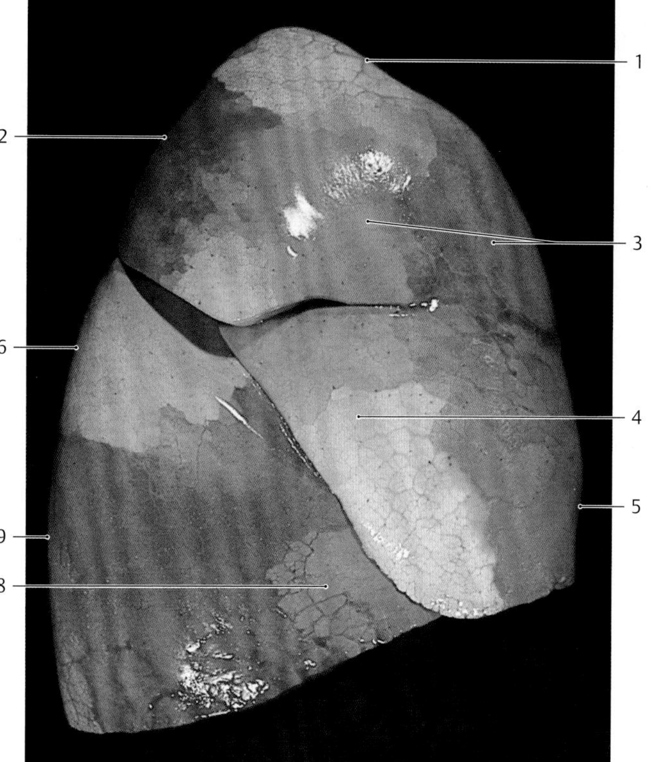


Fig. 5.20 **Right lung** (lateral aspect).

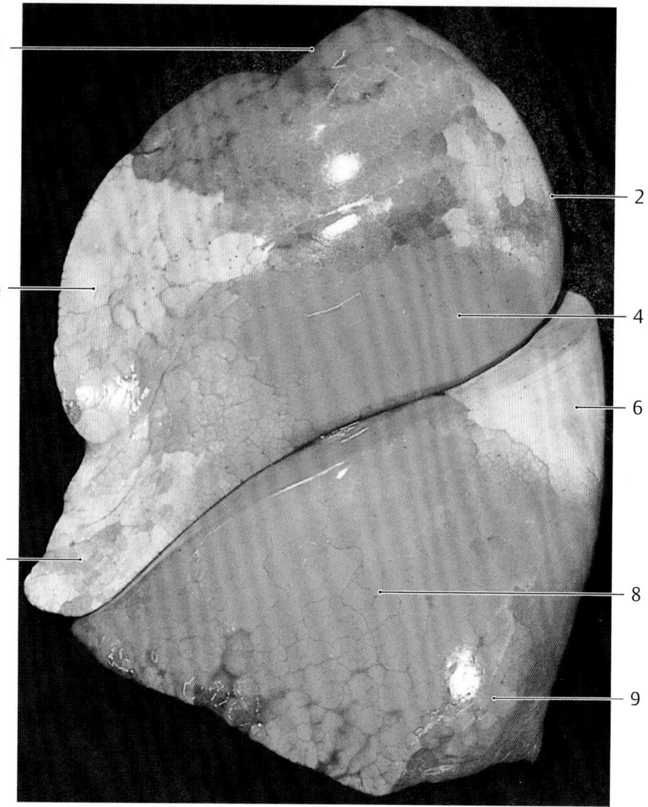


Fig. 5.21 **Left lung** (lateral aspect).

The bronchopulmonary segments of the lungs are differentiated by the various colors. Notice that there is no segment in the left lung that corresponds to the seventh segment of the right lung. (See corresponding schematic Fig. 5.22 on next page.)

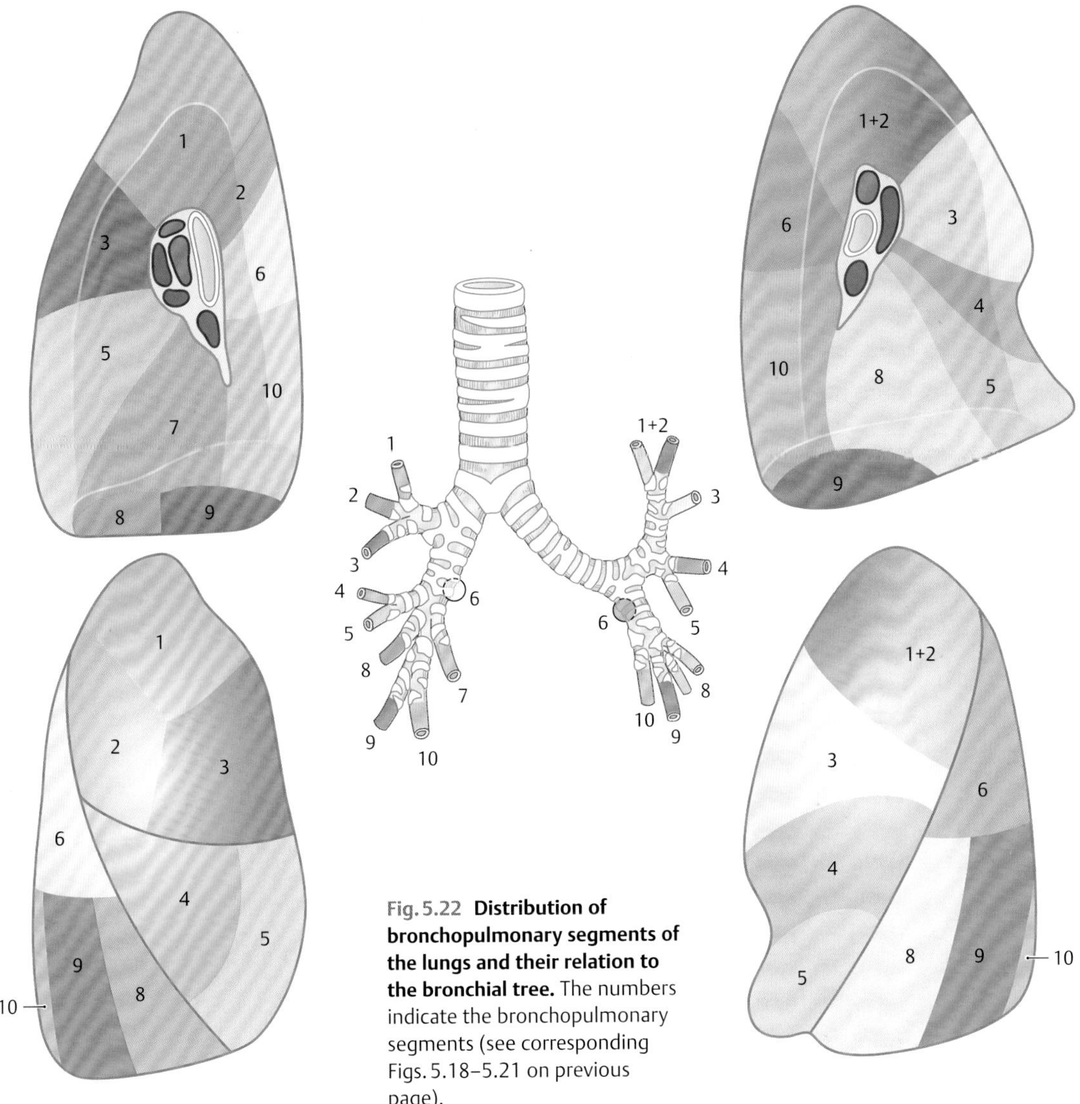


**Fig. 5.22 Distribution of bronchopulmonary segments of the lungs and their relation to the bronchial tree.** The numbers indicate the bronchopulmonary segments (see corresponding Figs. 5.18–5.21 on previous page).

The bronchopulmonary segments are morphologically and functionally separate, independent respiratory units of the lung tissue. Each segment is surrounded by connective tissue that is continuous with the visceral pleura. The segmental bronchi are centrally located in each segment and are closely accompanied by branches of the pulmonary arteries, whereas the tributaries of the pulmonary veins run **between** the segments. Thus, the veins serve two adjacent segments that drain for the most part into more than one vein. A bronchopulmonary segment is therefore not a complete vascular unit, but segmentation is the result of a specific architecture of the lung vasculature.

| Right Lung | | | Left Lung | | | |
|---|---|---|---|---|---|---|
| 1 | Apical segment | Superior lobar bronchus | 1+2 | Apicoposterior segment | Superior division | Superior lobar bronchus |
| 2 | Posterior segment | | | | | |
| 3 | Anterior segment | | 3 | Anterior segment | | |
| 4 | Lateral segment | Middle lobar bronchus | 4 | Superior lingular segment | Inferior division | |
| 5 | Medial segment | | 5 | Inferior lingular segment | | |
| 6 | Superior (apical) segment | Inferior lobar bronchus | 6 | Superior (apical) segment | Inferior lobar bronchus | |
| 7 | Medial basal segment | | 7 | Absent | | |
| 8 | Anterior basal segment | | 8 | Anteromedial basal segment | | |
| 9 | Lateral basal segment | | 9 | Lateral basal segment | | |
| 10 | Posterior basal segment | | 10 | Posterior basal segment | | |

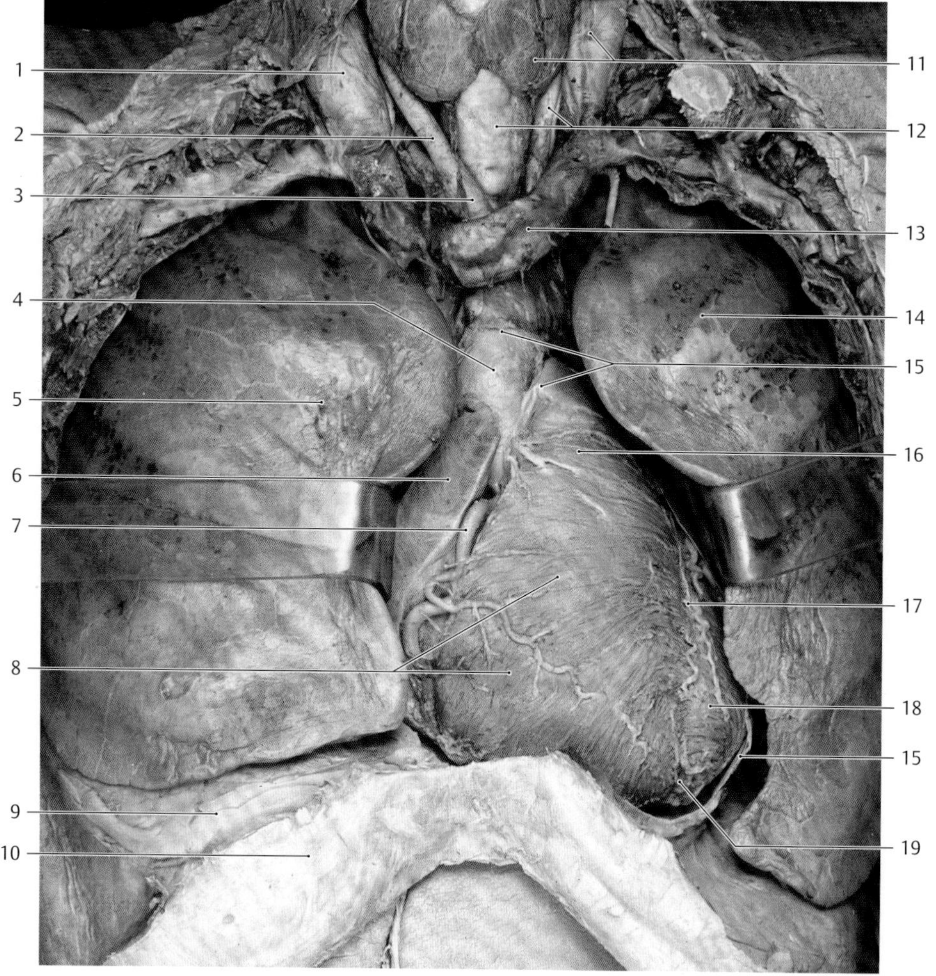


1 Internal jugular vein
2 Common carotid artery
3 Brachiocephalic trunk
4 Ascending aorta
5 Right lung
6 Right auricle
7 Right coronary artery
8 Myocardium of right ventricle
9 Diaphragm
10 Costal margin
11 Thyroid gland and internal jugular vein
12 Trachea and left common carotid artery
13 Left brachiocephalic vein
14 Left lung
15 Pericardium (cut edge)
16 Pulmonary trunk
17 Anterior interventricular artery
18 Myocardium of left ventricle
19 Apex of the heart

Fig. 5.23 **Heart and related vessels in situ** (anterior aspect). Myocardium and coronary arteries are displayed.

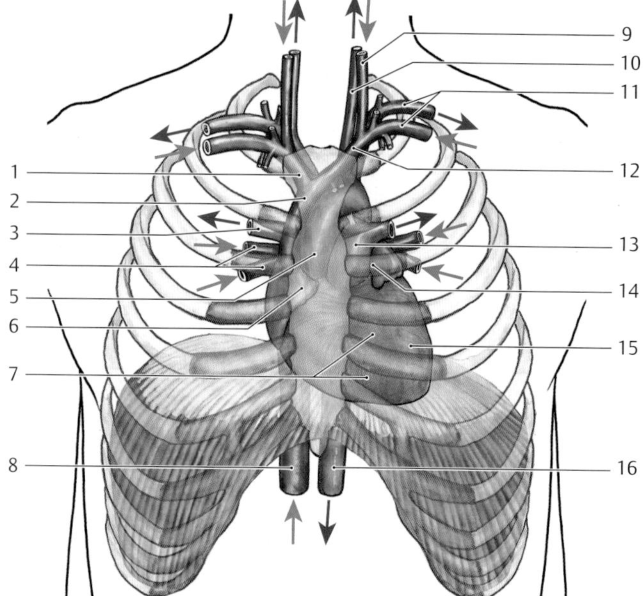


1 Right brachiocephalic vein
2 Superior vena cava
3 Right pulmonary artery
4 Right pulmonary veins
5 Ascending aorta
6 Right atrium
7 Right ventricle
8 Inferior vena cava
9 Left internal jugular vein
10 Left common carotid artery
11 Left axillary artery and vein
12 Left brachiocephalic vein
13 Pulmonary trunk
14 Left atrium
15 Left ventricle
16 Descending aorta

Fig. 5.24 **Position of heart and related vessels in the thoracic cavity** (anterior aspect). Blue = regions of heart and vessels with venous blood flow; red = regions of heart and vessels with arterial blood flow; blue arrows = veins; red arrows = arteries.

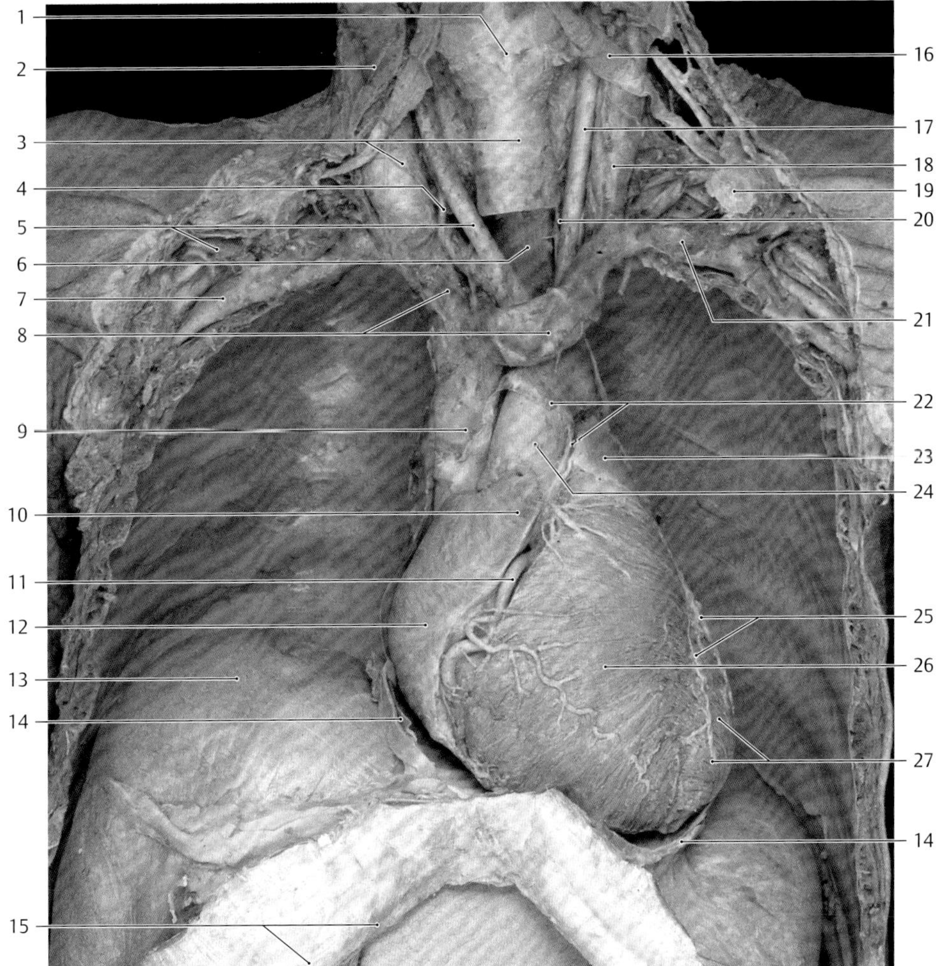


Fig. 5.25 **Heart and related vessels in situ** (anterior aspect). The anterior thoracic wall, pericardium, and epicardium have been removed and the trachea has been divided.

1 Larynx (thyroid cartilage)
2 Sternocleidomastoid muscle (divided)
3 Trachea (divided) and right internal jugular vein
4 Vagus nerve
5 Right common carotid artery and cephalic vein
6 Esophagus
7 Right axillary vein
8 Right and left brachiocephalic veins
9 Superior vena cava
10 Right auricle
11 Right coronary artery
12 Right atrium
13 Diaphragm
14 Pericardium (cut edges)
15 Costal margin
16 Omohyoid muscle
17 Left common carotid artery
18 Left internal jugular vein
19 Clavicle (divided)
20 Left recurrent laryngeal nerve
21 Subclavian vein
22 Pericardial reflection
23 Pulmonary trunk
24 Ascending aorta
25 Anterior interventricular sulcus and anterior interventricular branch of left coronary artery
26 Right ventricle
27 Left ventricle
28 Aortic valve
29 Tricuspid or right atrioventricular valve
30 Inferior vena cava
31 Pulmonary veins
32 Pulmonary valve
33 Left atrioventricular (bicuspid or mitral) valve

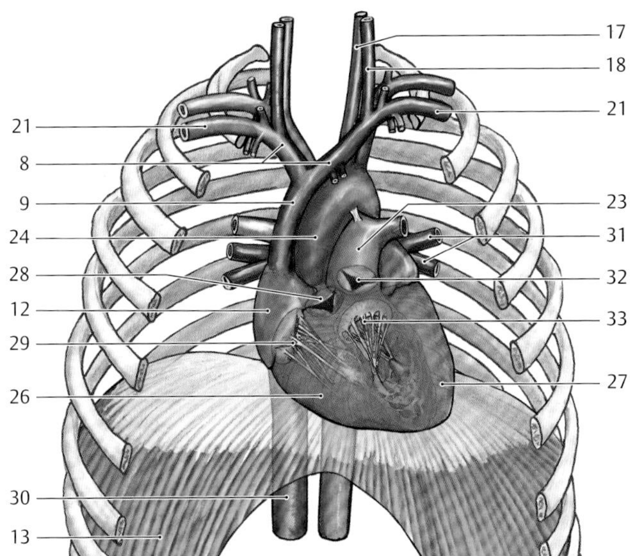


Fig. 5.26 **Heart and related vessels in situ** (anterior aspect). Position of the valves.

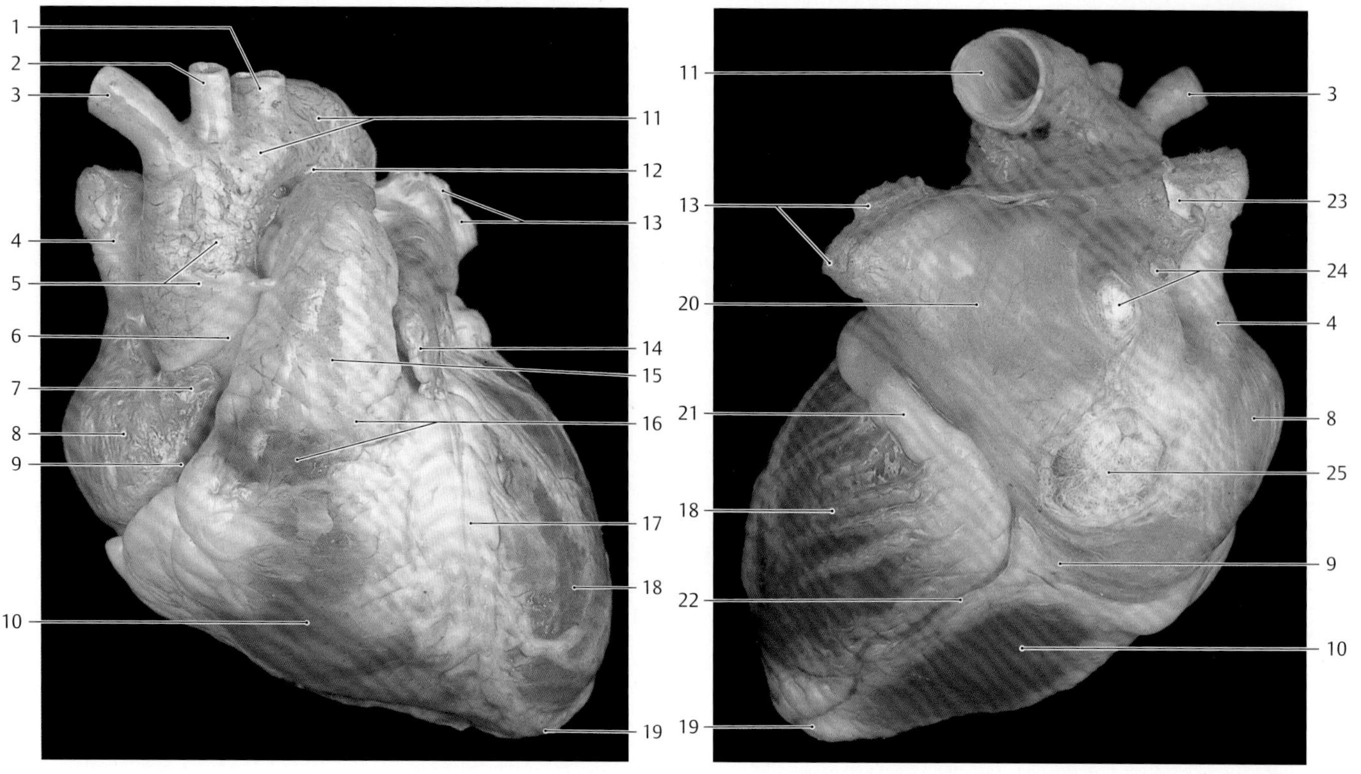

Fig. 5.27 **Heart** of 30-year-old woman (anterior aspect).

Fig. 5.28 **Heart** of 30-year-old woman (oblique-posterior aspect).

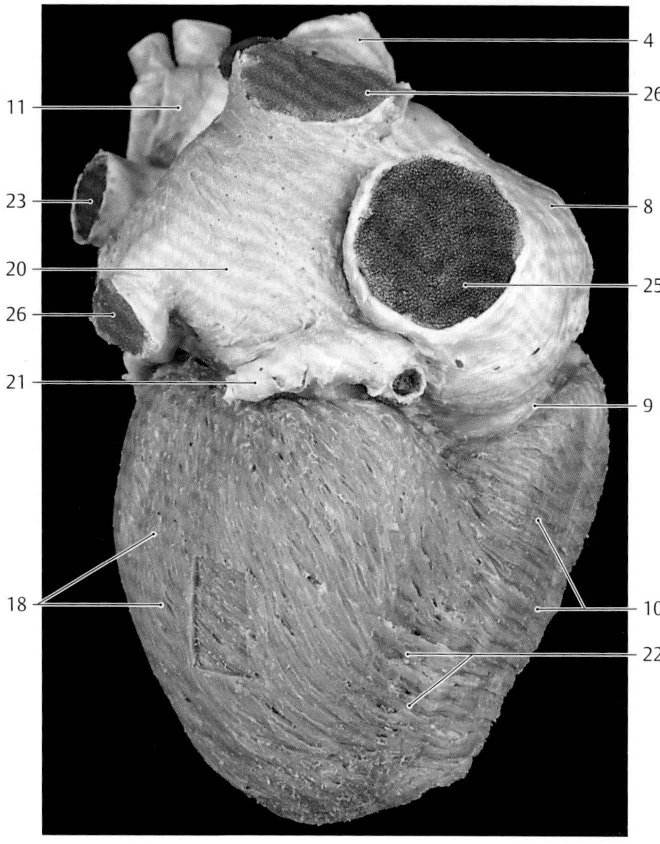

Fig. 5.29 **Heart** (posterior aspect). The myocardium of the left ventricle has been fenestrated to show the muscle fiber bundles of the deeper layer with their more circular course.

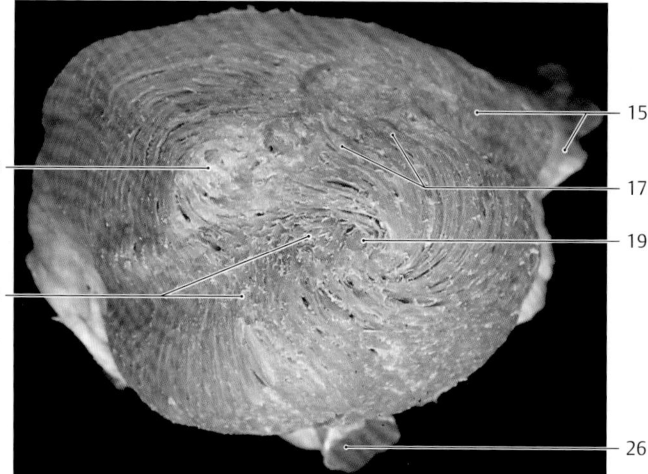

Fig. 5.30 **Vortex of cardiac muscle fibers** (inferior aspect).

1 Left subclavian artery
2 Left common carotid artery
3 Brachiocephalic trunk
4 Superior vena cava
5 Ascending aorta
6 Bulb of the aorta
7 Right auricle
8 Right atrium
9 Coronary sulcus
10 Right ventricle
11 Aortic arch
12 Ligamentum arteriosum
13 Left pulmonary veins
14 Left auricle
15 Pulmonary trunk
16 Sinus of pulmonary trunk
17 Anterior interventricular sulcus
18 Left ventricle
19 Apex of the heart
20 Left atrium
21 Epicardial fat overlying coronary sinus
22 Posterior interventricular sulcus
23 Pulmonary artery
24 Right pulmonary veins
25 Inferior vena cava
26 Pulmonary veins

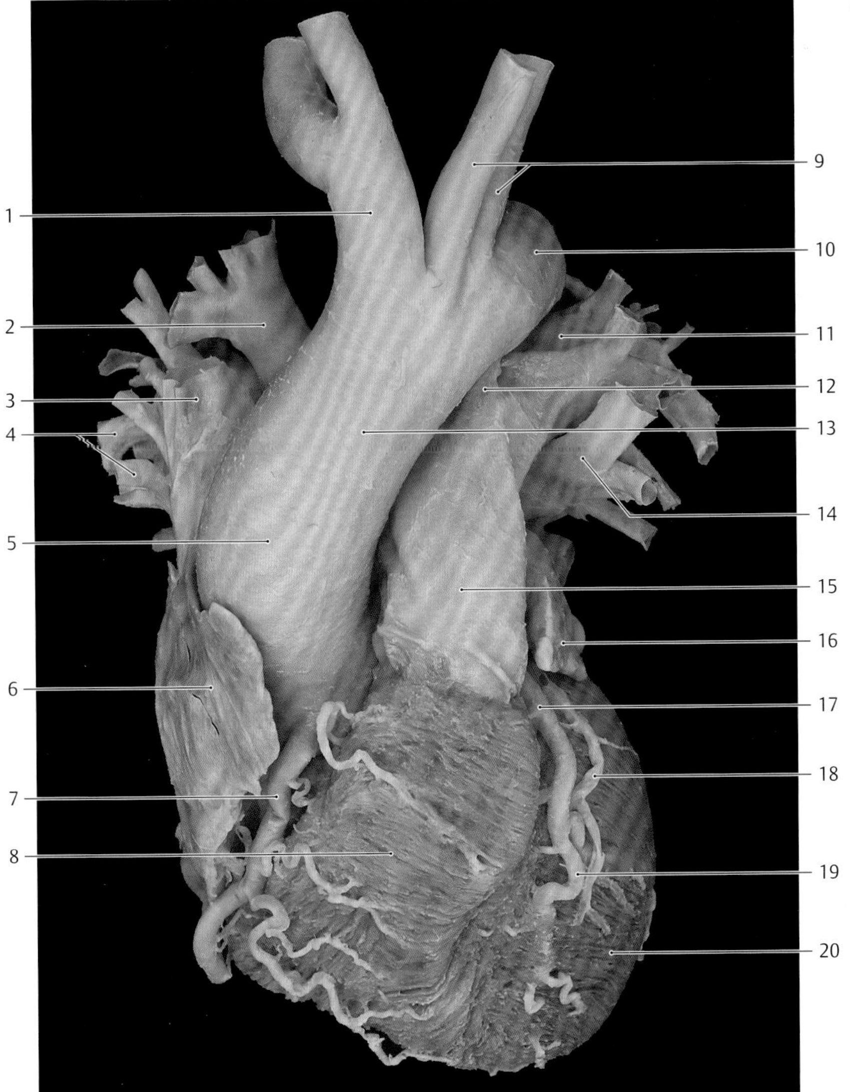


Fig. 5.31 **Heart with coronary arteries** (anterior aspect, systolic phase of heart action).

1 Brachiocephalic trunk
2 Right pulmonary artery
3 Superior vena cava
4 Right pulmonary veins
5 Ascending aorta
6 Right atrium
7 Right coronary artery
8 Right ventricle
9 Left common carotid artery and left subclavian artery
10 Descending aorta (thoracic part)
11 Ligamentum arteriosum (remnant of ductus arteriosus Botalli)
12 Left pulmonary artery
13 Aortic arch
14 Left pulmonary veins
15 Pulmonary trunk
16 Left atrium
17 Left coronary artery
18 Diagonal branch of anterior interventricular vein
19 Interventricular branch of left coronary artery
20 Left ventricle
21 Left brachiocephalic vein
22 Thoracic wall
23 Liver
24 Aortic valve
25 Chordae tendineae
26 Papillary muscles
27 Stomach

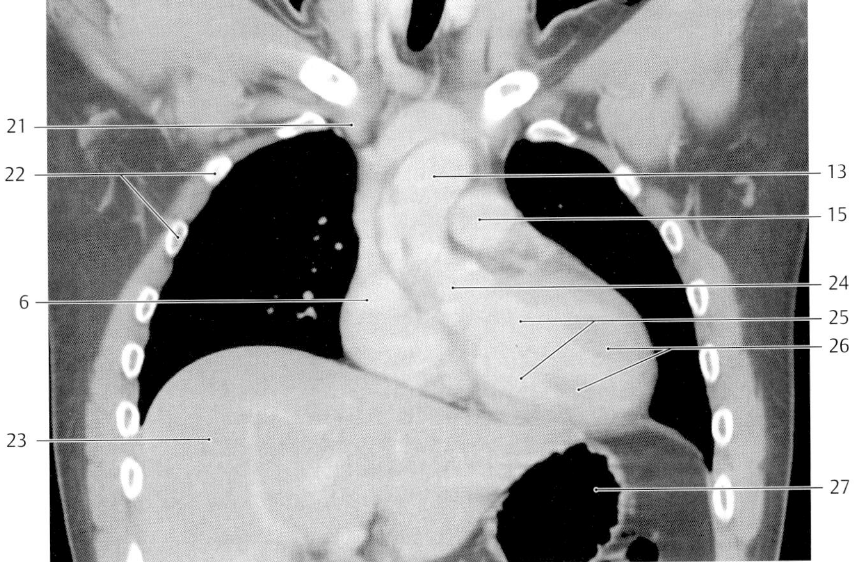


Fig. 5.32 **Coronal section through the thorax** at the level of the ascending aorta (CT scan). (Courtesy of Prof. Uder, Institute of Radiology, University Hospital Erlangen, Germany.)

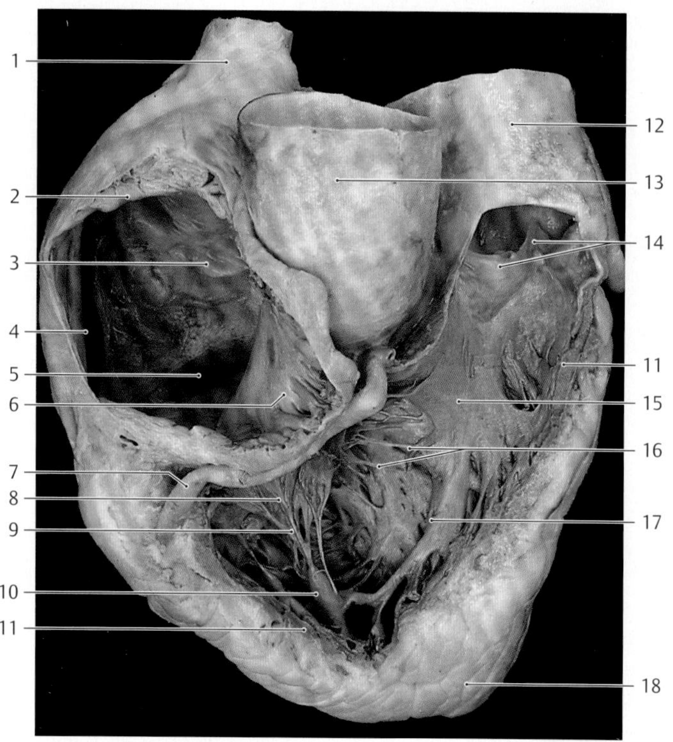


Fig. 5.33 **Right heart** (anterior aspect). Anterior wall of right atrium and ventricle removed.

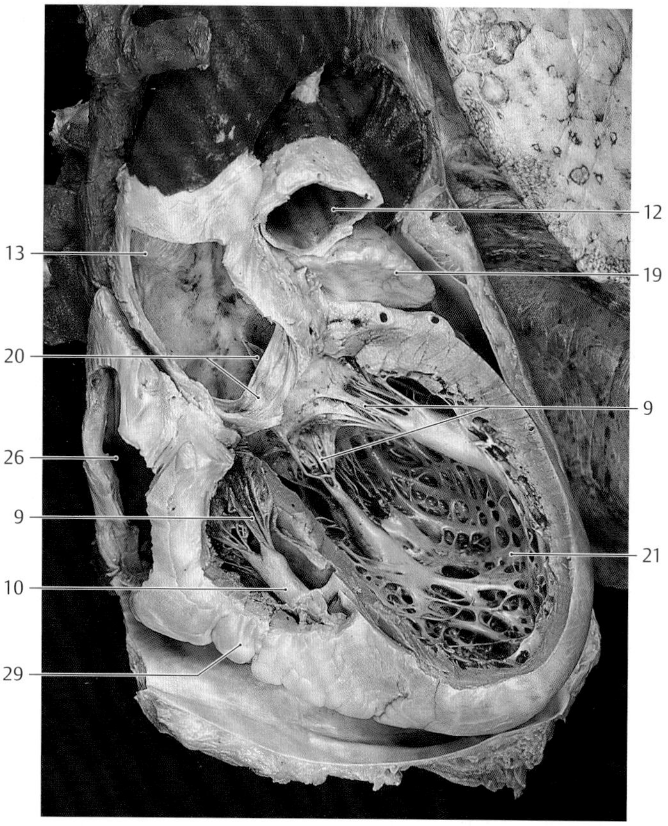

1 Superior vena cava
2 Crista terminalis
3 Fossa ovalis
4 Opening of inferior vena cava
5 Opening of coronary sinus
6 Right auricle
7 Right coronary artery and coronary sulcus
8 Anterior cusp of tricuspid valve
9 Tendinous cords
10 Anterior papillary muscle
11 Myocardium
12 Pulmonary trunk
13 Ascending aorta
14 Pulmonic valve
15 Conus arteriosus (interventricular septum)
16 Septal papillary muscles
17 Septomarginal trabecula or moderator band
18 Apex of heart
19 Left auricle
20 Aortic valve
21 Left ventricle
22 Pulmonary veins
23 Position of fossa ovalis
24 Left atrium
25 Left atrioventricular (bicuspid or mitral) valve
26 Right atrium
27 Pericardium
28 Posterior papillary muscle
29 Right ventricle
30 Interventricular septum

Fig. 5.34 **Heart, left ventricle with mitral valve, papillary muscles, and aortic valve.** Anterior portion of the heart removed.

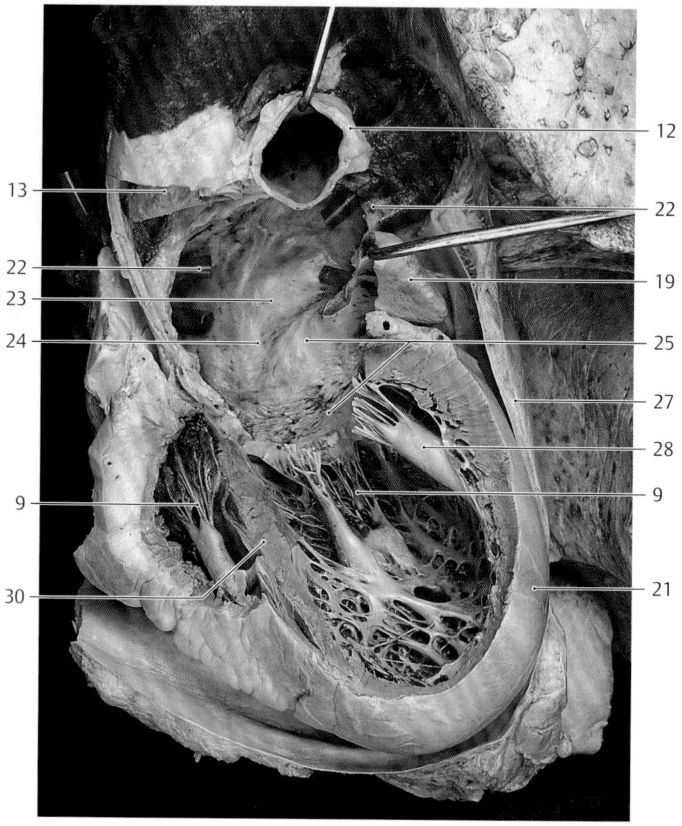

Fig. 5.35 **Heart, left ventricle with posterior part of mitral valve and papillary muscles.** Atrium opened.

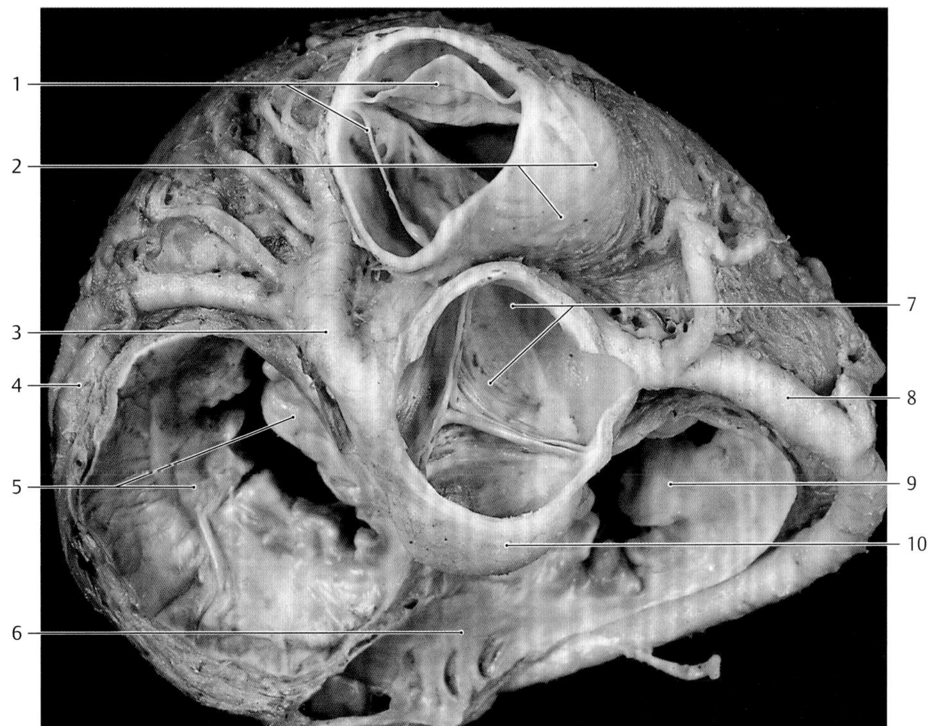


1 Pulmonic valve
2 Sinus of pulmonary trunk
3 Left coronary artery
4 Great cardiac vein
5 Left atrioventricular (mitral) valve
6 Coronary sinus
7 Aortic valve
8 Right coronary artery
9 Right atrioventricular (tricuspid) valve
10 Bulb of aorta
11 Anterior semilunar cusp of pulmonic valve
12 Left semilunar cusp of pulmonic valve
13 Right semilunar cusp of pulmonic valve
14 Left semilunar cusp of aortic valve
15 Right semilunar cusp of aortic valve
16 Posterior semilunar cusp of aortic valve
17 Pulmonary artery
18 Right atrium
19 Left atrium with pulmonary veins
20 Ascending aorta with aortic valve

Fig. 5.36 **Valves of the heart** (superior aspect). Left and right atria removed. Dissection of coronary arteries. Anterior wall of the heart at the top.

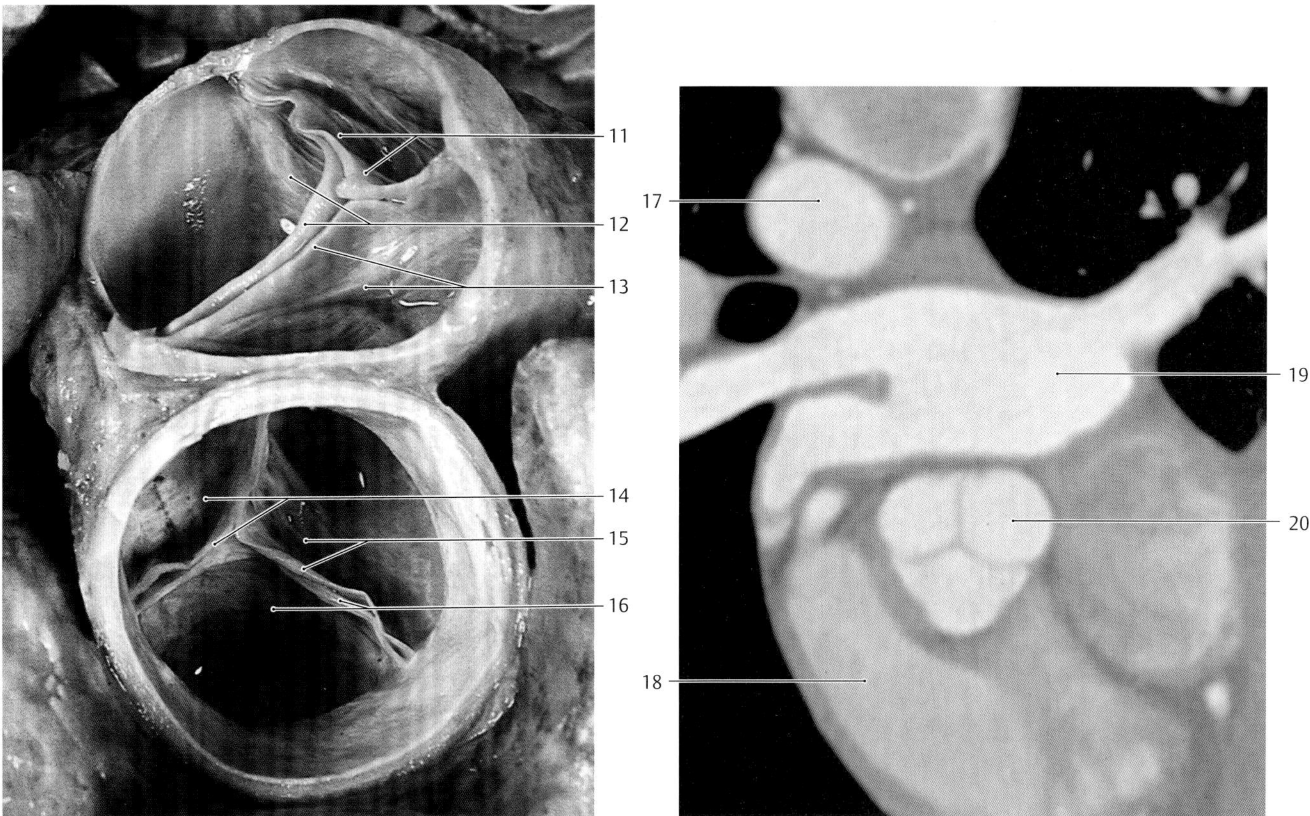


Fig. 5.37 **Pulmonic and aortic valves** (superior aspect). Both valves are closed. Anterior wall of the heart at the top.

Fig. 5.38 **Horizontal section through the heart** at the level of the aortic valve (CT scan). (Courtesy of Prof. Uder, Institute of Radiology, University Hospital Erlangen, Germany.)

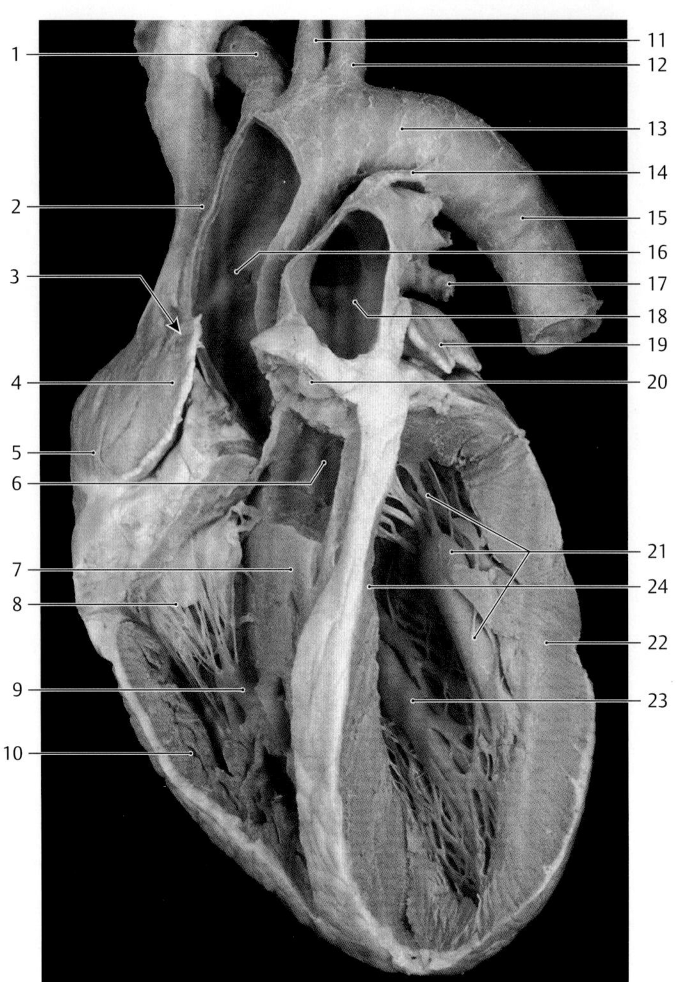


1 Brachiocephalic trunk
2 Superior vena cava
3 Sulcus terminalis
4 Right auricle
5 Right atrium
6 Aortic valve
7 Conus arteriosus (interventricular septum)
8 Right atrioventricular (tricuspid) valve
9 Anterior papillary muscle
10 Myocardium of right ventricle
11 Left common carotid artery
12 Left subclavian artery
13 Aortic arch
14 Ligamentum arteriosum (remnant of ductus arteriosus)
15 Thoracic aorta (descending aorta)
16 Ascending aorta
17 Left pulmonary vein
18 Pulmonary trunk
19 Left auricle
20 Pulmonic valve
21 Anterior papillary muscle with tendinous cords
22 Myocardium of left ventricle
23 Posterior papillary muscle
24 Interventricular septum
25 Brachiocephalic veins
26 Tendinous cords
27 Papillary muscles of right ventricle
28 Left atrium
29 Left atrioventricular (bicuspid or mitral) valve and tendinous cords
30 Apex of the heart
31 Left coronary artery
32 Left ventricle

Fig. 5.39 **Heart** (anterior aspect). Dissection of the four valves.

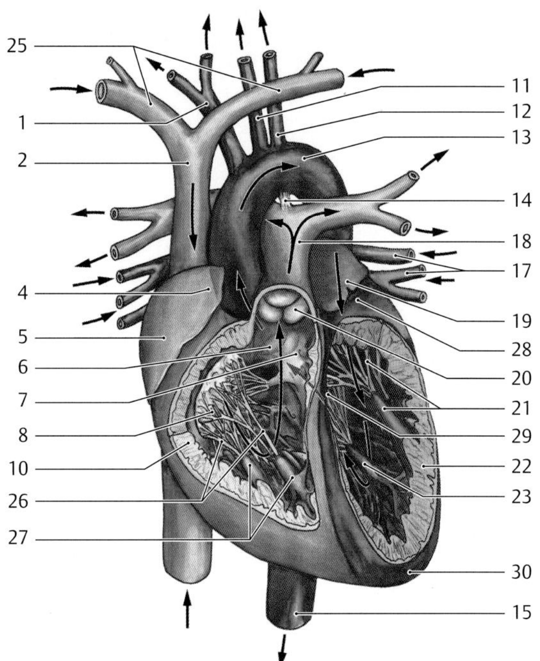


Fig. 5.40 **Circulation within the heart** (anterior aspect). Arrows = direction of blood flow.

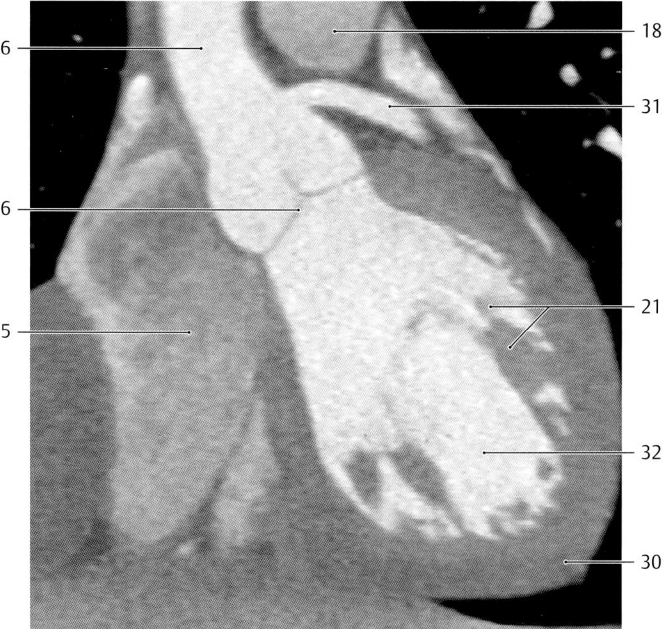


Fig. 5.41 **Frontal section through the heart** at the level of the left ventricle and ascending aorta (CT scan). (Courtesy of Prof. Uder, Institute of Radiology, University Hospital Erlangen, Germany.)

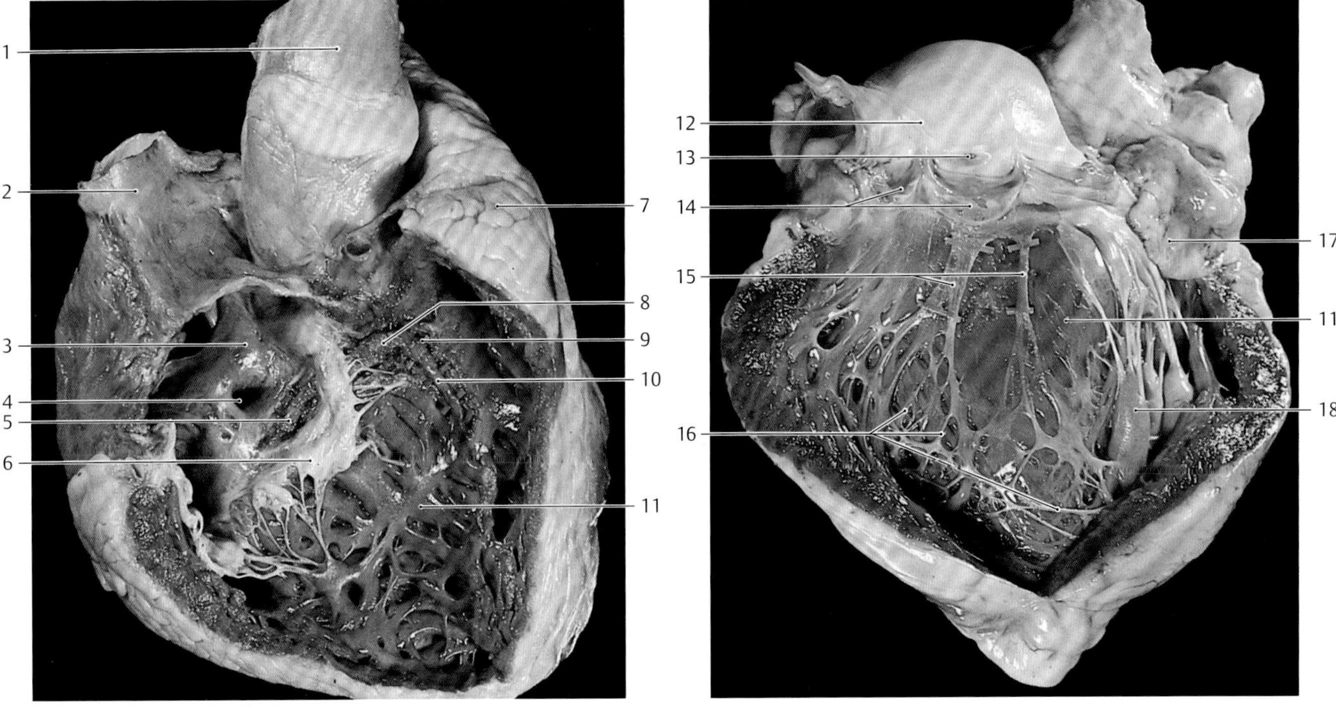


**Fig. 5.42 Right ventricle.** Dissection of atrioventricular node, atrioventricular bundle (bundle of His), and right limb or bundle branch of conducting system (probes).

**Fig. 5.43 Left ventricle.** Dissection of left limb or bundle branch of conducting system (probes).

1 Ascending aorta
2 Superior vena cava
3 Right atrium
4 Opening of coronary sinus
5 Atrioventricular node
6 Right atrioventricular valve
7 Pulmonary trunk
8 Atrioventricular bundle (bundle of His)
9 Bifurcation of atrioventricular bundle
10 Right bundle branch
11 Interventricular septum
12 Aortic sinus
13 Entrance of left coronary artery
14 Aortic valve
15 Branches of left bundle branch
16 Purkinje fibers
17 Left auricle
18 Anterior papillary muscles
19 Sulcus terminalis
20 Bulb of aorta
21 Sinu-atrial node (arrows)
22 Muscle fiber bundles of right atrium
23 Coronary sulcus (with right coronary artery)
24 Bundles of conducting system
25 Inferior vena cava
26 Papillary muscles with Purkinje fibers
27 Left atrium
28 Left bundle branch

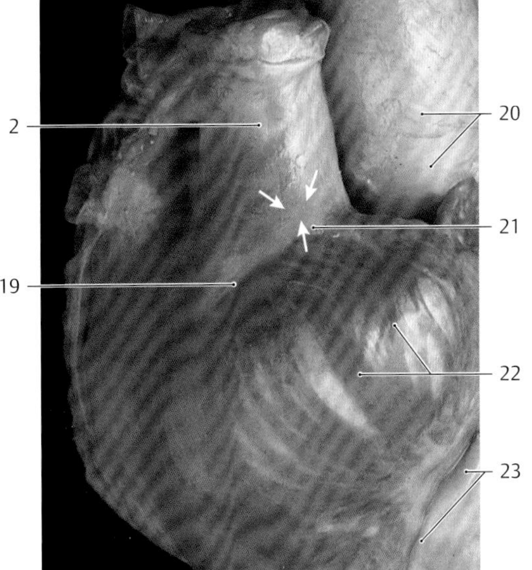


**Fig. 5.44 Right atrium.** Anterior wall, showing the location of the sinu-atrial node (arrows).

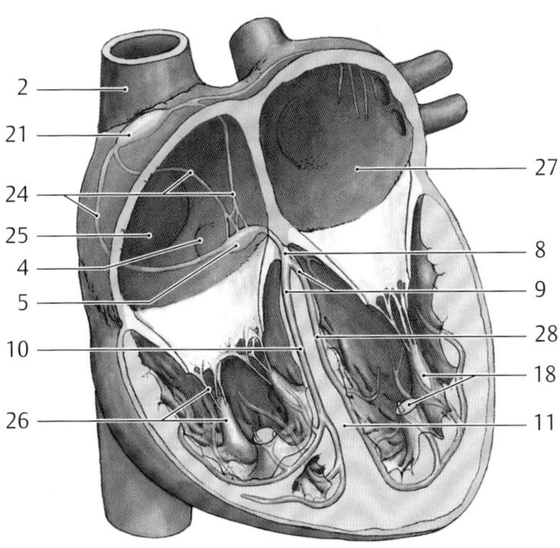


**Fig. 5.45 Conducting system** (yellow) **of the heart.**

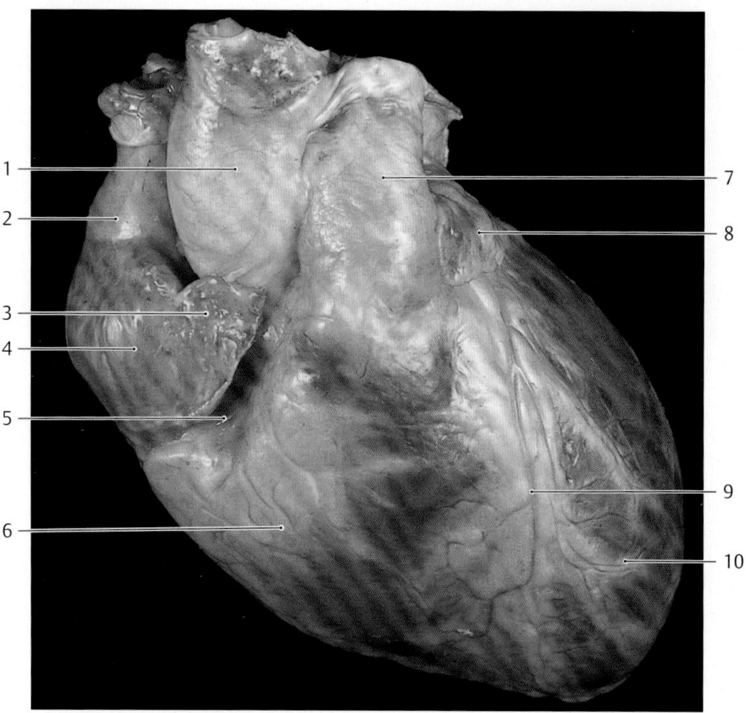


Fig. 5.46 **Heart, fixed in diastole** (anterior aspect). The ventricles are relaxed and the atria contracted.

1 Ascending aorta
2 Superior vena cava
3 Right auricle
4 Right atrium
5 Coronary sulcus
6 Right ventricle
7 Pulmonary trunk
8 Left auricle
9 Anterior interventricular sulcus
10 Left ventricle
11 Right pulmonary artery
12 Sulcus terminalis with sinu-atrial node
13 Line indicating plane of position of valves
14 Myocardium of right atrium
15 Inferior vena cava
16 Valve of pulmonary trunk
17 Right tricuspid valve
18 Myocardium of right ventricle

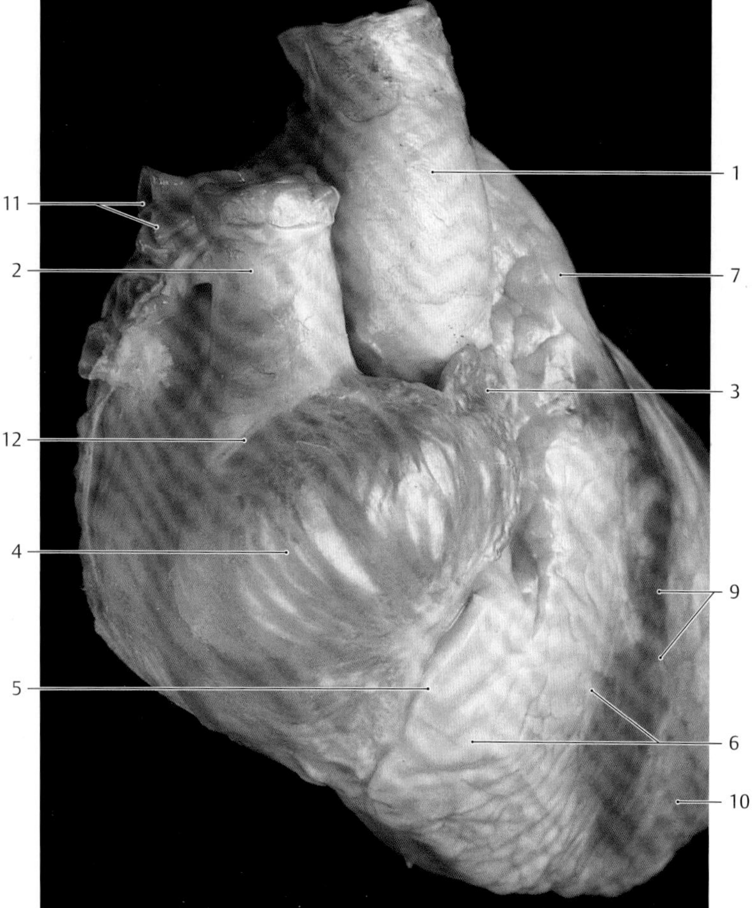


Fig. 5.47 **Heart, fixed in systole** (antero-lateral aspect). The ventricles are contracted and the atria dilated.

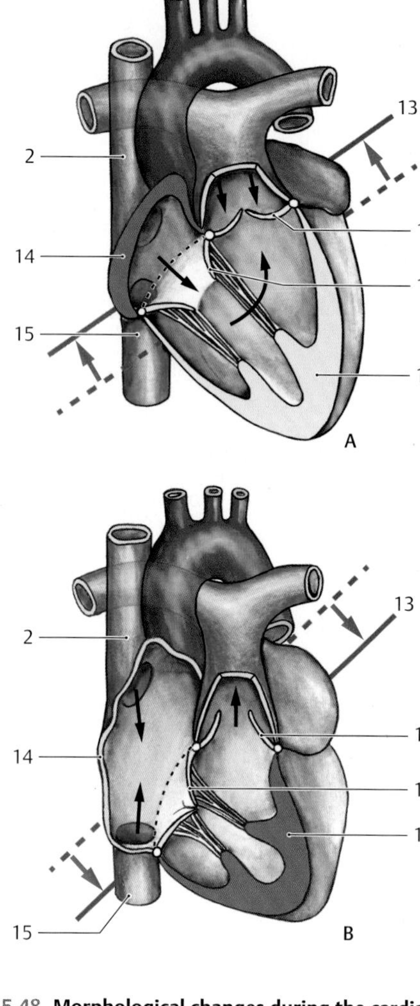


Fig. 5.48 **Morphological changes during the cardiac cycle.** Note the changes in the position of the valves (red arrows). Contracted portions of the heart are indicated in dark gray.

A = **Diastole:** muscles of the ventricles relaxed, atrioventricular valves open, semilunar valves closed
B = **Systole:** muscles of ventricles contracted, atrioventricular valves closed, semilunar valves open

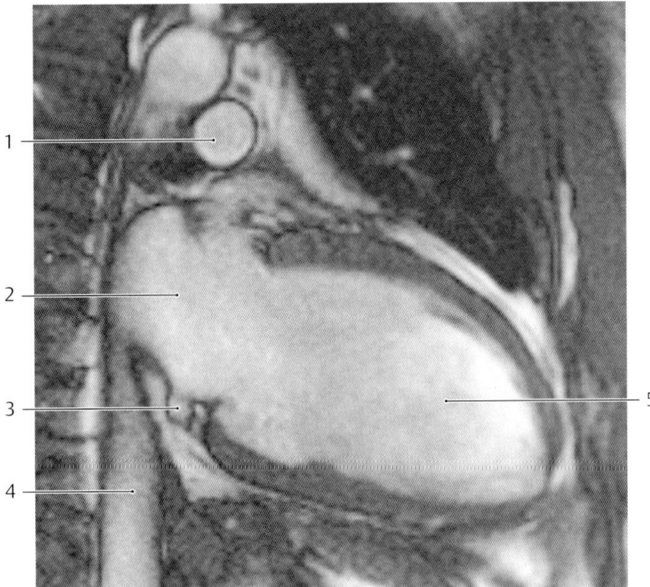


Fig. 5.49 **Coronal section through the thorax at the level of the left ventricle in dilation** (MRI scan). (Courtesy of Prof. Uder, Institute of Radiology, University Hospital Erlangen, Germany.)

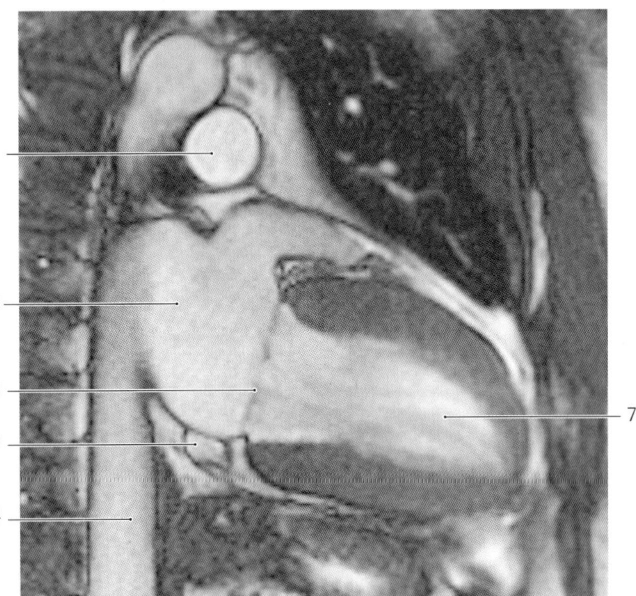


Fig. 5.50 **Coronal section through the thorax at the level of the left ventricle in contraction** (MRI scan). (Courtesy of Prof. Uder, Institute of Radiology, University Hospital Erlangen, Germany.)

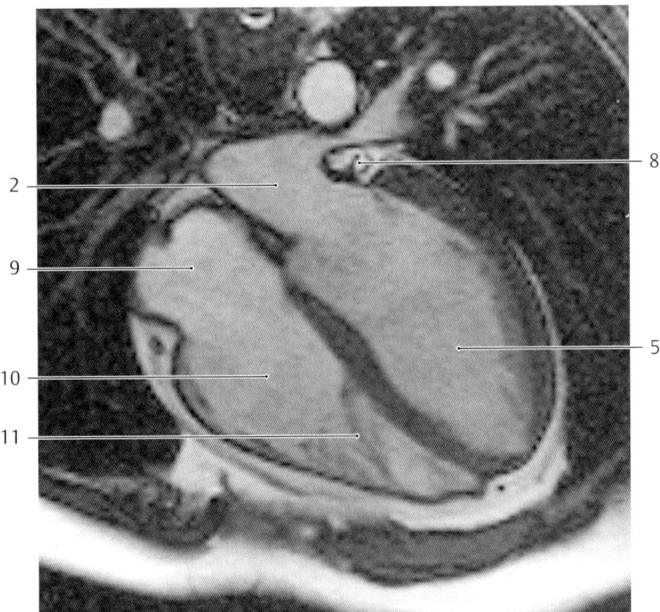


Fig. 5.51 **Coronal section through the human heart in the process of dilation** (MRI scan). (Courtesy of Prof. Uder, Institute of Radiology, University Hospital Erlangen, Germany.)

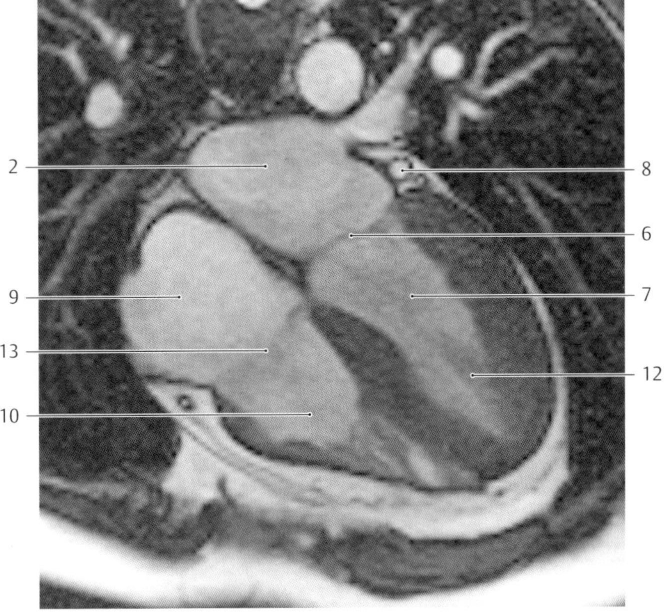


Fig. 5.52 **Coronal section through the human heart in the process of contraction** (MRI scan). (Courtesy of Prof. Uder, Institute of Radiology, University Hospital Erlangen, Germany.)

1 Pulmonary artery
2 Left atrium
3 Coronary sinus
4 Inferior vena cava
5 Left ventricle (dilated)
6 Left atrioventricular (mitral) valve
7 Left ventricle (contracted)
8 Great cardiac vein (left coronary vein)
9 Right atrium
10 Right ventricle
11 Septomarginal trabecula
12 Papillary muscle
13 Right atrioventricular (tricuspid) valve

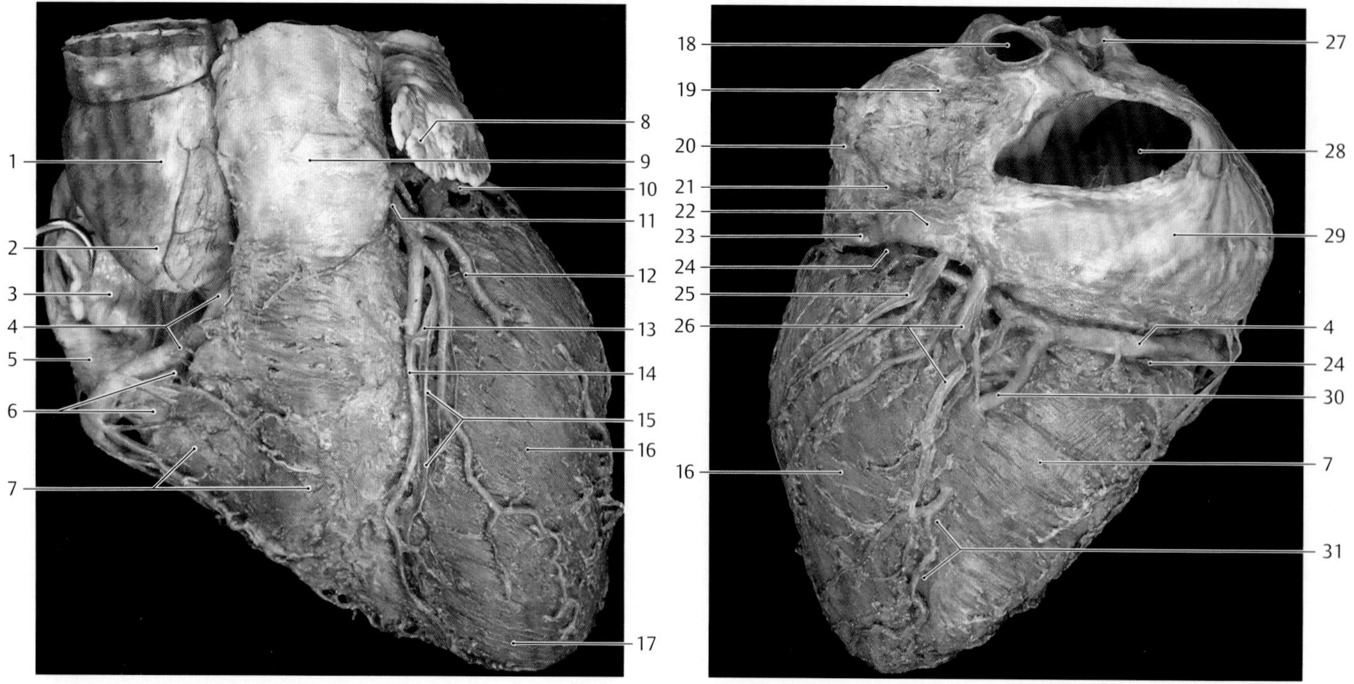


Fig. 5.53 **Coronary arteries** (anterior aspect). The epicardium and subepicardial fatty tissue have been removed. The arteries have been injected with red resin from the aorta.

Fig. 5.54 **Right coronary artery and veins of the heart** (posterior aspect). The epicardium and subepicardial fatty tissue have been removed. The arteries have been injected with red resin.

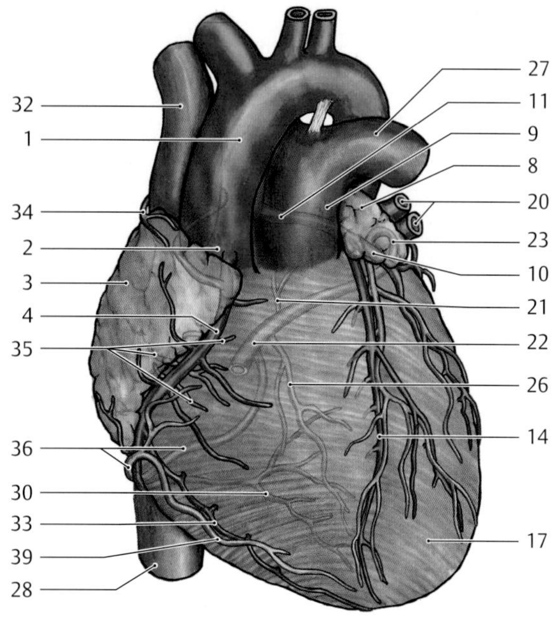


Fig. 5.55 **Coronary arteries and veins of the heart** (anterior aspect).

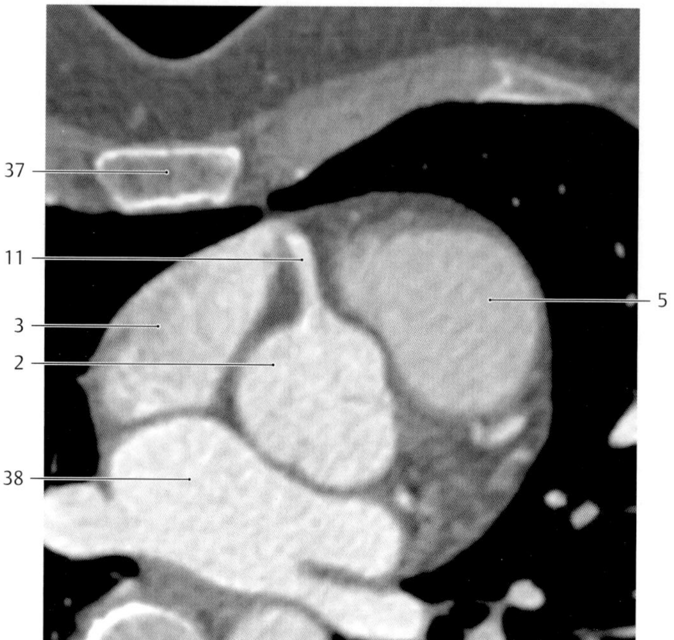


Fig. 5.56 **Horizontal section through heart and thoracic wall** at the level of the aortic bulb (CT scan). (Courtesy of Prof. Uder, Institute of Radiology, University Hospital Erlangen, Germany.)

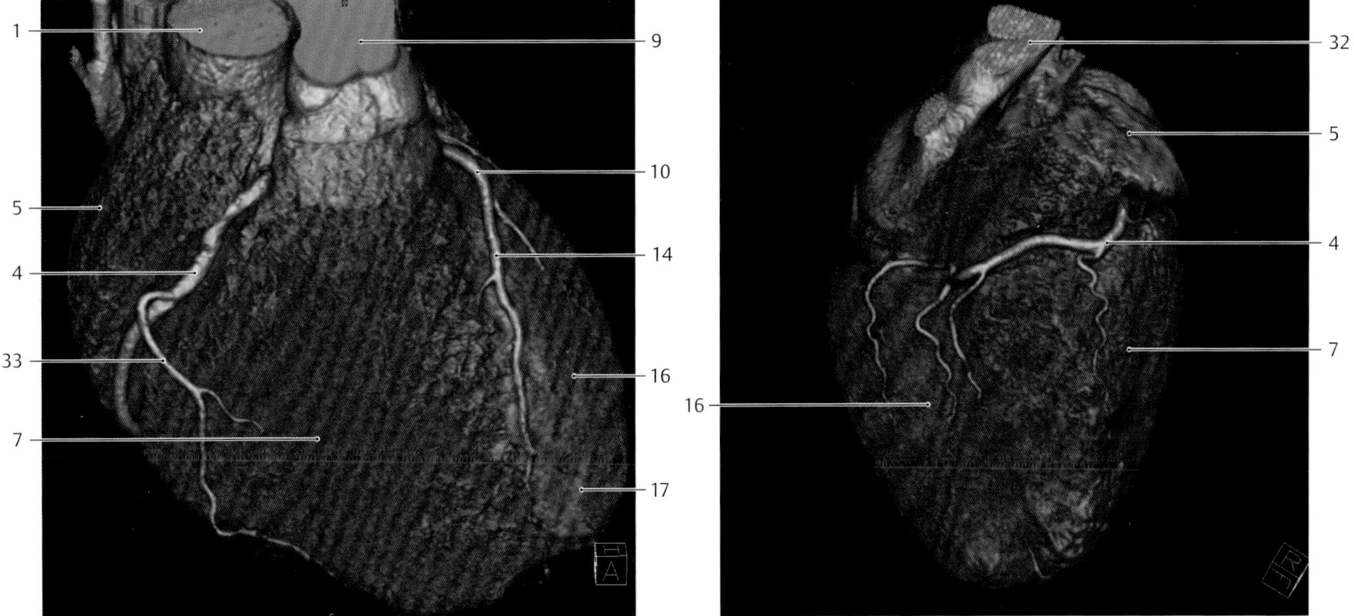


Fig. 5.57 **Coronary arteries** (anterior aspect; stereoscopic CT scan). (Courtesy of Prof. Uder, Institute of Radiology, University Hospital Erlangen, Germany.)

Fig. 5.58 **Coronary arteries** (posterior aspect; stereoscopic CT scan). (Courtesy of Prof. Uder, Institute of Radiology, University Hospital Erlangen, Germany.)

1 Ascending aorta
2 Aortic bulb and sinu-atrial branch of right coronary artery
3 Right auricle
4 Right coronary artery
5 Right atrium
6 Coronary sulcus
7 Right ventricle
8 Left auricle
9 Pulmonary trunk
10 Circumflex branch of left coronary artery
11 Left coronary artery
12 Diagonal branch of left coronary artery
13 Anterior interventricular vein
14 Anterior interventricular artery
15 Anterior interventricular sulcus
16 Left ventricle
17 Apex of the heart
18 Right pulmonary vein
19 Left atrium
20 Left pulmonary veins
21 Oblique vein of left atrium (Marshall's vein)
22 Coronary sinus
23 Great cardiac vein
24 Coronary sulcus (posterior part)
25 Posterior vein of left ventricle
26 Middle cardiac vein
27 Left pulmonary artery
28 Inferior vena cava
29 Right atrium
30 Posterior interventricular branch of right coronary artery
31 Posterior interventricular sulcus
32 Superior vena cava
33 Right marginal branch of right coronary artery
34 Branch of sinu-atrial node
35 Minimal cardiac veins
36 Small cardiac veins
37 Sternum
38 Left atrium with pulmonary veins
39 Right marginal vein

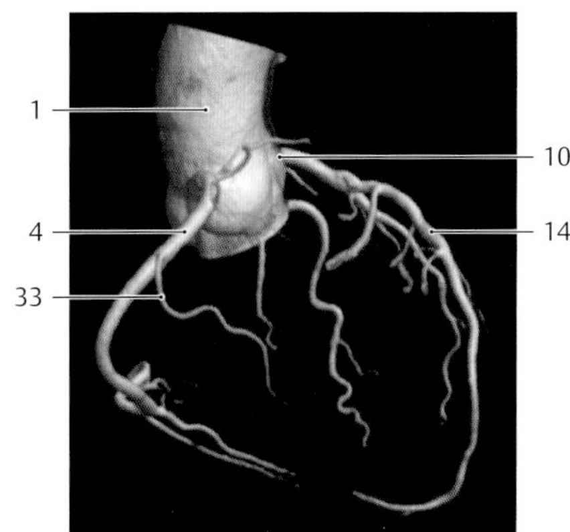


Fig. 5.59 **Coronary arteries** (stereoscopic CT scan). (Courtesy of Prof. Uder, Institute of Radiology, University Hospital Erlangen, Germany.)

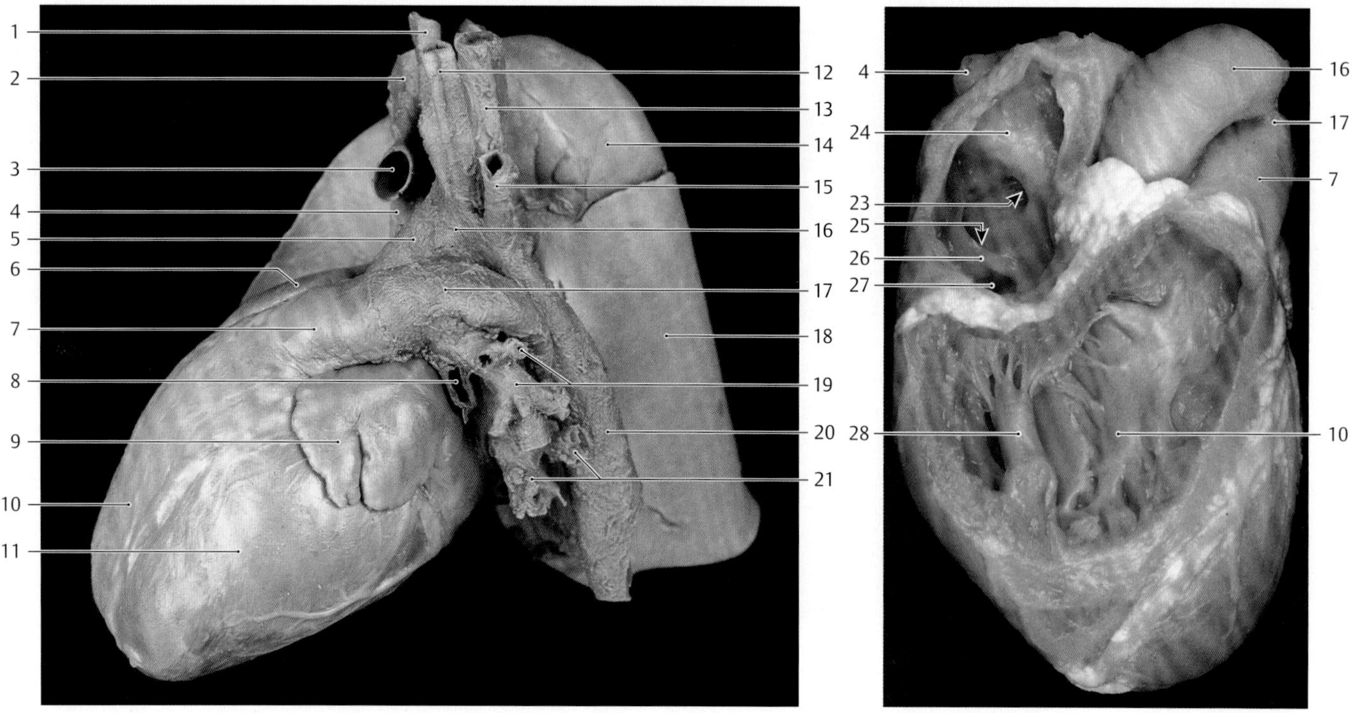


**Fig. 5.60** **Heart and right lung of the fetus** (viewed from left side). The left lung has been removed. Note the ductus arteriosus (Botalli).

**Fig. 5.61** **Heart of the fetus** (anterior aspect). Right atrium and ventricle have been opened.

| Shunts in the fetal circulation system | | | |
|---|---|---|---|
| 1. | Ductus venosus (of Arantius) | between umbilical vein and inferior vena cava | bypass of liver circulation |
| 2. | Foramen ovale | between right and left atria | bypass of pulmonary circulation |
| 3. | Ductus arteriosus (Botalli) | between pulmonary trunk and aorta | |

1 Right common carotid artery
2 Right brachiocephalic vein
3 Left brachiocephalic vein
4 Superior vena cava
5 Ascending aorta
6 Right auricle
7 Pulmonary trunk
8 Left primary bronchus
9 Left auricle
10 Right ventricle
11 Left ventricle
12 Left common carotid artery
13 Trachea
14 Superior lobe of right lung
15 Left subclavian artery
16 Aortic arch
17 Ductus arteriosus (Botalli)
18 Inferior lobe of right lung
19 Left pulmonary artery with branches to the left lung
20 Descending aorta
21 Left pulmonary veins
22 Inferior vena cava
23 Foramen ovale
24 Right atrium
25 Opening of inferior vena cava
26 Valve of inferior vena cava (Eustachian valve)
27 Opening of coronary sinus
28 Anterior papillary muscle of right ventricle

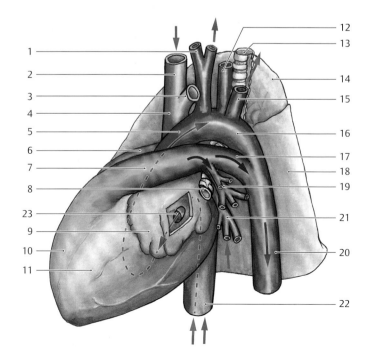

**Fig. 5.62** **Heart and right lung of the fetus** (see corresponding dissection in Fig. 5.60 above). Direction of blood flow indicated by arrows. Note the change in oxygenation of blood after ductus arteriosus entry into the aorta.

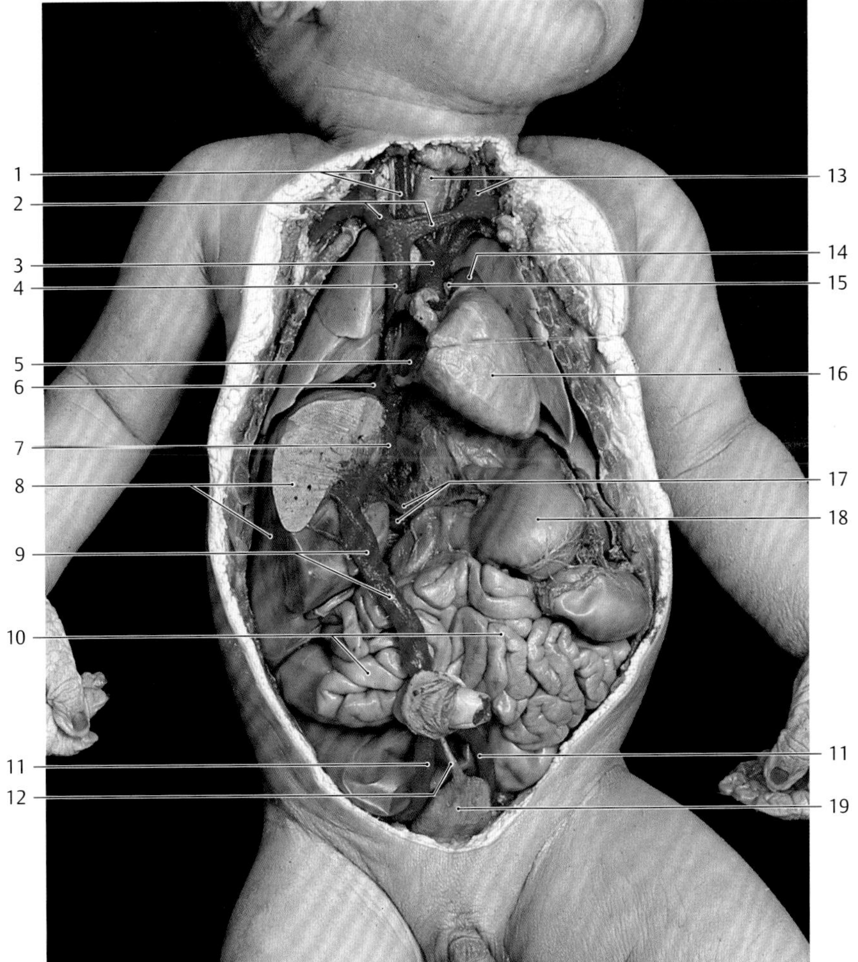


Fig. 5.63 **Thoracic and abdominal organs in the newborn** (anterior aspect). The right atrium has been opened to show the foramen ovale. The left lobe of the liver has been removed.

1 Internal jugular vein and right common carotid artery
2 Right and left brachiocephalic vein
3 Aortic arch
4 Superior vena cava
5 Foramen ovale
6 Inferior vena cava
7 Ductus venosus
8 Liver
9 Umbilical vein
10 Small intestine
11 Umbilical artery
12 Urachus
13 Trachea and left internal jugular vein
14 Left pulmonary artery
15 Ductus arteriosus (Botalli)
16 Right ventricle
17 Hepatic arteries (red) and portal vein (blue)
18 Stomach
19 Urinary bladder
20 Portal vein
21 Pulmonary veins
22 Descending aorta
23 Placenta

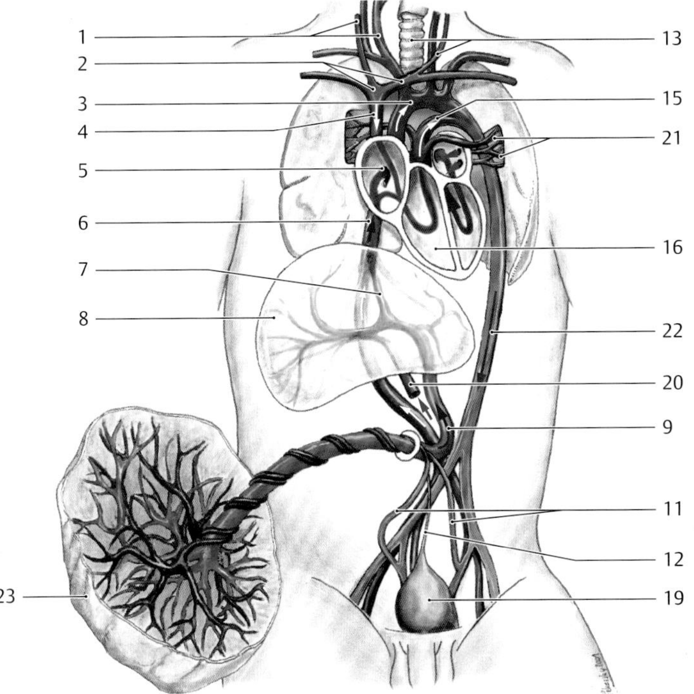


Fig. 5.64 **Fetal circulatory system.** The oxygen qradient is indicated by color.

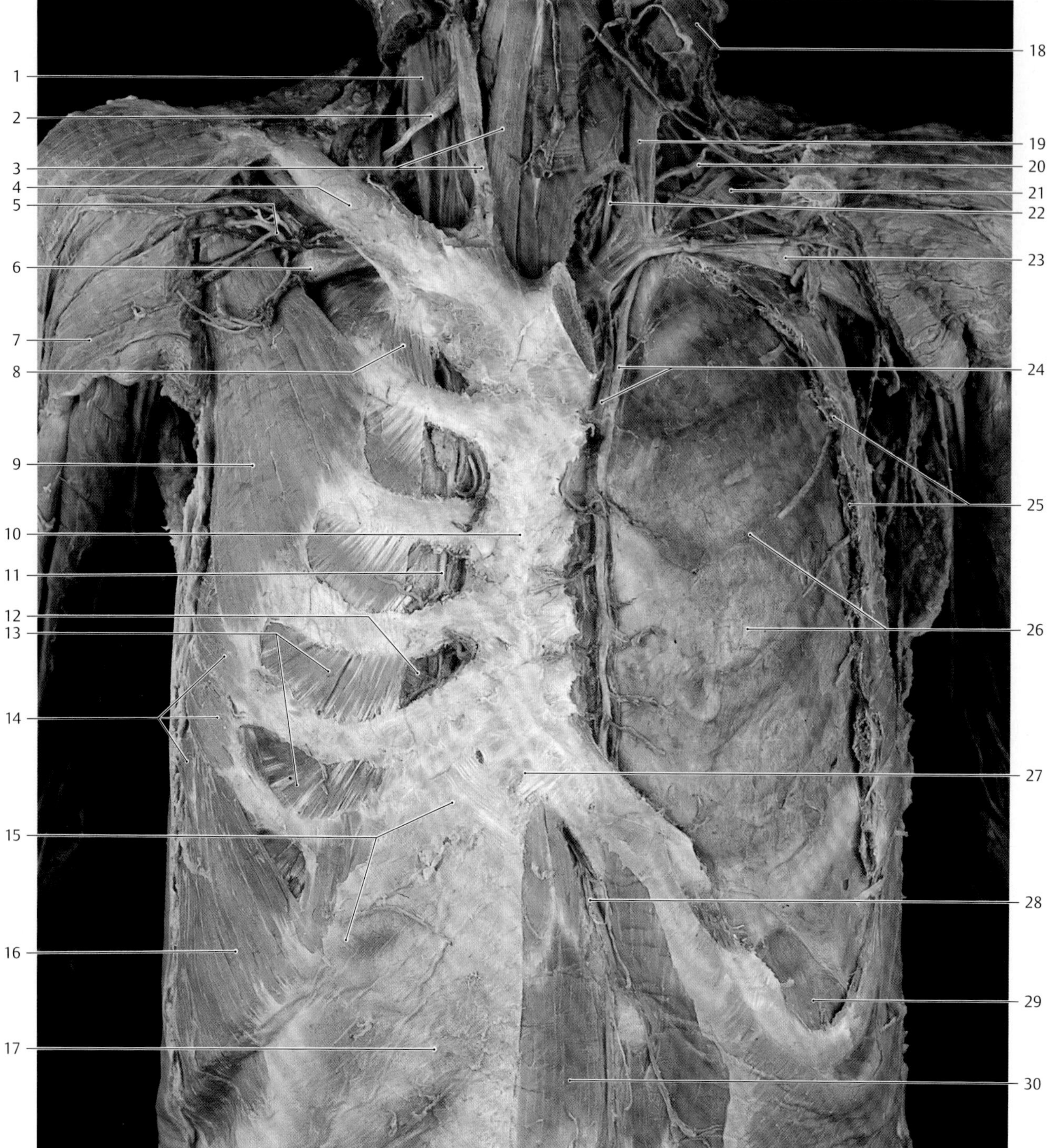


**Fig. 5.65 Thoracic organs** (anterior aspect). The left clavicle and ribs have been partially removed, and the right intercostal spaces have been opened to show the internal thoracic vein and artery.

1 Right internal jugular vein
2 Omohyoid muscle
3 Sternohyoid muscle and external jugular vein
4 Clavicle
5 Thoraco-acromial artery
6 Right subclavian vein
7 Pectoralis major muscle
8 External intercostal muscle
9 Pectoralis minor muscle
10 Body of sternum
11 Right internal thoracic artery and vein
12 Fascicles of transversus thoracis muscle
13 Internal intercostal muscles
14 Serratus anterior muscle
15 Costal margin
16 External abdominal oblique muscle
17 Anterior sheath of rectus abdominis muscle
18 Sternocleidomastoid muscle
19 Left internal jugular vein
20 Transverse cervical artery
21 Brachial plexus
22 Vagus nerve
23 Left axillary vein
24 Left internal thoracic artery and vein
25 Ribs and thoracic wall (cut)
26 Costal pleura
27 Xiphoid process
28 Superior epigastric artery
29 Diaphragm
30 Rectus abdominis muscle

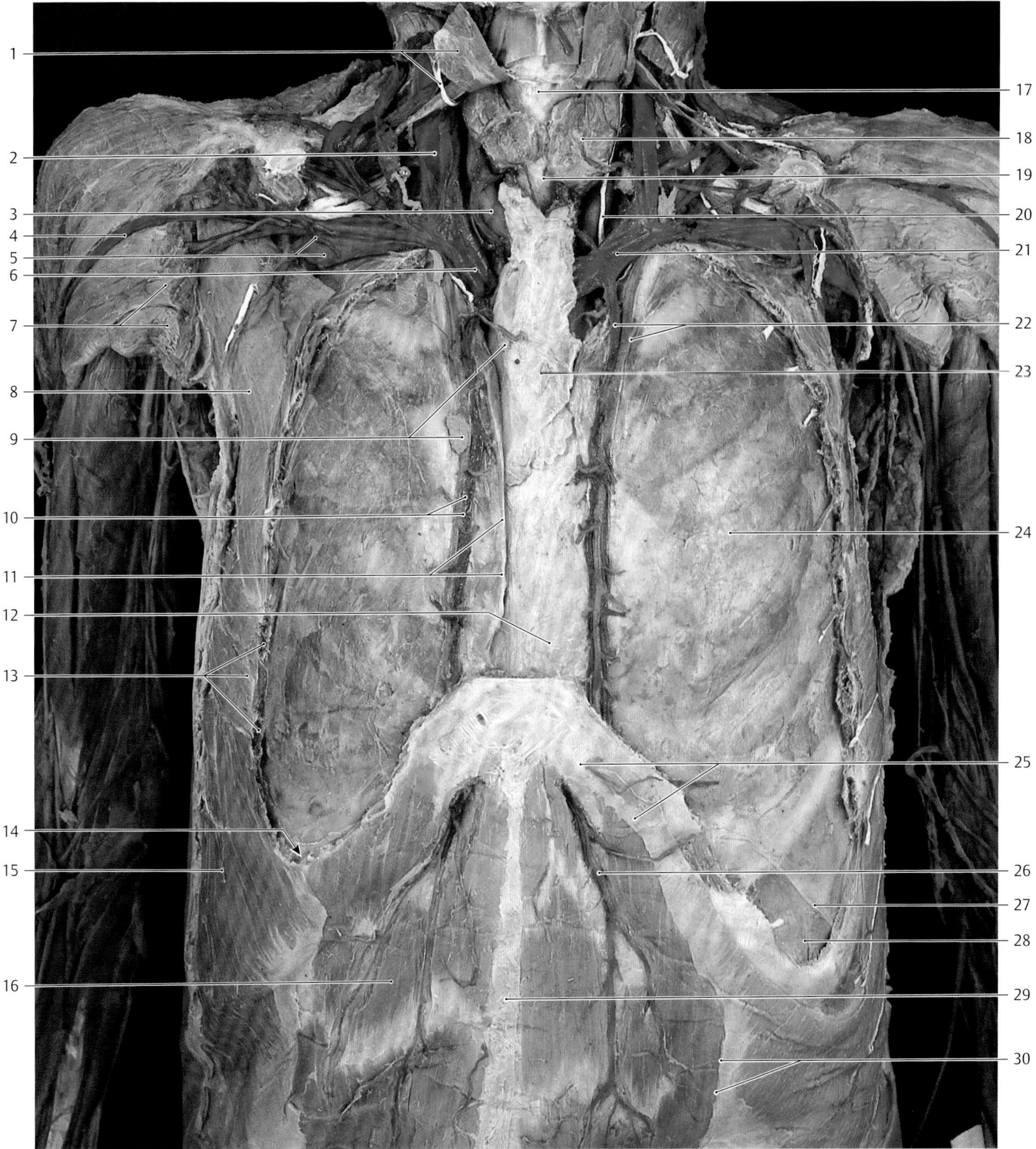


**Fig. 5.66 Thoracic organs** (anterior aspect). The ribs, clavicle, and sternum have been partly removed to show the anterior mediastinum and pleura. Red = arteries; blue = veins; green = lymph vessels and nodes.

1 Sternothyroid muscle and its nerve (a branch of the ansa cervicalis)
2 Right internal jugular vein
3 Right common carotid artery
4 Cephalic vein
5 Right subclavian vein
6 Right brachiocephalic vein
7 Pectoralis major muscle (divided)
8 Pectoralis minor muscle (divided)
9 Parasternal lymph nodes
10 Internal thoracic artery and vein
11 Anterior margin of costal pleura
12 Pericardium
13 Fifth and sixth ribs (divided) and serratus anterior muscle
14 Costodiaphragmatic recess
15 External abdominal oblique muscle
16 Rectus abdominis muscle
17 Larynx (thyroid cartilage)
18 Thyroid gland
19 Trachea
20 Left vagus nerve
21 Left brachiocephalic vein
22 Left internal thoracic artery and vein
23 Thymus
24 Costal pleura
25 Costal margin
26 Superior epigastric artery
27 Margin of costal pleura
28 Diaphragm
29 Linea alba
30 Cut edge of anterior sheath of rectus abdominis muscle

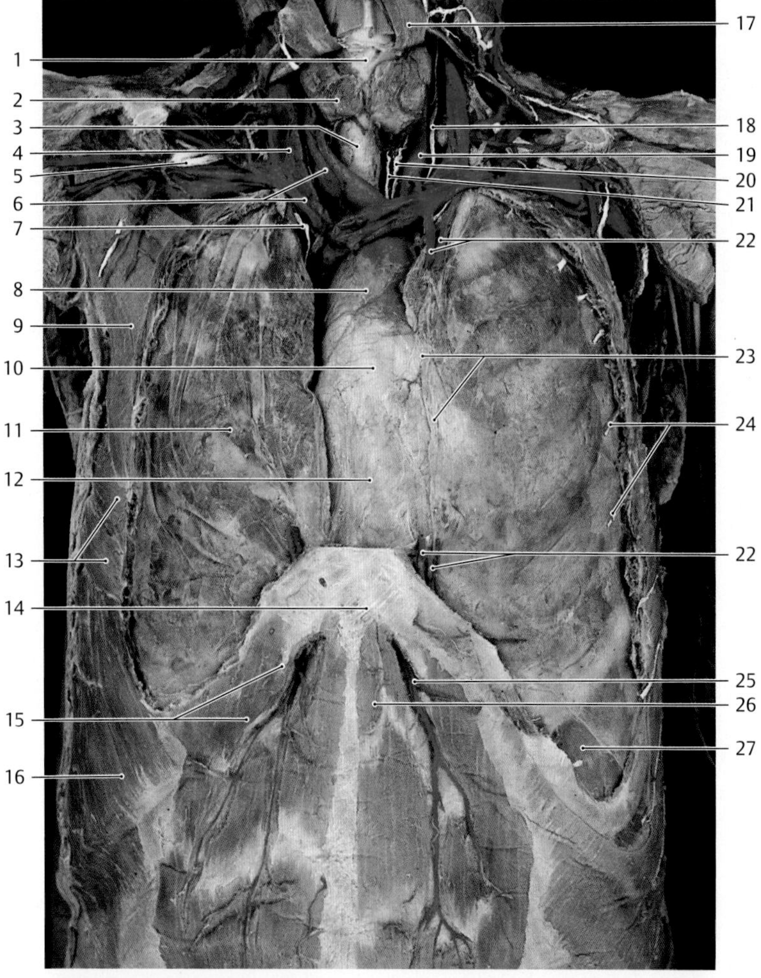


Fig. 5.67 **Thoracic organs** (anterior aspect). The internal thoracic vessels have been removed, and the anterior margins of the pleura and lungs have been slightly reflected to display the anterior and middle mediastinum, including the heart and great vessels. Red = arteries; blue = veins; green = lymph vessels and nodes.

1 Larynx (thyroid cartilage)
2 Thyroid gland
3 Trachea
4 Internal jugular vein
5 Brachial plexus
6 Right brachiocephalic vein and common carotid artery
7 Right phrenic nerve
8 Ascending aorta
9 Pectoralis minor muscle (divided)
10 Pulmonary trunk (covered by pericardium)
11 Costal pleura
12 Pericardium and heart
13 Serratus anterior muscle
14 Xiphoid process
15 Costal margin
16 External abdominal oblique muscle
17 Sternothyroid muscle (divided and reflected)
18 Vagus nerve
19 Left common carotid artery
20 Left sympathetic trunk
21 Left recurrent laryngeal nerve
22 Left internal thoracic artery and vein (divided)
23 Margin of costal pleura
24 Intercostal nerves and vessels
25 Superior epigastric artery
26 Rectus abdominis muscle
27 Diaphragm
28 Ansa cervicalis
29 Phrenic nerve and anterior scalene muscle
30 External jugular vein (divided)
31 Right subclavian vein
32 Right brachiocephalic vein
33 Internal thoracic artery (divided)
34 Internal thoracic vein (divided)
35 Right lung
36 Cricothyroid muscle
37 Omohyoid muscle
38 Thymus
39 Left lung

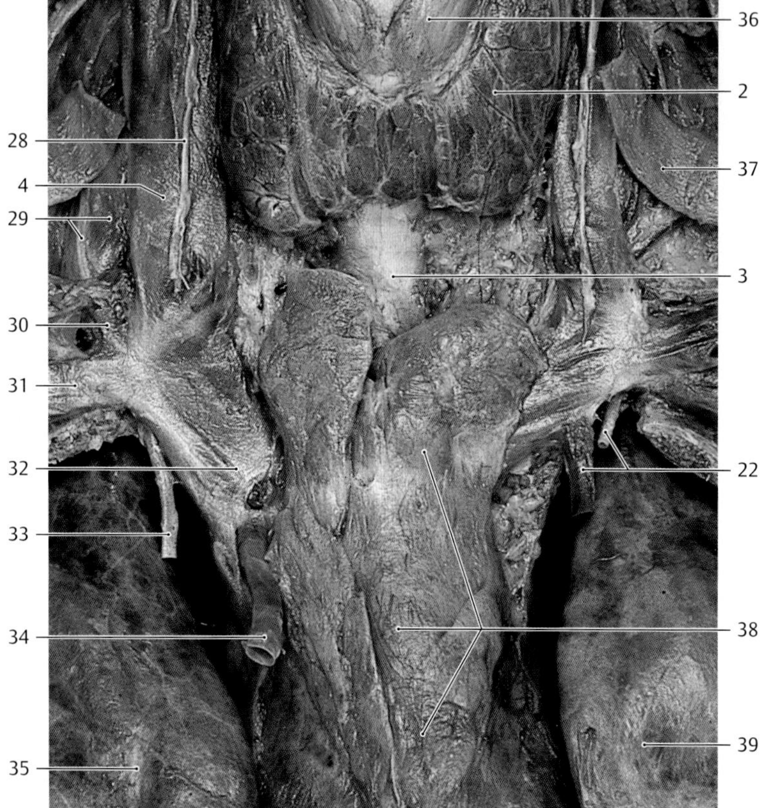


Fig. 5.68 **Thoracic organs** (anterior aspect, enlarged details). The position (above the heart) and size of the thymus are shown.

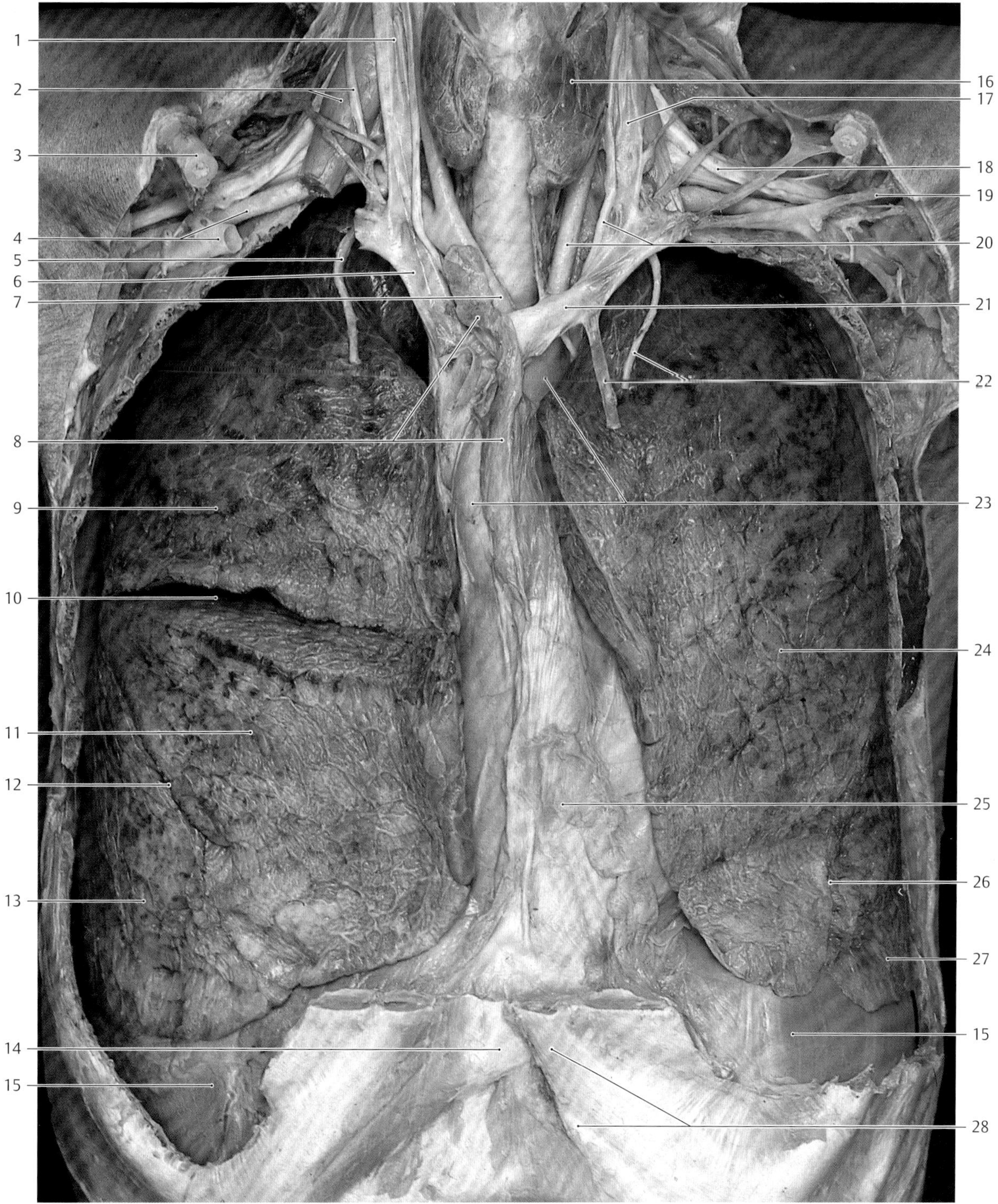


Fig. 5.69 **Thoracic organs** (anterior aspect). The pleura has been opened and the lungs exposed. Remnants of the thymus and pericardium are seen.

1 Right internal jugular vein
2 Phrenic nerve and anterior scalene muscle
3 Clavicle (divided)
4 Right subclavian artery and vein
5 Internal thoracic artery
6 Right brachiocephalic vein
7 Brachiocephalic trunk
8 Thymus (atrophic)
9 Upper lobe of right lung
10 Horizontal fissure of right lung (incomplete)
11 Middle lobe of right lung
12 Oblique fissure of right lung
13 Lower lobe of right lung
14 Xiphoid process
15 Diaphragm
16 Thyroid gland
17 Left internal jugular vein
18 Brachial plexus
19 Left cephalic vein
20 Left common carotid artery and vagus nerve
21 Left brachiocephalic vein
22 Internal thoracic artery and vein (divided)
23 Ascending aorta and aortic arch
24 Upper lobe of left lung
25 Pericardium
26 Oblique fissure of left lung
27 Lower lobe of left lung
28 Costal margin

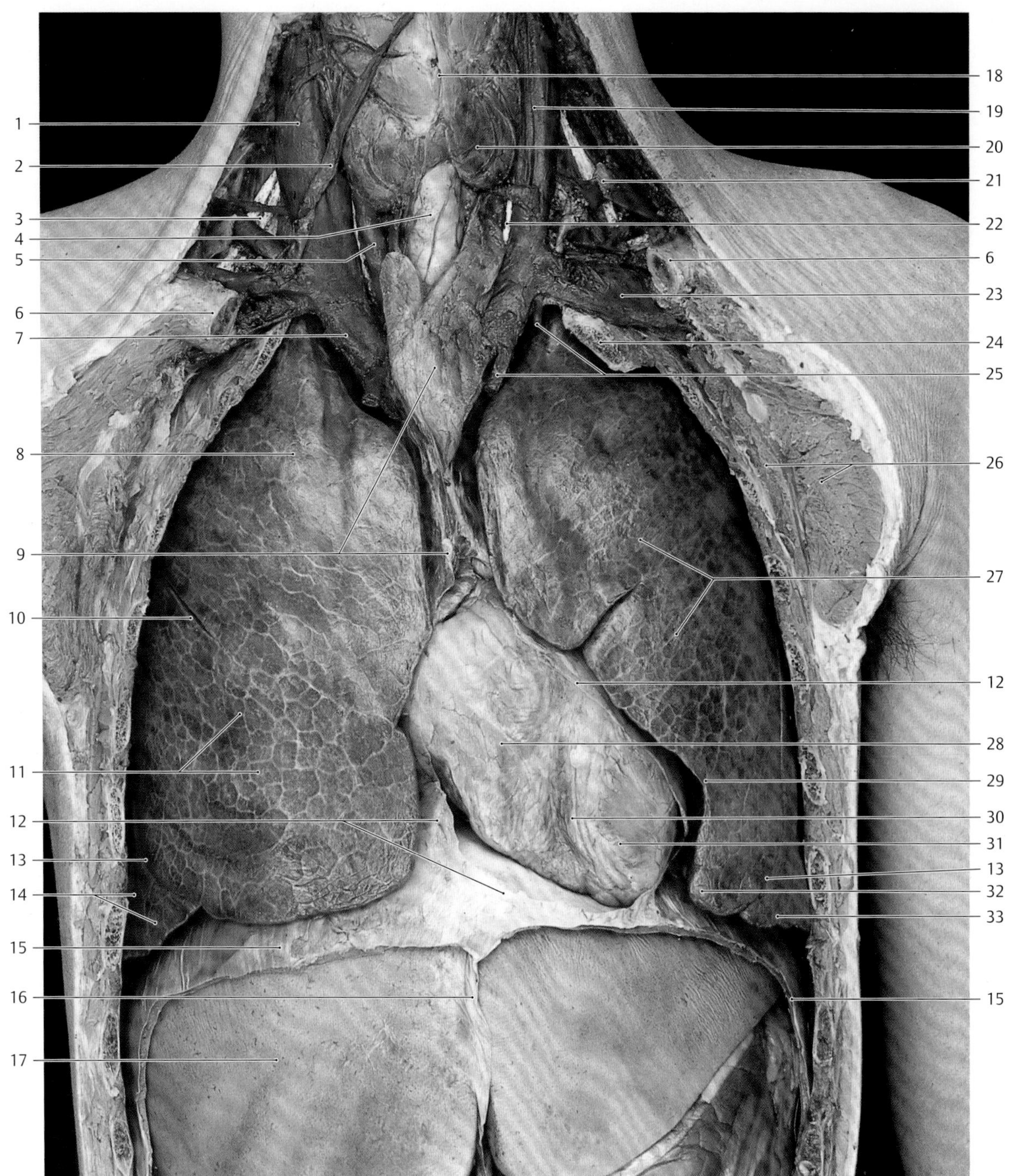


Fig. 5.70 **Thoracic organs** (anterior aspect). The thoracic wall, costal pleura, pericardium, and diaphragm have been partly removed. Red = arteries; blue = veins.

1 Internal jugular vein
2 External jugular vein (displaced medially)
3 Brachial plexus
4 Trachea
5 Right common carotid artery
6 Clavicle (divided)
7 Right brachiocephalic vein
8 Upper lobe of right lung
9 Thymus (atrophic)
10 Horizontal fissure of right lung
11 Middle lobe of right lung
12 Pericardium (cut edges)
13 Oblique fissure of lung
14 Lower lobe of right lung
15 Diaphragm
16 Falciform ligament
17 Liver
18 Location of larynx
19 Left internal jugular vein
20 Thyroid gland
21 Omohyoid muscle (divided)
22 Vagus nerve
23 Left subclavian vein
24 First rib (divided)
25 Internal thoracic artery and vein
26 Pectoralis major and pectoralis minor muscles (cut edges)
27 Upper lobe of left lung
28 Right ventricle
29 Cardiac notch of left lung
30 Interventricular sulcus of heart
31 Left ventricle
32 Lingula
33 Lower lobe of left lung

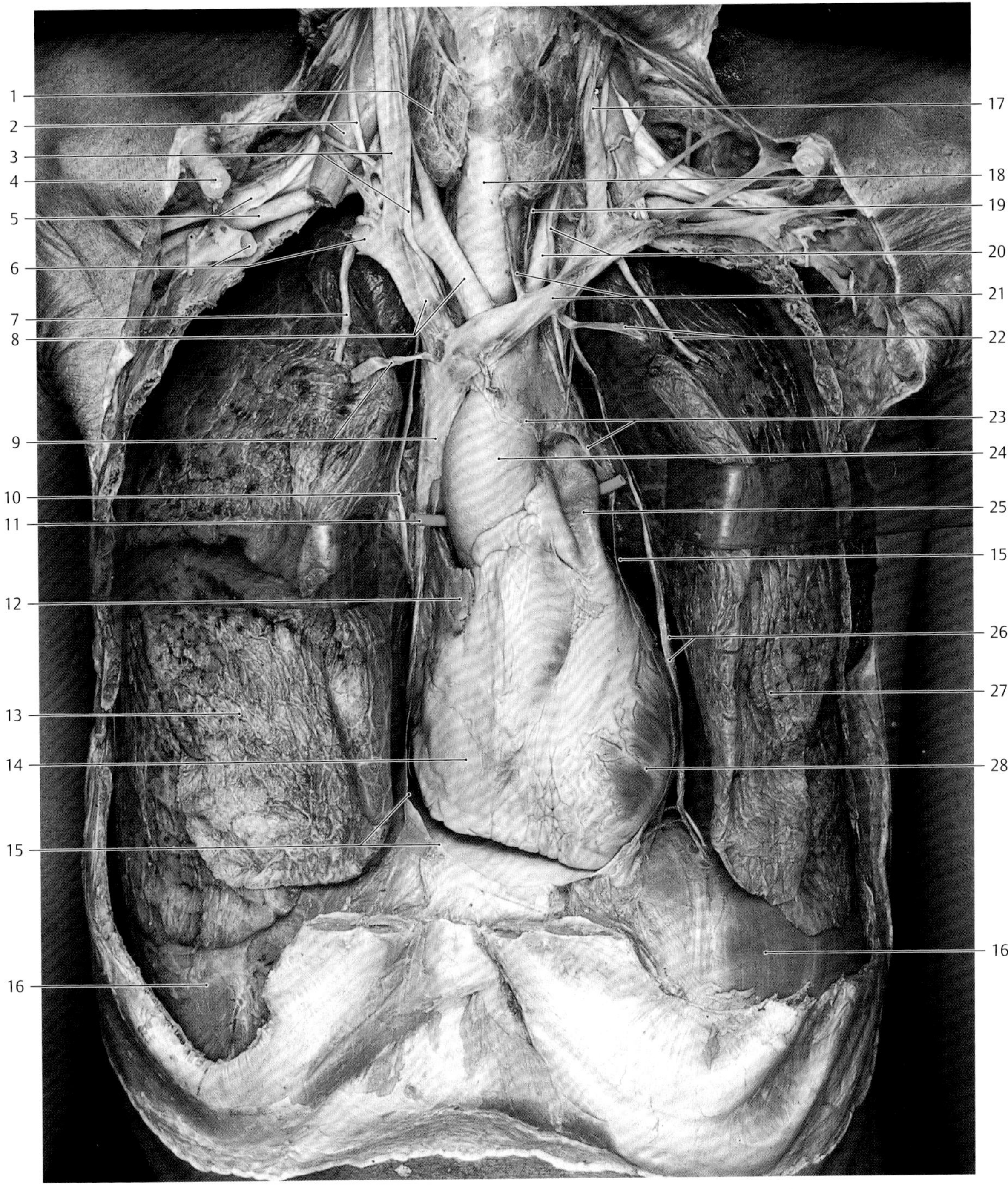


**Fig. 5.71 Thoracic organs** (anterior aspect). Position of the heart and middle mediastinum. The anterior wall of the thorax, the costal pleura, and the pericardium have been removed and the lungs slightly reflected.

1 Thyroid gland
2 Phrenic nerve and anterior scalene muscle
3 Vagus nerve and internal jugular vein
4 Clavicle (divided)
5 Brachial plexus and subclavian artery
6 Subclavian vein
7 Internal thoracic artery
8 Brachiocephalic trunk and right brachiocephalic vein
9 Superior vena cava and thymic vein
10 Right phrenic nerve
11 Transverse pericardial sinus (probe)
12 Right auricle
13 Middle lobe of right lung
14 Right ventricle
15 Cut edge of pericardium
16 Diaphragm
17 Internal jugular vein
18 Trachea
19 Left recurrent laryngeal nerve
20 Left common carotid artery and vagus nerve
21 Left brachiocephalic vein and inferior thyroid vein
22 Left internal thoracic artery and vein (divided)
23 Upper margin of pericardial sac
24 Ascending aorta
25 Pulmonary trunk
26 Left phrenic nerve and left pericardiacophrenic artery and vein
27 Upper lobe of left lung
28 Left ventricle

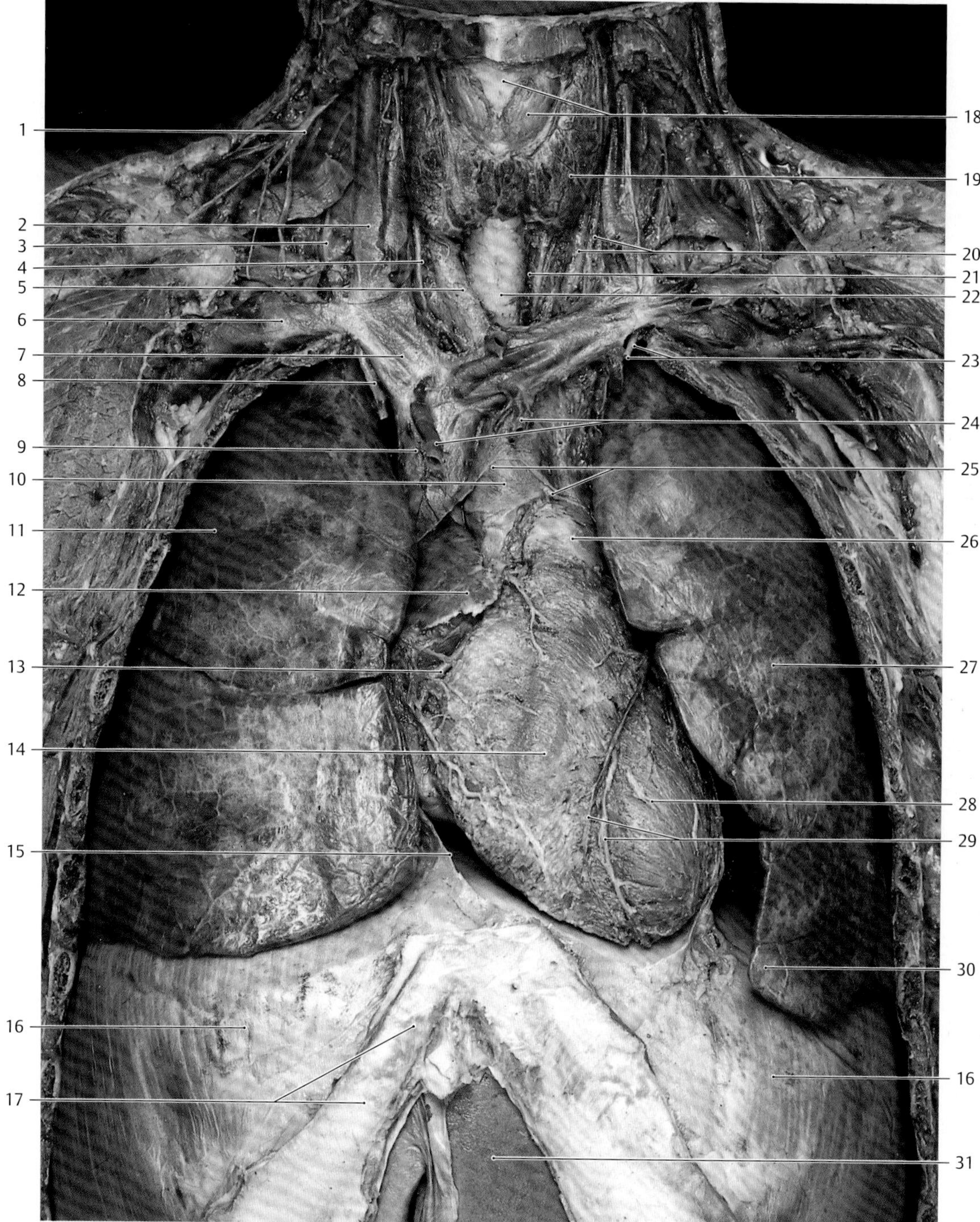


**Fig. 5.72 Thoracic organs** (anterior aspect). Position of the heart and dissection of coronary vessels in situ. The anterior wall of the thorax, costal pleura, and pericardium have been removed.

1 Intermediate supraclavicular nerve
2 Internal jugular vein
3 Right phrenic nerve
4 Right vagus nerve
5 Right common carotid artery
6 Right subclavian vein
7 Right brachiocephalic vein
8 Right internal thoracic artery
9 Superior vena cava
10 Ascending aorta
11 Right lung
12 Right atrium
13 Right coronary artery and small cardiac vein
14 Right ventricle
15 Cut edge of pericardium
16 Diaphragm
17 Costal margin
18 Larynx (cricothyroid muscle and thyroid cartilage)
19 Thyroid gland
20 Left common carotid artery and left vagus nerve
21 Left recurrent laryngeal nerve
22 Trachea
23 Left internal thoracic artery and vein (divided)
24 Thymic veins
25 Margin of pericardial sac
26 Pulmonary trunk
27 Left lung
28 Left ventricle
29 Anterior interventricular artery and vein
30 Lingula
31 Liver

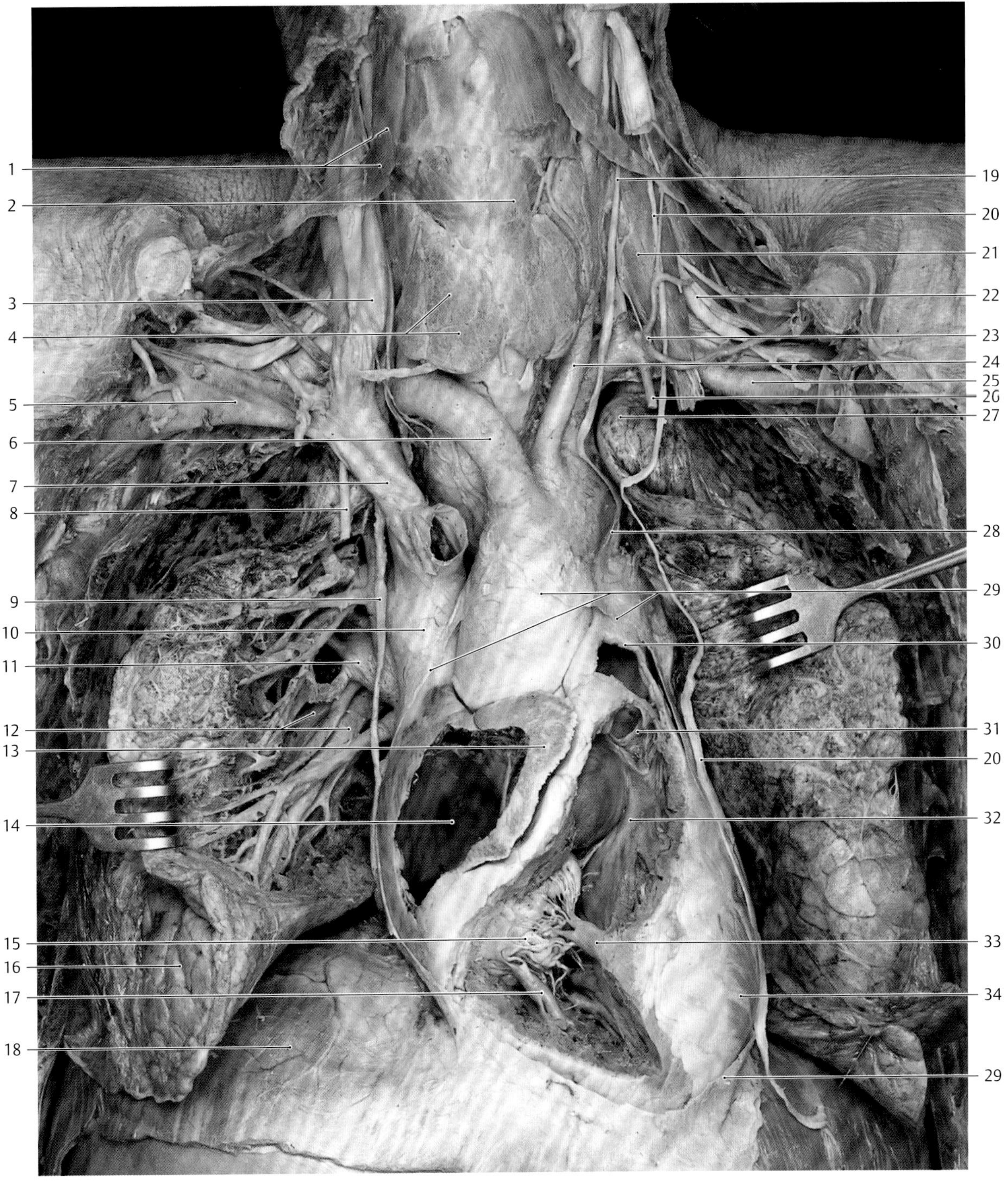


Fig. 5.73 **Thoracic organs** (anterior aspect). Heart with valves in situ. The anterior wall of the thorax, pleura, and anterior portion of the pericardium have been removed. The right atrium and ventricle have been opened to show the right atrioventricular and pulmonary valves.

1 Omohyoid muscle
2 Pyramidal lobe of thyroid gland
3 Internal jugular vein
4 Thyroid gland
5 Right subclavian vein
6 Brachiocephalic trunk
7 Right brachiocephalic vein
8 Right internal thoracic artery
9 Right phrenic nerve
10 Superior vena cava
11 Pulmonary vein
12 Branches of pulmonary artery
13 Right auricle
14 Right atrium
15 Right atrioventricular (tricuspid) valve
16 Right lung
17 Posterior papillary muscle
18 Diaphragm
19 Left vagus nerve
20 Left phrenic nerve
21 Anterior scalene muscle
22 Brachial plexus
23 Thyrocervical trunk
24 Left common carotid artery
25 Left subclavian artery
26 Left internal thoracic artery
27 Apex of left lung
28 Left recurrent laryngeal nerve
29 Cut edge of pericardium
30 Pulmonary trunk (fenestrated)
31 Pulmonic valve
32 Supraventricular crest
33 Anterior papillary muscle
34 Left ventricle

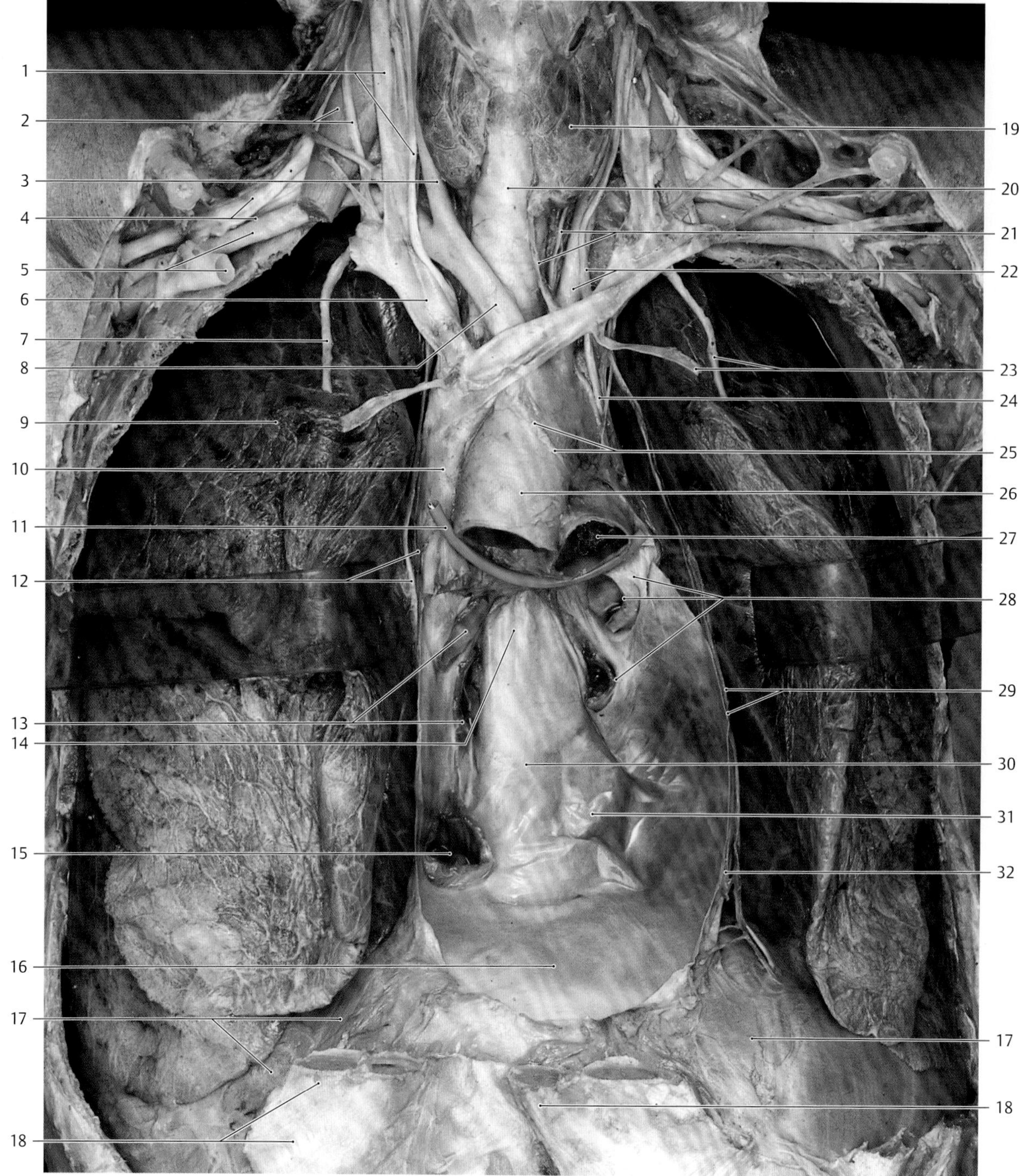


**Fig. 5.74 Thoracic organs** (anterior aspect). Pericardium and mediastinum. Anterior wall of thorax and heart have been removed and the lungs slightly reflected. Note the probe within the transverse pericardial sinus.

1 Right internal jugular vein and right vagus nerve
2 Right phrenic nerve and anterior scalene muscle
3 Right common carotid artery
4 Brachial plexus
5 Right subclavian artery and vein
6 Right brachiocephalic vein
7 Right internal thoracic artery (divided)
8 Brachiocephalic trunk
9 Upper lobe of right lung
10 Superior vena cava
11 Transverse pericardial sinus (probe)
12 Right phrenic nerve and right pericardiacophrenic artery and vein
13 Right pulmonary veins
14 Oblique sinus of pericardium
15 Inferior vena cava
16 Diaphragmatic part of pericardium
17 Diaphragm
18 Costal margin
19 Thyroid gland
20 Trachea
21 Left recurrent laryngeal nerve and inferior thyroid vein
22 Left common carotid artery and left vagus nerve
23 Left internal thoracic artery and vein (divided)
24 Vagus nerve at aortic arch
25 Cut edge of pericardium
26 Ascending aorta
27 Pulmonary trunk (divided)
28 Left pulmonary veins
29 Left phrenic nerve and left pericardiacophrenic artery and vein
30 Contour of esophagus beneath pericardium
31 Contour of aorta beneath pericardium
32 Pericardium (cut edge)

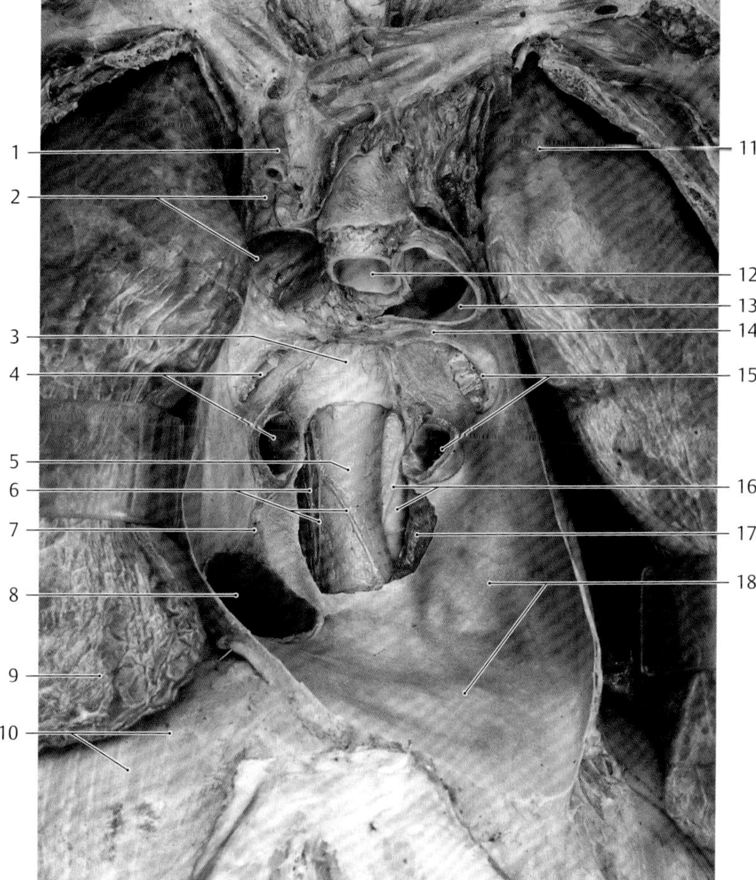


1 Internal thoracic vein
2 Superior vena cava
3 Oblique sinus of pericardium
4 Right pulmonary veins
5 Esophagus
6 Branches of right vagus nerve
7 Mesocardium
8 Inferior vena cava
9 Middle lobe of right lung
10 Diaphragm
11 Upper lobe of left lung
12 Ascending aorta
13 Pulmonary trunk
14 Transverse pericardial sinus
15 Left pulmonary veins
16 Descending aorta and left vagus nerve
17 Left lung (adjacent to pericardium)
18 Pericardium
19 Left subclavian artery
20 Vagus nerve
21 Left recurrent laryngeal nerve
22 Descending aorta
23 Pulmonary artery
24 Left atrium
25 Left ventricle
26 Coronary sinus
27 Left common carotid artery
28 Brachiocephalic trunk
29 Azygos arch
30 Right atrium
31 Right ventricle
32 Aortic arch

Fig. 5.75 **Pericardial sac** (anterior aspect). The heart has been removed, and the posterior wall of the pericardium has been opened to show the adjacent esophagus and aorta.

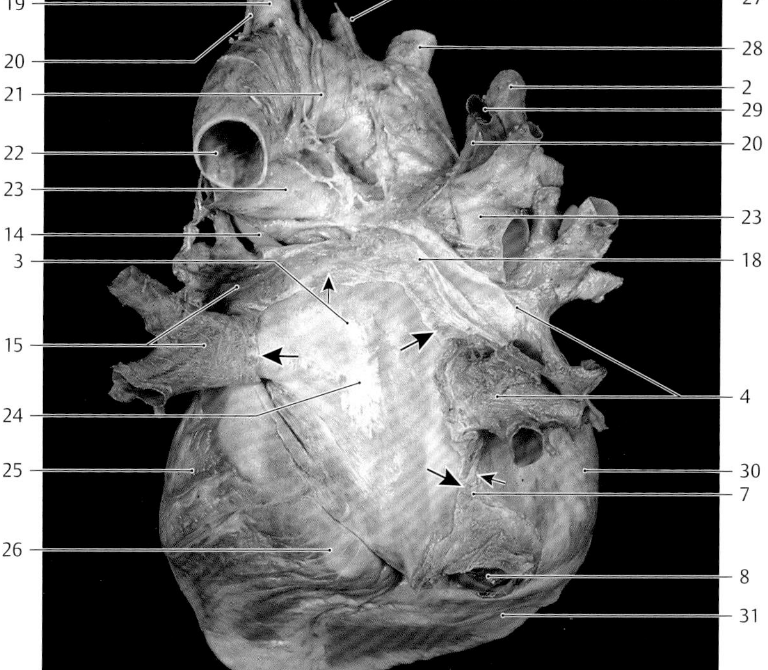


Fig. 5.76 **Heart with epicardium** (posterior aspect). Arrows = oblique sinus.

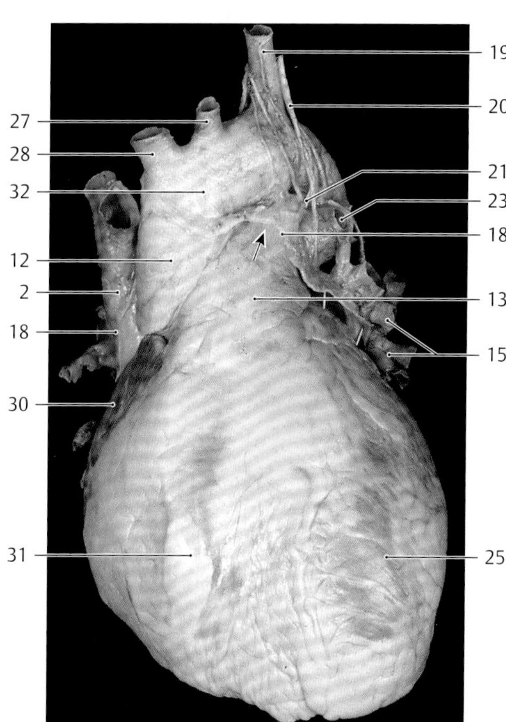


Fig. 5.77 **Heart with epicardium** (anterior aspect). Arrow = pericardial reflection.

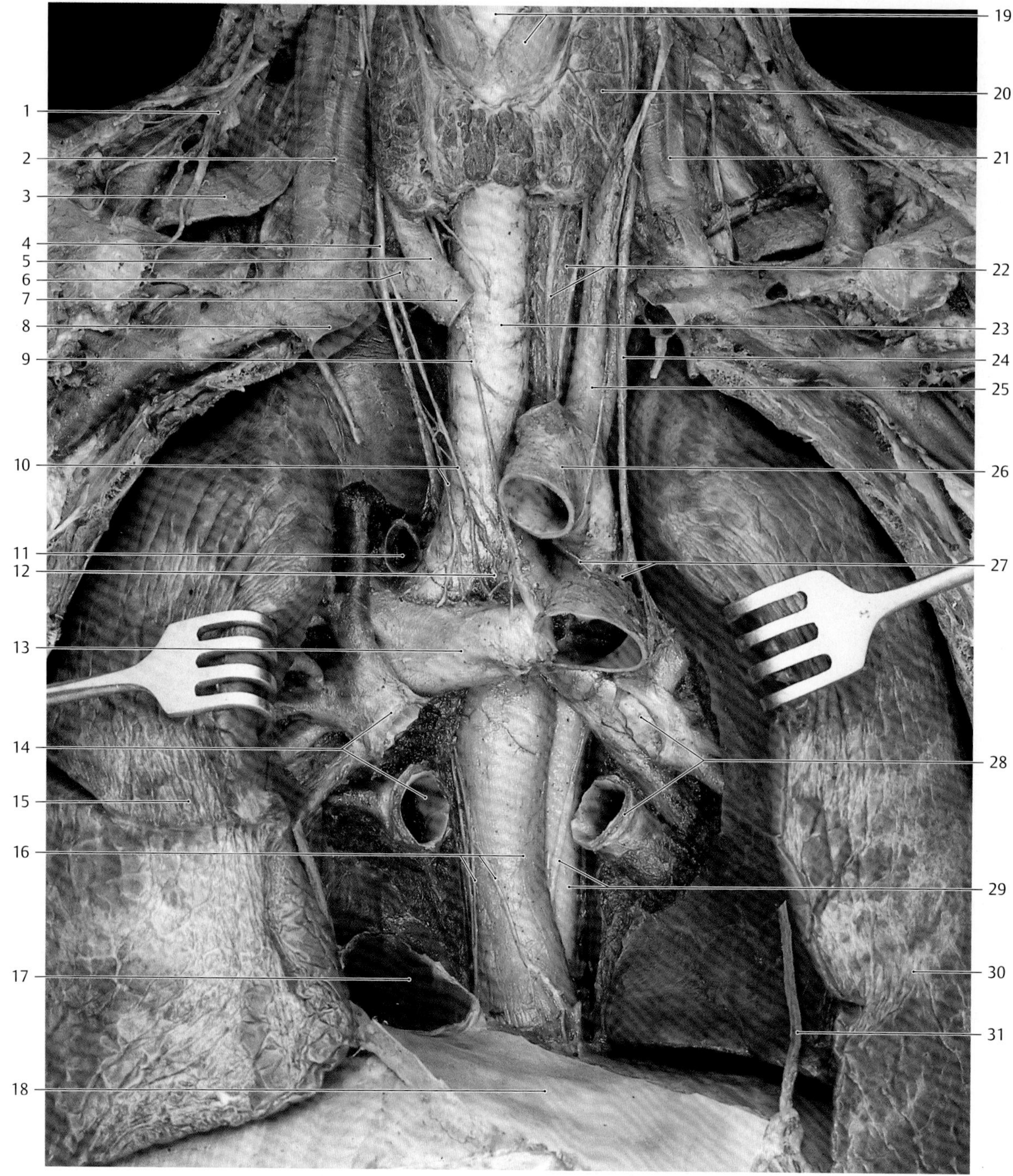


Fig. 5.78 **Posterior mediastinum** (anterior aspect). Heart and pericardium have been removed. Both lungs have been slightly reflected.

1 Supraclavicular nerves
2 Internal jugular vein
3 Omohyoid muscle
4 Right vagus nerve
5 Right common carotid artery
6 Right subclavian artery
7 Brachiocephalic trunk
8 Right brachiocephalic vein
9 Superior cervical cardiac branch of vagus nerve
10 Inferior cervical cardiac branches of vagus nerve
11 Azygos arch (divided)
12 Bifurcation of trachea
13 Right pulmonary artery
14 Right pulmonary veins
15 Right lung
16 Esophagus and branches of right vagus nerve
17 Inferior vena cava
18 Pericardium
19 Larynx (thyroid cartilage, cricothyroid muscle)
20 Thyroid gland
21 Internal jugular vein
22 Esophagus and left recurrent laryngeal nerve
23 Trachea
24 Left vagus nerve
25 Left common carotid artery
26 Aortic arch
27 Left recurrent laryngeal nerve branching off from vagus nerve
28 Left pulmonary veins
29 Thoracic aorta and left vagus nerve
30 Left lung
31 Left phrenic nerve (divided)

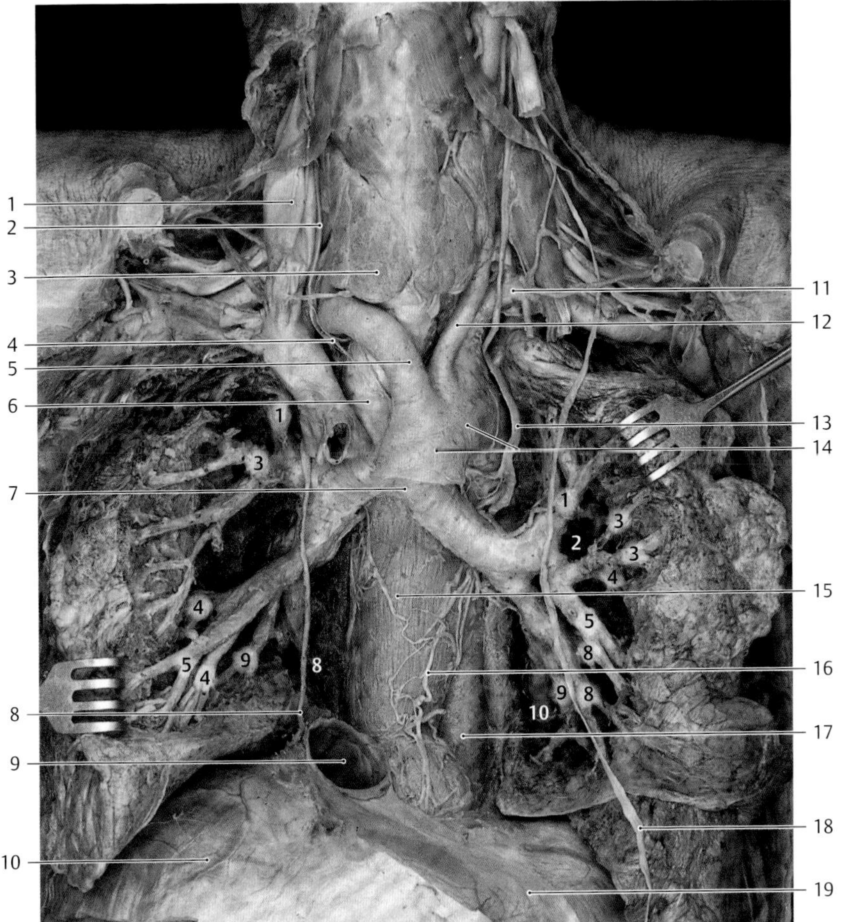


**Fig. 5.79 Bronchial tree in situ** (anterior aspect). Heart and pericardium have been removed. The bronchi of the bronchopulmonary segments have been dissected.
1–10 = numbers of segments (compare with figures on pages 222, 223, and 227).

1 Internal jugular vein
2 Right vagus nerve
3 Thyroid gland
4 Right recurrent laryngeal nerve
5 Brachiocephalic trunk
6 Trachea
7 Bifurcation of trachea
8 Right phrenic nerve
9 Inferior vena cava
10 Diaphragm
11 Left subclavian artery
12 Left common carotid artery
13 Left vagus nerve
14 Aortic arch
15 Esophagus
16 Esophageal plexus
17 Thoracic aorta
18 Left phrenic nerve
19 Pericardium at the central tendon of diaphragm
20 Superior vena cava
21 Pulmonary veins and left atrium

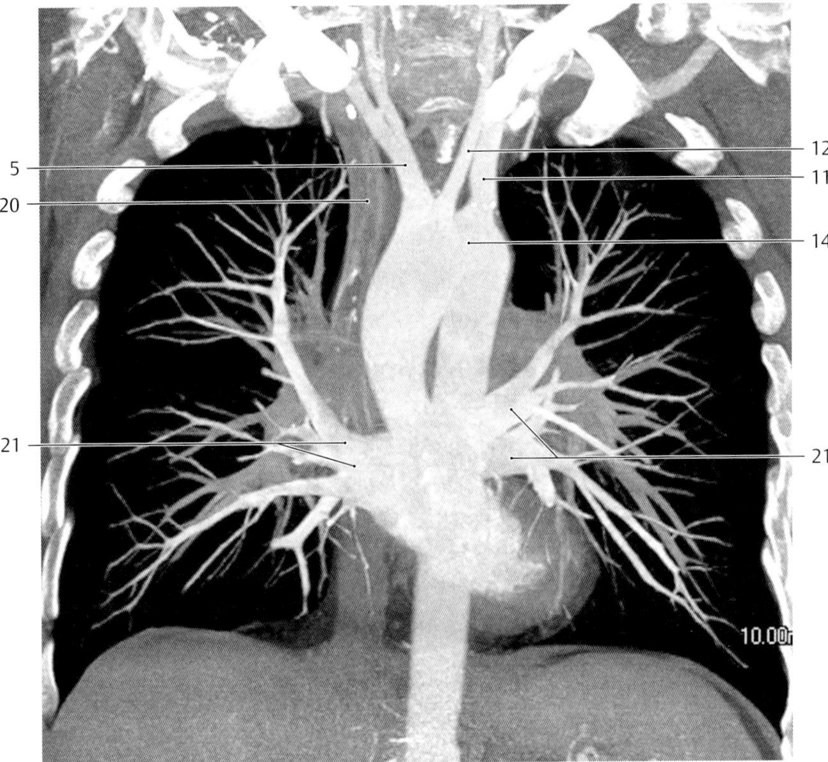


**Fig. 5.80 Frontal section through the thoracic cavity** showing the mediastinal vessels (CT scan). (Courtesy of Prof. Uder, Institute of Radiology, University Hospital Erlangen, Germany.)

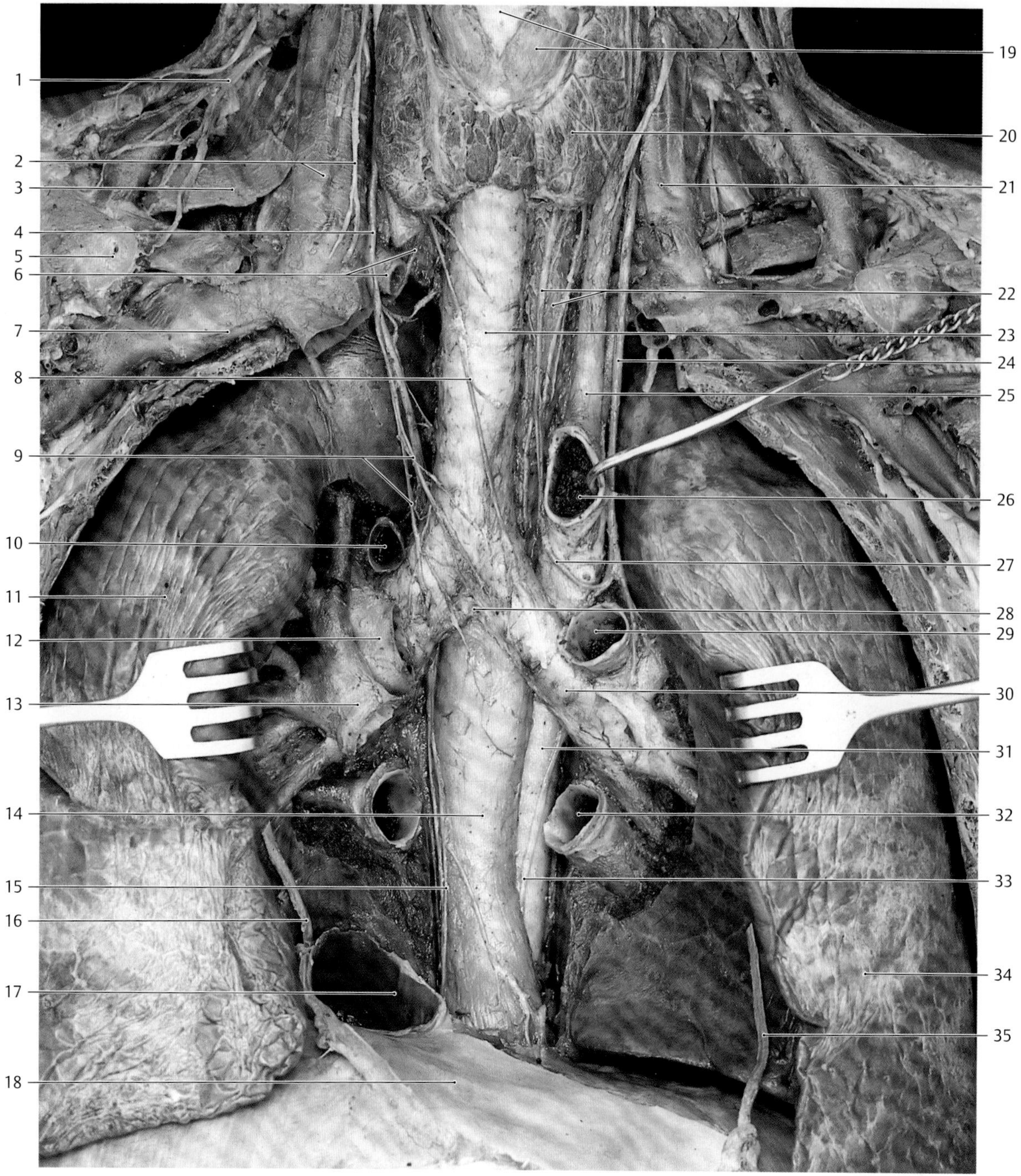


**Fig. 5.81 Posterior mediastinum** (anterior aspect). The heart with the pericardium has been removed, and the lungs and aortic arch have been slightly reflected to show the vagus nerves and their branches.

1 Supraclavicular nerves
2 Right internal jugular vein with ansa cervicalis
3 Omohyoid muscle
4 Right vagus nerve
5 Clavicle
6 Right subclavian artery and recurrent laryngeal nerve
7 Right subclavian vein
8 Superior cervical cardiac branch of vagus nerve
9 Inferior cervical cardiac branch of vagus nerve
10 Azygos arch (divided)
11 Right lung
12 Right pulmonary artery
13 Right pulmonary veins
14 Esophagus
15 Esophageal plexus
16 Right phrenic nerve (divided)
17 Inferior vena cava
18 Pericardium covering the diaphragm
19 Larynx (thyroid cartilage and cricothyroid muscle)
20 Thyroid gland
21 Left internal jugular vein
22 Esophagus and left recurrent laryngeal nerve
23 Trachea
24 Left vagus nerve
25 Left common carotid artery
26 Aortic arch
27 Left recurrent laryngeal nerve
28 Bifurcation of trachea
29 Left pulmonary artery
30 Left primary bronchus
31 Descending aorta
32 Left pulmonary veins
33 Branch of left vagus nerve
34 Left lung
35 Left phrenic nerve (divided)

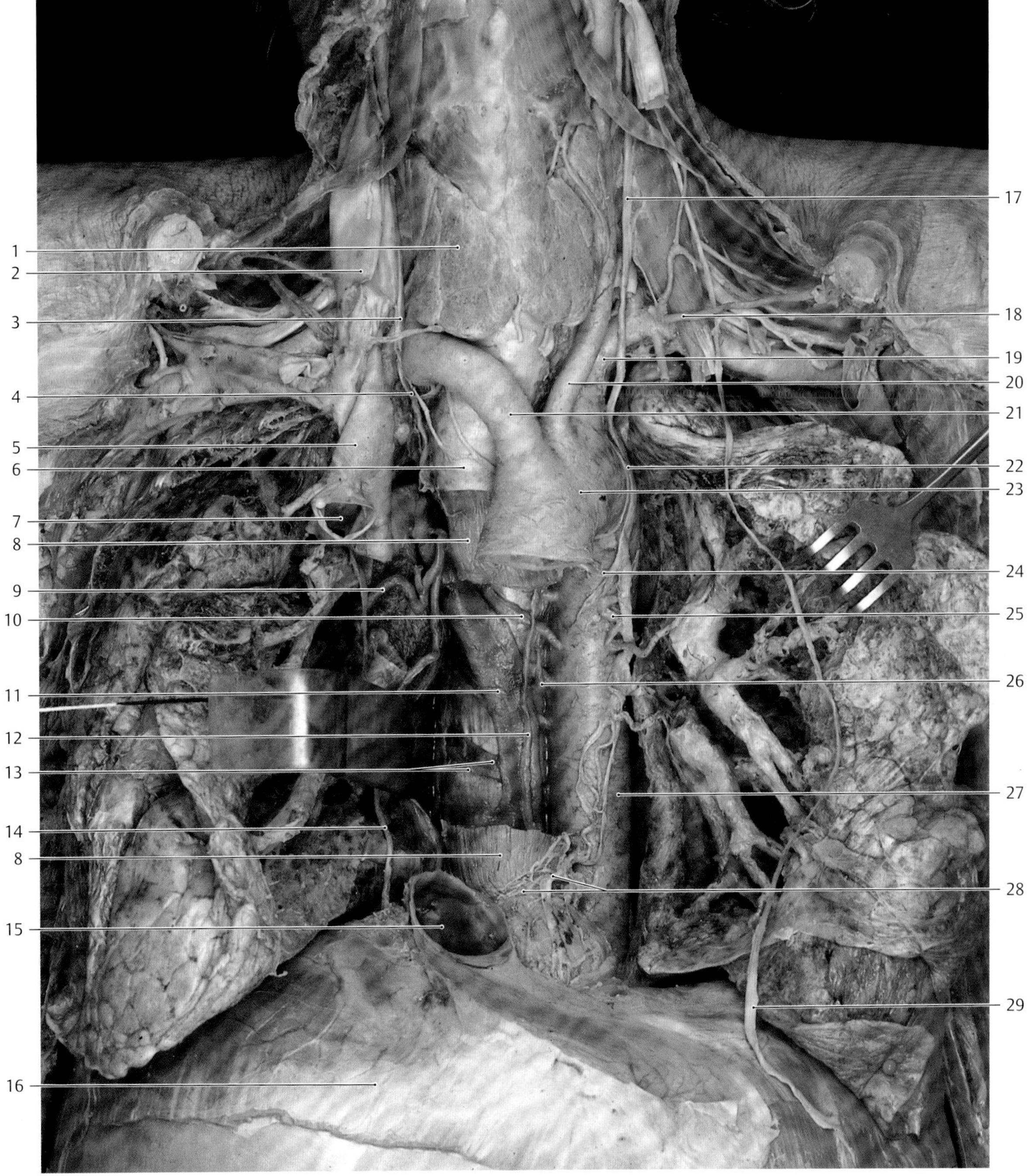


**Fig. 5.82 Posterior mediastinum** (anterior aspect). The heart and distal part of the esophagus have been removed to display the vessels and nerves of the posterior mediastinum.

1 Thyroid gland
2 Right internal jugular vein
3 Right vagus nerve
4 Point where right recurrent laryngeal nerve is branching off the vagus nerve
5 Right brachiocephalic vein
6 Trachea
7 Left brachiocephalic vein (reflected)
8 Esophagus
9 Right bronchial artery
10 Posterior intercostal artery
11 Azygos vein
12 Thoracic duct
13 Posterior intercostal artery and vein (in front of the vertebral column)
14 Right phrenic nerve
15 Inferior vena cava
16 Diaphragm
17 Left vagus nerve
18 Thyrocervical trunk
19 Left subclavian artery
20 Left common carotid artery
21 Brachiocephalic trunk
22 Left vagus nerve
23 Aortic arch
24 Left recurrent laryngeal nerve
25 Left bronchial artery
26 Lymph node
27 Thoracic aorta
28 Esophageal plexus
29 Left phrenic nerve

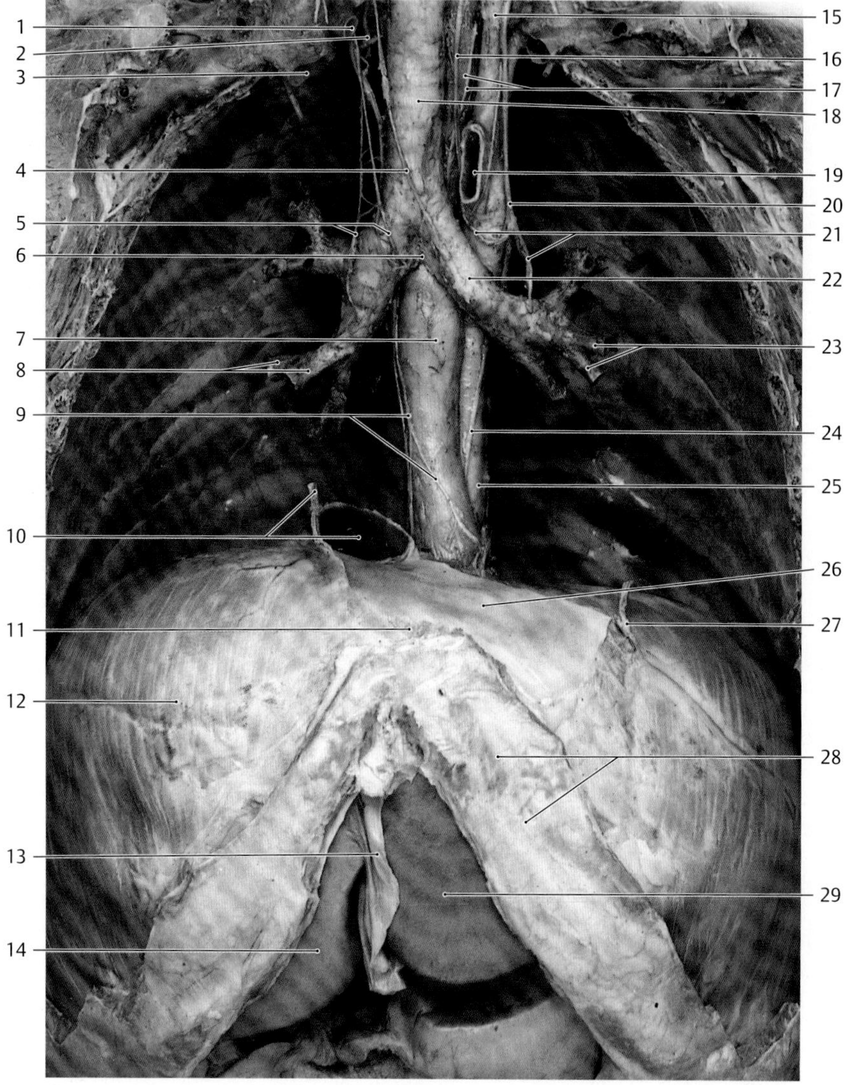


**Fig. 5.83 Posterior mediastinum and diaphragm** (anterior aspect). Heart and lungs have been removed, the costal margin remains in place. Note the different courses of left and right vagus.

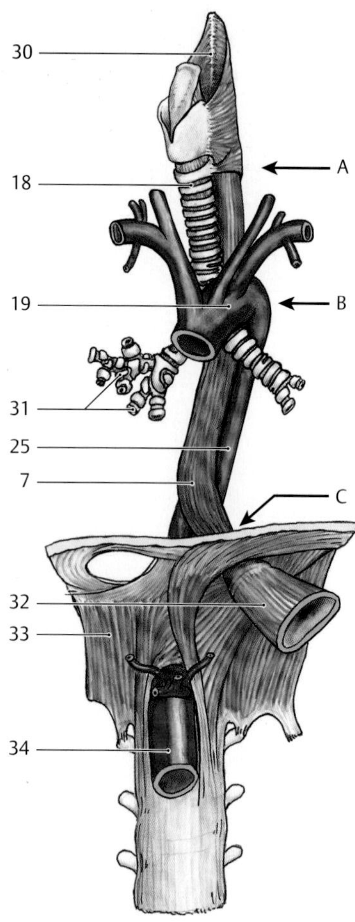


**Fig. 5.84 Posterior mediastinal organs with diaphragm** (anterior aspect). Three regions in which the esophagus is narrowed are shown.

A = Upper esophageal sphincter (at the level of the cricoid cartilage)
B = Middle esophageal sphincter (at the level of the aortic arch)
C = Lower esophageal sphincter (at the level of the diaphragm)

1 Right subclavian artery
2 Right recurrent laryngeal nerve
3 Right brachiocephalic vein
4 Superior cervical cardiac nerve
5 Inferior cervical cardiac nerves and pulmonary branches
6 Bifurcation of trachea
7 Esophagus (thoracic part)
8 Bronchi of lateral and medial segments of middle lobe
9 Esophageal plexus and branches of right vagus nerve
10 Inferior vena cava and right phrenic nerve (cut)
11 Sternal part of diaphragm
12 Costal part of diaphragm
13 Falciform ligament of liver
14 Liver (quadrate lobe)
15 Left common carotid artery
16 Left recurrent laryngeal nerve
17 Esophageal branches of left vagus nerve and esophagus
18 Trachea
19 Aortic arch
20 Left vagus nerve
21 Left recurrent laryngeal nerve with inferior cardiac nerve
22 Left primary bronchus
23 Superior and inferior lingular bronchi
24 Esophageal plexus of left vagus nerve
25 Descending aorta
26 Central tendon of diaphragm covered with pericardium
27 Left phrenic nerve (divided)
28 Costal margin
29 Liver (left lobe)
30 Pharynx
31 Secondary bronchi
32 Esophagus (abdominal part)
33 Diaphragm
34 Abdominal aorta

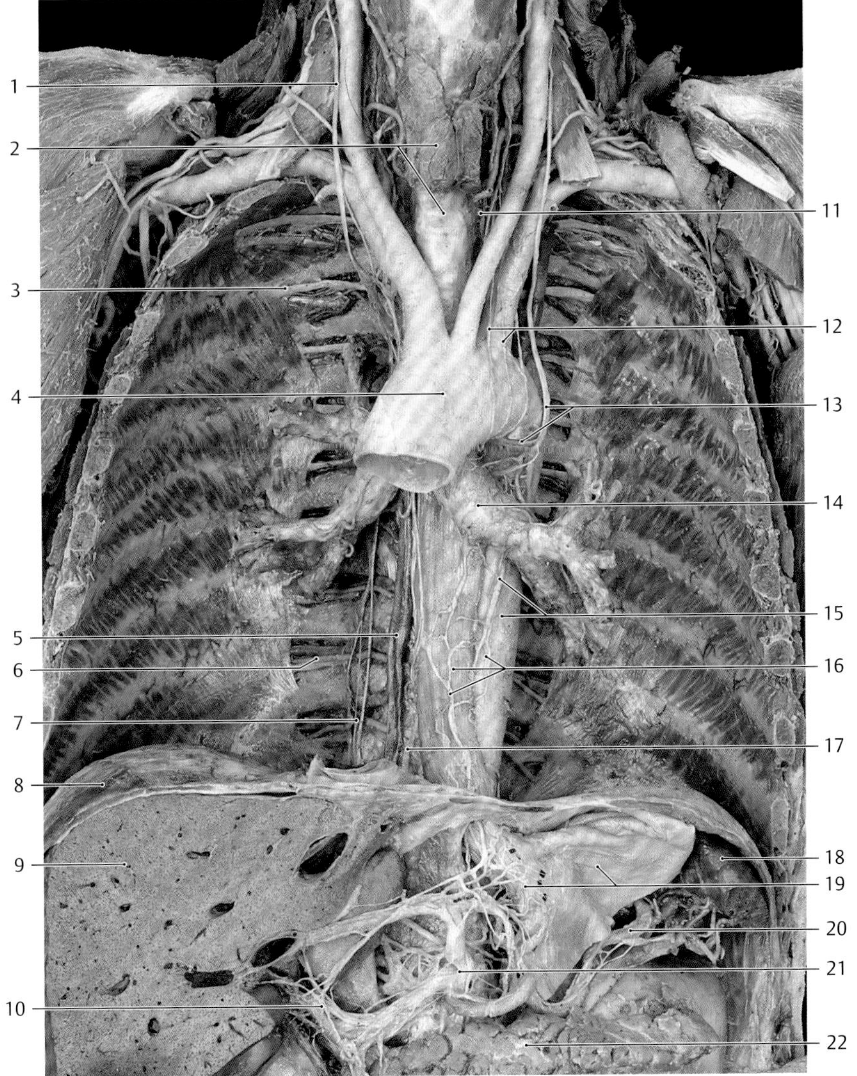


**Fig. 5.85 Posterior mediastinum** (anterior aspect). Dissection of thoracic aorta and esophagus with vagus nerve branches.

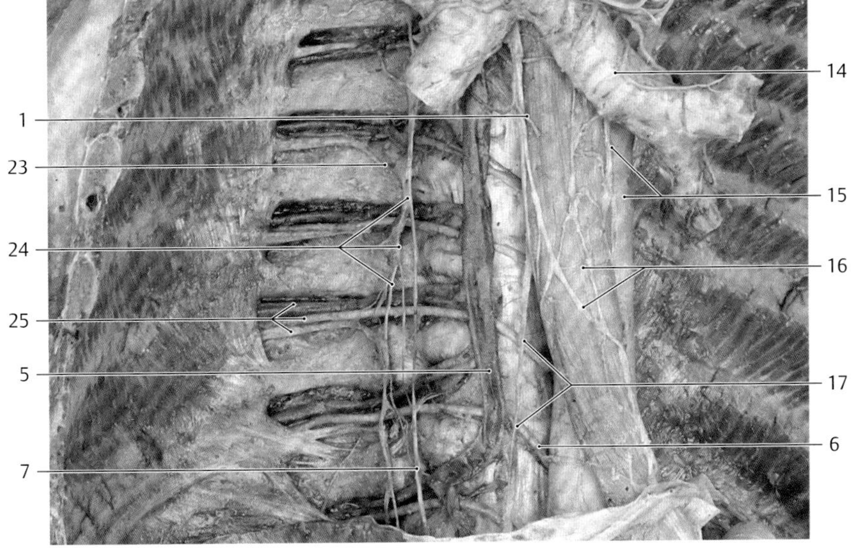


**Fig. 5.86 Inferior segment of posterior mediastinum** (anterior aspect).

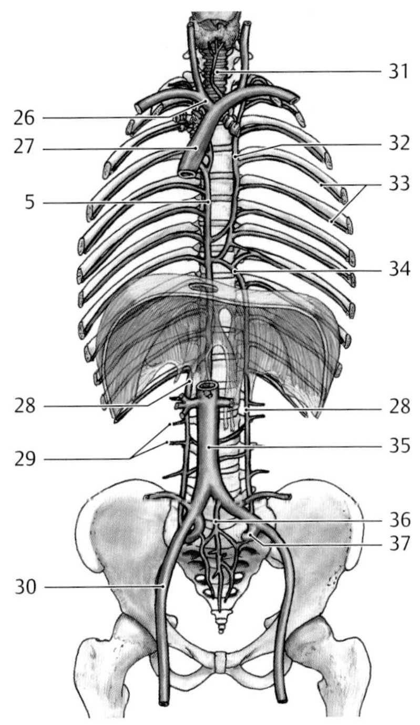


**Fig. 5.87 Veins of the posterior wall of thoracic and abdominal cavities** (anterior aspect).

1 Right vagus nerve
2 Thyroid gland and trachea
3 Intercostal nerve
4 Aortic arch
5 Azygos vein
6 Posterior intercostal artery
7 Greater splanchnic nerve
8 Diaphragm
9 Liver
10 Proper hepatic artery and hepatic plexus
11 Left recurrent laryngeal nerve
12 Inferior cervical cardiac nerves
13 Left vagus nerve and left recurrent laryngeal nerve
14 Left primary bronchus
15 Thoracic aorta and left vagus nerve
16 Esophagus and esophageal plexus
17 Thoracic duct
18 Spleen
19 Anterior gastric plexus and stomach (divided)
20 Splenic artery and splenic plexus
21 Celiac trunk and celiac plexus
22 Pancreas
23 Ramus communicans
24 Sympathetic trunk and sympathetic ganglion
25 Posterior intercostal vein and artery and intercostal nerve
26 Right brachiocephalic vein
27 Superior vena cava
28 Ascending lumbar vein
29 Lumbar veins
30 Right external iliac vein
31 Trachea
32 Accessory hemiazygos vein
33 Posterior intercostal veins
34 Hemiazygos vein
35 Inferior vena cava
36 Median sacral vein
37 Internal iliac vein

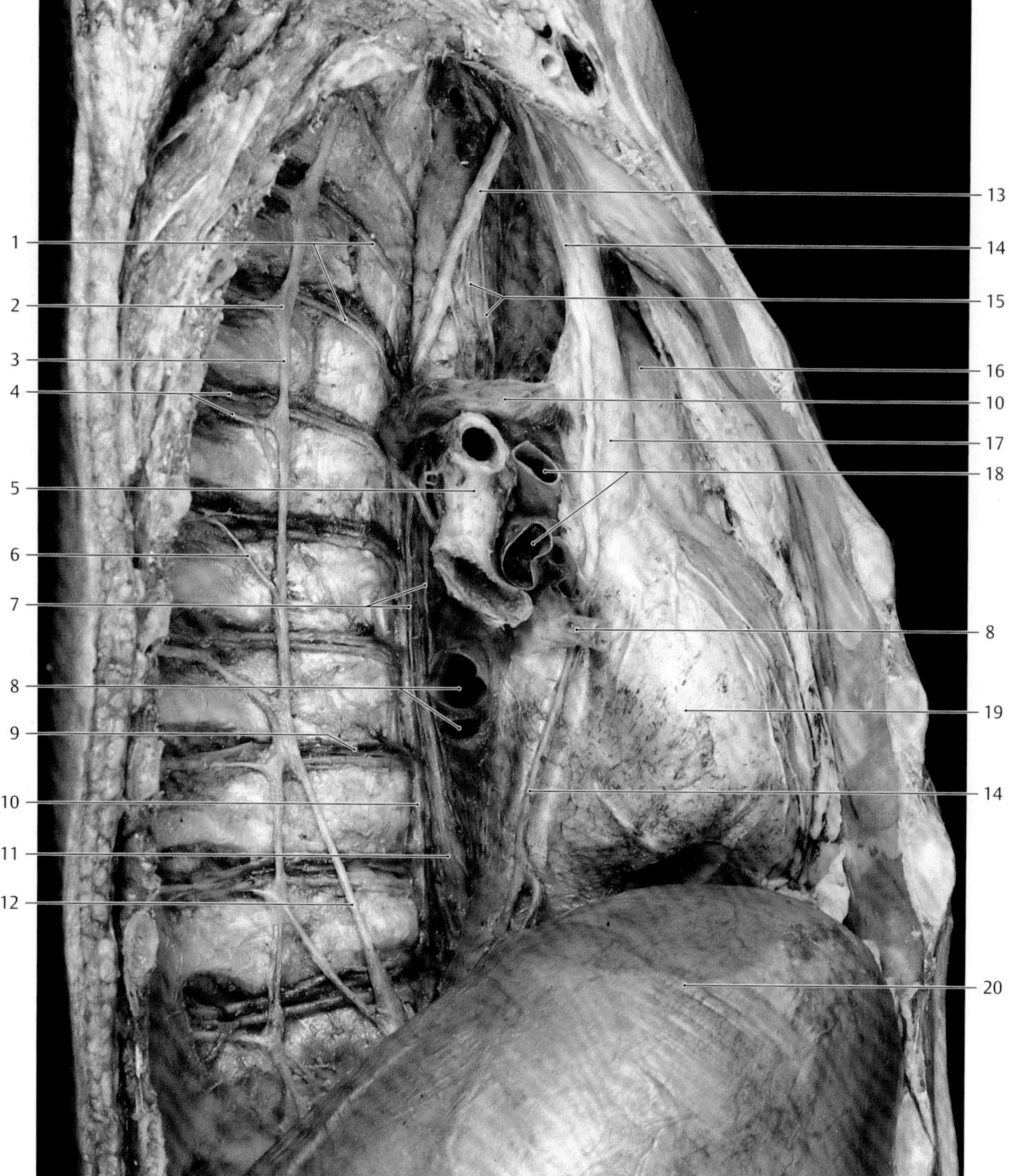


**Fig. 5.88 Posterior mediastinum** (right lateral aspect). Right lung and pleura of right half of the thorax have been removed.

1 Posterior intercostal arteries
2 Ganglion of sympathetic trunk
3 Sympathetic trunk
4 Vessels and nerves of the intercostal space (from above: posterior intercostal vein and artery and intercostal nerve)
5 Right primary bronchus
6 Ramus communicans of sympathetic trunk
7 Esophageal plexus (branches of right vagus nerve)
8 Pulmonary veins
9 Posterior intercostal vein
10 Azygos vein
11 Esophagus
12 Greater splanchnic nerve
13 Right vagus nerve
14 Right phrenic nerve
15 Inferior cervical cardiac branches of vagus nerve
16 Aortic arch
17 Superior vena cava
18 Right pulmonary artery
19 Heart with pericardium
20 Diaphragm

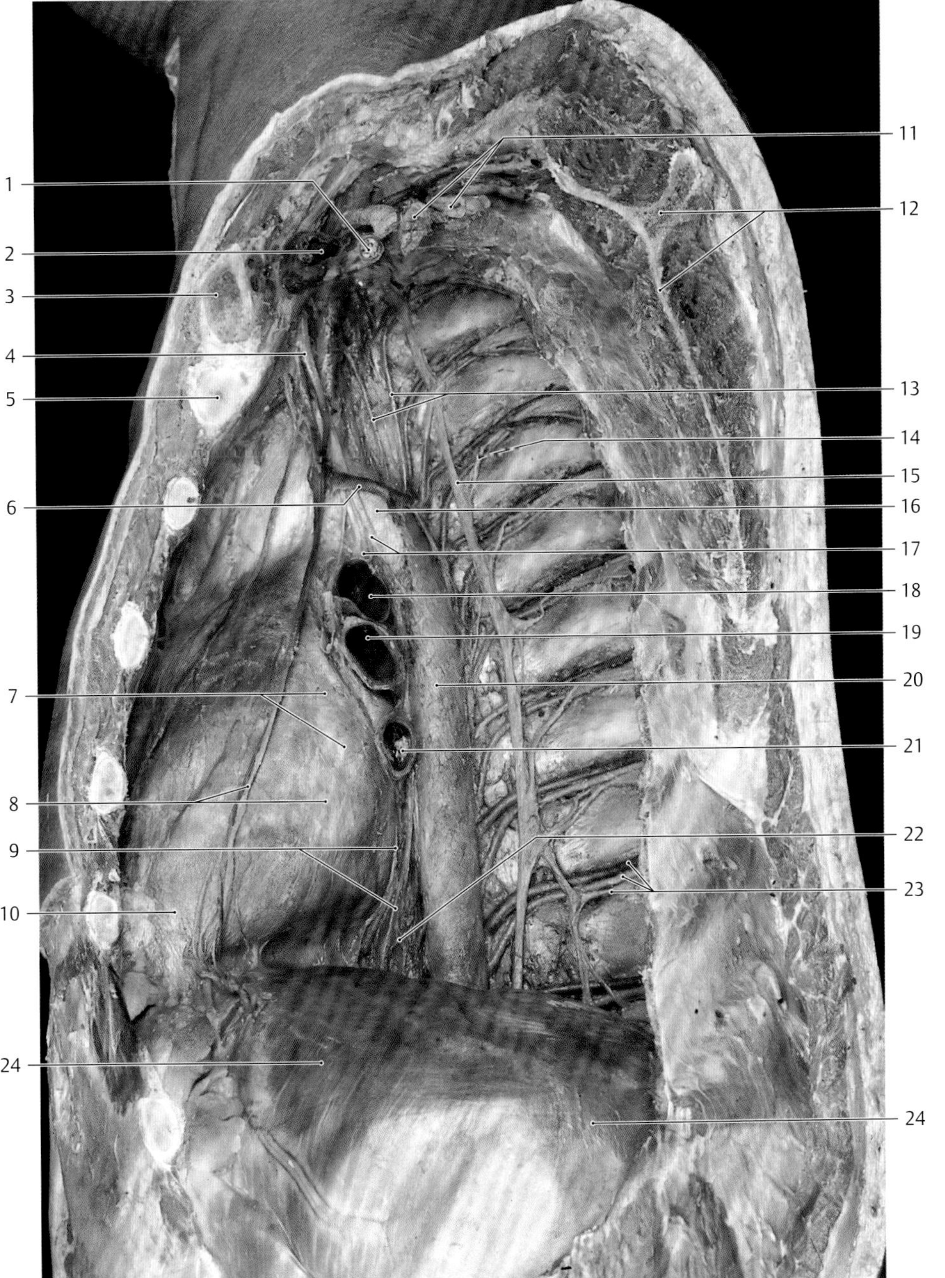


**Fig. 5.89 Posterior and superior mediastinum** (left lateral aspect). The heart with the pericardium is located in situ. Within the posterior mediastinum the descending thoracic aorta and the sympathetic trunk are shown.

**Fig. 5.90 Main branches of descending aorta** (anterior aspect).

1 Subclavian artery
2 Subclavian vein
3 Clavicle (divided)
4 Left vagus nerve
5 First rib (divided)
6 Left superior intercostal vein
7 Left atrium with pericardium
8 Left phrenic nerve and pericardiacophrenic artery and vein
9 Esophageal plexus (branches derived from left vagus nerve)
10 Apex of the heart with pericardium
11 Brachial plexus
12 Scapula (divided)
13 Posterior intercostal arteries
14 White ramus communicans of sympathetic trunk
15 Sympathetic trunk
16 Aortic arch
17 Left vagus nerve and left recurrent laryngeal nerve
18 Left pulmonary artery
19 Left primary bronchus
20 Thoracic aorta
21 Pulmonary vein
22 Esophagus (thoracic part)
23 Posterior intercostal artery and vein and intercostal nerve
24 Diaphragm
25 Common carotid artery
26 Subclavian artery
27 Highest intercostal artery
28 Bifurcation of trachea
29 Celiac trunk
30 Renal artery
31 Superior mesenteric artery
32 Inferior mesenteric artery
33 Common iliac artery

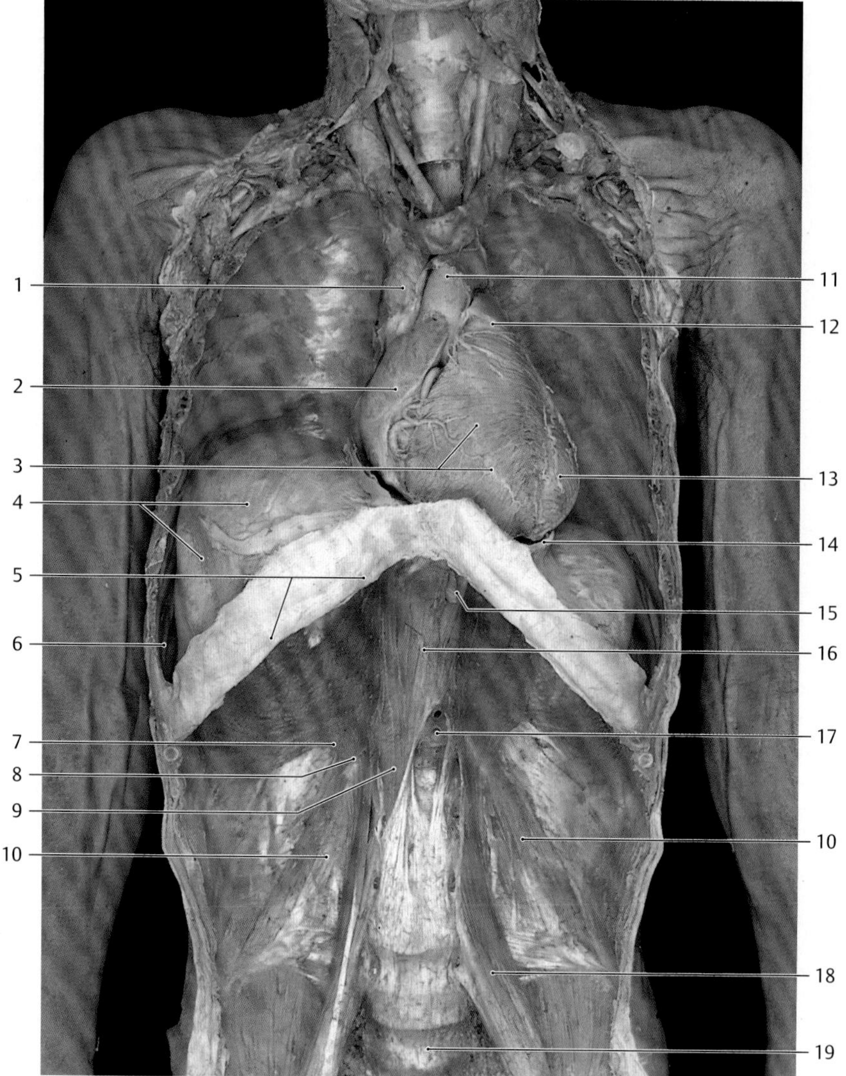


1 Superior vena cava
2 Right atrium
3 Right ventricle
4 Costal part of diaphragm
5 Costal margin
6 Position of costodiaphragmatic recess
7 Lateral arcuate ligament
8 Medial arcuate ligament
9 Right crus of lumbar part of diaphragm
10 Quadratus lumborum muscle
11 Ascending aorta
12 Pulmonary trunk
13 Left ventricle
14 Pericardium and diaphragm
15 Esophageal hiatus and abdominal part of esophagus (cut)
16 Lumbar part of diaphragm
17 Aortic hiatus
18 Psoas major muscle
19 Lumbar vertebrae

**Fig. 5.91 Diaphragm in situ** (anterior aspect). Anterior walls of the thoracic and abdominal cavities have been removed. The natural position of the heart above the central tendon on the diaphragm is shown.

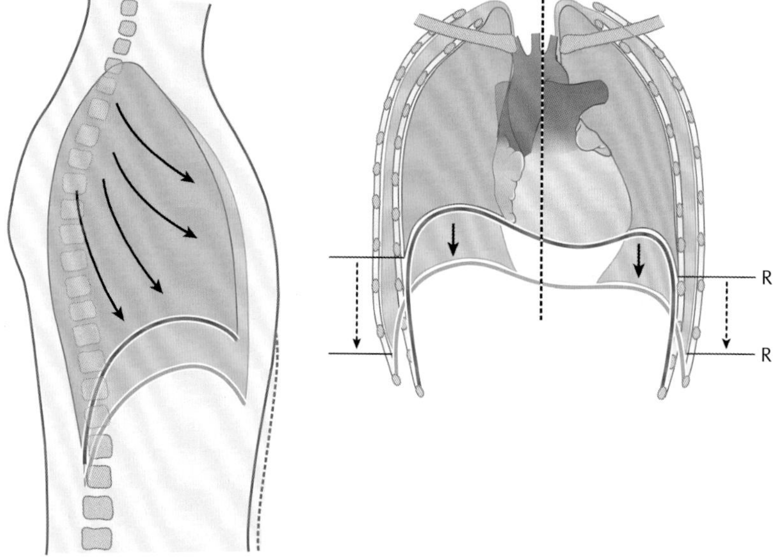


**Fig. 5.92 Changes in the position of the diaphragm and thoracic cage during respiration** (left [lateral aspect]; right [anterior aspect]). During inspiration the diaphragm moves downward and the lower part of the thoracic cage expands forward and laterally, causing the costodiaphragmatic recess (R) to enlarge (cf. dotted arrows).

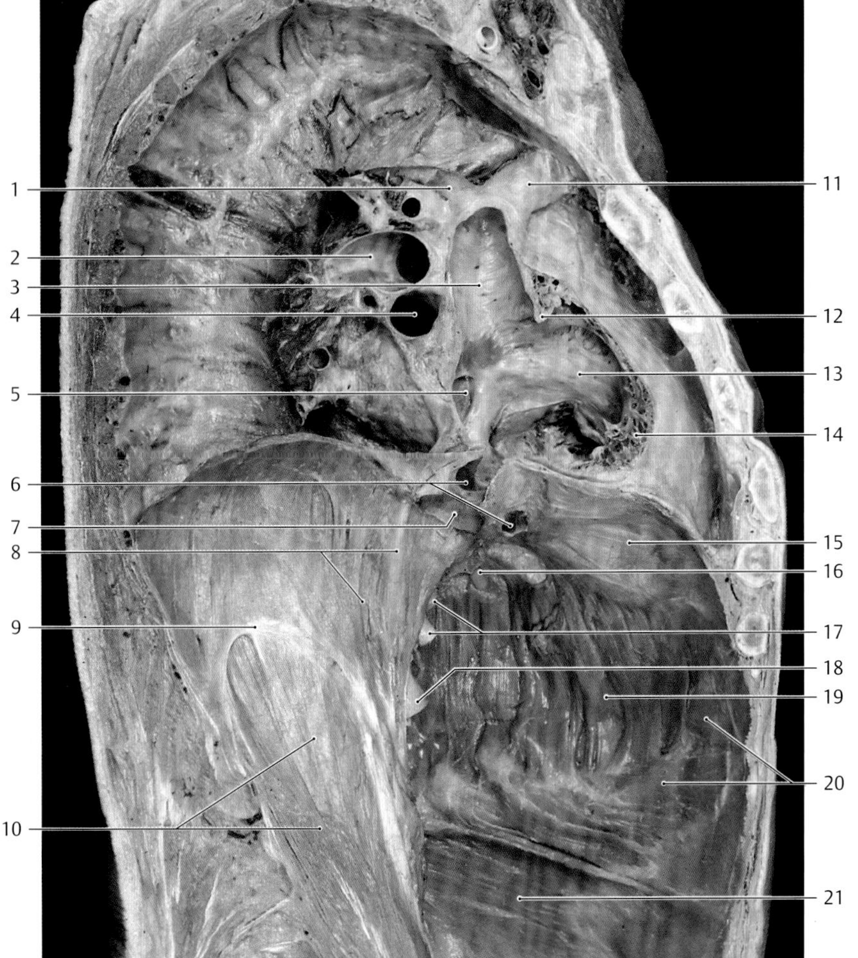


1 Azygos venous arch
2 Right pulmonary artery
3 Superior vena cava
4 Right pulmonary vein
5 Fossa ovalis
6 Hepatic veins
7 Inferior vena cava
8 Right crus of lumbar part of diaphragm
9 Medial arcuate ligament
10 Psoas major muscle
11 Left brachiocephalic vein
12 Crista terminalis
13 Right atrium
14 Right auricle
15 Central tendon of diaphragm
16 Esophagus
17 Celiac trunk and superior mesenteric artery
18 Aorta
19 Costal part of diaphragm
20 Costal margin
21 Transverse abdominal muscle

Fig. 5.93 **Diaphragm and thoracic organs.** Paramedian section to the right of the median plane through the thoracic and upper abdominal cavities. The plane passes through the superior and inferior vena cava just to the right of the vertebral bodies. Most of the heart remains in situ to the left of this plane (viewed from the right side).

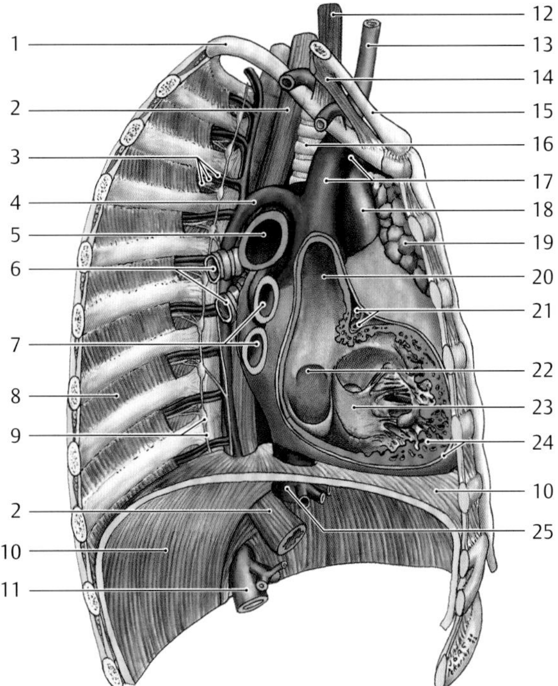


1 First rib
2 Esophagus
3 Intercostal artery, vein, and nerve
4 Azygos venous arch
5 Pulmonal artery
6 Right bronchi
7 Pulmonary veins
8 Internal intercostal muscle
9 Sympathetic trunk
10 Diaphragm
11 Abdominal aorta
12 Anterior scalene muscle
13 Internal jugular vein
14 Subclavius muscle
15 Clavicle
16 Trachea
17 Junction between superior vena cava and left brachiocephalic vein
18 Aorta
19 Remnants of thymus gland
20 Entrance of superior vena cava into the right atrium
21 Right coronary artery and vein
22 Fossa ovalis
23 Right atrioventricular valve and anterior papillary muscle
24 Right ventricle with pericardium
25 Inferior vena cava

Fig. 5.94 **Diaphragm and thoracic organs** (paramedian section). The heart is partly dissected.

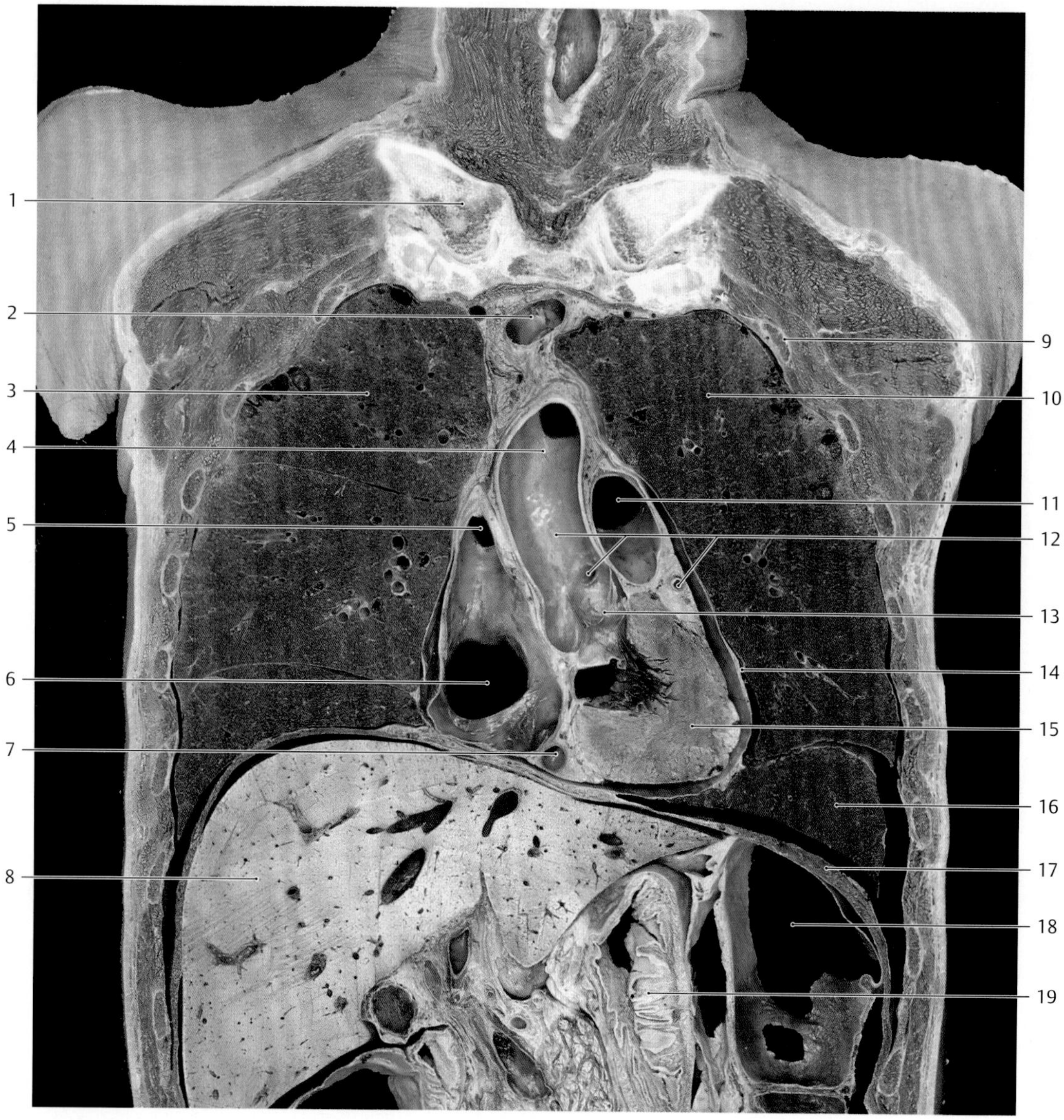

**Fig. 5.95 Coronal section through the thorax** at the level of the ascending aorta (anterior aspect).

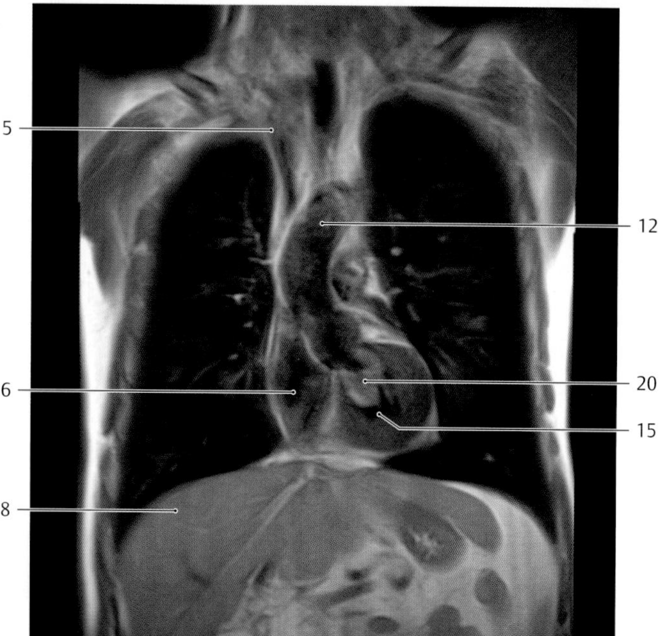


1 Clavicle
2 Left brachiocephalic vein
3 Upper lobe of right lung
4 Aortic arch
5 Superior vena cava
6 Right atrium (entrance of inferior vena cava)
7 Coronary sinus
8 Liver
9 Second rib
10 Upper lobe of left lung
11 Pulmonary trunk
12 Ascending aorta and left coronary artery
13 Aortic valve
14 Pericardium
15 Myocardium of left ventricle
16 Lower lobe of left lung
17 Diaphragm
18 Colic flexures
19 Stomach
20 Brachiocephalic trunk

**Fig. 5.96 Coronal section through the thorax** at the level of the ascending aorta (MRI scan). (Courtesy of Prof. Uder, Institute of Radiology, University Hospital Erlangen, Germany.)

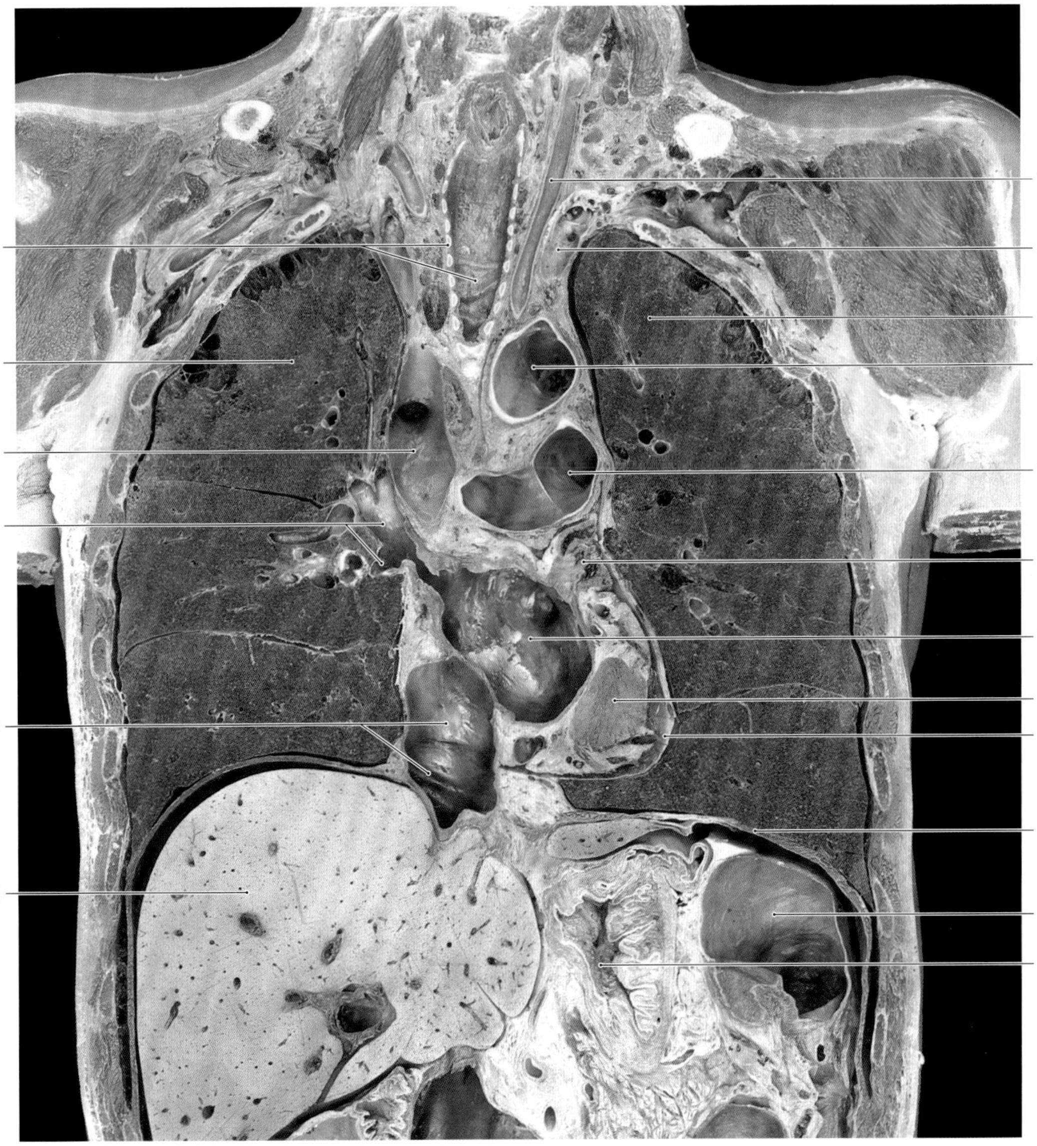

**Fig. 5.97 Coronal section through the thorax** at the level of superior and inferior vena cava (anterior aspect).

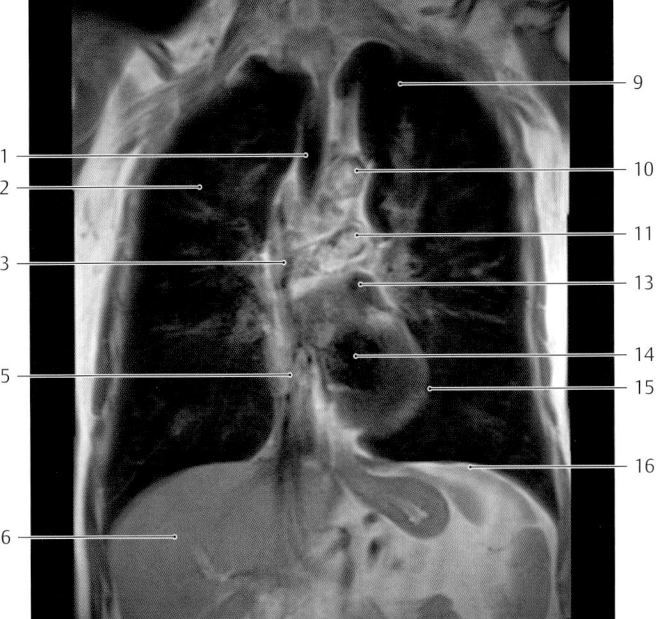


1 Trachea
2 Upper lobe of right lung
3 Superior vena cava
4 Right pulmonary veins
5 Inferior vena cava and right atrium
6 Liver
7 Left common carotid artery
8 Left subclavian vein
9 Upper lobe of left lung
10 Aortic arch
11 Left pulmonary artery
12 Left auricle
13 Left atrium with orifices of pulmonary veins
14 Left ventricle (myocardium)
15 Pericardium
16 Diaphragm
17 Left colic flexure
18 Stomach

**Fig. 5.98 Coronal section through the thorax** at the level of the superior vena cava (MRI scan). (Courtesy of Prof. Uder, Institute of Radiology, University Hospital Erlangen, Germany.)

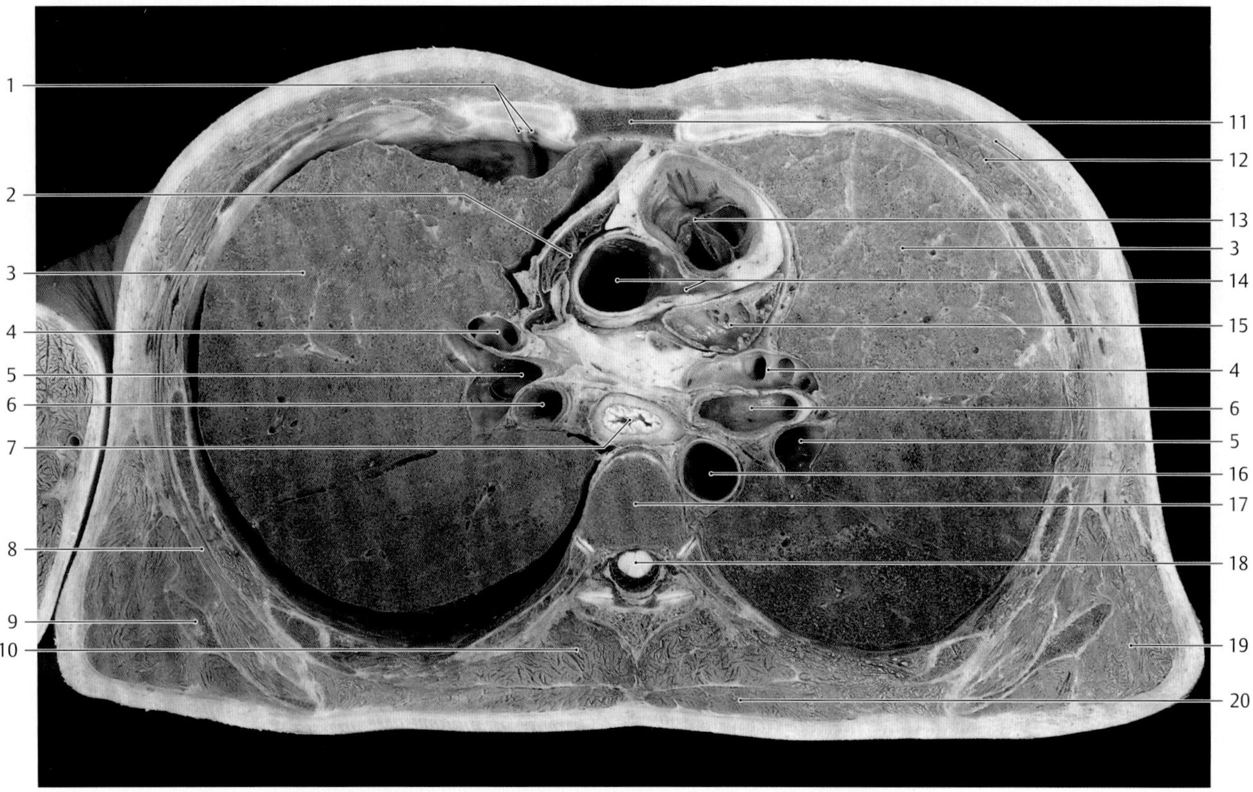


Fig. 5.99 **Horizontal section through the thorax.** Section 1 (from below).

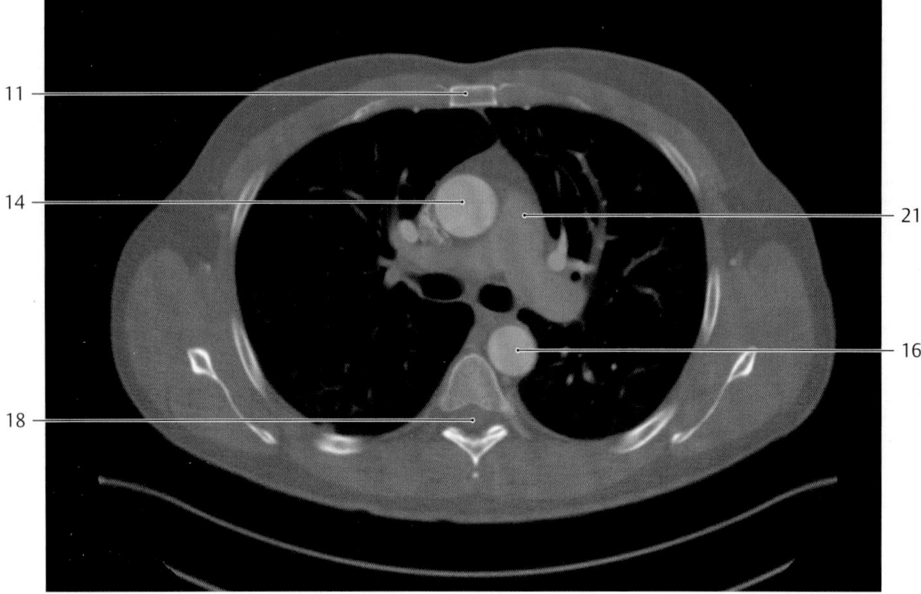


Fig. 5.100 **Horizontal section through the thorax** at the level of section 1 (MRI scan). (Courtesy of Prof. Uder, Institute of Radiology, University Hospital Erlangen, Germany.)

1 Internal thoracic artery and vein
2 Right atrium
3 Lung
4 Pulmonary artery
5 Pulmonary vein
6 Primary bronchus
7 Esophagus
8 Serratus anterior muscle
9 Scapula
10 Erector spinae muscle
11 Sternum
12 Pectoralis major and minor muscles
13 Conus arteriosus (right ventricle) and pulmonic valve
14 Ascending aorta and left coronary artery (Fig. 5.99 only)
15 Left atrium
16 Descending aorta
17 Thoracic vertebra
18 Spinal cord
19 Latissimus dorsi muscle
20 Trapezius muscle
21 Pulmonary trunk

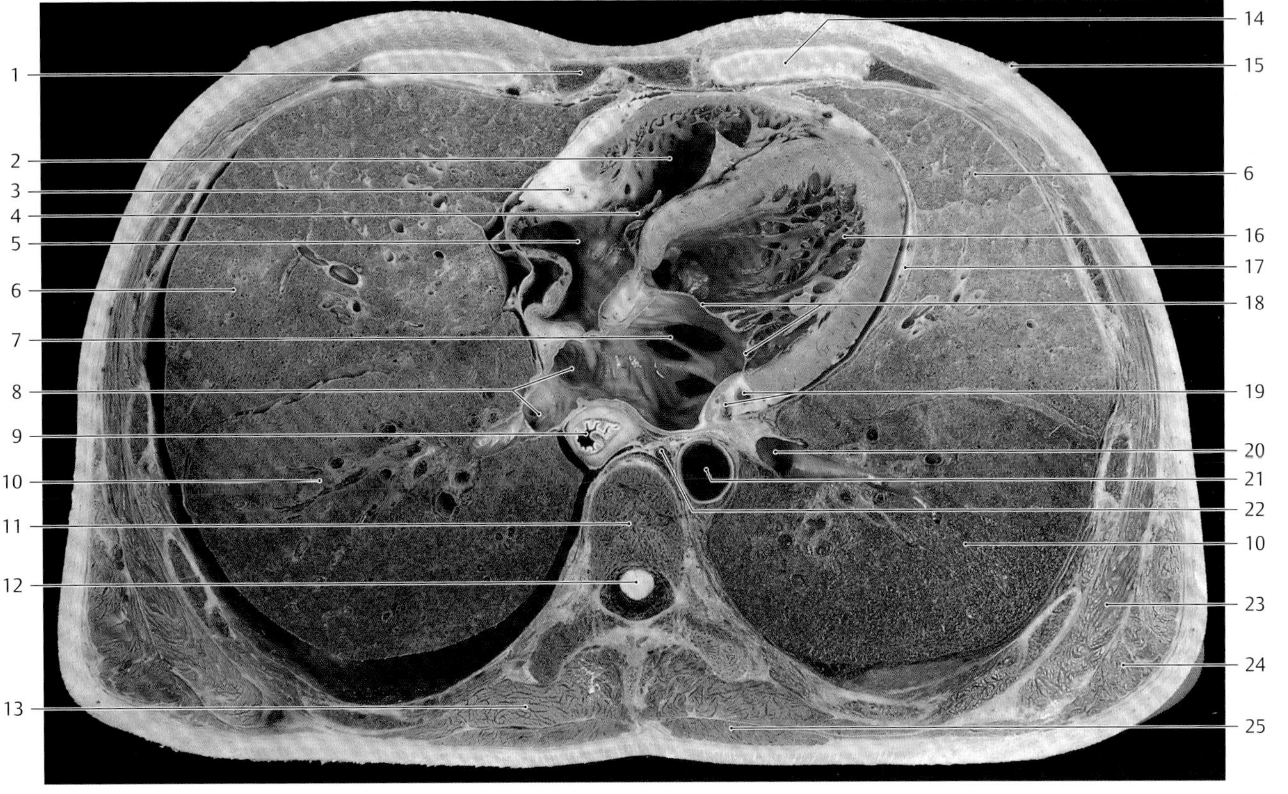


Fig. 5.101 **Horizontal section through the thorax.** Section 2 (from below).

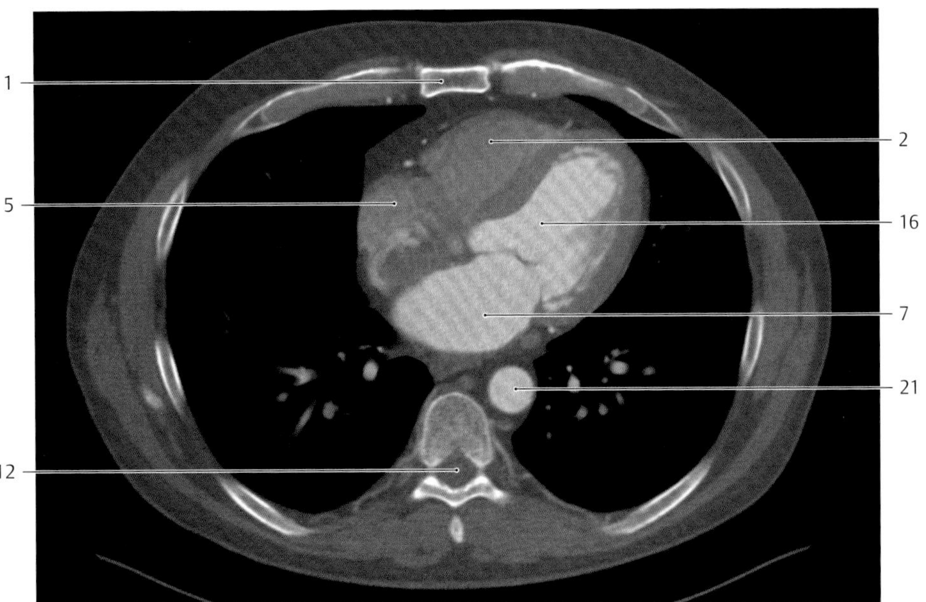


Fig. 5.102 **Horizontal section through the thorax** at the level of section 2 (MRI scan). (Courtesy of Prof. Uder, Institute of Radiology, University Hospital Erlangen, Germany.)

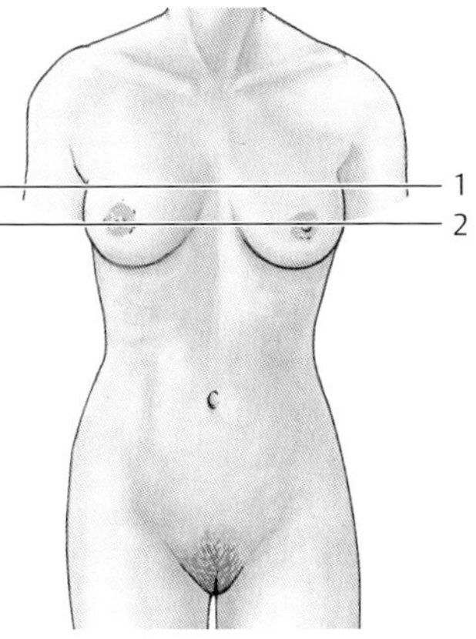


Fig. 5.103 **Horizontal section through the thorax.** Levels of the sections are indicated.

1 Sternum
2 Right ventricle
3 Right coronary artery
4 Right atrioventricular valve
5 Right atrium
6 Upper lobe of lung
7 Left atrium
8 Pulmonary veins
9 Esophagus
10 Lower lobe of lung
11 Thoracic vertebra
12 Spinal cord
13 Erector spinae muscle
14 Costal cartilage
15 Nipple
16 Left ventricle
17 Pericardium
18 Left atrioventricular valve
19 Left coronary artery and coronary sinus
20 Pulmonary vein
21 Descending aorta
22 Accessory hemiazygos vein
23 Serratus anterior muscle
24 Latissimus dorsi muscle
25 Trapezius muscle

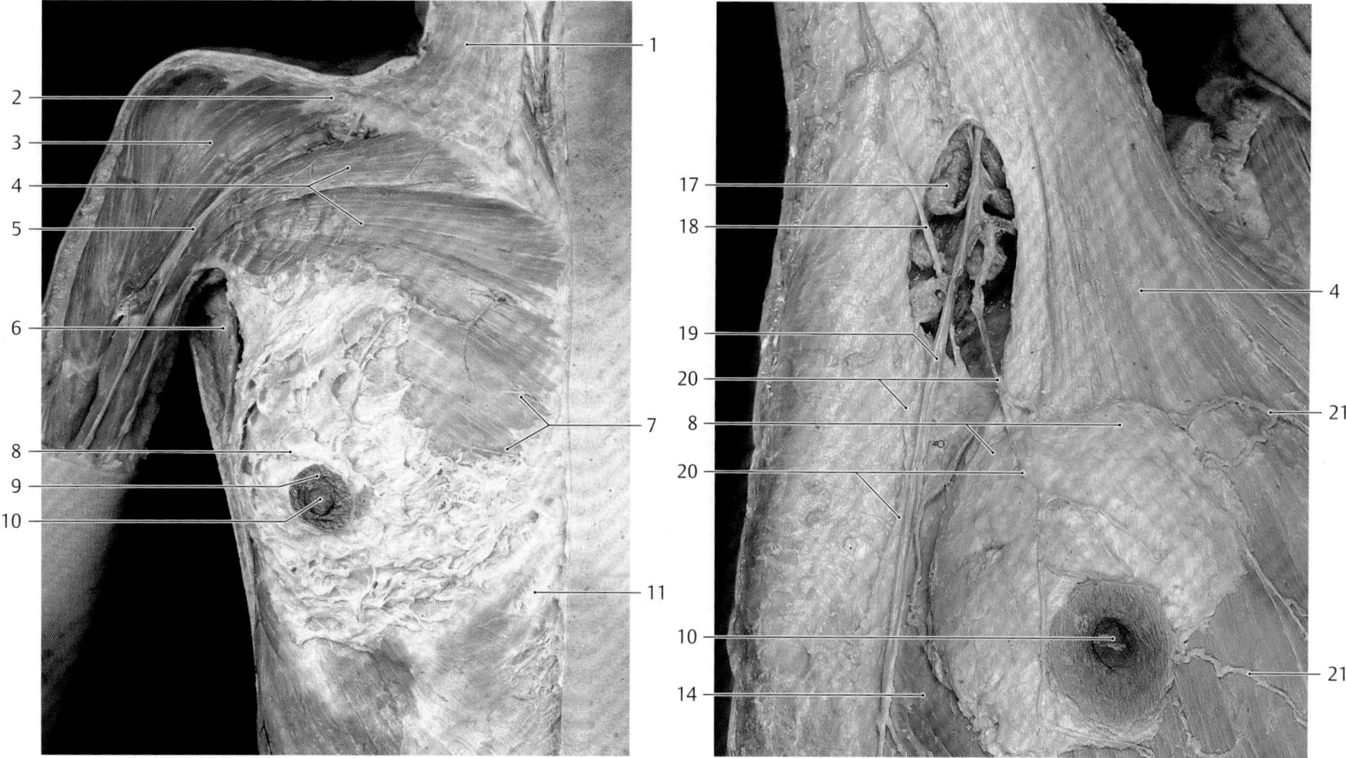


Fig. 5.104 **Dissection of mammary gland** (anterior aspect).

Fig. 5.105 **Dissection of mammary gland and axillary lymph nodes.**

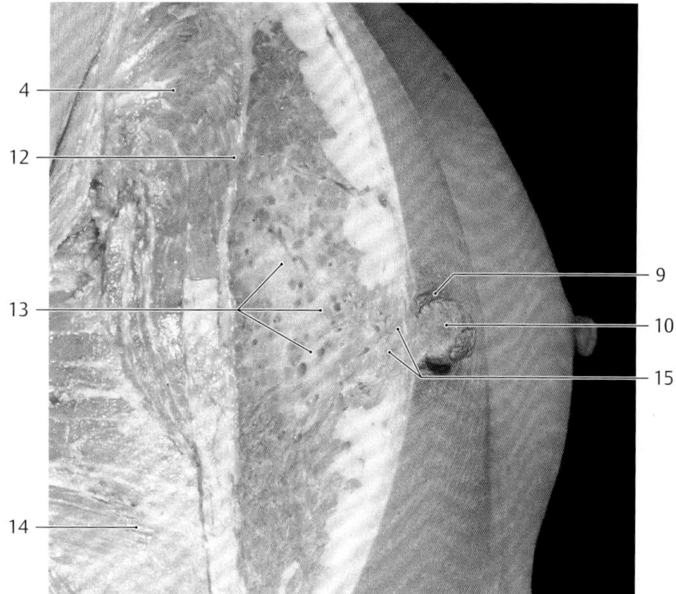


Fig. 5.106 **Mammary gland** of a pregnant female (sagittal section).

Fig. 5.107 **Lymphatics of the mammary gland.** Most lymph vessels drain into the axillary lymph nodes.

1 Platysma muscle
2 Clavicle
3 Deltoid muscle
4 Pectoralis major muscle
5 Deltopectoral groove and cephalic vein
6 Latissimus dorsi muscle
7 Medial mammarian branches of intercostal nerves
8 Breast tissue
9 Areola
10 Nipple (papilla)
11 Costal margin
12 Pectoral fascia
13 Mammary gland
14 Serratus anterior muscle (insertion)
15 Lactiferous sinus
16 Apical lymph nodes
17 Axillary lymph nodes
18 Intercostobrachial nerve
19 Lateral thoracic vein
20 Lymph vessels
21 Medial branches of intercostal arteries
22 Pectoralis minor muscle

# 6 Abdominal Organs

Internal Organs

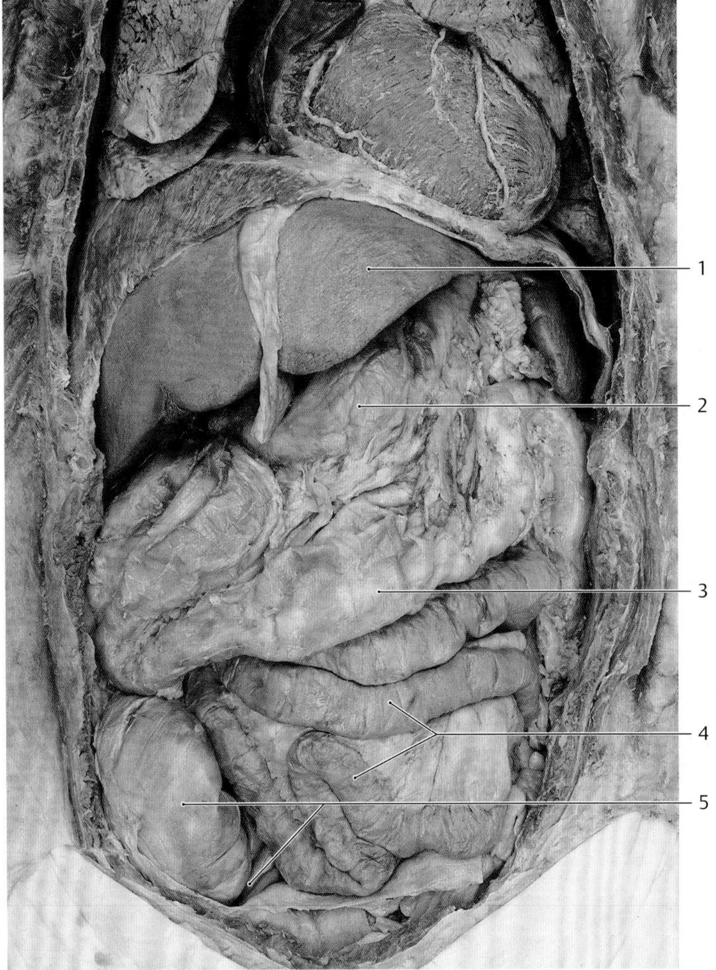


Fig. 6.1 **Abdominal organs in situ** (anterior aspect). The greater omentum has been partly removed or reflected.

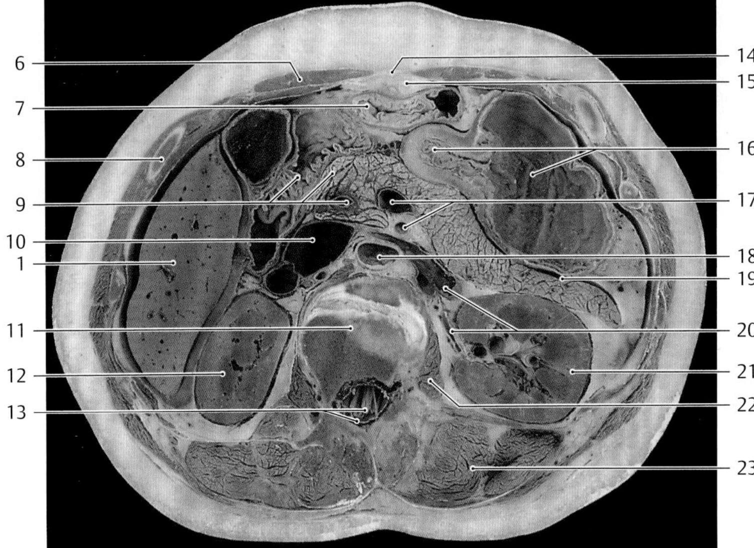


Fig. 6.2 **Horizontal section through the abdominal cavity** at the level of the second lumbar vertebra (from below).

1 Liver (left lobe)
2 Stomach
3 Transverse colon
4 Small intestine
5 Cecum with vermiform appendix
6 Rectus abdominis muscle
7 Small intestine and peritoneum
8 Rib (cut)
9 Bile duct, duodenum, and pancreas
10 Inferior vena cava
11 Body of second lumbar vertebra (L2)
12 Right kidney
13 Cauda equina and dura mater
14 Linea alba
15 Falciform ligament
16 Stomach and pylorus
17 Superior mesenteric artery and vein
18 Abdominal aorta
19 Pancreas adjacent to lesser sac (omental bursa)
20 Left renal artery and vein
21 Left kidney
22 Psoas major muscle
23 Deep muscles of the back

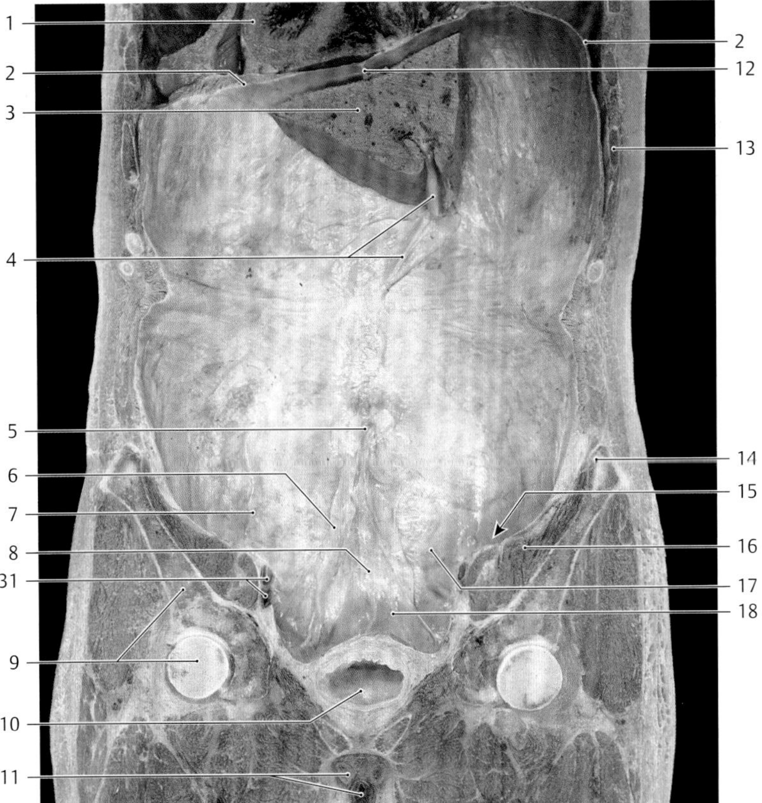


Fig. 6.3 **Anterior abdominal wall of the male.** Frontal section through pelvic cavity and hip joints (internal aspect).

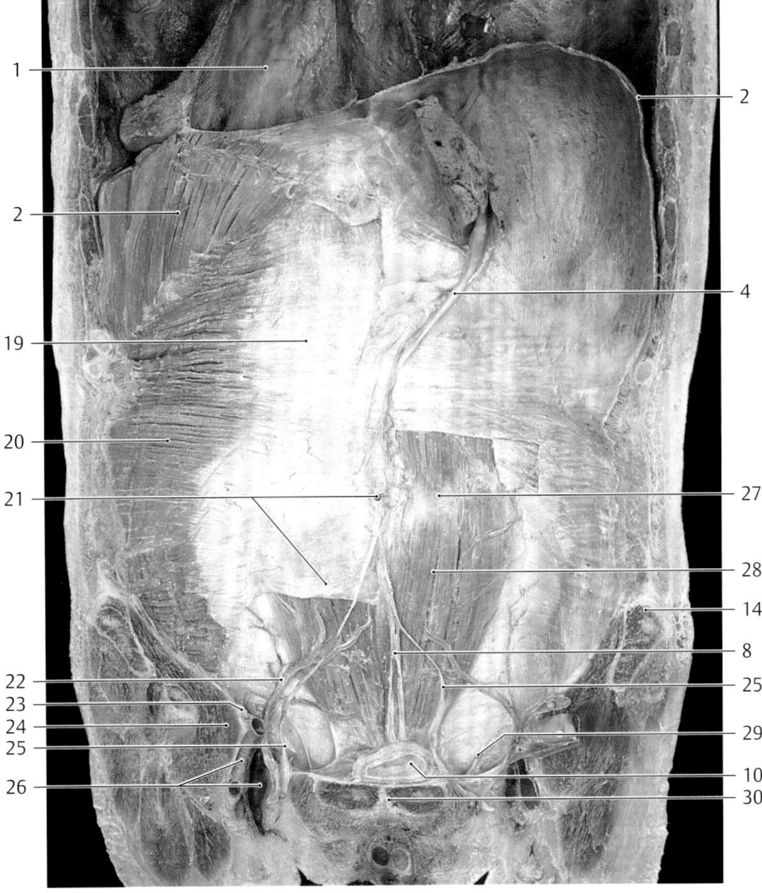


1 Left ventricle with pericardium
2 Diaphragm
3 Remnant of liver
4 Ligamentum teres (free margin of falciform ligament)
5 Site of umbilicus
6 Medial umbilical fold (containing the obliterated umbilical artery)
7 Lateral umbilical fold (containing inferior epigastric artery and vein)
8 Median umbilical fold (containing remnant of urachus)
9 Head of femur and pelvic bone
10 Urinary bladder
11 Root of penis
12 Falciform ligament of liver
13 Rib (divided)
14 Iliac crest (divided)
15 Site of deep inguinal ring and lateral inguinal fossa
16 Iliopsoas muscle (divided)
17 Medial inguinal fossa
18 Supravesical fossa
19 Posterior layer of rectus sheath
20 Transverse abdominal muscle
21 Umbilicus and arcuate line
22 Inferior epigastric artery
23 Femoral nerve
24 Iliopsoas muscle
25 Remnant of umbilical artery
26 Femoral artery and vein
27 Tendinous intersection of rectus abdominis muscle
28 Rectus abdominis muscle
29 Interfoveolar ligament
30 Pubic symphysis (divided)
31 External iliac artery and vein

Fig. 6.4 **Anterior abdominal wall of the male** (internal aspect). The peritoneum and parts of the posterior layer of the rectus sheath have been removed. Dissection of inferior epigastric arteries and veins.

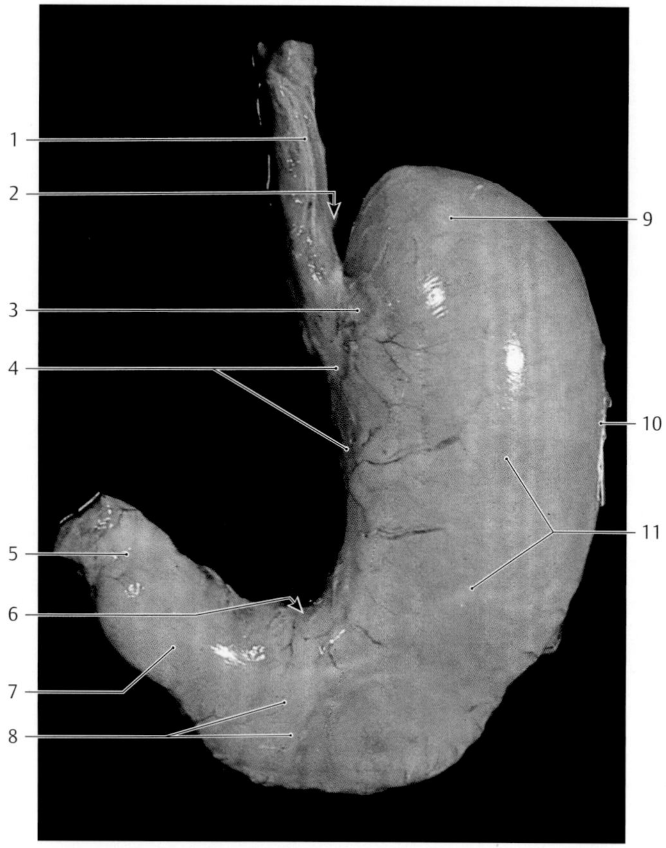

Fig. 6.5 **Stomach** (anterior aspect).

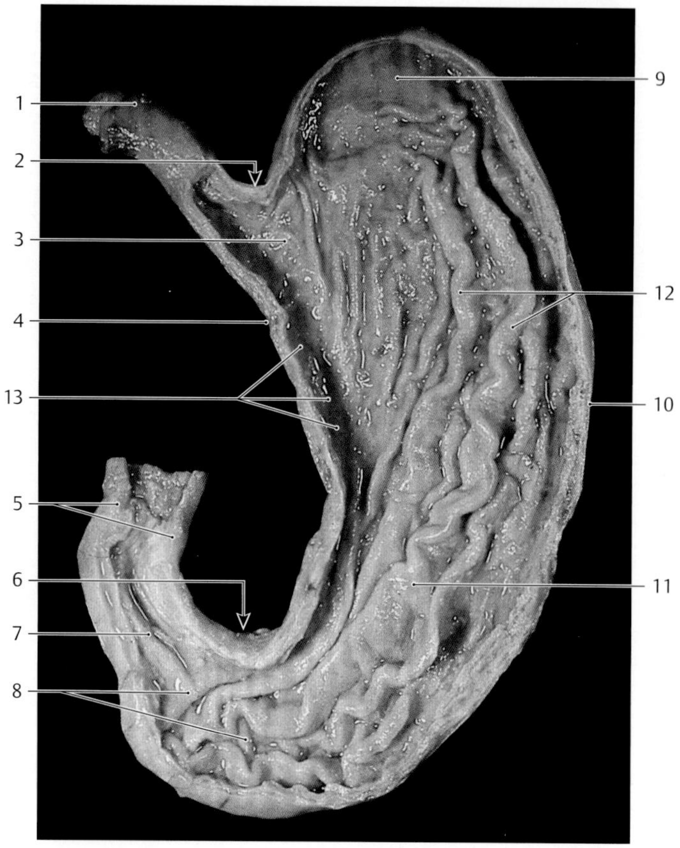

Fig. 6.6 **Mucosa of posterior wall of stomach** (anterior aspect).

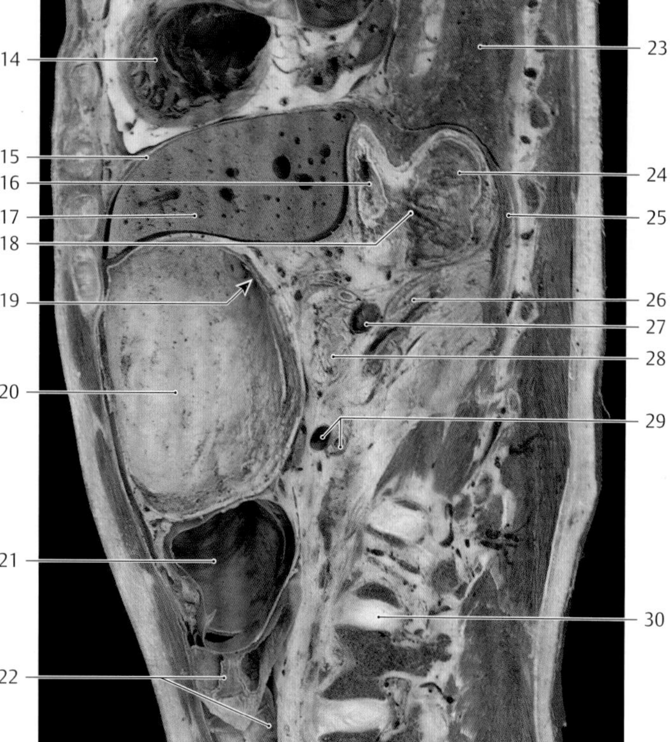


Fig. 6.7 **Position of the stomach** (parasagittal section through the upper part of the left abdominal cavity 3.5 cm lateral to the median plane).

1 Esophagus
2 Cardial notch
3 Cardial part of stomach
4 Lesser curvature of stomach
5 Pyloric sphincter
6 Angular notch (incisura angularis)
7 Pyloric canal
8 Pyloric antrum
9 Fundus of stomach
10 Greater curvature of stomach
11 Body of stomach
12 Folds of mucous membrane (gastric rugae)
13 Gastric canal
14 Right ventricle of heart
15 Diaphragm (cut edge)
16 Abdominal part of esophagus
17 Liver
18 Cardial part of stomach (cut edge)
19 Position of pyloric canal
20 Body of stomach
21 Transverse colon
22 Small intestine
23 Lung (cut edge)
24 Fundus of stomach (section)
25 Lumbar part of diaphragm (cut edge)
26 Suprarenal gland
27 Splenic vein
28 Pancreas
29 Superior mesenteric artery and vein
30 Intervertebral disc

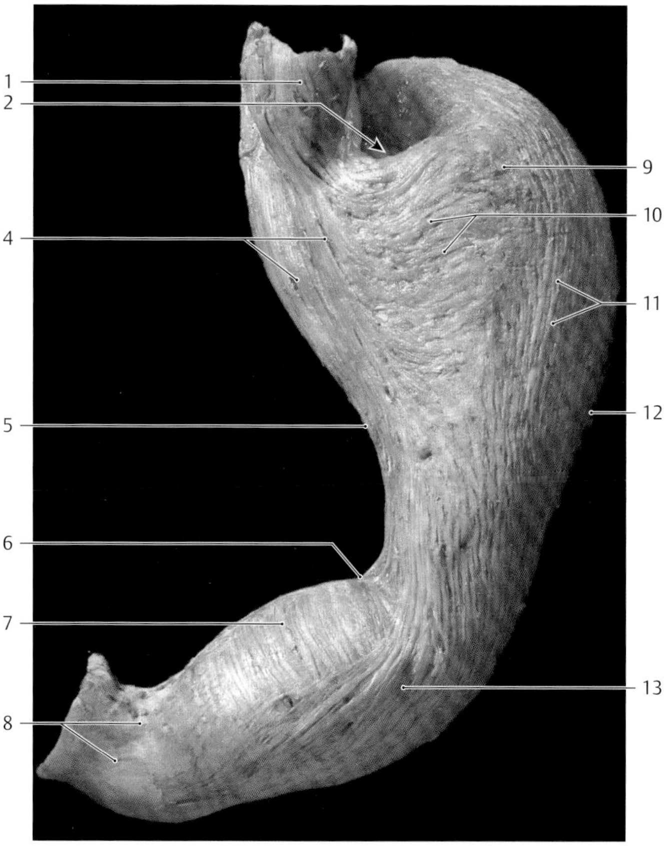

Fig. 6.8 **Muscular coat of stomach,** outer layer (anterior aspect).

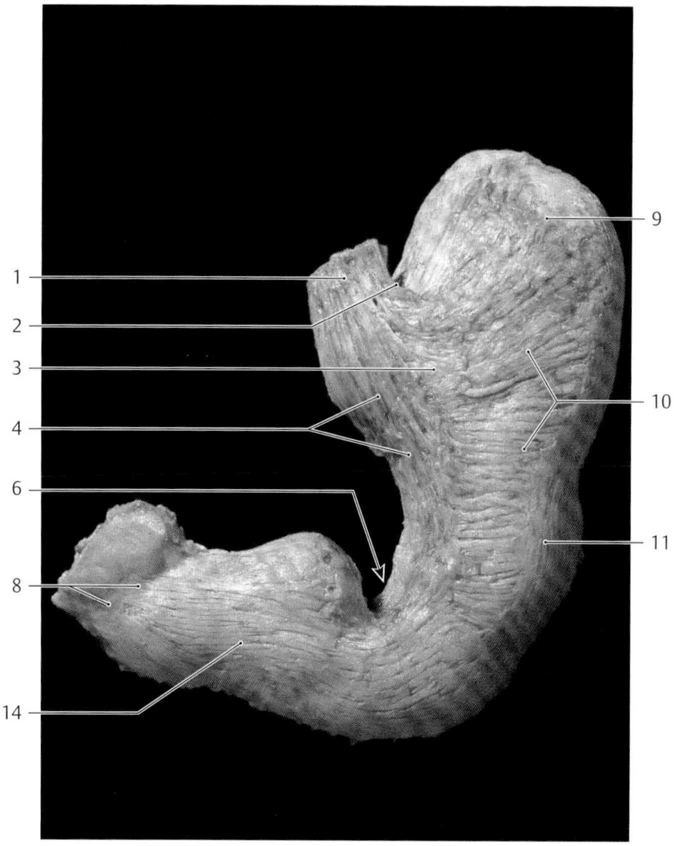

Fig. 6.9 **Muscular coat of stomach,** middle layer (anterior aspect).

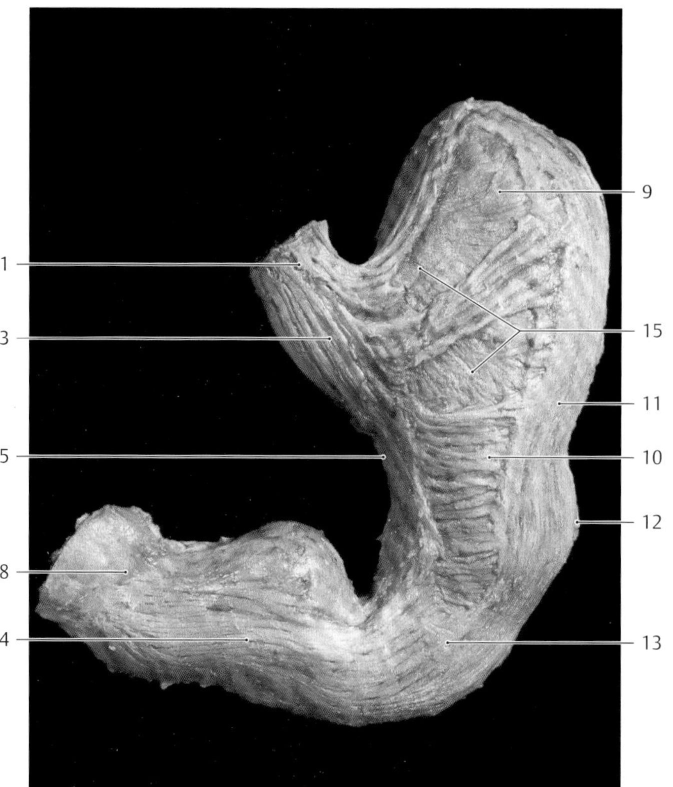


Fig. 6.10 **Muscular coat of stomach,** inner layer (anterior aspect).

1 Esophagus (abdominal part)
2 Cardial notch
3 Cardial part of stomach
4 Longitudinal muscle layer at lesser curvature of stomach
5 Lesser curvature
6 Incisura angularis
7 Circular muscle layer of pyloric part of stomach
8 Pyloric sphincter muscle
9 Fundus of stomach
10 Circular muscle layer of fundus of stomach
11 Longitudinal muscle layer of greater curvature of stomach
12 Greater curvature of stomach
13 Longitudinal muscle layer (transition from body to pyloric part of stomach)
14 Pyloric part of stomach
15 Oblique muscle fibers

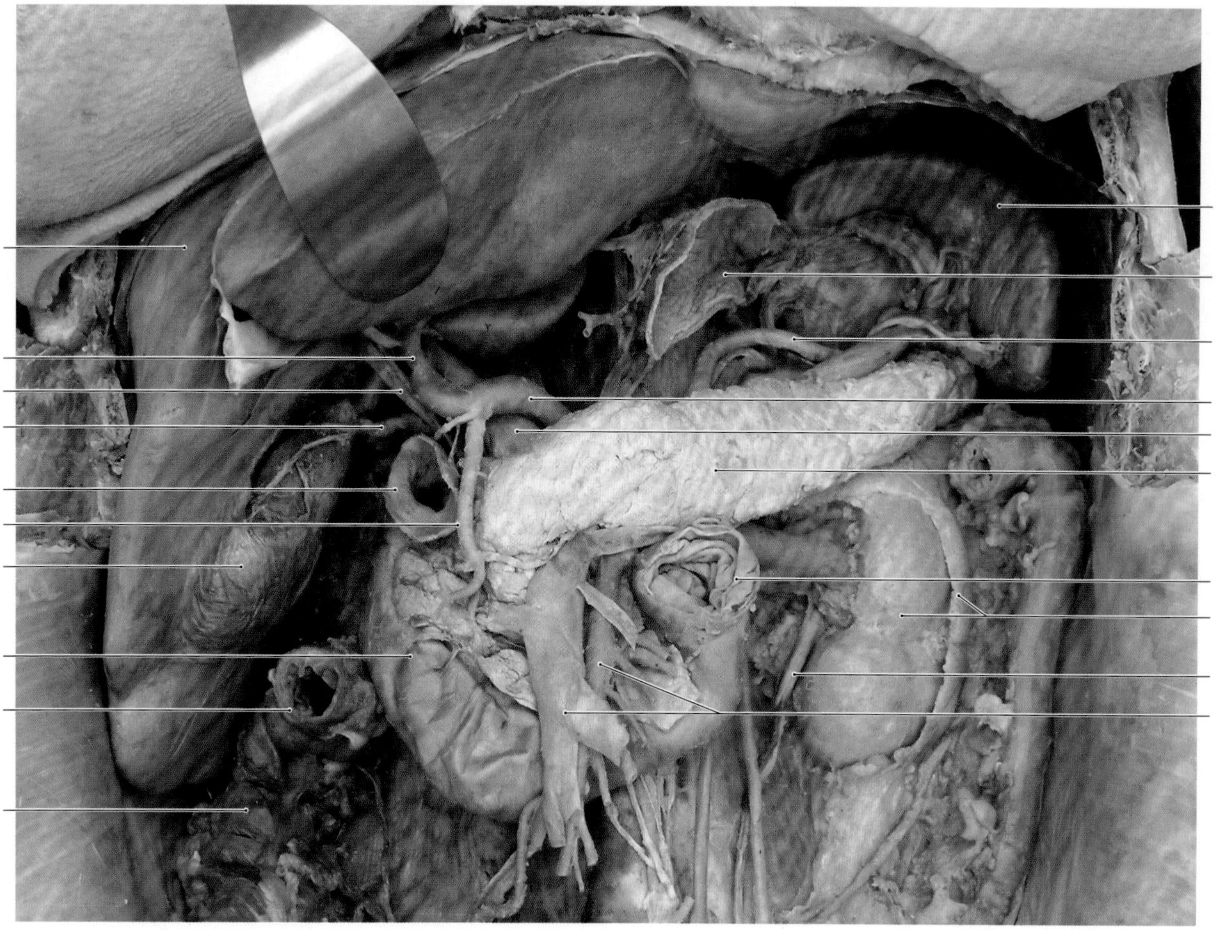

**Fig. 6.11 Upper abdominal region with pancreas, duodenum, spleen, and left kidney** (anterior aspect). The stomach and transverse colon have been removed and the liver elevated; the superior mesenteric vein is slightly enlarged.

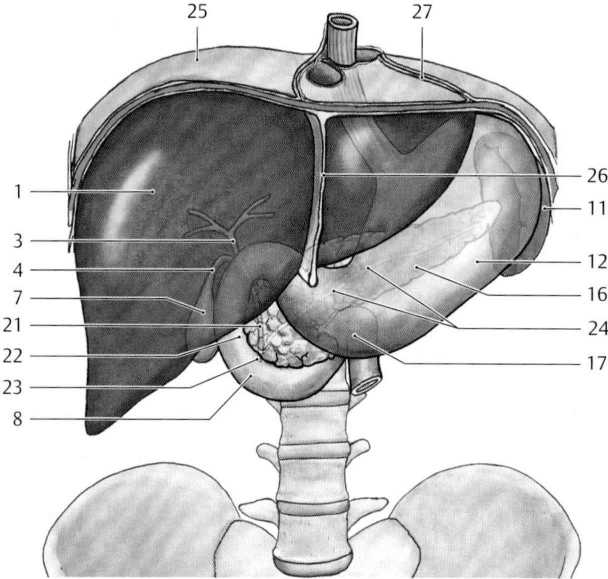


**Fig. 6.12 Pancreas, duodenum, liver, and extrahepatic bile ducts** (anterior aspect). The liver is shown here as slightly transparent. Morphologically, the liver can be divided into four lobes: the left and right lobes and the quadrate and caudate lobes (see additional figures on page 276). The falciform ligament separates the smaller left lobe from the larger right lobe.

1 Liver
2 Hepatic artery proper
3 Hepatic duct
4 Cystic duct
5 Pylorus
6 Gastroduodenal artery
7 Gallbladder
8 Duodenum
9 Right colic flexure
10 Ascending colon
11 Spleen
12 Stomach
13 Splenic artery
14 Common hepatic artery
15 Portal vein
16 Pancreas
17 Duodenojejunal flexure
18 Kidney (with capsula adiposa)
19 Ureter
20 Superior mesenteric artery and vein
21 Common bile duct
22 Minor duodenal papilla
23 Major duodenal papilla
24 Pancreatic duct
25 Peritoneum
26 Falciform ligament } of liver
27 Coronary ligament } of liver

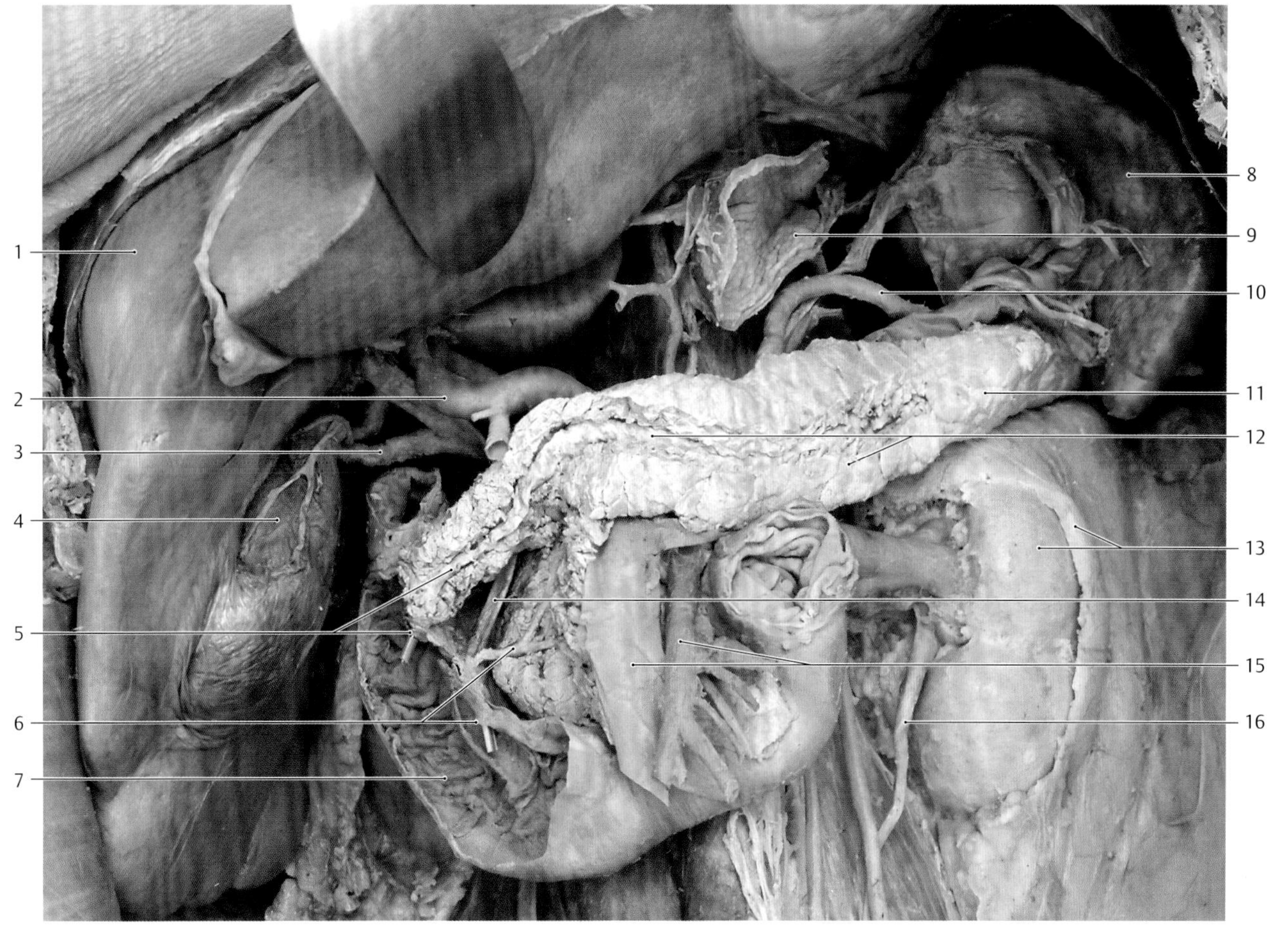

**Fig. 6.13 Upper abdominal region with pancreas, duodenum, spleen, and left kidney** (anterior aspect). The stomach and transverse colon have been removed and the duodenum fenestrated. The liver has been elevated to show the extrahepatic bile ducts. In this case, the accessory pancreatic duct represents the main excretory duct of the pancreas.

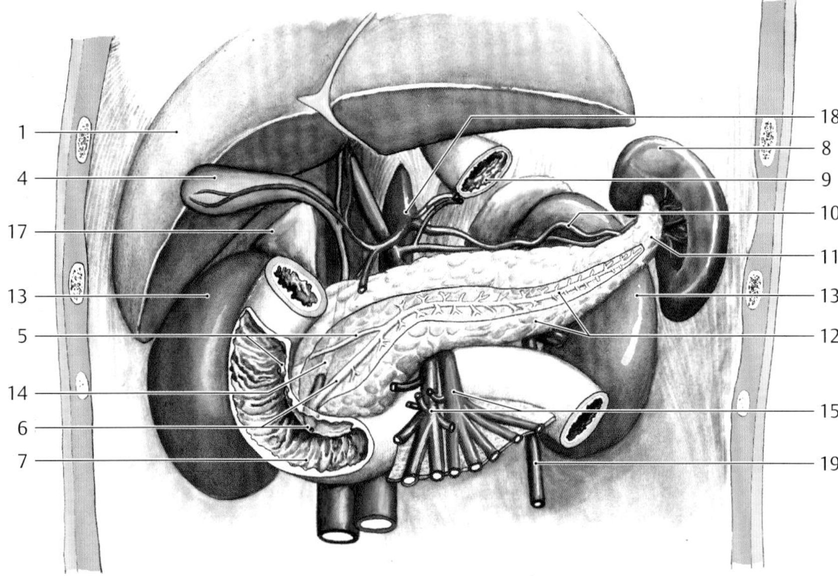


**Fig. 6.14 Upper abdominal organs** (anterior aspect). The schematic shows the most common situation of the pancreatic ducts.

1 Liver
2 Hepatic artery proper
3 Cystic duct
4 Gallbladder
5 Minor duodenal papilla and accessory pancreatic duct
6 Major duodenal papilla and pancreatic duct
7 Duodenum (fenestrated)
8 Spleen
9 Stomach
10 Splenic artery
11 Tail of pancreas
12 Pancreas (pancreatic duct and body of pancreas)
13 Kidney (with capsula adiposa in Fig. 6.13)
14 Common bile duct
15 Superior mesenteric artery and vein
16 Ureter
17 Suprarenal gland
18 Aorta with celiac trunk
19 Inferior mesenteric vein

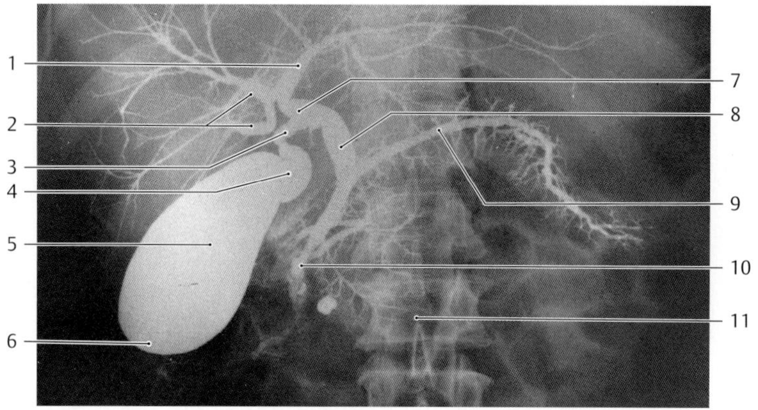


Fig. 6.15 **Bile ducts, gallbladder, and pancreatic duct** (antero-posterior direction, x-ray). (Courtesy of Prof. Uder, Institute of Radiology, University Hospital Erlangen, Germany.)

1 Left hepatic duct
2 Right hepatic duct
3 Cystic duct
4 Neck of gallbladder
5 Body of gallbladder
6 Fundus of gallbladder
7 Common hepatic duct
8 Common bile duct
9 Pancreatic duct
10 Major duodenal papilla
11 Second lumbar vertebra
12 Folds of mucous membrane of gallbladder
13 Muscular coat of gallbladder
14 Neck of gallbladder (opened)
15 Cystic duct with spiral fold
16 Minor duodenal papilla
17 Accessory pancreatic duct
18 Uncinate process
19 Plica circularis of duodenum (Kerckring's fold)
20 Head of pancreas
21 Body of pancreas
22 Tail of pancreas
23 Descending part of duodenum
24 Incisure of pancreas

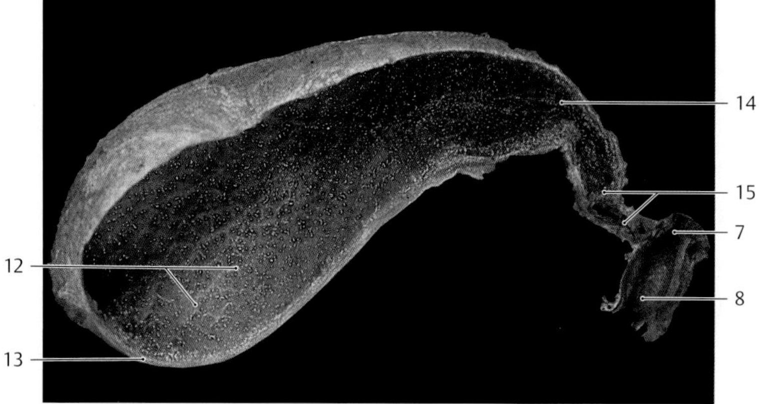


Fig. 6.16 **Isolated gallbladder and cystic duct** (anterior aspect). The gallbladder has been opened to display the mucous membrane.

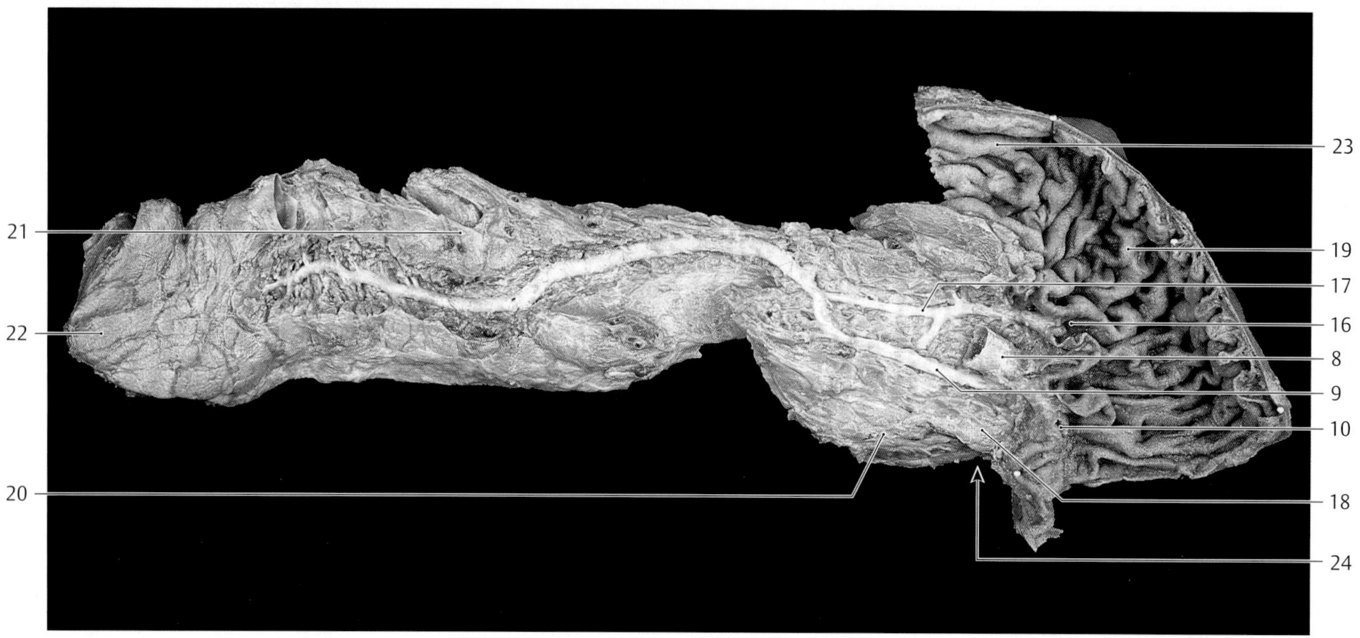


Fig. 6.17 **Pancreas with descending part of duodenum** (posterior aspect). The duodenum was opened to display the duodenal papillae. The pancreatic duct has been dissected and the common bile duct has been divided. The sphincter of Oddi is shown.

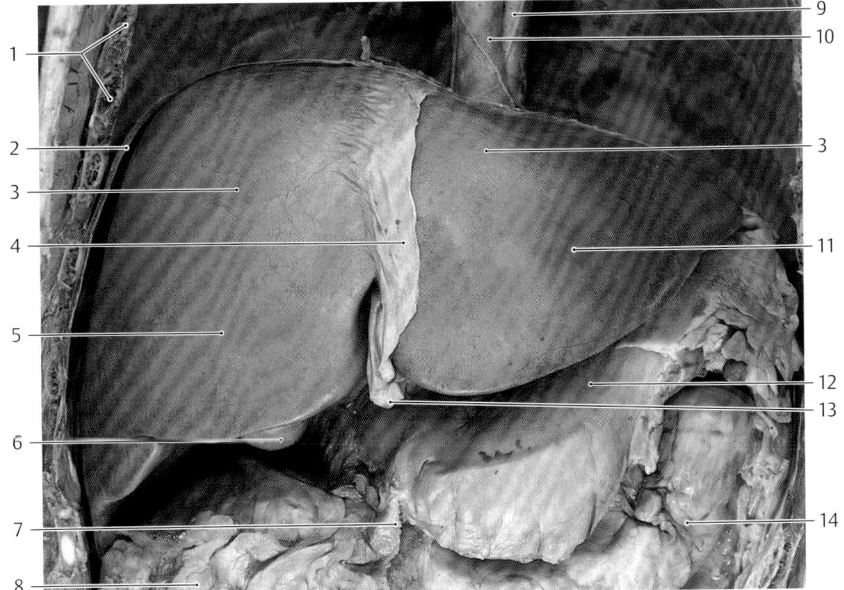


Fig. 6.18 **Liver in situ** (anterior aspect). Part of the diaphragm has been removed.

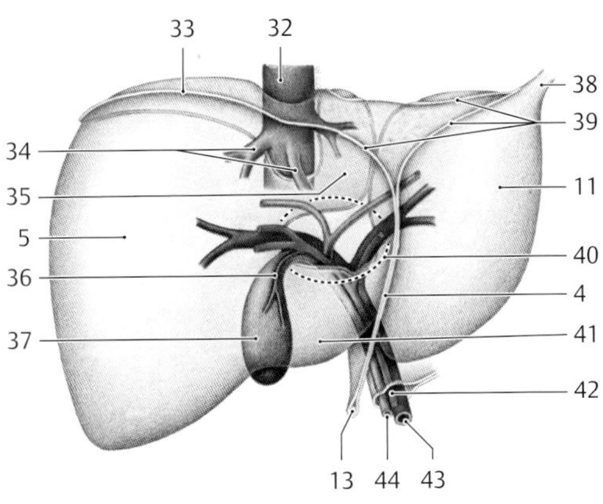


Fig. 6.19 **Liver and margins of peritoneal folds** (anterior aspect). The liver is shown as being transparent.

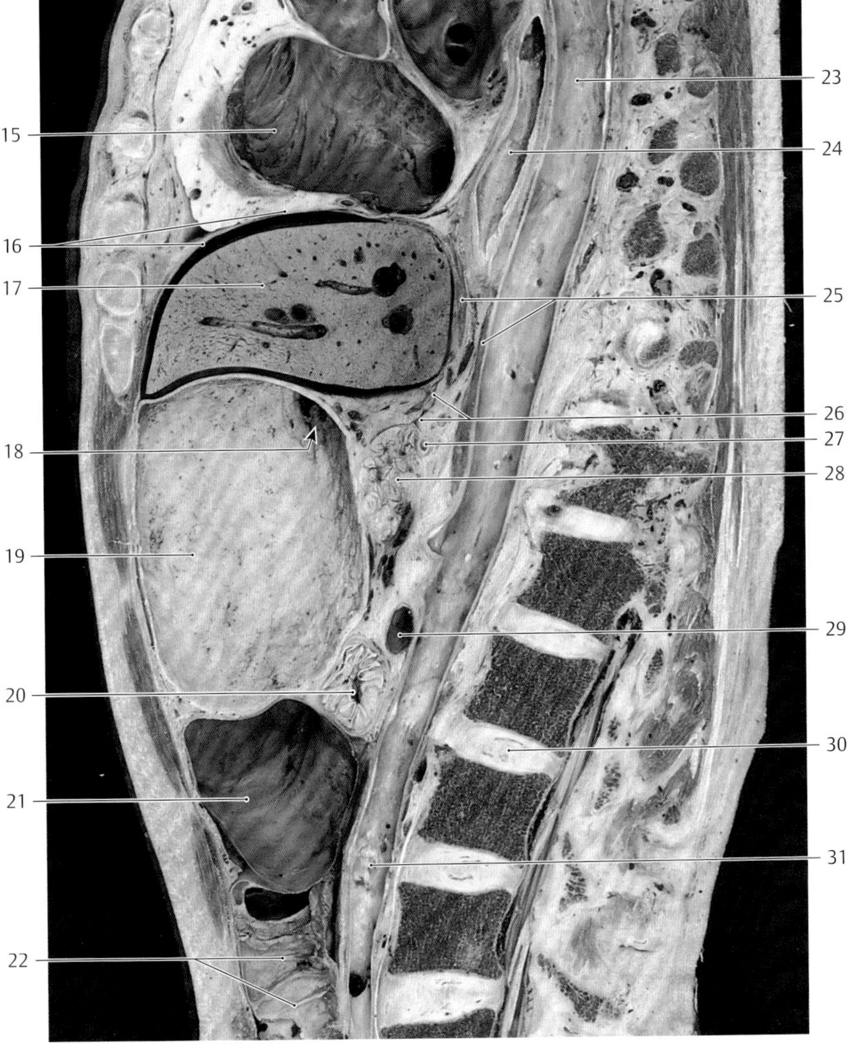


Fig. 6.20 **Liver in situ** (parasagittal section through the left side of the abdomen 2 cm lateral to the median plane).

1 Ribs (cut edges)
2 Diaphragm
3 Diaphragmatic surface of liver
4 Falciform ligament of liver
5 Right lobe of liver
6 Fundus of gallbladder
7 Gastrocolic ligament
8 Greater omentum
9 Aorta
10 Esophagus
11 Left lobe of liver
12 Stomach
13 Round ligament of the liver
14 Transverse colon
15 Right atrium of heart
16 Central tendon and sternal portion of diaphragm
17 Liver (cut edge)
18 Entrance to duodenum (pylorus)
19 Stomach
20 Duodenum
21 Transverse colon (divided, dilated)
22 Small intestine
23 Thoracic aorta (longitudinally divided)
24 Esophagus (longitudinally divided)
25 Esophageal hiatus of diaphragm
26 Omental bursa (lesser sac)
27 Splenic artery
28 Pancreas
29 Left renal vein
30 Intervertebral disc
31 Abdominal aorta (longitudinally divided)
32 Inferior vena cava
33 Peritoneum (cut edges)
34 Hepatic veins
35 Caudate lobe of liver
36 Cystic artery
37 Fundus of gallbladder
38 Appendix fibrosa (left triangular ligament)
39 Coronary ligament of liver
40 Porta hepatis
41 Quadrate lobe of liver
42 Hepatic artery proper } Portal triad
43 Portal vein
44 Common bile duct

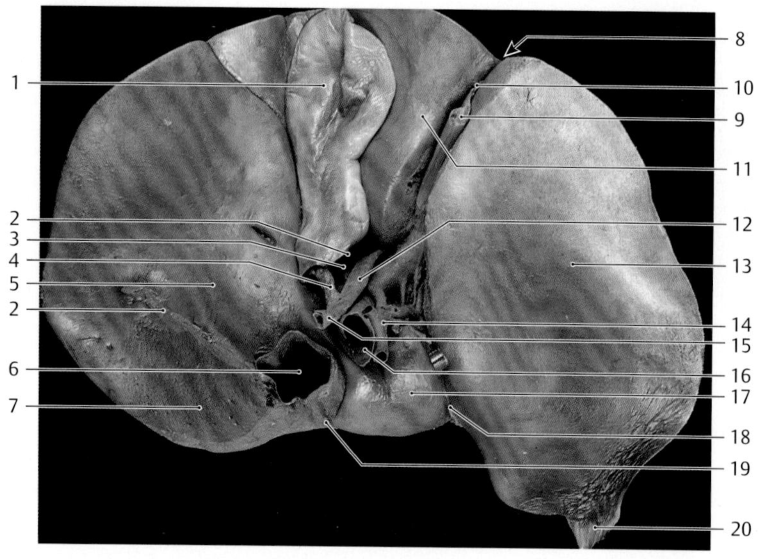


1 Fundus of gallbladder
2 Peritoneum (cut edges)
3 Cystic artery
4 Cystic duct
5 Right lobe of liver
6 Inferior vena cava
7 Bare area of liver
8 Notch for ligamentum teres and falciform ligament
9 Ligamentum teres
10 Falciform ligament of liver
11 Quadrate lobe of liver
12 Common hepatic duct
13 Left lobe of liver
14 Hepatic artery proper
15 Common bile duct
16 Portal vein
17 Caudate lobe of liver
18 Ligamentum venosum
19 Ligament of inferior vena cava
20 Appendix fibrosa (left triangular ligament)
21 Coronary ligament of liver
22 Hepatic veins
23 Porta hepatis
24 Hepatic arteries

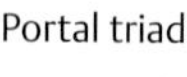

(14–16: Portal triad)

Fig. 6.21 **Liver** (inferior aspect). Dissection of porta hepatis. The gallbladder is partly collapsed. Ventral margin of liver above.

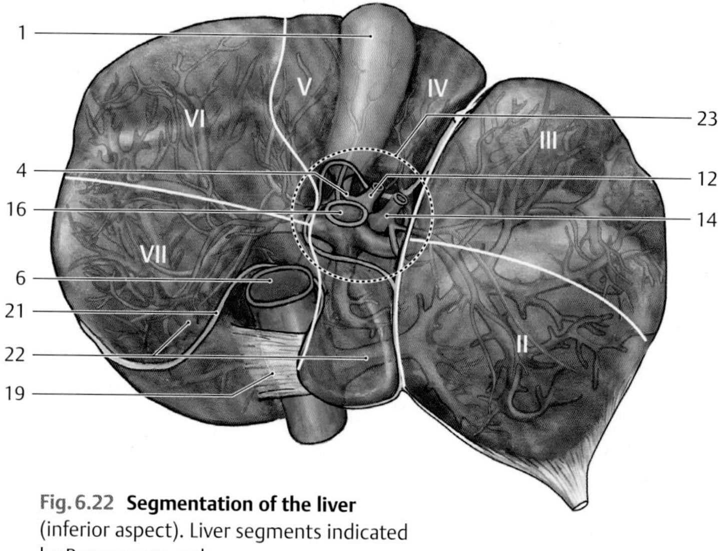


Fig. 6.22 **Segmentation of the liver** (inferior aspect). Liver segments indicated by Roman numerals.

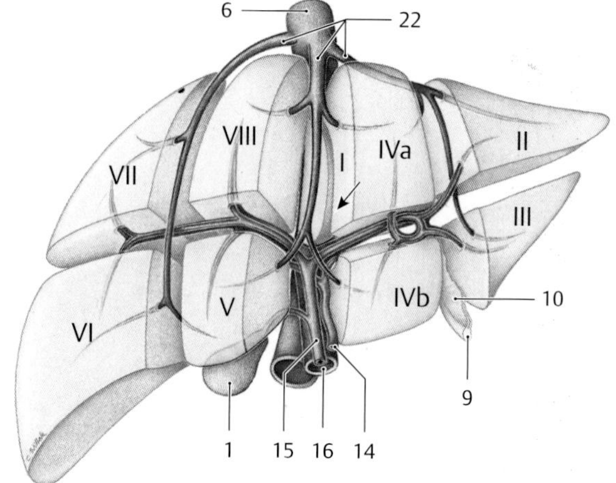


Fig. 6.23 **Segmentation of the liver** (anterior aspect). Liver segments indicated by Roman numerals.

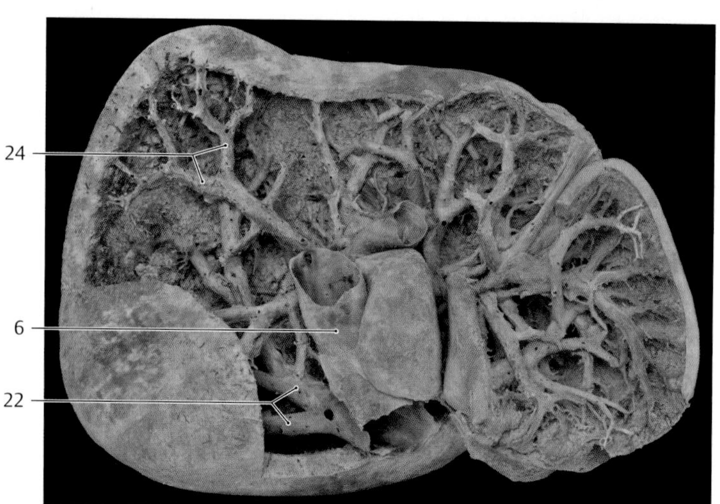


In visceral surgery, the eight functional segments of the liver are of great clinical relevance as they allow the resection of individual segments. The segmentation of the liver is not visible on its surface. Each of the eight functional segments is supplied by one branch of the portal triad (hepatic artery proper, common bile duct, and portal vein).

Fig. 6.24 **Segmentation of the liver** (inferior aspect). Dissection of the hepatic arteries and veins.

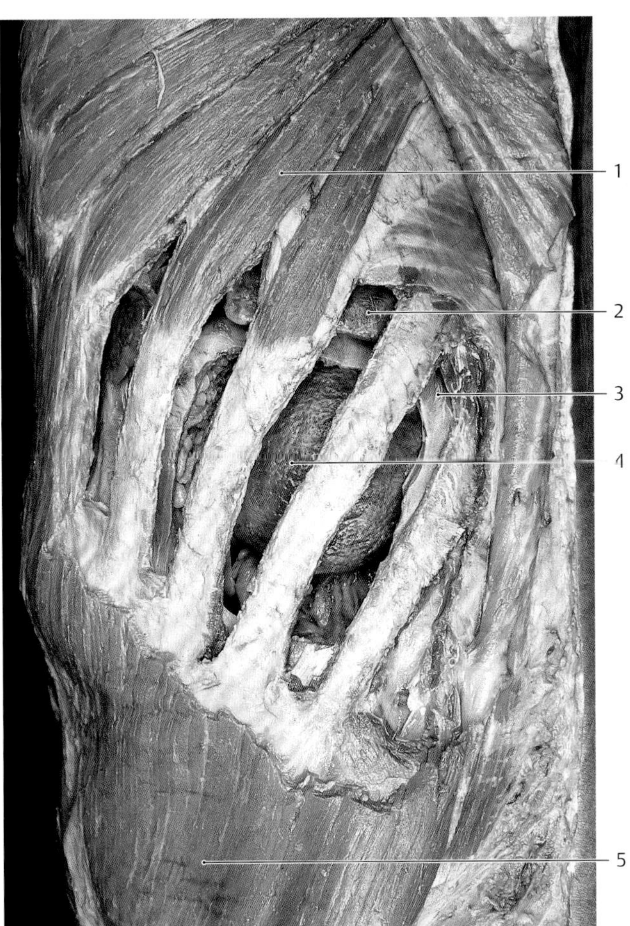


**Fig. 6.25 Spleen in situ** (left lateral aspect). The intercostal spaces and diaphragm have been fenestrated.

1 Serratus anterior muscle
2 Left lung
3 Diaphragm
4 Spleen
5 External abdominal oblique muscle
6 Gastrosplenic ligament
7 Splenic artery
8 Tail of pancreas
9 Superior border of spleen
10 Anterior border of spleen
11 Border of lung
12 Area of liver
13 Area of stomach
14 Tenth rib
15 Eleventh rib
16 Twelfth rib

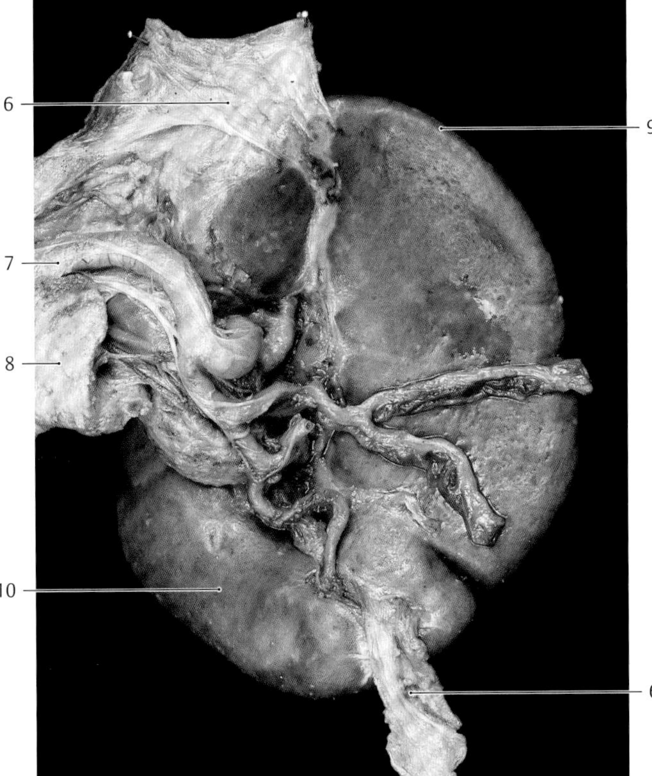


**Fig. 6.26 Spleen** (visceral surface). Hilum of spleen with vessels, nerves, and ligaments.

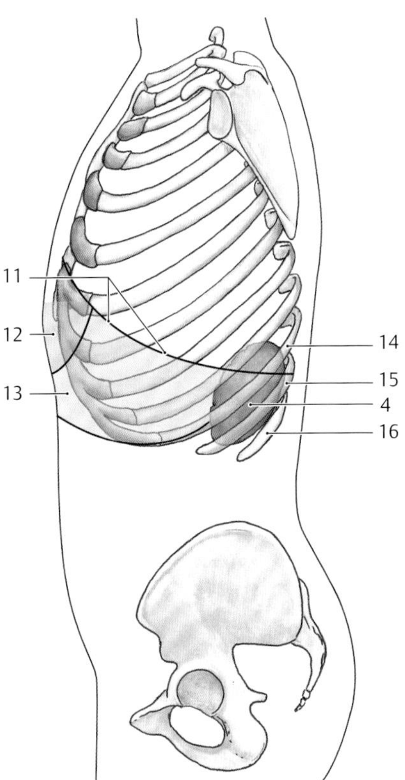


**Fig. 6.27 Location of the spleen** (left lateral aspect).

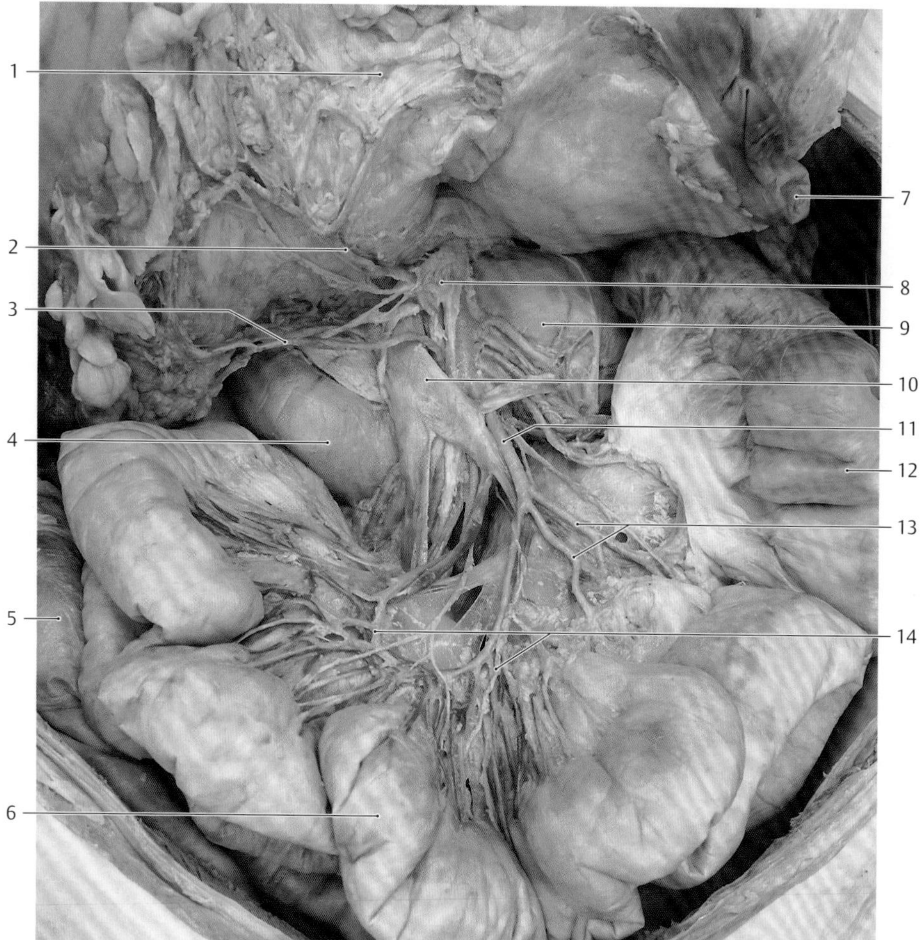


Fig. 6.28 **Vessels of upper abdominal organs and small intestine** (anterior aspect). Dissection of superior mesenteric artery and vein. Greater omentum and transverse colon are reflected.

1 Greater omentum
2 Middle colic artery
3 Right colic artery
4 Duodenum
5 Ascending colon
6 Ileum
7 Transverse colon
8 Celiac plexus
9 Duodenojejunal flexure
10 Superior mesenteric vein
11 Superior mesenteric artery
12 Jejunum
13 Jejunal arteries
14 Ileal arteries
15 Liver
16 Celiac trunk and abdominal aorta
17 Gallbladder
18 Pancreas
19 Ileocolic artery
20 Stomach
21 Spleen
22 Left colic flexure
23 Appendicular artery
24 Vermiform appendix
25 Spinal ganglion
26 Sympathetic ganglion
27 Intercostal artery and vein
28 Intercostal nerve
29 Splanchnic nerves
30 Sympathetic trunk
31 Rami communicantes
32 Right vagal trunk
33 Left vagal trunk
34 Diaphragm
35 Esophagus
36 Celiac trunk with celiac plexus
37 Renal plexus
38 Mesenteric plexus
39 Thoracic aorta

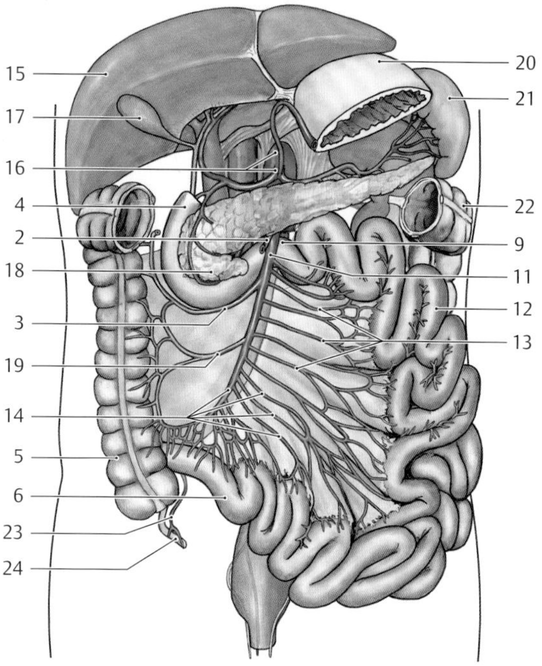

Fig. 6.29 **Arteries of upper abdominal organs and small intestine** (anterior aspect). Main branches of superior mesenteric artery.

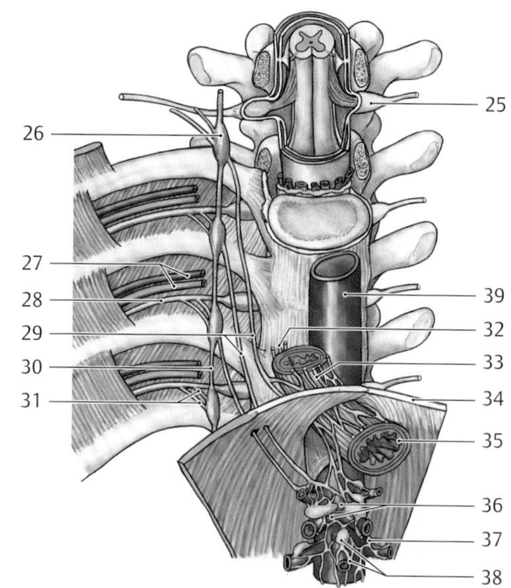


Fig. 6.30 **Branches of celiac, renal, and superior mesenteric nerve plexuses** run with the vessels to the organs they innervate.

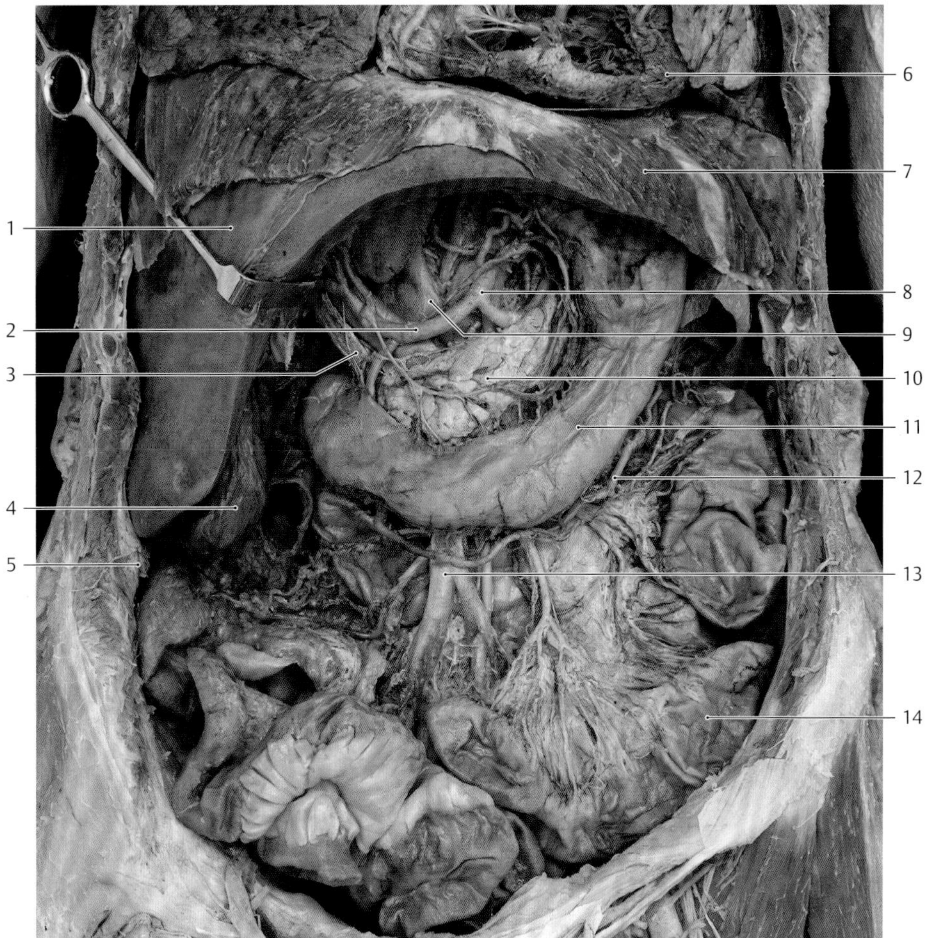


**Fig. 6.31 Vessels of upper abdominal organs and small intestine** (anterior aspect). Dissection of superior mesenteric vein. The liver has been dissected and elevated.

1 Liver
2 Common hepatic artery
3 Hepatic duct
4 Gallbladder
5 Major duodenal papilla
6 Apex of the heart
7 Diaphragm
8 Celiac trunk
9 Inferior vena cava
10 Pancreas
11 Stomach
12 Gastro-omental (gastro-epiploic) artery
13 Superior mesenteric vein
14 Small intestine
15 Jejunal vein
16 Superior mesenteric artery
17 Intestinal lymphatic vessels
18 Superior mesenteric plexus
19 Branches of superior mesenteric artery

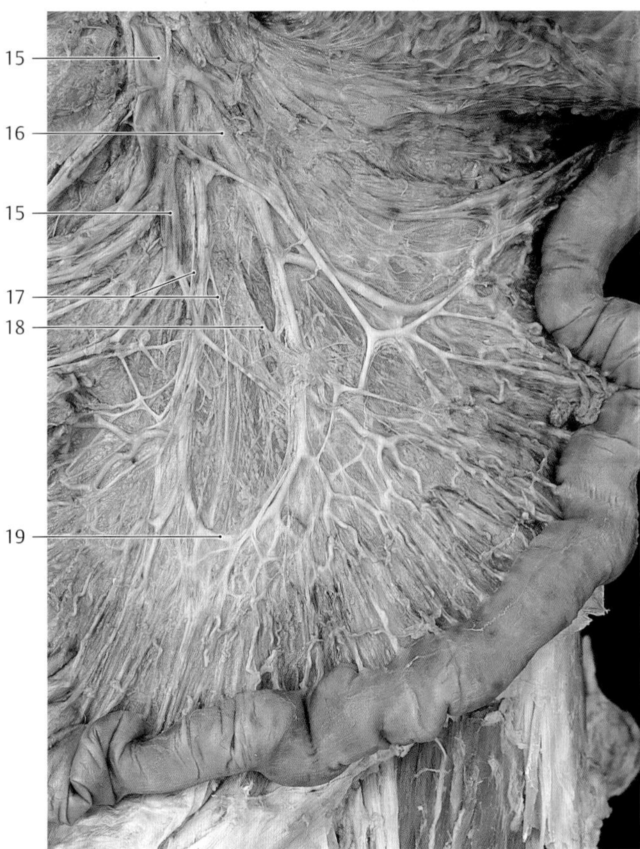


**Fig. 6.32 Blood and lymphatic vessels of the small intestine** (anterior aspect). Note the arterial arch of the mesenteric artery adjacent to the small intestine.

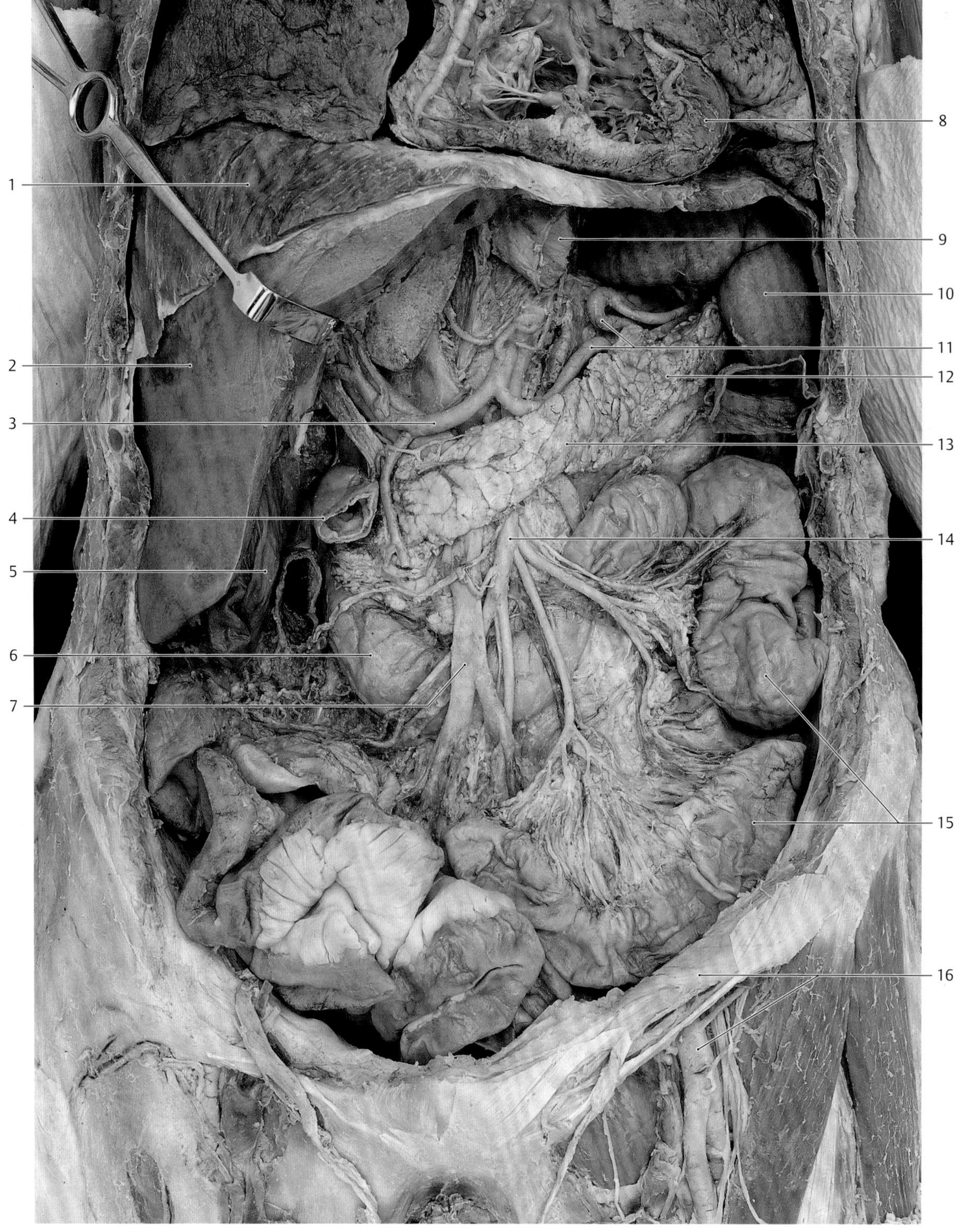


**Fig. 6.33 Vessels of upper abdominal organs and small intestine** (anterior aspect). The stomach and omentum majus have been removed. The liver is elevated.

1 Diaphragm
2 Liver
3 Common hepatic artery
4 Duodenum
5 Gallbladder
6 Inferior duodenal flexure
7 Superior mesenteric vein
8 Apex of the heart
9 Esophagus (abdominal part)
10 Spleen
11 Splenic artery
12 Tail of pancreas
13 Pancreas
14 Superior mesenteric artery
15 Small intestine
16 Inguinal ligament and femoral artery

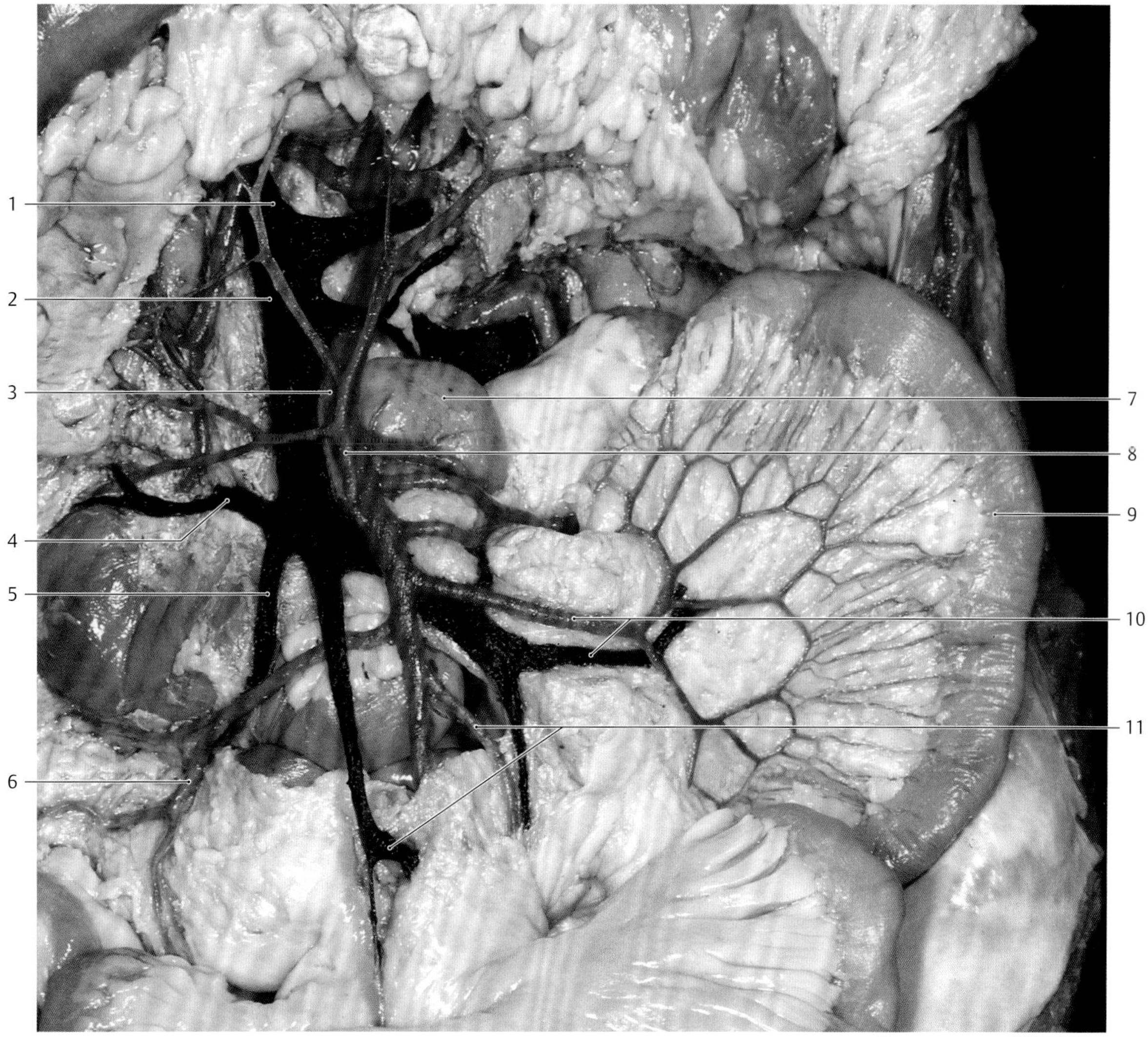

**Fig. 6.34 Dissection of portal venous system** (anterior aspect). Blue = tributaries of portal vein; red = branches of superior mesenteric artery.

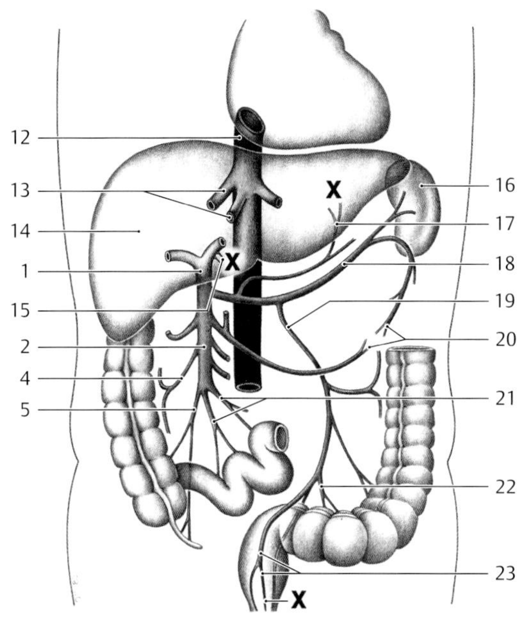


1 Portal vein
2 Superior mesenteric vein
3 Superior mesenteric artery
4 Right colic vein
5 Ileocolic vein
6 Ileocolic artery
7 Duodenojejunal flexure
8 Middle colic artery
9 Jejunum
10 Jejunal arteries and veins
11 Ileal arteries and veins
12 Inferior vena cava
13 Hepatic veins
14 Liver
15 Para-umbilical veins (located within the round ligament of the liver)
16 Spleen
17 Left gastric vein with esophageal branches
18 Splenic vein
19 Inferior mesenteric vein
20 Gastro-omental veins
21 Ileal veins
22 Sigmoid veins
23 Superior rectal vein

**Fig. 6.35 Main tributaries of portal vein** (anterior aspect). Blue = tributaries of portal vein; violet = inferior vena cava; X = sites of portocaval anastomoses.

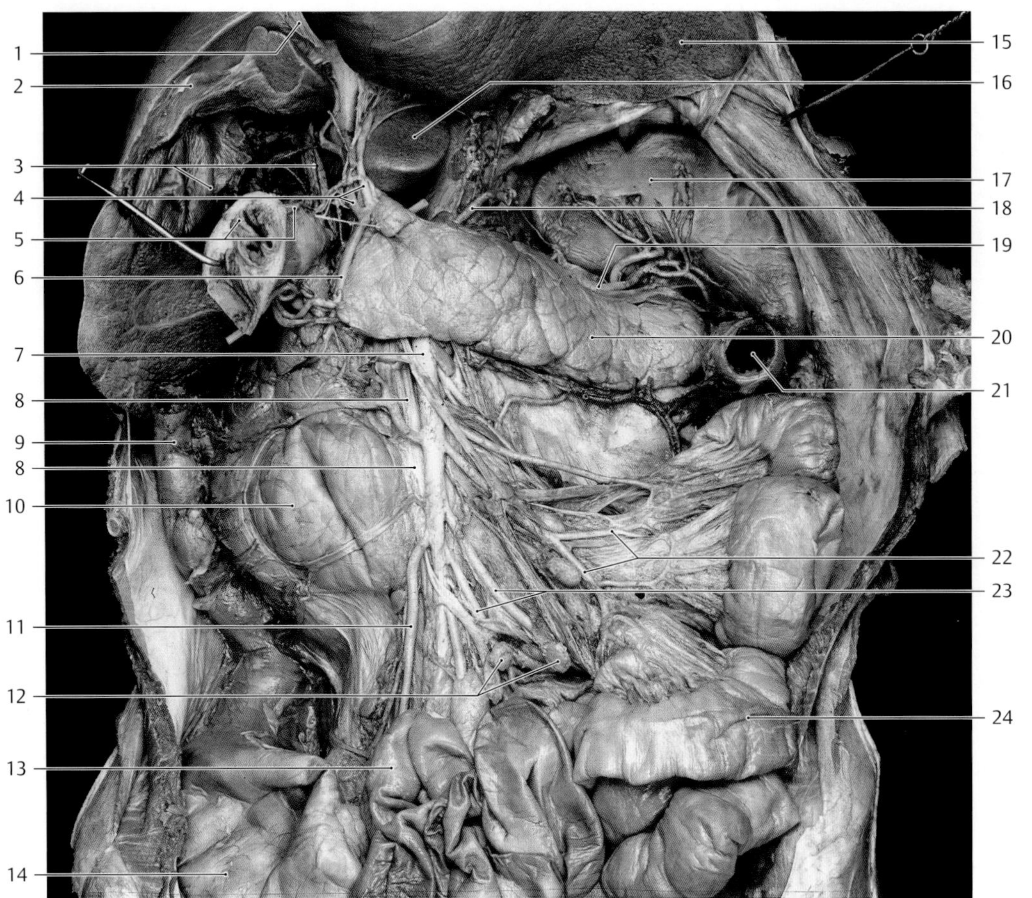


**Fig. 6.36 Superior mesenteric artery and vein in relation to pancreas and duodenum** (anterior aspect). The stomach and transverse colon have been removed and the liver elevated. Note the location of the spleen. A yellow probe has been inserted through the omental foramen.

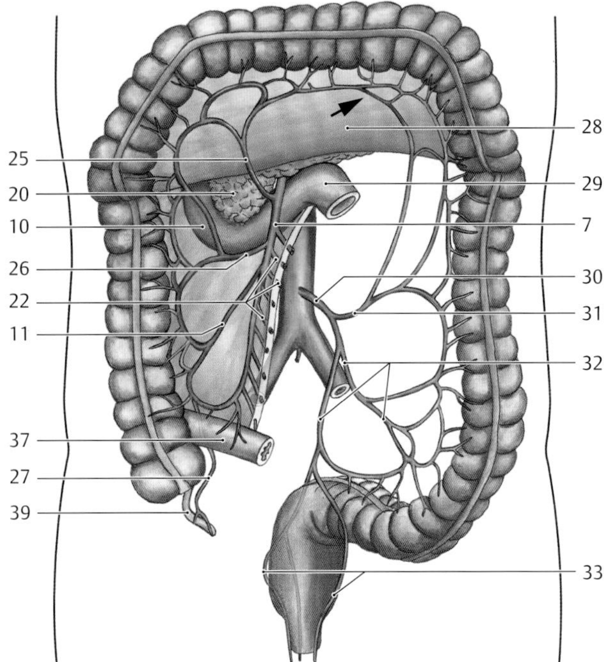


**Fig. 6.37 Main branches of superior and inferior mesenteric arteries** (anterior aspect). Arrow = Riolan's anastomosis.

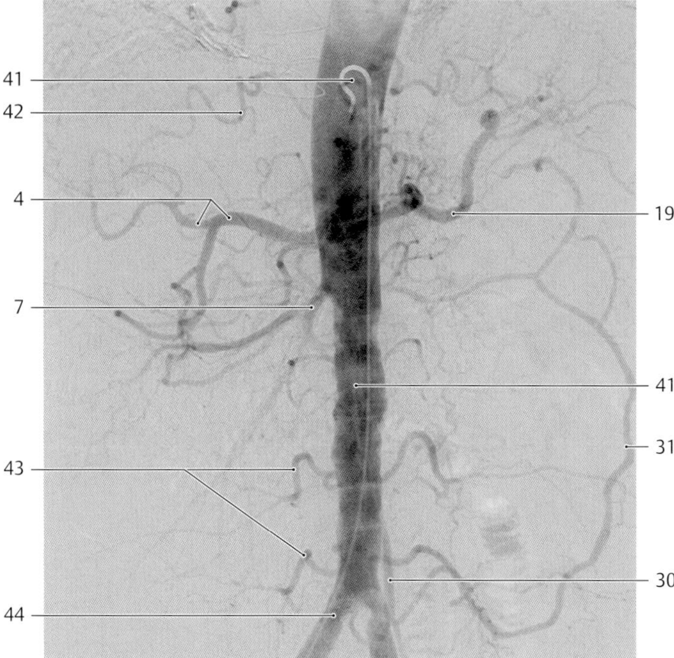


**Fig. 6.38 Arteriogram of abdominal aorta.** The distal portion of the aorta reveals sclerotic changes. (Courtesy of Dr. Wieners, Department of Radiology, Charité Universitätsmedizin Berlin, Germany.)

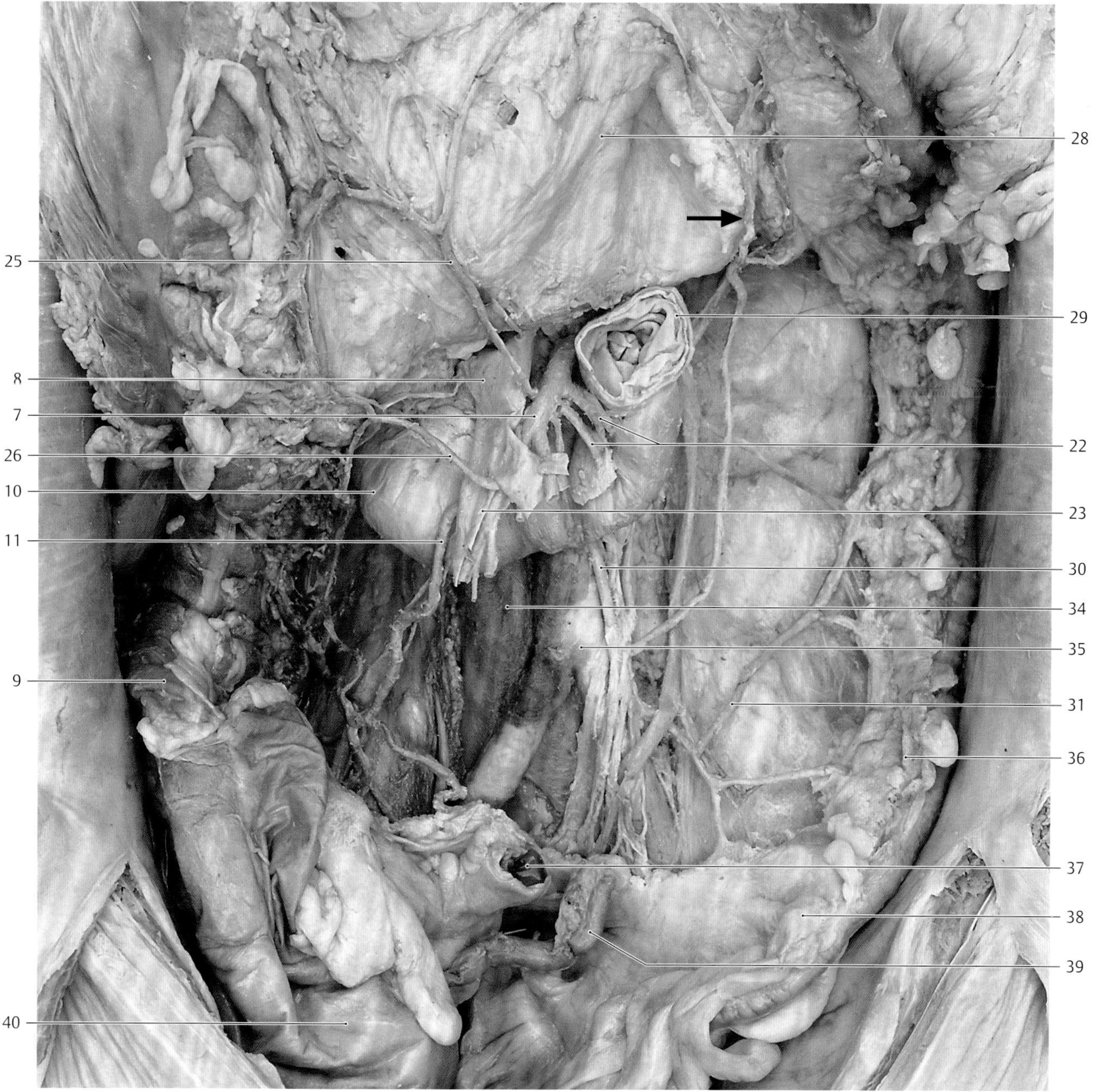


Fig. 6.39 **Vessels of the retroperitoneal organs** (anterior aspect). Dissection of the inferior mesenteric artery and its anastomosis with the middle colic artery (arrow = Riolan's anastomosis). The greater omentum and transverse colon have been reflected and the intestine partly removed. The normally retrocecally located vermiform appendix has been replaced anteriorly. The right common iliac artery is partly obstructed by a blood thrombus.

1 Round ligament of the liver
2 Liver
3 Gallbladder and common bile duct
4 Hepatic artery proper and portal vein
5 Right gastric artery and pylorus
6 Gastroduodenal artery
7 Superior mesenteric artery
8 Superior mesenteric vein
9 Ascending colon
10 Duodenum
11 Ileocolic artery
12 Lymph nodes
13 Ileum
14 Cecum
15 Left lobe of liver
16 Caudate lobe of liver
17 Spleen
18 Left gastric artery
19 Splenic artery
20 Pancreas
21 Left colic flexure (cut)
22 Jejunal arteries
23 Ileal arteries
24 Jejunum
25 Middle colic artery
26 Right colic artery
27 Appendicular artery
28 Transverse mesocolon
29 Duodenojejunal flexure
30 Inferior mesenteric artery
31 Left colic artery
32 Sigmoid arteries
33 Superior rectal arteries
34 Inferior vena cava
35 Abdominal aorta
36 Descending colon
37 Ileum
38 Sigmoid colon
39 Vermiform appendix
40 Cecum
41 Abdominal aorta
42 Superior suprarenal artery
43 Lumbal arteries
44 Common iliac artery

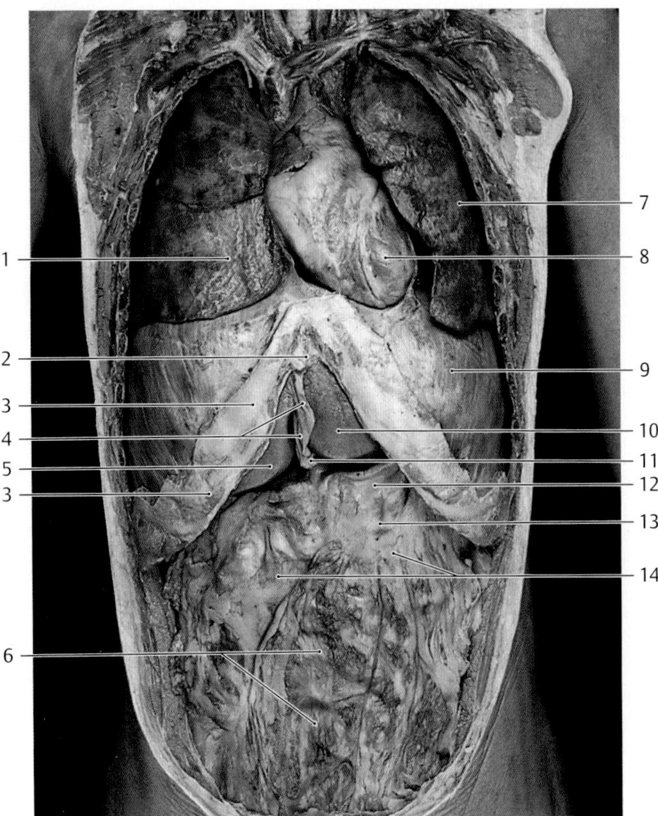


1 Middle lobe of right lung
2 Xiphoid process
3 Costal margin
4 Falciform ligament of liver
5 Quadrate lobe of liver
6 Greater omentum
7 Upper lobe of left lung
8 Heart
9 Diaphragm
10 Left lobe of liver
11 Ligamentum teres
12 Stomach
13 Gastrocolic ligament
14 Transverse colon
15 Taenia coli
16 Appendices epiploicae
17 Cecum
18 Taenia coli
19 Ileum
20 Transverse mesocolon
21 Jejunum
22 Sigmoid colon
23 Position of root of mesentery
24 Vermiform appendix
25 Duodenojejunal flexure
26 Mesentery

Fig. 6.40 **Abdominal organs** (anterior aspect). The anterior thoracic and abdominal walls have been removed.

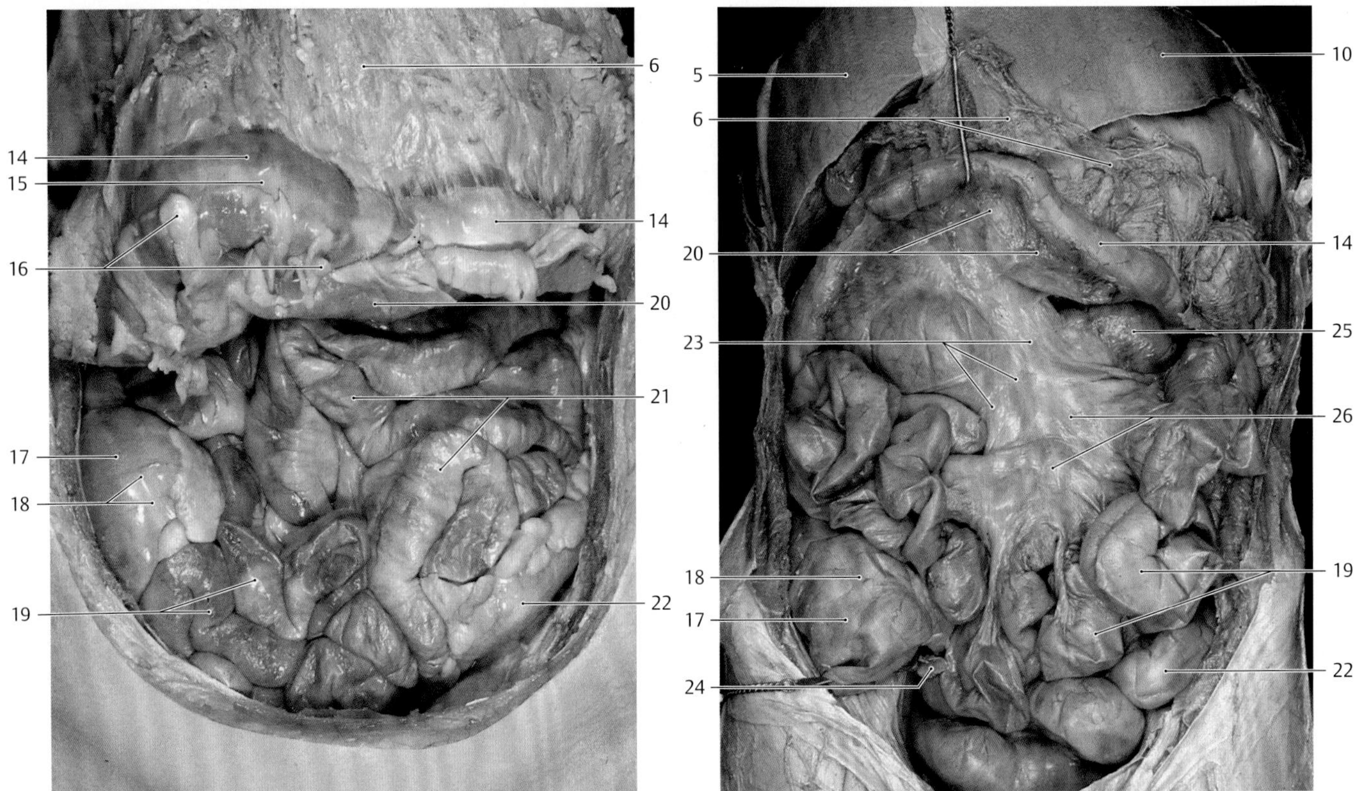


Fig. 6.41 **Abdominal organs** (anterior aspect). The greater omentum, which is fixed to the transverse colon, has been raised.

Fig. 6.42 **Abdominal organs** (anterior aspect). The transverse colon has been reflected.

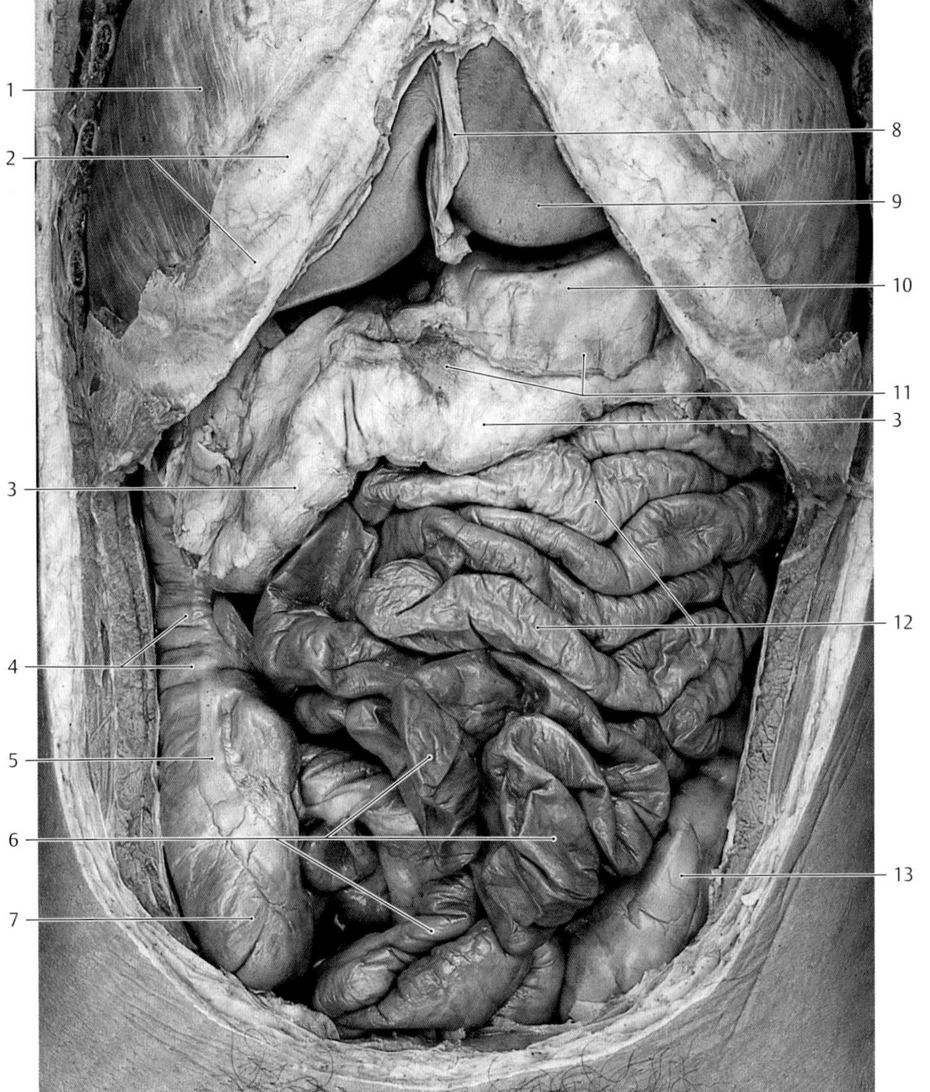


1 Diaphragm
2 Costal margin
3 Transverse colon
4 Ascending colon with haustra
5 Free taenia of cecum
6 Ileum
7 Cecum
8 Falciform ligament of liver
9 Liver
10 Stomach
11 Gastrocolic ligament
12 Jejunum
13 Sigmoid colon
14 Ileocecal valve
15 Ileal ostium
16 Frenulum of ileal opening
17 Ostium of vermiform appendix (probe in Fig. 6.44)
18 Ileocolic artery
19 Terminal ileum
20 Appendicular artery
21 Vermiform appendix
22 Meso-appendix
23 Mesentery

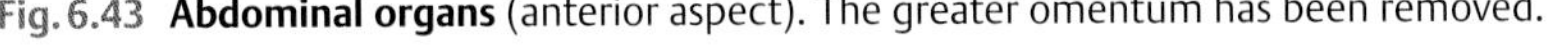

Fig. 6.43 **Abdominal organs** (anterior aspect). The greater omentum has been removed.

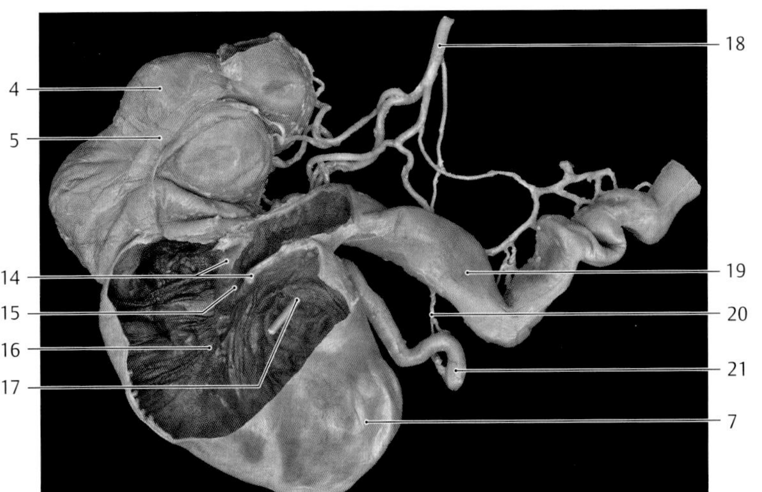


Fig. 6.44 **Ascending colon, cecum, and vermiform appendix.** The cecum has been opened. Note the probe in the entrance of the vermiform appendix.

a = retrocecal
b = paracolic
c = retro-ileal
d = pre-ileal
e = subcecal

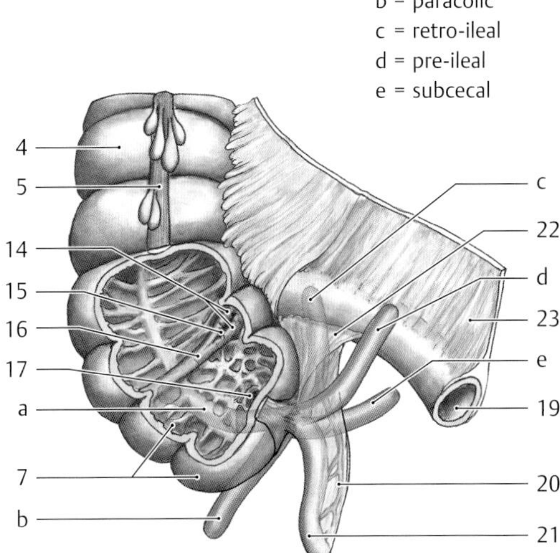


Fig. 6.45 **Variations in the position of the vermiform appendix.** The cecum has been opened to show the ileal opening.

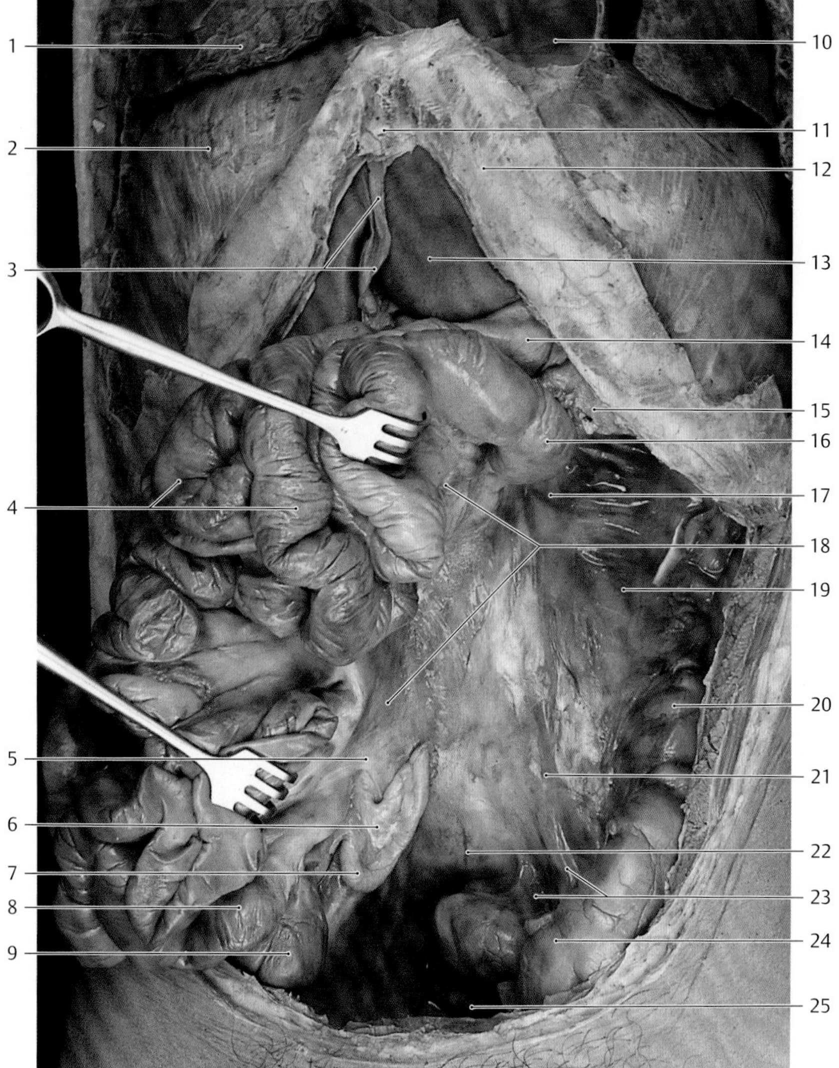


1 Lung
2 Diaphragm
3 Falciform ligament of liver
4 Jejunum
5 Ileocecal fold
6 Meso-appendix
7 Vermiform appendix
8 Terminal ileum
9 Cecum
10 Pericardial sac
11 Xiphoid process
12 Costal margin
13 Liver
14 Stomach
15 Transverse colon
16 Duodenojejunal flexure
17 Inferior duodenal fold
18 Mesentery
19 Position of left kidney
20 Descending colon
21 Position of left common iliac artery
22 Sacral promontory
23 Sigmoid mesocolon
24 Sigmoid colon
25 Rectum
26 Beginning of jejunum
27 Peritoneum of posterior abdominal wall
28 Transverse mesocolon
29 Superior duodenal fold
30 Superior duodenal recess
31 Retroduodenal recess
32 Free taenia of ascending colon
33 Ileocecal valve
34 Frenulum of ileocecal valve
35 Orifice of vermiform appendix (probe)
36 Ileocolic artery
37 Vermiform appendix with appendicular artery
38 Ascending colon

Fig. 6.46 **Abdominal organs with mesenteries** (anterior aspect). The small intestine has been reflected laterally to demonstrate the mesentery.

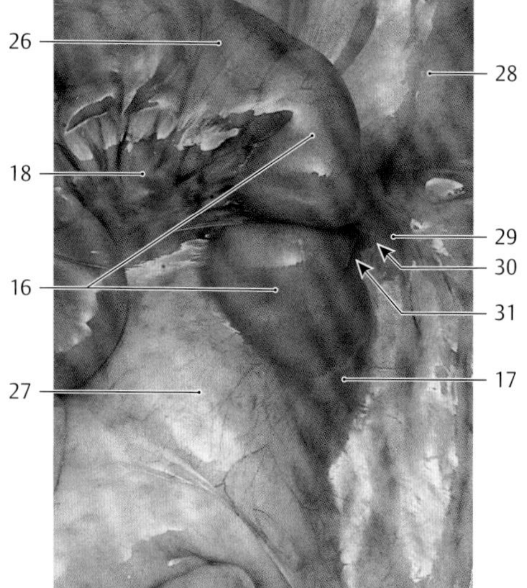


Fig. 6.47 **Duodenojejunal flexure** (detail).

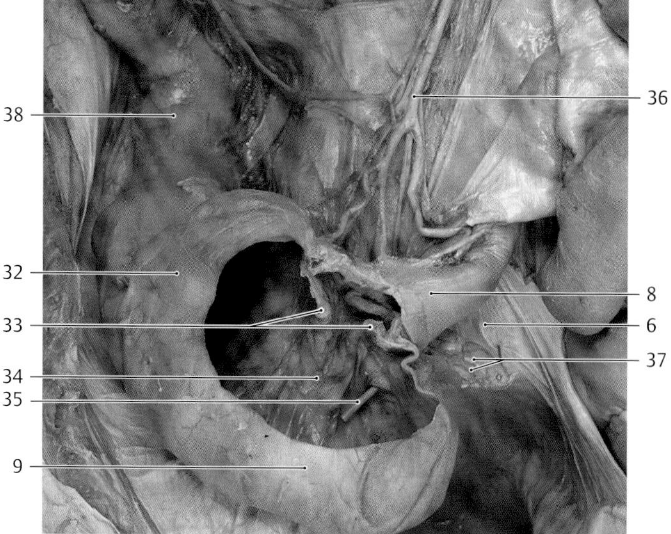


Fig. 6.48 **Ileocecal valve** (anterior aspect). Cecum and terminal part of the ileum have been opened.

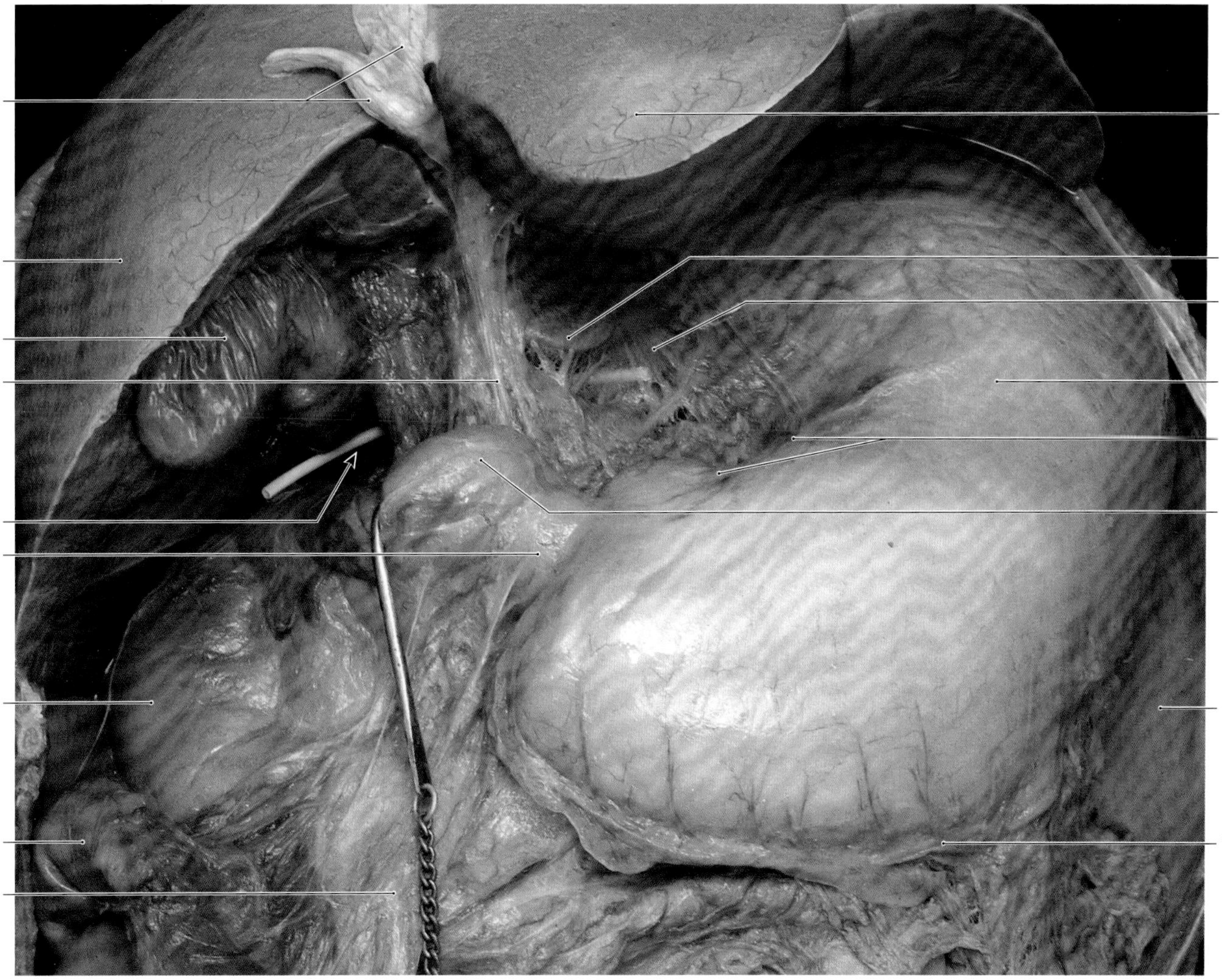

Fig. 6.49 **Upper abdominal organs** (anterior aspect). Thorax and anterior part of diaphragm have been removed and the liver raised to display the **lesser omentum**. A probe has been inserted into the epiploic foramen and lesser sac.

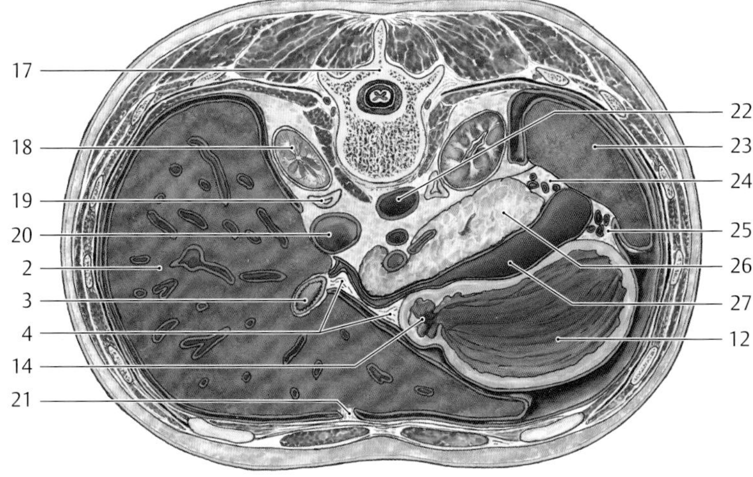


Fig. 6.50 **Horizontal section through the lesser sac** above the level of the epiploic foramen (superior aspect).

1 Falciform ligament and round ligament of the liver
2 Liver
3 Gallbladder (fundus)
4 Hepatoduodenal ligament
5 Epiploic foramen (probe)
6 Pylorus
7 Descending part of duodenum
8 Right colic flexure
9 Gastrocolic ligament
10 Caudate lobe of liver (behind lesser omentum)
11 Lesser omentum
12 Stomach
13 Lesser curvature of stomach
14 Superior part of duodenum
15 Diaphragm
16 Greater curvature of stomach with gastro-omental vessels
17 Twelfth thoracic vertebra
18 Right kidney
19 Right suprarenal gland
20 Inferior vena cava
21 Falciform ligament of liver
22 Abdominal aorta
23 Spleen
24 Lienorenal ligament
25 Gastrosplenic ligament
26 Pancreas
27 Lesser sac (omental bursa)

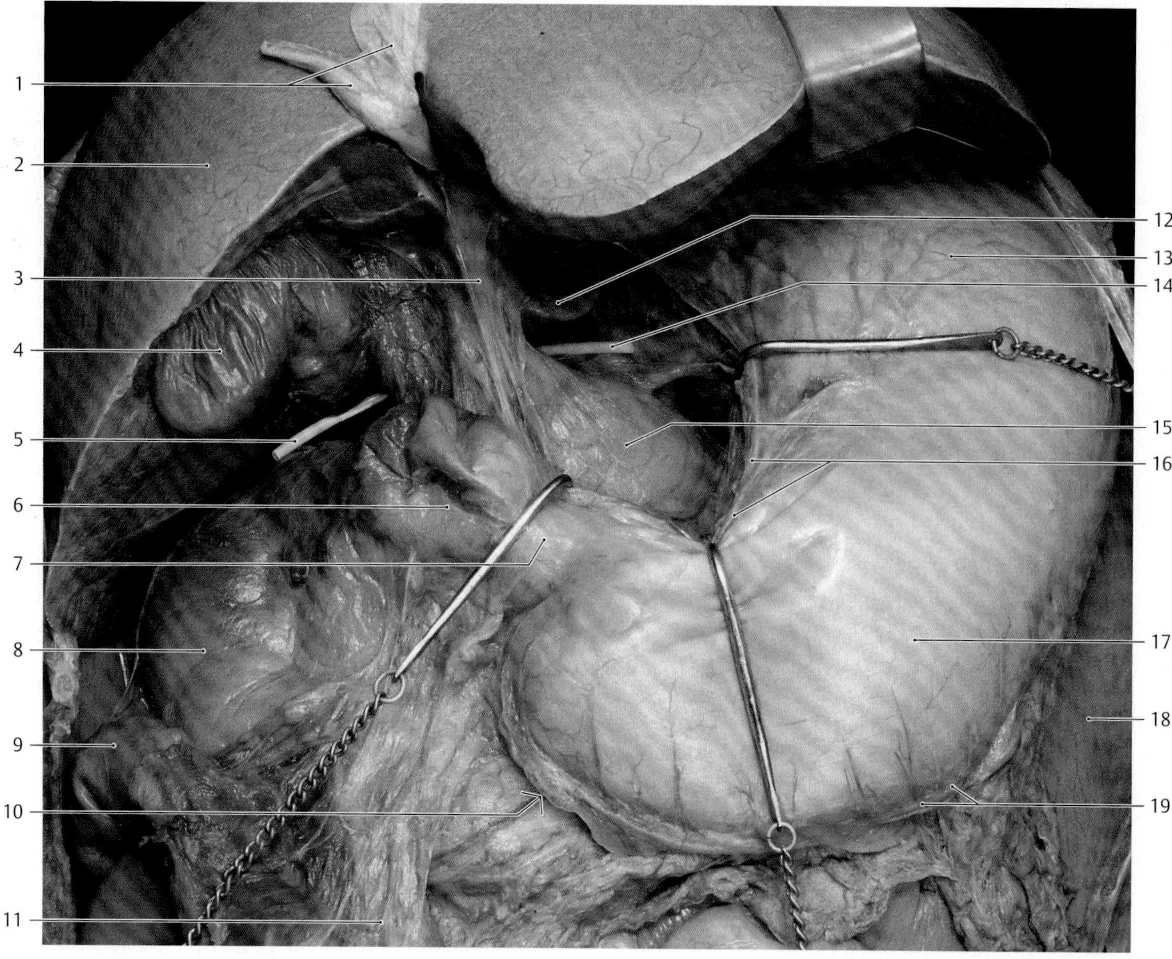


**Fig. 6.51 Upper abdominal organs** (anterior aspect). **Lesser sac.** The lesser omentum has been partly removed and the liver and stomach have been slightly reflected.

1 Falciform ligament and round ligament of the liver
2 Liver
3 Hepatoduodenal ligament
4 Gallbladder
5 Probe within the epiploic foramen
6 Superior part of duodenum
7 Pylorus
8 Descending part of duodenum
9 Right colic flexure
10 Gastrocolic ligament
11 Greater omentum
12 Caudate lobe of liver
13 Fundus of stomach
14 Probe at the level of the vestibule of lesser sac (through epiploic foramen)
15 Head of pancreas
16 Lesser curvature of stomach
17 Body of stomach
18 Diaphragm
19 Greater curvature with gastro-omental vessels
20 Head of pancreas and gastro-pancreatic fold
21 Spleen
22 Tail of pancreas
23 Left colic flexure
24 Root of transverse mesocolon
25 Transverse mesocolon
26 Gastrocolic ligament (cut edge)
27 Transverse colon
28 Umbilicus
29 Small intestine
30 Lesser omentum
31 Lesser sac (omental bursa)
32 Duodenum
33 Mesentery
34 Sigmoid colon

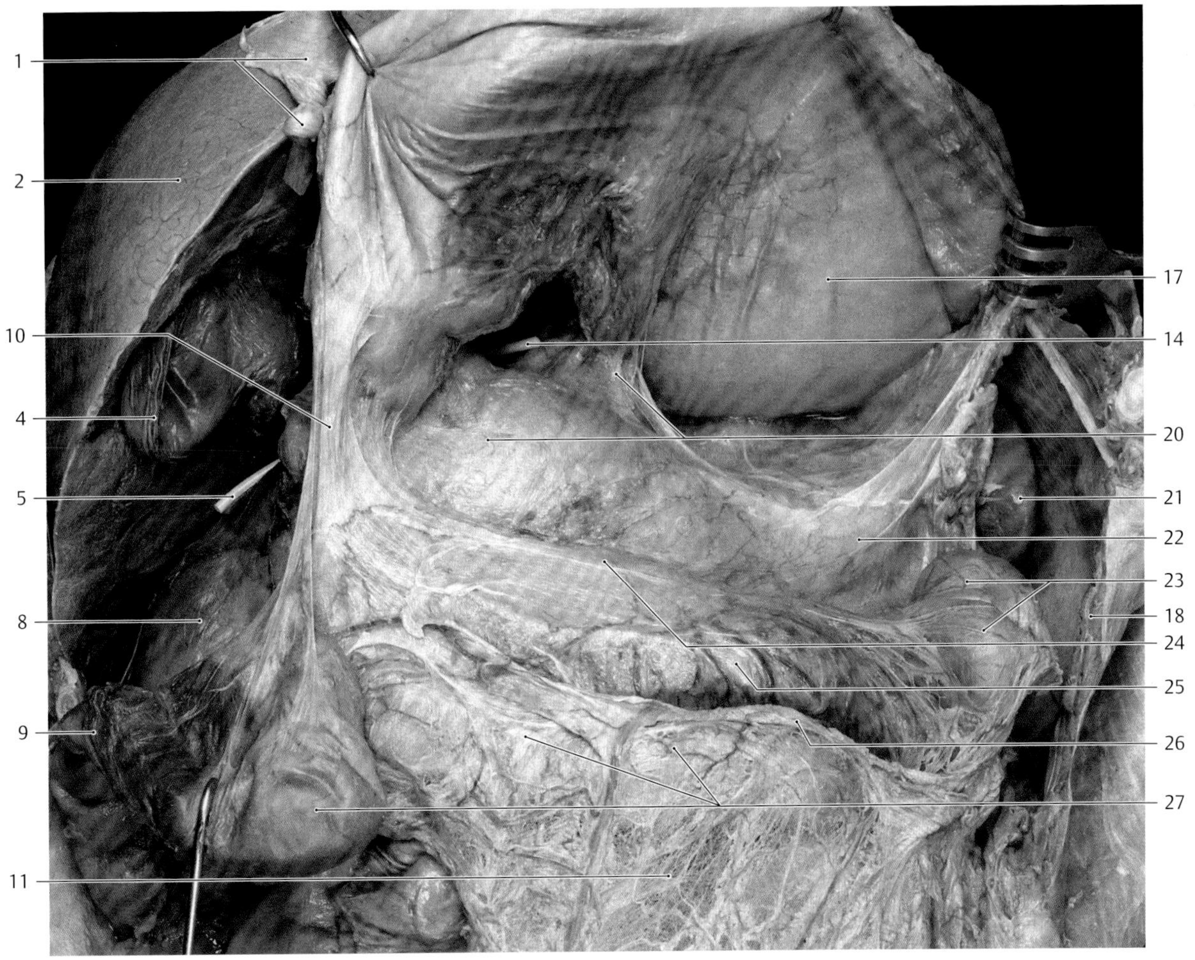

**Fig. 6.52 Upper abdominal organs** (anterior aspect). **Lesser sac.** The gastrocolic ligament has been divided and the whole stomach raised to display the posterior wall of the lesser sac.

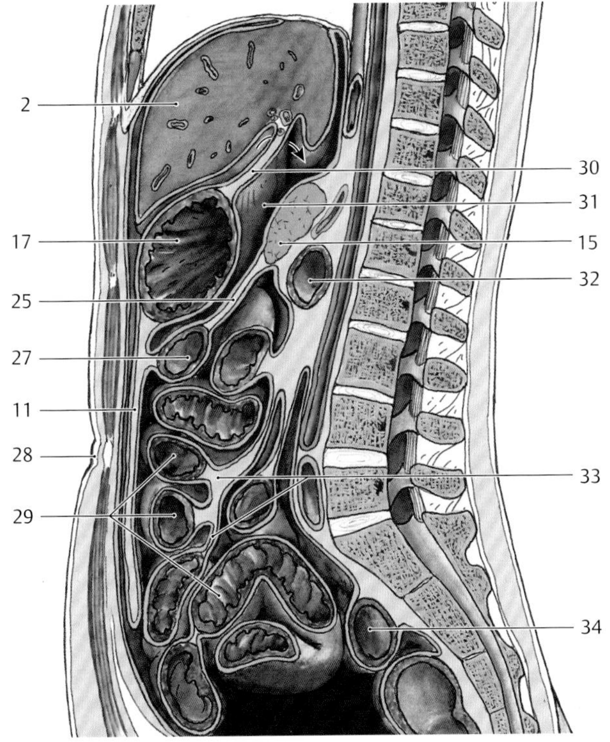


**Fig. 6.53 Midsagittal section through the abdominal cavity,** demonstrating the site of lesser sac. Blue = lesser sac (omental bursa); green = peritoneum; arrow = entrance to the lesser sac (epiploic foramen).

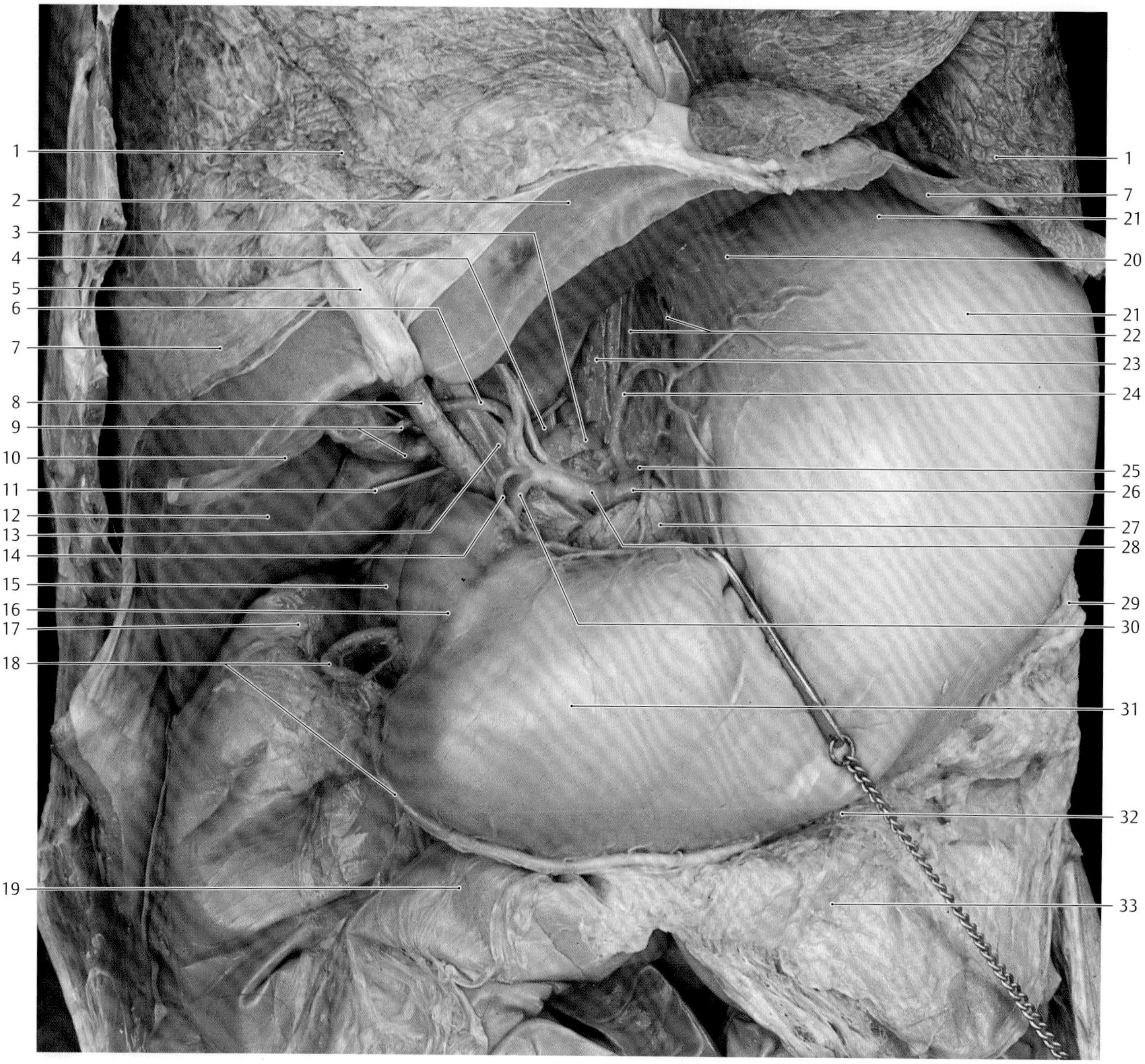

Fig. 6.54 **Upper abdominal organs** (anterior aspect). **Celiac trunk.** The lesser omentum has been removed and the lesser curvature of the stomach reflected to display the branches of the celiac trunk. The probe is situated within the epiploic foramen.

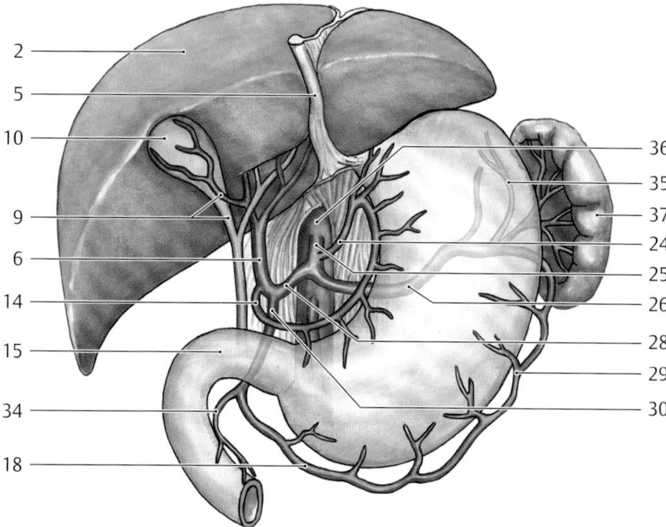


Fig. 6.55 **Arteries of upper abdominal organs and branches of celiac trunk.**

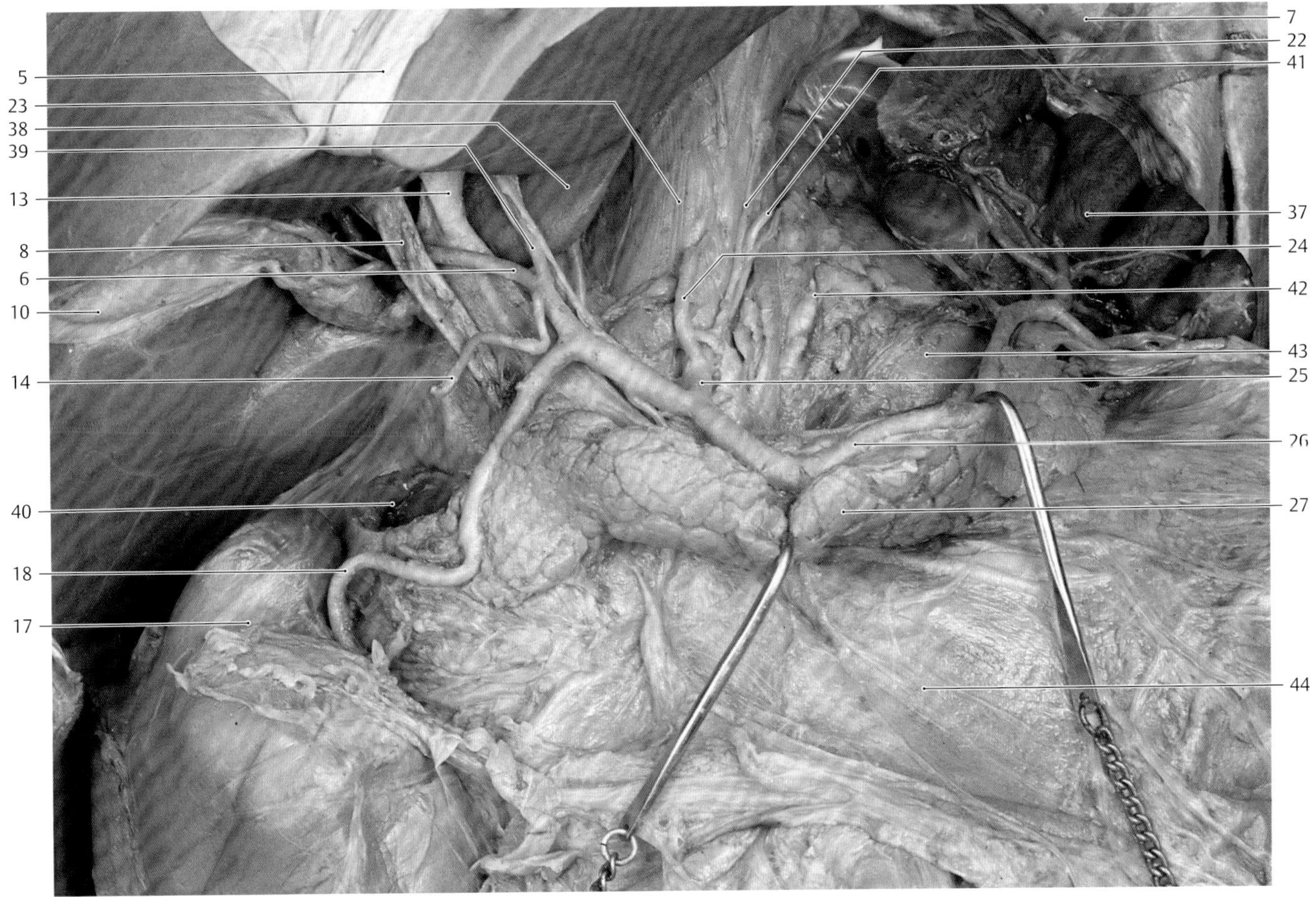


**Fig. 6.56 Upper abdominal organs** (anterior aspect). **Branches of celiac trunk; blood supply of liver, pancreas, and spleen.** The stomach, superior part of duodenum, and celiac ganglion have been removed to reveal the anterior aspect of the posterior wall of the lesser sac (omental bursa) and the vessels and ducts of the hepatoduodenal ligament. The pancreas has been slightly reflected anteriorly.

1 Lung
2 Liver (visceral surface)
3 Lymph node
4 Inferior vena cava
5 Ligamentum teres (reflected)
6 Right branch of hepatic artery proper
7 Diaphragm
8 Common hepatic duct (dilated)
9 Cystic duct and artery
10 Gallbladder
11 Probe within the epiploic foramen
12 Right lobe of liver
13 Portal vein
14 Right gastric artery
15 Duodenum
16 Pylorus
17 Right colic flexure
18 Right gastro-omental (gastro-epiploic) artery
19 Transverse colon
20 Abdominal part of esophagus (cardiac part of stomach)
21 Fundus of stomach
22 Esophageal branches of left gastric artery
23 Lumbar part of diaphragm
24 Left gastric artery
25 Celiac trunk
26 Splenic artery
27 Pancreas
28 Common hepatic artery
29 Left gastro-omental (gastro-epiploic) artery
30 Gastroduodenal artery
31 Pyloric part of stomach
32 Greater curvature of stomach
33 Gastrocolic ligament
34 Supraduodenal artery
35 Short gastric arteries
36 Aorta
37 Spleen
38 Caudate lobe of liver
39 Left branch of hepatic artery proper
40 Descending part of duodenum (cut)
41 Left inferior phrenic artery
42 Suprarenal gland
43 Kidney
44 Transverse mesocolon

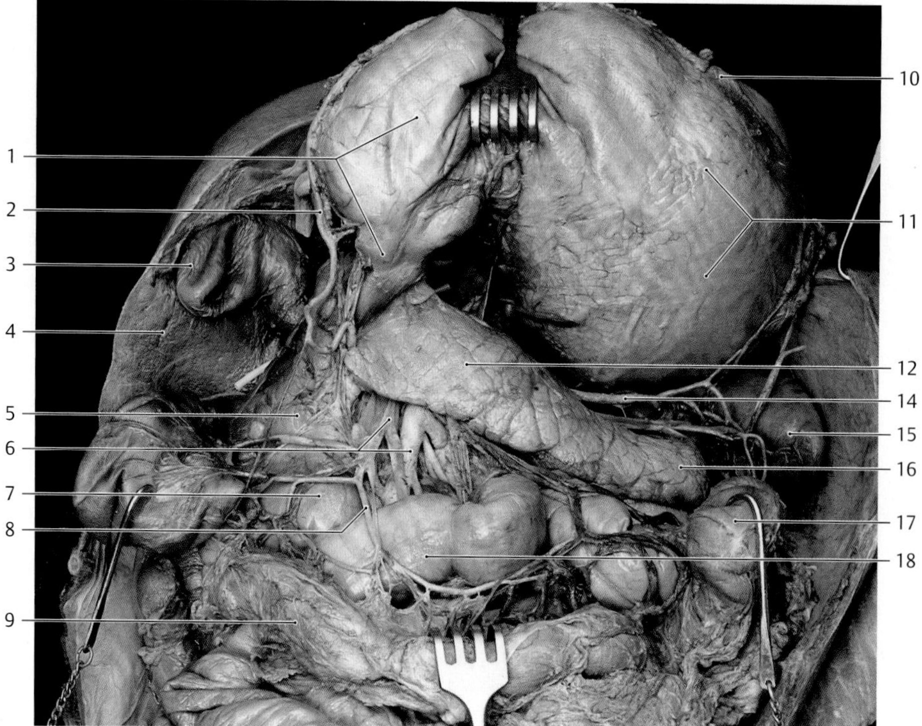


Fig. 6.57 **Posterior abdominal wall with pancreas and extrahepatic bile ducts in situ** (anterior aspect). The gastrocolic ligament has been divided and the transverse colon and the stomach replaced to display the pancreas and superior mesenteric vessels.

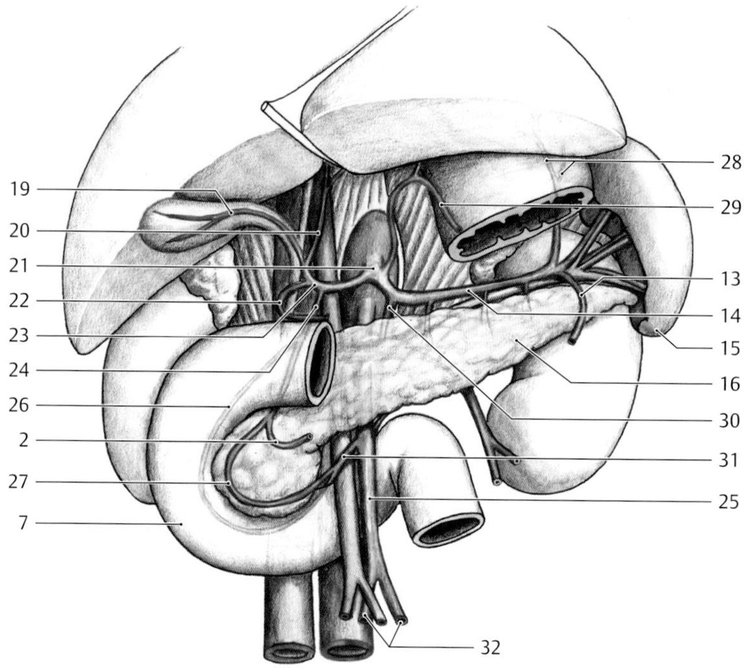


Fig. 6.58 **Blood supply of upper abdominal organs** (see corresponding Fig. 6.59 on next page). Note the branching of the celiac trunk.

1 Stomach (pyloric part) and pylorus
2 Right gastro-omental (gastro-epiploic) artery
3 Fundus of gallbladder
4 Liver (right lobe)
5 Head of pancreas
6 Superior mesenteric artery and vein
7 Duodenum
8 Middle colic artery
9 Transverse colon
10 Greater curvature of stomach (remnants of gastrocolic ligament)
11 Body of stomach
12 Body of pancreas
13 Left gastro-omental (gastro-epiploic) artery
14 Splenic artery
15 Spleen
16 Tail of pancreas
17 Left colic flexure
18 Jejunum
19 Cystic artery
20 Hepatic artery proper
21 Celiac trunk
22 Right gastric artery
23 Common hepatic artery
24 Gastroduodenal artery
25 Superior mesenteric artery
26 Superior posterior pancreaticoduodenal artery
27 Superior anterior pancreaticoduodenal artery
28 Short gastric arteries
29 Left gastric artery
30 Posterior pancreatic branch of splenic artery
31 Inferior pancreaticoduodenal artery
32 Jejunal arteries

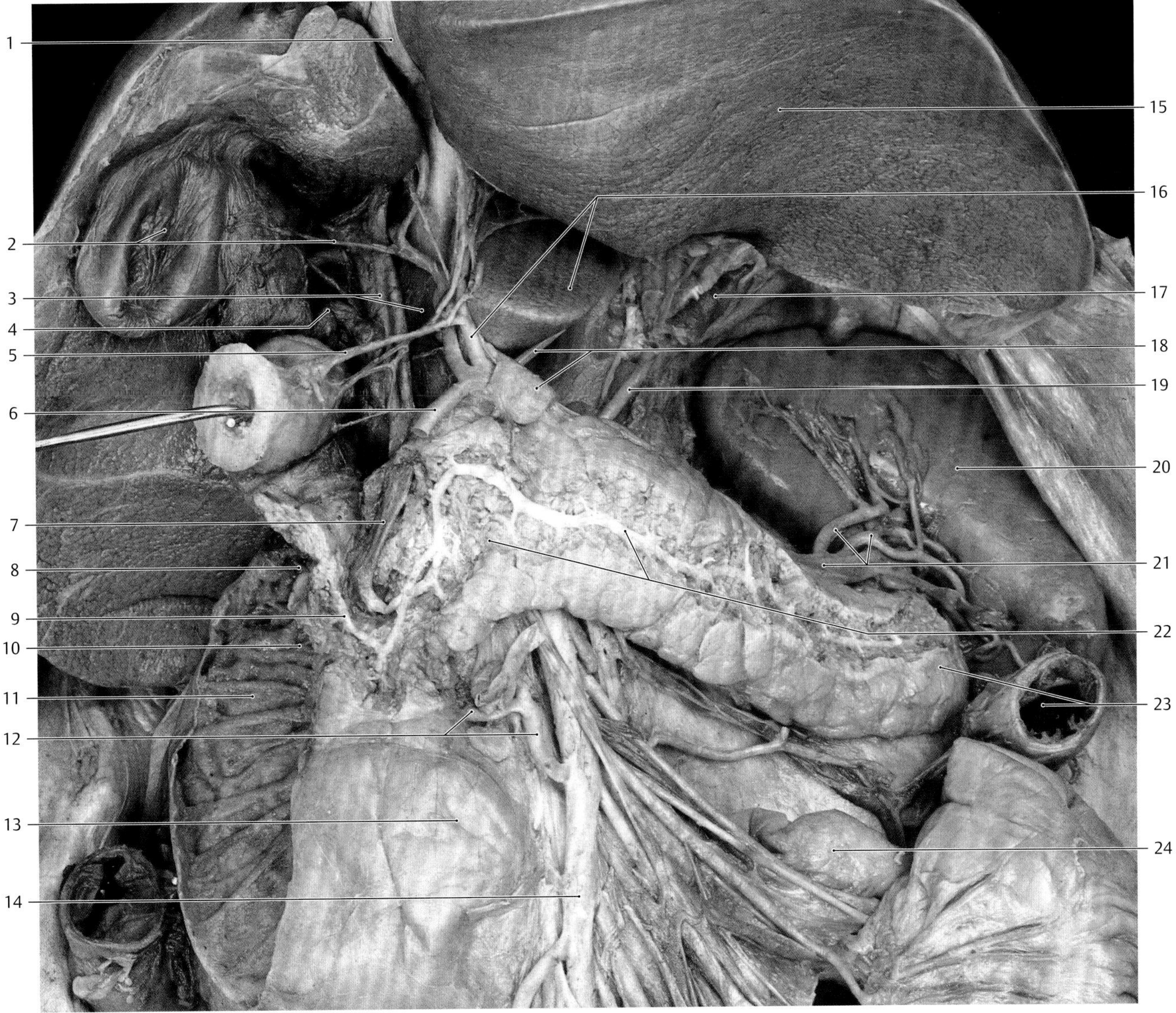


**Fig. 6.59 Posterior abdominal wall with pancreas, extrahepatic bile ducts, spleen, and liver with their vessels in situ** (anterior aspect). The stomach has been removed, the liver elevated, and the descending part of duodenum fenestrated to display the openings of the pancreatic ducts. The pancreatic ducts have been dissected. Note the location of superior mesenteric artery and vein between the duodenum and pancreas.

1 Round ligament of the liver
2 Gallbladder and cystic artery
3 Common hepatic duct and portal vein
4 Cystic duct
5 Right gastric artery (pylorus with superior part of duodenum, cut and reflected)
6 Gastroduodenal artery
7 Common bile duct
8 Probe within the minor duodenal papilla
9 Accessory pancreatic duct
10 Probe within the major duodenal papilla
11 Descending part of duodenum (opened)
12 Middle colic artery and inferior pancreaticoduodenal artery
13 Horizontal part of duodenum (distended)
14 Superior mesenteric artery
15 Liver (left lobe)
16 Caudate lobe of liver and hepatic artery proper
17 Abdominal part of esophagus (cut)
18 Probe in epiploic foramen and lymph node
19 Left gastric artery
20 Spleen
21 Splenic vein and branches of splenic artery
22 Main pancreatic duct and head of pancreas
23 Left colic flexure and tail of pancreas
24 Duodenojejunal flexure

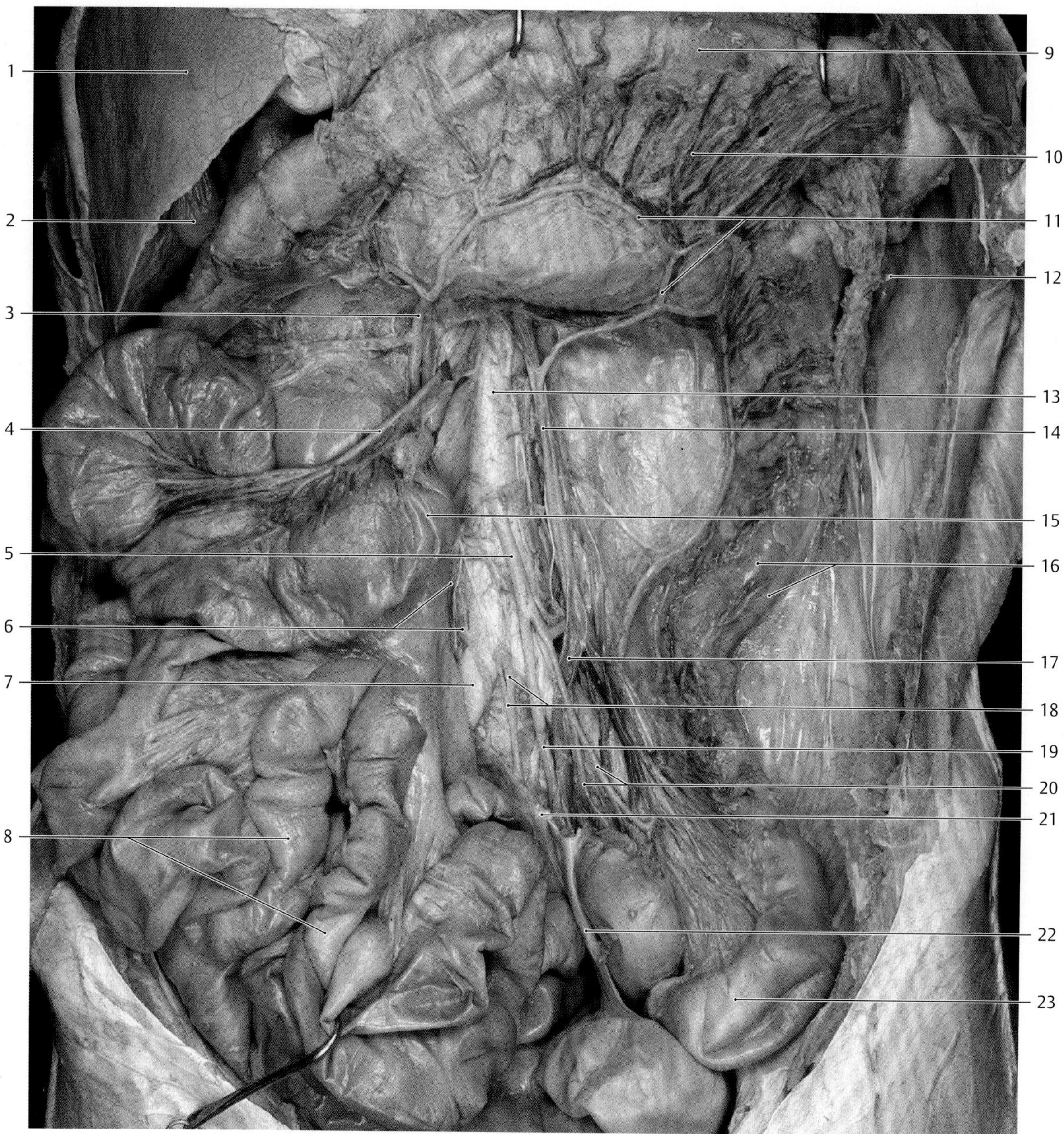


**Fig. 6.60 Lower abdominal organs** (anterior aspect). **Inferior mesenteric artery and autonomic plexus.** The transverse colon with the mesocolon has been raised and the small intestine reflected.

1 Liver
2 Gallbladder
3 Middle colic artery
4 Jejunal artery
5 Inferior mesenteric artery
6 Sympathetic nerves and ganglia
7 Right common iliac artery
8 Small intestine (ileum)
9 Transverse colon (reflected)
10 Transverse mesocolon
11 Anastomosis between middle and left colic artery
12 Spleen
13 Abdominal aorta
14 Left colic artery
15 Duodenojejunal flexure
16 Descending colon (free taenia of colon)
17 Inferior mesenteric vein
18 Superior hypogastric plexus
19 Superior rectal artery
20 Sigmoid arteries
21 Peritoneum (cut edge)
22 Sigmoid mesocolon
23 Sigmoid colon

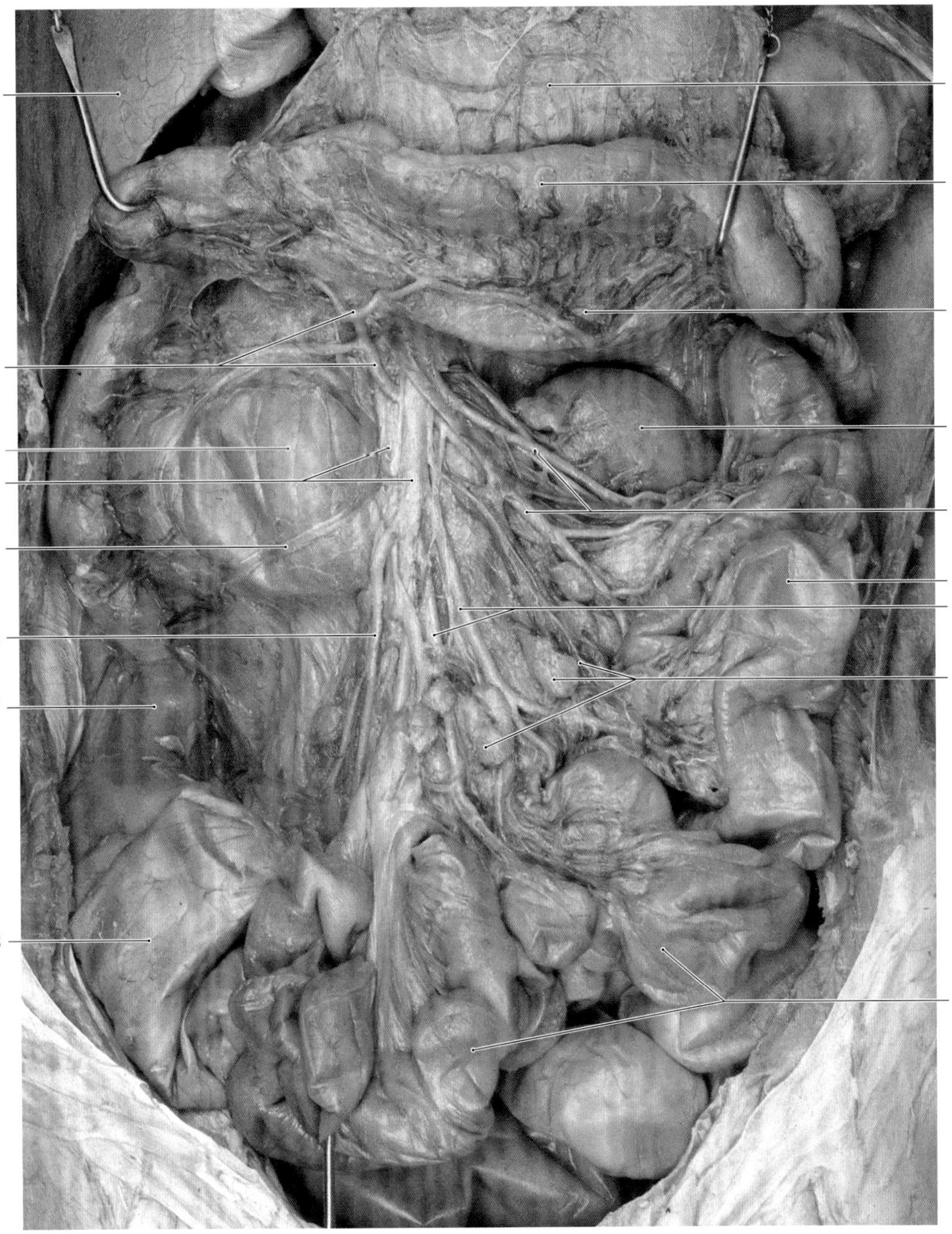

Fig. 6.61 **Lower abdominal organs** (anterior aspect). **Superior mesenteric artery and mesenteric lymph nodes.** The transverse colon has been reflected.

1 Liver
2 Middle colic artery
3 Horizontal part of duodenum (extended)
4 Superior mesenteric artery and vein
5 Right colic artery
6 Ileocolic artery
7 Ascending colon
8 Cecum
9 Greater omentum (reflected)
10 Transverse colon
11 Transverse mesocolon
12 Duodenojejunal flexure
13 Jejunal arteries
14 Jejunum
15 Ileal arteries
16 Mesenteric lymph nodes and lymph vessels
17 Ileum
18 Stomach
19 Head of pancreas
20 Portal vein
21 Descending colon

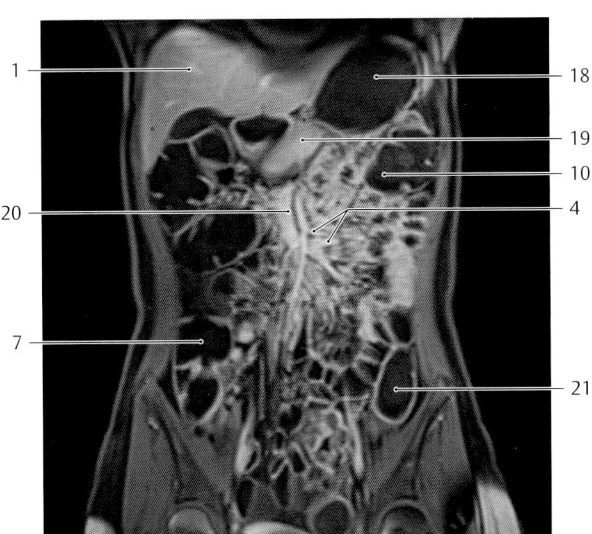


Fig. 6.62 **Frontal section through the abdominal cavity at the level of the root of the mesentery** (MRI, Sellink technique). (Courtesy of Prof. Uder, Institute of Radiology, University Hospital Erlangen, Germany.)

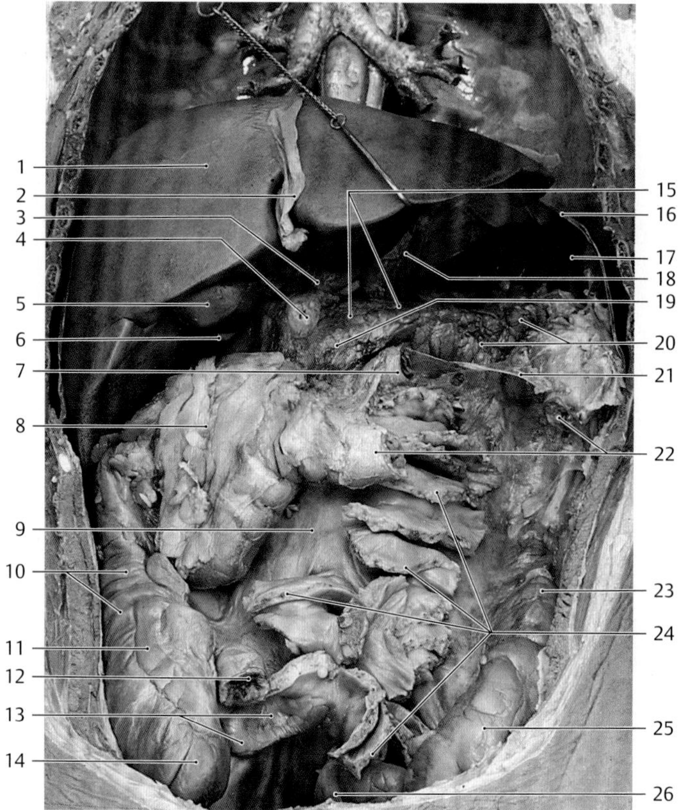


**Fig. 6.63 Abdominal cavity** after removal of stomach, jejunum, ileum, and part of the transverse colon. The liver has been slightly raised.

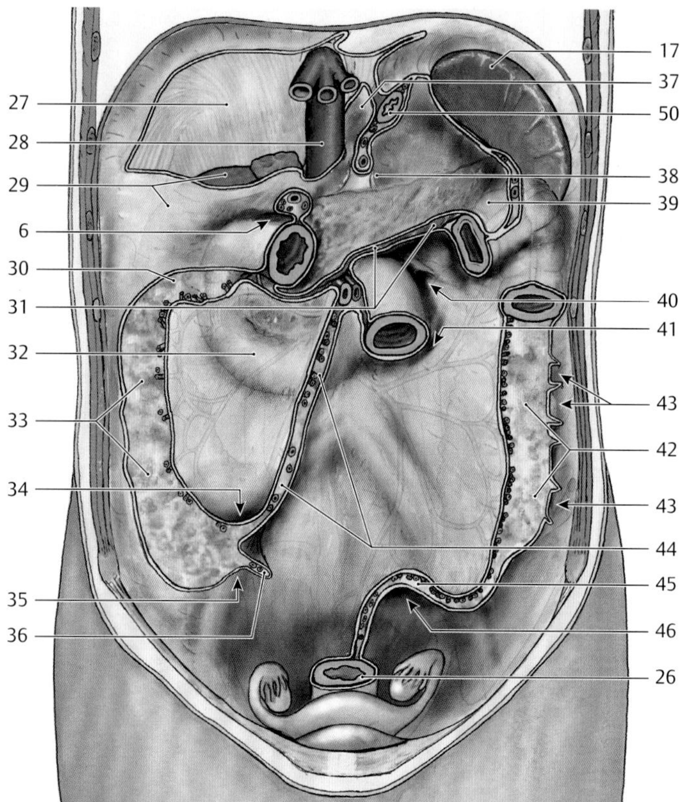


1 Liver
2 Falciform ligament
3 Hepatoduodenal ligament
4 Pylorus (divided)
5 Gallbladder
6 Probe within the epiploic foramen
7 Duodenojejunal flexure (divided)
8 Greater omentum
9 Root of mesentery
10 Ascending colon
11 Free colic taenia
12 End of ileum (divided)
13 Vermiform appendix with meso-appendix
14 Cecum
15 Pancreas and site of lesser sac (omental bursa)
16 Diaphragm
17 Spleen
18 Cardia (part of stomach, divided)
19 Head of pancreas
20 Body and tail of pancreas
21 Transverse mesocolon
22 Transverse colon (divided)
23 Descending colon
24 Cut edge of mesentery
25 Sigmoid colon
26 Rectum
27 Attachment of bare area of liver
28 Inferior vena cava
29 Kidney
30 Attachment of right colic flexure
31 Root of transverse mesocolon
32 Junction between descending and horizontal parts of duodenum
33 Bare surface for ascending colon
34 Ileocecal recess
35 Retrocecal recess
36 Root of meso-appendix
37 Superior recess } of lesser sac (omental bursa)
38 Isthmus (opening) } of lesser sac (omental bursa)
39 Splenic recess } of lesser sac (omental bursa)
40 Superior duodenal recess
41 Inferior duodenal recess
42 Bare surface for descending colon
43 Paracolic recesses
44 Root of mesentery
45 Root of mesosigmoid
46 Intersigmoid recess
47 Hepatic veins
48 Duodenojejunal flexure
49 Attachment of left colic flexure
50 Esophagus

**Fig. 6.64 Peritoneal reflections from organs and the position of the root of the mesentery and peritoneal recesses on the posterior abdominal wall.** Arrows = position of peritoneal recesses.

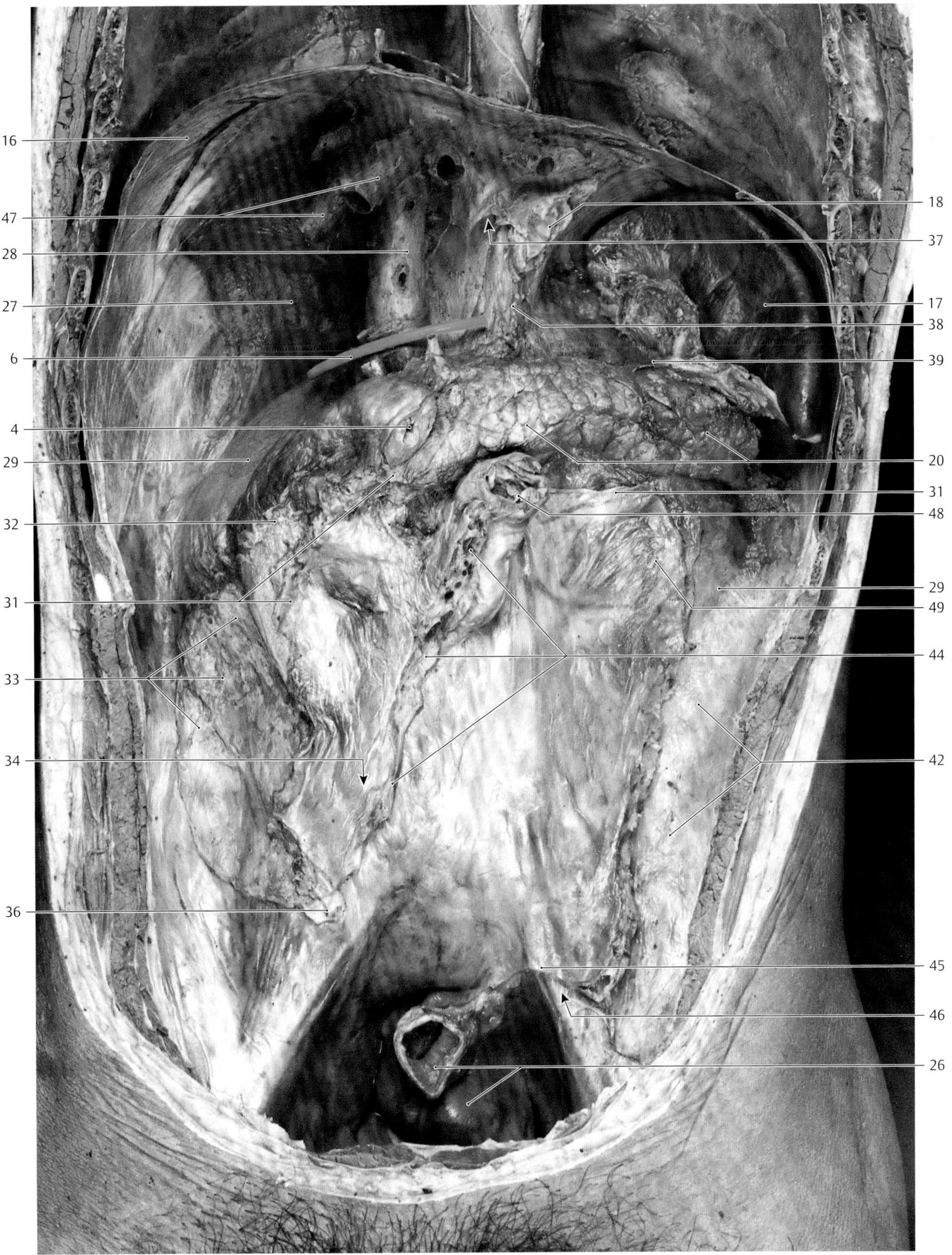


Fig. 6.65 **Peritoneal recesses on the posterior abdominal wall** (anterior aspect). The liver, stomach, jejunum, ileum, and colon have been removed. The duodenum, pancreas, and spleen have been left in place. Arrows = position of peritoneal recesses.

**Fig. 6.66 Horizontal section through the abdominal cavity.** Section 1 (from below).

1 Rectus abdominis muscle
2 Falciform ligament
3 Liver (right lobe)
4 Inferior vena cava
5 Diaphragm
6 Intervertebral disc
7 Liver (left lobe)
8 Rib
9 Liver (caudate lobe)
10 Abdominal (descending) aorta
11 Stomach
12 Spleen
13 Spinal cord
14 Erector spinae muscle

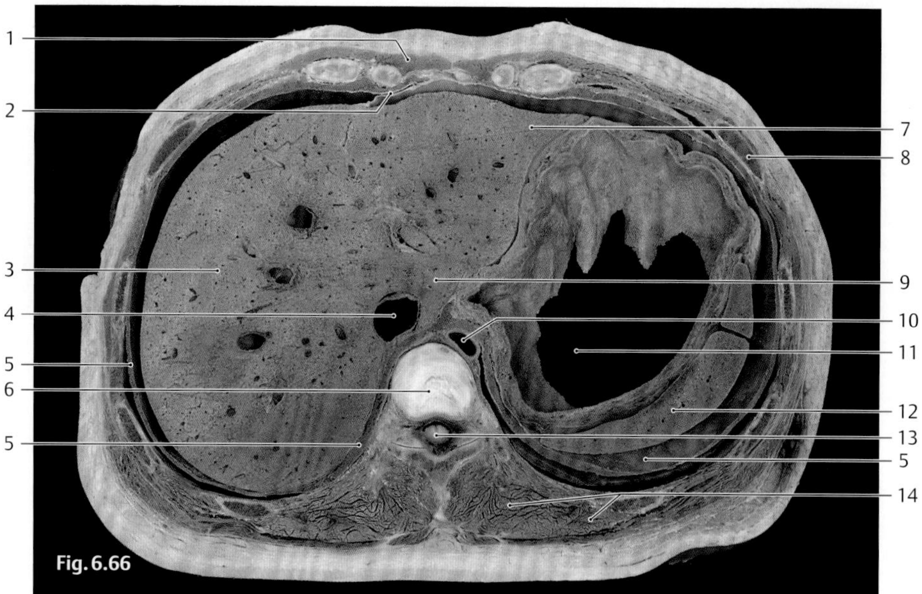


15 Rectus abdominis muscle
16 External abdominal oblique muscle
17 Transverse colon
18 Head of pancreas
19 Major duodenal papilla
20 Duodenum
21 Suprarenal gland and ureter
22 Kidney
23 Body of vertebra
24 Round ligament of liver
25 Small intestine
26 Superior mesenteric artery and vein
27 Psoas major muscle
28 Descending colon
29 Quadratus lumborum muscle
30 Cauda equina
31 Ileocecal valve

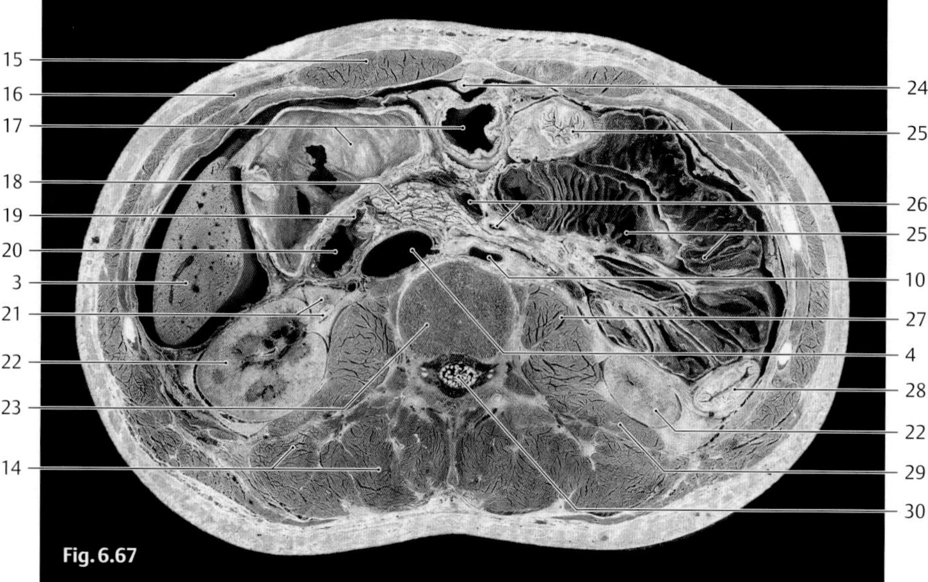


**Fig. 6.67 Horizontal section through the abdominal cavity** at the level of major duodenal papilla. Section 2 (from below).

32 Cecum
33 Common iliac artery and vein
34 Gluteus medius muscle
35 Vertebral canal and dura mater
36 Iliacus muscle
37 Ilium
38 Right renal vein
39 Common iliac arteries
40 Spinous process
41 Internal abdominal oblique muscle
42 Transverse abdominal muscle

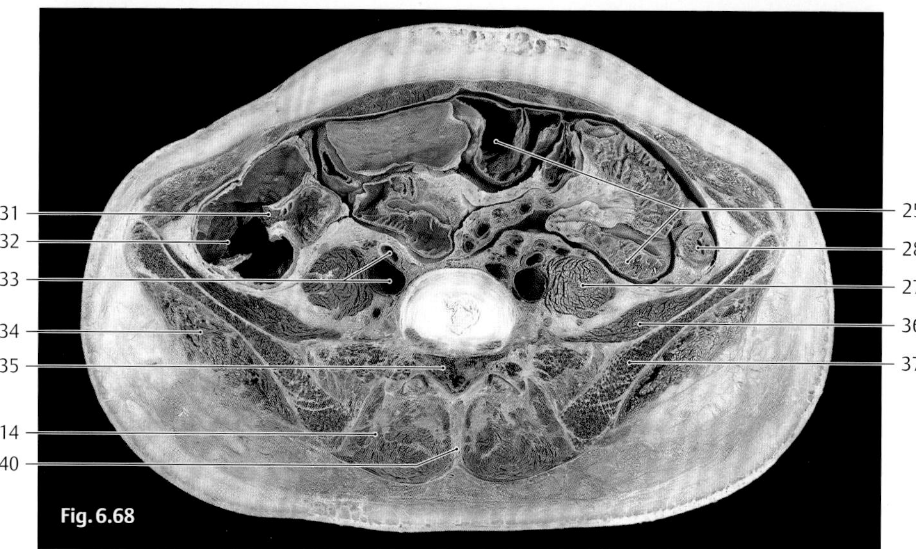


**Fig. 6.68 Horizontal section through the abdominal cavity.** Section 3 (from below).

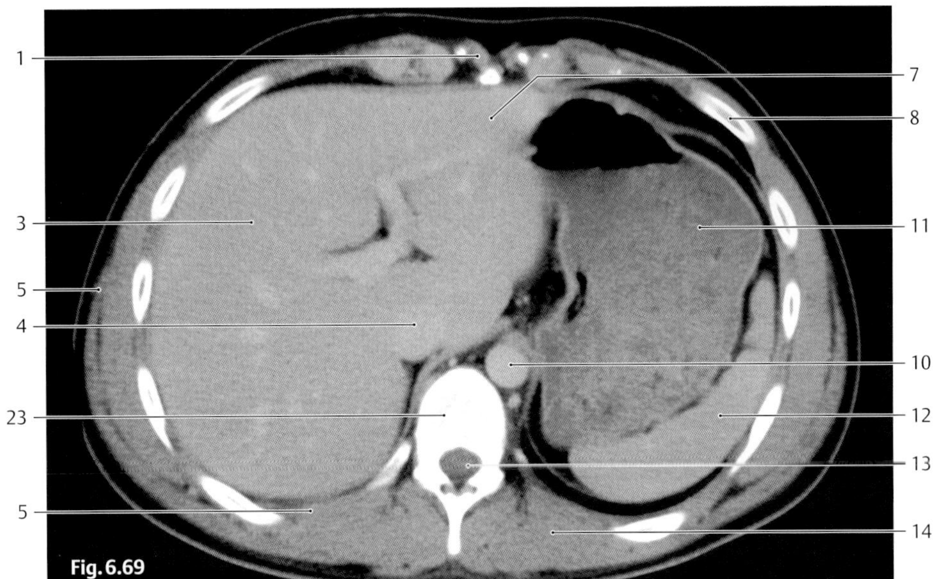


**Fig. 6.69 Horizontal section through the abdominal cavity** at the level of section 1 (CT scan). (Courtesy of Prof. Uder, Institute of Radiology, University Hospital Erlangen, Germany.)

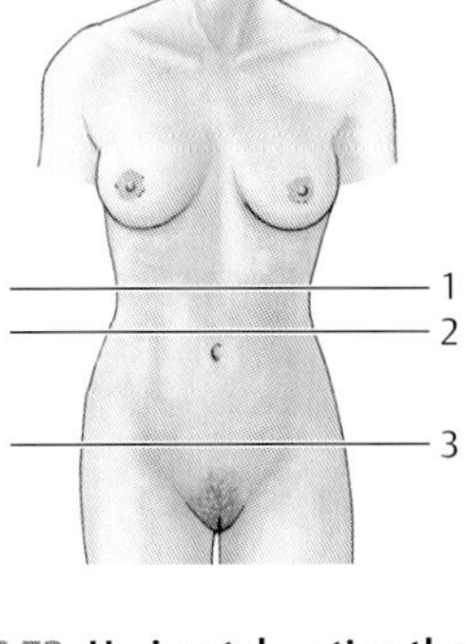


**Fig. 6.72 Horizontal section through the abdominal cavity.** Levels of the sections are indicated.

15
3
18
38
23
22
14
25
8
25
10
27
12
22
Fig. 6.70

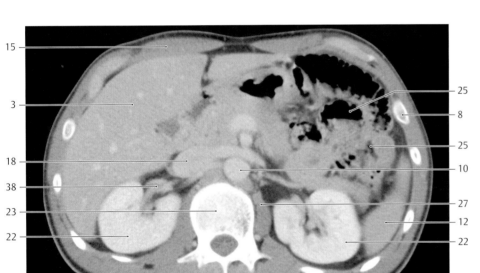

**Fig. 6.70 Horizontal section through the abdominal cavity** at the level of section 2 (CT scan). (Courtesy of Prof. Uder, Institute of Radiology, University Hospital Erlangen, Germany.)

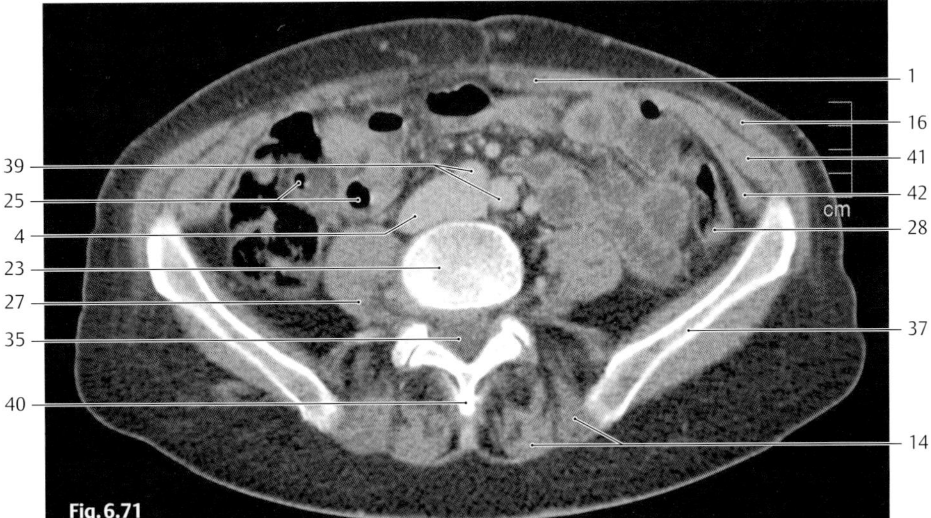


**Fig. 6.71 Horizontal section through the abdominal cavity** at the level of section 3 (CT scan). (Courtesy of Prof. Uder, Institute of Radiology, University Hospital Erlangen, Germany.)

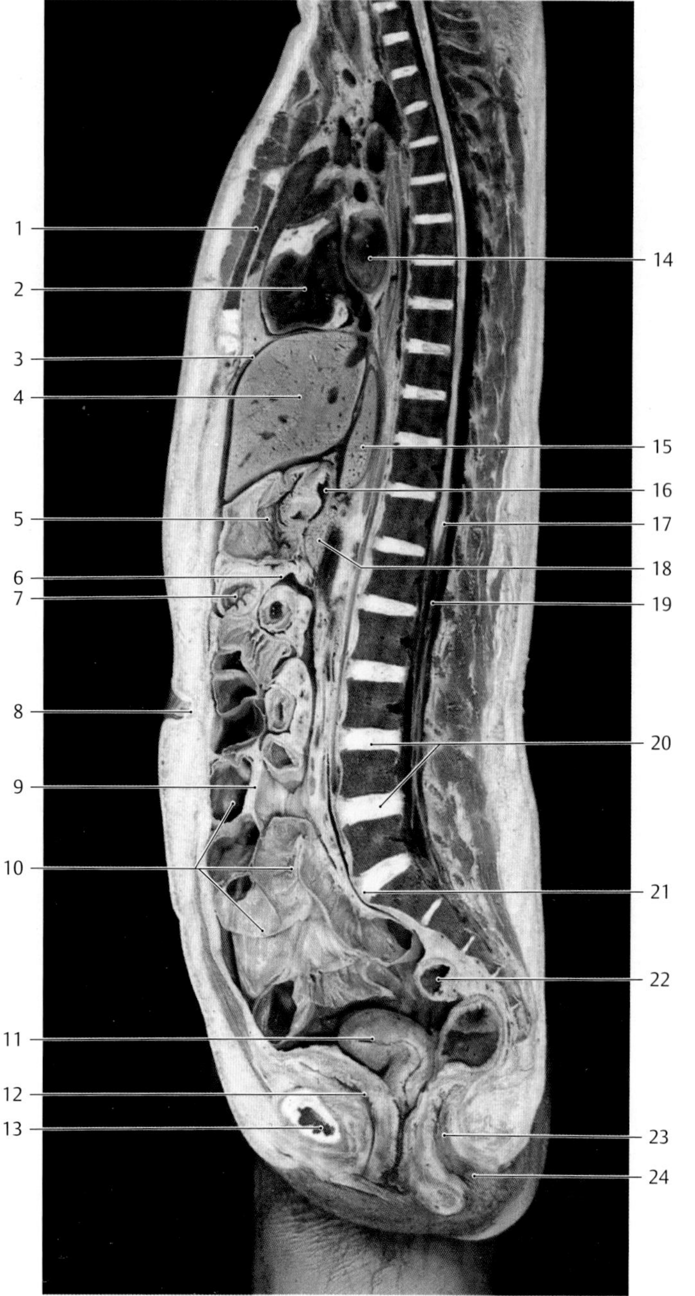


Fig. 6.73 **Midsagittal section through the female trunk.**

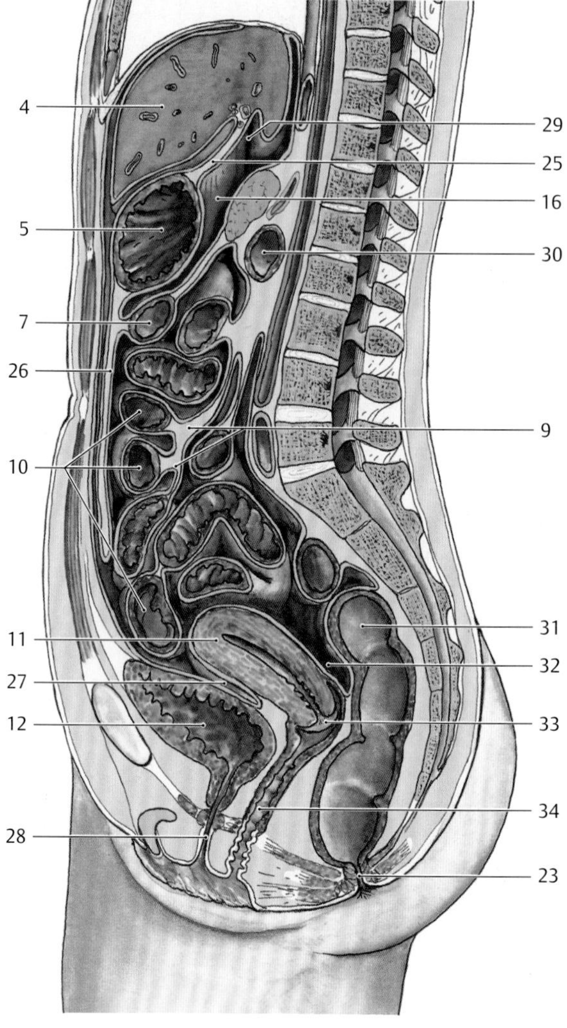


Fig. 6.74 **Midsagittal section through the female trunk.** Blue = lesser sac (omental bursa); green = peritoneum.

1 Sternum
2 Right ventricle of heart
3 Diaphragm
4 Liver
5 Stomach
6 Transverse mesocolon
7 Transverse colon
8 Umbilicus
9 Mesentery
10 Small intestine
11 Uterus
12 Urinary bladder
13 Pubic symphysis
14 Left atrium of heart
15 Caudate lobe of liver
16 Lesser sac (omental bursa)
17 Conus medullaris
18 Pancreas
19 Cauda equina
20 Intervertebral discs (lumbar vertebral column)
21 Sacral promontory
22 Sigmoid colon
23 Anal canal
24 Anus
25 Lesser omentum
26 Greater omentum
27 Vesico-uterine pouch
28 Urethra
29 Epiploic (omental) foramen
30 Duodenum
31 Rectum
32 Recto-uterine pouch
33 Vaginal part of cervix of uterus
34 Vagina

# 7 Retroperitoneal Organs

Internal Organs

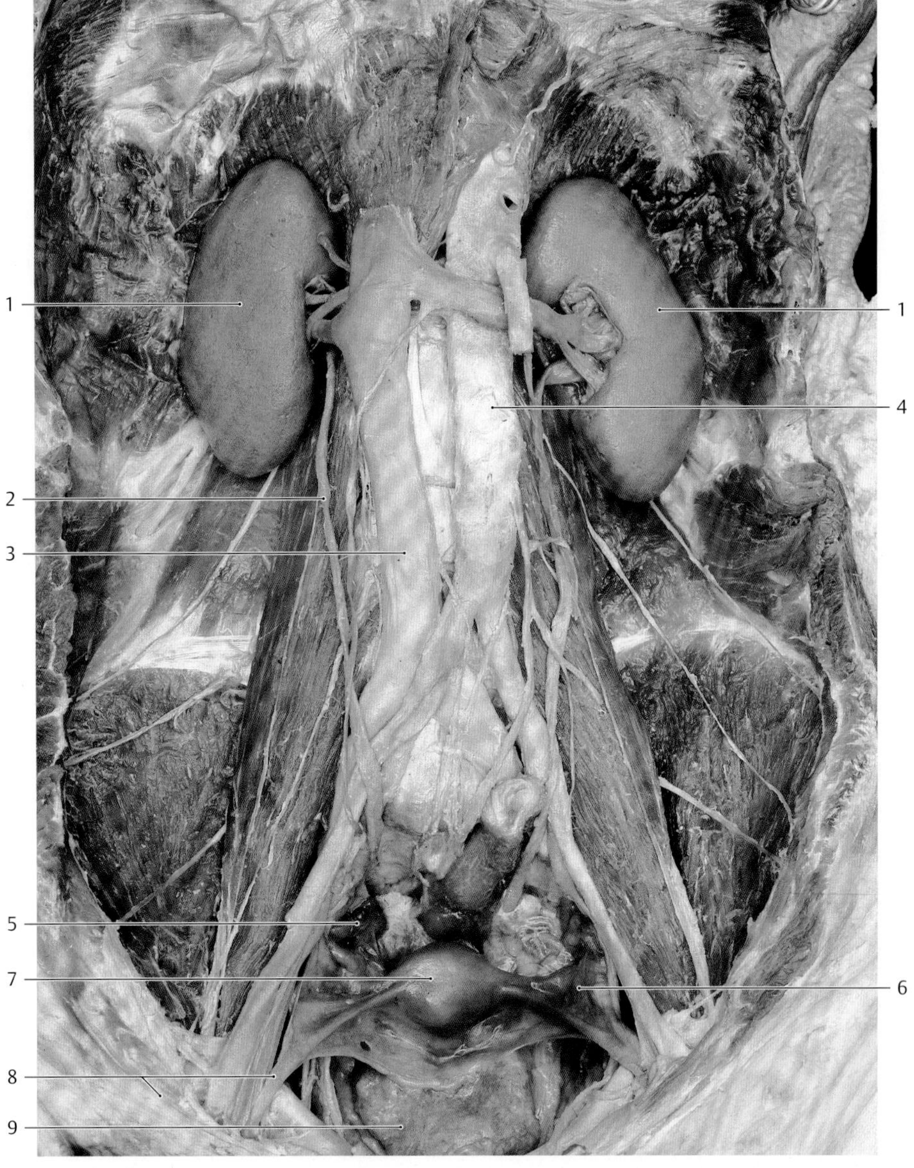


**Fig. 7.1 Retroperitoneal organs of the female in situ** (anterior aspect). View of the female pelvis showing the uterus with uterine ligaments, ovary, and urinary bladder.

1 Kidney
2 Ureter
3 Inferior vena cava
4 Abdominal aorta
5 Ovary
6 Uterine tube
7 Uterus
8 Round ligament of uterus and inguinal canal
9 Urinary bladder

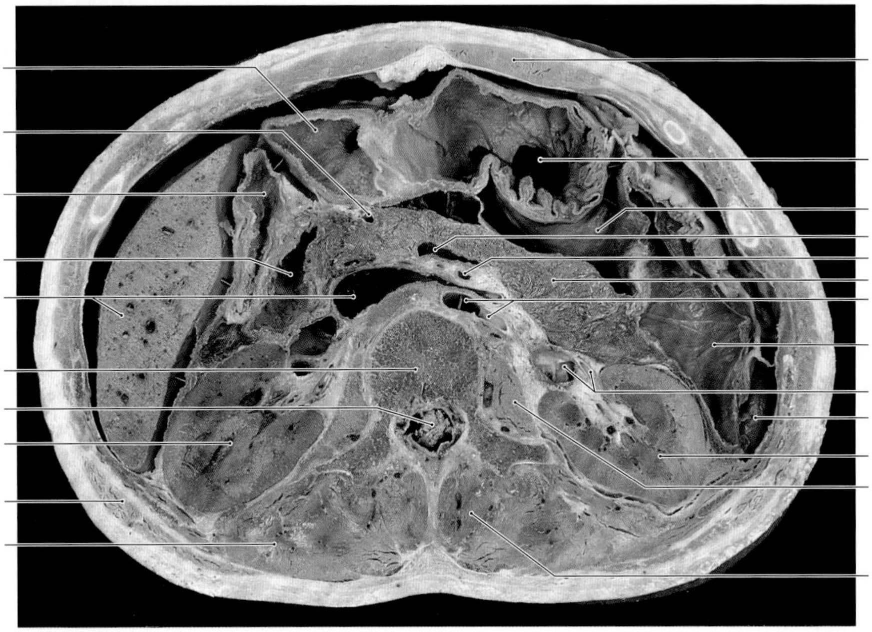

1 Pyloric antrum
2 Gastroduodenal artery
3 Descending part of duodenum
4 Vestibule of lesser sac (omental bursa)
5 Inferior vena cava and liver
6 Body of first lumbar vertebra
7 Cauda equina
8 Right kidney
9 Latissimus dorsi muscle
10 Iliocostalis muscle
11 Rectus abdominis muscle
12 Stomach
13 Lesser sac (omental bursa)
14 Splenic vein
15 Superior mesenteric artery
16 Pancreas
17 Aorta and left renal artery
18 Transverse colon
19 Renal artery and vein
20 Spleen
21 Left kidney
22 Psoas major muscle
23 Multifidus muscle

**Fig. 7.2 Horizontal section through the abdominal cavity** at the level of the first lumbar vertebra (from below).

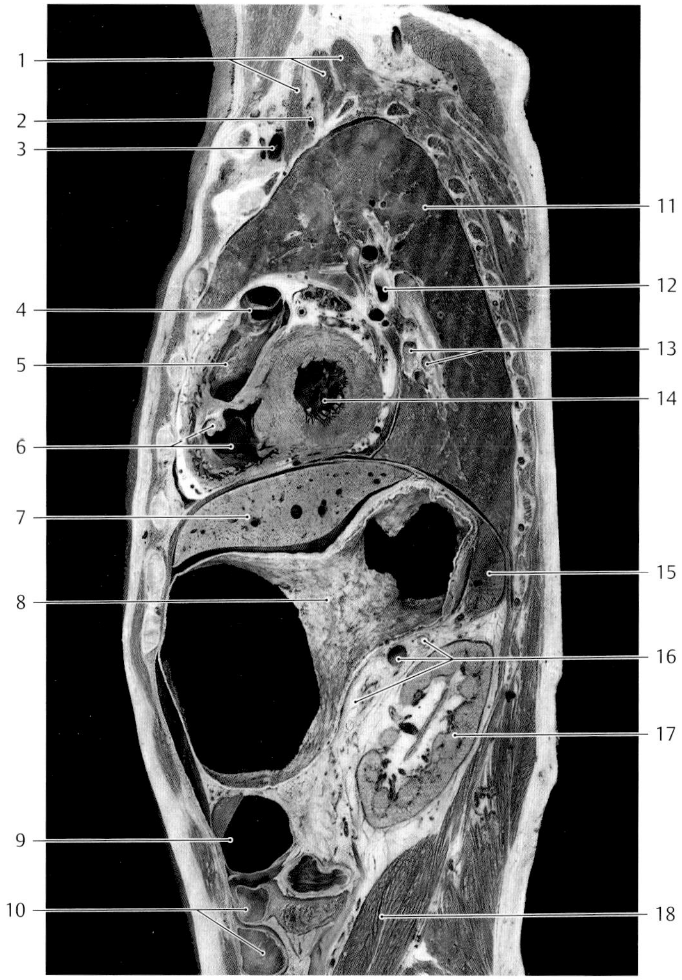

Fig. 7.3 **Parasagittal section through thoracic and abdominal cavities** at the level of the left kidney 5.5 cm left to the median plane.

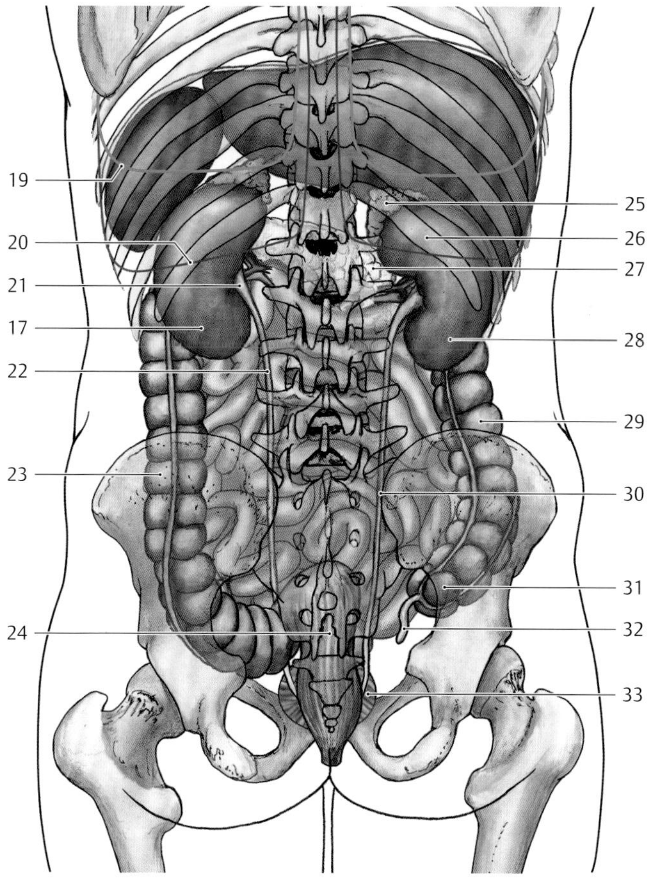

Fig. 7.4 **Positions of urinary organs** (posterior aspect). Notice that the upper part of the kidney reaches the level of the margin of the pleura and lung.

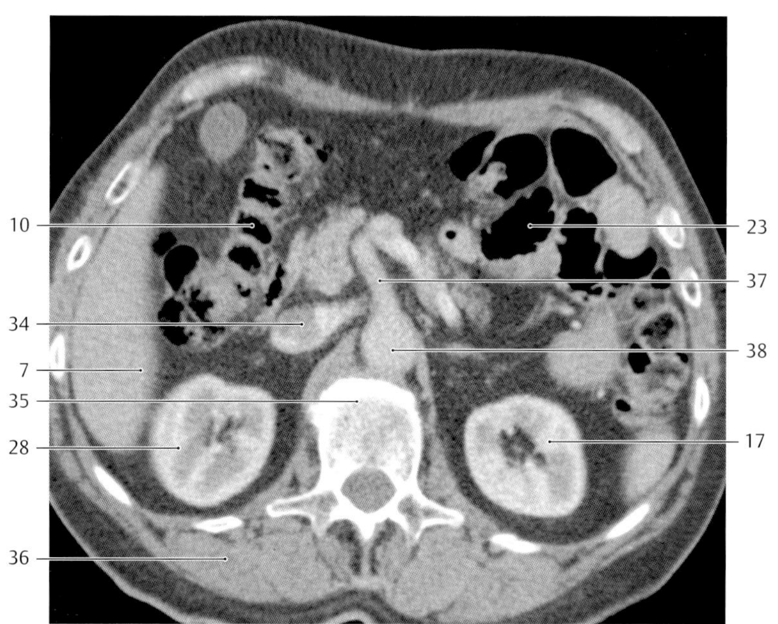


Fig. 7.5 **Horizontal section through the abdominal cavity** (CT scan). (Courtesy of Prof. Uder, Institute of Radiology, University Hospital Erlangen, Germany.)

1 Anterior, middle, and posterior scalene muscles
2 Left subclavian artery
3 Left subclavian vein
4 Pulmonic valve
5 Arterial cone
6 Right ventricle of heart
7 Liver
8 Stomach
9 Transverse colon
10 Small intestine
11 Left lung
12 Left main bronchus
13 Branches of pulmonary vein
14 Left ventricle of heart
15 Spleen
16 Splenic artery and vein, and pancreas
17 Left kidney
18 Psoas major muscle
19 Margin of lung
20 Margin of pleura
21 Renal pelvis
22 Left ureter
23 Descending colon
24 Rectum
25 Suprarenal gland
26 Twelfth rib
27 Pancreas
28 Right kidney
29 Ascending colon
30 Right ureter
31 Cecum
32 Vermiform appendix
33 Urinary bladder
34 Inferior vena cava
35 Body of lumbar vertebra (L1)
36 Iliocostal muscle
37 Superior mesenteric artery
38 Abdominal aorta

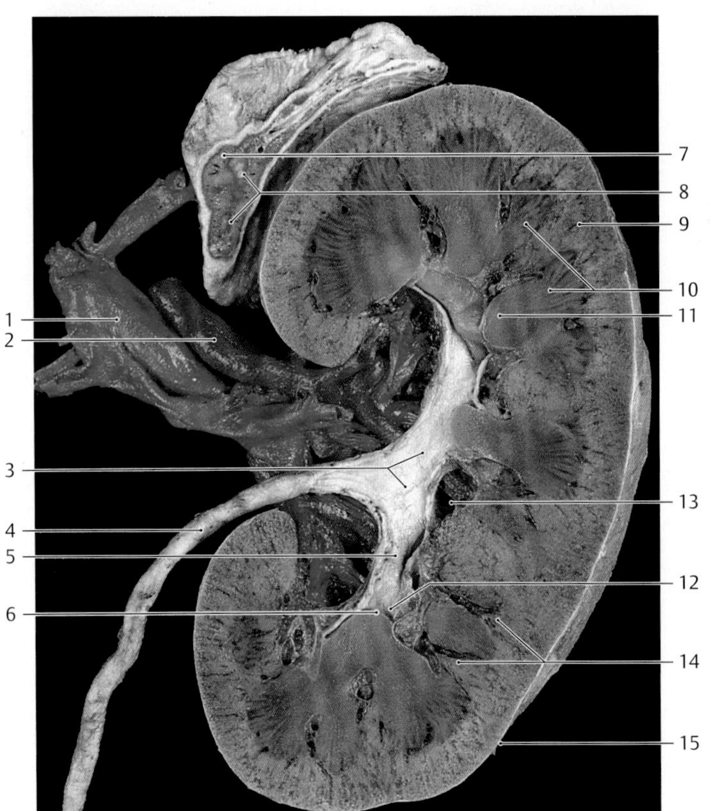


Fig. 7.6 **Coronal section through right kidney and suprarenal gland** (posterior aspect). The renal pelvis has been opened and the fatty tissue removed to display the renal vessels.

1 Renal vein
2 Renal artery
3 Renal pelvis
4 Abdominal part of ureter
5 Major renal calyx
6 Cribriform area of renal papilla
7 Cortex of suprarenal gland
8 Medulla of suprarenal gland
9 Cortex of kidney
10 Medulla of kidney
11 Renal papilla
12 Minor renal calyx
13 Renal sinus
14 Renal columns
15 Fibrous capsule of kidney

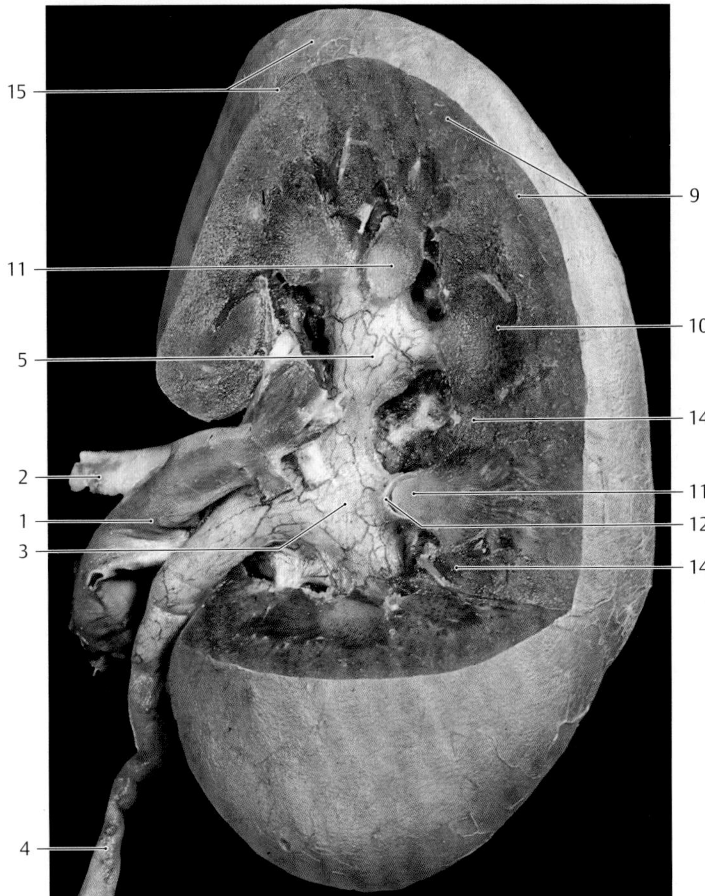


Fig. 7.7 **Right kidney** (posterior aspect). Partial coronal section to expose the internal aspect of the kidney.

Each kidney can be divided into five segments, which are supplied by individual interlobar arteries known as end arteries. Thus, obstruction leads to infarcts that clearly mark the segment borders. There are four segments on the anterior surface of the kidney, and only three on the posterior surface (1, 4, and 5).

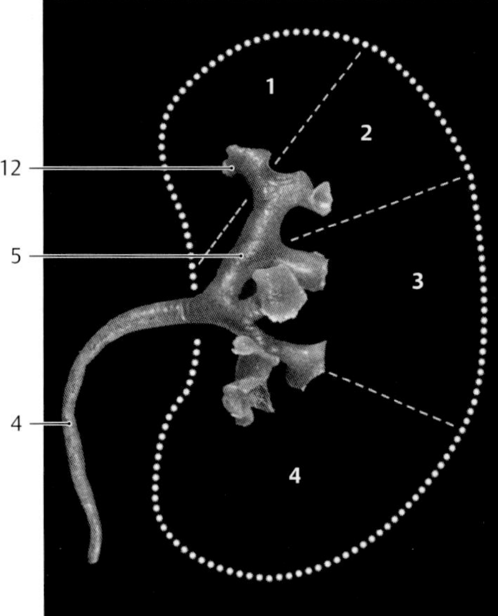


Fig. 7.8 **Cast of renal pelvis and calices.**
1–4 = Renal segments on anterior surface.

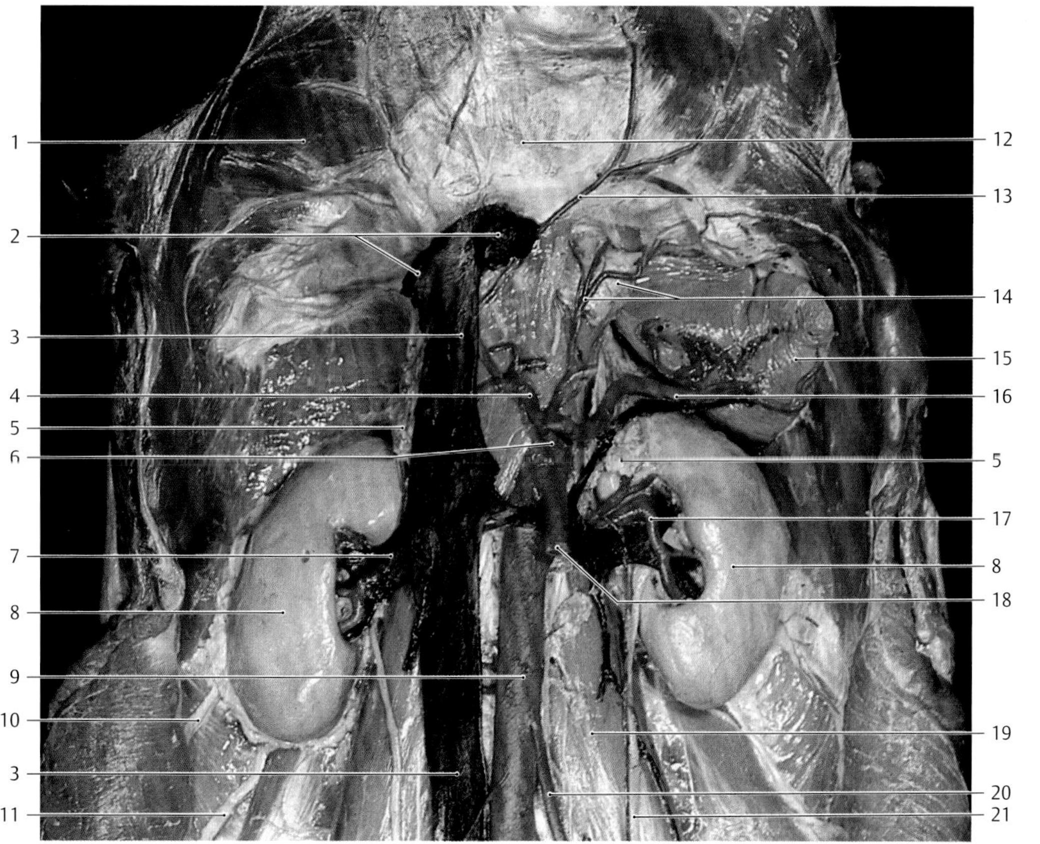


Fig. 7.9 **Retroperitoneal organs, kidneys, and suprarenal glands in situ** (anterior aspect). Red = arteries; blue = veins.

1 Diaphragm
2 Hepatic veins
3 Inferior vena cava
4 Common hepatic artery
5 Suprarenal gland
6 Celiac trunk
7 Right renal vein
8 Kidney
9 Abdominal aorta
10 Subcostal nerve
11 Iliohypogastric nerve
12 Central tendon of diaphragm
13 Inferior phrenic artery
14 Cardiac part of stomach
15 Spleen
16 Splenic artery
17 Superior renal artery
18 Superior mesenteric artery
19 Psoas major muscle
20 Inferior mesenteric artery
21 Ureter
22 Glomerulus
23 Afferent arteriole of glomerulus
24 Glomeruli
25 Radiating cortical artery
26 Subcortical or arcuate artery
27 Subcortical or arcuate vein
28 Interlobular vein
29 Interlobular artery
30 Vessels of renal capsule
31 Efferent arteriole of glomerulus
32 Vasa recta of renal medulla
33 Spiral arteries of renal pelvis

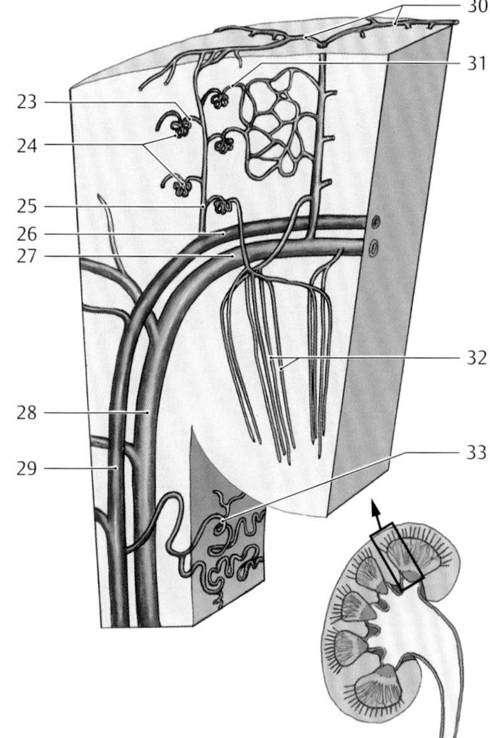


Fig. 7.10 **Architecture of the vascular system of the kidney.**

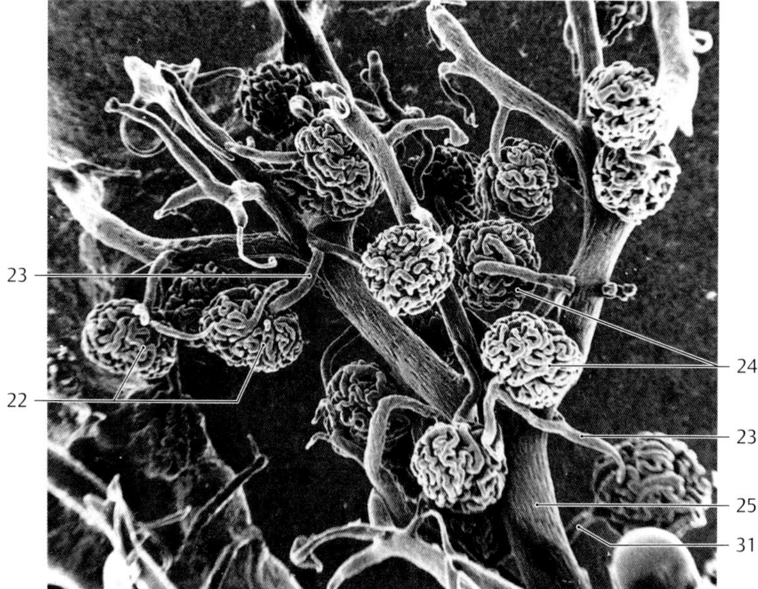


Fig. 7.11 **Electron micrograph showing glomeruli and associated arteries** (×210).

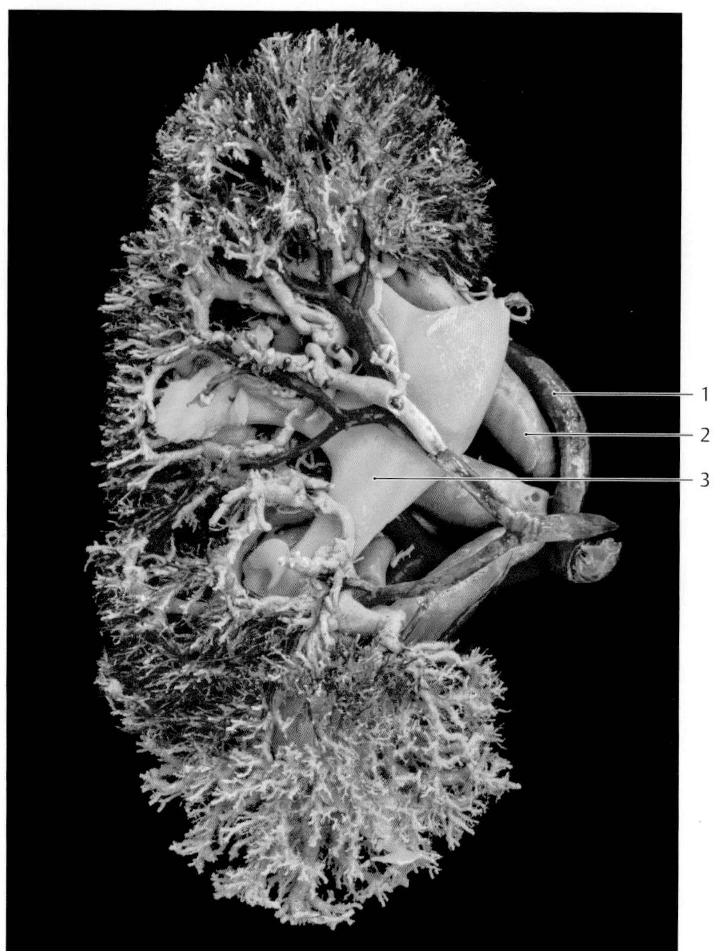


Fig. 7.12 **Cast of renal pelvis with arteries and veins.**

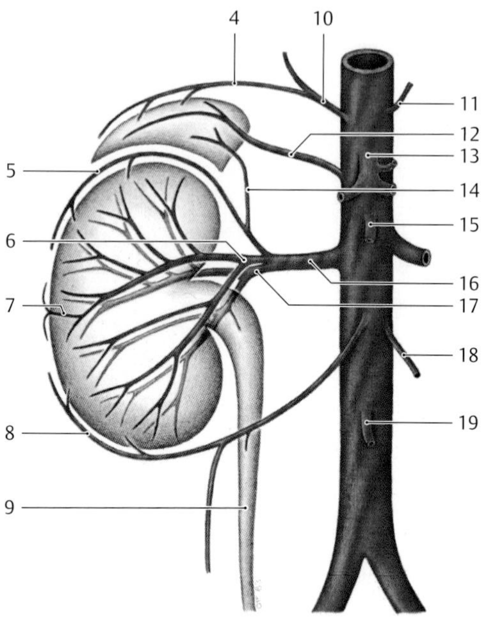


Fig. 7.13 **Arteries of kidney and suprarenal gland.**

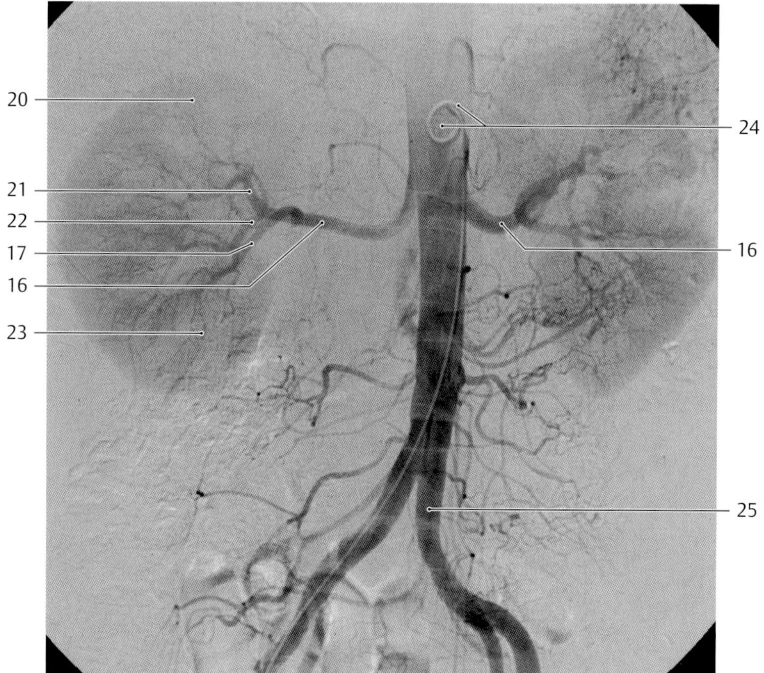


Fig. 7.14 **Arteriograph of abdominal aorta with renal arteries and renal vessels.** (Courtesy of Dr. Wieners, Department of Radiology, Charité Universitätsmedizin Berlin, Germany.)

1 Branches of renal artery
2 Branches of renal vein
3 Renal pelvis
4 Superior suprarenal artery
5 Upper capsular artery
6 Anterior branch of renal artery
7 Perforating artery
8 Lower capsular artery
9 Ureter
10 Right inferior phrenic artery
11 Left inferior phrenic artery
12 Middle suprarenal artery
13 Celiac trunk
14 Inferior suprarenal artery
15 Superior mesenteric artery
16 Renal artery
17 Posterior branch of renal artery
18 Left testicular (or ovarian) artery
19 Inferior mesenteric artery
20 Upper pole of kidney
21 Anterior superior segmental artery of renal artery
22 Anterior segmental artery of renal artery
23 Lower pole of kidney
24 Abdominal aorta (with catheter)
25 Common iliac artery

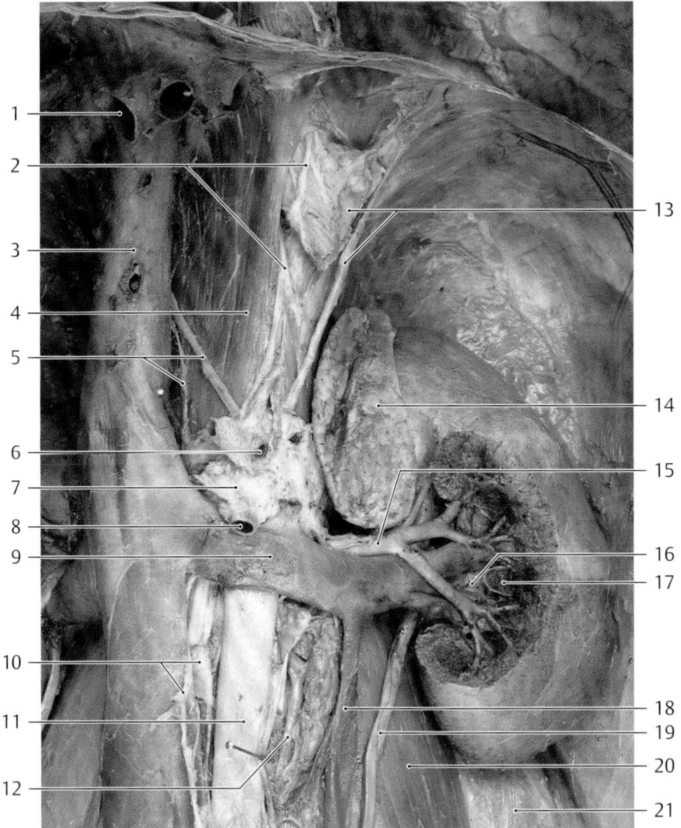


Fig. 7.15 **Left kidney and suprarenal gland in situ.** The anterior cortical layer of the kidney has been removed to display the renal pelvis and papillae.

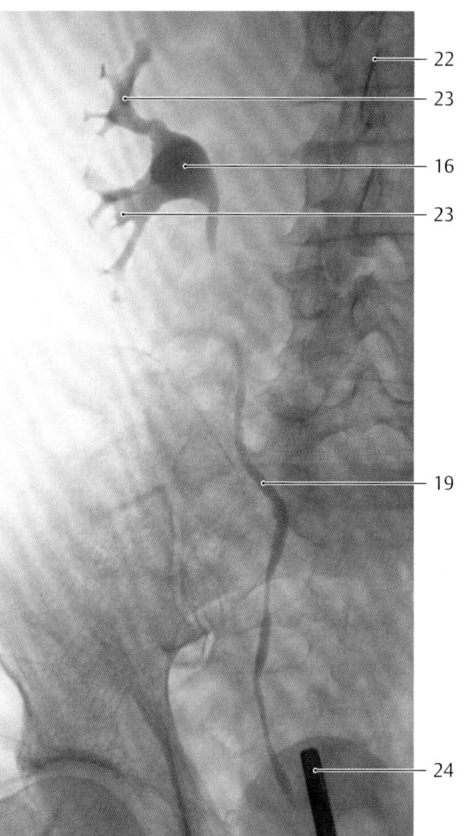


Fig. 7.16 **Renal pelvis with calices and ureter** (retrograde injection, x-ray). (Courtesy of Prof. Herrlinger, Fürth, Germany.)

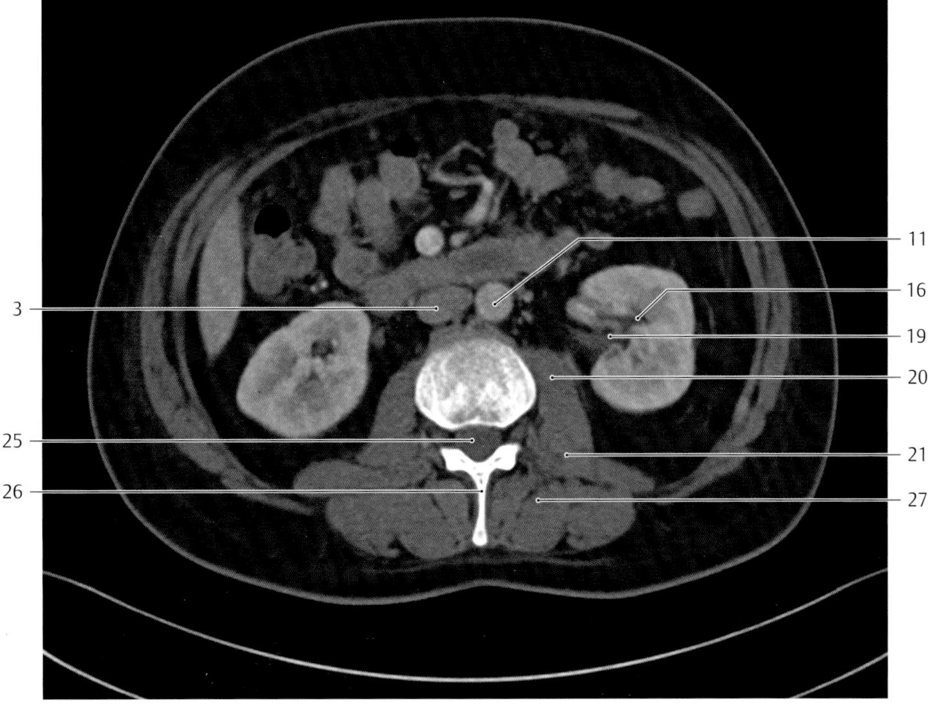


Fig. 7.17 **Horizontal section through the abdominal cavity at the level of the first lumbar vertebra** (CT scan). Section of renal pelvis and ureter. (Courtesy of Prof. Uder, Institute of Radiology, University Hospital Erlangen, Germany.)

1 Hepatic vein
2 Anterior and posterior vagal trunk
3 Inferior vena cava
4 Lumbar part of diaphragm
5 Right greater and lesser splanchnic nerves
6 Celiac trunk
7 Celiac ganglion and plexus
8 Superior mesenteric artery
9 Left renal vein
10 Right sympathetic trunk and ganglion
11 Abdominal aorta
12 Left sympathetic trunk
13 Esophagus (cut) and left greater splanchnic nerve
14 Left suprarenal gland
15 Left renal artery
16 Renal pelvis
17 Renal papilla with minor calyx
18 Left testicular vein
19 Ureter
20 Psoas major muscle
21 Quadratus lumborum muscle
22 Lumbar vertebra (L2)
23 Renal calyx
24 Catheter
25 Spinal cord
26 Spinous process of lumbar vertebra
27 Erector spinae muscle

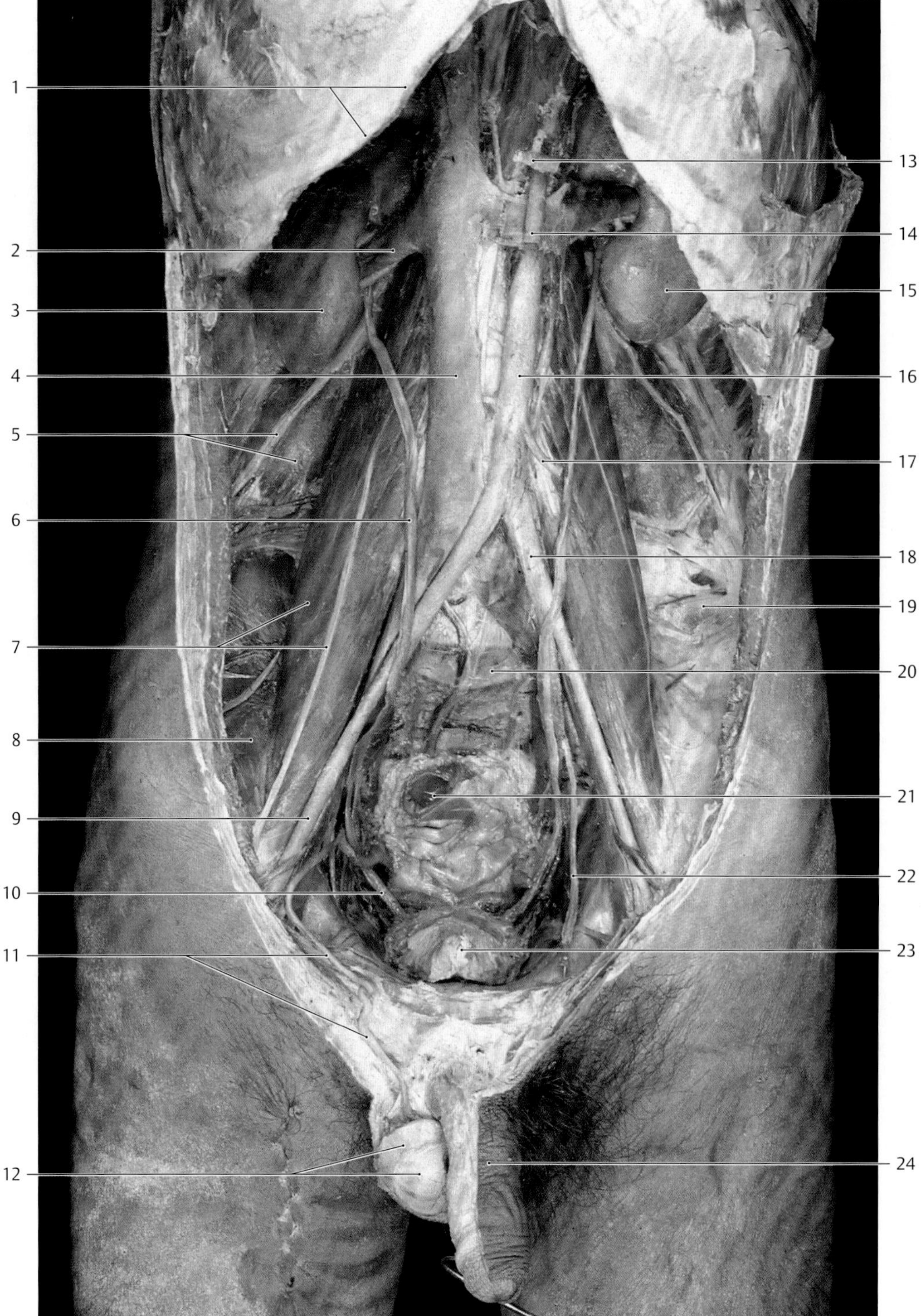


Fig. 7.18 **Urinary system in the male** (anterior aspect). The peritoneum has been removed.

1 Costal arch
2 Right renal vein
3 Right kidney
4 Inferior vena cava
5 Iliohypogastric nerve and quadratus lumborum muscle
6 Ureter (abdominal part)
7 Psoas major muscle and genitofemoral nerve
8 Iliacus muscle
9 External iliac artery
10 Ureter (pelvic part)
11 Ductus deferens
12 Testis and epididymis
13 Celiac trunk
14 Superior mesenteric artery
15 Left kidney
16 Abdominal aorta
17 Inferior mesenteric artery
18 Common iliac artery
19 Iliac crest
20 Sacral promontory
21 Rectum (cut)
22 Medial umbilical ligament
23 Urinary bladder
24 Penis

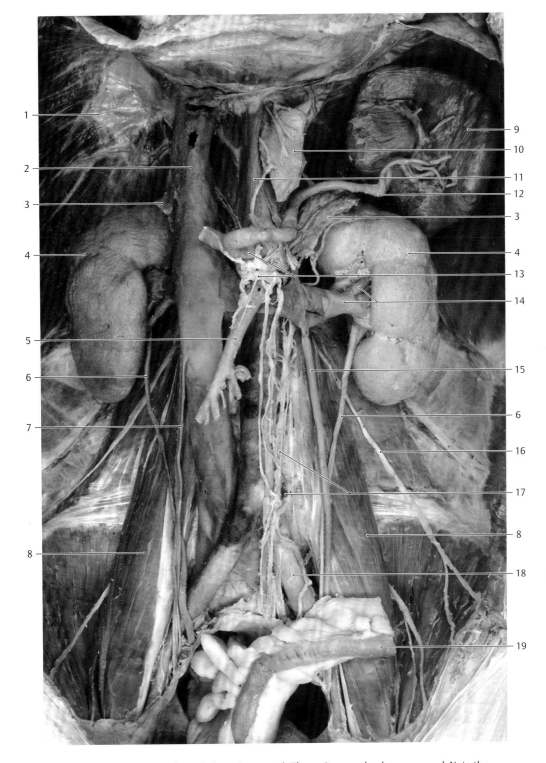


Fig. 7.19 **Urinary system in the male** (anterior aspect). The peritoneum has been removed. Note the autonomic plexus and ganglia at the abdominal aorta.

1 Diaphragm
2 Inferior vena cava
3 Suprarenal gland
4 Kidney
5 Superior mesenteric artery
6 Ureter
7 Right spermatic vein
8 Psoas major muscle
9 Spleen
10 Cardiac part of stomach
11 Abdominal aorta
12 Splenic artery
13 Celiac trunk and celiac ganglion
14 Renal artery and vein
15 Left spermatic vein
16 Ilio-inguinal nerve
17 Superior hypogastric plexus and ganglion
18 Left common iliac artery
19 Sigmoid colon

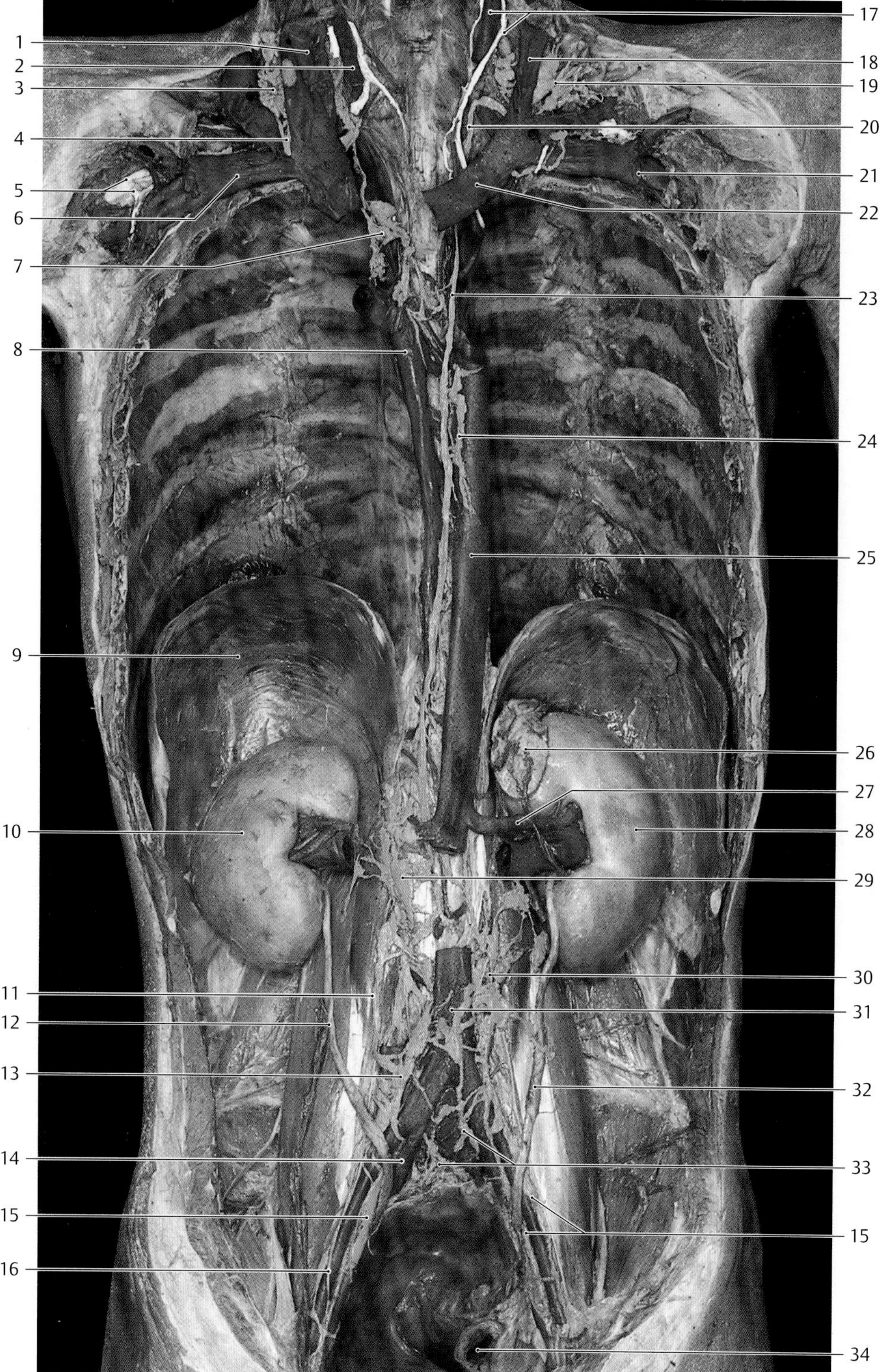


1 Internal jugular vein
2 Right common carotid artery and right vagus nerve
3 Jugulo-omohyoid lymph node
4 Right lymphatic duct
5 Subclavian trunk
6 Right subclavian vein
7 Bronchomediastinal trunk
8 Azygos vein
9 Diaphragm
10 Right kidney
11 Right lumbar trunk
12 Right ureter
13 Common iliac lymph nodes
14 Right internal iliac artery
15 External iliac lymph nodes
16 Right external iliac artery
17 Left common carotid artery and left vagus nerve
18 Internal jugular vein
19 Deep cervical lymph nodes
20 Thoracic duct entering left jugular angle
21 Left subclavian vein
22 Left brachiocephalic vein
23 Thoracic duct
24 Mediastinal lymph nodes
25 Thoracic aorta
26 Left suprarenal gland
27 Left renal artery
28 Left kidney
29 Cisterna chyli
30 Lumbar lymph nodes
31 Abdominal aorta
32 Left ureter
33 Sacral lymph nodes
34 Rectum (cut edge)
35 Aortic arch
36 Superior vena cava
37 Intercostal vein
38 Left jugular trunk
39 Left subclavian artery
40 Quadratus lumborum muscle
41 Psoas major muscle
42 Parotid lymph nodes
43 Axillary lymph nodes

Fig. 7.20 **Lymph vessels and lymph nodes of the posterior wall of thoracic and abdominal cavities** (anterior aspect). Green = lymph vessels and nodes; blue = veins; red = arteries; white = nerves.

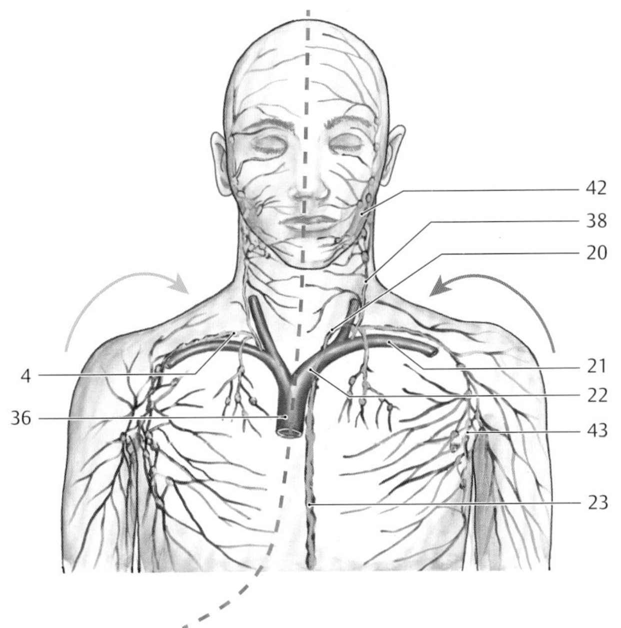


Fig. 7.21 **Lymph vessels and lymph nodes of the upper part of the body.** Lymph of the right arm, the right side of the head and neck, and the right breast passes into the right venous angle (between the internal jugular vein and the subclavian vein). Lymph from all other regions passes through the thoracic duct into the left venous angle. Dotted red line = border between irrigation areas of the right and left part of the body.

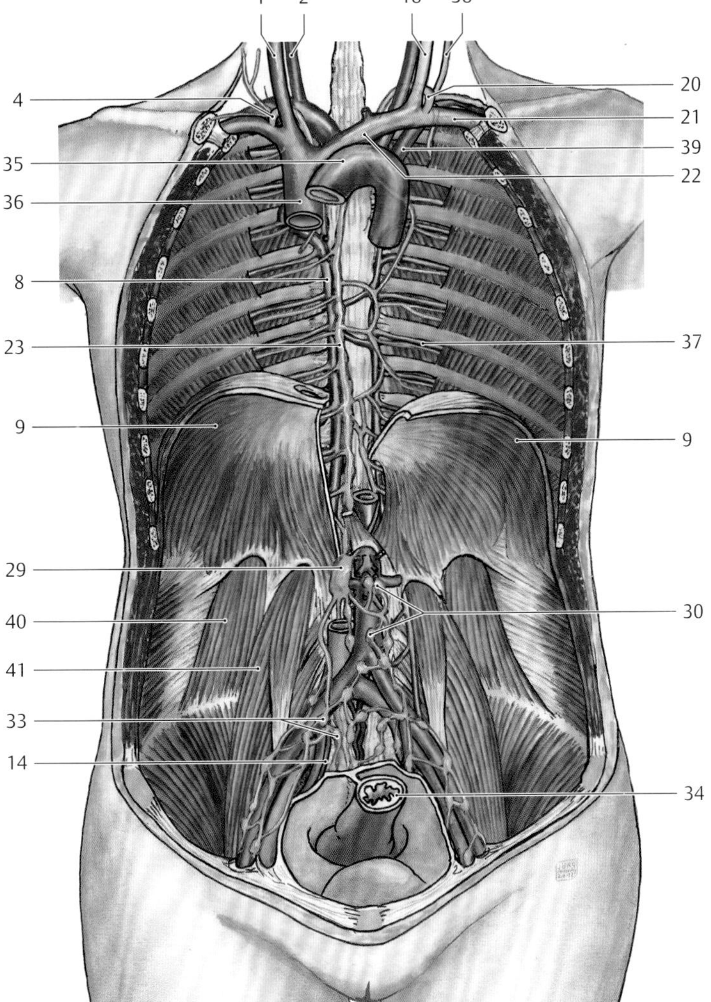


Fig. 7.22 **Lymph vessels and lymph nodes of the posterior wall of thoracic and abdominal cavities** (anterior aspect). Note the course of the thoracic duct from the cisterna chyli to the left venous angle. The lymph vessels of the intercostal spaces communicate mainly with the thoracic duct.

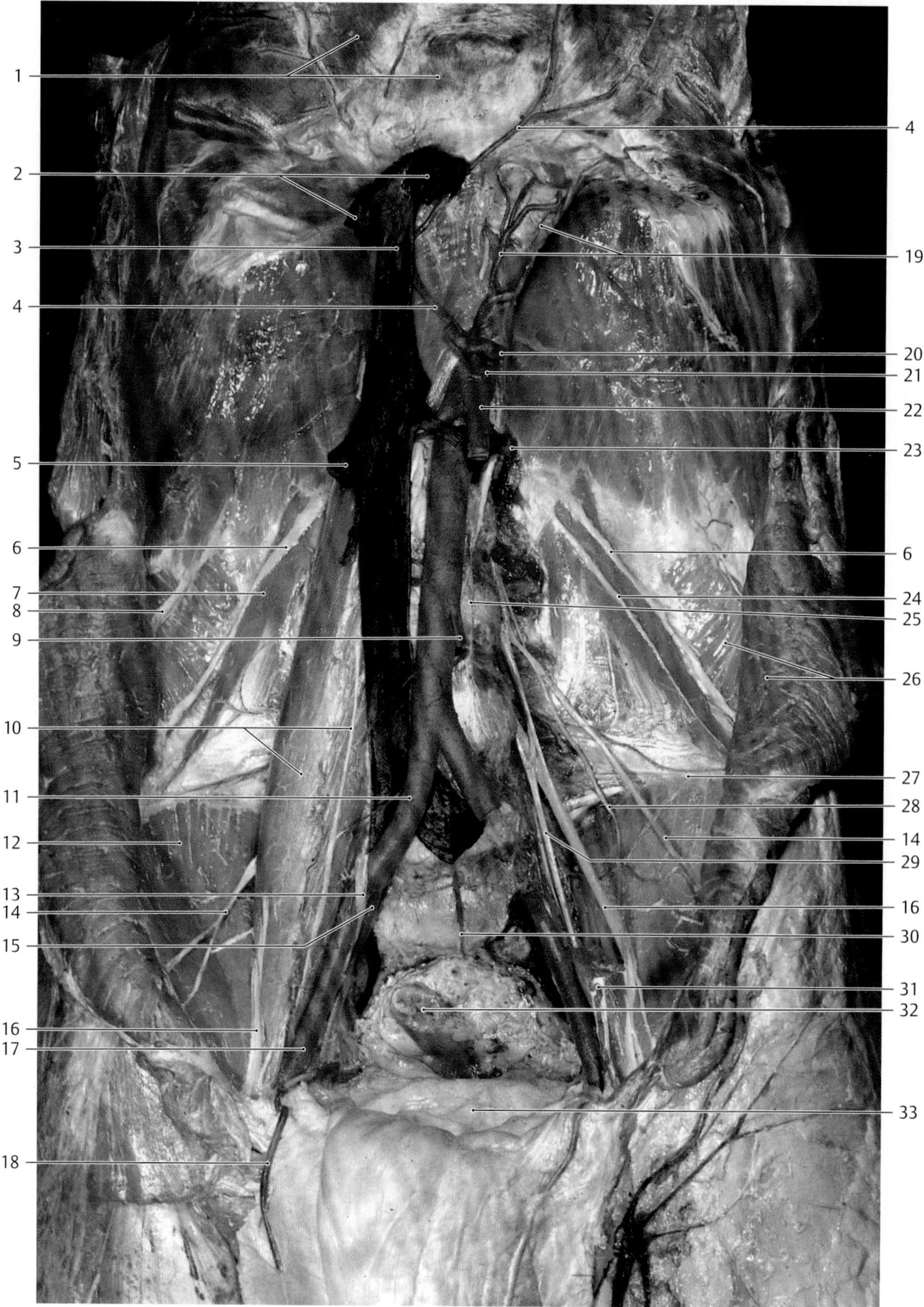


Fig. 7.23 **Vessels and nerves within the retroperitoneal space** (anterior aspect). Part of the left psoas major muscle has been removed to display the lumbar plexus. Red = arteries; blue = veins.

1 Diaphragm
2 Hepatic veins
3 Inferior vena cava
4 Inferior phrenic artery
5 Right renal vein
6 Iliohypogastric nerve
7 Quadratus lumborum muscle
8 Subcostal nerve
9 Inferior mesenteric artery
10 Right genitofemoral nerve and psoas major muscle
11 Common iliac artery
12 Iliacus muscle
13 Right ureter (divided)
14 Lateral femoral cutaneous nerve
15 Internal iliac artery
16 Femoral nerve
17 External iliac artery
18 Inferior epigastric artery
19 Cardiac part of stomach and esophageal branches of left gastric artery
20 Splenic artery
21 Celiac trunk
22 Superior mesenteric artery
23 Left renal artery
24 Ilio-inguinal nerve
25 Sympathetic trunk
26 Transverse abdominal muscle
27 Iliac crest
28 Left genitofemoral nerve
29 Left obturator nerve
30 Median sacral artery
31 Psoas major muscle (divided) with supplying artery
32 Rectum (cut)
33 Urinary bladder

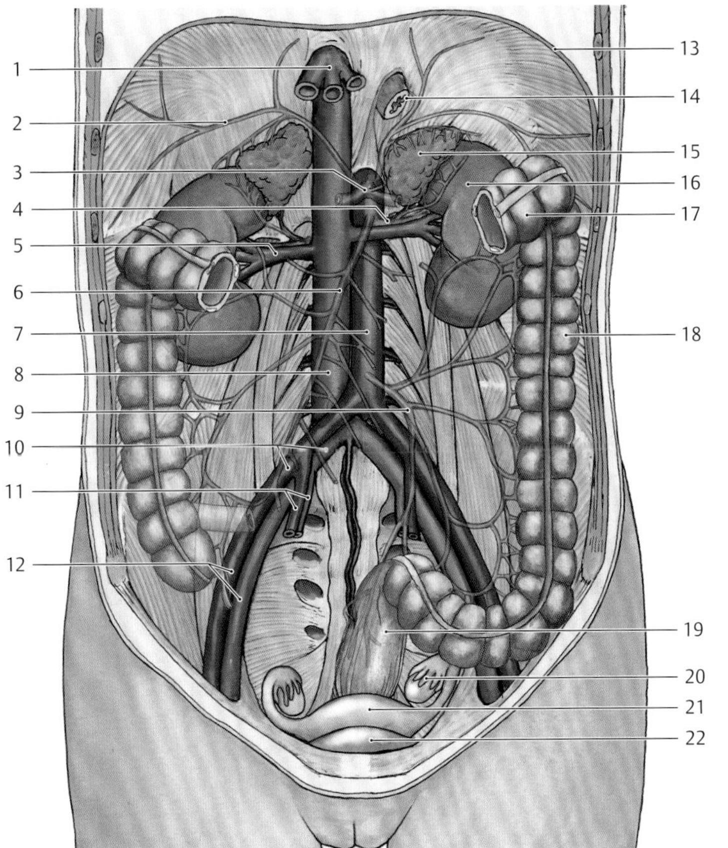


Fig. 7.24 **Vessels of the retroperitoneal region** and the course of the superior and inferior mesenteric arteries that supply the ascending and descending parts of the colon.

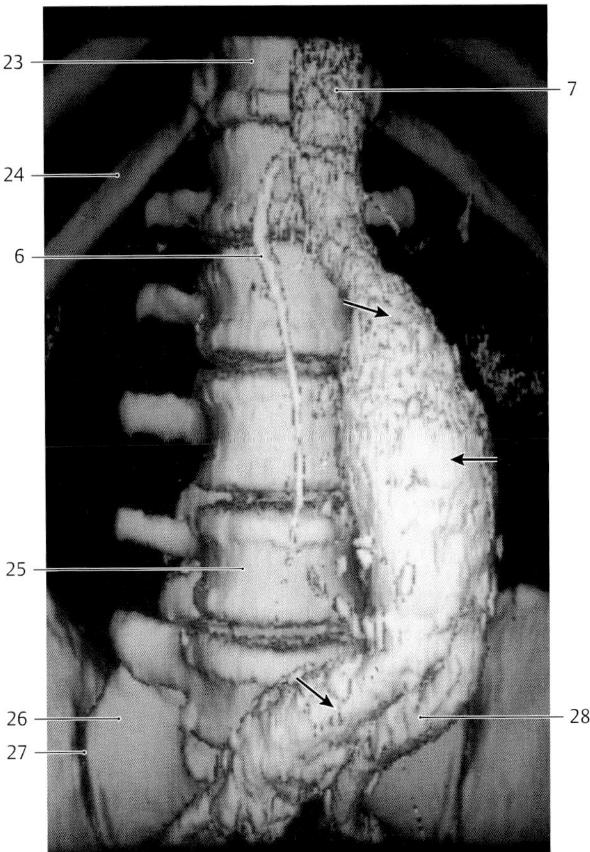


Fig. 7.25 **Abdominal aorta showing an infrarenal aneurysm** (3-D reconstruction). Arrows = involvement of both iliac arteries. (Courtesy of Prof. Rupprecht, Neumarkt, Germany.)

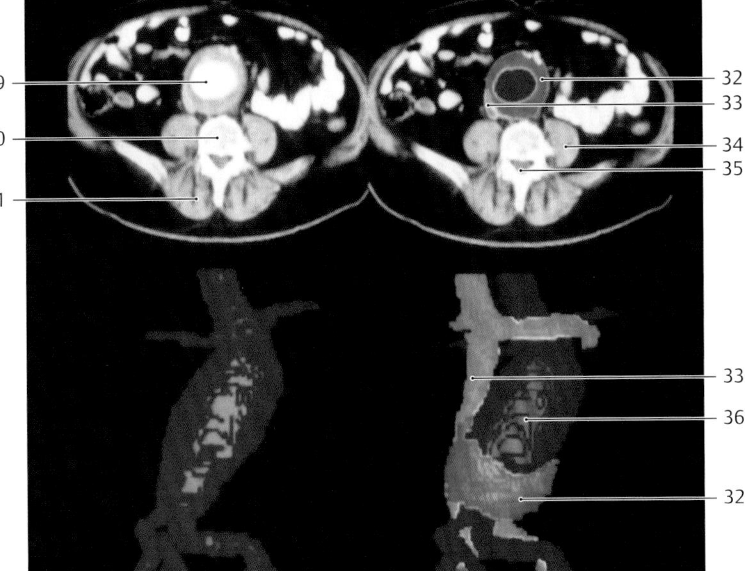


Fig. 7.26 **Abdominal aorta with an aneurysm,** after injection of contrast medium. Above = horizontal sections through the abdominal cavity showing different contrast medium concentrations within the aorta and the aneurysm; below = 3-D reconstruction of the aneurysm; red = aorta; green = thrombotic areas; blue = inferior vena cava (partly compressed). (Courtesy of Prof. Rupprecht, Neumarkt, Germany.)

1 Hepatic veins
2 Inferior phrenic artery
3 Celiac trunk
4 Left renal artery
5 Right renal vein
6 Superior mesenteric artery
7 Aorta (abdominal part)
8 Inferior vena cava
9 Inferior mesenteric artery
10 Common iliac artery and vein
11 Internal iliac artery and vein
12 External iliac artery and vein
13 Diaphragm
14 Esophagus
15 Suprarenal gland
16 Kidney
17 Transverse colon
18 Descending colon
19 Rectum
20 Ovary with infundibulum of uterine tube
21 Uterus
22 Urinary bladder
23 Twelfth thoracic vertebra (T12)
24 Twelfth rib (rib XII)
25 Fourth lumbar vertebra (L4)
26 Sacrum
27 Sacro-iliac articulation
28 Left common iliac artery (included into the aneurysm)
29 Aorta with aneurysm
30 Body of lumbar vertebra
31 Erector spinae muscle
32 Thrombotic part of the aneurysm (green)
33 Inferior vena cava (compressed, blue)
34 Iliopsoas muscle
35 Vertebral canal
36 Aneurysm of the aorta (red)

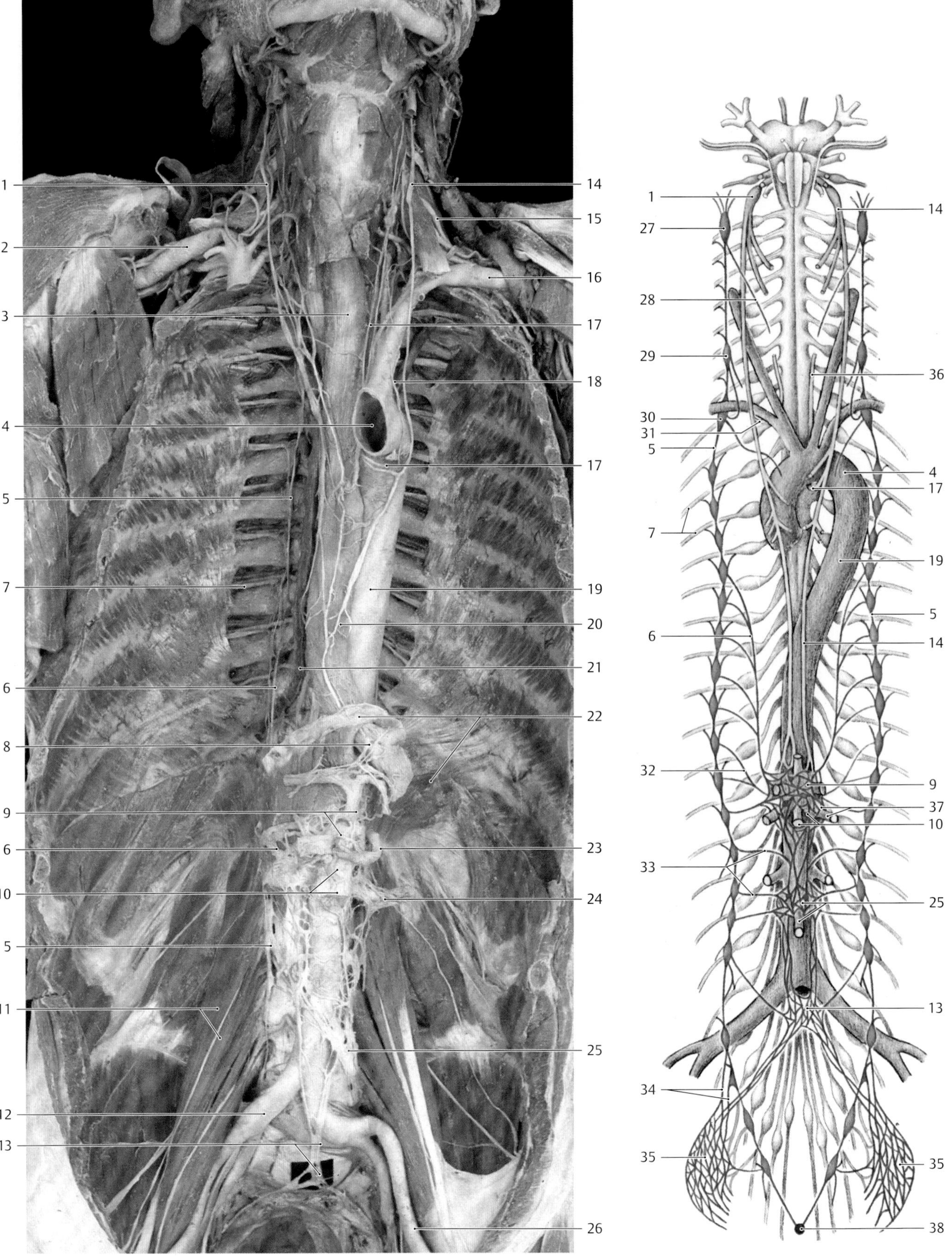


Fig. 7.27 **Posterior wall of thoracic and abdominal cavities with sympathetic trunk, vagus nerve, and autonomic ganglia** (anterior aspect). The thoracic and abdominal organs have been removed, except for the esophagus and aorta.

Fig. 7.28 **Organization of autonomic nervous system.** Yellow = parasympathetic nerves; green = sympathetic nerves.

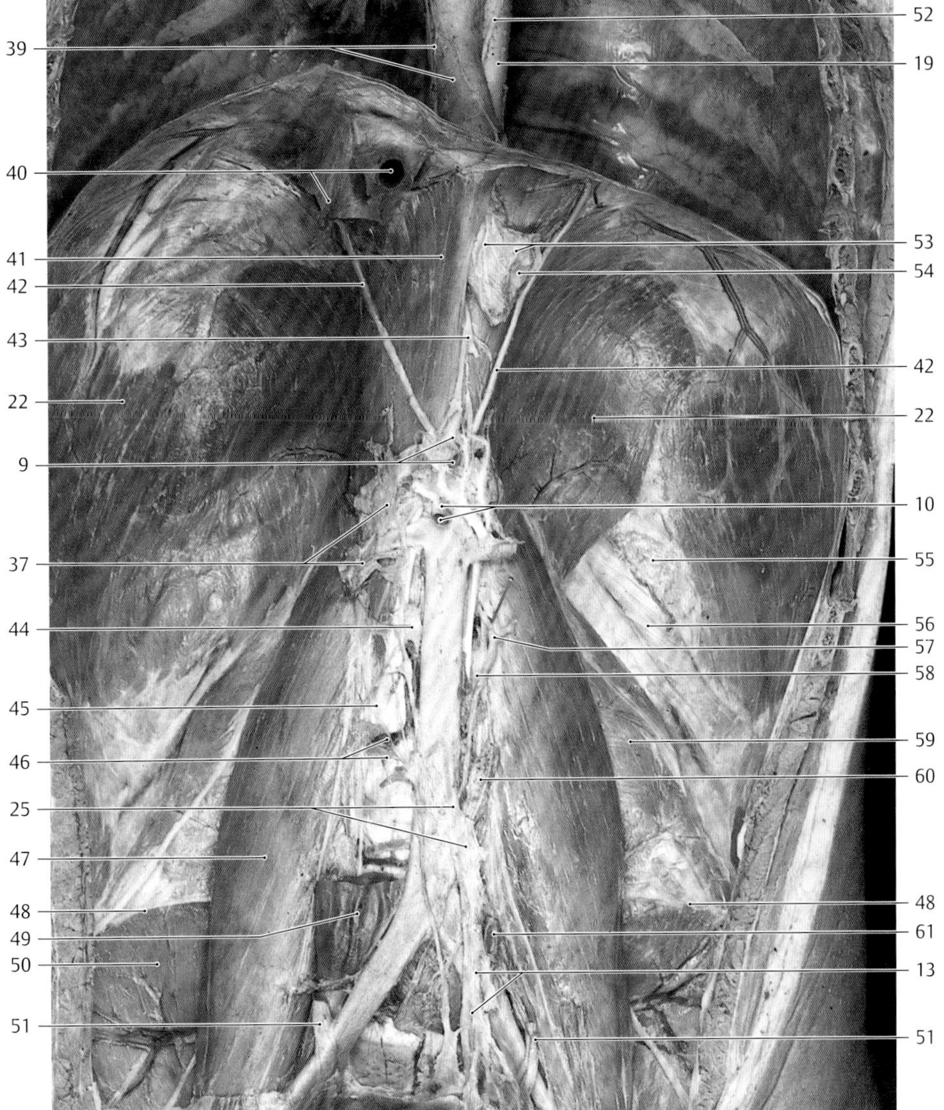


Fig. 7.29 **Ganglia and plexus of the autonomic nervous system within the retroperitoneal space** (anterior aspect). The kidneys and the inferior vena cava with its tributaries have been removed.

1 Right vagus nerve
2 Right subclavian artery
3 Esophagus
4 Aortic arch
5 Sympathetic trunk
6 Greater splanchnic nerve
7 Intercostal nerve
8 Abdominal part of esophagus and vagal trunk
9 Celiac trunk with celiac ganglion
10 Superior mesenteric artery and ganglion
11 Psoas major muscle and genitofemoral nerve
12 Common iliac artery
13 Superior hypogastric plexus and ganglion
14 Left vagus nerve
15 Brachial plexus
16 Left subclavian artery
17 Left recurrent laryngeal nerve
18 Inferior cervical cardiac nerve
19 Thoracic aorta
20 Esophageal plexus
21 Azygos vein
22 Diaphragm
23 Splenic artery
24 Left renal artery and plexus
25 Inferior mesenteric ganglion and artery
26 Left external iliac artery
27 Superior cervical ganglion of sympathetic trunk
28 Superior cardiac branch of sympathetic trunk
29 Middle cervical ganglion of sympathetic trunk
30 Inferior cervical ganglion of sympathetic trunk
31 Right recurrent laryngeal nerve
32 Lesser splanchnic nerve
33 Lumbar splanchnic nerves
34 Sacral splanchnic nerves
35 Inferior hypogastric ganglion and plexus
36 Left recurrent laryngeal nerve
37 Aorticorenal plexus and renal artery
38 Ganglion impar
39 Esophagus with branches of vagus nerve
40 Hepatic veins
41 Right crus of diaphragm
42 Inferior phrenic artery
43 Right vagus nerve entering the celiac ganglion
44 Right lumbar lymph trunk
45 Lumbar part of right sympathetic trunk
46 Lumbar artery and vein
47 Psoas major muscle
48 Iliac crest
49 Inferior vena cava
50 Iliacus muscle
51 Ureter
52 Left vagus nerve forming the esophageal plexus
53 Left vagus nerve forming the gastric plexus
54 Esophagus continuing into the cardiac part of stomach
55 Lumbocostal triangle
56 Position of twelfth rib
57 Left lumbar lymph trunk
58 Ganglion of sympathetic trunk
59 Quadratus lumborum muscle
60 Lumbar part of left sympathetic trunk
61 Iliac lymph vessels

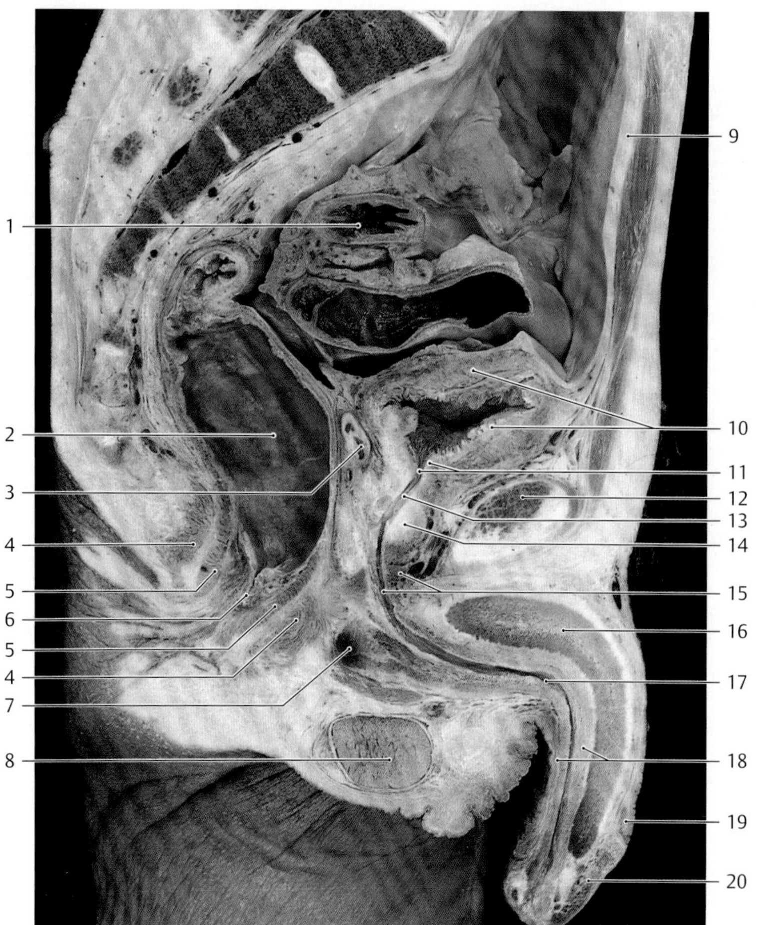


Fig. 7.30 **Male urogenital system** (midsagittal section through the pelvic cavity).

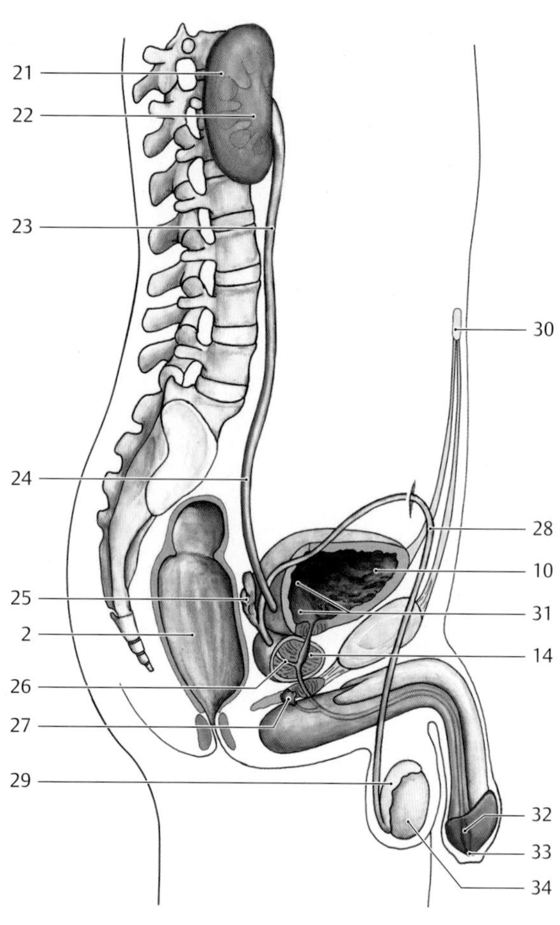


Fig. 7.31 **Male urogenital system** (lateral aspect).

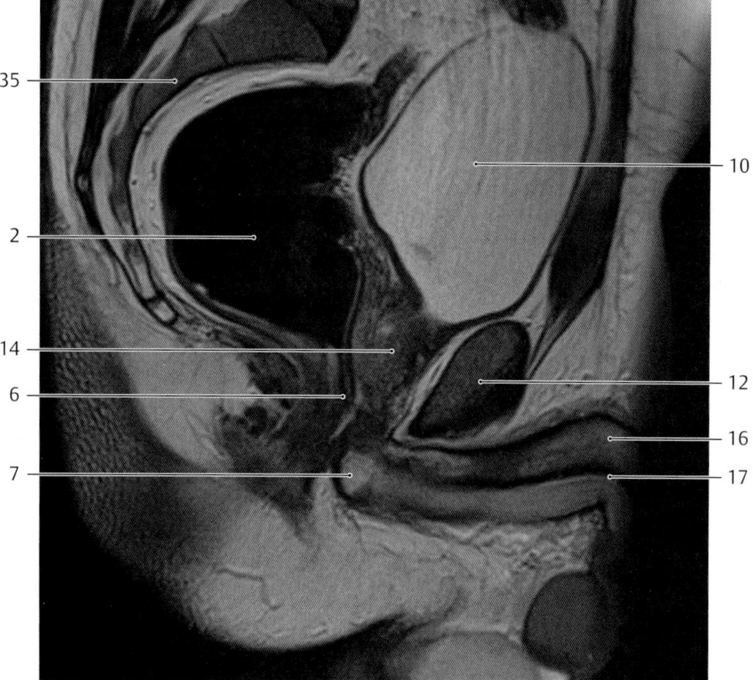


Fig. 7.32 **Midsagittal section through the pelvic cavity in the male** (MRI scan). (Courtesy of Prof. Uder, Institute of Radiology, University Hospital Erlangen, Germany.)

1 Sigmoid colon
2 Ampulla of rectum
3 Ampulla of ductus deferens
4 External anal sphincter muscle
5 Internal anal sphincter muscle
6 Anal canal
7 Bulb of penis
8 Testis (cut surface)
9 Median umbilical ligament
10 Urinary bladder
11 Internal urethral orifice and sphincter
12 Pubic symphysis
13 Prostatic part of urethra
14 Prostate gland
15 Membranous part of urethra and external urethral sphincter
16 Corpus cavernosum of penis
17 Spongy urethra
18 Corpus spongiosum of penis
19 Foreskin (prepuce)
20 Glans penis
21 Kidney
22 Renal pelvis
23 Abdominal part of ureter
24 Pelvic part of ureter
25 Seminal vesicle
26 Ejaculatory duct
27 Bulbo-urethral gland (Cowper's gland)
28 Ductus deferens
29 Epididymis
30 Umbilicus
31 Trigone of urinary bladder and ureteric orifice
32 Navicular fossa of urethra
33 External urethral orifice
34 Testis
35 Sacrum

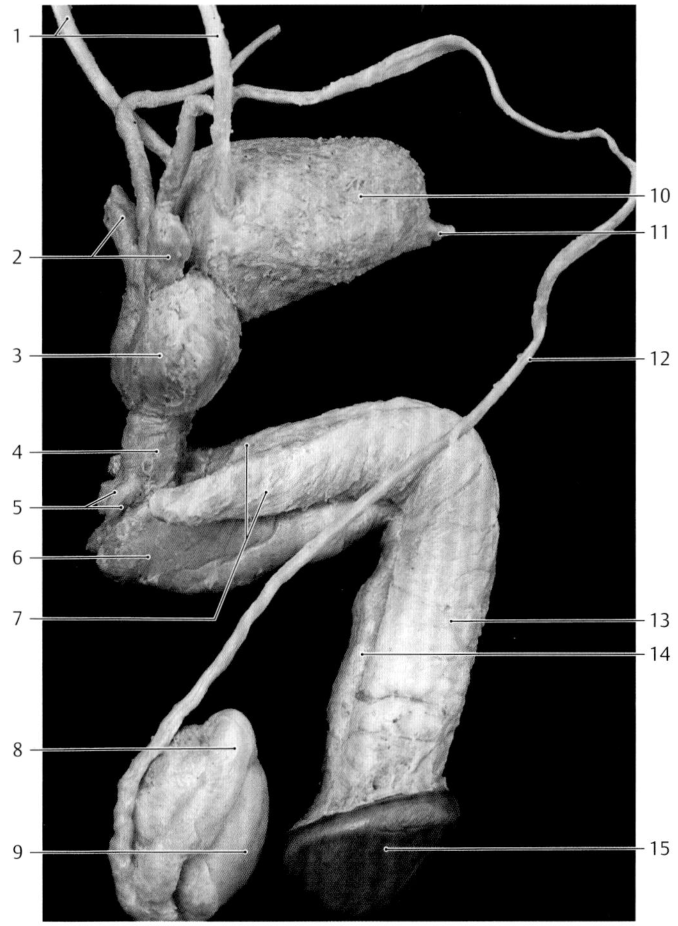

**Fig. 7.33 Male genital organs, isolated** (right lateral aspect).

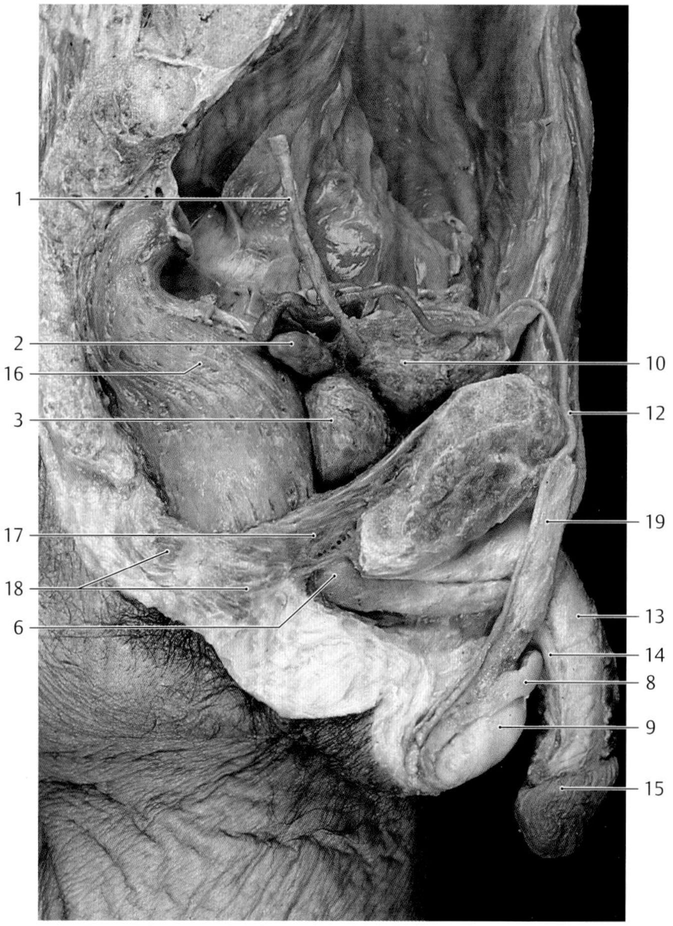

**Fig. 7.34 Male genital organs in situ** (right lateral aspect).

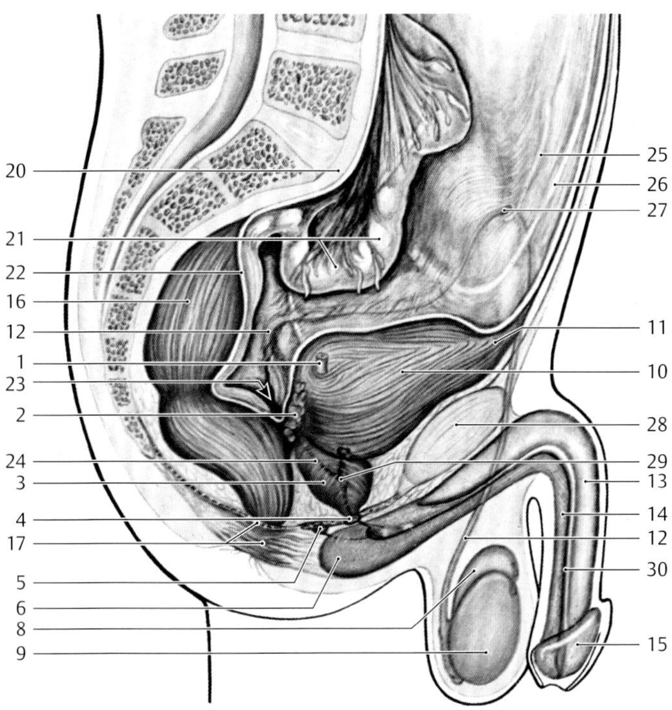

**Fig. 7.35 Positions of male genital organs** (right lateral aspect).

1 Ureter
2 Seminal vesicle
3 Prostate gland
4 Urogenital diaphragm and membranous part of urethra
5 Bulbo-urethral gland (Cowper's gland)
6 Bulb of penis
7 Left and right crus penis
8 Epididymis
9 Testis
10 Urinary bladder
11 Apex of urinary bladder
12 Ductus deferens
13 Corpus cavernosum of penis
14 Corpus spongiosum of penis
15 Glans penis
16 Ampulla of rectum
17 Levator ani muscle
18 Anal canal and external anal sphincter muscle
19 Spermatic cord (cut)
20 Sacral promontory
21 Sigmoid colon
22 Peritoneum (cut edge)
23 Rectovesical pouch
24 Ejaculatory duct
25 Lateral umbilical fold
26 Medial umbilical fold
27 Deep inguinal ring and ductus deferens
28 Pubic symphysis
29 Prostatic part of urethra
30 Spongy urethra

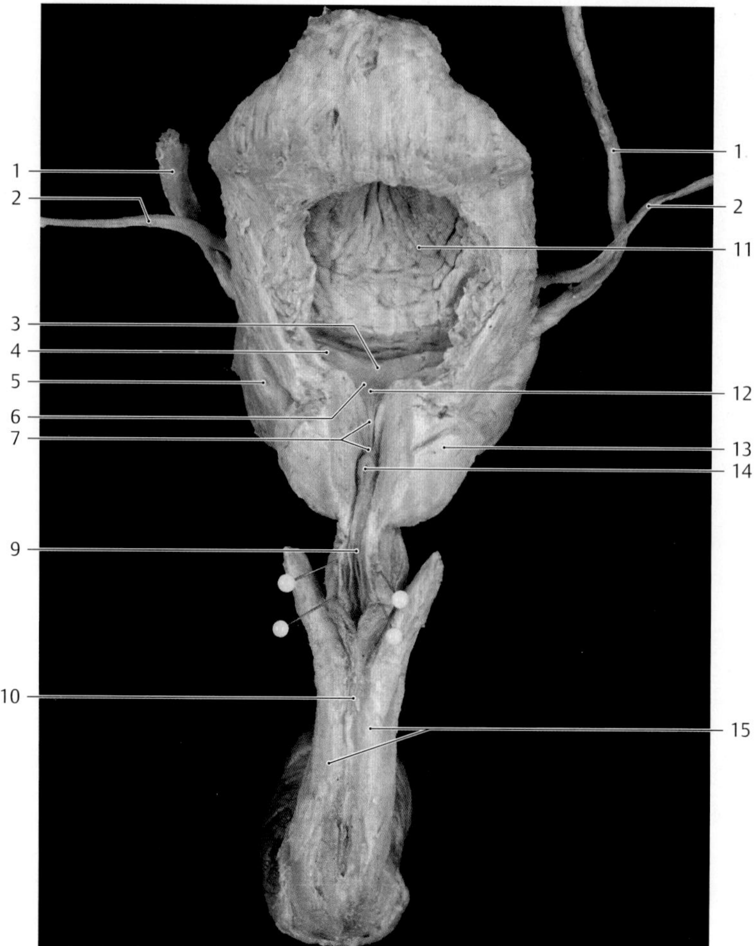


1 Ureter
2 Ductus deferens
3 Interureteric fold
4 Ureteric orifice
5 Seminal vesicle
6 Trigone of urinary bladder
7 Prostatic urethra with seminal colliculus and urethral crest
8 Deep transverse perineal muscle
9 Membranous urethra
10 Spongy urethra
11 Mucous membrane of urinary bladder
12 Internal urethral orifice and uvula of urinary bladder
13 Prostate
14 Prostatic utricle
15 Right and left corpus cavernosum of penis
16 Ejaculatory duct
17 Sphincter urethrae muscle
18 Sphincter muscle of urinary bladder
19 Bulbo-urethral gland (Cowper's gland)
20 Crus penis
21 Orifices of bulbo-urethral glands
22 Glans penis
23 Ureteric orifices

Fig. 7.36 **Male genital organs and urinary bladder, isolated** (anterior aspect). The urinary bladder, prostate, and urethra have been opened and the urinary bladder contracted.

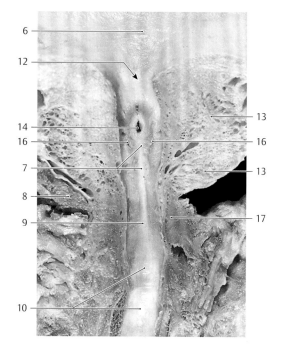

Fig. 7.37 **Posterior half of male urethra and prostate** in continuity with the neck of the urinary bladder (anterior aspect).

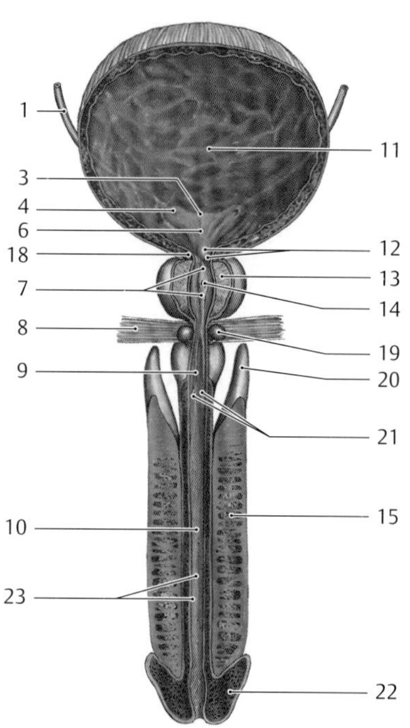


Fig. 7.38 **Male genital organs and urinary bladder** (anterior aspect). The urinary bladder, urethra, and penis have been dissected.

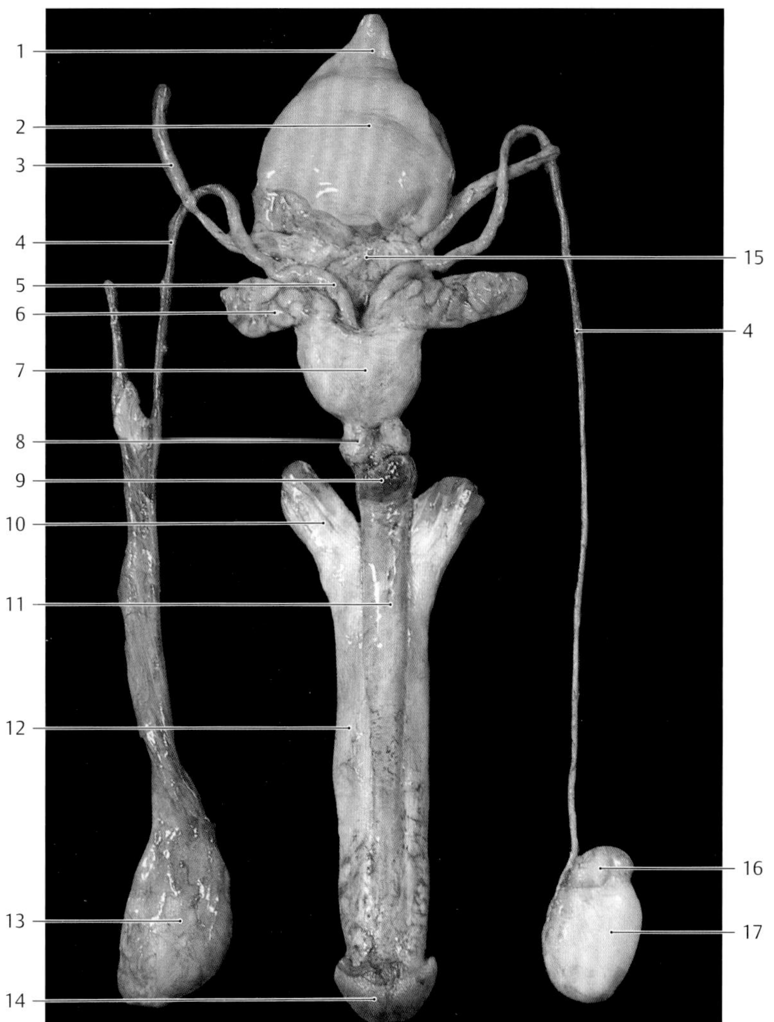


1 Apex of urinary bladder with urachus
2 Urinary bladder
3 Ureter
4 Ductus deferens
5 Ampulla of ductus deferens
6 Seminal vesicle
7 Prostate
8 Bulbo-urethral gland (Cowper's gland)
9 Bulb of penis
10 Crus penis
11 Corpus spongiosum of penis
12 Corpus cavernosum of penis
13 Testis and epididymis with coverings
14 Glans penis
15 Fundus of urinary bladder
16 Head of epididymis
17 Testis
18 Mucous membrane of bladder
19 Trigone of bladder
20 Ureteric orifice
21 Internal urethral orifice
22 Seminal colliculus
23 Prostate
24 Prostatic urethra
25 Membranous urethra
26 Spongy (penile) urethra
27 Skin of penis
28 Deep dorsal vein of penis (unpaired)
29 Dorsal artery of penis (paired)
30 Tunica albuginea of corpora cavernosa
31 Septum of penis
32 Deep artery of penis
33 Tunica albuginea of corpus spongiosum
34 Deep fascia of penis

Fig. 7.39 **Male genital organs and urinary bladder, isolated** (posterior aspect).

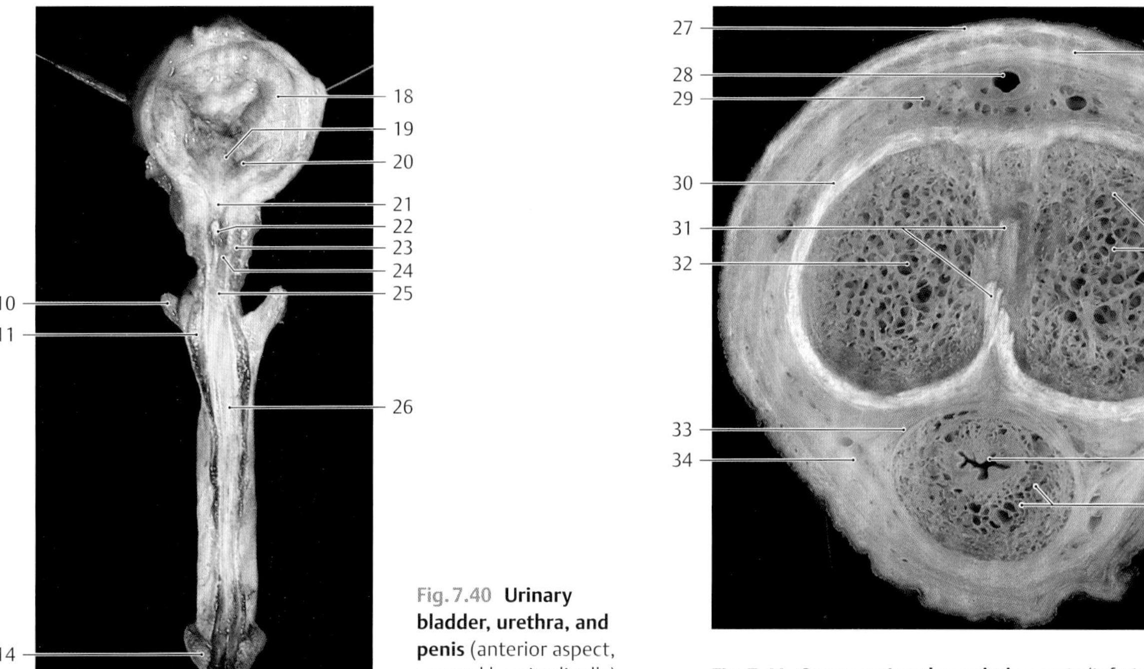


Fig. 7.40 **Urinary bladder, urethra, and penis** (anterior aspect, opened longitudinally).

Fig. 7.41 **Cross section through the penis** (inferior aspect).

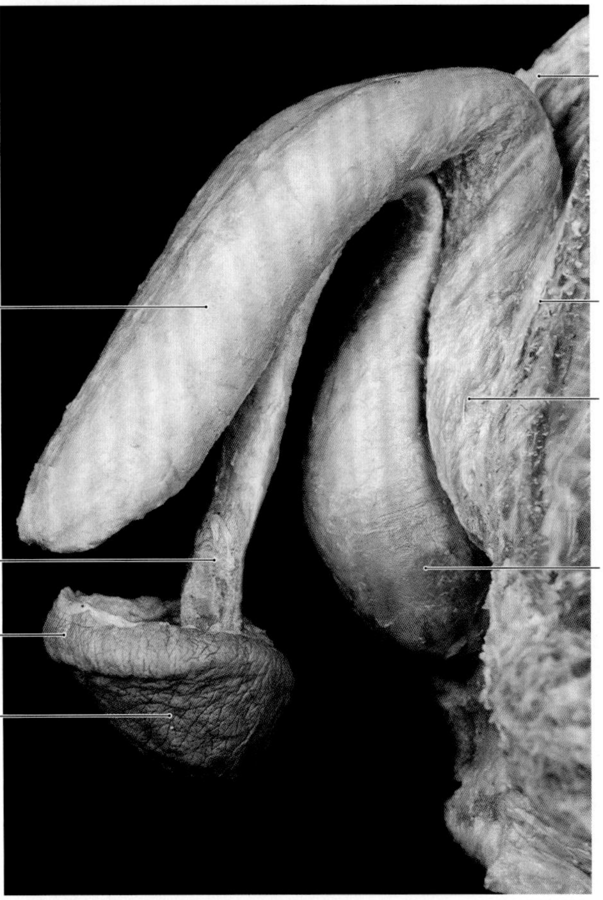

Fig. 7.42 **Male external genital organs** (oblique-lateral aspect). The corpus spongiosum of the penis with the glans penis has been isolated and reflected.

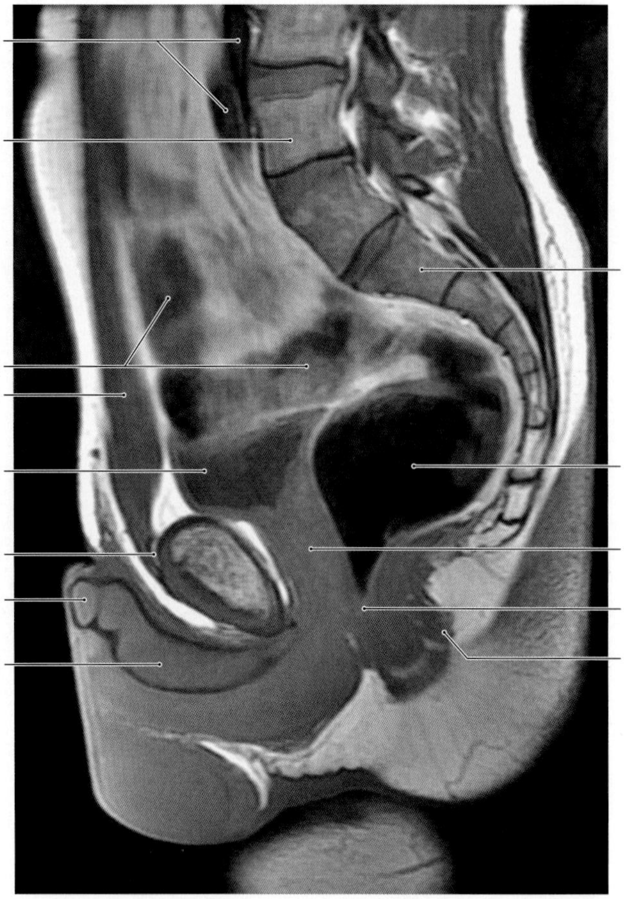

Fig. 7.43 **Sagittal section through the pelvic cavity with the male genital organs** (MRI scan). (Heuck A, et al. MRT-Atlas des muskuloskelettalen Systems. Stuttgart, Germany: Schattauer, 2009.)

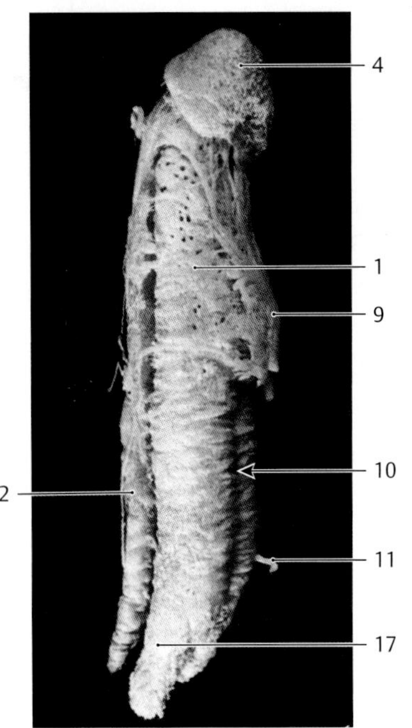


Fig. 7.44 **Resin cast of an erect penis.**

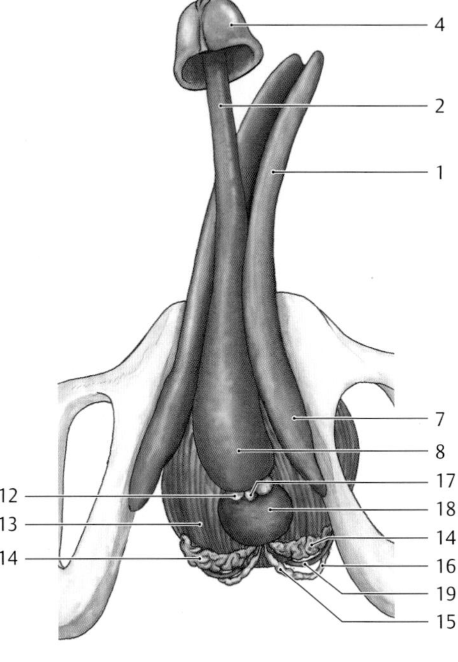


Fig. 7.45 **Male external genital organs and accessory glands.**

1 Corpus cavernosum of penis
2 Corpus spongiosum of penis
3 Corona of glans penis
4 Glans penis
5 Suspensory ligament of penis
6 Pubis (inferior pubic ramus, dissected)
7 Crus penis
8 Bulb of penis
9 Dorsal vein of penis
10 Septum pectiniforme
11 Dorsal artery of penis
12 Bulbo-urethral gland (Cowper's gland)
13 Urinary bladder
14 Seminal vesicle
15 Ampulla of ductus deferens
16 Ductus deferens
17 Membranous urethra
18 Prostate
19 Ureter
20 Common iliac artery and vein
21 Fifth lumbar vertebral body
22 Intestinal loops
23 Rectus abdominis muscle
24 Pubic symphysis
25 Root of penis
26 Sacrum
27 Ampulla of rectum
28 Anal canal
29 External anal sphincter muscle

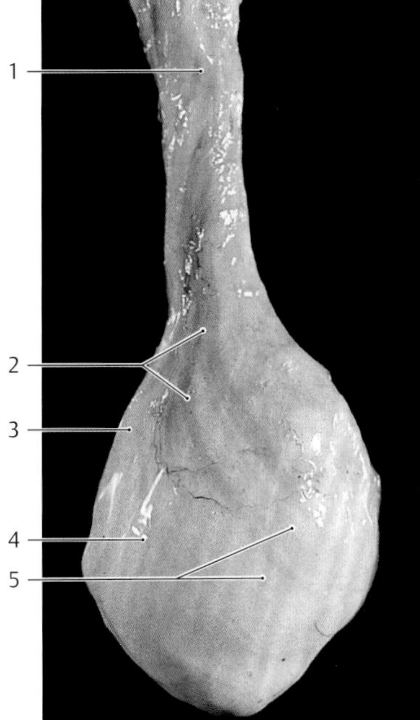


Fig. 7.46 **Testis and epididymis** with investing layers (lateral aspect).

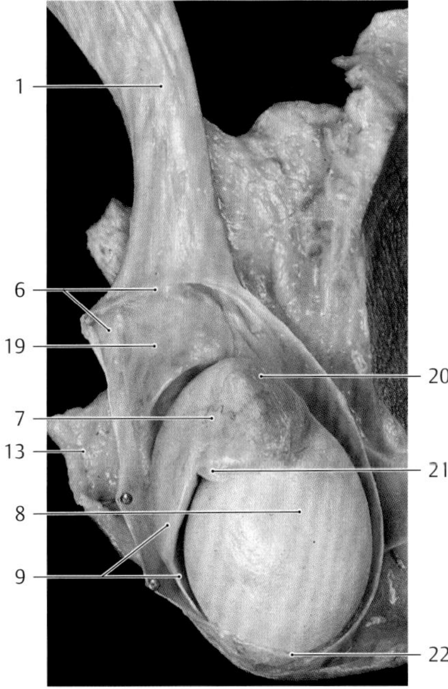


Fig. 7.47 **Testis and epididymis** (lateral aspect). The tunica vaginalis has been opened.

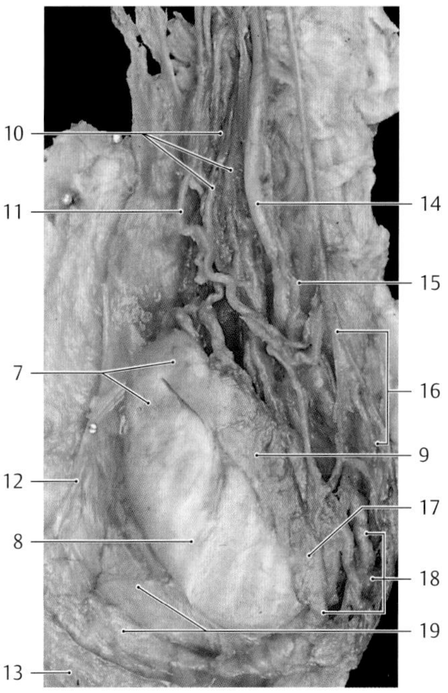


Fig. 7.48 **Testis, epididymis, and spermatic cord** (left side, postero-lateral aspect). Dissection of spermatic cord and ductus deferens.

1 Spermatic cord covered with cremasteric fascia
2 Cremaster muscle
3 Position of epididymis
4 Internal spermatic fascia
5 Position of testis
6 Internal spermatic fascia with adjacent investing layers of testis (cut surface)
7 Head of epididymis
8 Testis with tunica vaginalis (visceral layer)
9 Body of epididymis
10 Pampiniform venous plexus (anterior veins)
11 Testicular artery
12 Tunica vaginalis (parietal layer, cut edge)
13 Skin and dartos muscle (reflected)
14 Ductus deferens
15 Artery of ductus deferens
16 Posterior veins of pampiniform plexus
17 Tail of epididymis
18 Transition of epididymal duct to ductus deferens and venous plexus
19 Parietal layer of tunica vaginalis
20 Appendix of epididymis
21 Appendix of testis
22 Gubernaculum testis

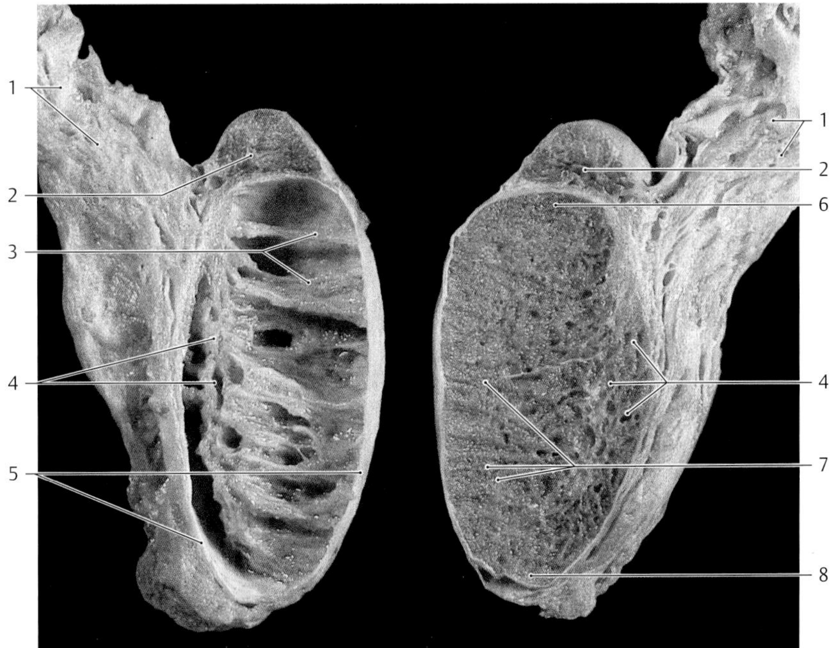


1 Spermatic cord (cut surface)
2 Head of epididymis (cut surface)
3 Septa of testis
4 Mediastinum testis
5 Tunica albuginea
6 Superior pole of testis
7 Convoluted seminiferous tubules
8 Inferior pole of testis

Fig. 7.49 **Longitudinal section through testis and epididymis.** The left figure shows the testicular septa after removal of the seminiferous tubules.

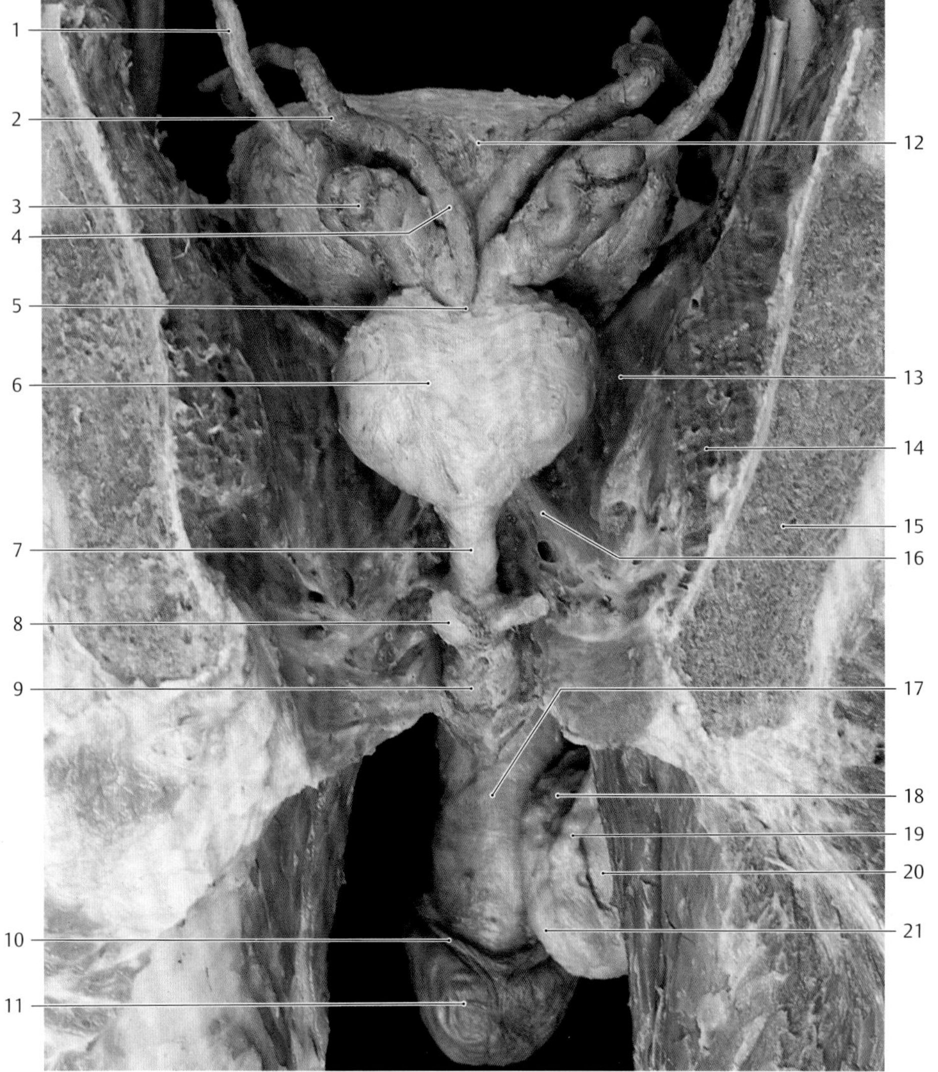


Fig. 7.50 **Accessory glands of male genital organs.** Coronal section through the pelvic cavity. Posterior aspect of urinary bladder, prostate, and seminal vesicles.

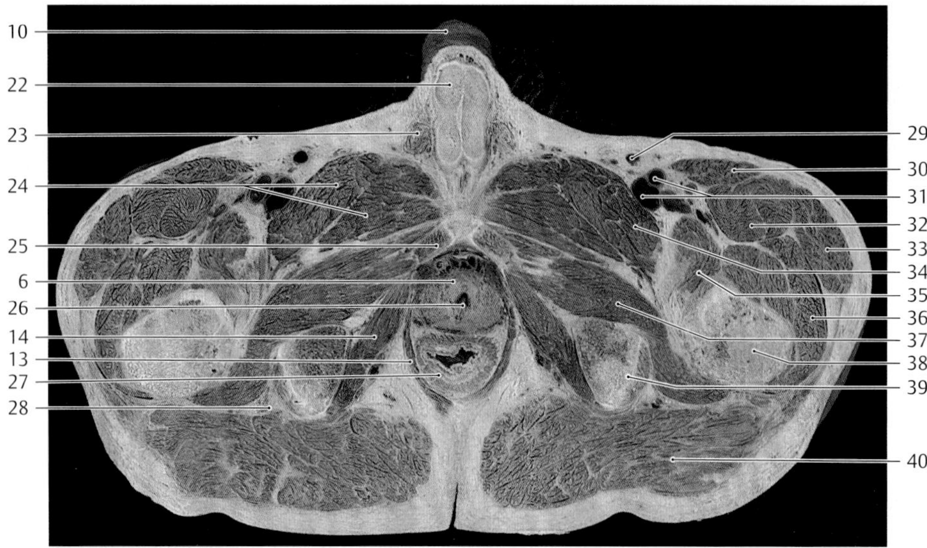


Fig. 7.51 **Horizontal section through the pelvic cavity in the male** at the level of the prostate.

1 Ureter
2 Ductus deferens
3 Seminal vesicle
4 Ampulla of ductus deferens
5 Ejaculatory duct (proximal portion)
6 Prostate
7 Membranous urethra
8 Bulbo-urethral gland (Cowper's gland)
9 Bulb of penis
10 Penis
11 Glans penis
12 Urinary bladder
13 Levator ani muscle
14 Obturator internus muscle
15 Pelvic bone (cut edge)
16 Puboprostatic ligament
17 Corpus spongiosum of penis
18 Head of epididymis
19 Beginning of ductus deferens
20 Testis
21 Tail of epididymis
22 Corpus cavernosum of penis
23 Spermatic cord
24 Pectineus and adductor muscles
25 Pubis
26 Prostatic part of urethra (seminal colliculus)
27 Rectum
28 Sciatic nerve
29 Great saphenous vein
30 Sartorius muscle
31 Femoral artery and vein
32 Rectus femoris muscle
33 Tensor fasciae latae muscle
34 Pectineus muscle
35 Iliopsoas muscle
36 Vastus lateralis muscle
37 Obturator externus muscle
38 Femur
39 Ischial tuberosity
40 Gluteus maximus muscle

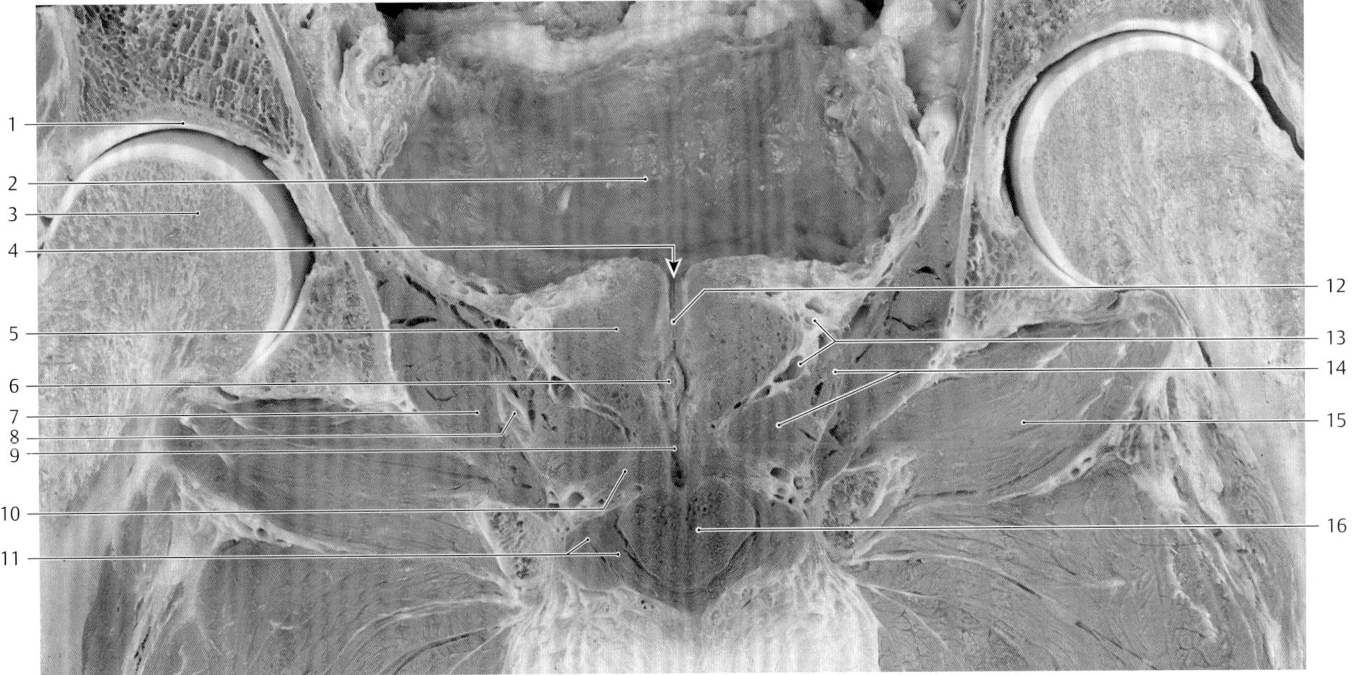


Fig. 7.52 **Coronal section through the pelvic cavity in the male** at the level of prostate and hip joint (anterior aspect).

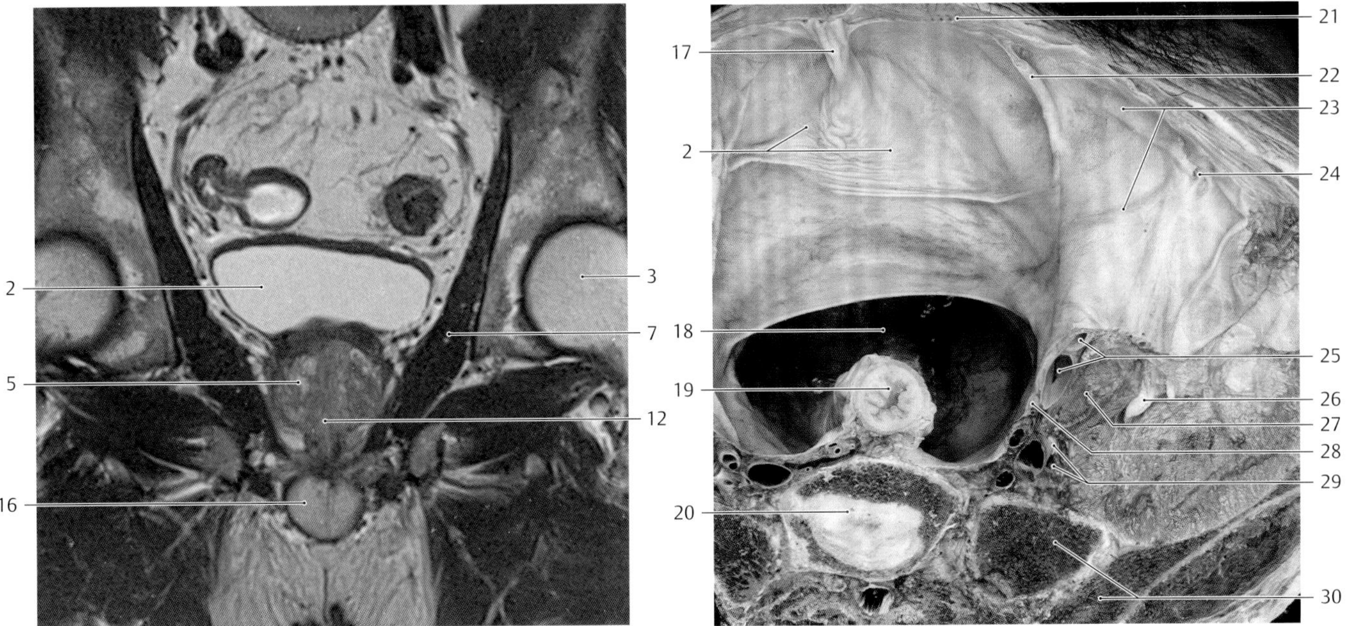


Fig. 7.53 **Coronal section through the pelvic cavity in the male** (MRI scan). (Courtesy of Prof. Uder, Institute of Radiology, University Hospital Erlangen, Germany.)

Fig. 7.54 **Pelvic cavity in the male** (from above).

1 Acetabulum of hip joint
2 Urinary bladder
3 Head of femur
4 Internal urethral orifice
5 Prostate
6 Seminal colliculus
7 Obturator internus muscle
8 Ischiorectal fossa
9 Membranous urethra
10 Deep transverse perineal muscle
11 Crus penis and ischiocavernosus muscle
12 Prostatic part of urethra
13 Prostatic plexus
14 Levator ani muscle
15 Obturator externus muscle
16 Bulb of penis
17 Median umbilical fold with remnant of urachus
18 Rectovesical pouch
19 Rectum
20 Sacrum
21 Inferior epigastric artery
22 Medial umbilical fold with remnant of umbilical artery
23 Deep inguinal ring and ductus deferens
24 Deep iliac circumflex artery
25 External iliac artery and vein
26 Femoral nerve
27 Iliopsoas muscle
28 Ureter
29 Obturator nerve and internal iliac artery
30 Ilium and sacrum

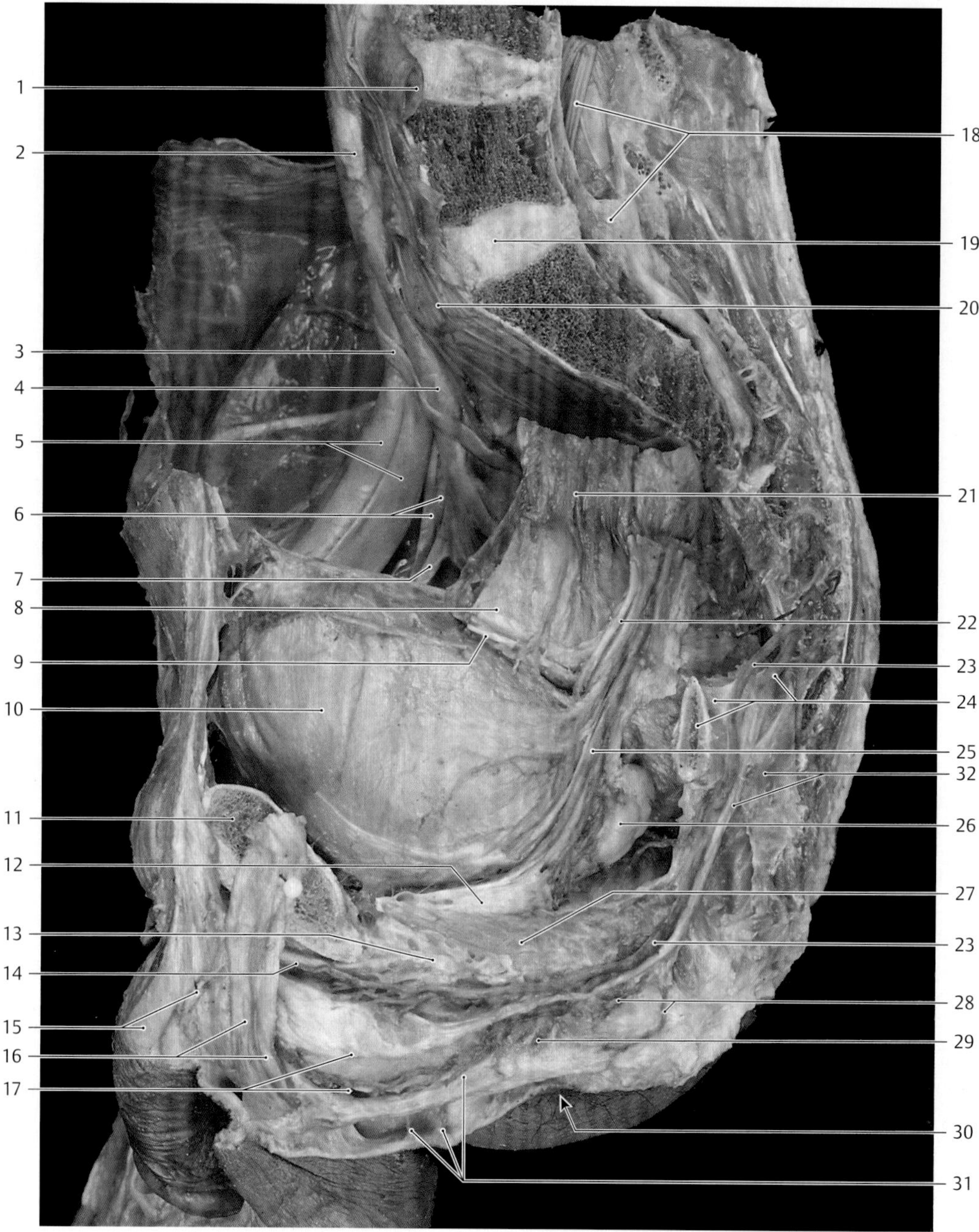


**Fig. 7.55 Vessels of the pelvic cavity in the male** (right half, parasagittal section). The arteries have been injected with red resin. The parietal layer of peritoneum has been removed. The urinary bladder is filled to a great extent.

1 Left common iliac artery
2 Right common iliac artery
3 Right ureter
4 Right internal iliac artery
5 Right external iliac artery and vein
6 Right obturator artery and nerve
7 Umbilical artery
8 Sigmoid and superior vesical artery
9 Left ductus deferens
10 Urinary bladder
11 Pubis (cut)
12 Prostate
13 Vesicoprostatic venous plexus
14 Deep dorsal vein of penis and dorsal artery of penis
15 Penis and superficial dorsal vein
16 Spermatic cord and testicular artery
17 Bulb of penis and deep artery of penis
18 Cauda equina and dura mater (divided)
19 Intervertebral disc between fifth lumbar vertebra and sacrum
20 Sacral promontory
21 Mesosigmoid
22 Left ureter
23 Left internal pudendal artery
24 Ischial spine (cut), sacrospinal ligament, and inferior gluteal artery
25 Left inferior vesical artery
26 Seminal vesicle
27 Levator ani muscle
28 Branches of inferior rectal artery
29 Perineal artery
30 Anus
31 Posterior scrotal branches
32 Pudendal nerve and sacrotuberous ligament

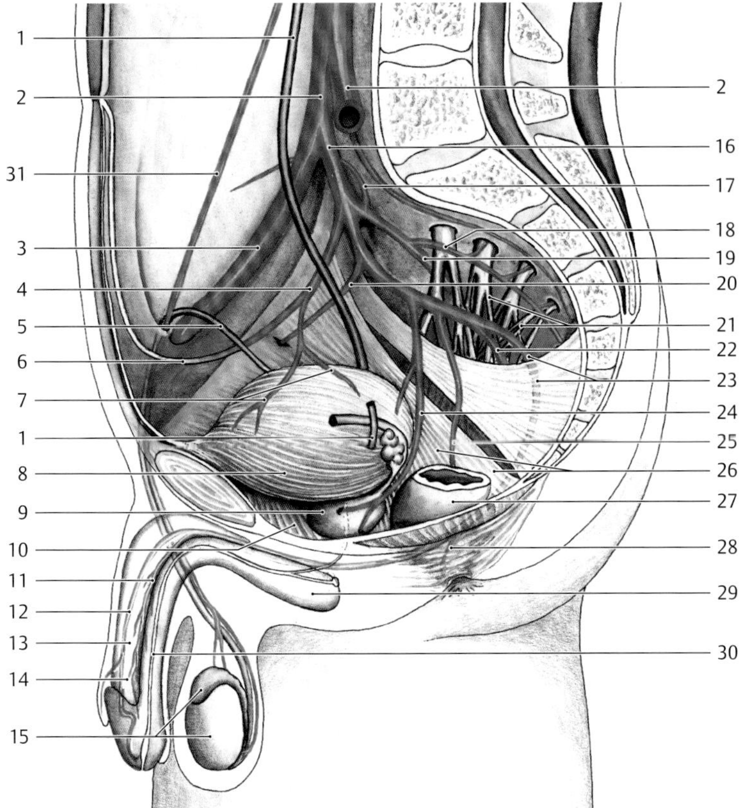


Fig. 7.56 **Main branches of internal iliac artery in the male** (lateral aspect).

1 Ureter
2 Common iliac artery
3 External iliac artery
4 Umbilical artery
5 Ductus deferens
6 Medial umbilical ligament
7 Branches of superior vesical artery
8 Urinary bladder (vesica urinaria)
9 Prostate
10 Urogenital diaphragm
11 Deep artery of penis
12 Dorsal artery of penis
13 Penis
14 Cavernous body of penis
15 Testis and epididymis
16 Internal iliac artery
17 Iliolumbar artery
18 Lateral sacral artery
19 Superior gluteal artery
20 Obturator artery
21 Plexus sacralis
22 Inferior gluteal artery
23 Internal pudendal artery
24 Inferior vesical artery
25 Middle rectal artery
26 Levator ani muscle
27 Rectum
28 Inferior rectal artery
29 Spongy part of penis
30 Urethra (spongy part)
31 External iliac artery
32 Artery of bulb of penis
33 Septum of penis

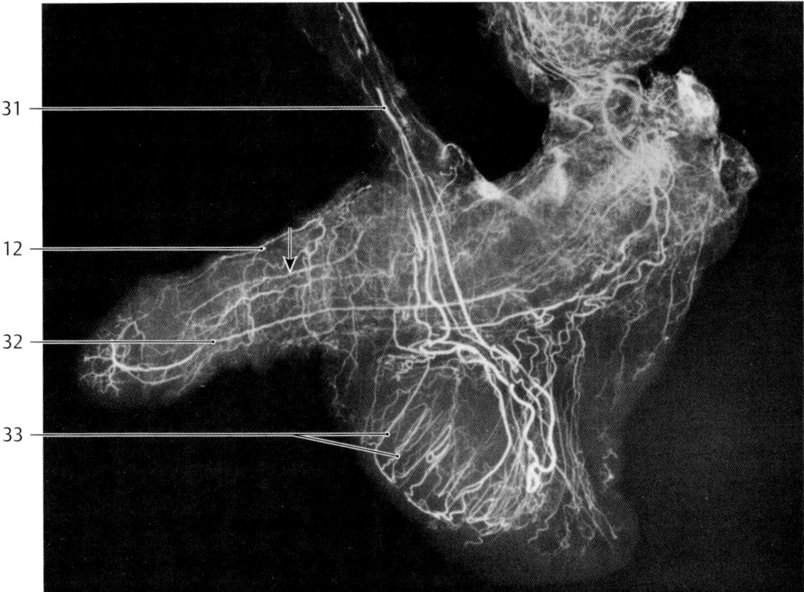


Fig. 7.57 **Arteriograph of male genital organs** (lateral aspect).
Arrow = helicine artery.

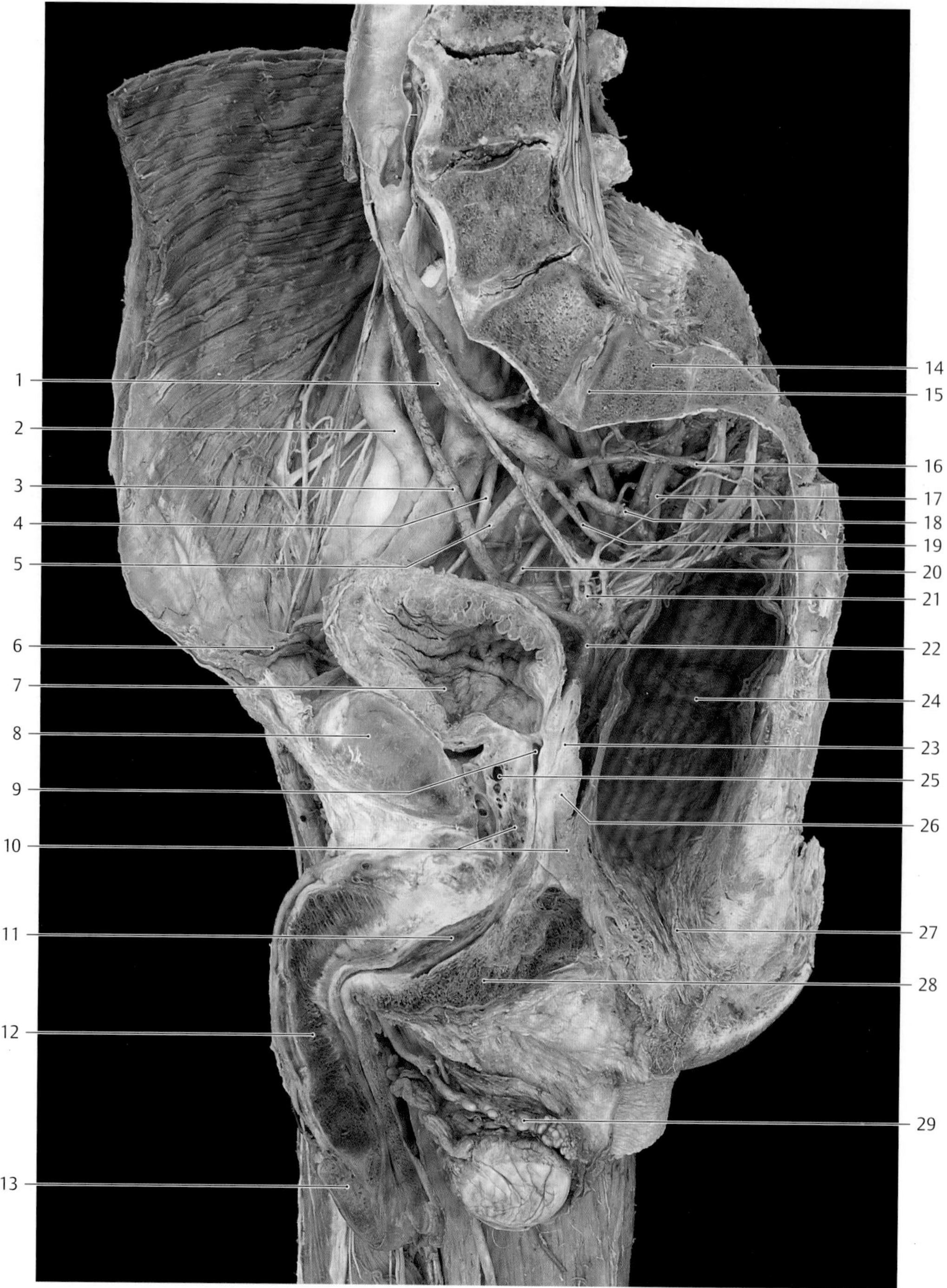


Fig. 7.58 **Vessels of the pelvic cavity in the male** (medial aspect, midsagittal section). The gluteus maximus muscle has been removed.

1 Internal iliac artery
2 External iliac artery
3 Ureter
4 Obturator nerve
5 Umbilical artery
6 Deep inguinal ring
7 Urinary bladder (vesica urinaria)
8 Symphysis
9 Prostatic part of urethra
10 Sphincter muscle of urethra
11 Urethra (spongy part)
12 Cavernous body of penis
13 Glans penis
14 Sacrum
15 Promontory
16 Lateral sacral artery
17 Plexus sacralis
18 Inferior gluteal artery
19 Internal pudendal artery
20 Obturator artery
21 Inferior hypogastric plexus
22 Ductus deferens
23 Seminal vesicle (vesicula seminalis)
24 Rectum
25 Prostatic venous plexus
26 Prostate
27 Anal canal
28 Spongy part of penis
29 Pampiniform plexus

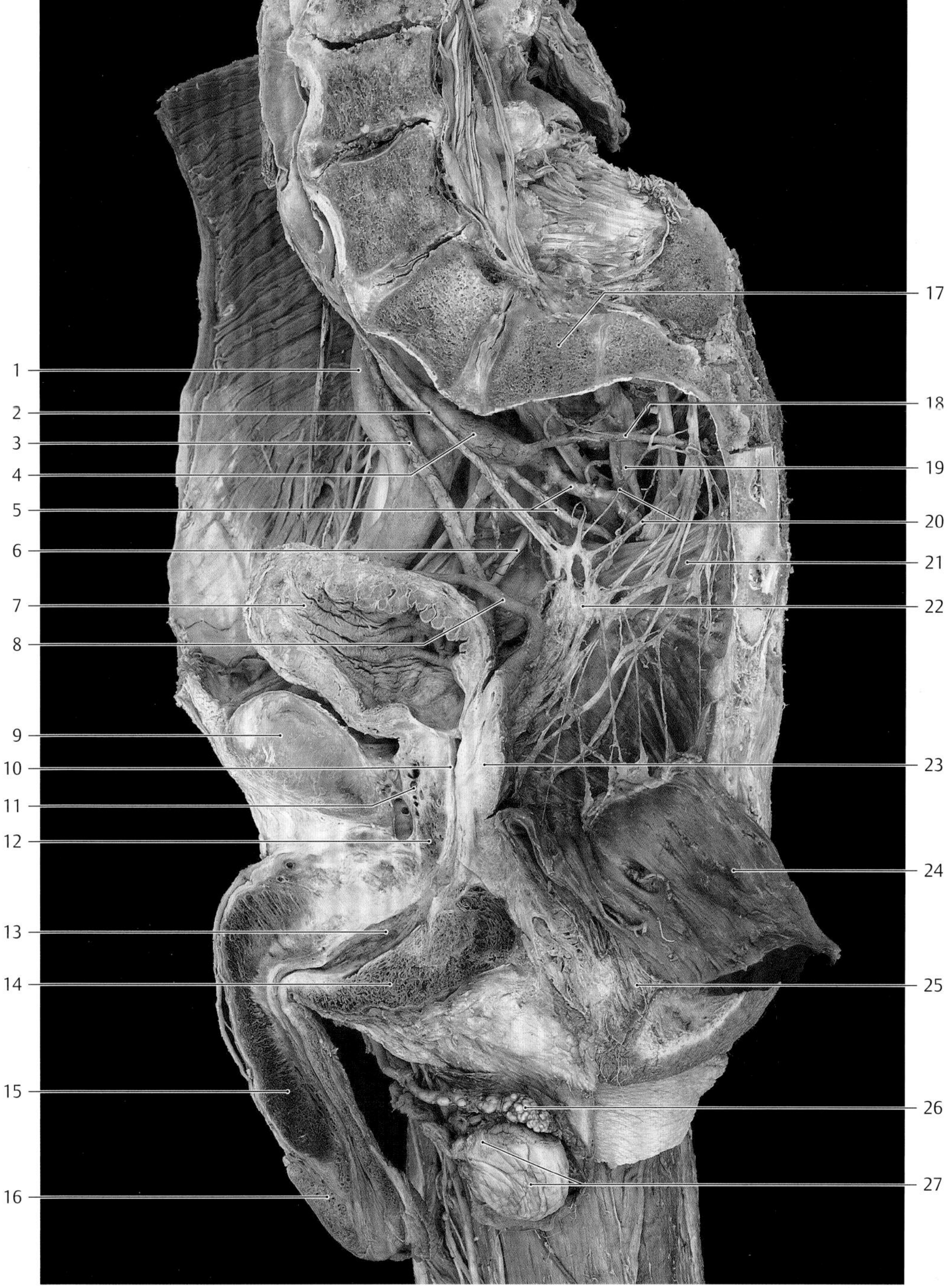


Fig. 7.59 **Vessels and nerves of the pelvic cavity in the male** (medial aspect, midsagittal section). The rectum has been reflected to display the inferior hypogastric plexus. The gluteus maximus muscle has been removed.

1 External iliac artery
2 Right hypogastric nerve
3 Ureter
4 Internal iliac artery
5 Inferior gluteal artery and internal pudendal artery
6 Obturator artery
7 Urinary bladder
8 Ductus deferens
9 Symphysis pubica
10 Prostatic part of urethra
11 Prostatic venous plexus
12 Sphincter urethrae muscle
13 Spongy part of urethra
14 Corpus spongiosum penis
15 Corpus cavernosum penis
16 Glans penis
17 Sacrum
18 Lateral sacral artery
19 Sacral plexus
20 Pelvic splanchnic nerves (nervi erigentes)
21 Levator ani muscle
22 Inferior hypogastric plexus (pelvic plexus)
23 Prostate
24 Rectum (reflected)
25 Anal canal and external anal sphincter muscle
26 Pampiniform plexus continuous with testicular vein
27 Testis and epididymis

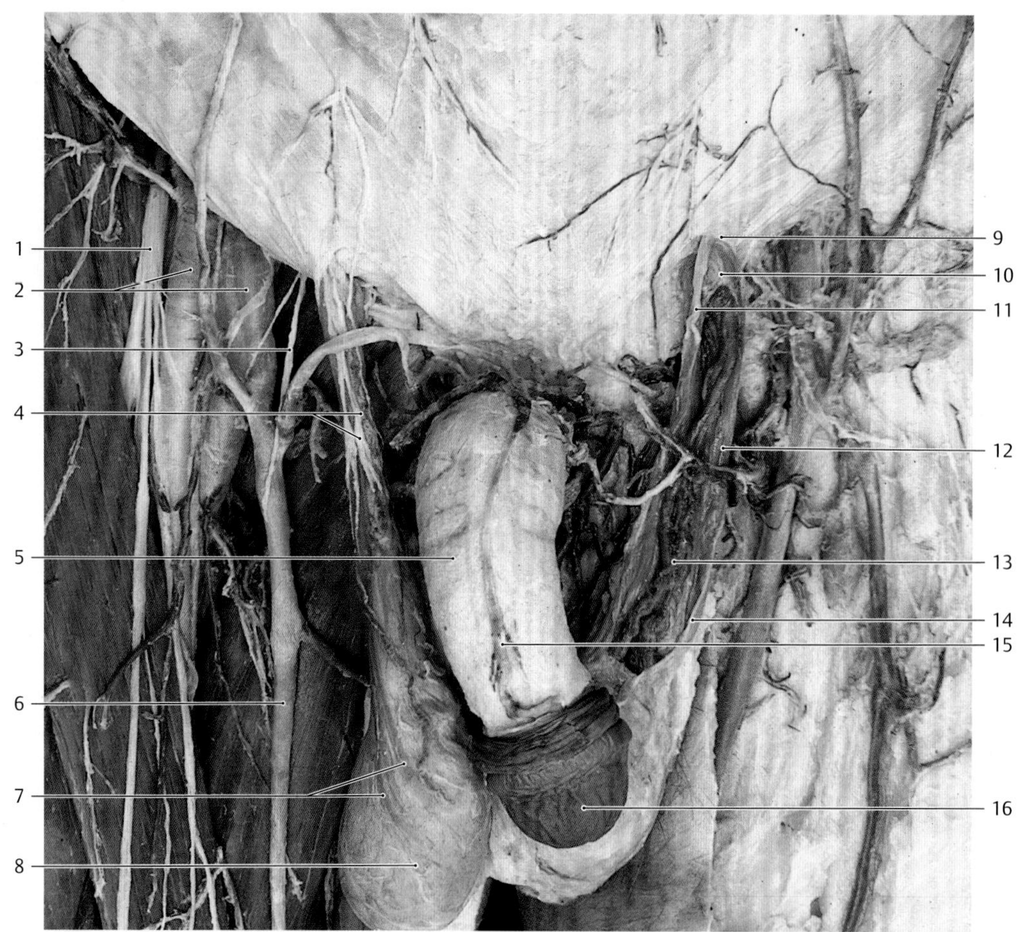


Fig. 7.60 **Male external genital organs with penis, testis, and spermatic cord,** superficial layer (anterior aspect).

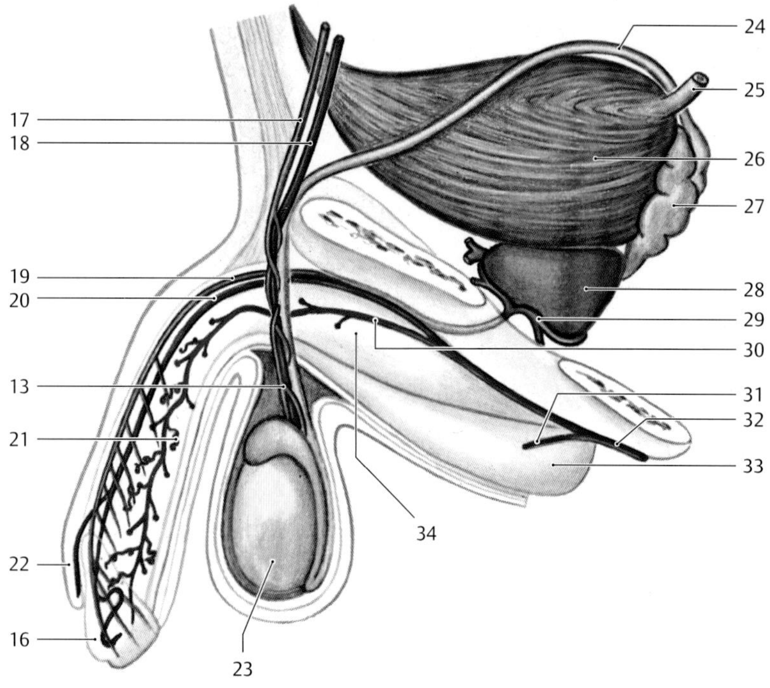


Fig. 7.61 **Vessels of male genital organs** (lateral aspect).

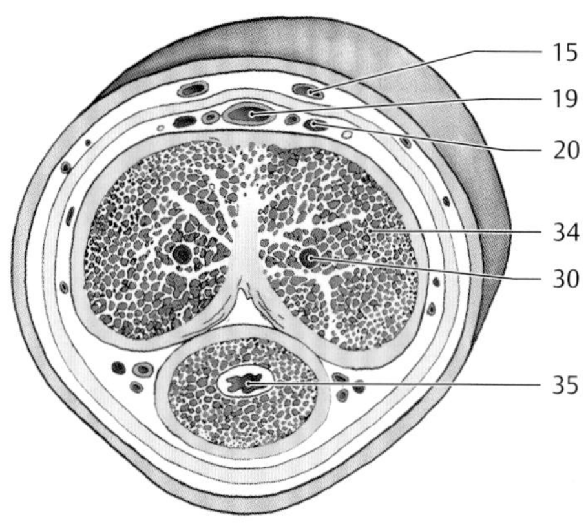


Fig. 7.62 **Vessels of male genital organs** (cross section through the penis).

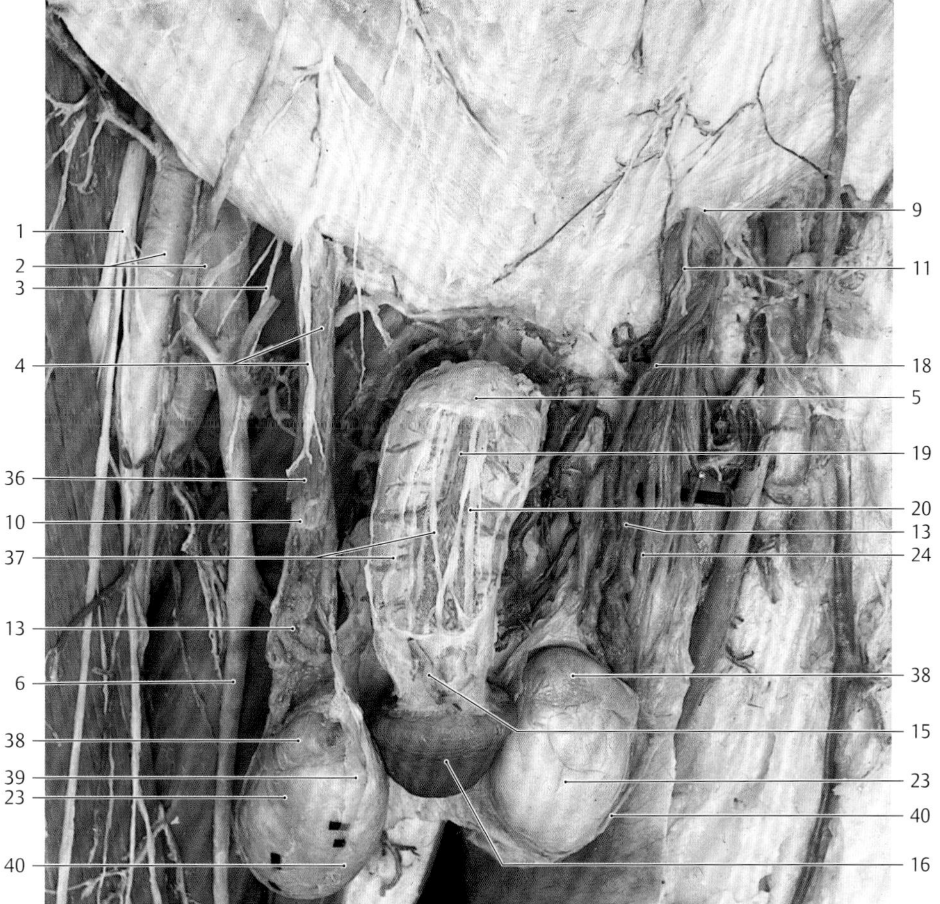


Fig. 7.63 **Male external genital organs with penis, testis, and spermatic cord,** deeper layer (anterior aspect). The deep fascia of the penis has been opened to display the dorsal nerves and vessels.

1 Femoral nerve
2 Femoral artery and vein
3 Femoral branch of genitofemoral nerve
4 Spermatic cord with genital branch of genitofemoral nerve
5 Penis with deep fascia
6 Great saphenous vein
7 Cremaster muscle
8 Testis with cremaster muscle
9 Superficial inguinal ring
10 Internal spermatic fascia (cut edge)
11 Ilio-inguinal nerve
12 Left spermatic cord
13 Pampiniform venous plexus
14 External spermatic fascia
15 Superficial dorsal vein of penis
16 Glans penis
17 Testicular vein
18 Testicular artery
19 Deep dorsal vein of penis
20 Dorsal artery of penis
21 Helicine arteries
22 Prepuce
23 Testis with tunica albuginea
24 Ductus deferens
25 Ureter
26 Urinary bladder
27 Seminal vesicle
28 Prostate
29 Vesicoprostatic venous plexus
30 Deep artery of penis
31 Artery of bulb of penis
32 Internal pudendal artery
33 Corpus spongiosum of penis
34 Corpus cavernosum of penis
35 Urethra
36 Cremasteric fascia with cremaster muscle
37 Dorsal nerve of penis
38 Epididymis
39 Tunica vaginalis (visceral layer)
40 Tunica vaginalis (parietal layer)
41 Inguinal ligament
42 Femoral cutaneous nerve
43 Deep inguinal ring
44 Ductus deferens and testicular artery
45 Hiatus saphenous
46 Epididymis

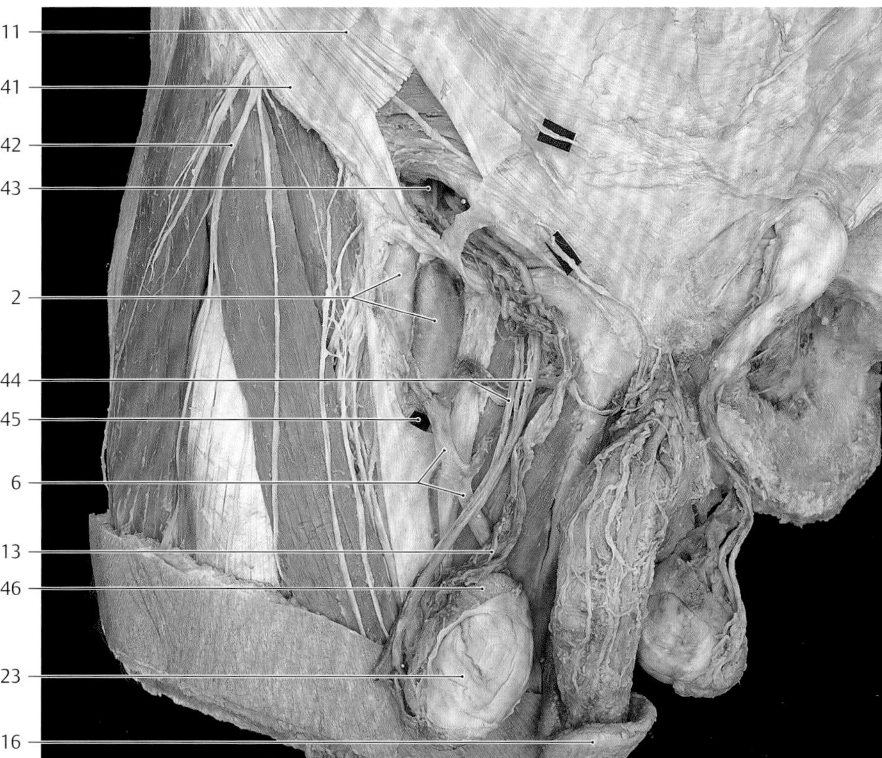


Fig. 7.64 **Male external genital organs and inguinal region** (anterior aspect). Dissection of the inguinal canal, ductus deferens, and testicular artery.

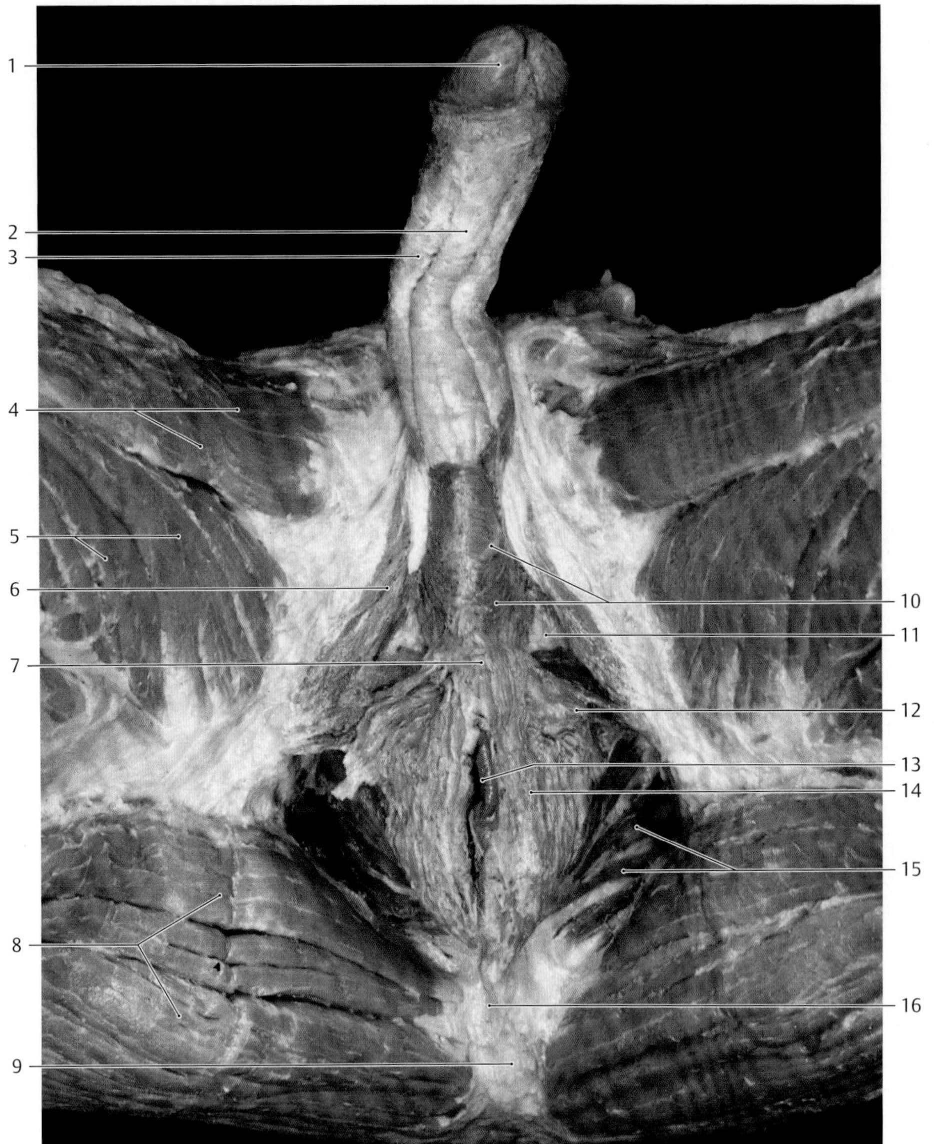


Fig. 7.65 **Urogenital diaphragm and external genital organs in the male** with muscles of the pelvic floor (from below).

1 Glans penis
2 Corpus spongiosum of penis
3 Corpus cavernosum of penis
4 Gracilis muscle
5 Adductor muscles
6 Ischiocavernosus muscle overlying crus of penis
7 Central tendon of the perineum
8 Gluteus maximus muscle
9 Coccyx
10 Bulbospongiosus muscle
11 Deep transverse perineal muscle covered by inferior fascia of urogenital diaphragm
12 Superficial transverse perineal muscle
13 Anus
14 External anal sphincter muscle
15 Levator ani muscle
16 Anococcygeal ligament
17 Testis
18 Urethra
19 Deep dorsal vein of penis
20 Dorsal artery of penis
21 Deep transverse perineal muscle
22 Obturator internus muscle
23 Sacrotuberal ligament

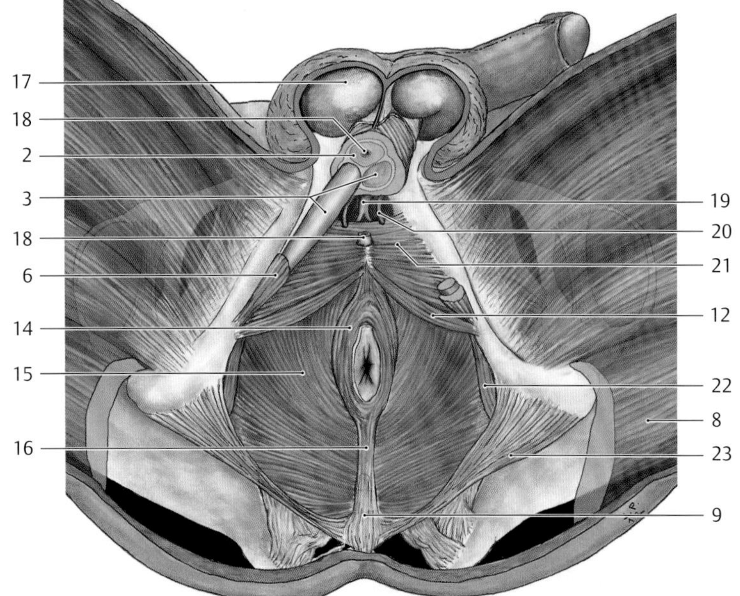


Fig. 7.66 **Urogenital and anal regions in the male** (from below). Muscles of the urogenital and pelvic diaphragms.

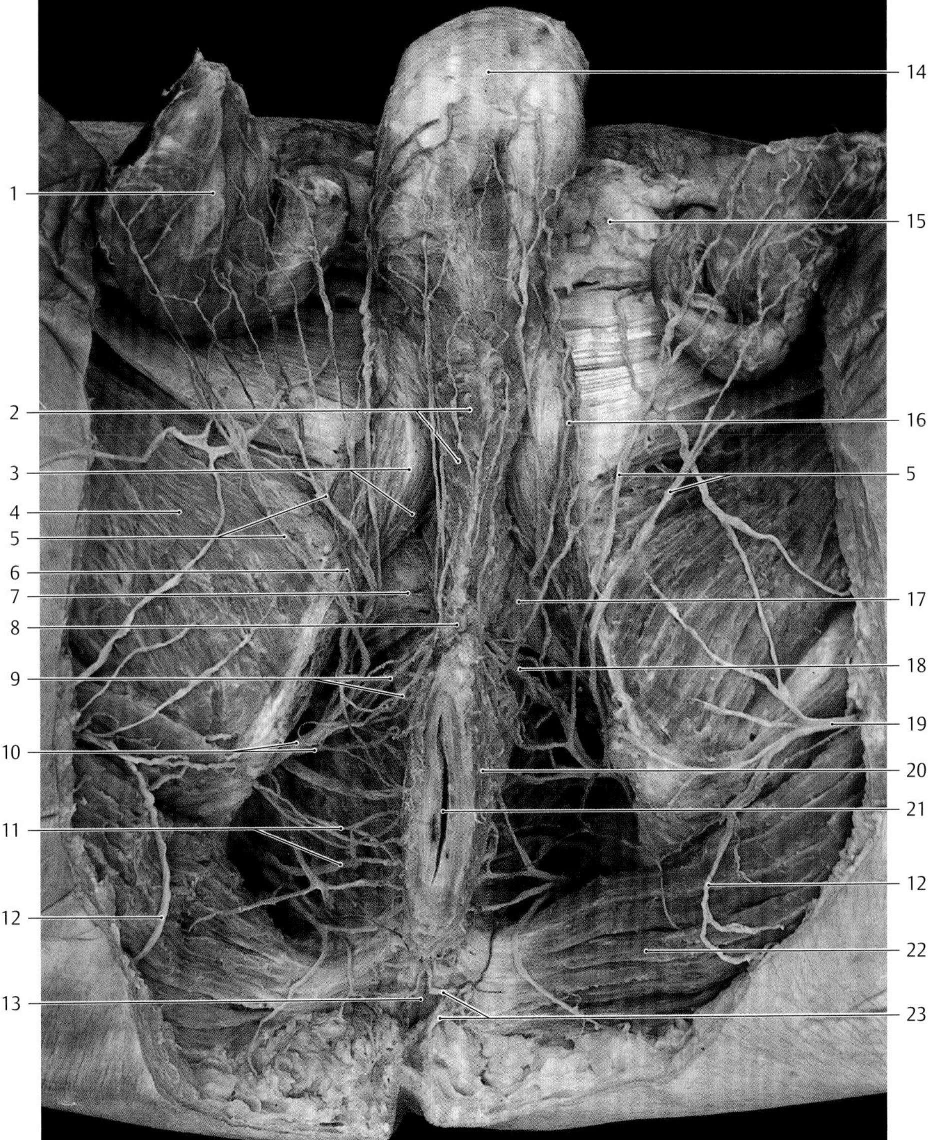


**Fig. 7.67 Urogenital diaphragm and external genital organs in the male** with vessels and nerves (from below). The testes have been reflected laterally.

1 Right testis (reflected laterally and upward)
2 Bulbospongiosus muscle
3 Ischiocavernosus muscle
4 Adductor magnus muscle
5 Posterior scrotal nerves and superficial perineal arteries
6 Posterior scrotal artery and vein
7 Right artery of bulb of penis
8 Central tendon of the perineum
9 Perineal branches of pudendal nerve
10 Pudendal nerve and internal pudendal artery
11 Inferior rectal arteries and nerves
12 Inferior cluneal nerves
13 Coccyx (location)
14 Penis
15 Left testis (reflected laterally)
16 Left posterior scrotal artery
17 Deep transverse perineal muscle
18 Left artery of bulb of penis
19 Branch of posterior femoral cutaneous nerve
20 External anal sphincter muscle
21 Anus
22 Gluteus maximus muscle
23 Anococcygeal nerves
24 Acetabulum (femur removed)
25 Ligament of femoral head
26 Body of ischium (cut)
27 Sciatic nerve
28 Coccygeus muscle
29 Levator ani muscle
(a) Iliococcygeus muscle
(b) Pubococcygeus muscle
(c) Puborectalis muscle
30 Prostatic venous plexus
31 Pubis
32 Testis

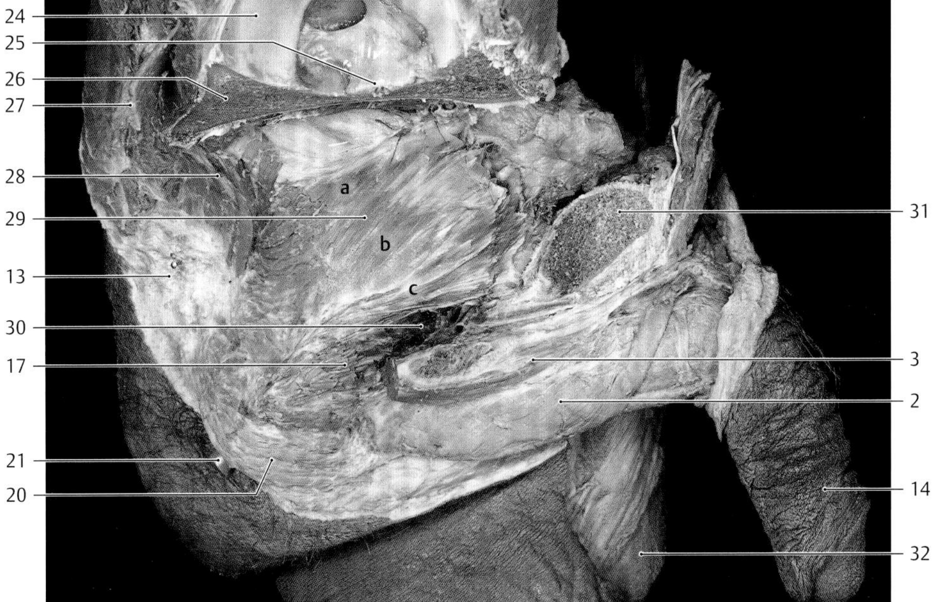


**Fig. 7.68 Pelvic diaphragm and external genital organs in the male** (lateral aspect). The right half of the pelvis including the obturator internus muscle and femur have been removed to display the right half of the levator ani muscle.

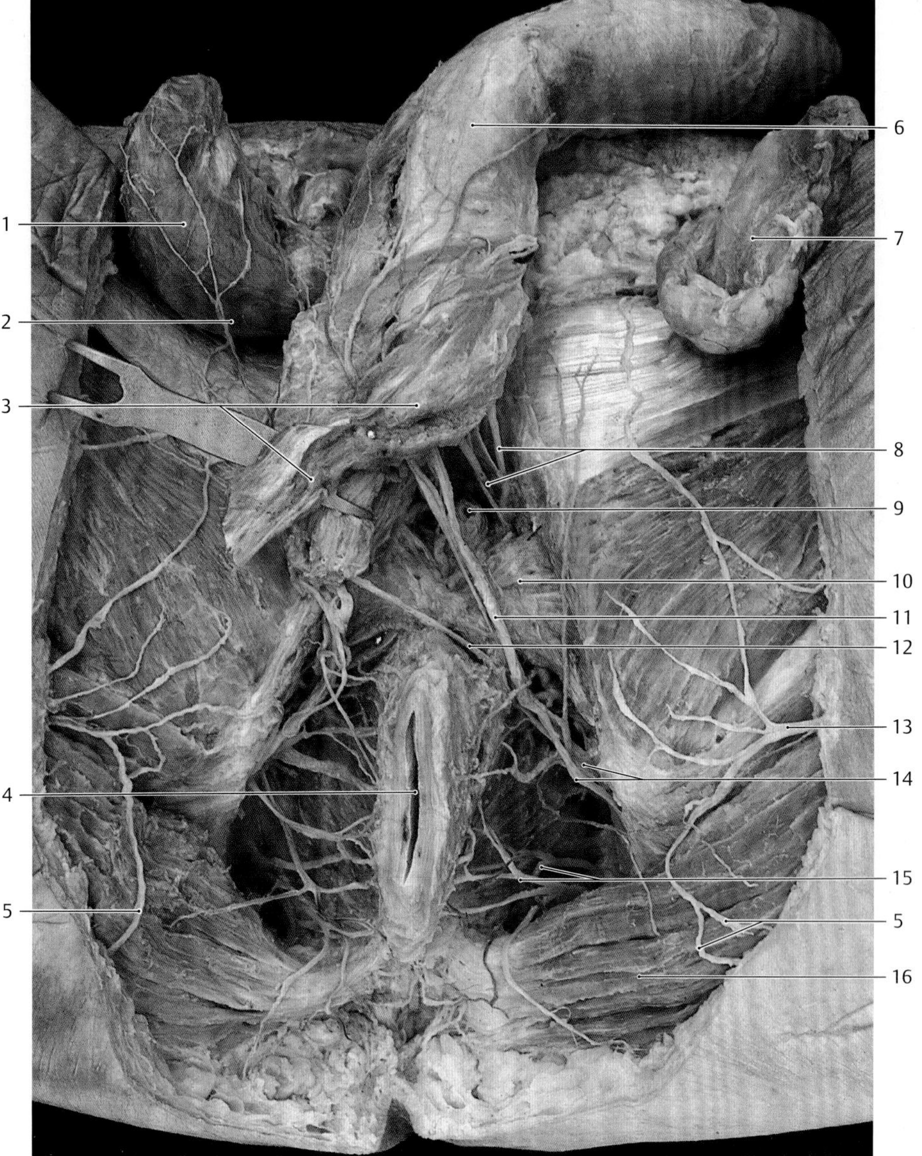


**Fig. 7.69 Urogenital diaphragm and external genital organs in the male** (from below). The left crus penis has been isolated and reflected laterally together with the bulb of the penis. The urethra has been cut.

1 Right testis (reflected)
2 Posterior scrotal nerves
3 Left crus penis with ischio-cavernosus muscle
4 Anus
5 Inferior cluneal nerves
6 Penis
7 Left testis (reflected)
8 Dorsal artery and nerve of penis
9 Urethra
10 Deep transverse perineal muscle
11 Perineal branches of pudendal nerve
12 Artery of bulb of penis (reflected)
13 Branch of posterior femoral cutaneous nerve
14 Internal pudendal artery and pudendal nerve
15 Inferior rectal arteries and nerves
16 Gluteus maximus muscle
17 Dorsal nerve of penis
18 Posterior femoral cutaneous nerve
19 Perineal and anal branches of pudendal nerve
20 Pudendal nerve
21 Inferior rectal nerves
22 Bulbospongiosus muscle
23 Ischiocavernosus muscle
24 Dorsal artery of penis
25 Perineal artery
26 External anal sphincter muscle
27 Internal pudendal artery and vein
28 Inferior rectal arteries

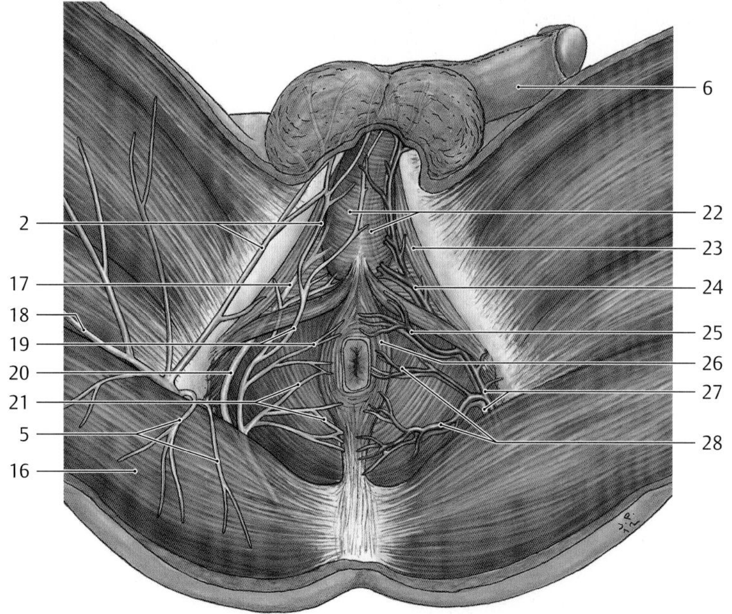


**Fig. 7.70 Urogenital and anal regions in the male** (from below). Right side = nerves; left side = arteries and veins.

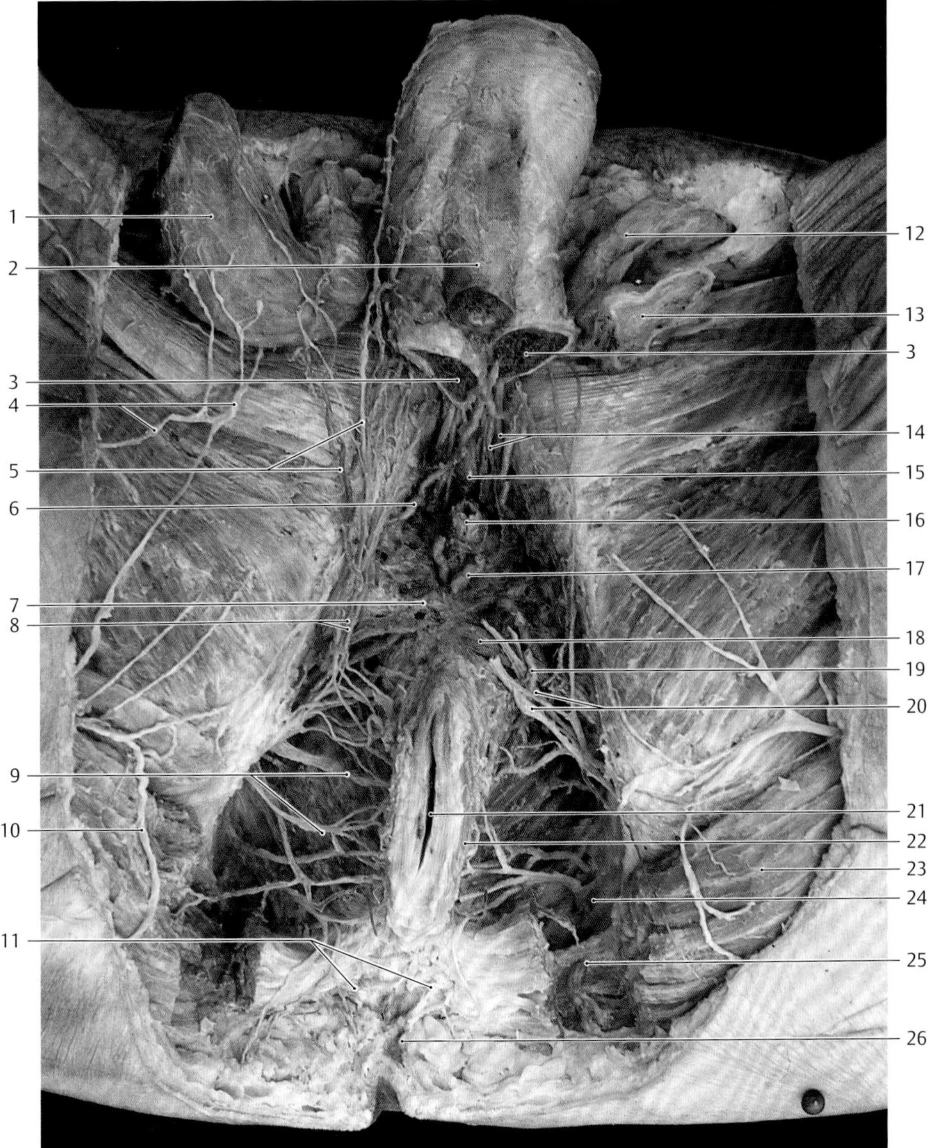


**Fig. 7.71 Urogenital diaphragm and external genital organs in the male** (from below). Dissection of the urogenital diaphragm. The root of the penis has been cut.

1 Right testis (reflected)
2 Corpus spongiosum of penis
3 Corpus cavernosum of penis
4 Perineal branch of posterior femoral cutaneous nerve
5 Posterior scrotal arteries and nerves
6 Deep artery of penis
7 Deep transverse perineal muscle
8 Right perineal nerves
9 Inferior rectal nerves
10 Inferior cluneal nerve
11 Anococcygeal nerves
12 Left spermatic cord
13 Left testis (cut surface)
14 Dorsal artery and nerve of penis
15 Deep dorsal vein of penis
16 Urethra (cut)
17 Artery of bulb of penis
18 Superficial transverse perineal muscle
19 Left artery of bulb of penis
20 Perineal branch of pudendal nerve
21 Anus
22 External anal sphincter muscle
23 Gluteus maximus muscle
24 Obturator fascia with Alcock's canal for pudendal nerve, and internal pudendal artery and vein
25 Sacrotuberous ligament
26 Coccyx
27 Urogenital diaphragm with perineal membrane
28 Perineal fascia (superficial investing fascia of perineum)

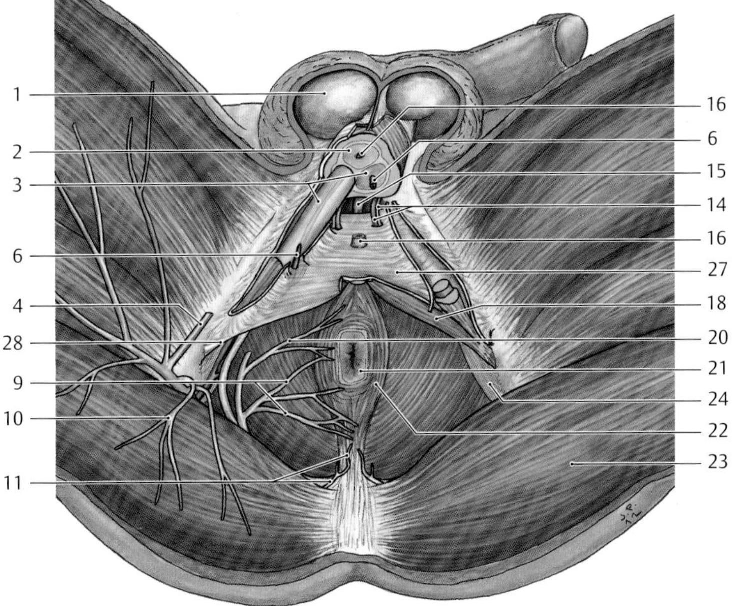


**Fig. 7.72 Urogenital and anal regions in the male** (from below). Muscles of urogenital and pelvic diaphragms. On the left side, the fascia covering the ischiocavernosus muscle and the corpus cavernosum of the penis has been removed. Light blue = perineal fascia and membrane.

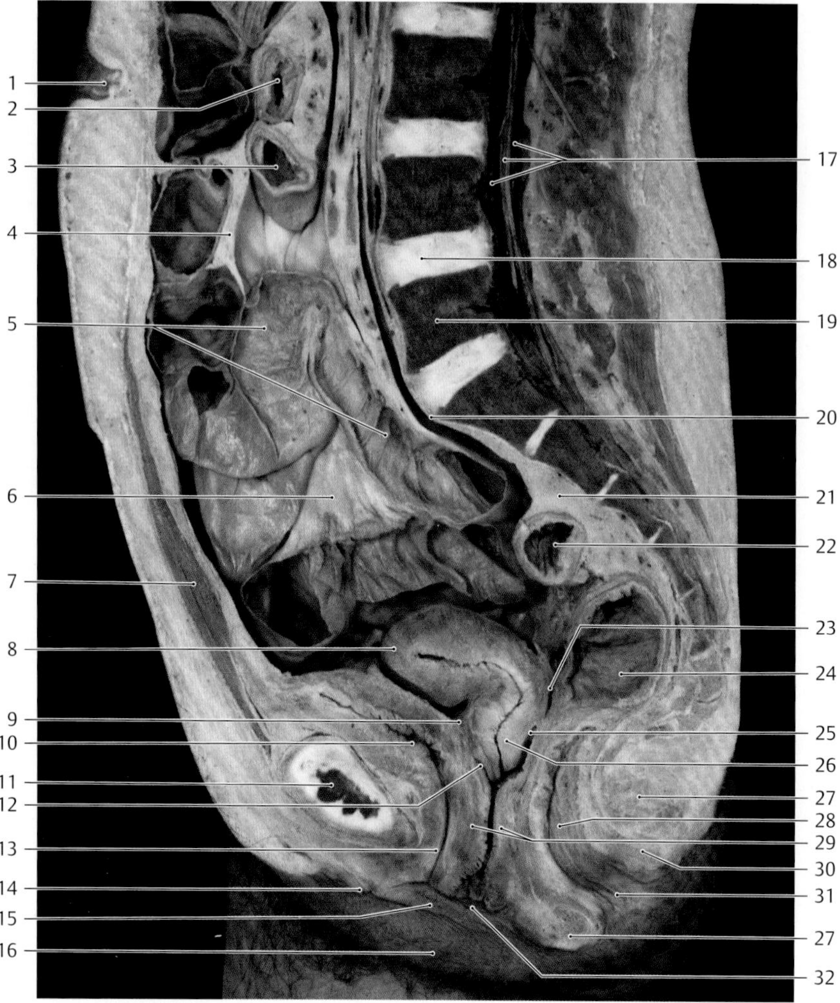


1 Umbilicus
2 Duodenum
3 Ascending part of duodenum
4 Root of mesentery
5 Small intestine
6 Mesentery
7 Rectus abdominis muscle
8 Uterus
9 Vesico-uterine pouch
10 Urinary bladder (collapsed)
11 Pubic symphysis
12 Anterior fornix of vagina
13 Urethra
14 Clitoris
15 Labium minus
16 Labium majus
17 Vertebral canal with cauda equina
18 Intervertebral disc
19 Body of fifth lumbar vertebra (L5)
20 Sacral promontory
21 Mesosigmoid
22 Sigmoid colon
23 Recto-uterine pouch (of Douglas)
24 Ampulla of rectum
25 Posterior fornix of vagina
26 Cervix of uterus
27 External anal sphincter muscle
28 Anal canal
29 Vagina
30 Internal anal sphincter muscle
31 Anus
32 Hymen
33 Abdominal aorta
34 Discus intervertebralis, promontory
35 Sacrum
36 Rectum

Fig. 7.73 **Female urogenital system** (midsagittal section through the pelvic cavity). The urinary bladder is empty; the position and shape of the uterus are normal.

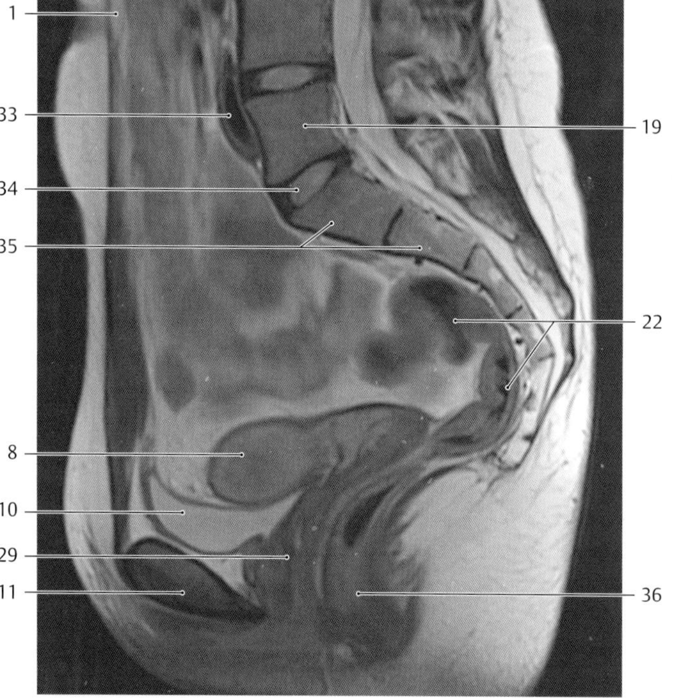


Fig. 7.74 **Sagittal section through the pelvic cavity of a young female.** The uterus reveals an extreme anteflexion (MRI scan). (Courtesy of Prof. Uder, Institute of Radiology, University Hospital Erlangen, Germany.)

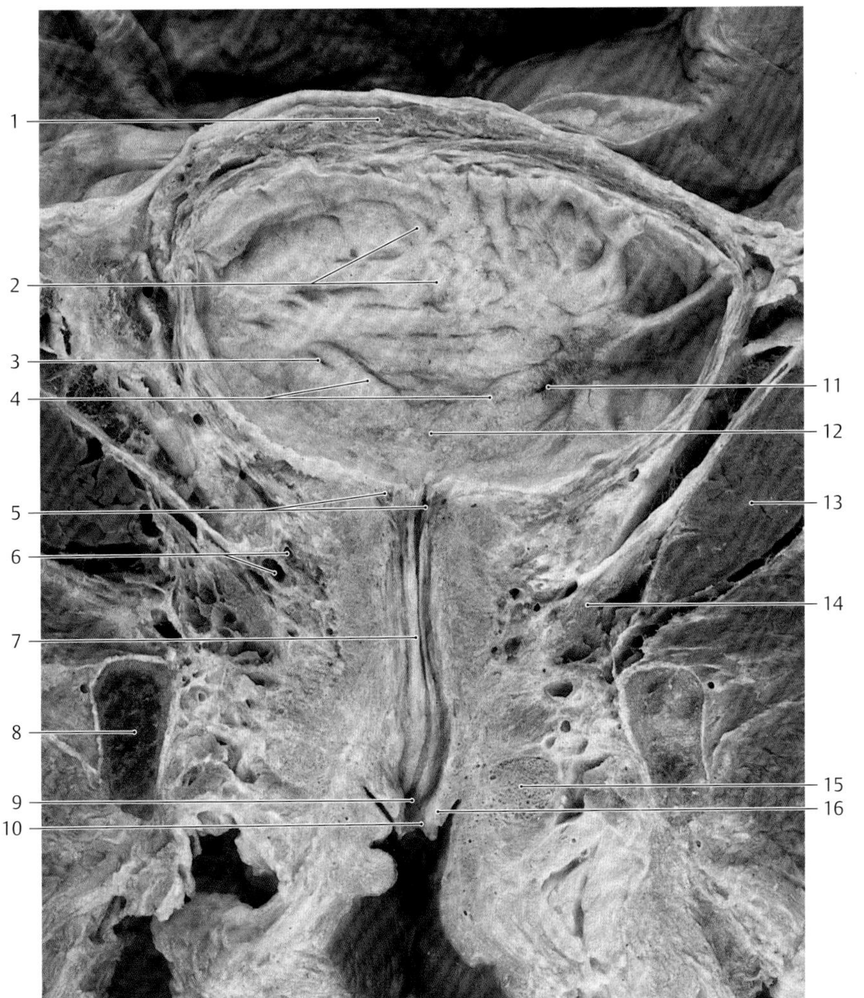


1 Muscular coat of urinary bladder
2 Folds of mucous membrane of urinary bladder
3 Right ureteric orifice
4 Interureteric fold
5 Internal urethral orifice
6 Vesico-uterine venous plexus
7 Urethra
8 Pubis (cut edge)
9 External urethral orifice
10 Vestibule of vagina
11 Left ureteric orifice
12 Trigone of bladder
13 Obturator internus muscle
14 Levator ani muscle
15 Bulb of vestibule
16 Left labium minus
17 Umbilicus
18 Sigmoid colon
19 Median umbilical fold with urachus
20 Infundibulum of uterine tube
21 Fimbriae of uterine tube
22 Ovary
23 Uterine tube (isthmus)
24 Uterus
25 Round ligament of uterus
26 Vesico-uterine pouch
27 Urinary bladder
28 Vagina
29 Pubic symphysis
30 Clitoris
31 Body of fifth lumbar vertebra (L5)
32 Sacral promontory
33 Right ureter
34 Peritoneum (cut edge)
35 Left ureter
36 Recto-uterine pouch (of Douglas)
37 Rectal ampulla
38 Kidney

**Fig. 7.75 Coronal section through the urinary bladder and urethra in the female** (anterior aspect).

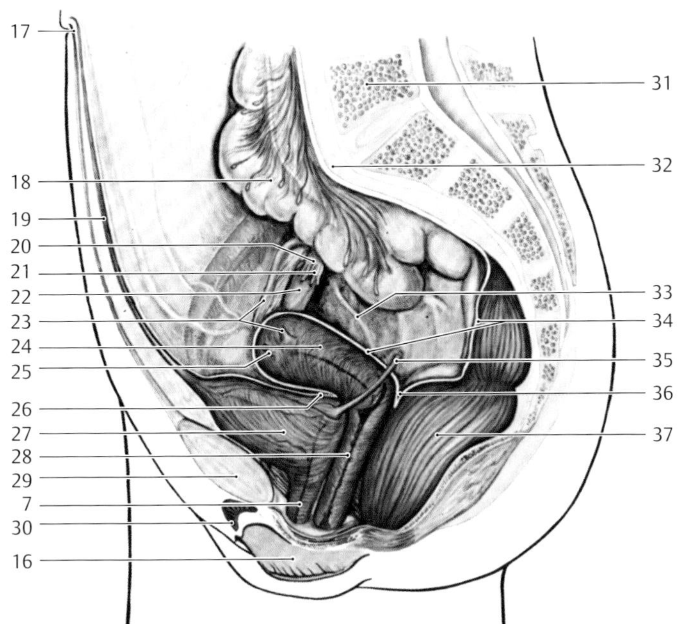


**Fig. 7.76 Position of female genital organs** (medial aspect).

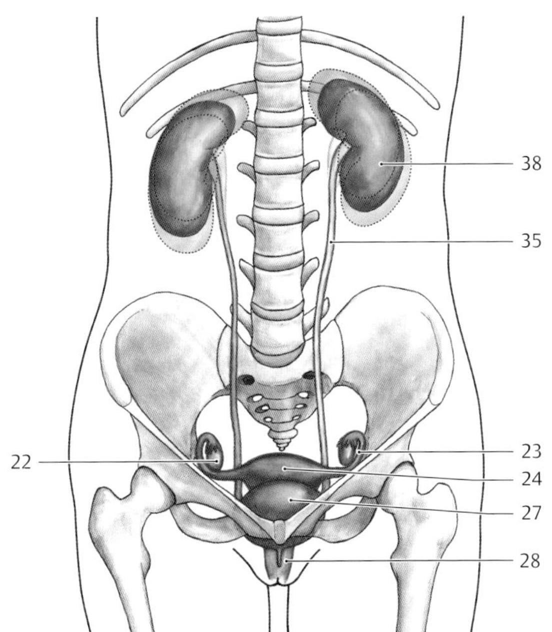


**Fig. 7.77 Position of kidneys, urinary, and genital organs in the female** (anterior aspect). The excursions of the kidneys are indicated.

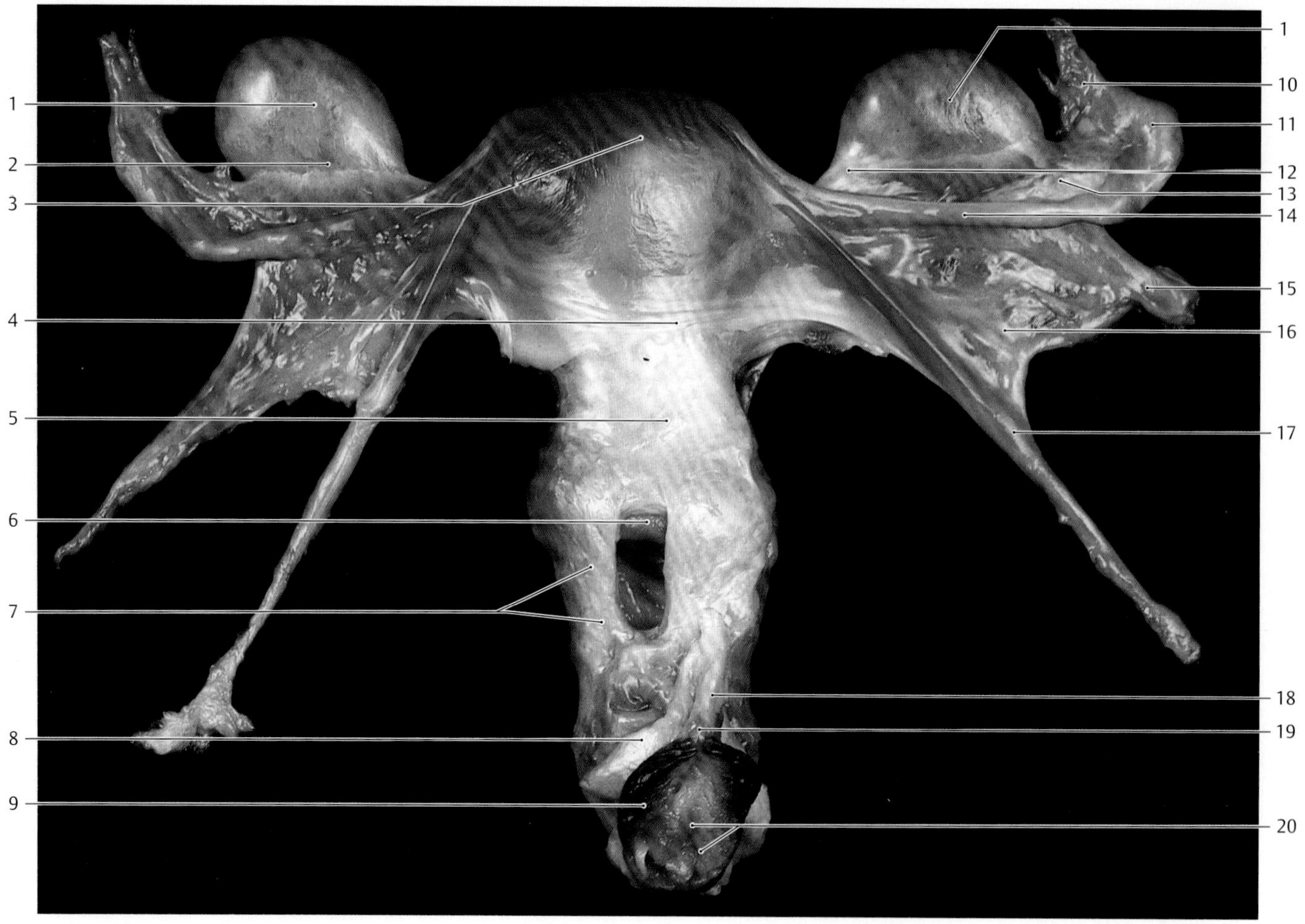

Fig. 7.78 **Female genital organs, isolated** (anterior aspect). The anterior wall of the vagina has been opened to display the vaginal portion of the cervix.

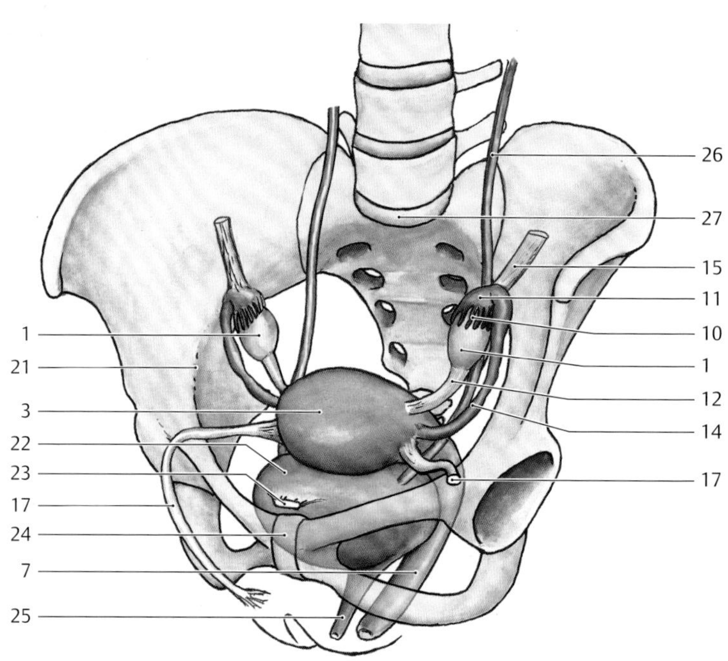


Fig. 7.79 **Position of female internal genital organs** (oblique-anterior aspect).

1 Ovary
2 Mesovarium
3 Fundus of uterus
4 Vesico-uterine pouch
5 Cervix of uterus
6 Vaginal portion of cervix
7 Vagina
8 Crus of clitoris
9 Labium minus
10 Fimbriae of uterine tube
11 Infundibulum of uterine tube
12 Ligament of the ovary
13 Mesosalpinx
14 Uterine tube
15 Suspensory ligament of ovary (caudally displaced)
16 Broad ligament of uterus
17 Round ligament of uterus
18 Corpus cavernosum of clitoris
19 Glans of clitoris
20 Hymen and vaginal orifice
21 Linea terminalis
22 Urinary bladder
23 Medial umbilical ligament
24 Pubic symphysis
25 Urethra
26 Ureter
27 Promontory

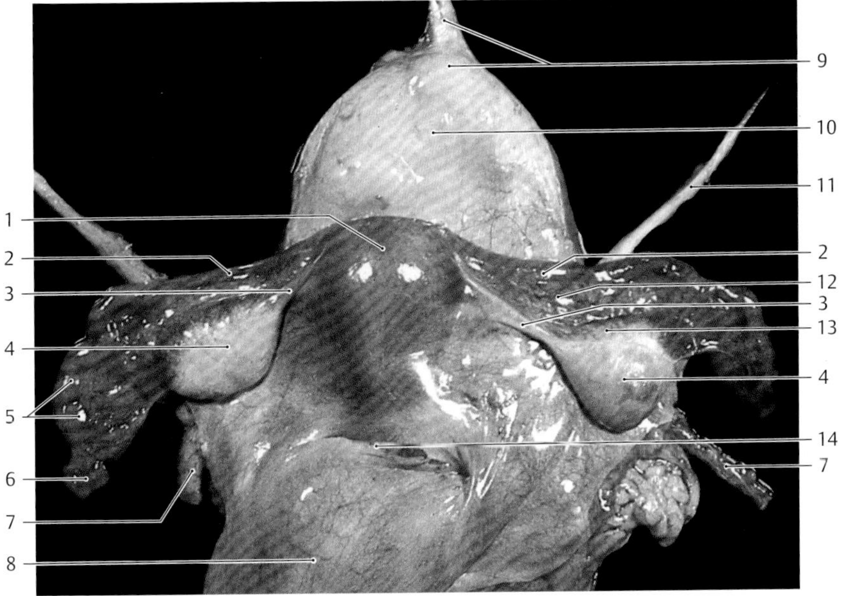


Fig. 7.80 **Female genital organs, isolated** (supero-posterior aspect).

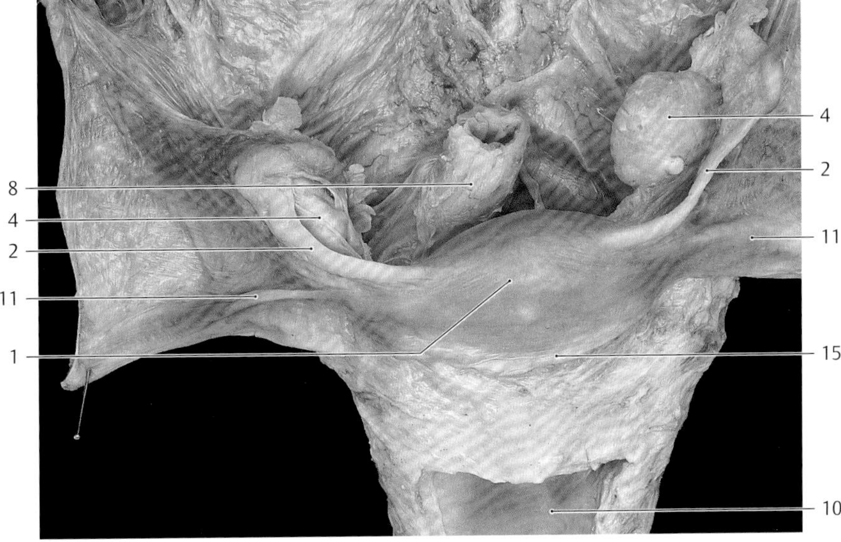


Fig. 7.81 **Uterus and related organs, isolated** (superior aspect). The left ovary is enlarged.

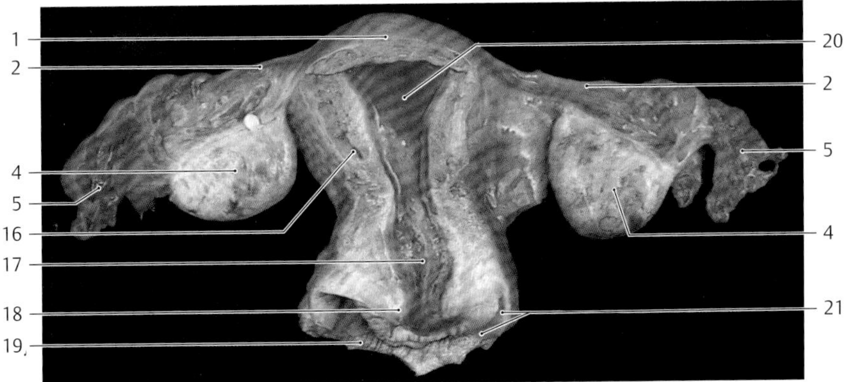


Fig. 7.82 **Uterus and related organs, isolated** (posterior aspect). The posterior wall of the uterus has been opened.

1 Fundus of uterus
2 Uterine tube
3 Ligament of the ovary
4 Ovary
5 Infundibulum of uterine tube
6 Fimbriae of uterine tube
7 Ureter
8 Rectum
9 Apex of urinary bladder and median umbilical ligament
10 Urinary bladder (fenestrated in the dissection in the middle)
11 Round ligament of uterus
12 Mesosalpinx
13 Mesovarium
14 Recto-uterine pouch (of Douglas)
15 Vesico-uterine pouch
16 Body of uterus
17 Cervix of uterus
18 Vaginal portion of cervix of uterus
19 Vagina
20 Mucous membrane of uterus congestion
21 Anterior fornix of vagina

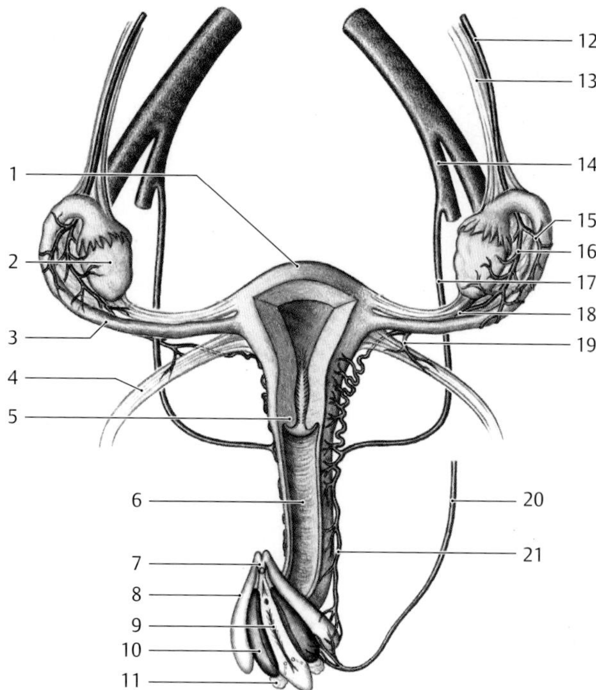


**Fig. 7.83 Arteries of female genital organs.**

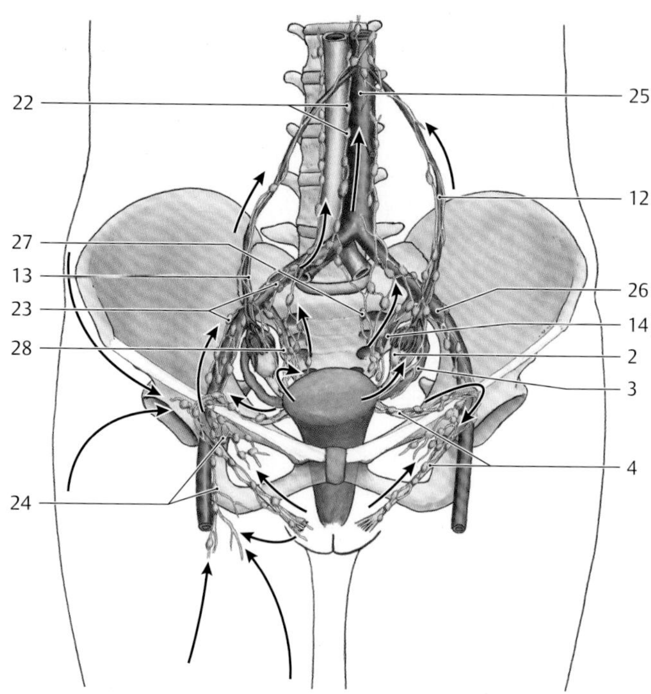


**Fig. 7.84 Main drainage routes of lymph vessels of uterus and related organs** (indicated by arrows).

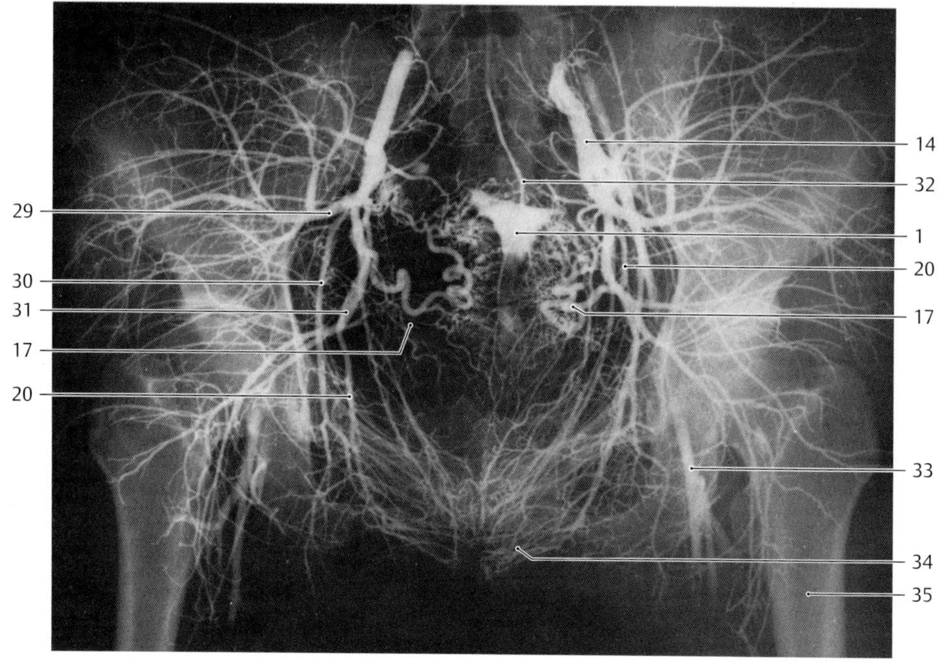


**Fig. 7.85 Arteriograph of pelvic vessels in the female** (antero-posterior direction).

1 Uterus
2 Ovary
3 Uterine tube
4 Round ligament of uterus
5 Vaginal portion of cervix of uterus
6 Vagina
7 Clitoris
8 Corpus cavernosum of clitoris
9 Vaginal orifice
10 Bulb of vestibule
11 Greater vestibular gland
12 Ovarian artery
13 Suspensory ligament of ovary
14 Internal iliac artery
15 Tubal branch of ovarian artery
16 Ovarian branch of ovarian artery
17 Uterine artery
18 Ovarian branch of uterine artery
19 Artery of round ligament
20 Internal pudendal artery
21 Vaginal artery
22 Lumbar lymph nodes
23 External iliac lymph nodes
24 Inguinal lymph nodes
25 Abdominal aorta
26 External iliac artery
27 Sacral lymph nodes
28 Internal iliac lymph nodes
29 Superior gluteal artery
30 Obturator artery
31 Inferior gluteal artery
32 Middle sacral artery
33 Femoral artery
34 Vessels of labium majus
35 Femur

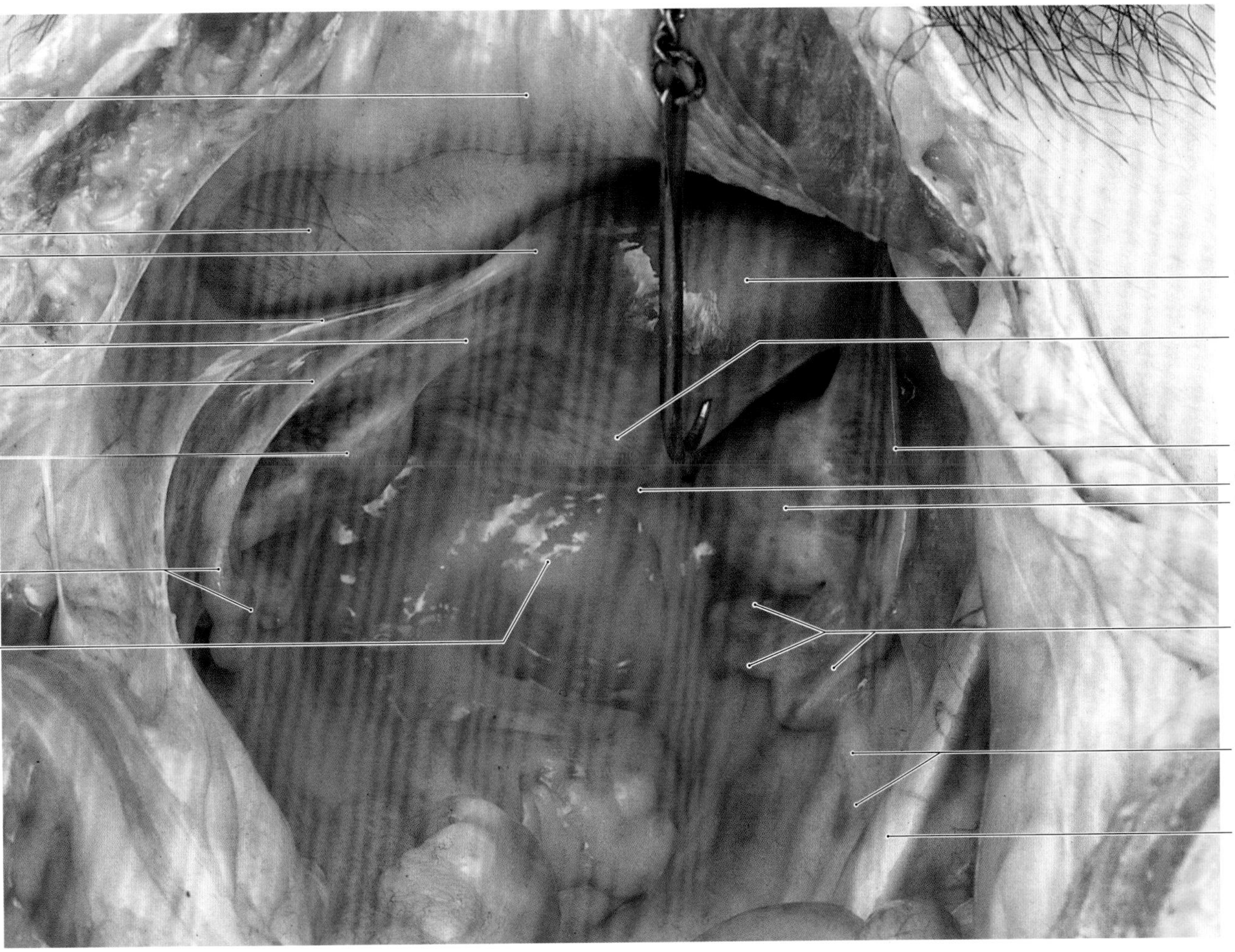

Fig. 7.86 **Female internal genital organs.** View of the pelvic cavity (superior aspect). The uterus has been reflected to the right.

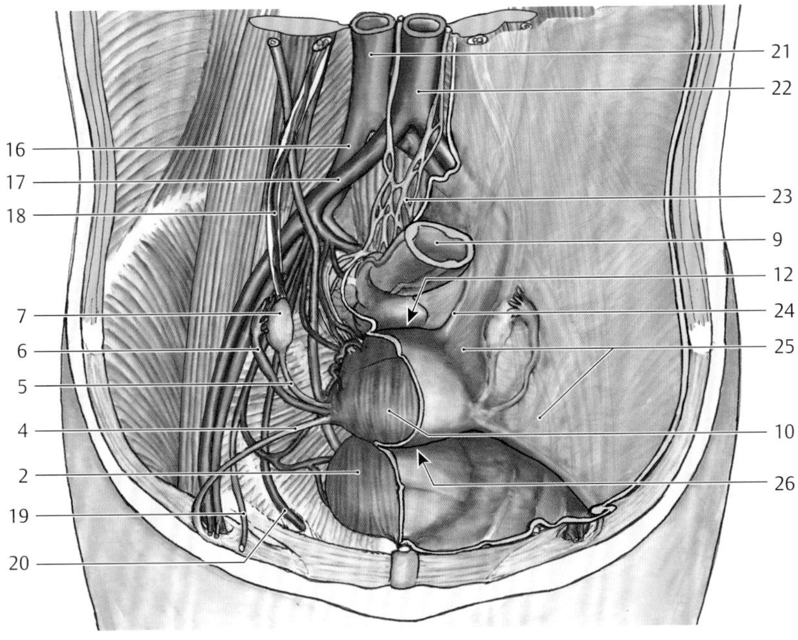


Fig. 7.87 **Pelvic cavity in the female showing uterus and related organs** (antero-superior aspect). The peritoneal cover has been removed on the right side. Arrows = vesico-uterine and recto-uterine pouches.

1 Median umbilical fold with urachus
2 Urinary bladder
3 Insertion of uterine tube at fundus of uterus
4 Round ligament of uterus
5 Ligament of ovary
6 Uterine tube (isthmus)
7 Ovary
8 Ampulla of uterine tube
9 Rectum
10 Uterus
11 Vagina
12 Recto-uterine pouch (of Douglas)
13 Fimbriae of uterine tube
14 Suspensory ligament of ovary
15 Right common iliac artery (covered by peritoneum)
16 Common iliac vein
17 Common iliac artery
18 Ovarian artery and vein
19 Umbilical fold
20 Obturator artery
21 Inferior vena cava
22 Abdominal aorta
23 Superior hypogastric plexus
24 Recto-uterine fold
25 Broad ligament of uterus
26 Vesico-uterine pouch

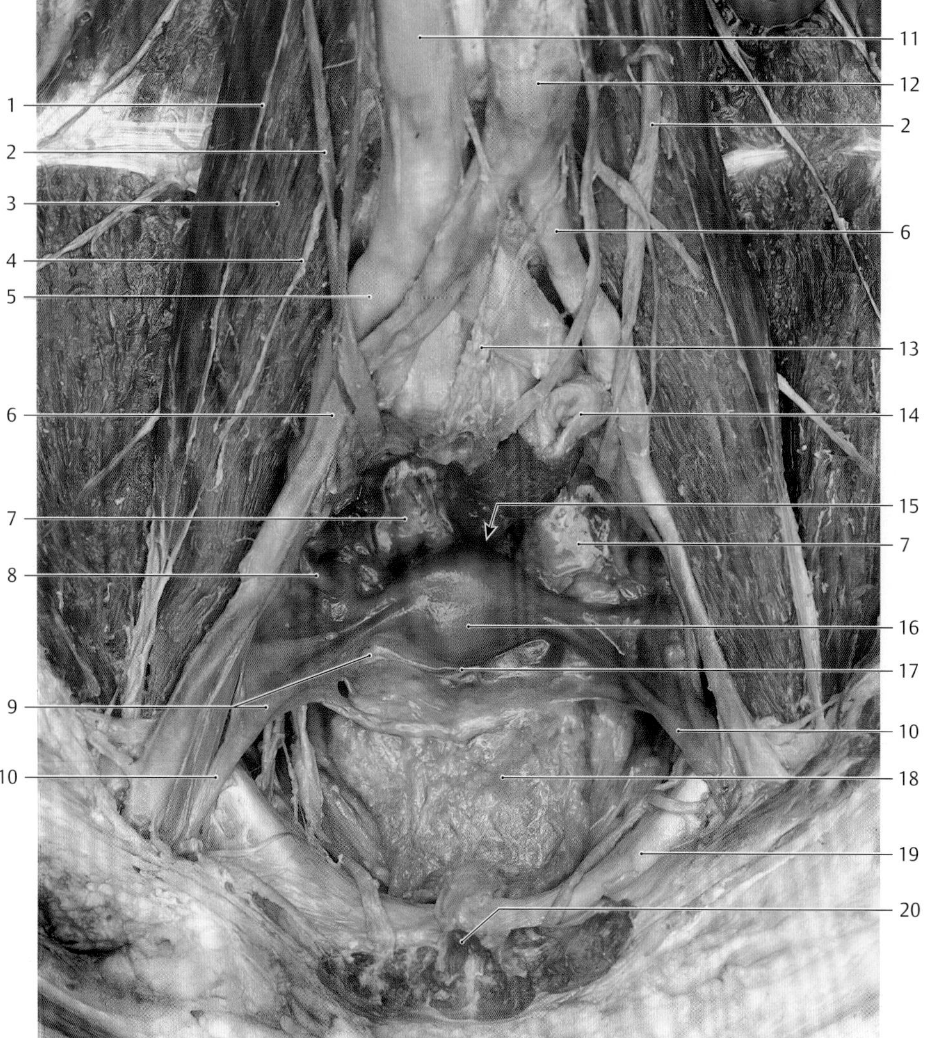


Fig. 7.88 **Pelvic cavity in the female showing uterus and related organs** (superior aspect). The peritoneum has been mostly removed.

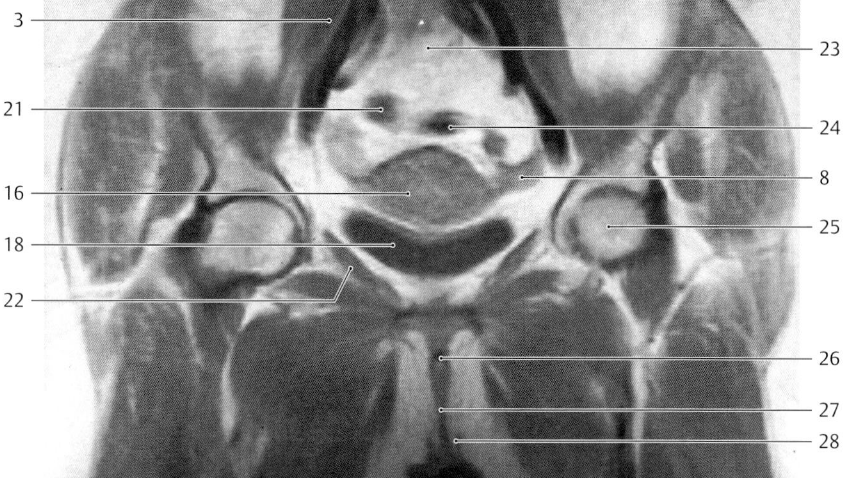


Fig. 7.89 **Horizontal section through the pelvic cavity in the female** (MRI scan). (Courtesy of Prof. Uder, Institute of Radiology, University Hospital Erlangen, Germany.)

1 Ilio-inguinal nerve
2 Ureter
3 Psoas major muscle
4 Genitofemoral nerve
5 Common iliac vein
6 Common iliac artery
7 Ovary
8 Uterine tube
9 Peritoneum
10 Round ligament of uterus
11 Inferior vena cava
12 Abdominal aorta
13 Superior hypogastric plexus
14 Rectum
15 Recto-uterine pouch (of Douglas)
16 Uterus
17 Vesico-uterine pouch
18 Urinary bladder
19 Iliac crest
20 Pubic symphysis
21 Rectal ampulla
22 Obturator internus muscle
23 Promontorium
24 Sigmoid colon
25 Head of femur
26 Urethra
27 Vagina
28 Labium minus

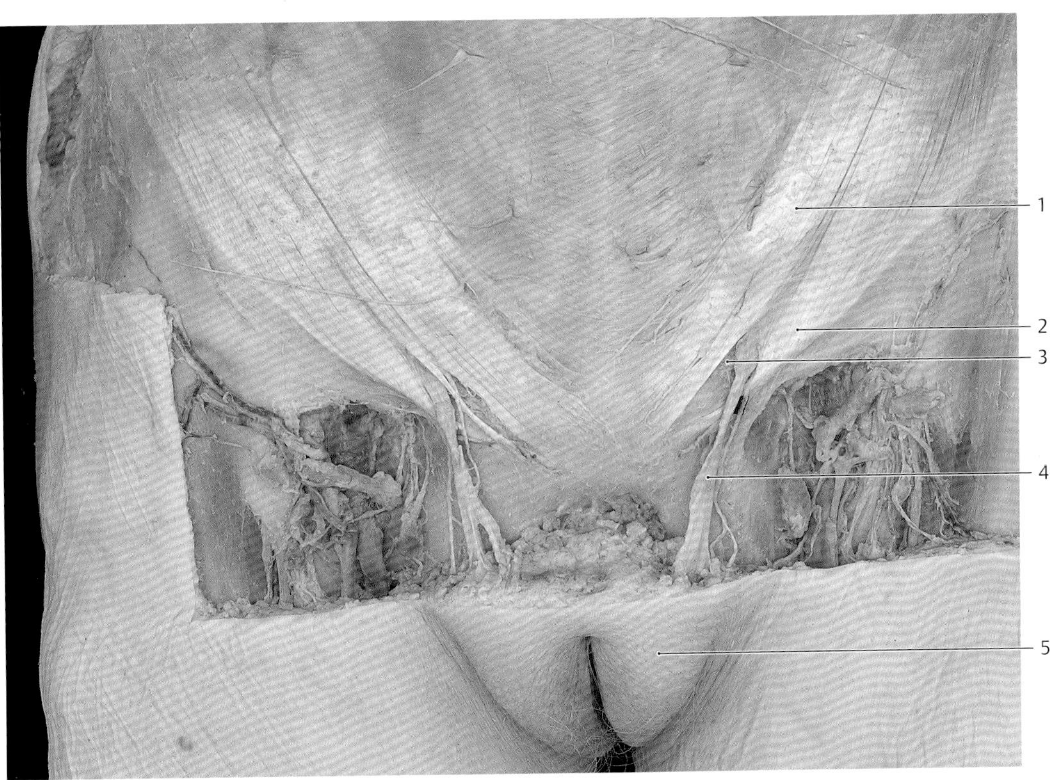


1 Medial crus of superficial inguinal ring
2 Lateral crus of superficial inguinal ring
3 Superficial inguinal ring
4 Round ligament of uterus
5 Outer labia (labium majus)
6 Rectus abdominis muscle and inferior epigastric artery
7 Deep inguinal ring with ilio-inguinal nerve
8 Inguinal ligament
9 Femoral nerve
10 Femoral artery

Fig. 7.90 **Inguinal region and external genital organs in the female** (anterior aspect). Dissection of the inguinal canal and round ligament of uterus of a child.

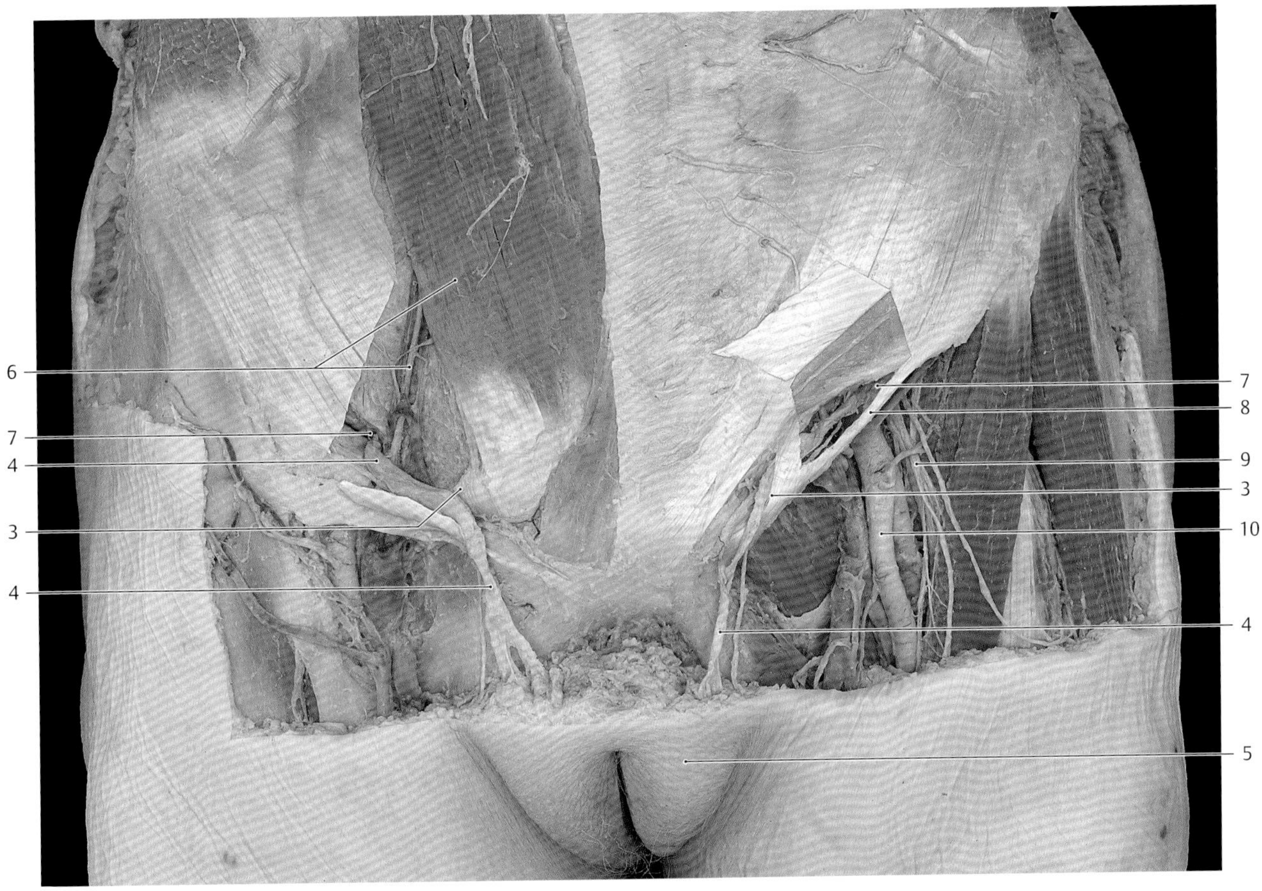

Fig. 7.91 **Inguinal region and external genital organs in the female** (anterior aspect). The inguinal canal has been opened. The round ligament of uterus and the ilio-inguinal nerve have been dissected.

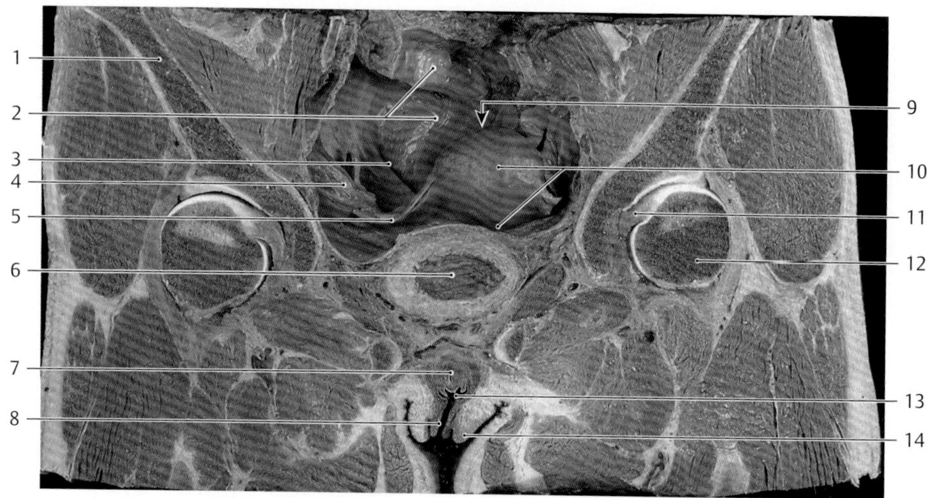


Fig. 7.92 **Coronal section through the pelvic cavity of the female** at the level of the hip joints.

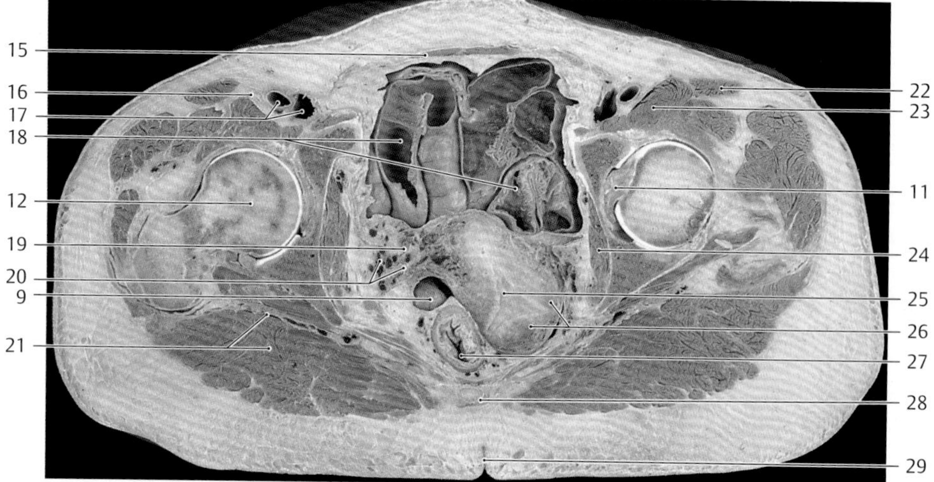


Fig. 7.93 **Horizontal section through the pelvic cavity of the female** at the level of the uterus (inferior aspect). The uterus has been retroverted to the left.

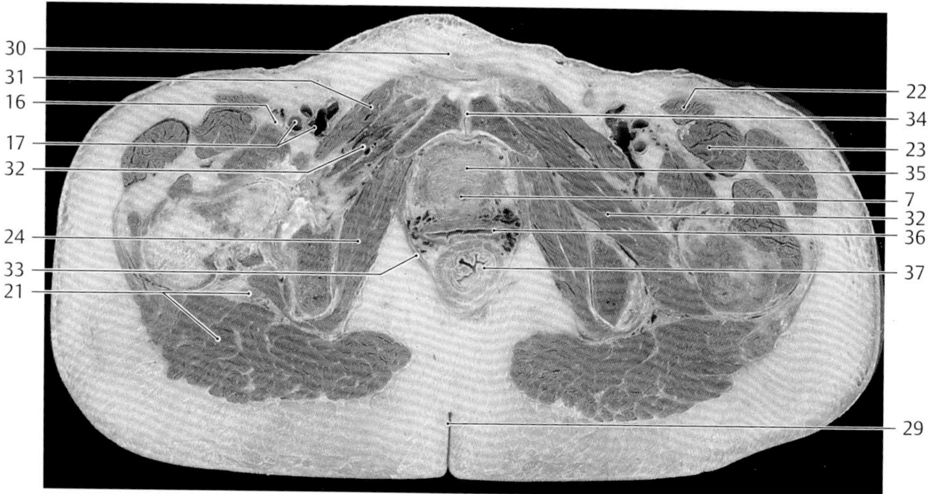


Fig. 7.94 **Horizontal section through the pelvic cavity of the female** at the level of the urethral sphincter muscle and vagina (inferior aspect).

1 Ilium
2 Rectum
3 Recto-uterine fold
4 Ovary
5 Uterine tube
6 Urinary bladder
7 Urethra
8 Labium minus
9 Recto-uterine pouch
10 Uterus and vesico-uterine pouch
11 Ligament of the head of femur
12 Head of femur
13 Vestibule of vagina
14 Labium majus
15 Pyramidalis muscle
16 Femoral nerve
17 Femoral artery and vein
18 Small intestine
19 Broad ligament of uterus
20 Uterine venous plexus
21 Sciatic nerve and gluteus maximus muscle
22 Sartorius muscle
23 Iliopsoas muscle
24 Obturator internus muscle
25 Endometrium
26 Myometrium
27 Rectal ampulla
28 Coccyx
29 Anal cleft
30 Mons pubis
31 Pectineus muscle
32 Obturator externus muscle
33 Levator ani muscle
34 Pubic symphysis
35 Urethral sphincter muscle (base of urinary bladder)
36 Vagina
37 Rectum (anal canal)

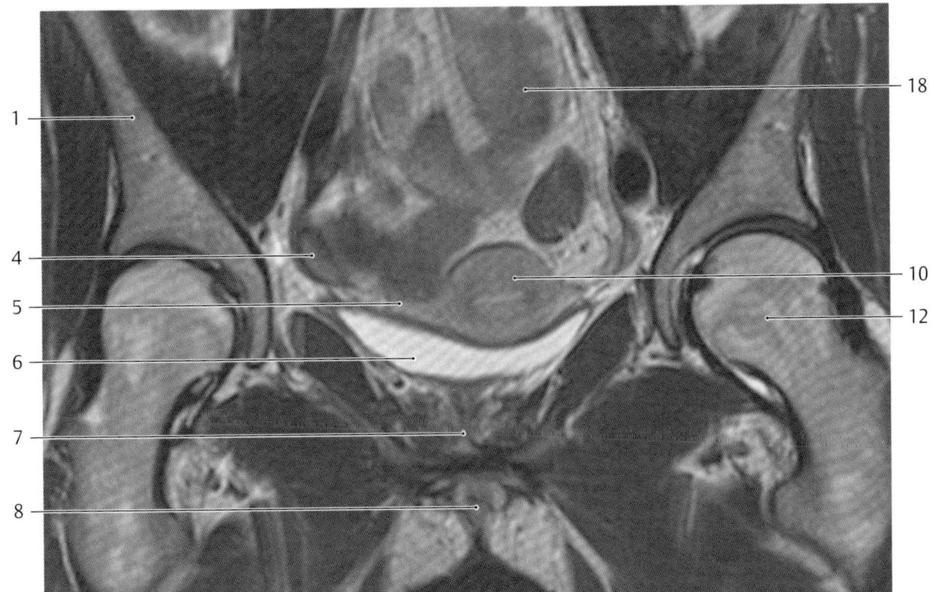


Fig. 7.95 **Coronal section through the pelvic cavity of the female** at the level of the hip joints (MRI scan). (Courtesy of Prof. Uder, Institute of Radiology, University Hospital Erlangen, Germany.)

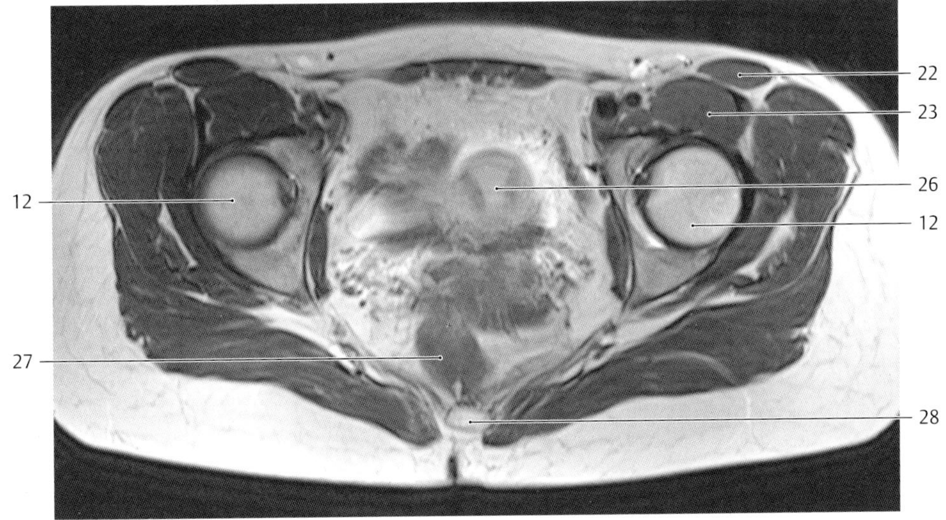


Fig. 7.96 **Horizontal section through the pelvic cavity of the female** at the level of the uterus (MRI scan). (Courtesy of Prof. Uder, Institute of Radiology, University Hospital Erlangen, Germany.)

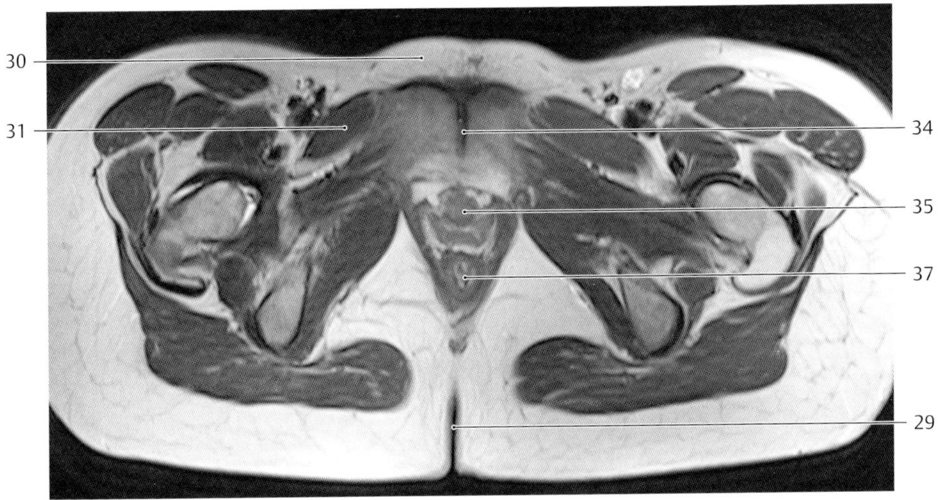


Fig. 7.97 **Horizontal section through the pelvic cavity of the female** at the level of the urethral sphincter muscle and vagina (MRI scan). (Courtesy of Prof. Uder, Institute of Radiology, University Hospital Erlangen, Germany.)

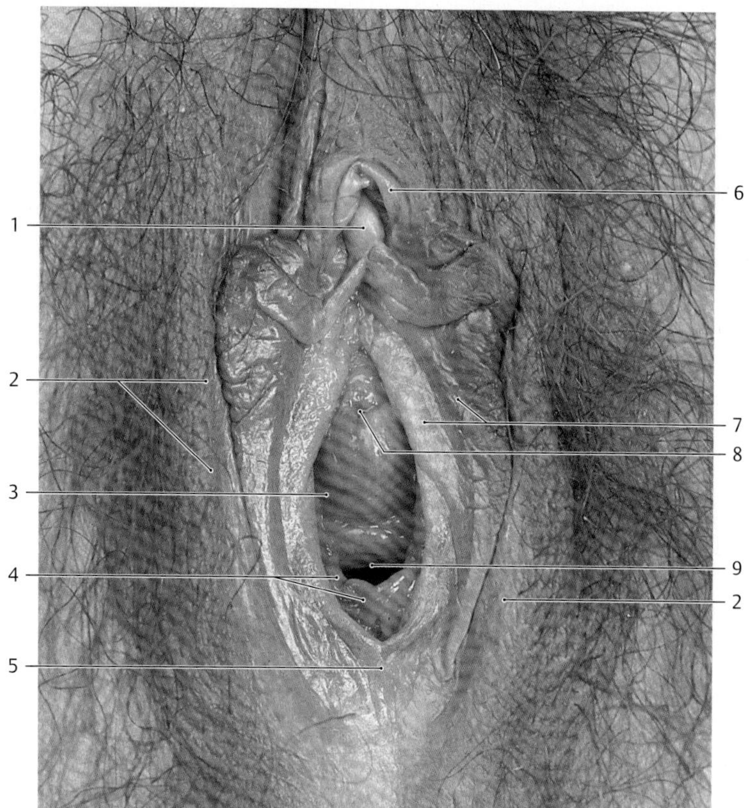


**Fig. 7.98 Female external genital organs in situ** (anterior aspect). Labia reflected.

1 Glans of clitoris
2 Labium majus
3 Vestibule of vagina
4 Hymen
5 Posterior labial commissure
6 Prepuce of clitoris
7 Labium minus
8 External urethral orifice
9 Vaginal orifice
10 Body of clitoris
11 Crus of clitoris
12 Bulb of vestibule with bulbo-spongiosus muscle
13 Frenulum of clitoris
14 Greater vestibular gland
15 Ureter
16 Adnexa of uterus
17 Cavernous body of clitoris
18 Anus and internal anal sphincter
19 Urachus
20 Urinary bladder
21 Infundibulum of uterine tube
22 Ovary
23 Uterine tube
24 Suspensory ligament of ovary
25 Perineal body
26 External anal sphincter

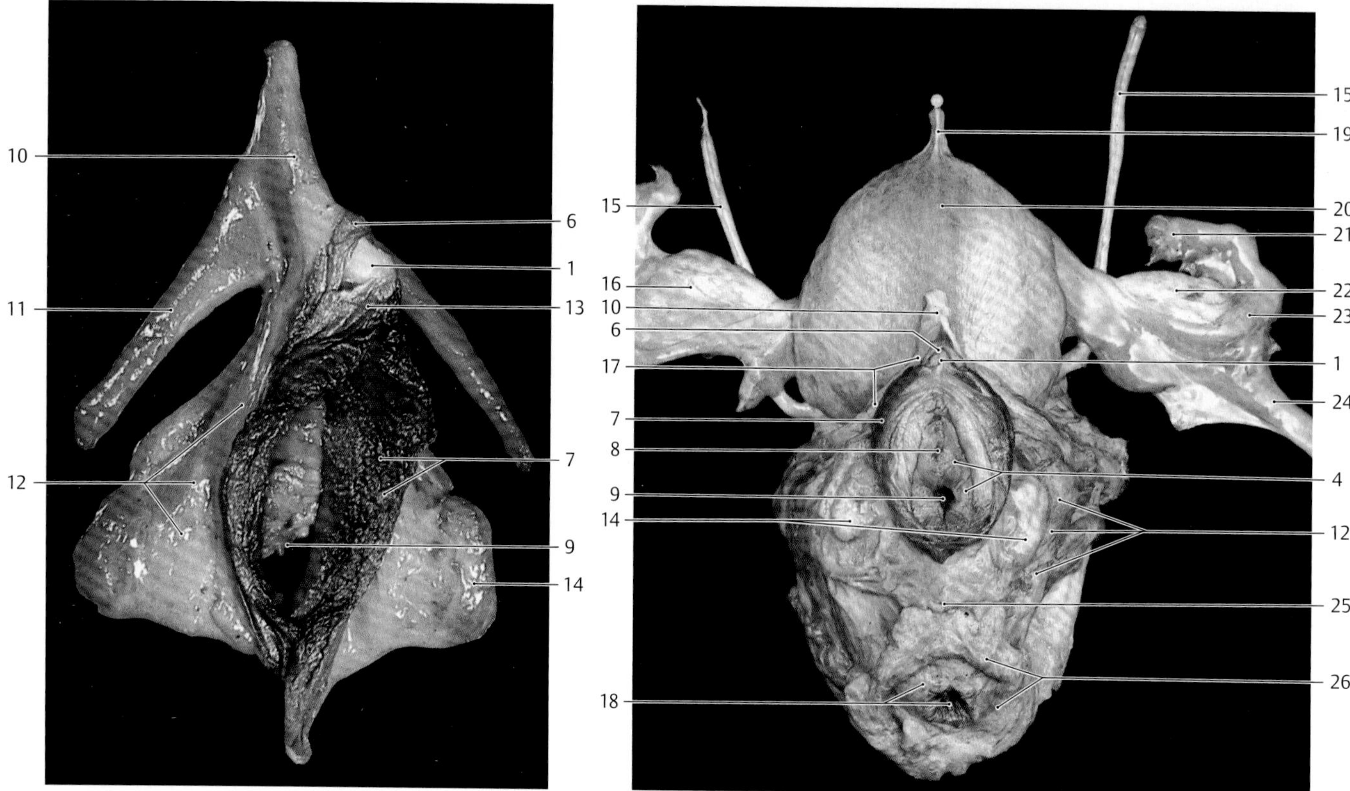


**Fig. 7.99 Cavernous tissue of female external genital organs,** isolated (anterior aspect).

**Fig. 7.100 Female external genital organs** in relation to internal genital organs and urinary system, isolated (anterior aspect).

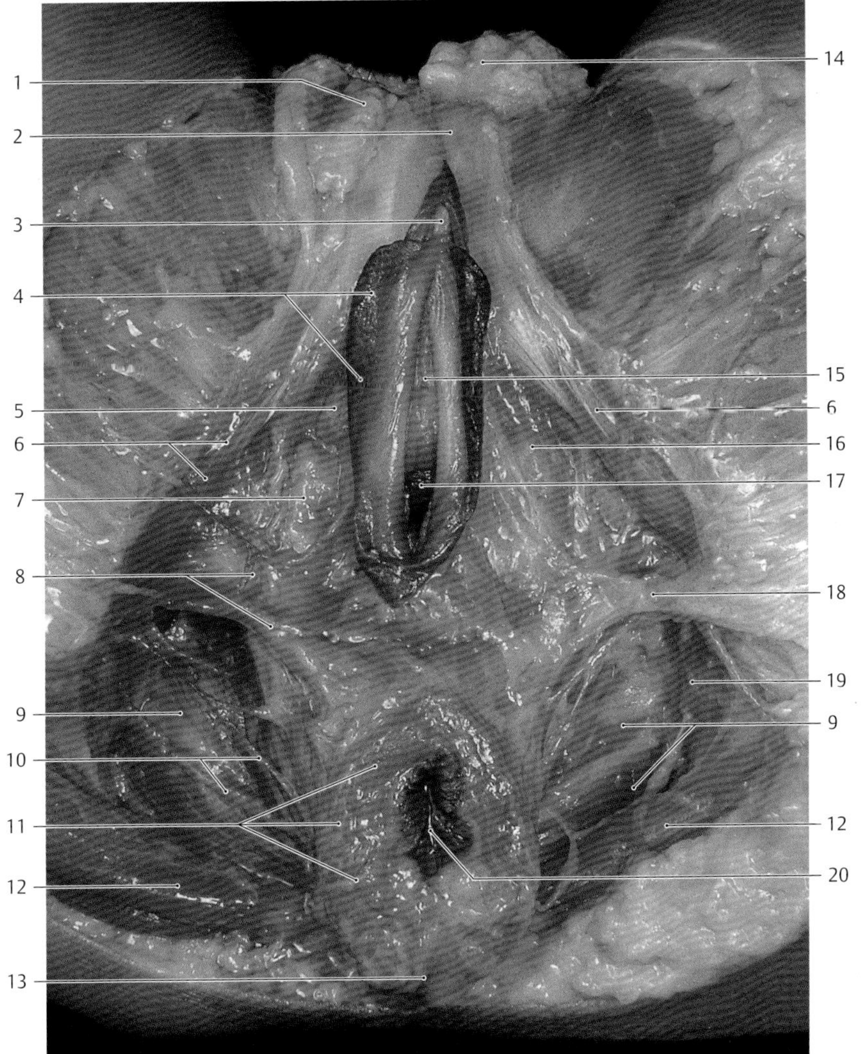


**Fig. 7.101 External genital organs and urogenital diaphragm in the female,** superficial layer (inferior aspect).

1 Fatty tissue encasing round ligament of uterus
2 Position of pubic symphysis
3 Clitoris
4 Labium minus
5 Bulb of vestibule
6 Ischiocavernosus muscle
7 Greater vestibular gland
8 Perineal branches of pudendal nerve
9 Levator ani muscle
10 Inferior rectal nerves
11 External anal sphincter muscle
12 Gluteus maximus muscle
13 Coccyx
14 Fatty tissue of mons pubis
15 External orifice of urethra
16 Urogenital diaphragm with fascia of deep transverse perineal muscle
17 Vaginal orifice
18 Superficial transverse perineal muscle
19 Obturator internus muscle
20 Anus
21 Suspensory ligament of clitoris
22 Glans of clitoris
23 Crus of clitoris
24 Perineal body
25 Prepuce of clitoris
26 Frenulum of clitoris
27 Posterior commissure of labia

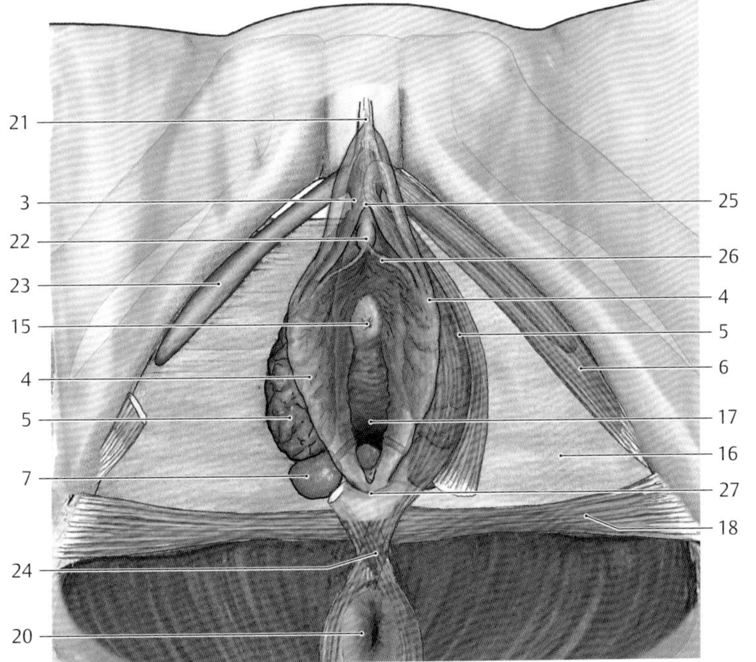


**Fig. 7.102 External genital organs with cavernous tissue in the female** (inferior aspect). Blue = cavernous tissue of clitoris and bulb of vestibule.

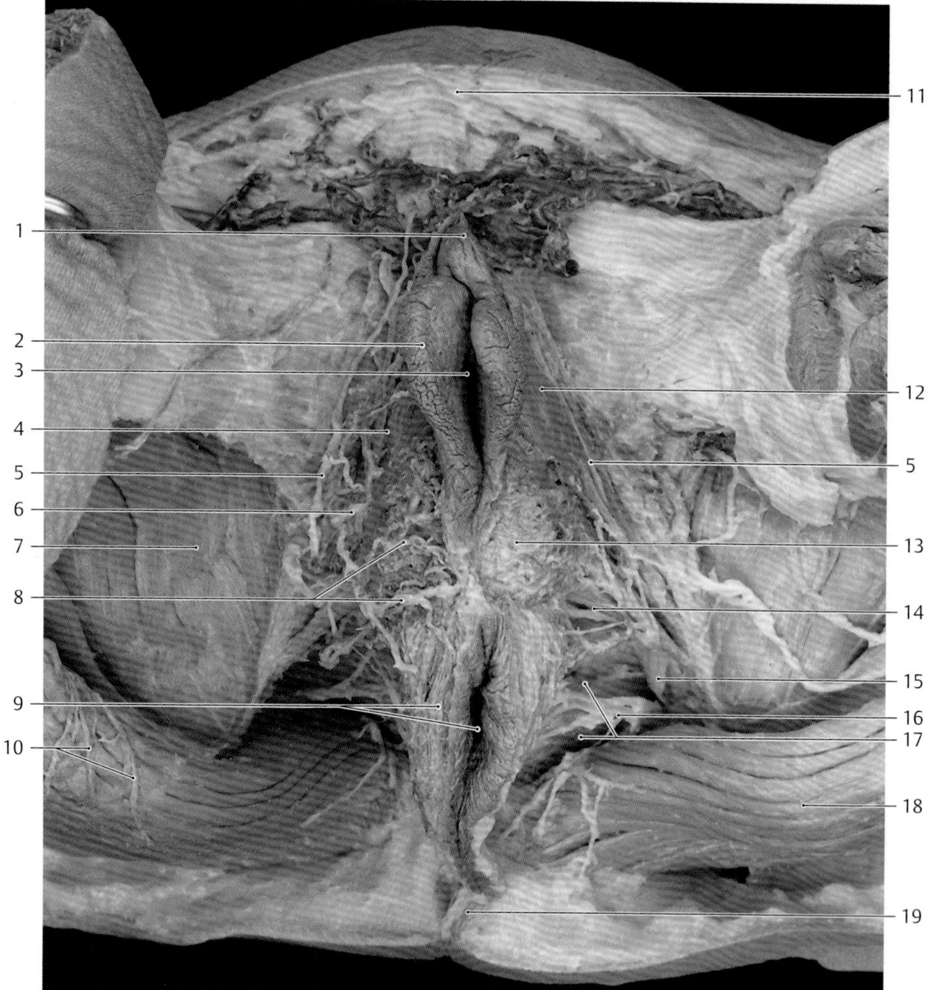


Fig. 7.103 **External genital organs and urogenital diaphragm in the female,** deeper layer (inferior aspect). On the right side, the bulb of the vestibule has been removed.

1 Prepuce of clitoris
2 Labium minus
3 Vaginal orifice
4 Deep transverse perineal muscle
5 Dorsal nerve of clitoris
6 Posterior labial nerves
7 Great adductor muscle
8 Perineal branch of pudendal nerve
9 Anus and external anal sphincter muscle
10 Inferior cluneal nerves
11 Mons pubis
12 Crus of clitoris with ischiocavernosus muscle
13 Bulb of vestibule
14 Superficial transverse perineal muscle
15 Pudendal nerve and internal pudendal artery
16 Inferior rectal nerves
17 Levator ani muscle
18 Gluteus maximus muscle
19 Anococcygeal ligament
20 External urethral orifice

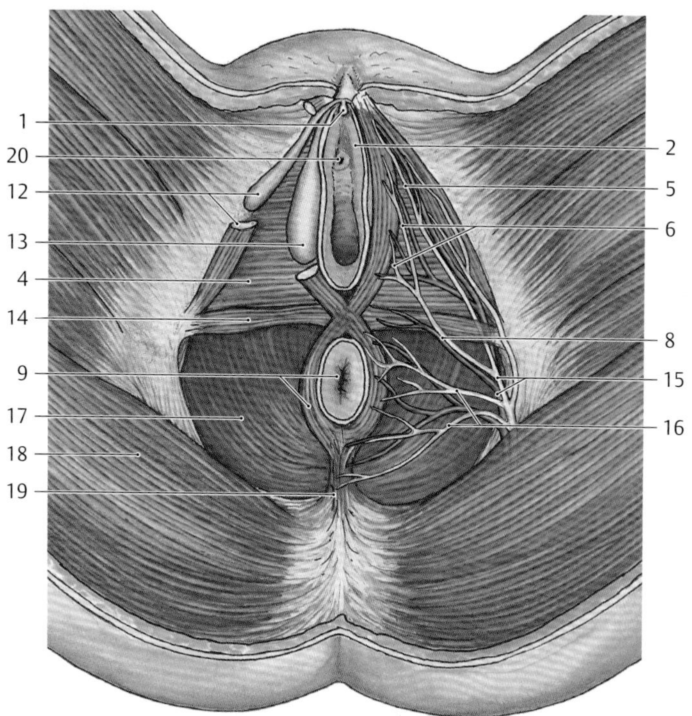


Fig. 7.104 **Urogenital and pelvic diaphragms in the female** (inferior aspect). Muscles, nerves, and arteries have been displayed. The bulb of the vestibule has been partly removed.

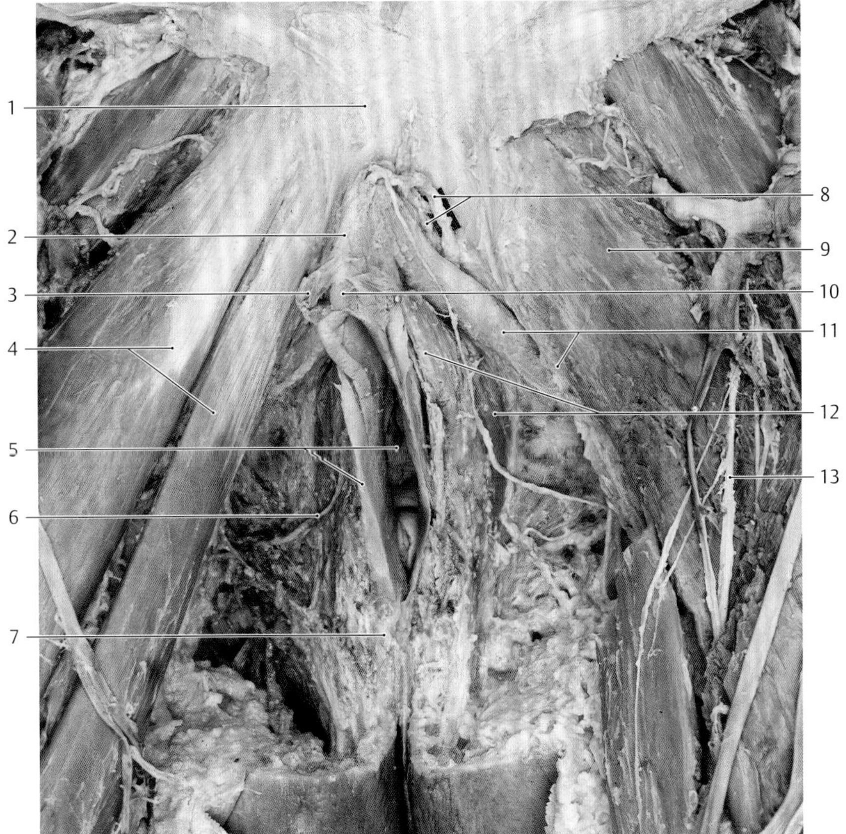


**Fig. 7.105 External genital organs in the female** (anterior aspect). The clitoris has been dissected and slightly reflected to the right. The prepuce of the clitoris has been divided to display the glans.

1 Position of pubic symphysis
2 Body of clitoris
3 Prepuce of clitoris
4 Adductor longus and gracilis muscles
5 External orifice of vagina and labium minus
6 Posterior labial nerve
7 Perineal body
8 Deep artery of clitoris and dorsal nerve of clitoris
9 Adductor brevis muscle
10 Glans of clitoris
11 Crus of clitoris and ischiocavernosus muscle
12 Bulb of vestibule and bulbospongiosus muscle
13 Anterior branch of obturator nerve
14 Clitoris
15 Labium minus
16 Vaginal orifice
17 Posterior labial nerves
18 Perineal branches of pudendal nerve
19 External anal sphincter muscle
20 Anus
21 Crus of clitoris and ischiocavernosus muscle
22 Bulb of vestibule
23 Dorsal artery of clitoris
24 Superficial transverse perineal muscle
25 Perineal branch of posterior femoral cutaneous nerve
26 Levator ani muscle
27 Internal pudendal artery
28 Inferior rectal nerves
29 Gluteus maximus muscle
30 Anococcygeal ligament

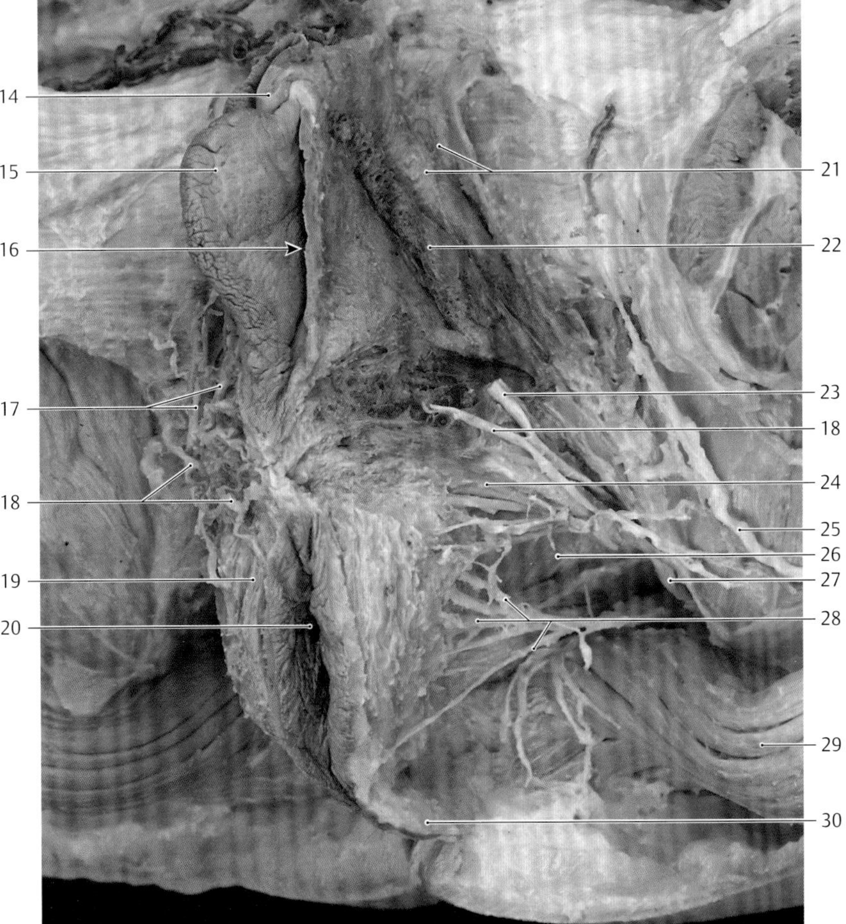


**Fig. 7.106 External genital organs and urogenital diaphragm in the female** (latero-inferior aspect). The bulb of the vestibule has been partly removed. The left labium minus has been cut away.

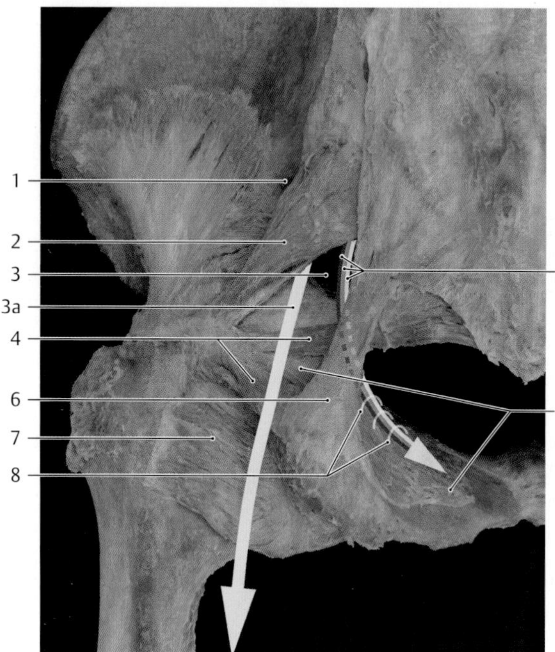


**Fig. 7.107 Course of pudendal nerve, and internal pudendal artery and vein (small arrows) in the female lesser pelvis** (posterior aspect). The vessels and nerves leave the lesser pelvis through the infrapiriform foramen and curve around the ischial spine through the lesser sciatic foramen (see Fig. 7.109) into the anterior part of the pelvis onto the obturator internus muscle. Large yellow arrow = indicated course of the sciatic nerve.

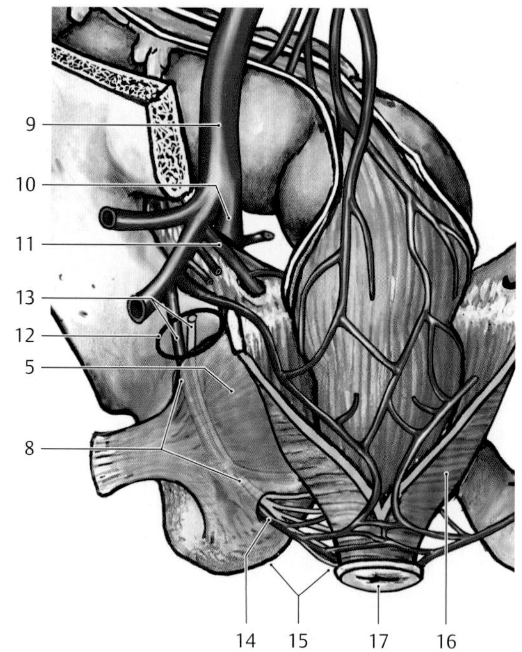


**Fig. 7.108 Ischio-anal fossa between internal obturator muscle and levator ani muscle with pudendal nerve and internal pudendal artery** (posterior aspect). The veins are not shown. After entering the lesser pelvis through the lesser sciatic foramen (see Fig. 7.107) the pudendal nerve accompanies the internal pudendal artery and vein in the Alcock's canal along the lateral wall of the ischio-anal fossa and runs through the fossa to the anus and the external genital organs.

1 Suprapiriform foramen (see table on p. 196)
2 Piriform muscle
3 Infrapiriform foramen (see table on p. 196)
3a Sciatic nerve
3b Pudendal artery, vein, and nerve
4 Gemelli muscles
5 Obturator internus muscle
6 Sacrotuberous ligament
7 Quadratus femoris muscle
8 Pudendal canal (Alcock's canal)
9 Internal iliac artery
10 External iliac artery
11 Obturator artery
12 Level of infrapiriform foramen
13 Pudendal artery and nerve
14 Middle rectal artery
15 Ischioanal fossa
16 Levator ani muscle
17 Anus
18 Sacrospinous ligament
19 Lesser sciatic foramen
20 External iliac artery
21 Tendinous arch of levator ani
22 Pubic symphysis
23 Sacral plexus

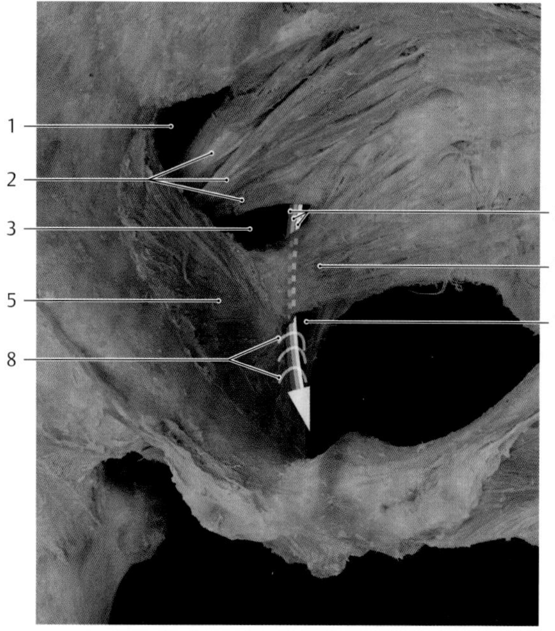


**Fig. 7.109 Course of pudendal artery, vein, and nerve through Alcock's canal** (internal aspect of Fig. 7.107). Note the passage of the pudendal nerve and accompanying vessels (arrows) through the lesser sciatic foramen into the Alcock's canal within the obturator fascia (see Fig. 7.108).

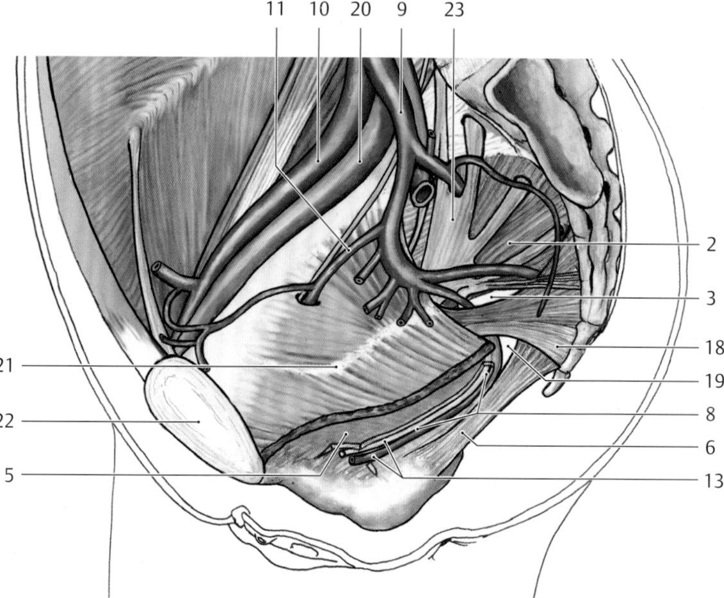


**Fig. 7.110 Alcock's canal** (latero-internal aspect). Branches of iliac veins are not shown. The pelvis has been removed between the pubic symphysis and the iliosacral joint to show the Alcock's canal.

# 8 Head and Neck

Head, Neck, and Brain

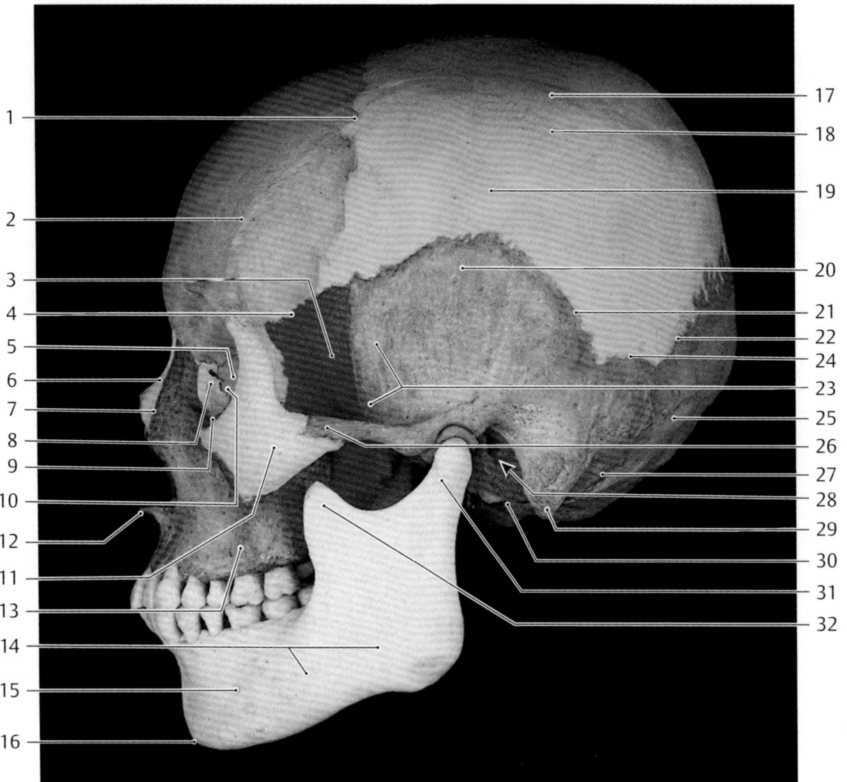


1 Coronal suture
2 Frontal bone
3 Sphenoid bone
4 Sphenofrontal suture
5 Ethmoid bone
6 Nasal bone
7 Nasomaxillary suture
8 Lacrimal bone
9 Lacrimomaxillary suture
10 Ethmoidolacrimal suture
11 Zygomatic bone
12 Anterior nasal spine
13 Maxilla
14 Mandible
15 Mental foramen
16 Mental protuberance
17 Superior temporal line
18 Inferior temporal line
19 Parietal bone
20 Temporal bone
21 Squamous suture
22 Lambdoid suture
23 Temporal fossa
24 Parietomastoid suture
25 Occipital bone
26 Zygomatic arch
27 Occipitomastoid suture
28 External acoustic meatus
29 Mastoid process
30 Tympanic portion of temporal bone
31 Condylar process of mandible
32 Coronoid process of mandible

**Fig. 8.1 General architecture of the skull** (lateral aspect). The different bones are indicated in color (see corresponding table below).

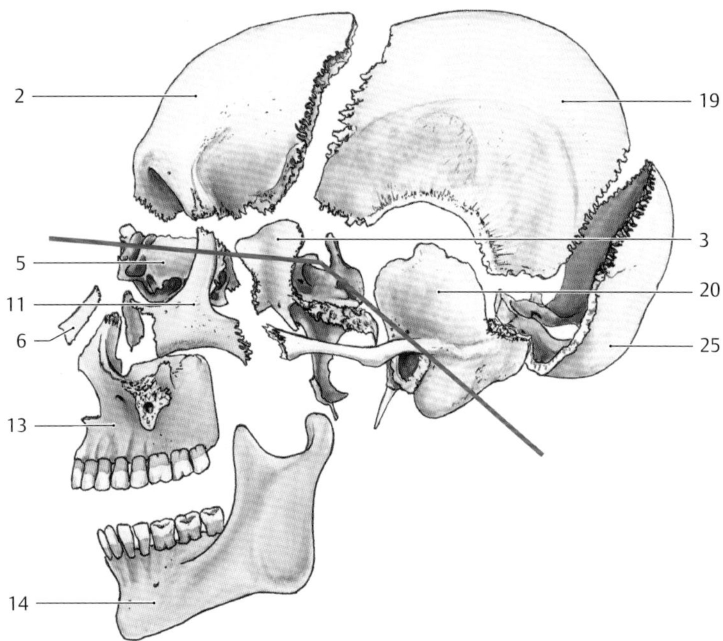


**Fig. 8.2 Disarticulated skull** (lateral aspect). Blue = facial bones; red line = angle of the clivus.

| No. | Bone | Group | Division |
|---|---|---|---|
| 2 | Frontal bone (orange) | Cranial bones | Neurocranium |
| 19 | Parietal bone (light yellow) | Cranial bones | Neurocranium |
| 3 | Greater wing of sphenoid bone (red) | Cranial bones | Neurocranium |
| 25 | Squamous part of occipital bone (blue) | Cranial bones | Neurocranium |
| 20 | Squamous part of temporal bone (brown) | Cranial bones | Neurocranium |
| 5 | Ethmoid bone (dark green) | Base of skull | Neurocranium |
| 3 | Sphenoid bone (red) | Base of skull | Neurocranium |
| | Temporal bone excluding squamous part (brown) | Base of skull | Neurocranium |
| 30 | Tympanic portion of temporal bone (dark brown) | Base of skull | Neurocranium |
| | Occipital bone excluding squamous part (blue) | Base of skull | Neurocranium |
| 6 | Nasal bone (white) | Facial bones | Viscerocranium |
| 8 | Lacrimal bone (light yellow) | Facial bones | Viscerocranium |
| | Inferior nasal concha | Facial bones | Viscerocranium |
| | Vomer | Facial bones | Viscerocranium |
| 11 | Zygomatic bone (dark yellow) | Facial bones | Viscerocranium |
| | Palatine bone | Facial bones | Viscerocranium |
| 13 | Maxilla (violet) | Facial bones | Viscerocranium |
| 14 | Mandible (white) | Facial bones | Viscerocranium |
| | Malleus, Incus, Stapes – within petrous portion of temporal bone | Auditory ossicles | Viscerocranium |
| | Hyoid | | Viscerocranium |

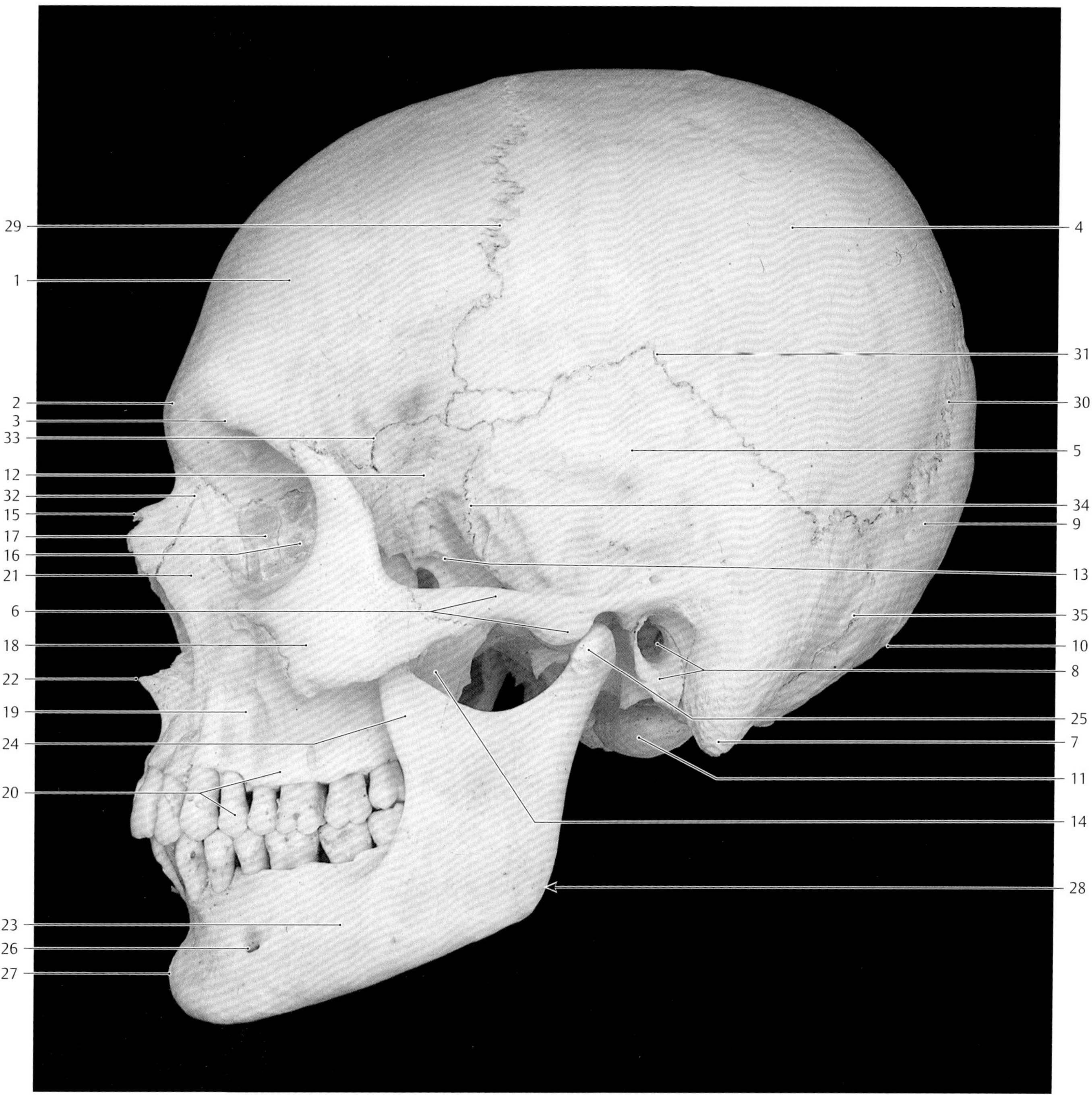


Fig. 8.3 **Lateral aspect of the skull.**

1 Frontal bone
2 Glabella
3 Supra-orbital margin
4 Parietal bone
5 Temporal bone (squamous part)
6 Zygomatic process (articular tubercle)
7 Mastoid process
8 Tympanic part (tympanic plate) and external acoustic meatus
9 Occipital bone (squamous part)
10 External occipital protuberance
11 Occipital condyle
12 Sphenoid bone
13 Infratemporal crest of sphenoid
14 Pterygoid process (lateral pterygoid plate)
15 Nasal bone
16 Ethmoid bone (orbital part)
17 Lacrimal bone
18 Zygomatic bone
19 Maxilla (body)
20 Alveolar process and teeth
21 Frontal process
22 Anterior nasal spine
23 Mandible (body)
24 Coronoid process
25 Condylar process
26 Mental foramen
27 Mental protuberance
28 Angle of the mandible

**Sutures**

29 Coronal suture
30 Lambdoid suture
31 Squamous suture
32 Nasomaxillary suture
33 Frontosphenoid suture
34 Sphenosquamosal suture
35 Occipitomastoid suture

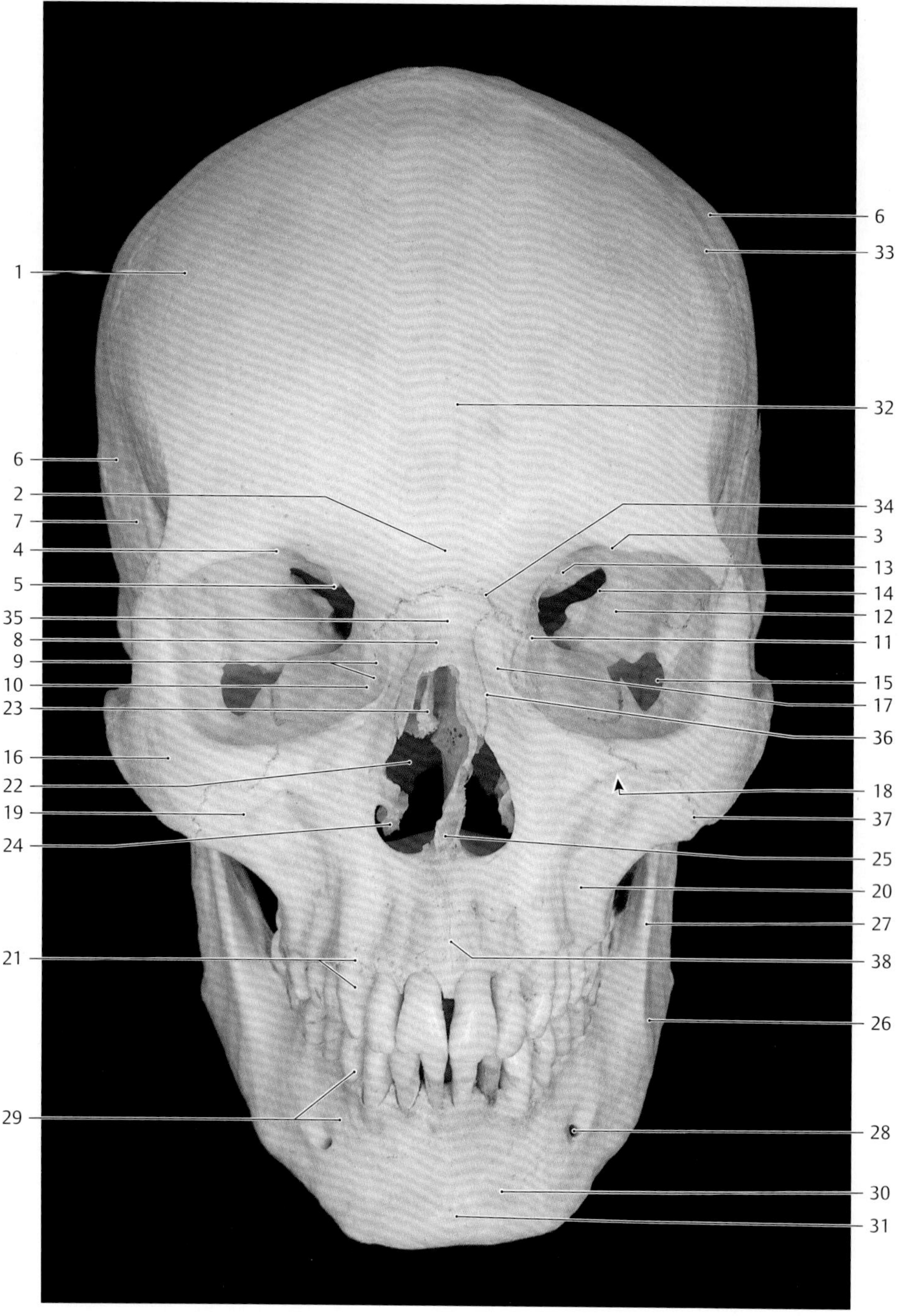


1 Frontal bone
2 Glabella
3 Supra-orbital margin
4 Supra-orbital notch
5 Trochlear spine
6 Parietal bone
7 Temporal bone
8 Nasal bone

**Orbit**
9 Lacrimal bone
10 Posterior lacrimal crest
11 Ethmoid bone

**Sphenoid bone**
12 Greater wing of sphenoid bone
13 Lesser wing of sphenoid bone
14 Superior orbital fissure
15 Inferior orbital fissure
16 Zygomatic bone

**Maxilla**
17 Frontal process
18 Infra-orbital foramen
19 Zygomatic process
20 Body of maxilla
21 Alveolar process with teeth

**Nasal cavity**
22 Anterior nasal aperture
23 Middle nasal concha
24 Inferior nasal concha
25 Nasal septum, vomer

**Mandible**
26 Body of mandible
27 Ramus of mandible
28 Mental foramen
29 Alveolar part with teeth
30 Base of mandible
31 Mental protuberance

**Sutures**
32 Frontal suture
33 Coronal suture
34 Frontonasal suture
35 Internasal suture
36 Nasomaxillary suture
37 Zygomaticomaxillary suture
38 Intermaxillary suture

Fig. 8.4 **Anterior aspect of the skull.**

The skull comprises a mosaic of numerous complicated bones that form the cranial cavity protecting the brain **(neurocranium)** and several cavities such as the nasal and oral cavities in the facial region. The neurocranium consists of large bony plates that develop directly from the surrounding sheets of connective tissue **(desmocranium)**.

The bones of the skull base are formed out of cartilaginous tissue **(chondrocranium)**, which ossifies secondarily. The **visceral skeleton,** which in fish gives rise to the gills, has in higher vertebrates been transformed into the bones of the masticatory and auditory apparatus (maxilla, mandible, auditory ossicles, and hyoid bone).

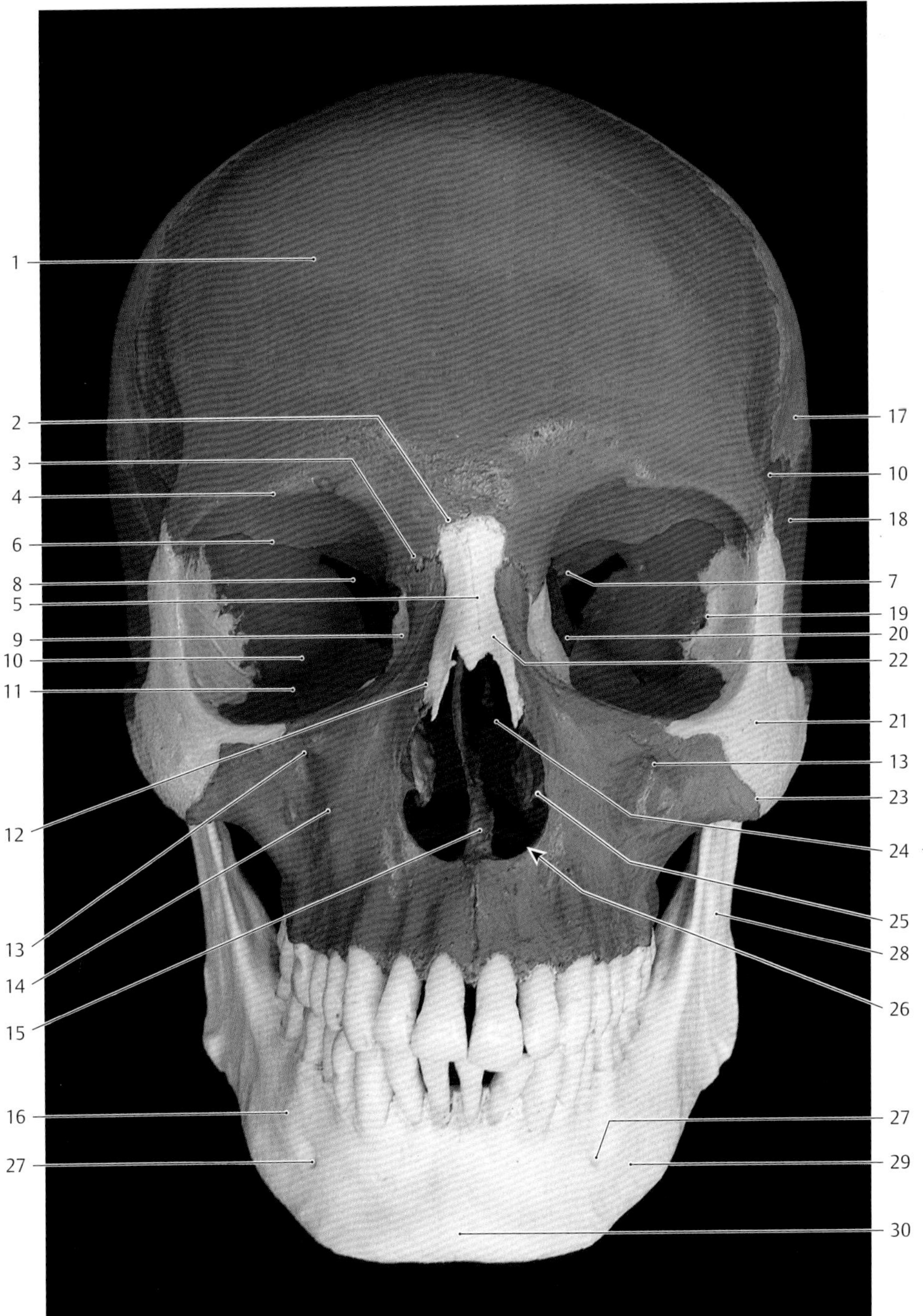


1 Frontal bone
2 Frontonasal suture
3 Frontomaxillary suture
4 Supra-orbital margin
5 Internasal suture
6 Sphenofrontal suture
7 Optic canal in lesser wing of sphenoid bone
8 Superior orbital fissure
9 Lacrimal bone
10 Sphenoid bone (greater wing)
11 Inferior orbital fissure
12 Nasomaxillary suture
13 Infra-orbital foramen
14 Maxilla
15 Vomer
16 Body of mandible
17 Parietal bone
18 Temporal bone
19 Sphenozygomatic suture
20 Ethmoid bone
21 Zygomatic bone
22 Nasal bone
23 Zygomaticomaxillary suture
24 Middle nasal concha
25 Inferior nasal concha
26 Anterior nasal aperture
27 Mental foramen
28 Ramus of mandible
29 Base of mandible
30 Mental protuberance

**Bones**

| | | |
|---|---|---|
| Brown | = | frontal bone |
| Light green | = | parietal bone |
| Dark brown | = | temporal bone |
| Red | = | sphenoid bone |
| Yellow | = | zygomatic bone |
| Dark green | = | ethmoid bone |
| Yellow | = | lacrimal bone |
| Orange | = | vomer |
| Violet | = | maxilla |
| White | = | nasal bone |
| White | = | mandible |

Fig. 8.5 **Anterior aspect of the skull** (individual bones indicated by color).

The following series of figures are arranged so that the mosaic-like pattern of the skull becomes understandable. It starts with the bones of the **skull base** (sphenoid and occipital bones) to which the other bones are added step by step. The facial skeleton is built up by the ethmoid bone to which the palatine bone and maxilla are attached laterally; the small nasal and lacrimal bones fill the remaining spaces. Cartilages remain only in the external part of the nose.

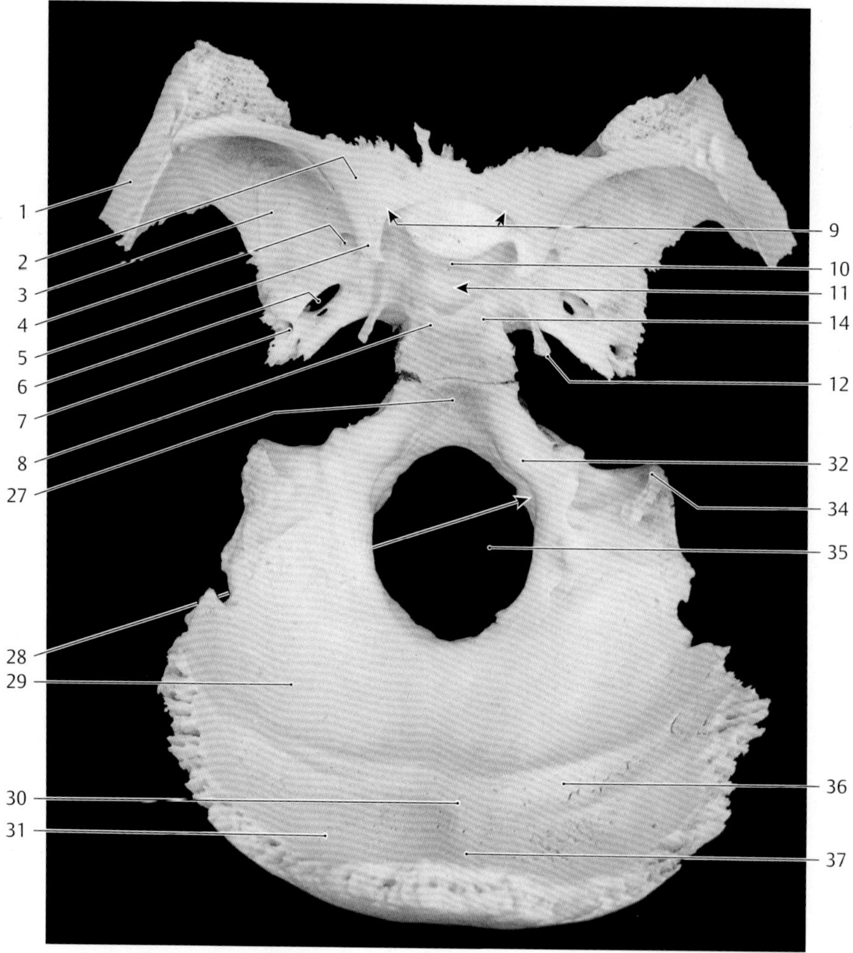


Fig. 8.6 **Sphenoid and occipital bones** (from above).

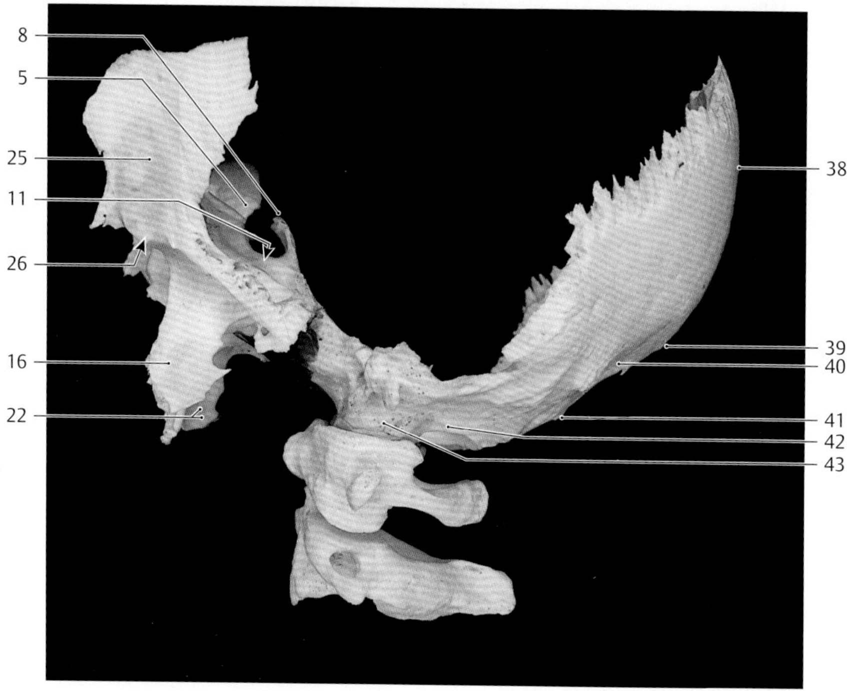


Fig. 8.7 **Sphenoid and occipital bones** connected to the atlas and axis (first and second cervical vertebrae) (left lateral view).

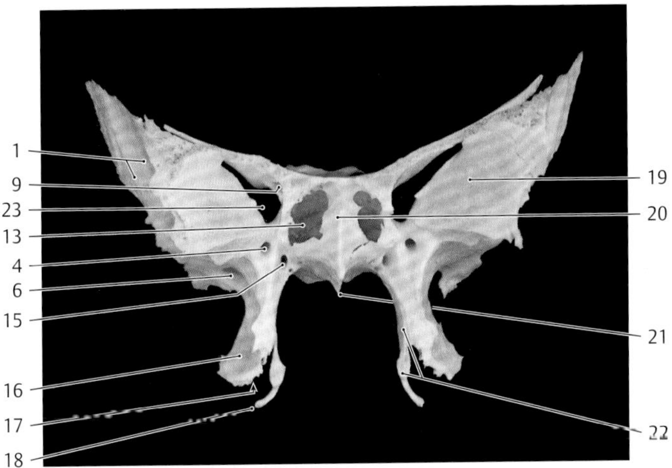


Fig. 8.8 **Sphenoid bone** (anterior aspect).

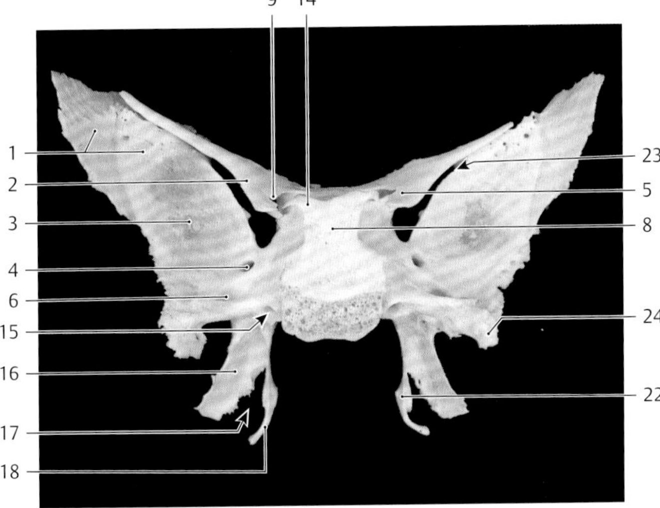


Fig. 8.9 **Sphenoid bone** (posterior aspect).

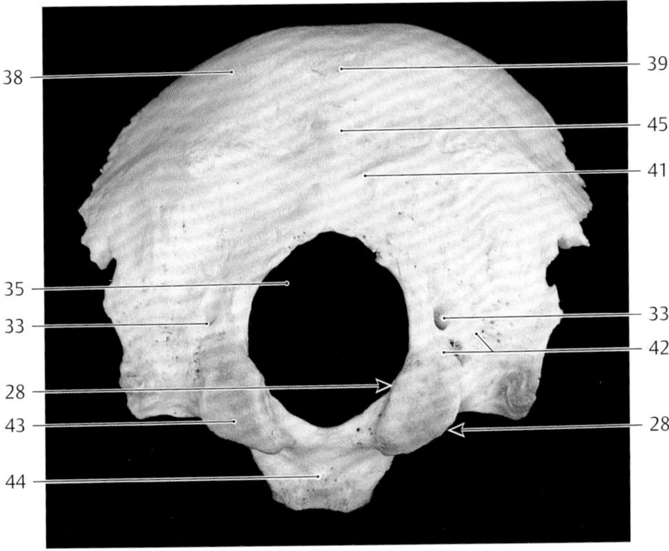


Fig. 8.10 **Occipital bone** (from below).

**Sphenoid bone**

1 Greater wing
2 Lesser wing
3 Cerebral or superior surface of greater wing
4 Foramen rotundum
5 Anterior clinoid process
6 Foramen ovale
7 Foramen spinosum
8 Dorsum sellae
9 Optic canal
10 Chiasmatic groove (sulcus chiasmatis)
11 Hypophysial fossa (sella turcica)
12 Lingula
13 Opening of sphenoidal sinus
14 Posterior clinoid process
15 Pterygoid canal
16 Lateral pterygoid plate of pterygoid process
17 Pterygoid notch
18 Pterygoid hamulus
19 Orbital surface of greater wing
20 Sphenoidal crest
21 Sphenoidal rostrum
22 Medial pterygoid plate
23 Superior orbital fissure
24 Spine of sphenoid
25 Temporal surface of greater wing
26 Infratemporal crest

**Occipital bone**

27 Clivus with basilar part of occipital bone
28 Hypoglossal canal
29 Fossa for cerebellar hemisphere
30 Internal occipital protuberance
31 Fossa for cerebral hemisphere
32 Jugular tubercle
33 Condylar canal
34 Jugular process
35 Foramen magnum
36 Groove for transverse sinus
37 Groove for superior sagittal sinus
38 Squamous part of the occipital bone
39 External occipital protuberance
40 Superior nuchal line
41 Inferior nuchal line
42 Condylar fossa
43 Condyle
44 Pharyngeal tubercle
45 External occipital crest

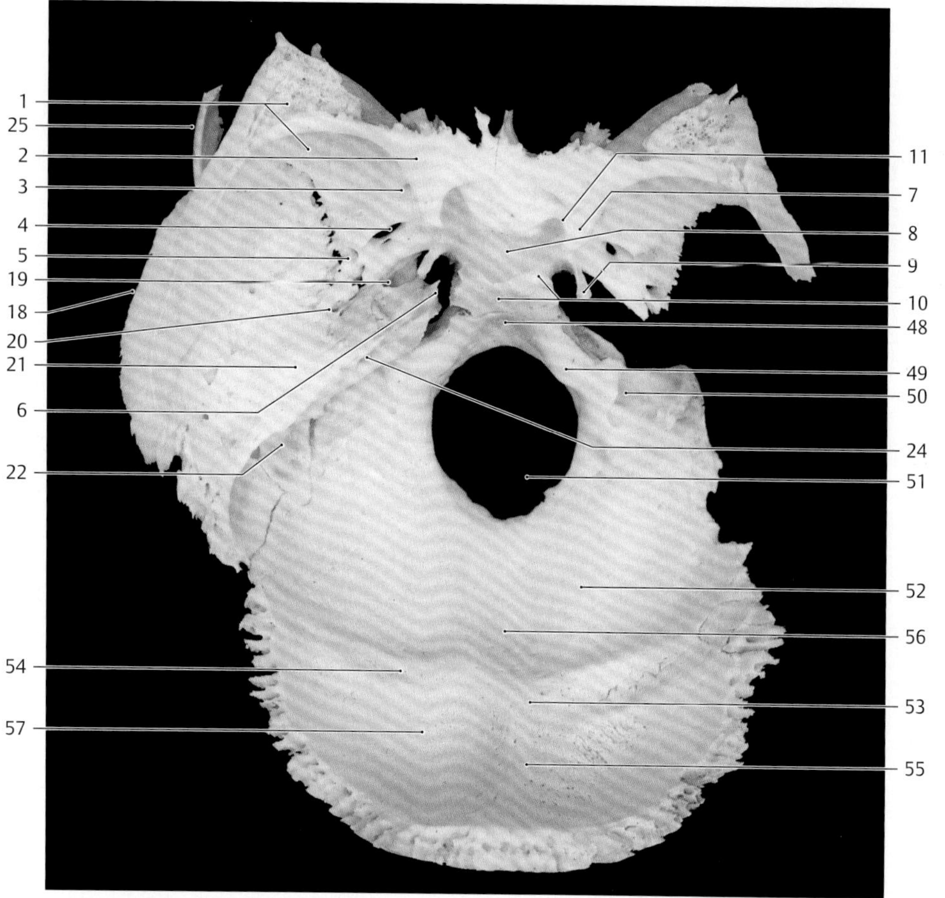


Fig. 8.11 **Sphenoid, occipital, and left temporal bones** (from above). Internal aspect of the base of the skull. The left temporal bone has been added to the preceding figure.

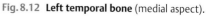

**Sphenoid bone**

1 Greater wing
2 Lesser wing
3 Foramen rotundum
4 Foramen ovale
5 Foramen spinosum
6 Foramen lacerum
7 Anterior clinoid process
8 Hypophysial fossa (sella turcica)
9 Lingula
10 Dorsum sellae and posterior clinoid process
11 Optic canal
12 Sphenoidal rostrum
13 Medial pterygoid plate
14 Lateral pterygoid plate
15 Pterygoid hamulus
16 Infratemporal crest
17 Body of the sphenoid bone

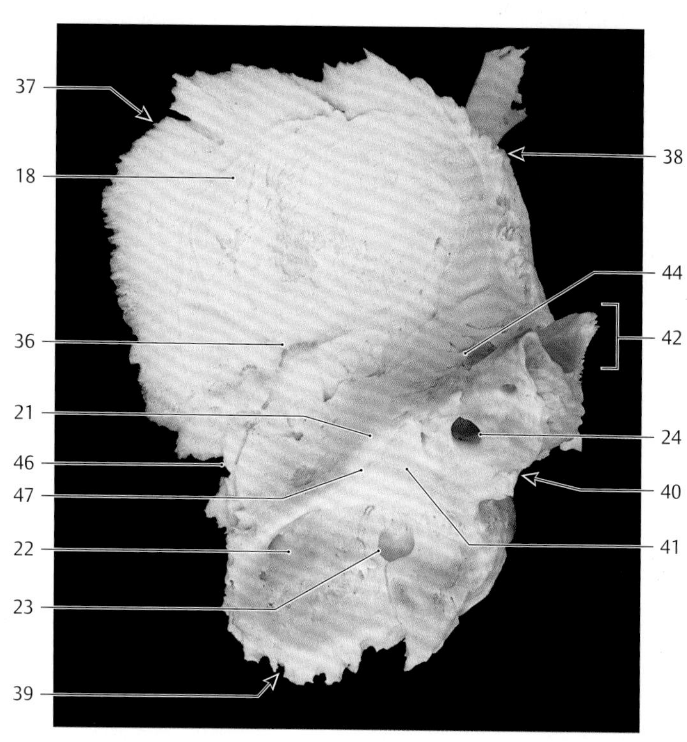


Fig. 8.12 **Left temporal bone** (medial aspect).

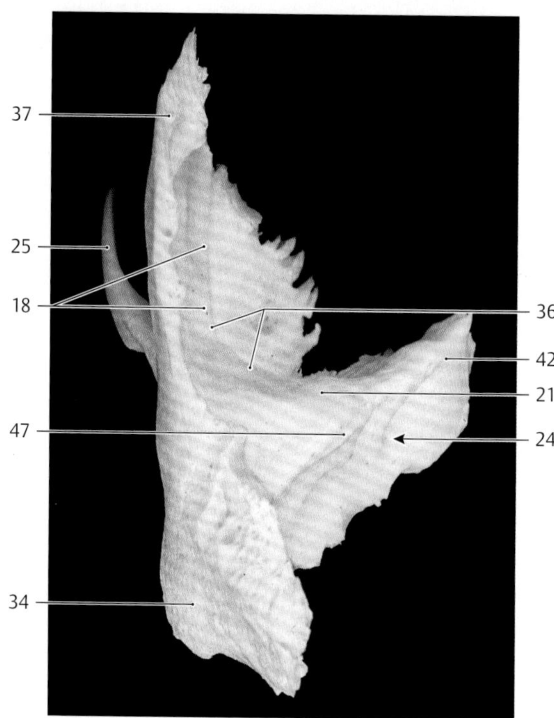


Fig. 8.13 **Left temporal bone** (from above).

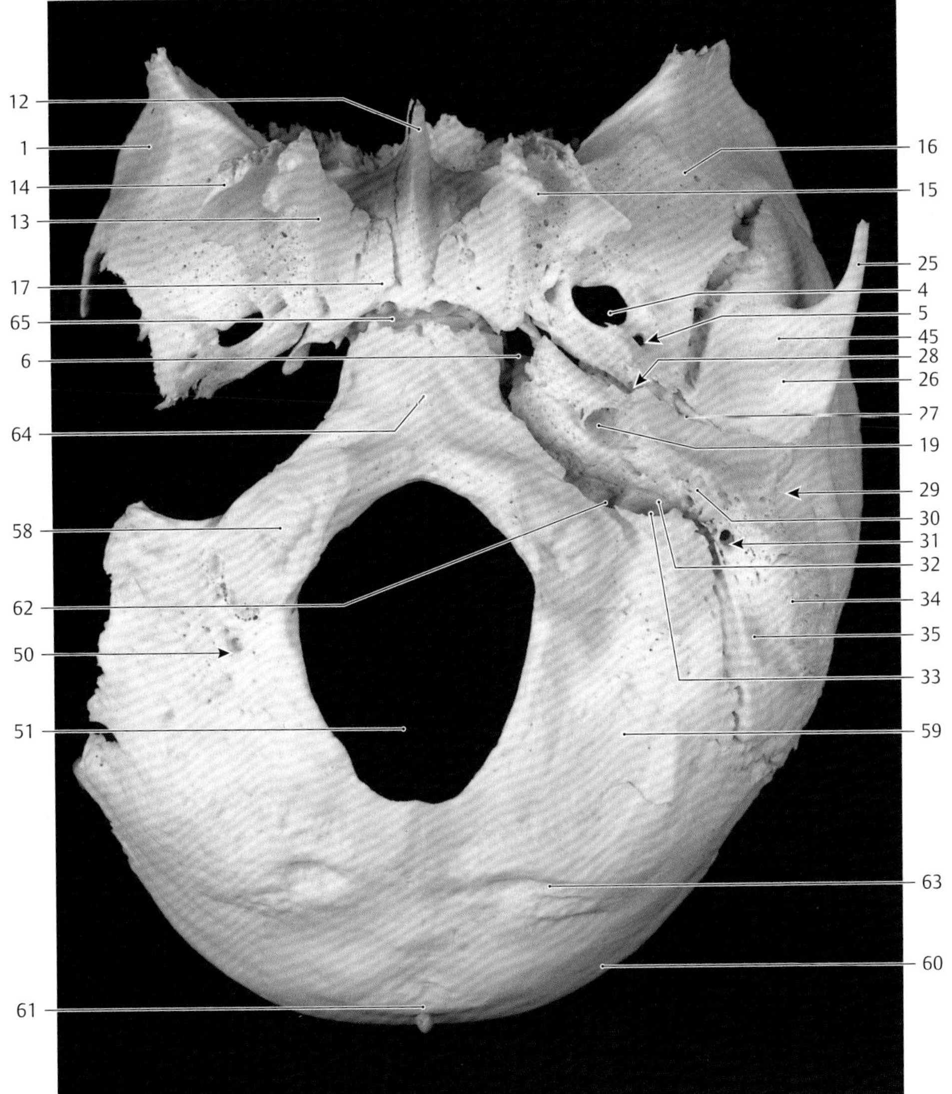


Fig. 8.14 **Sphenoid, occipital, and left temporal bones.** Base of the skull (external aspect).

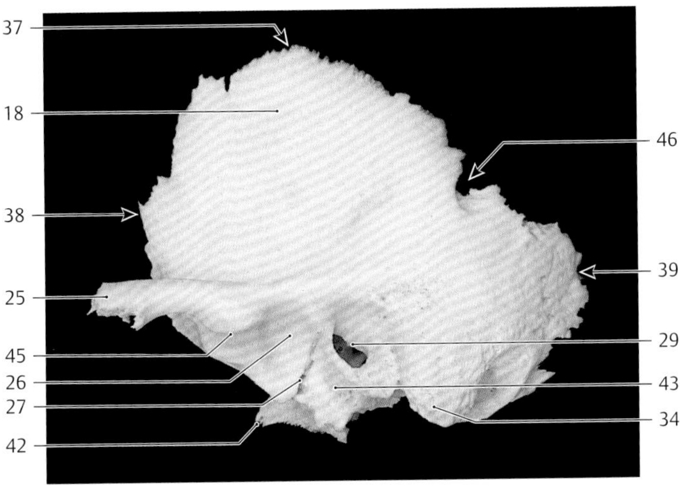


Fig. 8.15 **Left temporal bone** (lateral aspect).

**Temporal bone**

18 Squamous part
19 Carotid canal
20 Hiatus of facial canal (for the greater petrosal nerve)
21 Arcuate eminence
22 Groove for the sigmoid sinus
23 Mastoid foramen
24 Internal acoustic meatus
25 Zygomatic process
26 Mandibular fossa
27 Petrotympanic fissure
28 Canalis musculotubarius (bony part of auditory tube)
29 External acoustic meatus
30 Styloid process (remnant only)
31 Stylomastoid foramen
32 Mastoid canaliculus
33 Jugular fossa
34 Mastoid process
35 Mastoid notch
36 Groove for middle meningeal vessels
37 Parietal margin
38 Sphenoidal margin
39 Occipital margin
40 Cochlear canaliculus
41 Aqueduct of the vestibule
42 Apex of the petrous part
43 Tympanic part
44 Trigeminal impression
45 Articular tubercle
46 Parietal notch
47 Groove for the superior petrosal sinus

**Occipital bone**

48 Clivus
49 Jugular tubercle
50 Condylar canal
51 Foramen magnum
52 Lower part of squamous occipital bone (cerebellar fossa)
53 Internal occipital protuberance
54 Groove for the transverse sinus
55 Groove for the superior sagittal sinus
56 Internal occipital crest
57 Upper part of squamous occipital bone (cerebral fossa)
58 Condyle
59 Nuchal plane
60 Superior nuchal line
61 External occipital protuberance
62 Jugular foramen
63 Inferior nuchal line
64 Pharyngeal tubercle
65 Spheno-occipital synchondrosis

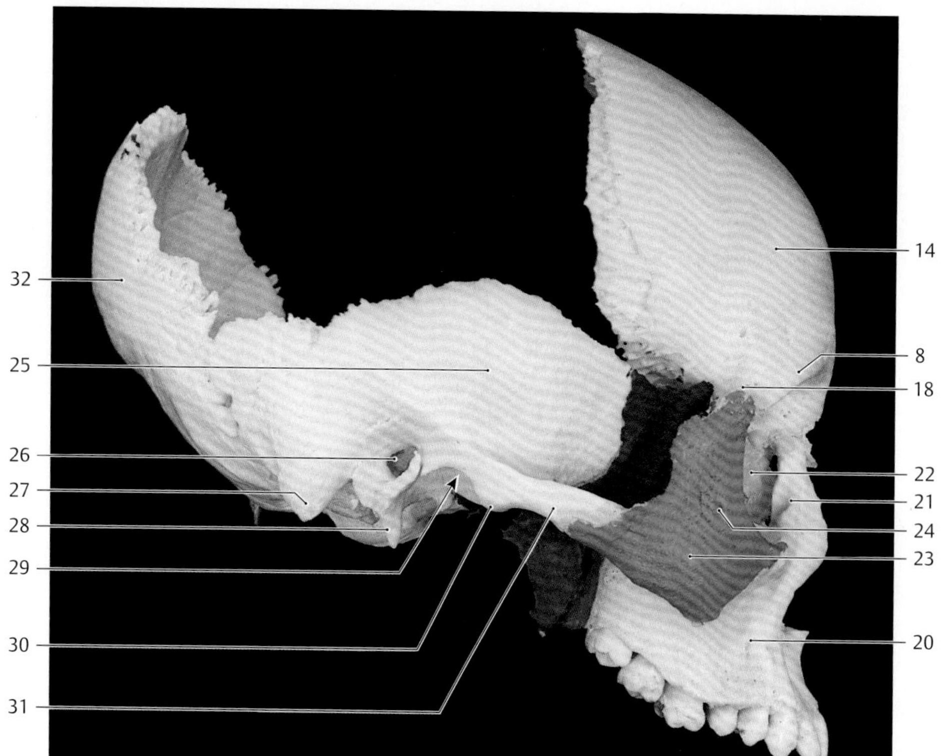


Fig. 8.16 **Part of a disarticulated skull** (right lateral aspect). The frontal bone and the maxilla are connected with the temporal bone by the zygomatic bone (orange). Black = sphenoid bone; red = palatine bone; yellow = lacrimal bone.

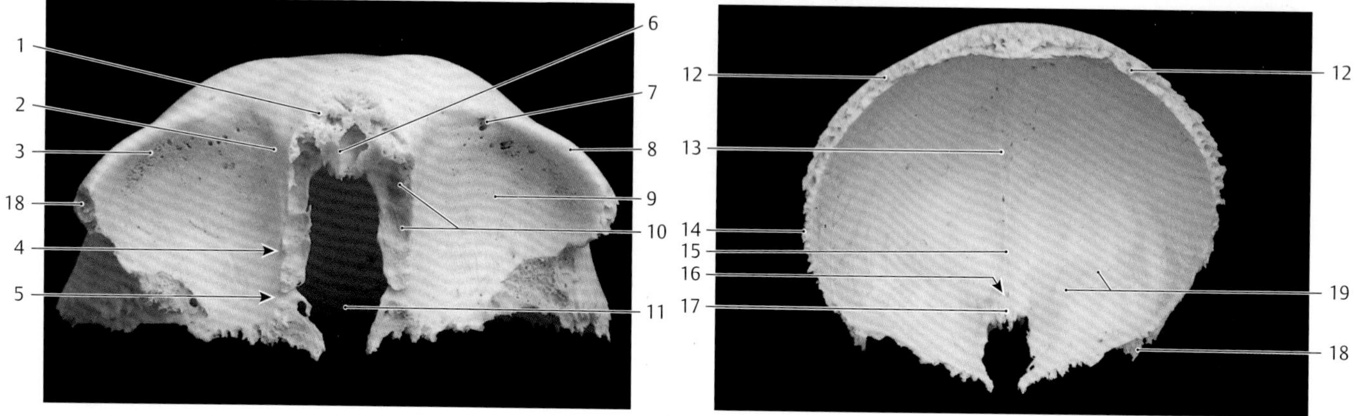


Fig. 8.17 **Frontal bone** (inferior aspect). The ethmoidal foveolae cover the ethmoidal cavities of the ethmoid bone.

Fig. 8.18 **Frontal bone** (posterior aspect).

**Frontal bone**

1 Nasal margin
2 Trochlear fossa
3 Fossa for lacrimal gland
4 Anterior ethmoidal foramen
5 Posterior ethmoidal foramen
6 Nasal spine
7 Supra-orbital notch
8 Supra-orbital margin
9 Orbital plate
10 Roofs of the ethmoidal air cells
11 Ethmoidal notch
12 Parietal margin
13 Groove for superior sagittal sinus
14 Squamous part of frontal bone
15 Frontal crest
16 Foramen cecum
17 Nasal spine
18 Zygomatic process of frontal bone
19 Juga cerebralia

**Facial bones**

20 Maxilla
21 Frontal process of maxilla
22 Lacrimal bone (yellow)
23 Zygomatic bone (orange)
24 Zygomaticofacial foramen

**Temporal bone**

25 Squamous part of temporal bone
26 External acoustic meatus
27 Mastoid process
28 Styloid process
29 Mandibular fossa
30 Articular tubercle
31 Zygomatic process

**Occipital bone**

32 Squamous part of occipital bone

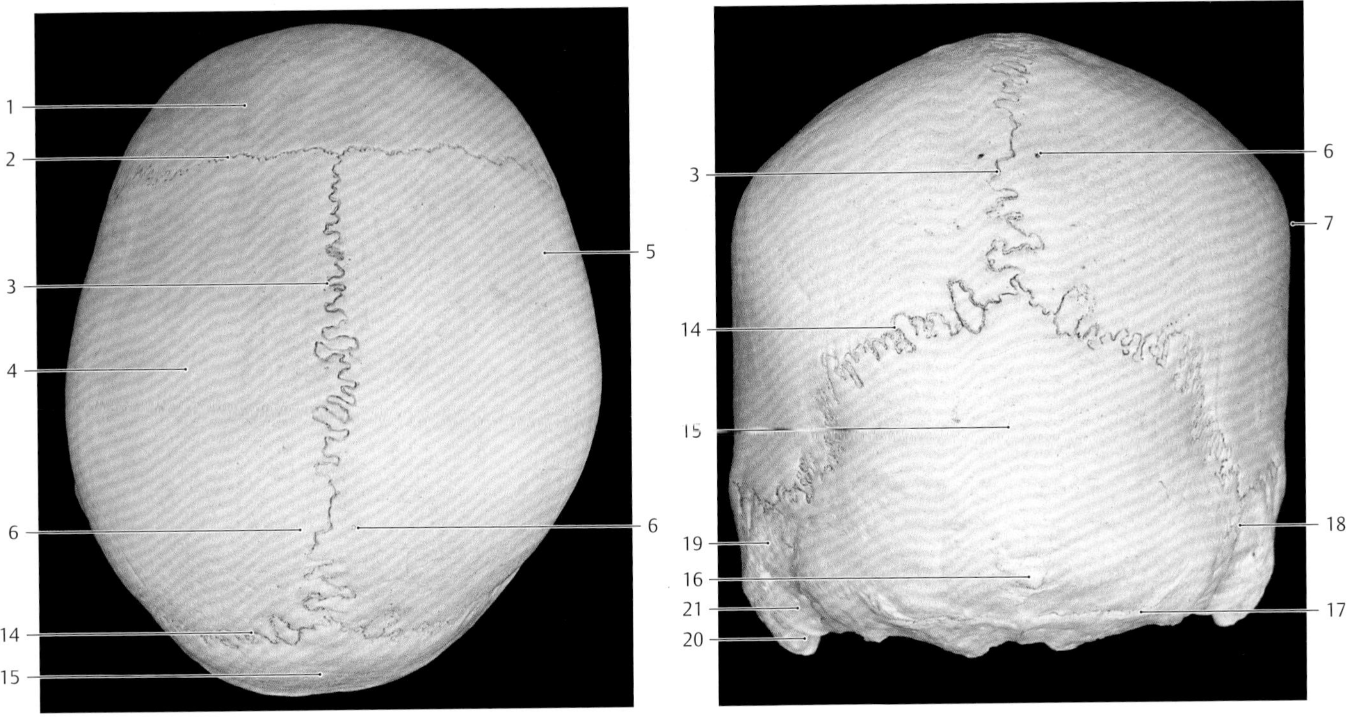


Fig. 8.19 **Calvaria** (superior aspect).

Fig. 8.20 **Calvaria** (posterior aspect).

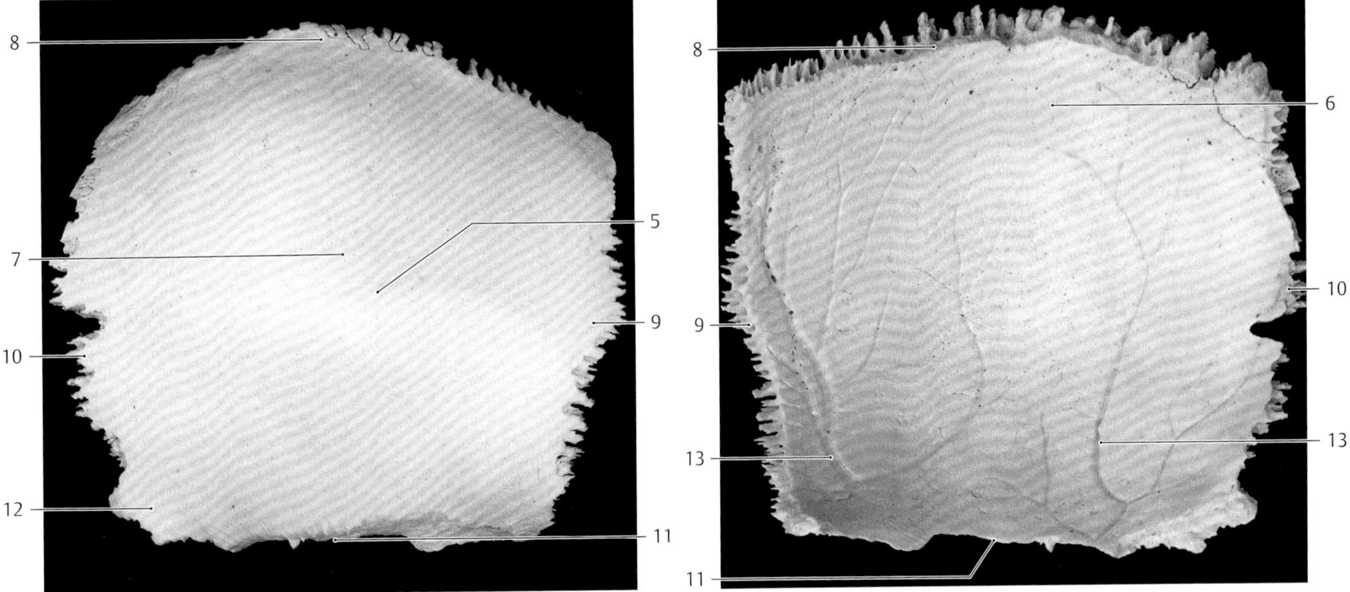


Fig. 8.21 **Left parietal bone** (external aspect).

Fig. 8.22 **Left parietal bone** (internal aspect).

1 Frontal bone
2 Coronal suture
3 Sagittal suture
4 Parietal bone
5 Superior temporal line
6 Parietal foramen
7 Parietal tuber or eminence
8 Sagittal margin
9 Occipital margin
10 Frontal margin
11 Squamous margin
12 Sphenoidal angle
13 Groove for middle meningeal artery
14 Lambdoid suture
15 Occipital bone
16 External occipital protuberance
17 Inferior nuchal line
18 Occipitomastoid suture
19 Temporal bone
20 Mastoid process
21 Mastoid notch

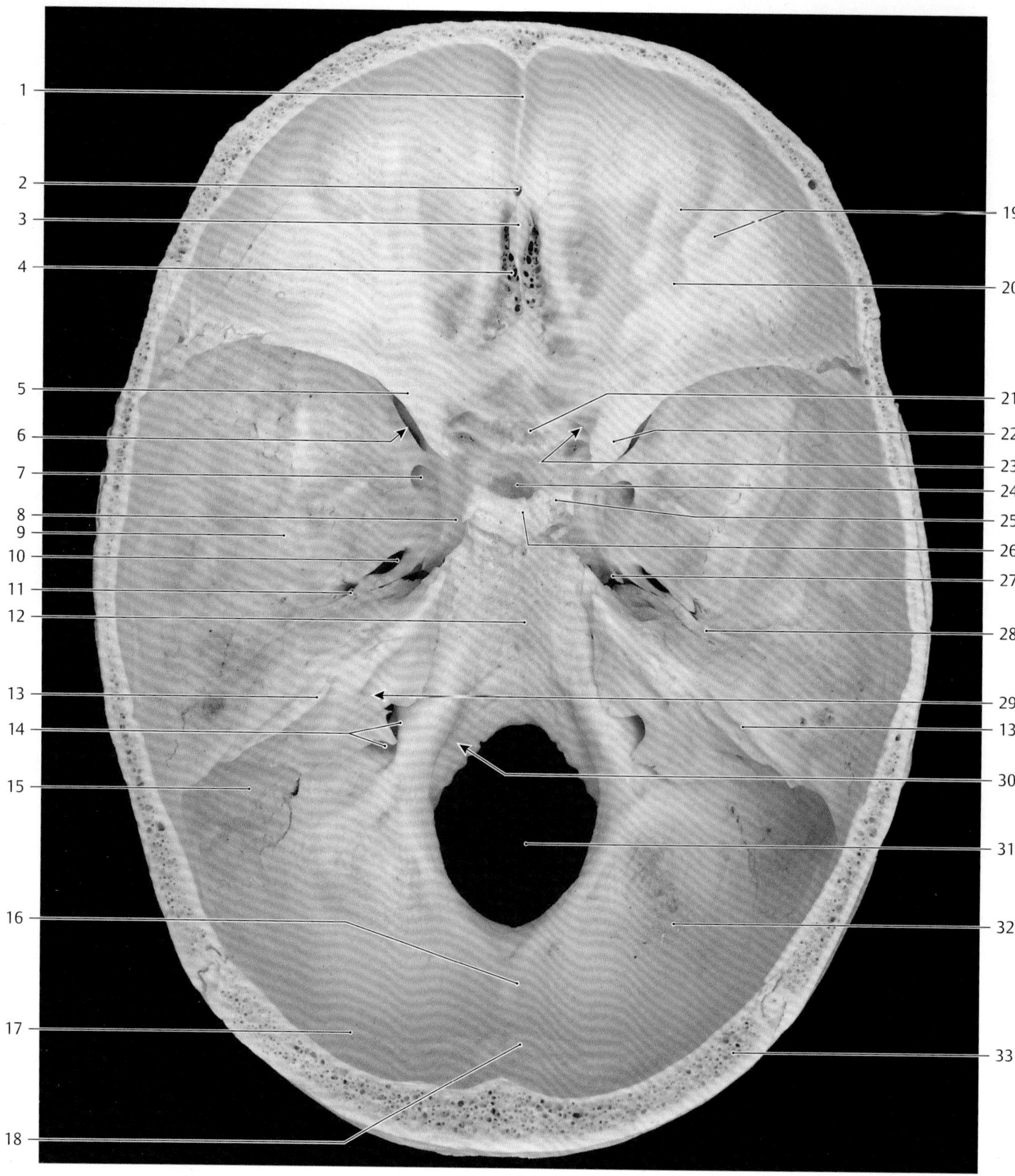


Fig. 8.23 **Base of the skull,** calvaria removed (internal aspect).

1 Frontal crest
2 Foramen cecum
3 Crista galli
4 Cribriform plate of ethmoid bone
5 Lesser wing of sphenoid bone
6 Superior orbital fissure
7 Foramen rotundum
8 Carotid sulcus
9 Middle cranial fossa
10 Foramen ovale
11 Foramen spinosum
12 Clivus
13 Groove for superior petrosal sinus
14 Jugular foramen
15 Groove for sigmoid sinus
16 Internal occipital crest
17 Groove for transverse sinus
18 Internal occipital protuberance
19 Digitate impressions
20 Anterior cranial fossa
21 Chiasmatic sulcus
22 Anterior clinoid process
23 Optic canal
24 Sella turcica (hypophysial fossa)
25 Posterior clinoid process
26 Dorsum sellae
27 Foramen lacerum
28 Groove for greater petrosal nerve
29 Internal acoustic meatus
30 Hypoglossal canal
31 Foramen magnum
32 Posterior cranial fossa
33 Diploë

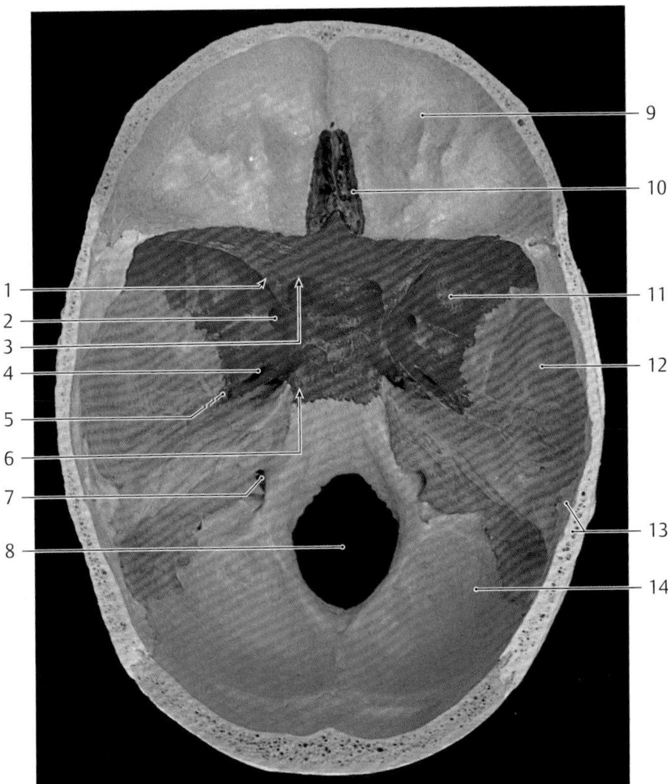

**Canals, fissures, and foramina of the base of the skull**

1 Superior orbital fissure
2 Foramen rotundum
3 Optic canal
4 Foramen ovale
5 Foramen spinosum
6 Internal acoustic meatus
7 Jugular foramen
8 Foramen magnum

**Bones**

9 Frontal bone (orange)
10 Ethmoid bone (dark green)
11 Sphenoid bone (red)
12 Temporal bone (brown)
13 Parietal bone (yellow)
14 Occipital bone (blue)

Fig. 8.24 **Base of the skull** (internal aspect, superior view). The individual bones are indicated by different colors.

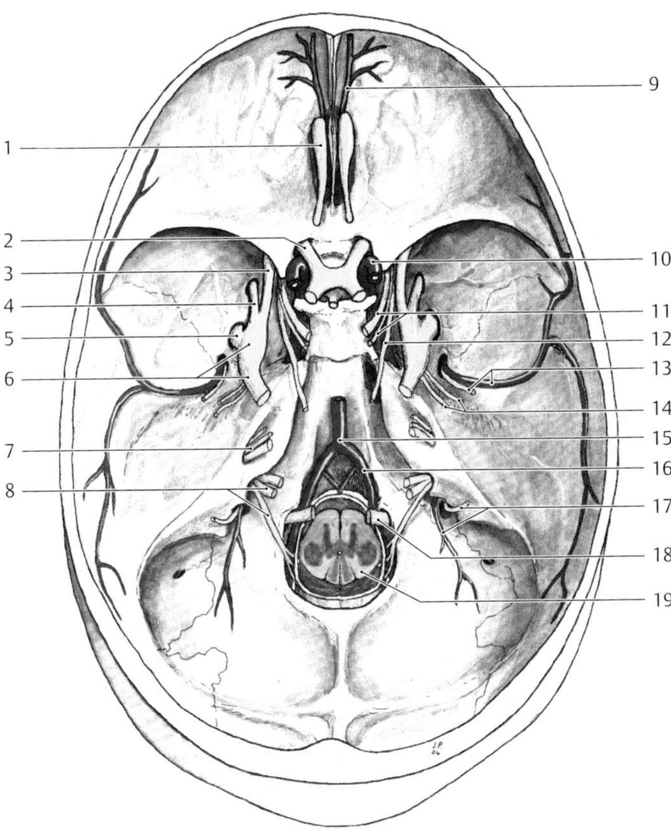

1 Olfactory bulb
2 Optic nerve (CN II)
3 Ophthalmic nerve (CN $V_1$)
4 Maxillary nerve (CN $V_2$)
5 Mandibular nerve (CN $V_3$)
6 Trigeminal nerve (CN V) with trigeminal ganglion
7 Facial nerve (CN VII) and vestibulocochlear nerve (CN VIII)
8 Glossopharyngeal nerve (CN IX), vagus nerve (CN X) and accessory nerve (CN XI)
9 Anterior meningeal artery
10 Internal carotid artery
11 Oculomotor nerve (CN III) and trochlear nerve (CN IV)
12 Abducent nerve (CN VI)
13 Middle meningeal artery and meningeal branch of mandibular nerve
14 Greater and lesser petrosal nerves
15 Basilar artery
16 Vertebral artery
17 Posterior meningeal artery and recurrent meningeal nerve
18 Hypoglossal nerve (CN XII)
19 Medulla oblongata

Fig. 8.25 **Base of the skull** with cranial nerves and meningeal arteries (internal aspect).

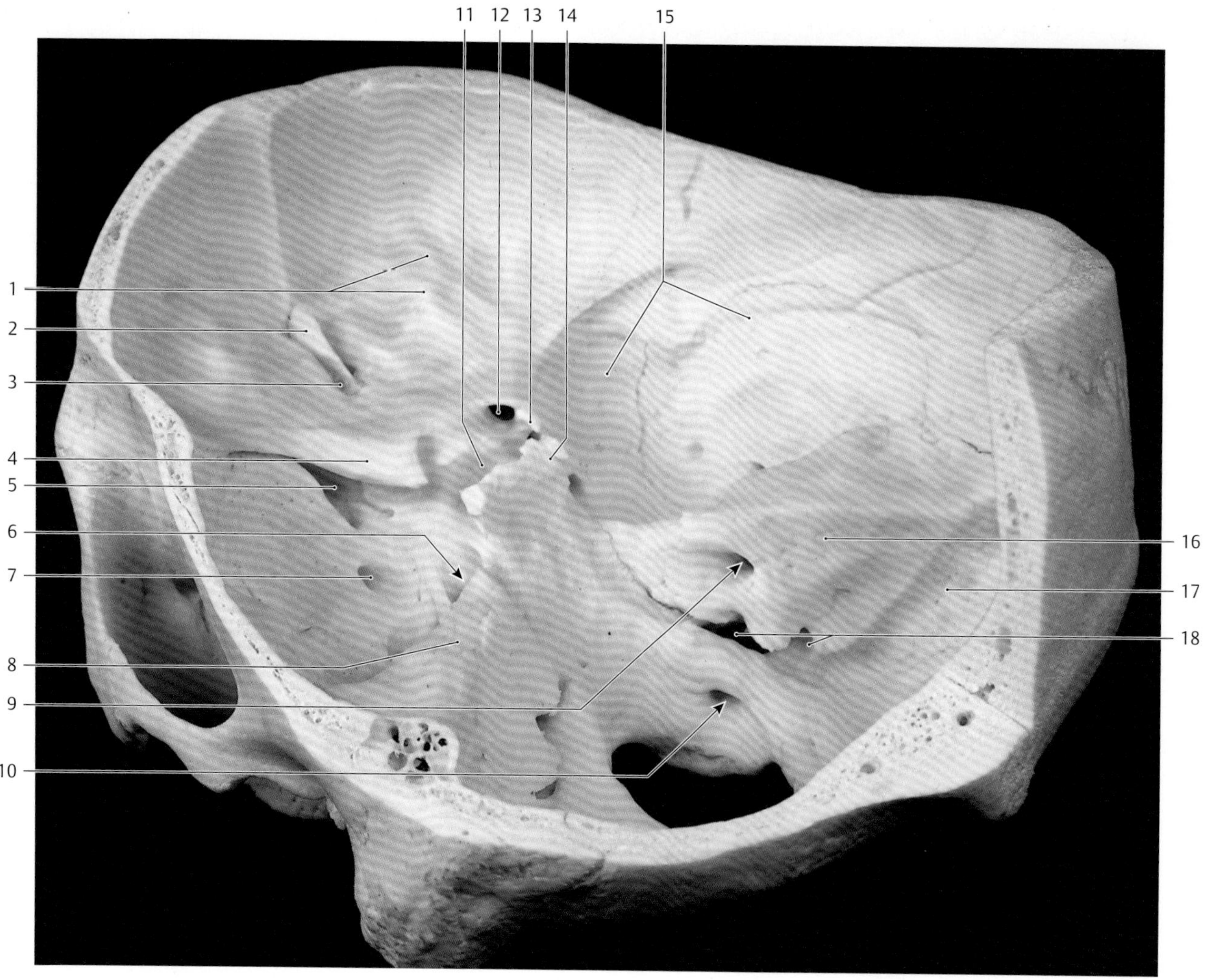


Fig. 8.26 **Base of the skull** (internal aspect, oblique-lateral view from left side). See corresponding table below for cranial nerves and vessels and related foramina.

| | Cranial nerves and vessels | Related foramina | Related regions |
|---|---|---|---|
| **Anterior cranial fossa** | Olfactory nerves (CN I),<br>Anterior ethmoidal artery, vein, and nerve,<br>Anterior meningeal artery | Lamina cribrosa | Nasal cavity |
| **Middle cranial fossa** | Optic nerve (CN II), Ophthalmic artery | Optic canal | Orbit |
| | Oculomotor nerve (CN III), Trochlear nerve (CN IV),<br>Abducent nerve (CN VI), Ophthalmic nerve (CN $V_1$),<br>Superior ophthalmic vein | Superior orbital fissure | Orbit |
| | Maxillary nerve (CN $V_2$) | Foramen rotundum | Pterygopalatine fossa |
| | Mandibular nerve (CN $V_3$) | Foramen ovale | Infratemporal fossa |
| | Middle meningeal artery,<br>Meningeal branch of mandibular nerve (CN $V_3$) | Foramen spinosum | Infratemporal fossa |
| | Internal carotid artery | Carotid canal | Cavernous sinus,<br>Base of skull |
| **Posterior cranial fossa** | Facial nerve (CN VII), Vestibulocochlear nerve (CN VIII),<br>Artery and vein of the labyrinth | Internal acoustic meatus, Stylomastoid foramen, Facial canal | Inner ear, Face |
| | Glossopharyngeal nerve (CN IX), Vagus nerve (CN X),<br>Accessory nerve (CN XI), Internal jugular vein,<br>Posterior meningeal artery | Jugular foramen | Parapharyngeal region |
| | Hypoglossal nerve (CN XII) | Hypoglossal canal | Tongue |
| | Accessory nerve (CN XI, spinal root), Vertebral arteries,<br>Anterior and posterior spinal arteries, Medulla oblongata | Foramen magnum | Base of skull |

1 Digitate impressions (frontal bone)
2 Crista galli
3 Cribriform plate
4 Lesser wing of sphenoid bone
5 Superior orbital fissure
6 Foramen lacerum
7 Foramen rotundum
8 Trigeminal impression
9 Internal acoustic meatus
10 Hypoglossal canal
11 Hypophysial fossa (sella turcica)
12 Optic canal
13 Anterior clinoid process
14 Dorsum sellae (posterior clinoid process)
15 Greater wing of sphenoid bone, groove for middle meningeal artery
16 Petrous part of temporal bone
17 Groove for sigmoid sinus
18 Jugular foramen

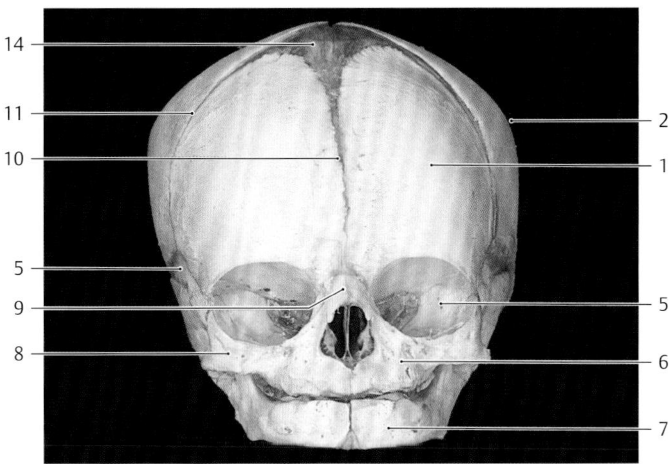


Fig. 8.27 **Skull of the newborn** (anterior aspect).

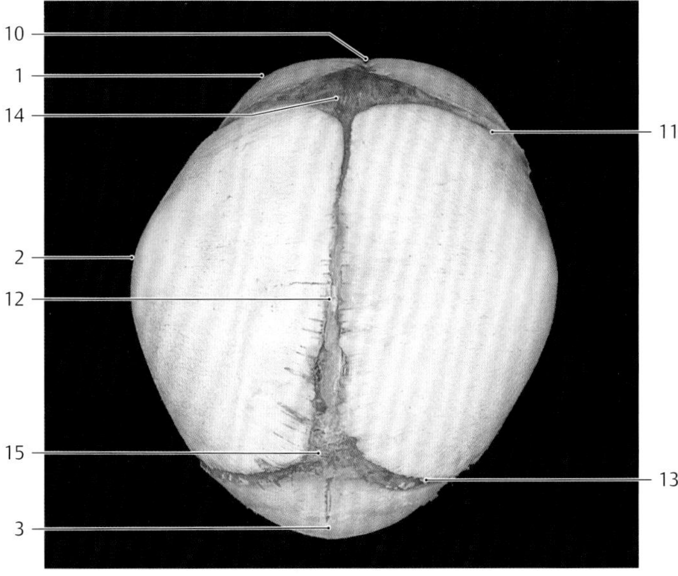


Fig. 8.28 **Skull of the newborn** (superior aspect). Calvaria.

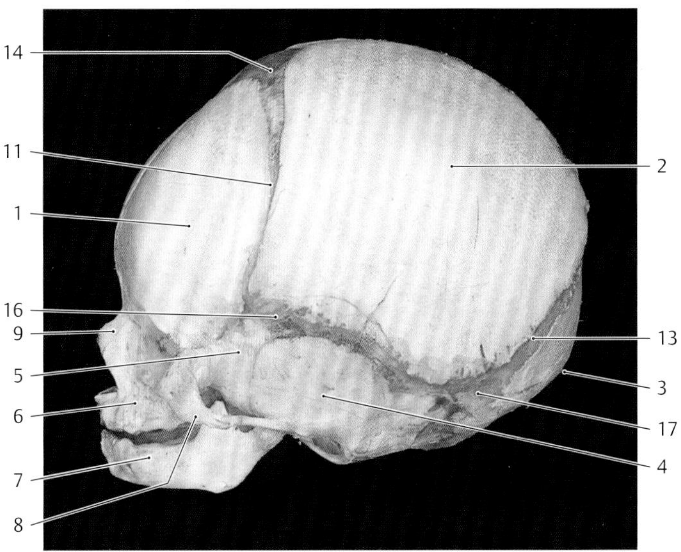


Fig. 8.29 **Skull of the newborn** (lateral aspect).

**Cranial skeleton**
1 Frontal tuber or eminence
2 Parietal tuber or eminence
3 Occipital tuber or eminence
4 Squamous part of temporal bone
5 Greater wing of sphenoid bone

**Facial skeleton**
6 Maxilla
7 Mandible
8 Zygomatic bone
9 Nasal bone

**Sutures and fontanelles**
10 Frontal suture
11 Coronal suture
12 Sagittal suture
13 Lambdoid suture
14 Anterior fontanelle
15 Posterior fontanelle
16 Sphenoidal (anterolateral) fontanelle
17 Mastoid (posterolateral) fontanelle

**Base of the skull**
18 Frontal bone
19 Ethmoid bone
20 Sphenoid bone
21 Hypophysial fossa (sella turcica)
22 Dorsum sellae
23 Temporal bone
24 Mastoid (posterolateral) fontanelle
25 Occipital bone

In the newborn, the facial skeleton, in contrast to the cranial skeleton, appears relatively small. There are no teeth presenting. The bones of the cranium are separated by wide fontanelles.

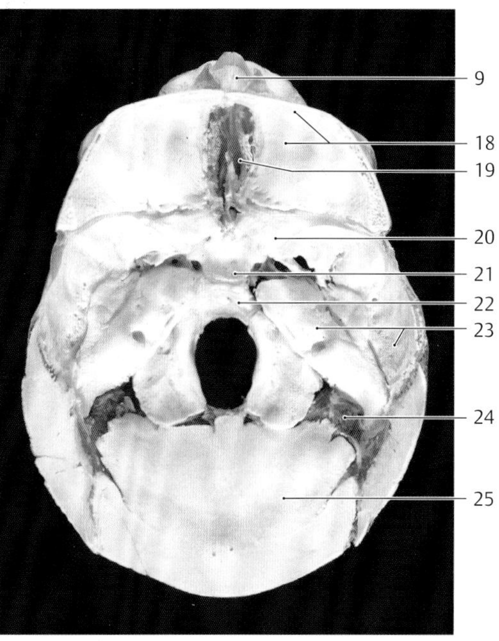


Fig. 8.30 **Base of the skull of the newborn** (internal aspect).

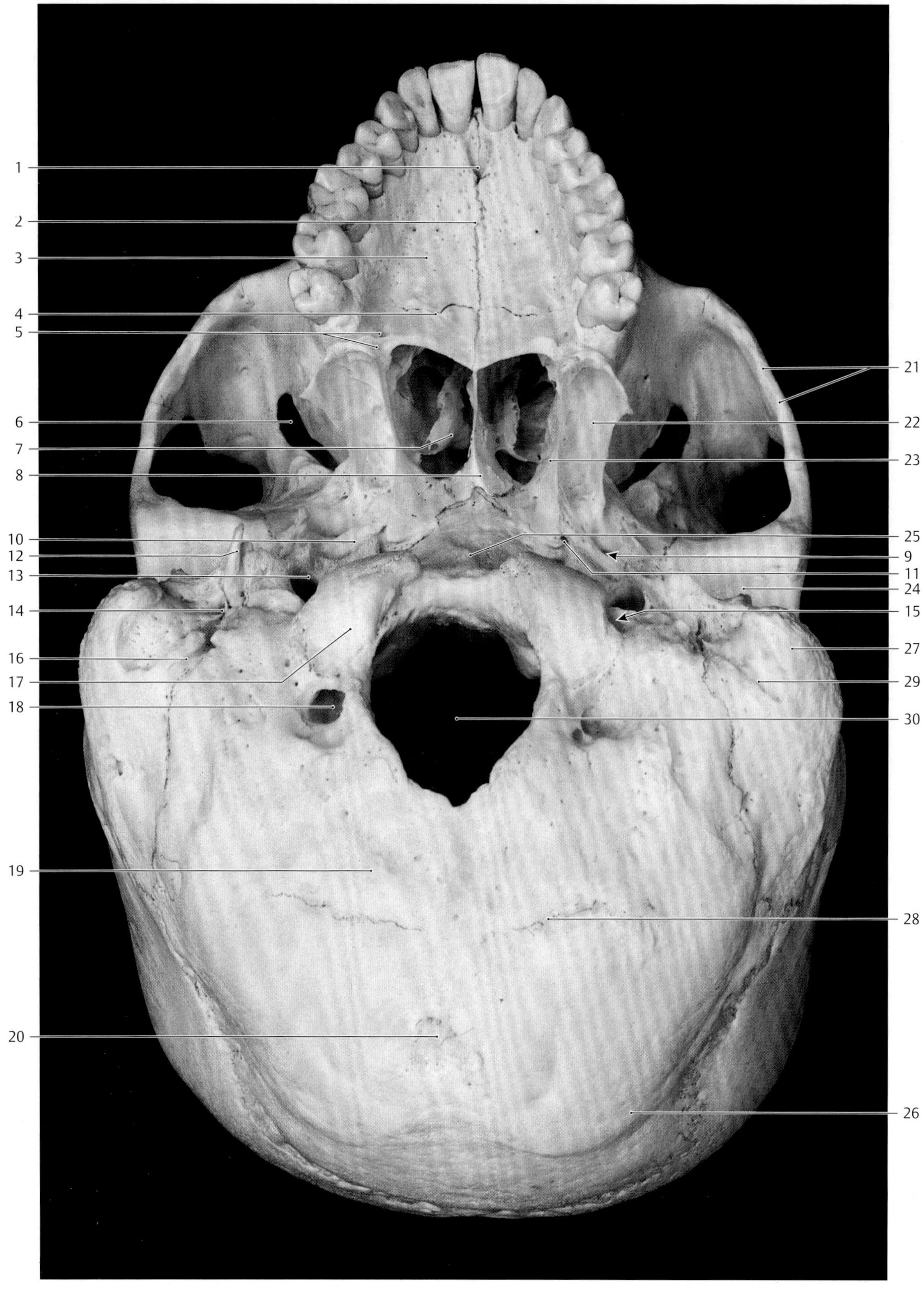


Fig. 8.31 **Base of the skull** (inferior aspect).

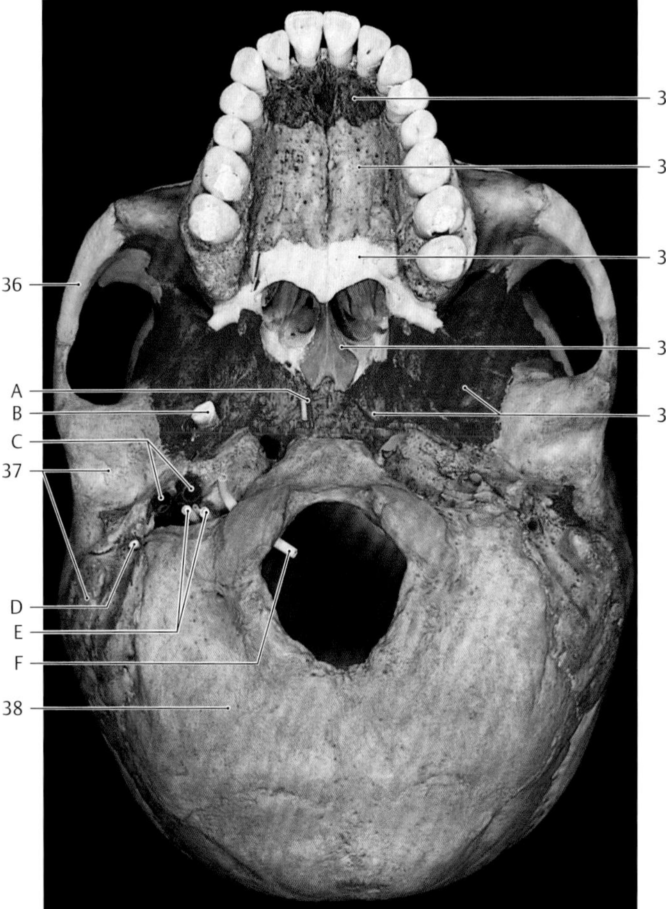


Fig. 8.32 **Base of the skull** (from below). The individual bones are indicated by different colors.

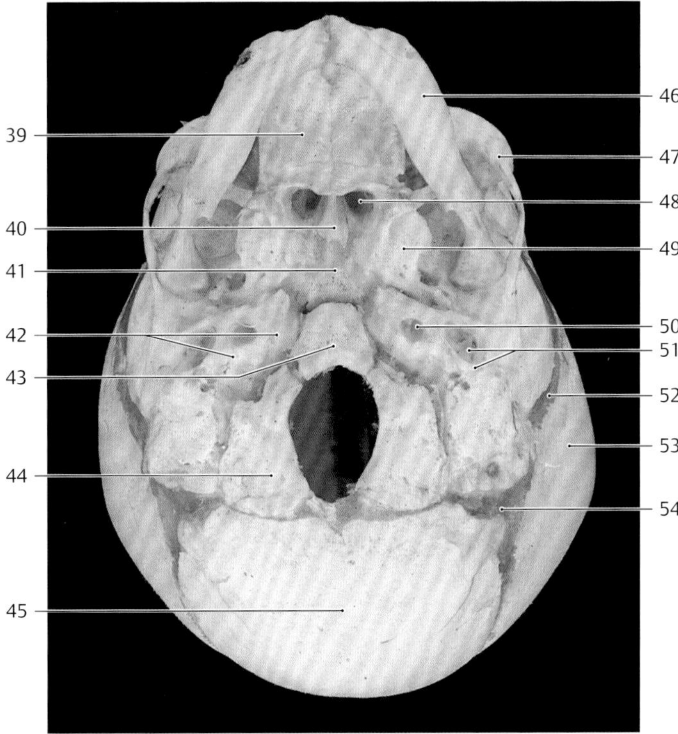


Fig. 8.33 **Skull of the newborn** (inferior aspect).

A = Pterygoid canal
B = Foramen ovale
C = Internal carotid artery within carotid canal and internal jugular vein within the venous part of jugular foramen
D = Stylomastoid foramen (facial nerve)
E = Jugular foramen (glossopharyngeal, vagus, and accessory nerves)
F = Hypoglossal canal (hypoglossal nerve)

1 Incisive canal
2 Median palatine suture
3 Palatine process of maxilla
4 Palatomaxillary suture
5 Greater and lesser palatine foramina
6 Inferior orbital fissure
7 Middle concha (process of ethmoid bone)
8 Vomer
9 Foramen ovale
10 Groove for auditory tube
11 Pterygoid canal
12 Styloid process
13 Carotid canal
14 Stylomastoid foramen
15 Jugular foramen
16 Groove for occipital artery
17 Occipital condyle
18 Condylar canal
19 Nuchal plane
20 External occipital protuberance
21 Zygomatic arch
22 Lateral pterygoid plate
23 Medial pterygoid plate
24 Mandibular fossa
25 Pharyngeal tubercle
26 Superior nuchal line
27 Mastoid process
28 Inferior nuchal line
29 Mastoid notch
30 Foramen magnum

**Bones**

31 Incisive bone or premaxilla (dark violet)
32 Maxilla (violet)
33 Palatine bone (white)
34 Vomer (orange)
35 Sphenoid bone (red)
36 Zygomatic bone (yellow)
37 Temporal bone (brown)
38 Occipital bone (blue)
39 Palatine process of maxilla
40 Vomer
41 Sphenoid bone
42 Petrous part of temporal bone
43 Basilar part } of occipital bone
44 Lateral part } of occipital bone
45 Squamous part } of occipital bone
46 Mandible
47 Zygomatic arch
48 Choana
49 Pterygoid process of sphenoid bone
50 Carotid canal
51 External acoustic meatus (tympanic anulus)
52 Sphenoidal fontanelle
53 Parietal bone
54 Mastoid fontanelle

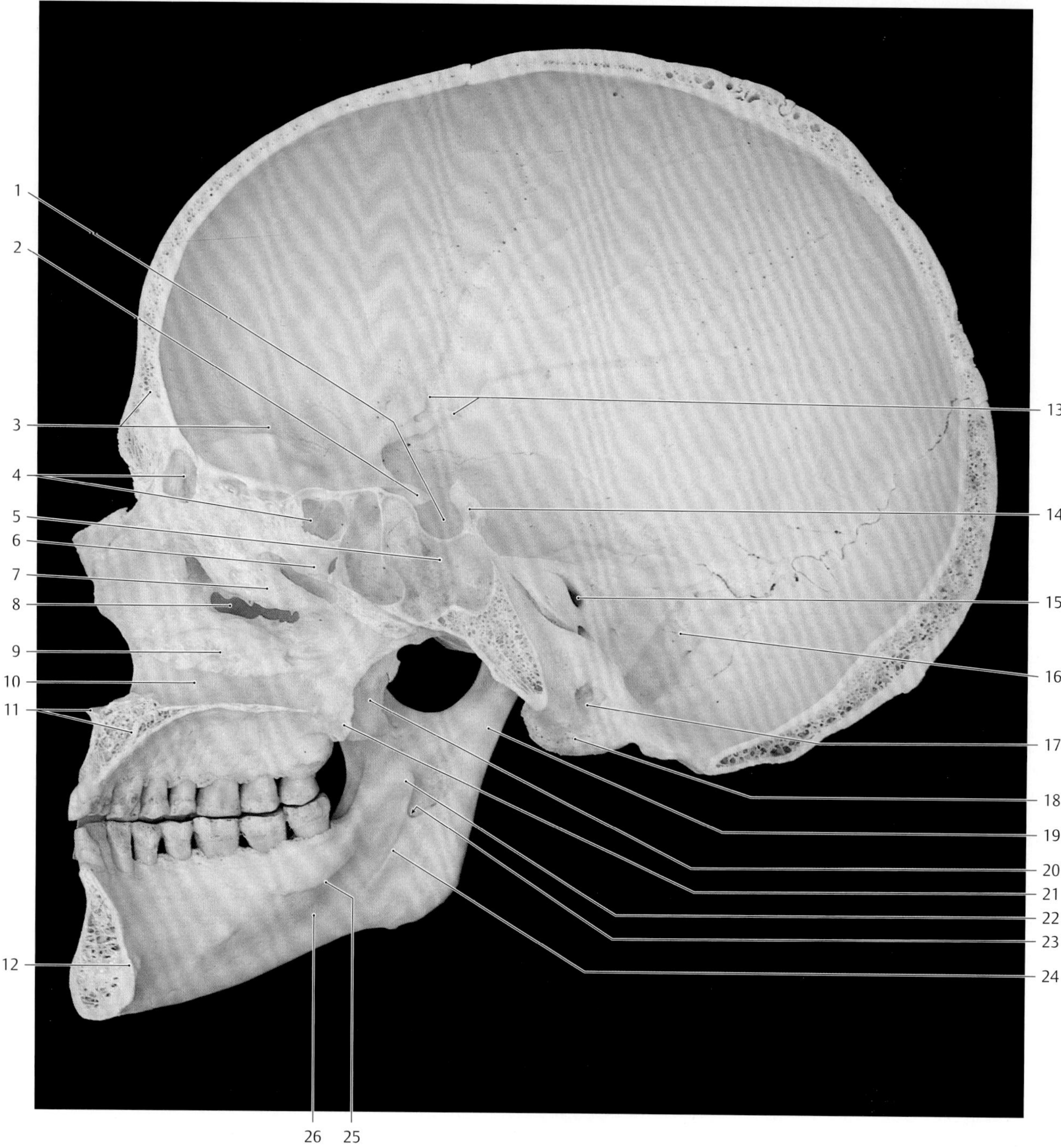


Fig. 8.34 **Median section through the skull,** right half (internal aspect).

1 Hypophysial fossa (sella turcica)
2 Anterior clinoid process
3 Frontal bone
4 Ethmoidal air cells
5 Sphenoidal sinus
6 Superior concha
7 Middle concha
8 Maxillary hiatus
9 Inferior concha
10 Inferior meatus
11 Anterior nasal spine and maxilla
12 Mental spine or genial tubercle
13 Groove for middle meningeal artery
14 Dorsum sellae
15 Internal acoustic meatus
16 Groove for sigmoid sinus
17 Hypoglossal canal
18 Occipital condyle
19 Condylar process
20 Lateral pterygoid plate of pterygoid process
21 Medial pterygoid plate
22 Lingula of mandible
23 Mandibular foramen
24 Mylohyoid groove
25 Mylohyoid line
26 Submandibular fovea

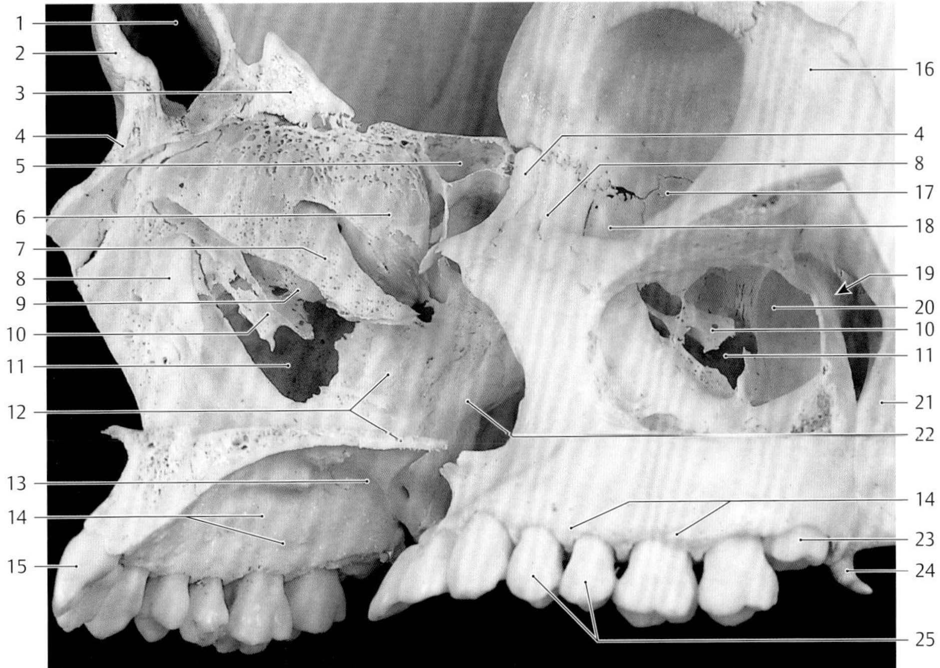

1 Frontal sinus
2 Frontal bone
3 Crista galli
4 Nasal bone
5 Sphenoidal sinus
6 Superior concha } of ethmoid bone
7 Middle concha } of ethmoid bone
8 Frontal process of maxilla
9 Ethmoidal bulla
10 Uncinate process
11 Maxillary hiatus
12 Palatine bone
13 Greater palatine foramen
14 Alveolar process of maxilla
15 Central incisor
16 Zygomatic bone
17 Ethmoid bone
18 Lacrimal bone
19 Pterygopalatine fossa
20 Maxillary sinus
21 Lateral pterygoid plate
22 Medial pterygoid plate
23 Third molar tooth
24 Pterygoid hamulus
25 Two premolar teeth

Fig. 8.35 **Facial part of the skull (viscerocranium),** divided in two halves (lateral and medial aspect). The right inferior concha has been removed to show the maxillary hiatus. The left maxillary sinus has been opened.

**Bones**

1 Frontal bone (yellow)
2 Nasal bone (white)
3 Ethmoid bone (dark green)
4 Lacrimal bone (yellow)
5 Inferior nasal concha (pink)
6 Palatine bone (white)
7 Maxilla (violet)
8 Mandible (white)
9 Parietal bone (light green)
10 Temporal bone (brown)
11 Sphenoid bone (red)
12 Petrous part of temporal bone (brown)
13 Occipital bone (blue)
14 Ala of vomer (light brown)

Fig. 8.36 **Median section through the skull.** The nasal septum has been removed. The individual bones are indicated by different colors.

Because of the upright posture that the human developed in the course of evolution, the cranial cavity greatly increased in size, whereas the facial skeleton decreased. As a result, the base of the skull developed an angulation of about 120° between the clivus and the cribriform plate (see Fig. 8.2 on page 350). The hypophysial fossa containing the pituitary gland lies at the angle formed between these two planes.

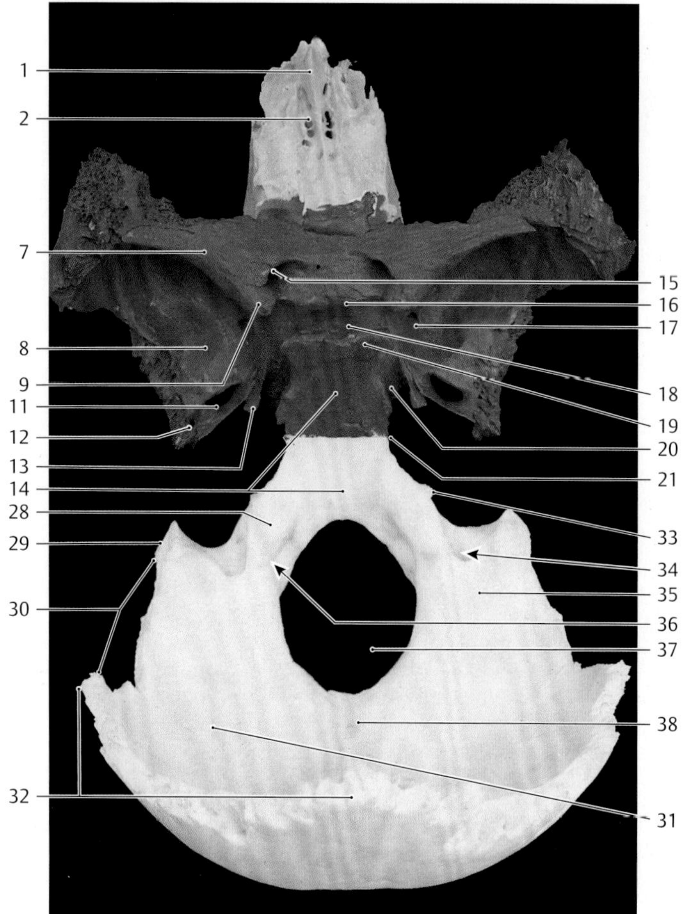


Fig. 8.37 **Part of a disarticulated base of the skull.** Ethmoid, sphenoid, and occipital bones (from above). Green = sphenoid bone; yellow = ethmoid bone.

**Ethmoid bone**

1 Crista galli
2 Cribriform plate
3 Ethmoidal air cells
4 Middle concha
5 Perpendicular plate (part of nasal septum)
6 Orbital plate

**Sphenoid bone**

7 Lesser wing
8 Greater wing
9 Anterior clinoid process
10 Posterior clinoid process
11 Foramen ovale
12 Foramen spinosum
13 Lingula of the sphenoid bone
14 Clivus
15 Optic canal
16 Tuberculum sellae
17 Foramen rotundum (right side)
18 Hypophysial fossa (sella turcica)
19 Dorsum sellae
20 Carotid sulcus
21 Spheno-occipital synchondrosis
22 Lateral pterygoid plate
23 Greater wing of sphenoid bone (orbital surface)
24 Greater wing of sphenoid bone (maxillary surface)
25 Foramen rotundum (left side)
26 Superior orbital fissure
27 Infratemporal crest of the greater wing

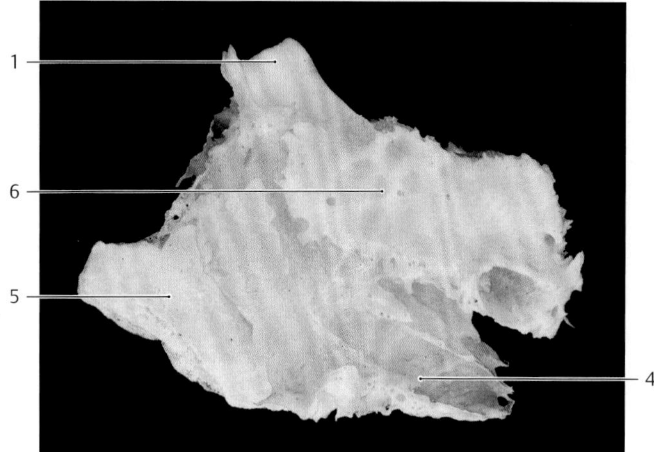


Fig. 8.38 **Ethmoid bone** (lateral aspect), posterior portion to the right.

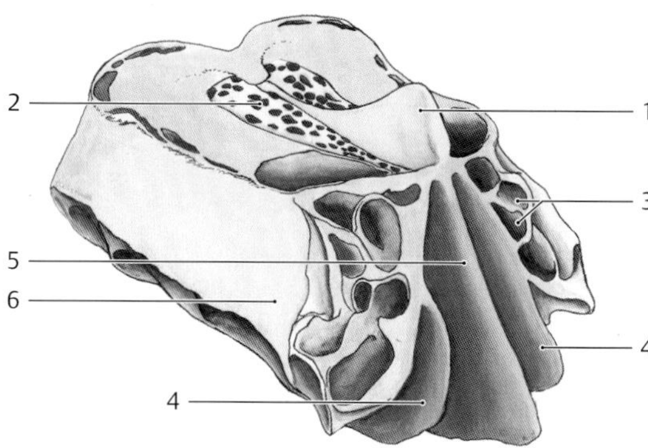


Fig. 8.39 **Ethmoid bone** (anterior aspect).

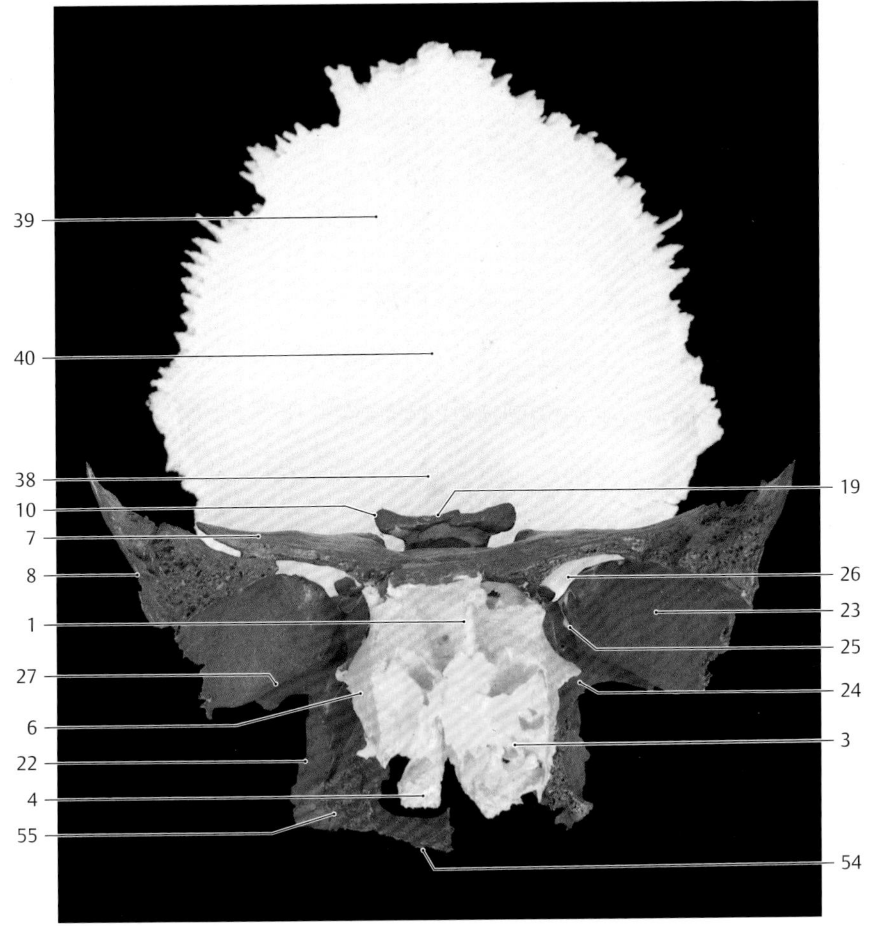


Fig. 8.40 **Part of a disarticulated base of the skull** (anterior aspect). Green = sphenoid bone; yellow = ethmoid bone; red = palatine bone.

**Occipital bone**
28 Jugular tubercle
29 Jugular process
30 Mastoid margin
31 Posterior cranial fossa
32 Lambdoid margin
33 Intrajugular process
34 Condylar canal
35 Lateral part of occipital bone
36 Hypoglossal canal
37 Foramen magnum
38 Internal occipital crest
39 Squamous part of occipital bone
40 Internal occipital protuberance

**Maxilla**
41 Orbital surface
42 Infra-orbital groove
43 Maxillary tuberosity with foramina
44 Frontal process
45 Nasolacrimal groove
46 Infra-orbital margin
47 Anterior nasal spine
48 Zygomatic process
49 Alveolar process

**Palatine bone**
50 Orbital process
51 Sphenopalatine notch
52 Sphenoidal process
53 Perpendicular plate
54 Horizontal plate
55 Pyramidal process

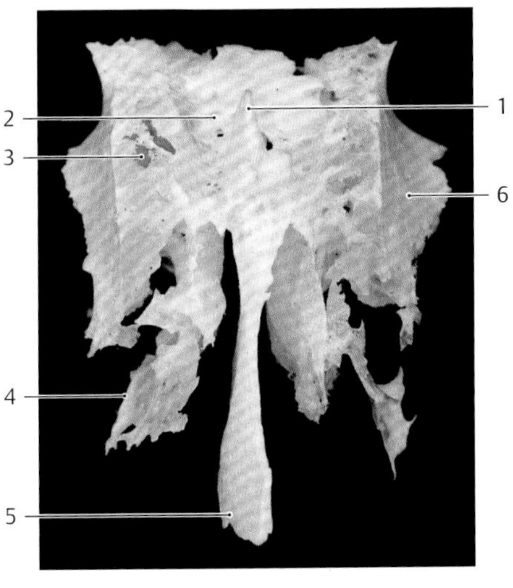


Fig. 8.41 **Ethmoid bone** (anterior aspect).

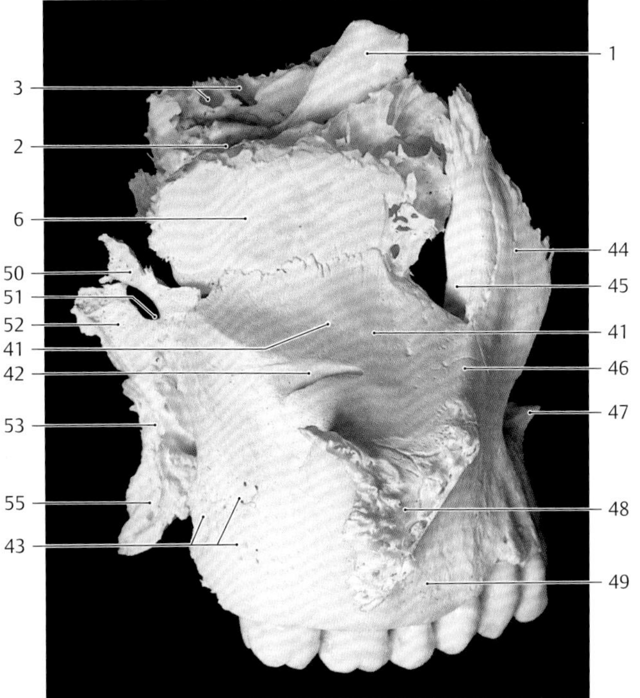


Fig. 8.42 **Right maxilla, ethmoidal, and palatine bones** (lateral aspect).

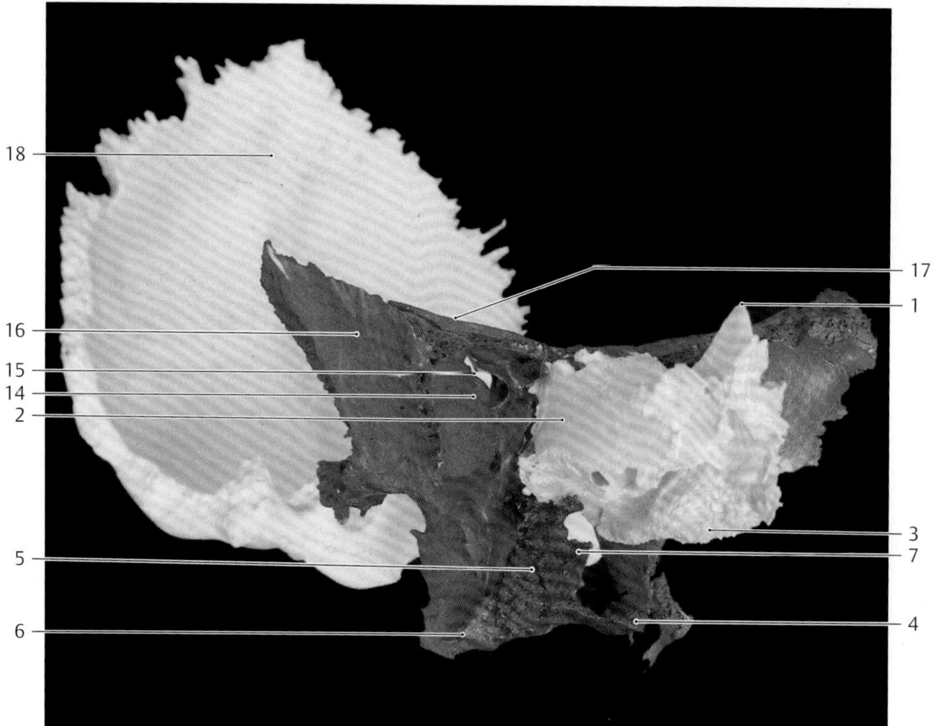


Fig. 8.43 **Part of a disarticulated base of the skull,** similar to the preceding figures, but with palatine bone. Green = sphenoid bone; yellow = ethmoid bone; red = palatine bone.

**Ethmoid bone**

1 Crista galli
2 Orbital plate
3 Middle concha

**Palatine bone**

4 Horizontal plate of palatine bone
5 Greater palatine canal
6 Pyramidal process
7 Maxillary process
8 Orbital process
9 Sphenopalatine notch
10 Perpendicular plate of palatine bone
11 Conchal crest
12 Nasal crest
13 Sphenoidal process

**Sphenoid bone**

14 Greater wing
15 Superior orbital fissure
16 Greater wing (orbital surface)
17 Lesser wing

**Occipital bone**

18 Squamous part of occipital bone

**Maxilla**

19 Maxillary tuberosity
20 Frontal process
21 Orbital surface
22 Infra-orbital margin
23 Infra-orbital groove
24 Zygomatic process
25 Alveolar process

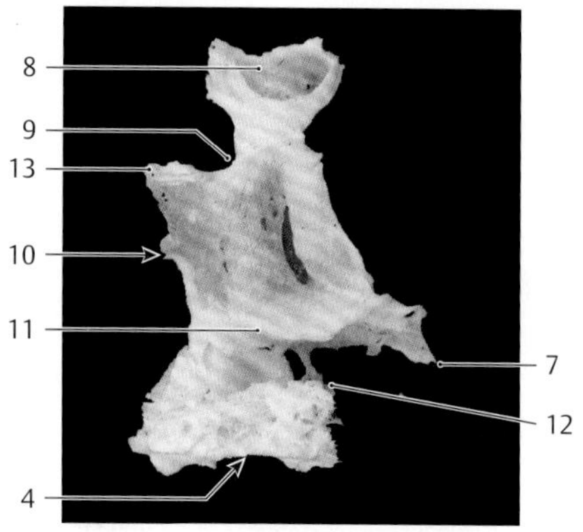

Fig. 8.44 **Left palatine bone** (medial aspect, posterior aspect to the left).

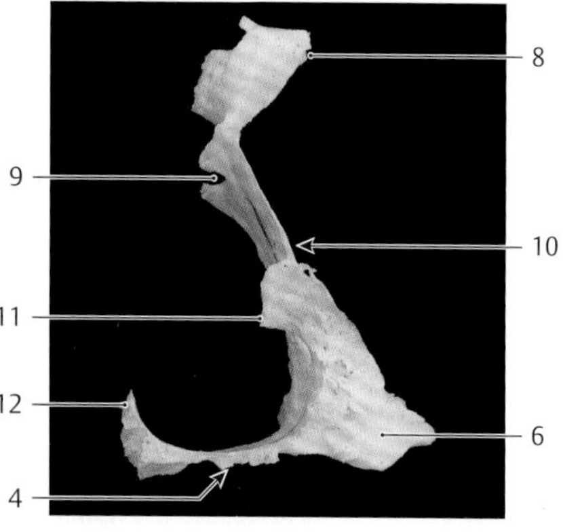


Fig. 8.45 **Left palatine bone** (anterior aspect).

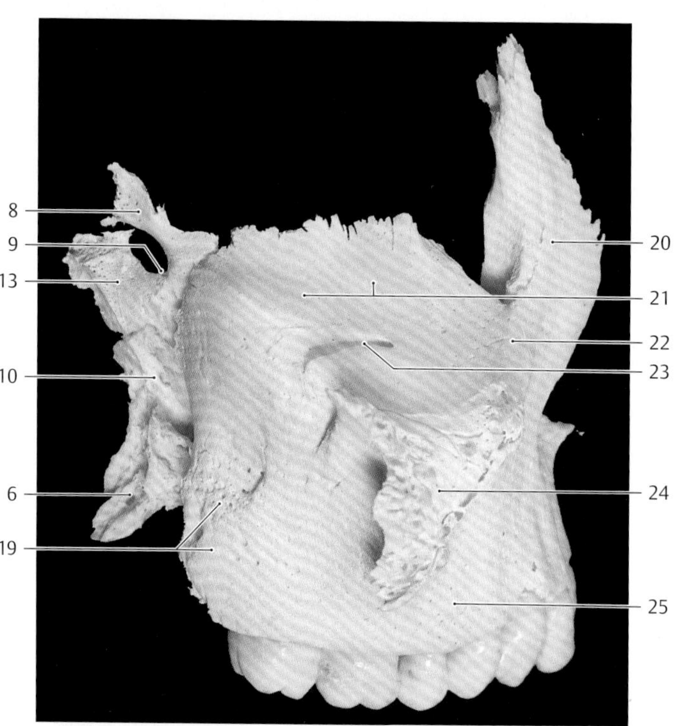


Fig. 8.46 **Right maxilla and palatine bone** (lateral aspect).

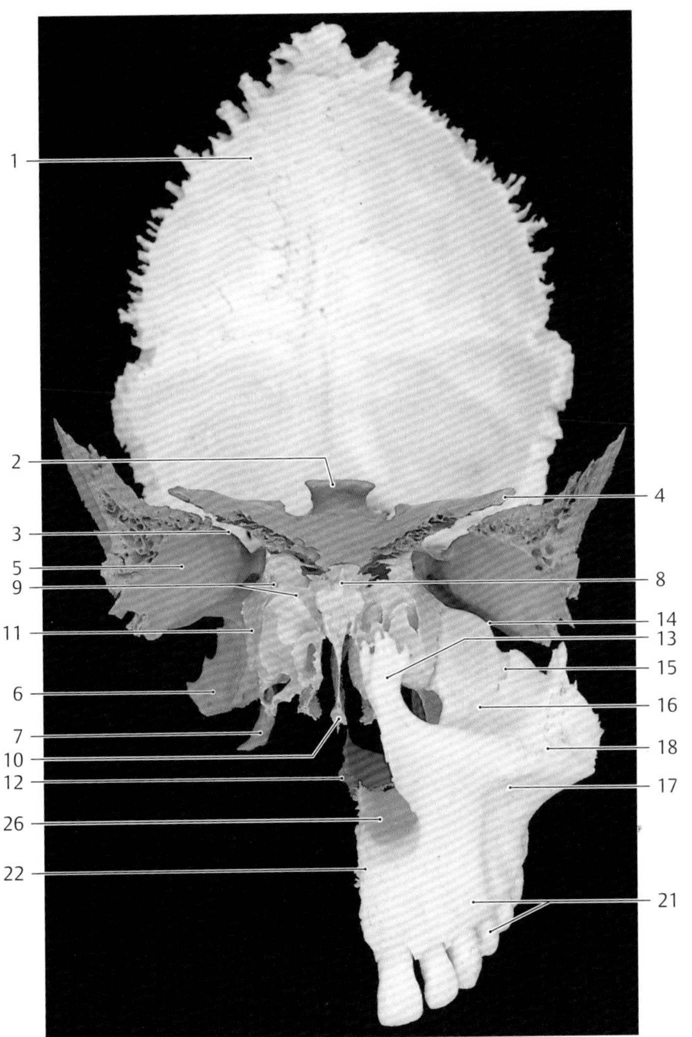


Fig. 8.47 **Part of a disarticulated base of the skull** (anterior aspect). The left **maxilla** is added to the preceding specimen.

**Occipital bone**
1 Squamous part

**Sphenoid bone**
2 Dorsum sellae
3 Superior orbital fissure
4 Lesser wing
5 Greater wing (orbital surface)
6 Lateral pterygoid plate
7 Medial pterygoid plate

**Ethmoid bone**
8 Crista galli
9 Ethmoidal air cells
10 Perpendicular plate
11 Orbital plate

**Palatine bone**
12 Horizontal plate (nasal crest)

**Maxilla**
13 Frontal process
14 Inferior orbital fissure
15 Infra-orbital groove
16 Orbital surface
17 Infra-orbital foramen
18 Zygomatic process
19 Anterior lacrimal crest
20 Canine fossa
21 Alveolar process with teeth
22 Anterior nasal spine
23 Juga alveolaria (elevations formed by roots of teeth)
24 Lacrimal groove
25 Maxillary tuberosity with alveolar foramina
26 Palatine process of maxilla

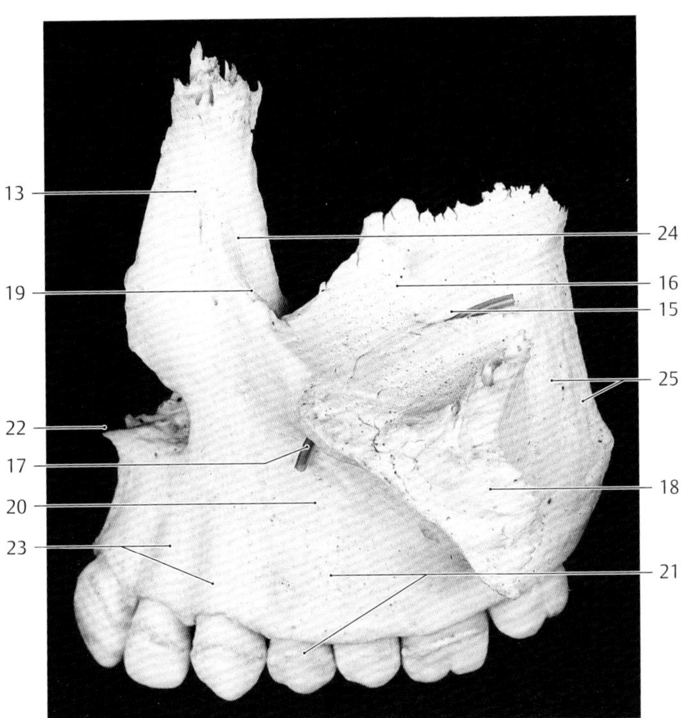


Fig. 8.48 **Left maxilla** (lateral aspect). Probe = infra-orbital canal.

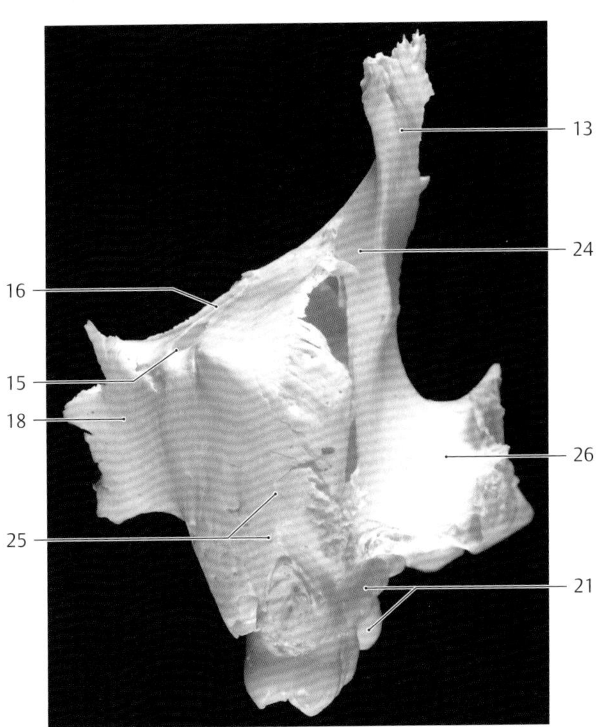


Fig. 8.49 **Left maxilla** (posterior aspect).

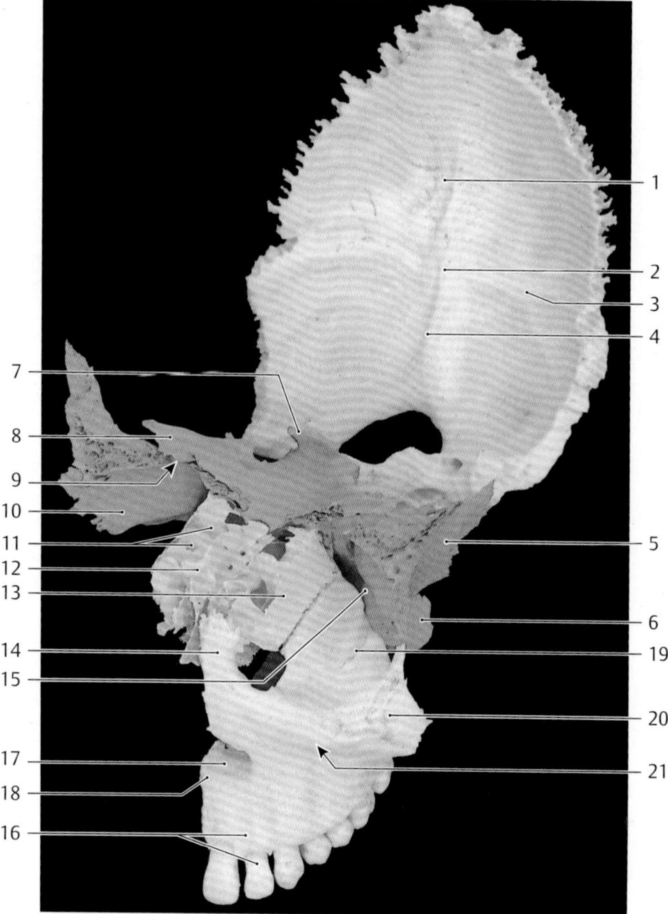


Fig. 8.50 **Part of a disarticulated base of the skull** (antero-lateral aspect). Mosaic of the facial bones. Green = sphenoid bone; yellow = ethmoid bone; red = palatine bone.

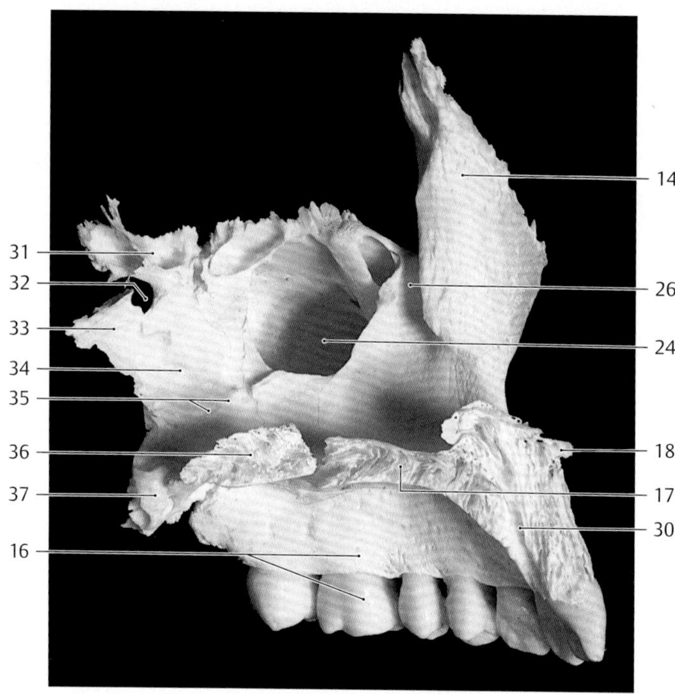


Fig. 8.51 **Left maxilla and palatine bone** (medial aspect).

**Occipital bone**
1 Groove for superior sagittal sinus
2 Internal occipital protuberance
3 Groove for transverse sinus
4 Internal occipital crest

**Sphenoid bone**
5 Greater wing (temporal surface)
6 Lateral pterygoid plate
7 Dorsum sellae
8 Lesser wing
9 Superior orbital fissure
10 Greater wing (orbital surface)

**Ethmoid bone**
11 Ethmoidal air cells
12 Crista galli
13 Orbital plate

**Maxilla**
14 Frontal process
15 Inferior orbital fissure
16 Alveolar process with teeth
17 Palatine process
18 Anterior nasal spine
19 Infra-orbital groove
20 Zygomatic process
21 Location of infra-orbital foramen
22 Middle nasal meatus
23 Inferior nasal meatus
24 Maxillary hiatus (leading to maxillary sinus)
25 Third molar
26 Lacrimal groove
27 Conchal crest
28 Body of maxilla (nasal surface)
29 Nasal crest
30 Incisive canal

**Palatine bone**
31 Orbital process
32 Sphenopalatine notch
33 Sphenoidal process
34 Perpendicular plate
35 Conchal crest
36 Horizontal plate
37 Pyramidal process

**Frontal bone**
38 Squamous part
39 Supra-orbital foramen
40 Frontal notch
41 Frontal spine

**Inferior nasal concha**
42 Inferior nasal concha with maxillary process

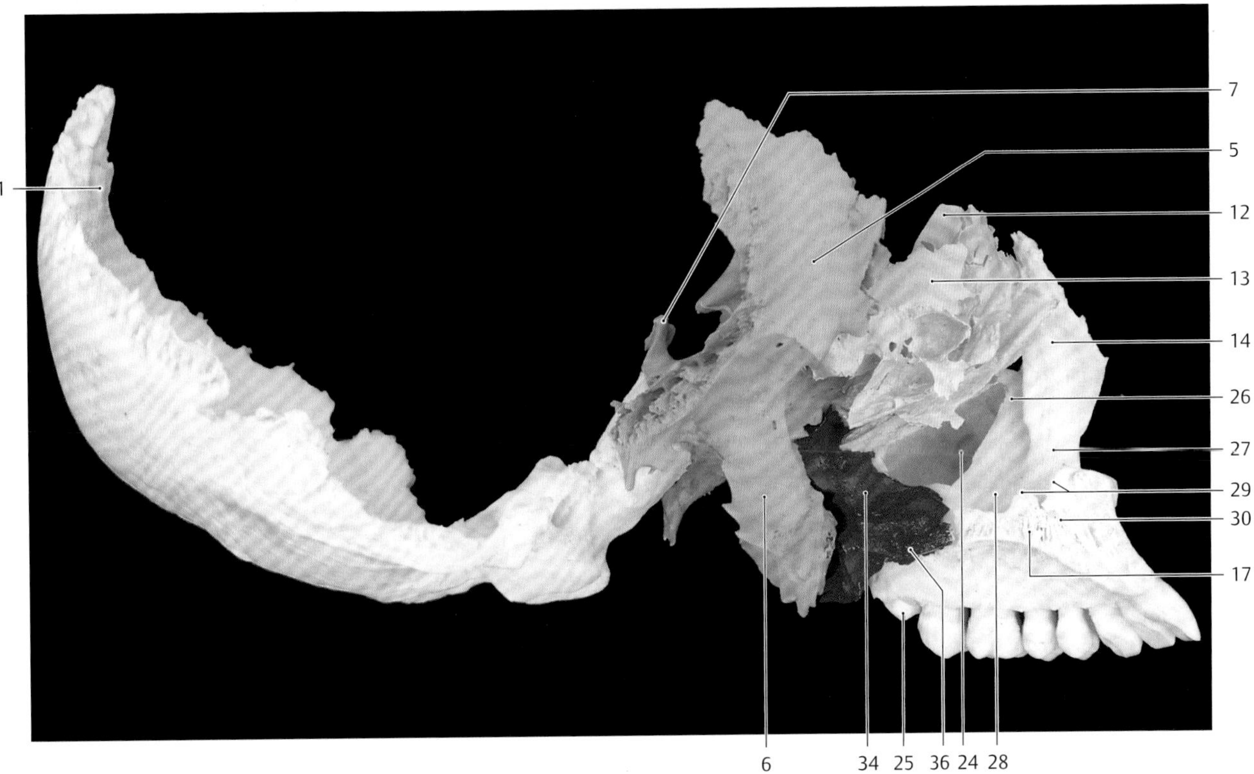


Fig. 8.52 **Part of a disarticulated base of the skull** (medial aspect). Green = sphenoid bone; yellow = ethmoid bone; red = palatine bone; natural colored = left maxilla.

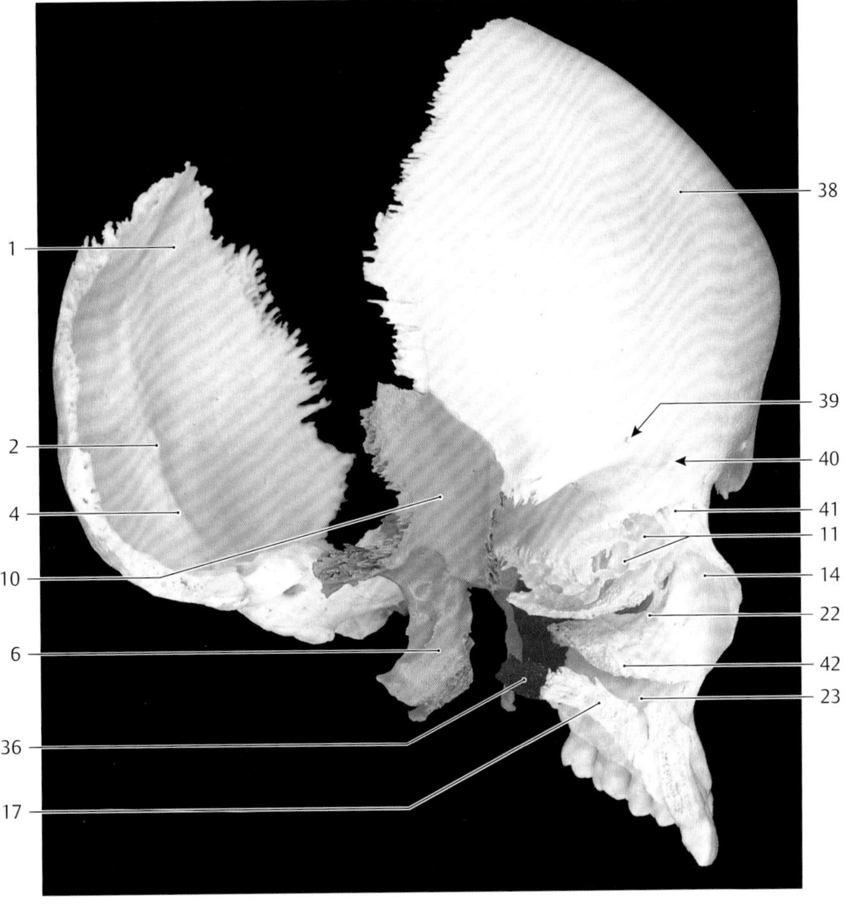


Fig. 8.53 **Part of a disarticulated base of the skull** (oblique-lateral aspect). The same specimen as shown in Figure 8.52 above but with frontal bone.

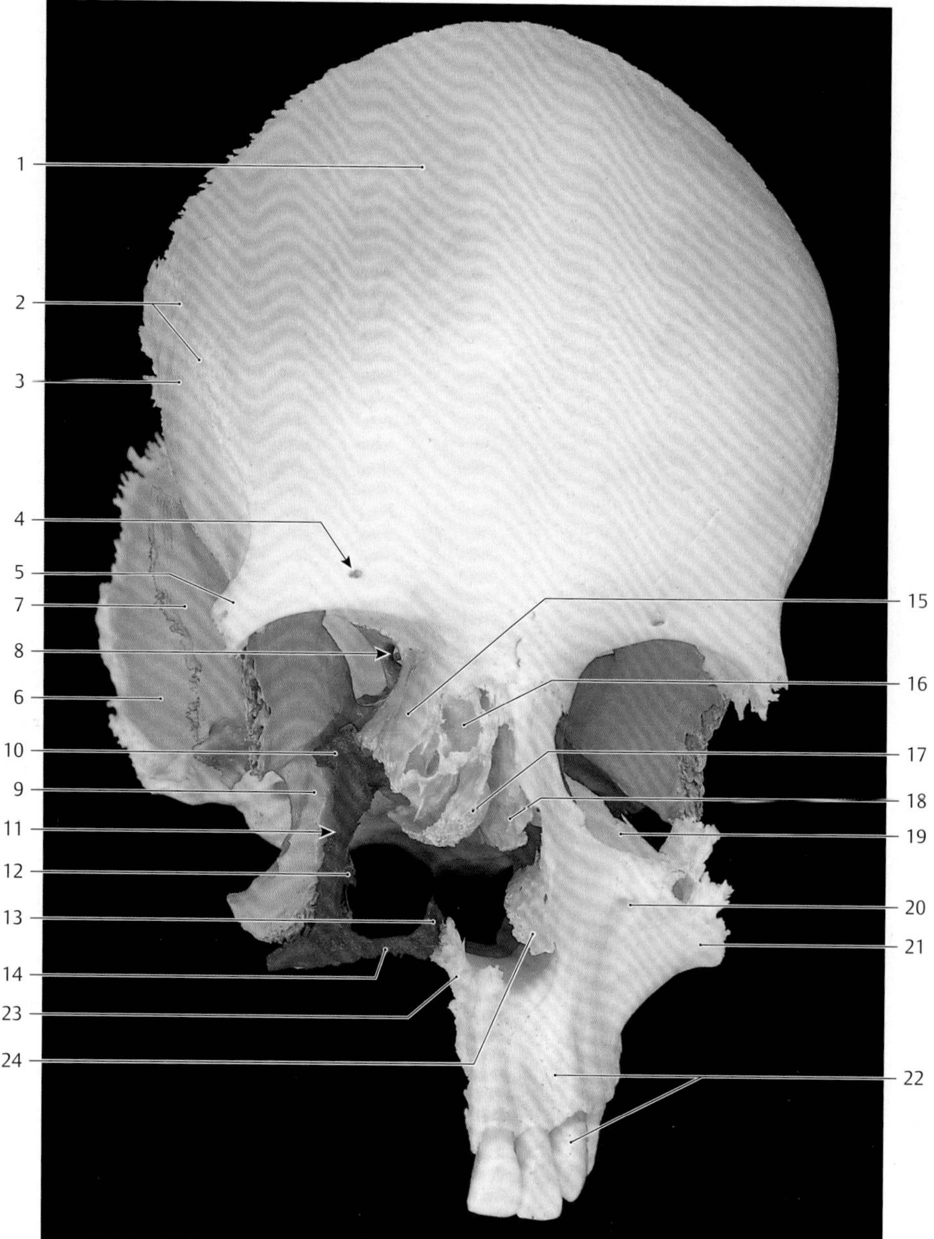


Fig. 8.54 **Part of a disarticulated skull** showing connection of the palatine bone and the maxilla with the ethmoid bone and sphenoid bone (anterior aspect). Red = palatine bone; yellow = ethmoid bone; green = sphenoid bone.

**Frontal bone**
1 Squamous part
2 Inferior temporal line
3 Temporal surface
4 Supra-orbital foramen
5 Zygomatic process

**Occipital bone**
6 Squamous part

**Sphenoid bone**
7 Greater wing (temporal surface)
8 Optic canal within the lesser wing
9 Lateral pterygoid plate

**Palatine bone**
10 Orbital process
11 Perpendicular plate
12 Conchal crest
13 Nasal crest
14 Horizontal plate

**Ethmoid bone**
15 Orbital plate
16 Ethmoidal air cell
17 Middle concha
18 Perpendicular plate (part of bony nasal septum)

**Maxilla**
19 Infra-orbital groove
20 Infra-orbital foramen
21 Zygomatic process
22 Alveolar process with teeth
23 Palatine process

**Left inferior nasal concha**
24 Anterior part of inferior concha

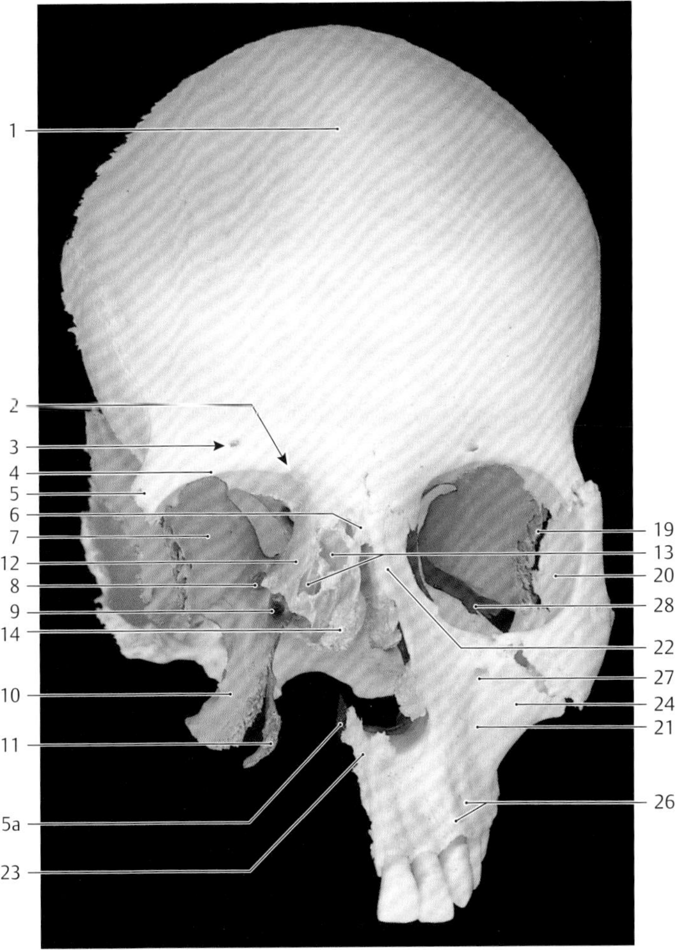


Fig. 8.55 **Part of a disarticulated skull** showing the connection of the maxilla with the frontal and zygomatic bones (anterior aspect). Yellow = ethmoid bone; red = palatine bone; green = sphenoid bone.

**Frontal bone**
1 Squamous part
2 Frontal notch
3 Supra-orbital foramen
4 Supra-orbital margin
5 Zygomatic process
6 Frontal spine

**Sphenoid bone**
7 Greater wing (orbital surface)
8 Foramen rotundum
9 Pterygoid or Vidian canal
10 Lateral pterygoid plate
11 Medial pterygoid plate

**Ethmoid bone**
12 Orbital plate
13 Ethmoidal air cells
14 Middle concha

**Palatine bone**
15 Horizontal plate
15a Nasal crest
16 Pyramidal process
17 Lesser palatine foramen
18 Greater palatine foramen

**Zygomatic bone**
19 Frontal process
20 Orbital surface

**Maxilla**
21 Canine fossa
22 Frontal process
23 Palatine process
24 Zygomatic process
25 Alveolar process and teeth
26 Juga alveolaria
27 Infra-orbital foramen
28 Infra-orbital groove
29 Anterior nasal aperture
30 Anterior nasal spine

**Incisive bone**
31 Central incisor and incisive bone or premaxilla
32 Incisive fossa

**Vomer**
33 Ala of the vomer

**Sutures and choanae**
34 Median palatine suture
35 Transverse palatine suture
36 Choanae

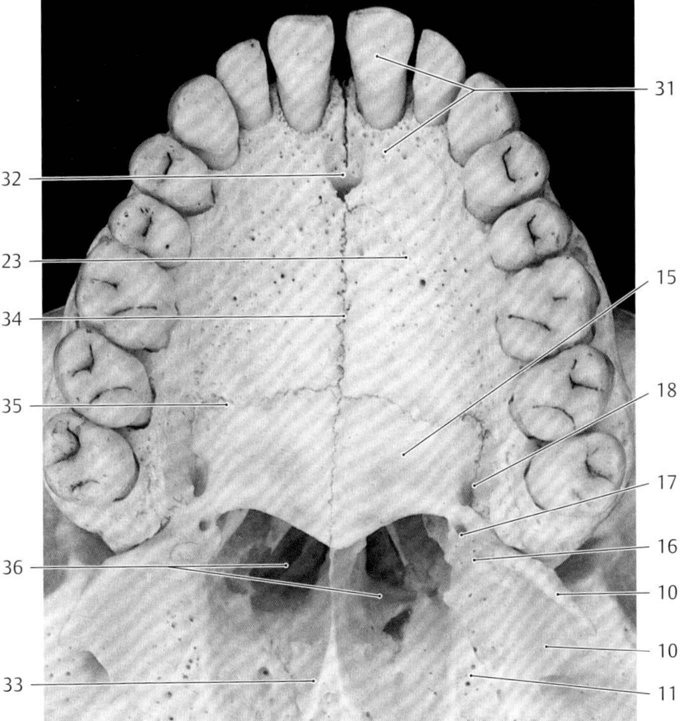


Fig. 8.56 **Bony palate and teeth of the maxillae** (from below).

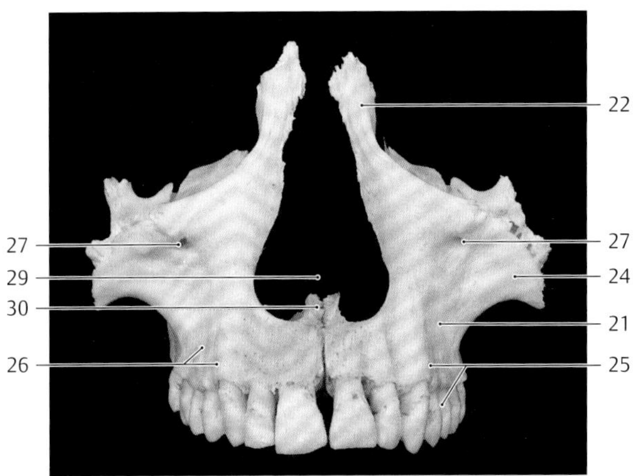


Fig. 8.57 **Anterior view of both maxillae** forming the anterior bony aperture of the nose.

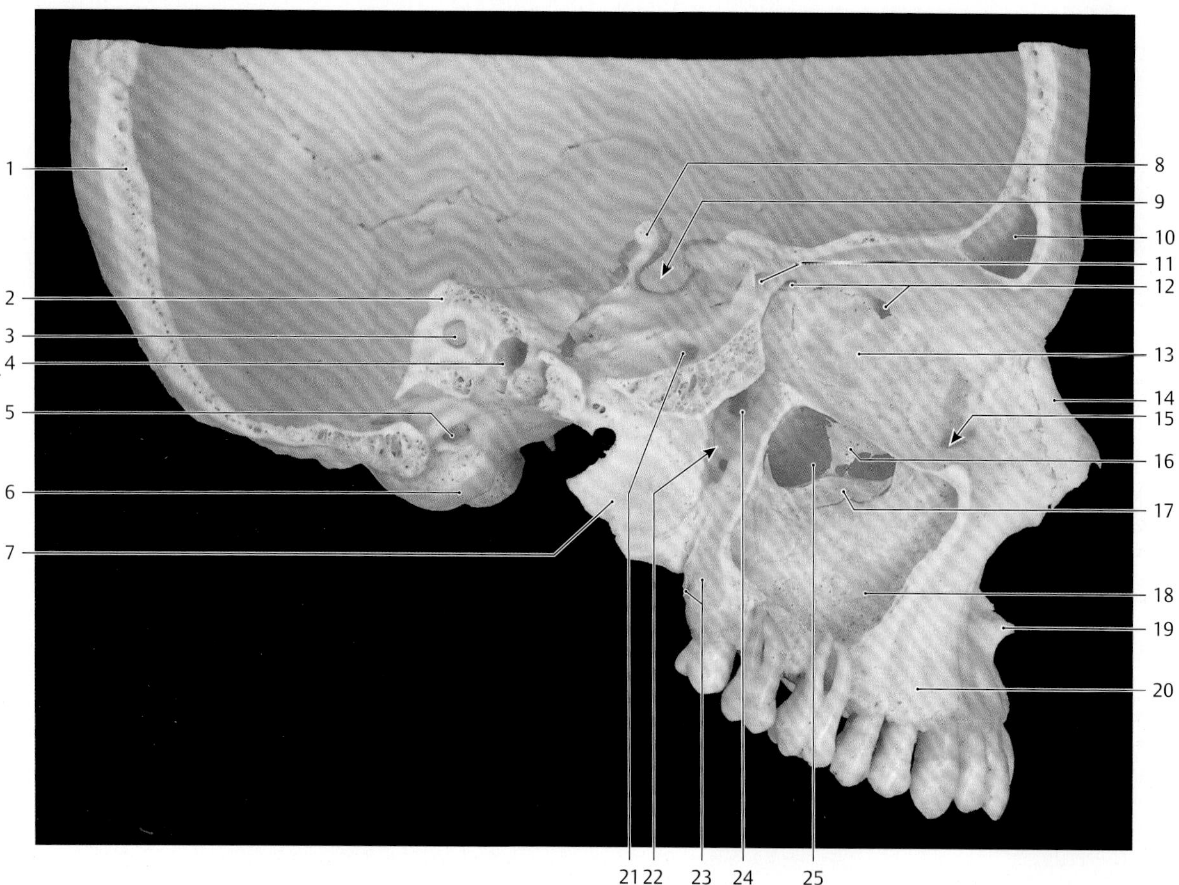


**Fig. 8.58 Pterygopalatine fossa, maxillary sinus, and orbit.** Paramedian section through the skull (right side, lateral aspect). The frontal and maxillary sinuses have been opened.

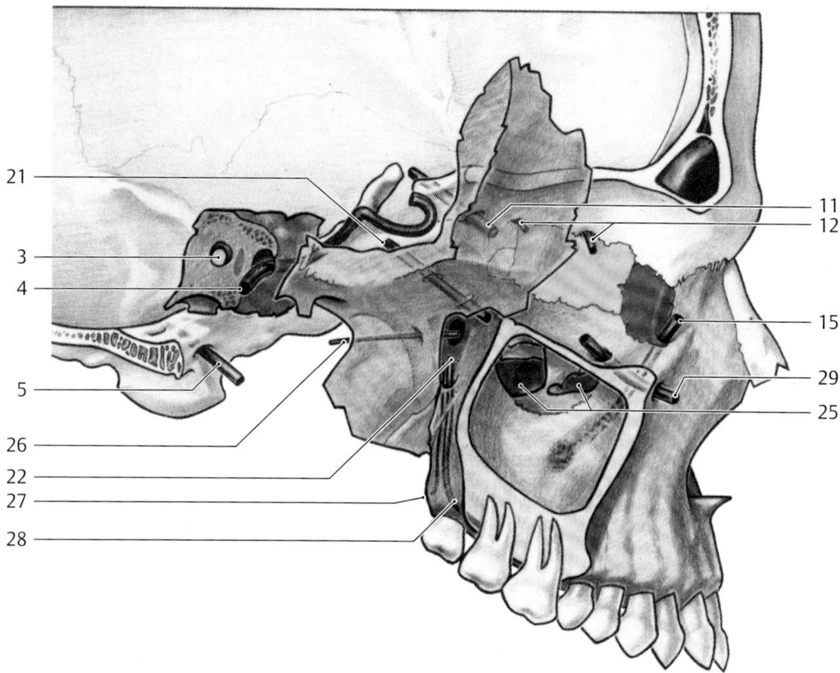


**Fig. 8.59 Illustration of canals and foramina connected with the right orbit and pterygopalatine fossa** (see corresponding Fig. 8.58 above). The greater wing of the sphenoid bone is shown as being transparent. Brown = temporal bone; yellow = ethmoid bone; green = sphenoid bone; red = lacrimal bone; light red = inferior nasal concha; violet = maxilla; red = palatine bone.

1 Occipital bone
2 Temporal bone (petrous part)
3 Internal acoustic meatus
4 Carotid canal
5 Hypoglossal canal
6 Occipital condyle
7 Lateral plate of pterygoid process
8 Dorsum of sella turcica
9 Sella turcica
10 Frontal sinus
11 Optic canal
12 Posterior and anterior ethmoidal foramina
13 Orbital plate of ethmoid bone
14 Nasal bone
15 Nasolacrimal canal
16 Uncinate process
17 Inferior nasal concha (maxillary process)
18 Maxillary sinus
19 Anterior nasal spine
20 Alveolar process of maxilla
21 Foramen rotundum
22 Pterygopalatine fossa
23 Tuberosity of maxilla with alveolar foramina
24 Sphenopalatine foramen
25 Maxillary hiatus
26 Pterygoid or Vidian canal
27 Lesser palatine canal
28 Greater palatine canal
29 Infra-orbital canal

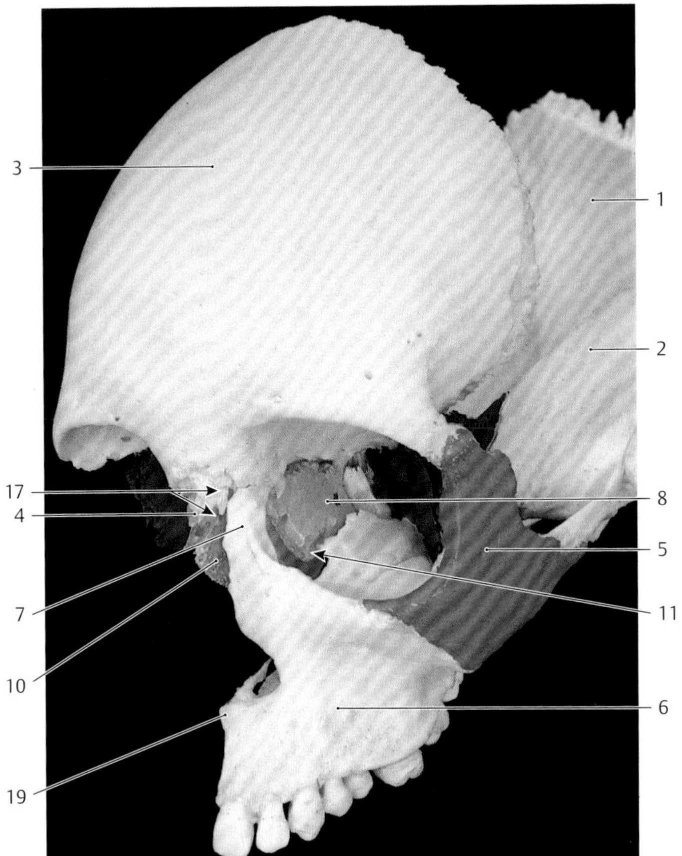


Fig. 8.60 **Part of a disarticulated skull** (antero-lateral aspect). Orange = zygomatic bone; yellow = ethmoid bone; dark green = sphenoid bone; arrows = locations of the lacrimal bone (11) and the nasal bone (17).

1 Occipital bone
2 Temporal bone
3 Frontal bone
4 Nasal spine of frontal bone
5 Zygomatic bone
6 Maxilla
7 Frontal process of maxilla
8 Ethmoid bone
9 Orbital plate of ethmoid bone
10 Perpendicular plate of ethmoid bone
11 Site of lacrimal bone
12 Lacrimal groove of lacrimal bone
13 Posterior lacrimal crest
14 Fossa for lacrimal sac
15 Lacrimal hamulus
16 Nasolacrimal canal
17 Site of nasal bone
18 Nasal foramina of nasal bone
19 Anterior nasal spine of maxilla
20 Vomer
21 Greater wing of sphenoid bone
22 Anterior and posterior ethmoidal foramina
23 Optic canal
24 Superior orbital fissure
25 Inferior orbital fissure
26 Infra-orbital groove
27 Infra-orbital foramen

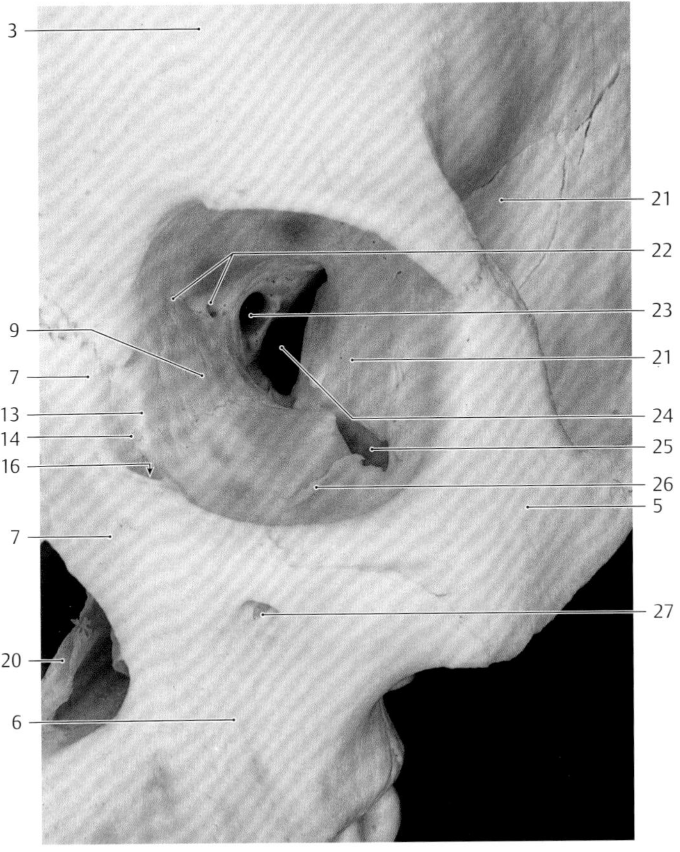


Fig. 8.61 **Left orbit** (anterior aspect).

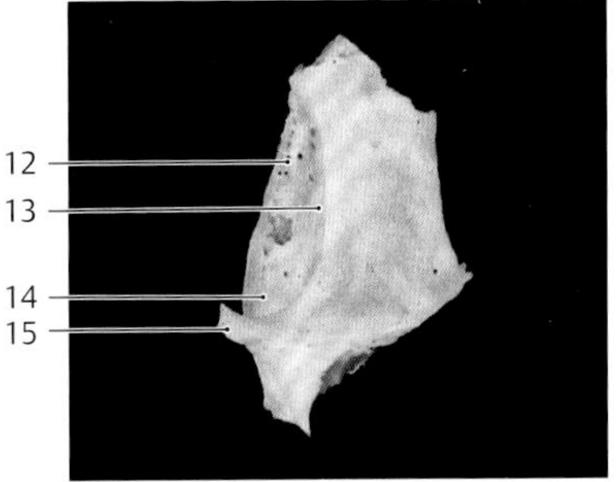


Fig. 8.62 **Left lacrimal bone** (anterior aspect).

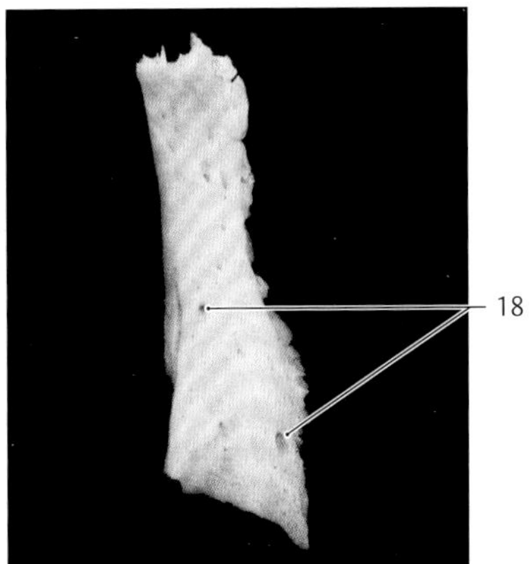


Fig. 8.63 **Left nasal bone** (anterior aspect).

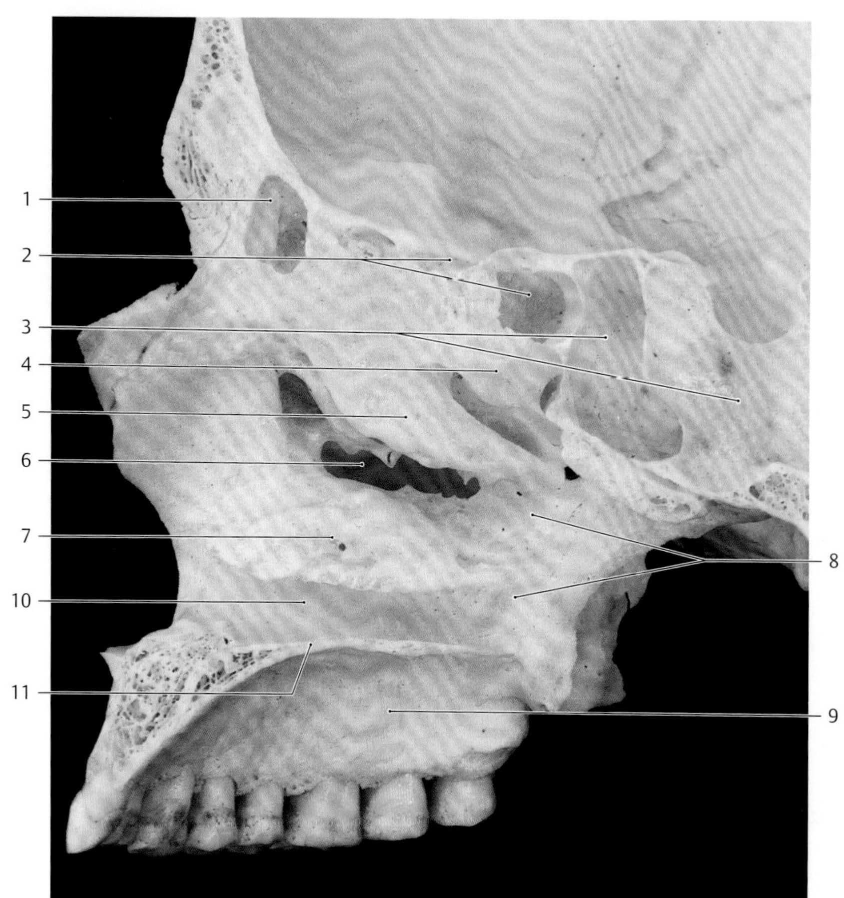


1 Frontal sinus
2 Ethmoidal air cells
3 Sphenoidal sinus
4 Superior nasal concha
5 Middle nasal concha
6 Maxillary hiatus
7 Inferior nasal concha
8 Palatine bone
9 Maxilla
10 Inferior meatus
11 Palatine process of the maxilla

Fig. 8.64 **Lateral wall of the nasal cavity.** Median section through the skull.

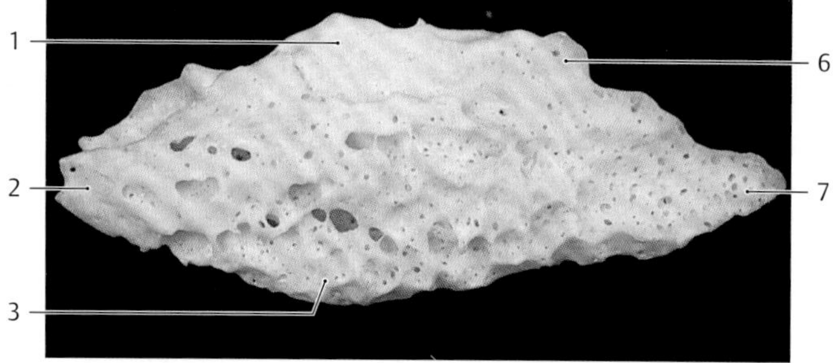


Fig. 8.65 **Right inferior nasal concha** (medial aspect). Anterior part to the left.

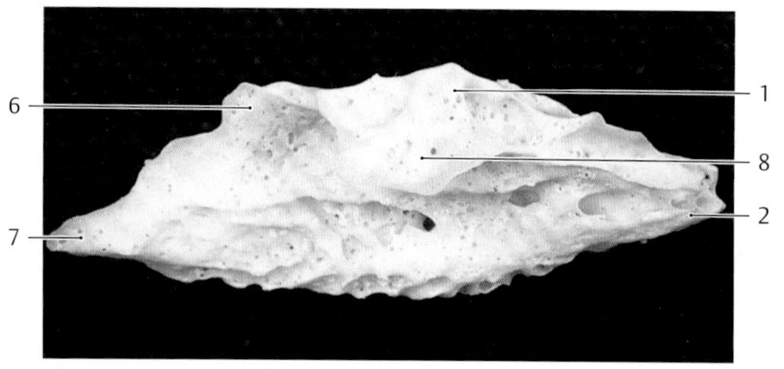


Fig. 8.66 **Right inferior nasal concha** (lateral aspect). Anterior part to the right.

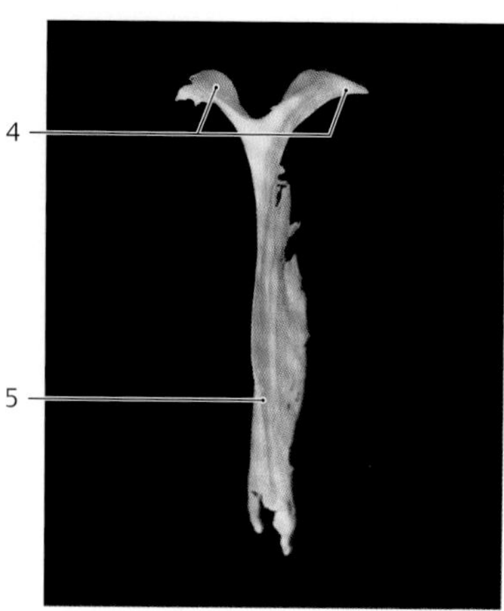


Fig. 8.67 **Vomer** (posterior aspect).

**Inferior concha and vomer**

1 Ethmoidal process
2 Anterior part of concha
3 Inferior border
4 Ala of vomer
5 Posterior border of nasal septum
6 Lacrimal process
7 Posterior part of concha
8 Maxillary process

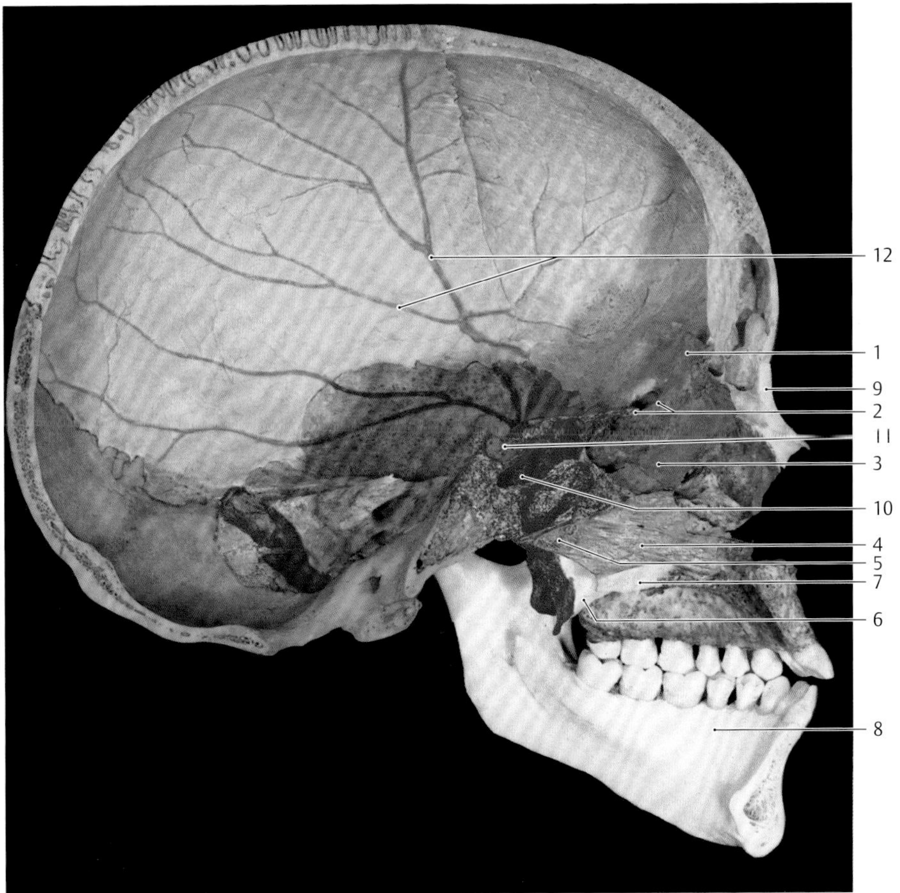


Fig. 8.68 **Paramedian sagittal section through the skull including the nasal septum.**

1 Crista galli
2 Cribriform plate of ethmoid bone
3 Perpendicular plate of ethmoid bone
4 Vomer
5 Ala of the vomer
6 Palatine bone (perpendicular process)
7 Palatine bone (horizontal plate)
8 Mandible
9 Nasal bone
10 Sphenoidal sinus
11 Hypophysial fossa (sella turcica)
12 Grooves for the middle meningeal artery

**Cartilages of the nose**
13 Lateral nasal cartilage
14 Greater alar cartilage
15 Lesser alar cartilages
16 Septal cartilage
17 Location of nasal bone

| | | |
|---|---|---|
| Blue | = | Occipital bone |
| Light green | = | Parietal bone |
| Yellow | = | Frontal bone |
| Dark brown | = | Temporal bone |
| Red | = | Sphenoid bone |
| Dark green | = | Ethmoid bone |
| Light blue | = | Nasal bone |
| Pink | = | Inferior concha |
| Orange | = | Vomer |
| Violet | = | Maxilla |
| White | = | Palatine bone |
| White | = | Mandible |

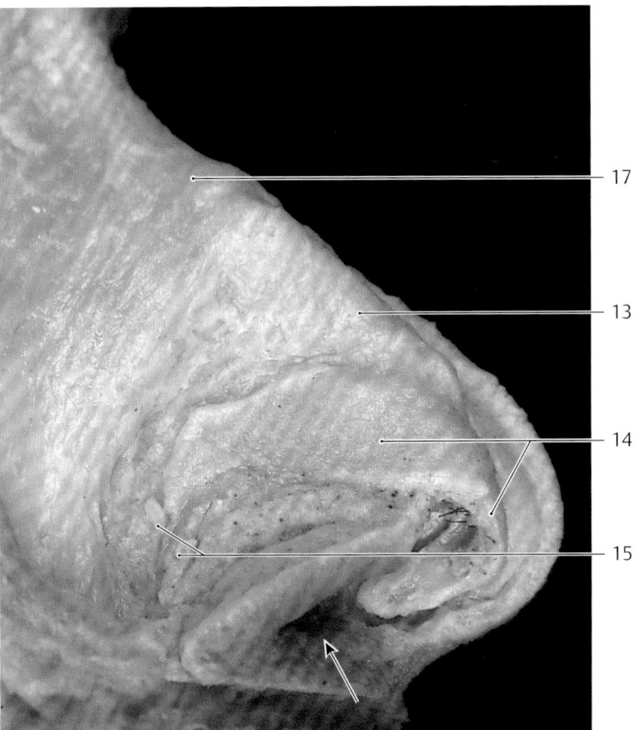


Fig. 8.69 **Cartilages of the nose** (right anterior aspect). Arrow = nostril, framed by nasal wing.

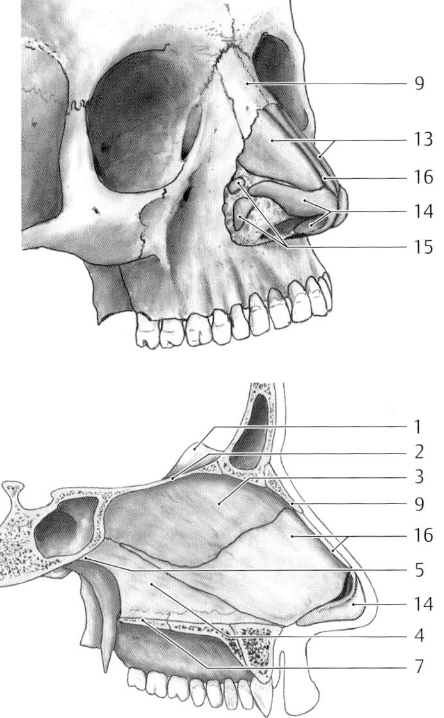


Fig. 8.70 **Shape of the cartilages of the nose.**

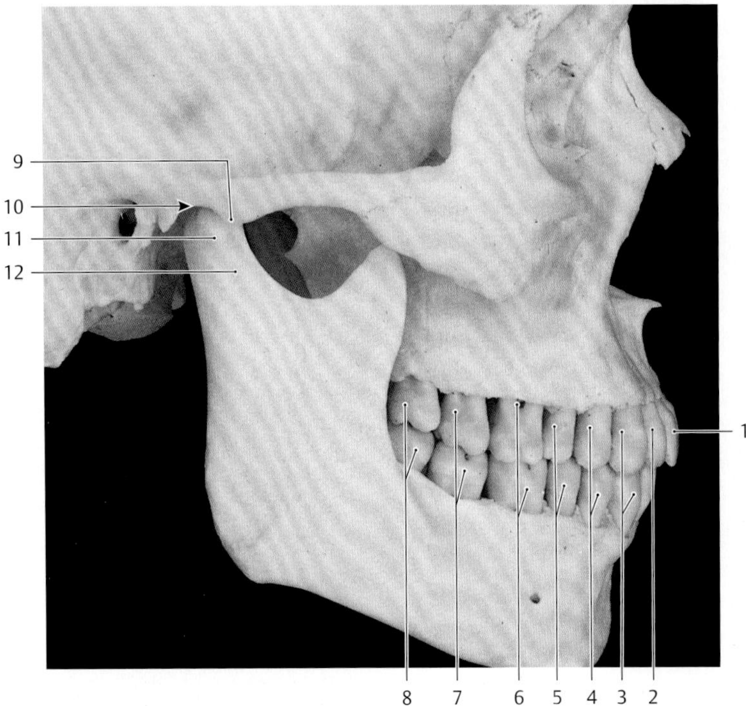


Fig. 8.71 **Normal position of the teeth.** Dentition in centric occlusion (lateral aspect).

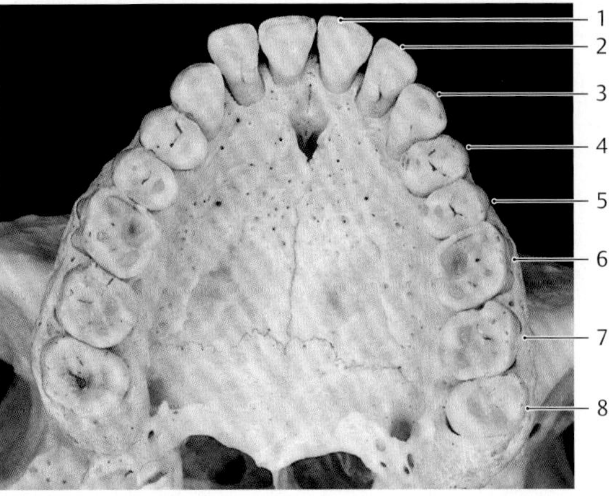


Fig. 8.72 **Upper teeth of the adult** (inferior aspect).

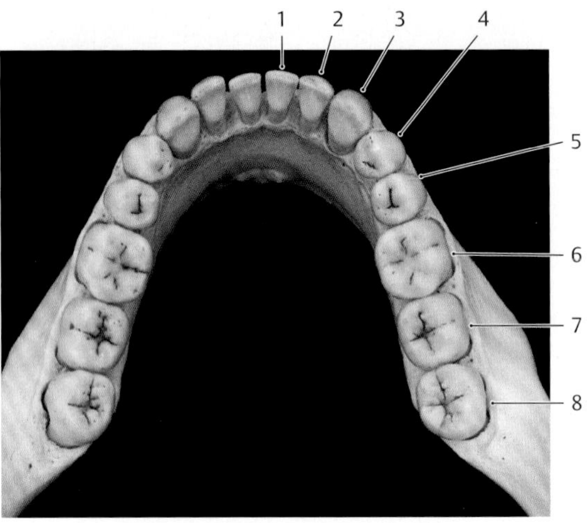


Fig. 8.73 **Lower teeth of the adult** (superior aspect).

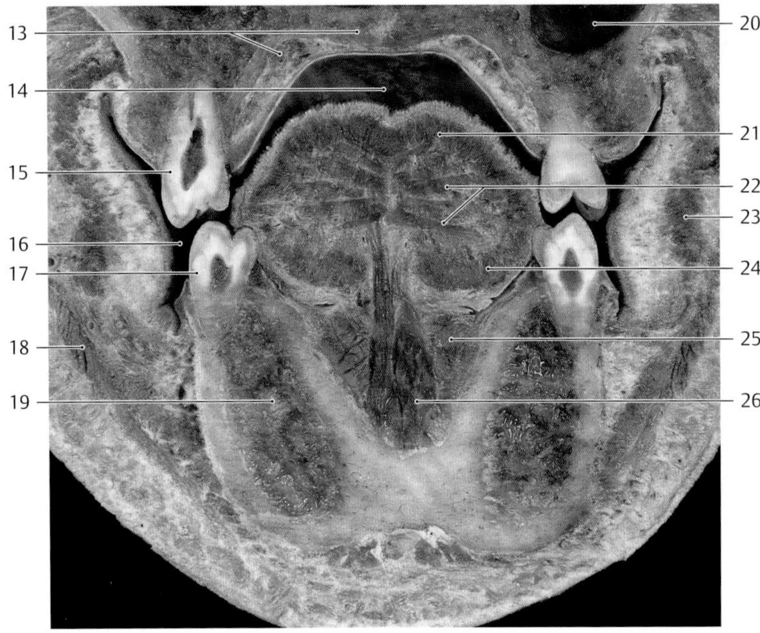


Fig. 8.74 **Coronal section through the oral cavity** (anterior aspect).

1 Central incisor
2 Lateral incisor
3 Canines
4 First premolars or bicuspids
5 Second premolars or bicuspids
6 First molars
7 Second molars
8 Third molars
9 Articular tubercle
10 Mandibular fossa
11 Head of mandible
12 Condylar process
13 Hard palate and palatine glands
14 Oral cavity
15 Upper molar
16 Oral vestibule
17 Lower molar
18 Platysma muscle
19 Mandible
20 Maxillary sinus
21 Superior longitudinal muscle of tongue
22 Transverse muscle of tongue
23 Buccinator muscle
24 Inferior longitudinal muscle of tongue
25 Sublingual gland
26 Genioglossus muscle

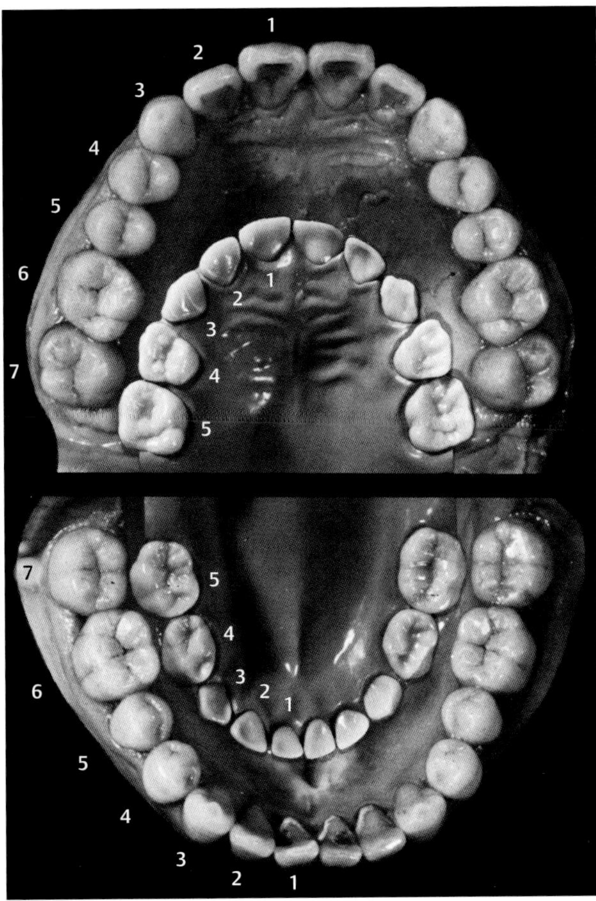


Fig. 8.75 **Comparison of the deciduous and permanent teeth.** Notice that the breadth of the alveolar arch of the child's mandible and maxilla holding the deciduous teeth is nearly the same as the comparable portion in the jaws of the adult. Note the emergence of the third molars. The numbers of the teeth correspond to the numbers in the Figure 8.77 below.

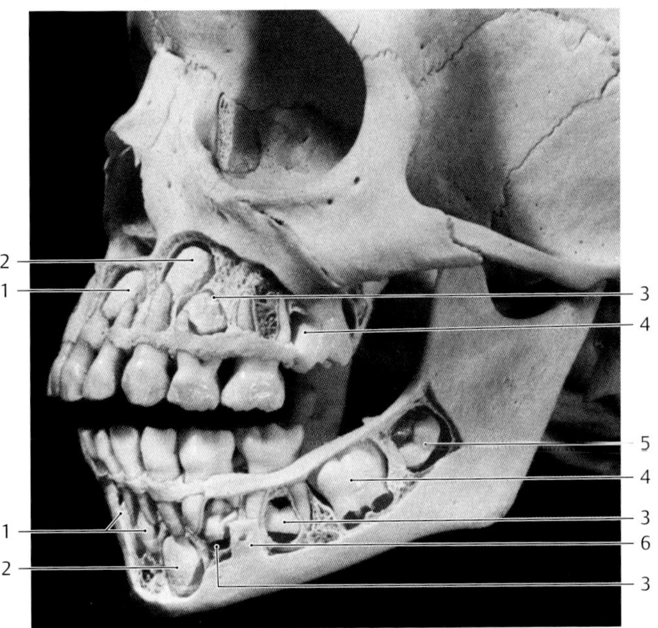


Fig. 8.76 **Deciduous teeth in a child's skull.** The developing crowns of the permanent teeth are displayed in their crypts in the maxilla and mandible.

1 Permanent incisors
2 Permanent cuspid (canine)
3 Premolars
4 First permanent molar
5 Second permanent molar
6 Mental foramen

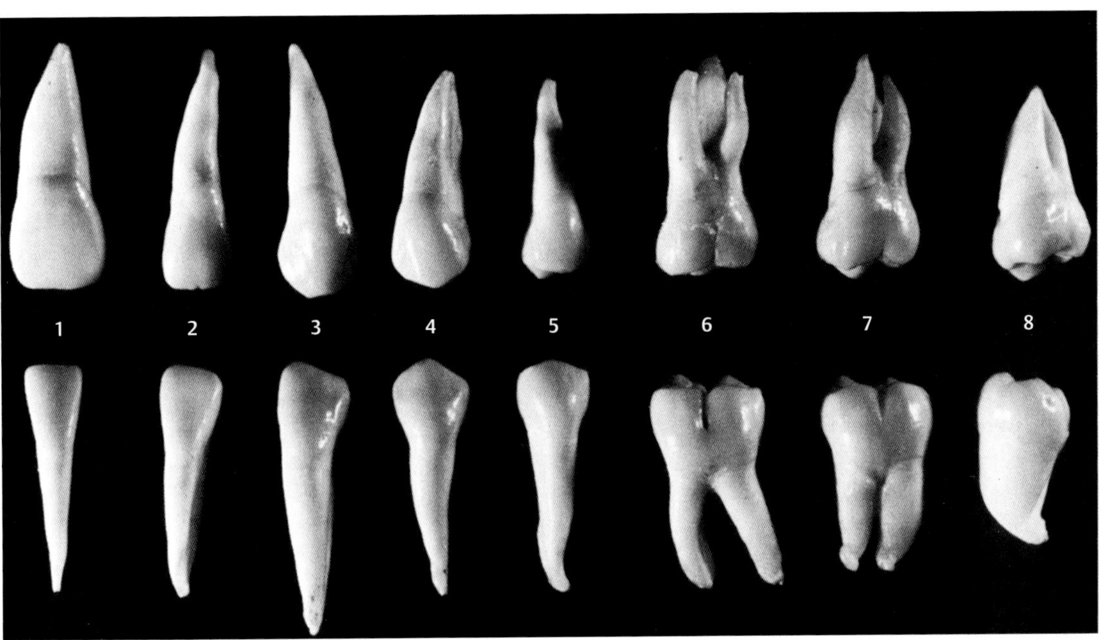


Fig. 8.77 **Isolated teeth of the alveolar part of the maxilla** (top row) and the **mandible** (lower row), labial surface of the teeth.

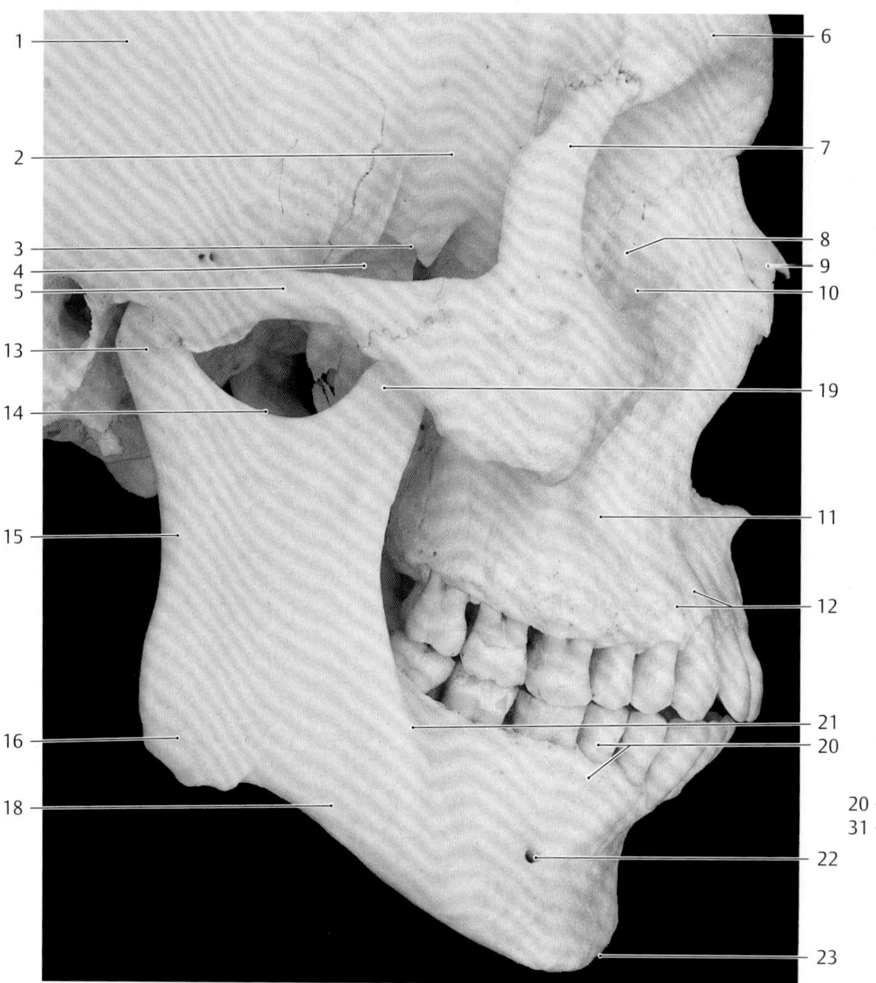


Fig. 8.78 **Lateral aspect of the facial bones.** Mandible and teeth in the position of occlusion. Upper and lower jaw occluded.

Fig. 8.79 **Mandible of the adult** (anterior aspect).

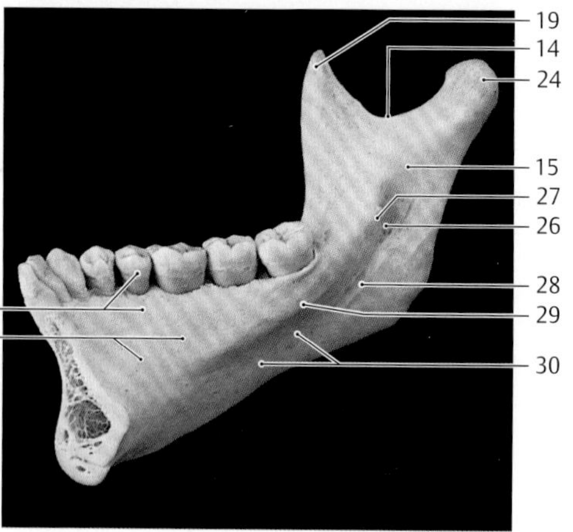


Fig. 8.80 **Right half of the mandible** (medial aspect).

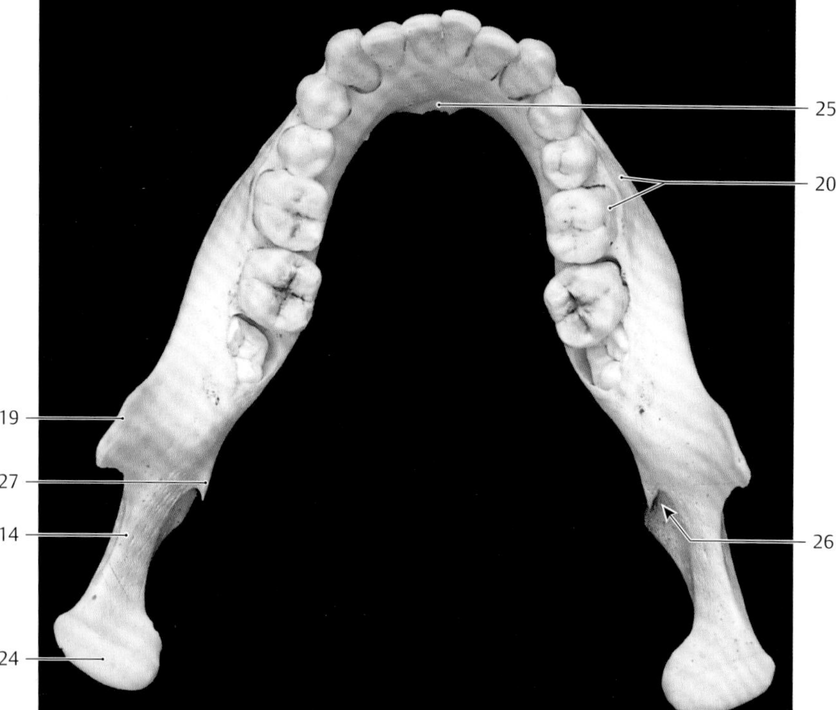


Fig. 8.81 **Mandible of the adult** (superior aspect).

1 Temporal bone
2 Temporal fossa (greater wing of sphenoid bone)
3 Infratemporal crest
4 Infratemporal fossa
5 Zygomatic arch
6 Frontal bone
7 Zygomatic bone (frontal process)
8 Lacrimal bone
9 Nasal bone
10 Lacrimal groove
11 Maxilla (canine fossa)
12 Alveolar process of maxilla

**Mandible**
13 Condylar process
14 Mandibular notch
15 Ramus of the mandible
16 Masseteric tuberosity
17 Angle of the mandible
18 Body of the mandible
19 Coronoid process
20 Alveolar process including teeth
21 Oblique line
22 Mental foramen
23 Mental protuberance
24 Head of the mandible
25 Genial tubercle or mental spine
26 Mandibular foramen (entrance to mandibular canal)
27 Lingula
28 Mylohyoid sulcus
29 Mylohyoid line
30 Submandibular fossa
31 Sublingual fossa

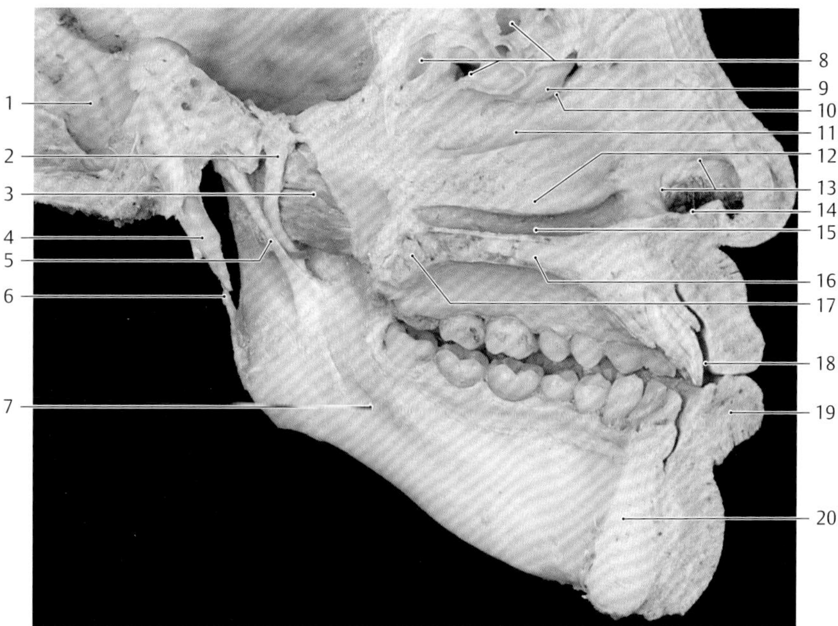


Fig. 8.82 **Ligaments of temporomandibular joint.** Left half of the head (medial aspect).

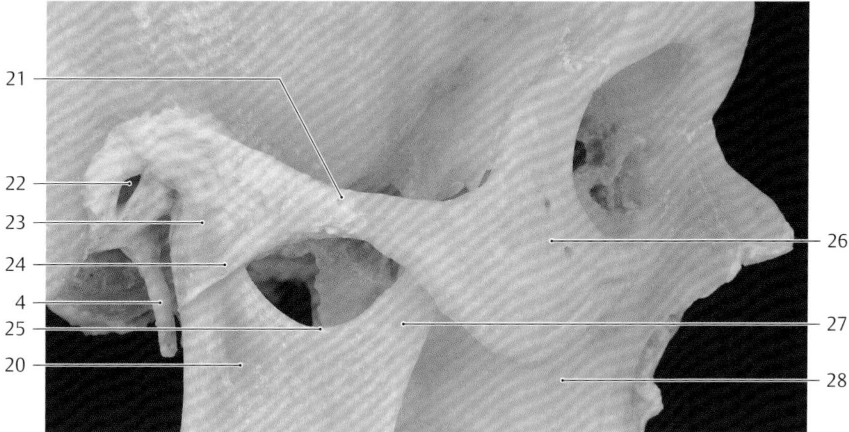


Fig. 8.83 **Temporomandibular joint with ligaments** (lateral aspect).

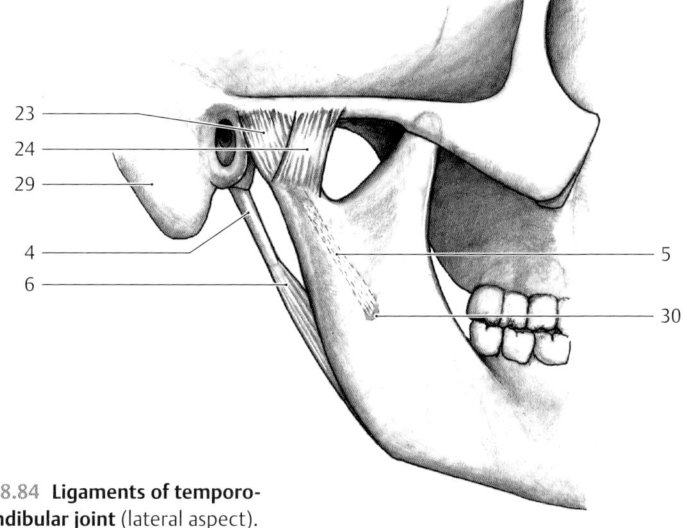


Fig. 8.84 **Ligaments of temporomandibular joint** (lateral aspect).

1 Groove for sigmoid sinus
2 Mandibular nerve
3 Lateral pterygoid muscle
4 Styloid process
5 Sphenomandibular ligament
6 Stylomandibular ligament
7 Mylohyoid groove
8 Ethmoidal air cells
9 Ethmoidal bulla
10 Hiatus semilunaris
11 Middle meatus
12 Inferior nasal concha
13 Limen nasi
14 Vestibule with hairs
15 Inferior meatus
16 Hard palate
17 Soft palate
18 Vestibule of oral cavity
19 Lower lip
20 Mandible
21 Zygomatic arch
22 External acoustic meatus
23 Articular capsule
24 Lateral ligament
25 Mandibular notch
26 Zygomatic bone
27 Coronoid process
28 Maxilla
29 Mastoid process
30 Mandibular foramen

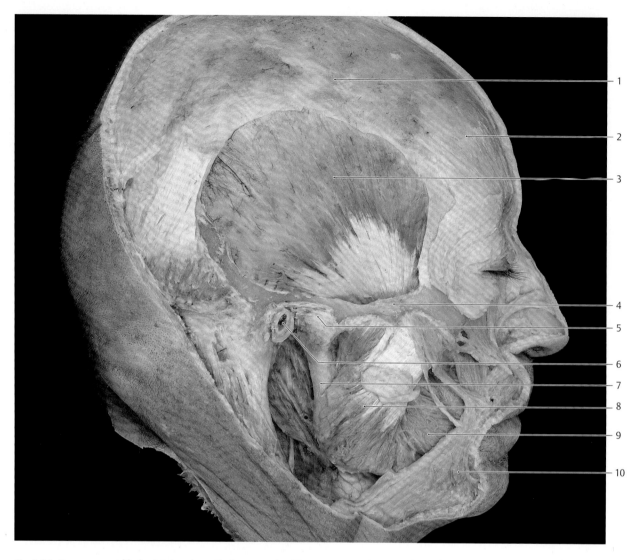

Fig. 8.85 **Temporomandibular joint and masticatory muscles.** The masseter and temporal muscles are shown.

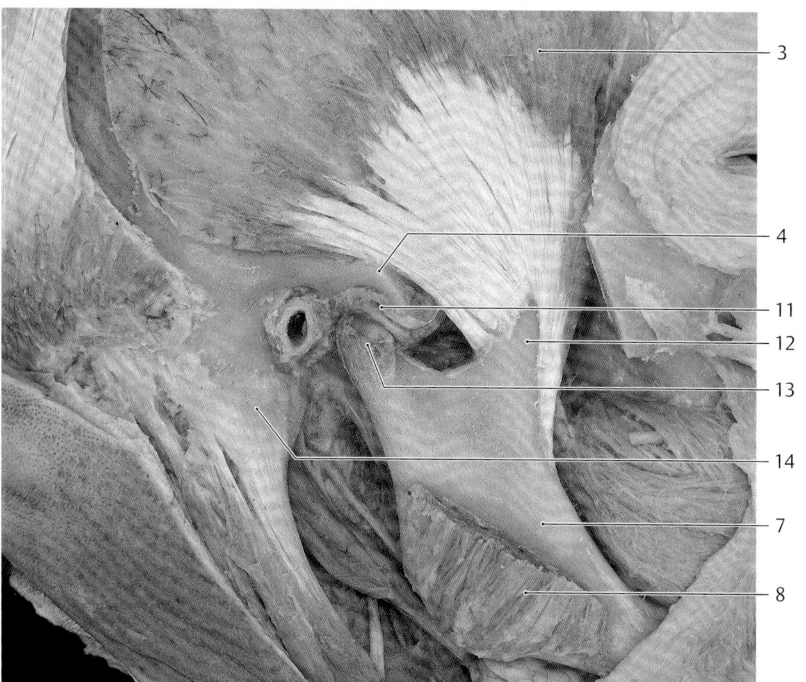


1 Galea aponeurotica
2 Frontal belly of occipitofrontalis muscle
3 Temporal muscle
4 Zygomatic arch
5 Temporomandibular joint
6 External acoustic meatus
7 Mandible
8 Masseter muscle
9 Buccinator muscle
10 Platysma muscle
11 Articular disc of temporomandibular joint
12 Coronoid process of mandible
13 Condylar process of mandible
14 Mastoid process

Fig. 8.86 **Temporal muscle** with insertion at the mandible and the temporomandibular joint. The zygomatic arch and masseter muscle have been partly removed.

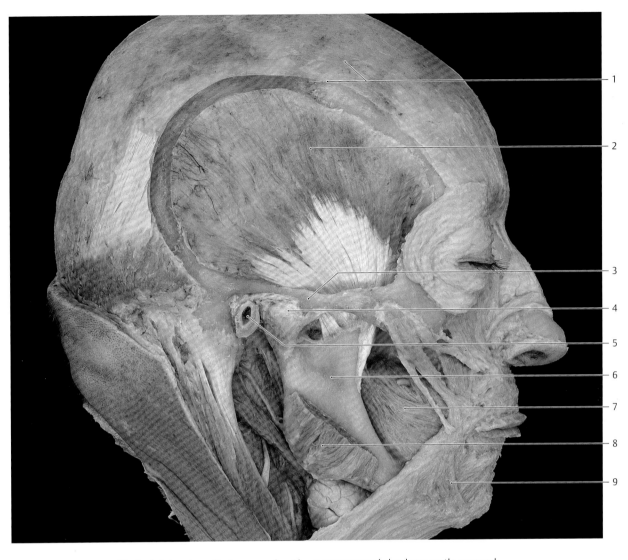

Fig. 8.87 **Temporomandibular joint and masticatory muscles.** The masseter muscle has been partly removed.

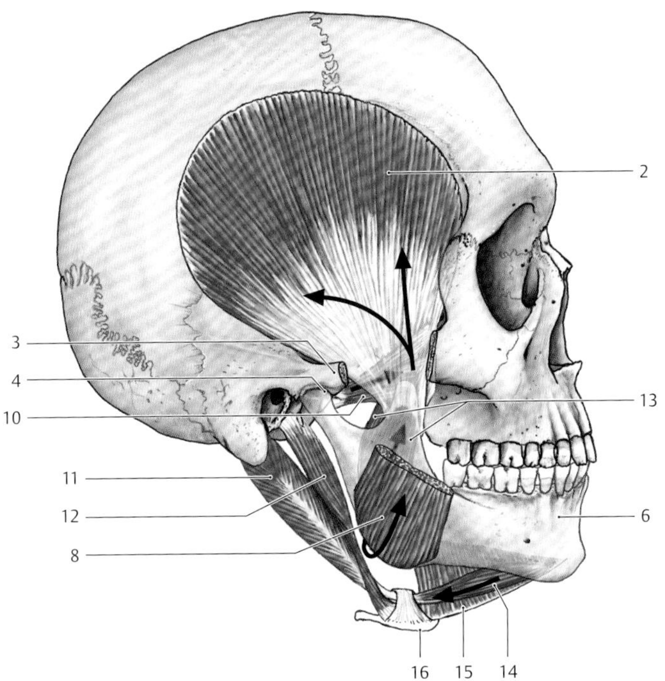


1 Galea aponeurotica
2 Temporal muscle
3 Zygomatic arch
4 Temporomandibular joint
5 External acoustic meatus
6 Mandible
7 Buccinator muscle
8 Masseter muscle (cut)
9 Platysma muscle
10 Lateral pterygoid muscle
11 Posterior belly of digastric muscle
12 Stylohyoid muscle
13 Medial pterygoid muscle
14 Anterior belly of digastric muscle
15 Mylohyoid muscle
16 Hyoid bone

Fig. 8.88 **Effect of the masticatory muscles on the temporomandibular joint** (arrows).

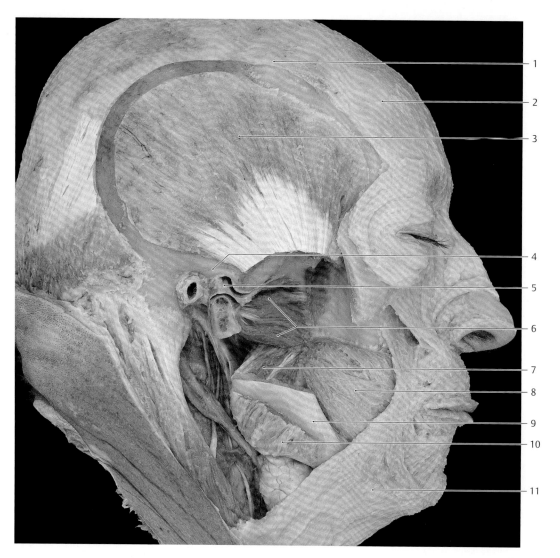

1 Galea aponeurotica
2 Frontal belly of occipitofrontalis muscle
3 Temporal muscle
4 Zygomatic arch
5 Articular disc of temporomandibular joint
6 Lateral pterygoid muscle
7 Medial pterygoid muscle
8 Buccinator muscle
9 Mandible
10 Masseter muscle
11 Platysma muscle
12 Temporomandibular joint
13 External acoustic meatus

**Fig. 8.89 Temporomandibular joint and masticatory muscles.** The zygomatic arch and part of the mandible have been removed to reveal the medial and lateral pterygoid muscles.

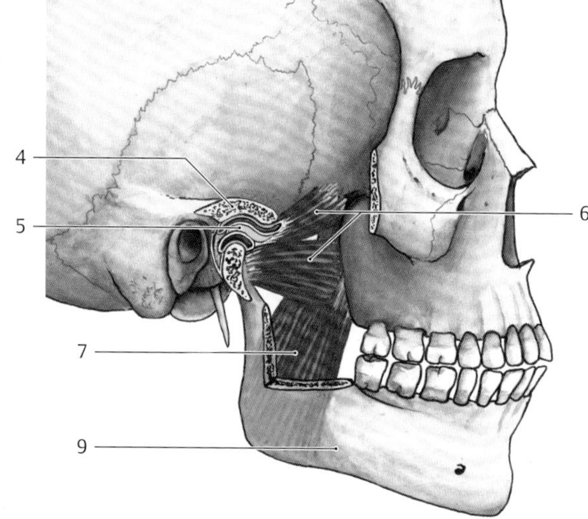


**Fig. 8.90 Medial and lateral pterygoid muscles** and their connections with the articular disc of the temporomandibular joint.

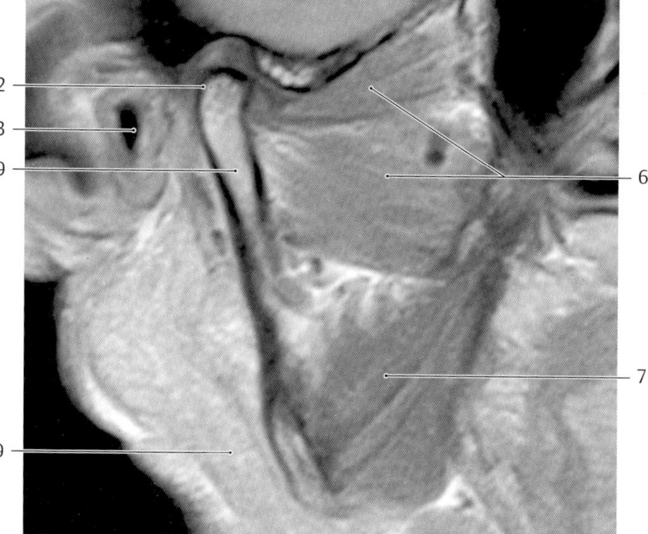


**Fig. 8.91 Temporomandibular joint and masticatory muscles** (sagittal section, MRI scan). (Courtesy of Prof. Uder, Institute of Radiology, University Hospital Erlangen, Germany.)

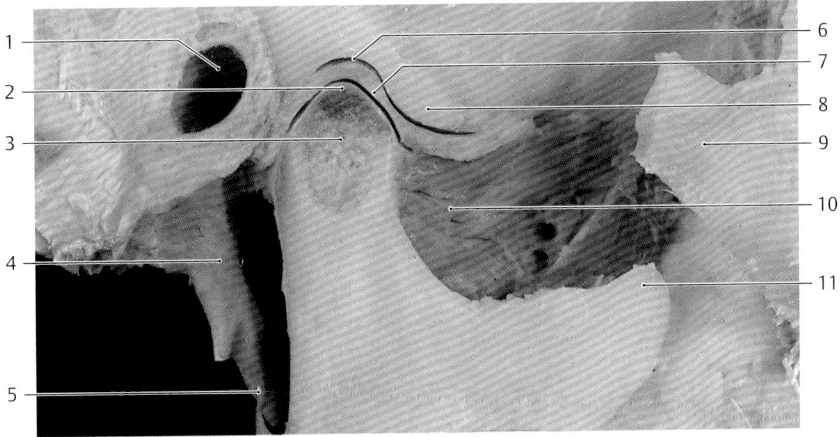


Fig. 8.92 **Temporomandibular joint** (sagittal section).

1 External acoustic meatus
2 Articular cartilage of condylar process
3 Condylar process of mandible
4 Styloid process
5 Stylomandibular ligament
6 Mandibular fossa
7 Articular disc
8 Articular tubercle
9 Zygomatic bone
10 Lateral pterygoid muscle
11 Coronoid process of mandible
12 Posterior belly of digastric muscle
13 Masseter muscle
14 Temporal muscle
15 Medial pterygoid muscle
16 Parotid duct
17 Buccinator muscle
18 Mandible
19 Mandibular foramen

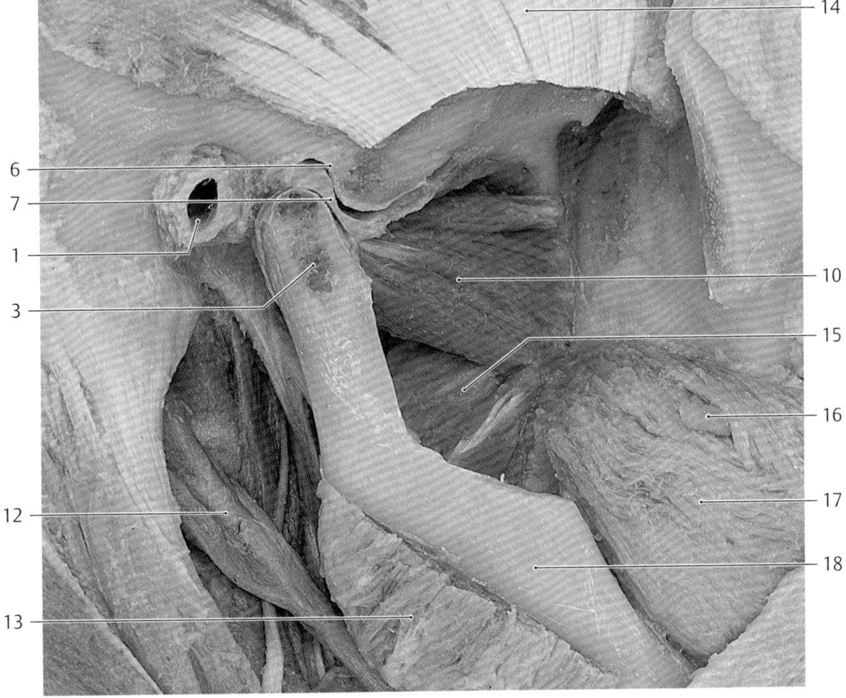


Fig. 8.93 **Temporomandibular joint.** Dissection of the articular disc and the related muscles (lateral aspect).

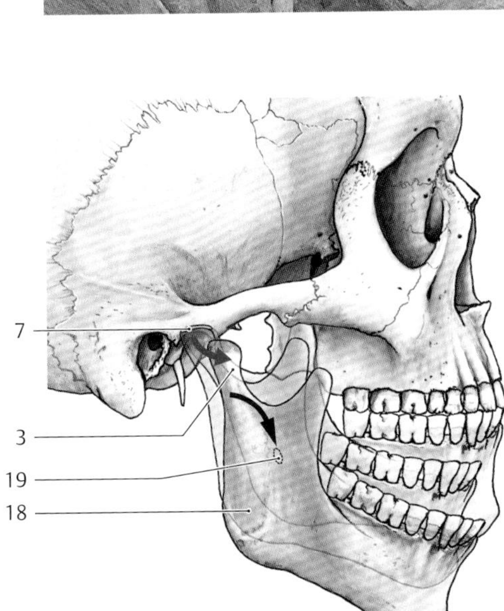


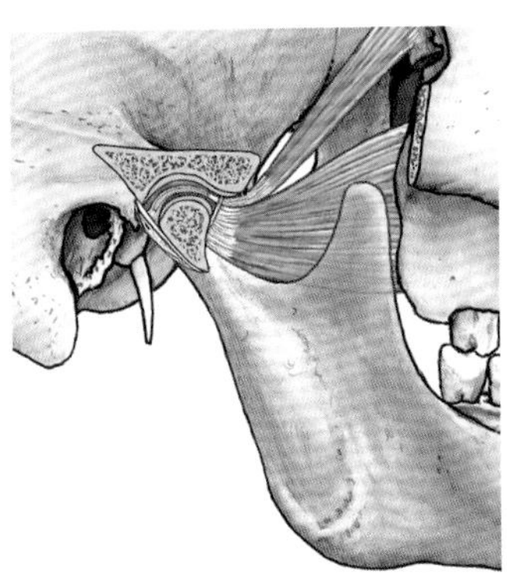

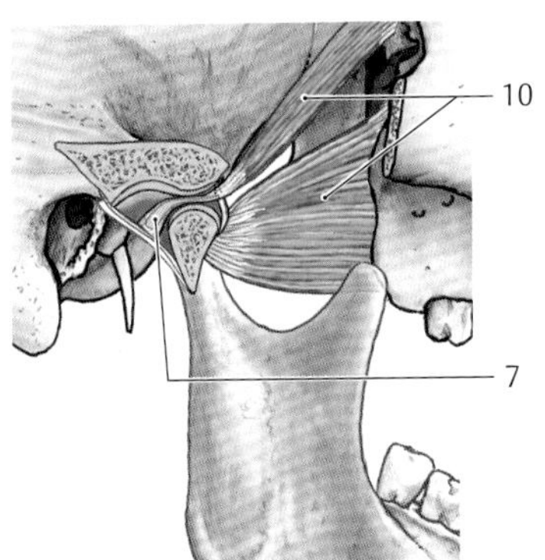


Fig. 8.94 **Movements of the temporomandibular joint and the related lateral pterygoid muscles.**

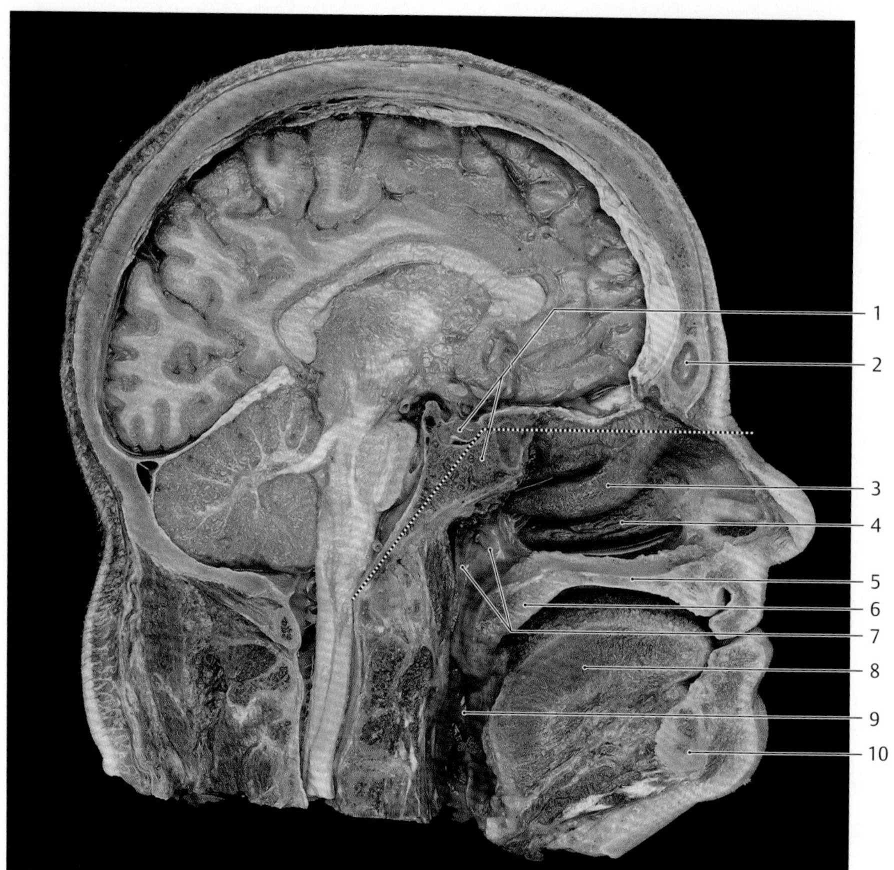


**Fig. 8.95 Median sagittal section through the head.** The palate separates the nasal and oral cavities. The base of the skull forms an angle of about 150° at the sella turcica (dotted line).

1 Hypophysis within hypophysial fossa
2 Frontal sinus
3 Middle nasal concha
4 Inferior nasal concha
5 Hard palate
6 Soft palate
7 Pharynx with auditory tube
8 Tongue
9 Pharynx with palatine tonsil
10 Mandible
11 Larynx

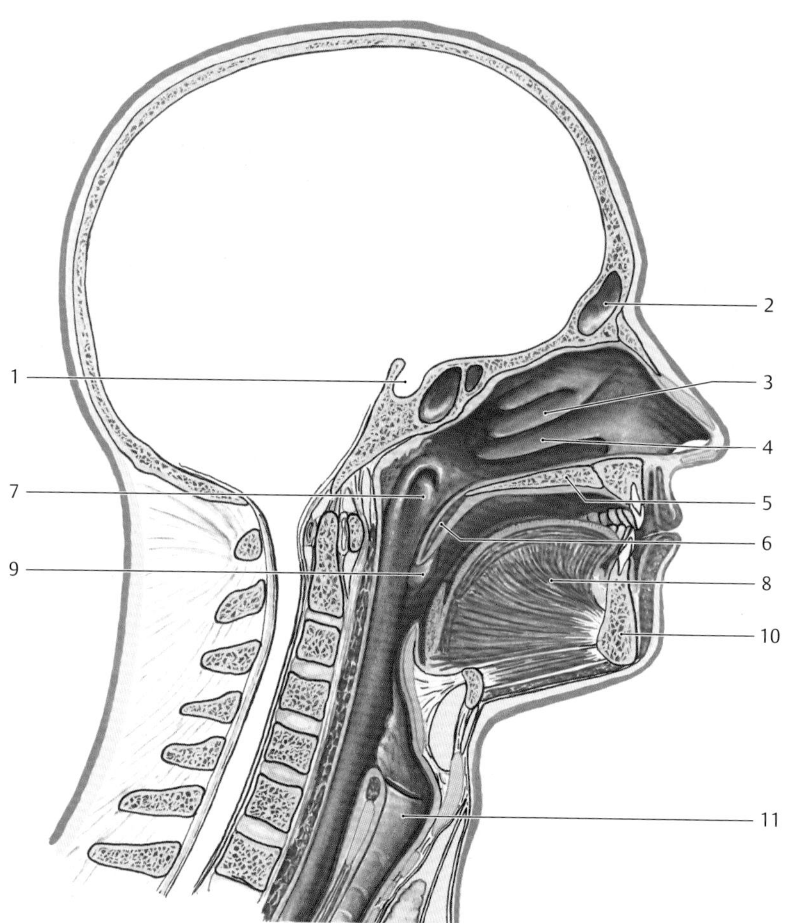


**Fig. 8.96 Median sagittal section through the head.** The tongue has been disposed to show the connection of the oral cavity with the pharynx and the position of the palatine tonsil.

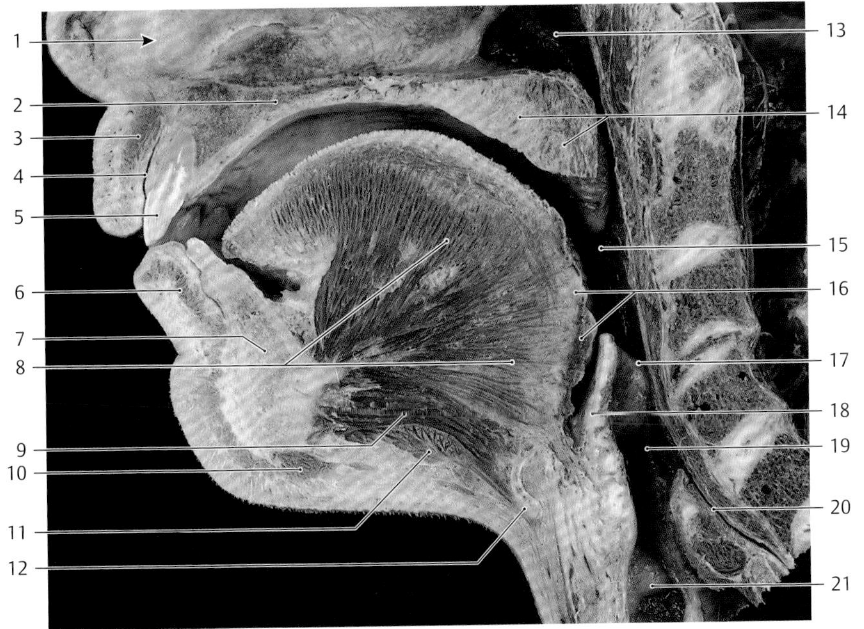


1 Nasal cavity
2 Hard palate
3 Upper lip and orbicularis oris muscle
4 Vestibule of oral cavity
5 First incisor
6 Lower lip and orbicularis oris muscle
7 Mandible
8 Genioglossus muscle
9 Geniohyoid muscle
10 Anterior belly of diagastric muscle
11 Mylohyoid muscle
12 Hyoid bone
13 Nasopharynx
14 Soft palate and uvula
15 Oropharynx
16 Root of tongue and lingual tonsil
17 Laryngopharynx
18 Epiglottis
19 Ary-epiglottic fold
20 Laryngopharynx continuous with esophagus
21 Larynx

**Fig. 8.97 Median sagittal section through the oral cavity and pharynx.**

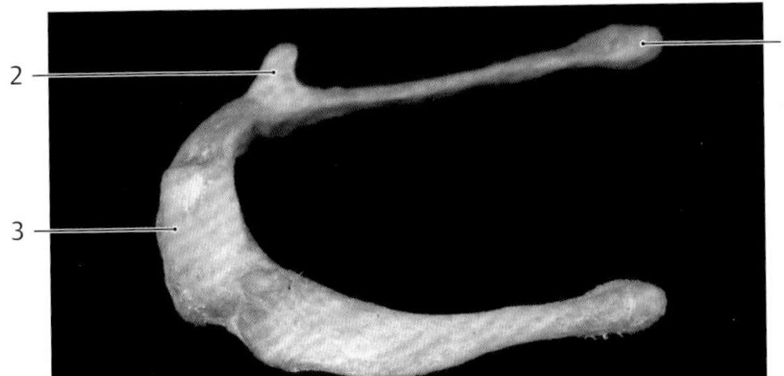


**Fig. 8.98 Hyoid bone** (oblique-lateral aspect).

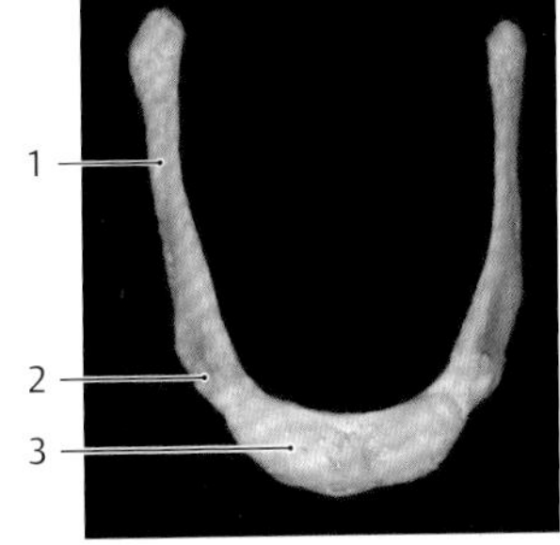


1 Greater cornu } of hyoid bone
2 Lesser cornu } of hyoid bone
3 Body } of hyoid bone

**Fig. 8.99 Hyoid bone** (anterior aspect).

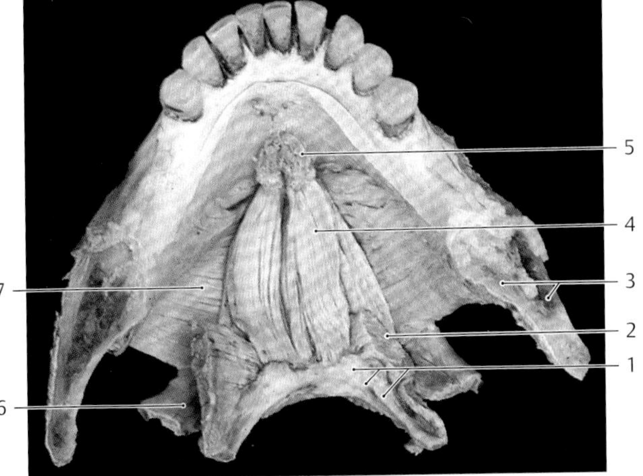


**Fig. 8.100 Muscles of the floor of the oral cavity** (superior aspect).

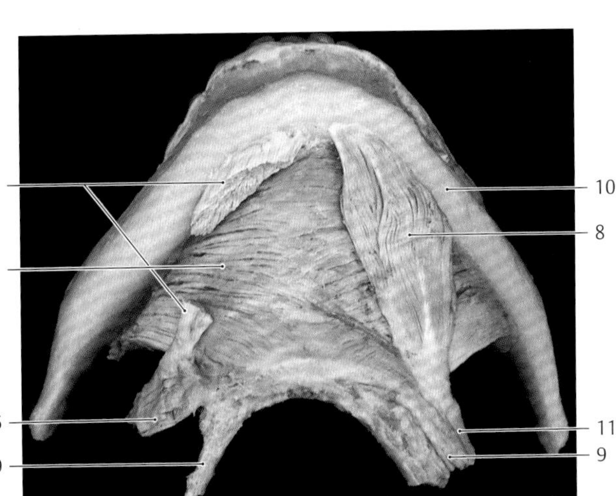


**Fig. 8.101 Muscles of the floor of the oral cavity** (inferior aspect). Cut on the base.

1 Lesser cornu and body of hyoid bone
2 Hyoglossus muscle (divided)
3 Ramus of mandible and inferior alveolar nerve
4 Geniohyoid muscle
5 Genioglossus muscle (divided)
6 Stylohyoid muscle (divided)
7 Mylohyoid muscle
8 Anterior belly of digastric muscle
9 Hyoid bone
10 Mandible
11 Intermediate tendon of digastric muscle

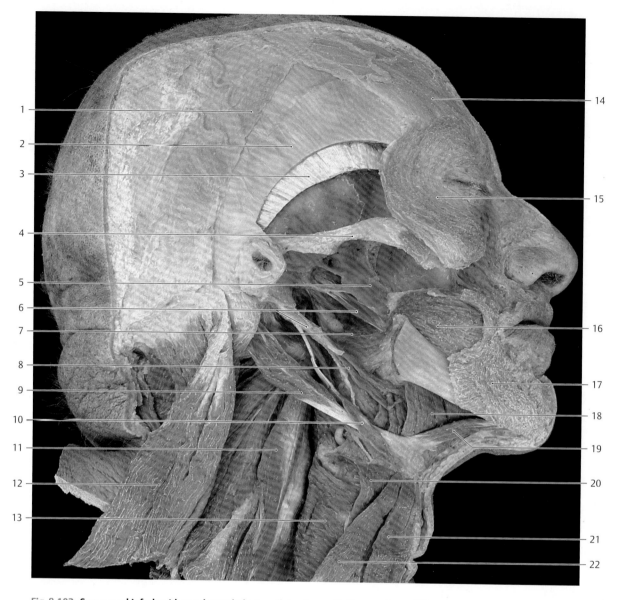

Fig. 8.102 **Supra- and infrahyoid muscles and pharynx** (lateral aspect). Ramus of mandible, pterygoid muscles, and insertion of temporal muscle removed.

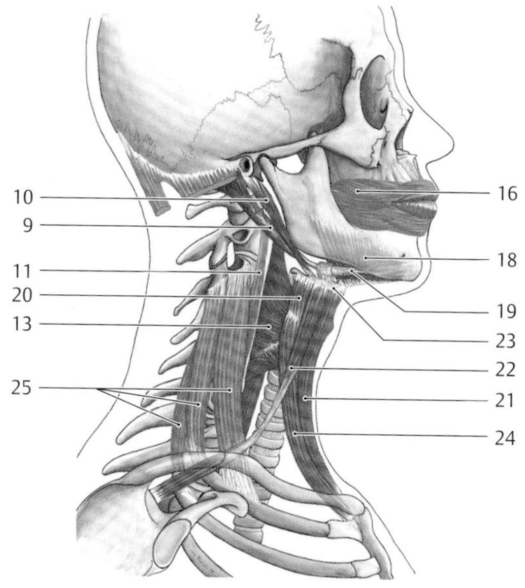


1 Galea aponeurotica
2 Temporal fascia
3 Tendon of temporal muscle
4 Zygomatic arch
5 Lateral pterygoid plate
6 Tensor veli palatini muscle (styloid process)
7 Superior constrictor muscle of pharynx
8 Styloglossus muscle
9 Posterior belly of digastric muscle
10 Stylohyoid muscle
11 Longus capitis muscle
12 Sternocleidomastoid muscle (reflected)
13 Inferior constrictor of pharynx
14 Frontal belly of occipito-frontalis muscle
15 Orbital part of orbicularis oculi muscle
16 Buccinator muscle
17 Depressor anguli oris muscle
18 Mylohyoid muscle
19 Anterior belly of digastric muscle
20 Thyrohyoid muscle
21 Sternohyoid muscle
22 Omohyoid muscle
23 Hyoid bone
24 Sternothyroid muscle
25 Scalene muscles

Fig. 8.103 **Supra- and infrahyoid muscles** (lateral aspect).

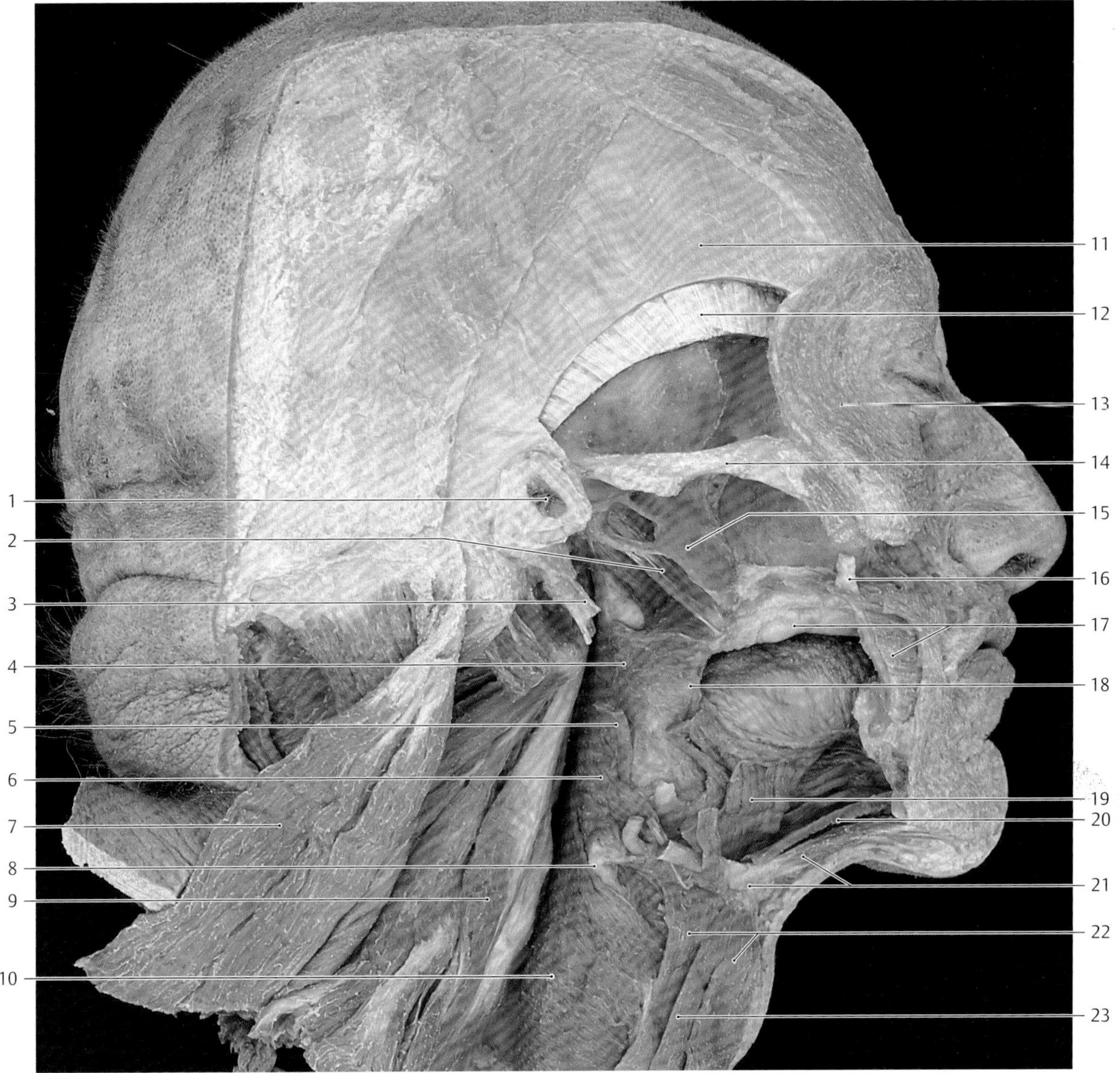


Fig. 8.104 **Supra- and infrahyoid muscles and pharynx** (lateral aspect). The buccinator muscle has been removed and the oral cavity opened.

1 External acoustic meatus
2 Tensor veli palatini muscle
3 Styloid process
4 Superior constrictor muscle of pharynx
5 Stylopharyngeus muscle (divided)
6 Middle constrictor muscle of pharynx
7 Sternocleidomastoid muscle
8 Greater horn of hyoid bone
9 Longus capitis muscle
10 Inferior constrictor muscle of pharynx
11 Temporal fascia
12 Tendon of temporal muscle
13 Orbicularis oculi muscle
14 Zygomatic arch
15 Lateral pterygoid plate
16 Parotid duct
17 Gingiva of upper jaw (without teeth) and buccinator muscle (divided)
18 Pterygomandibular raphe
19 Hyoglossus muscle
20 Mylohyoid muscle
21 Anterior belly of digastric muscle (hyoid bone)
22 Sternohyoid and thyrohyoid muscles
23 Omohyoid muscle

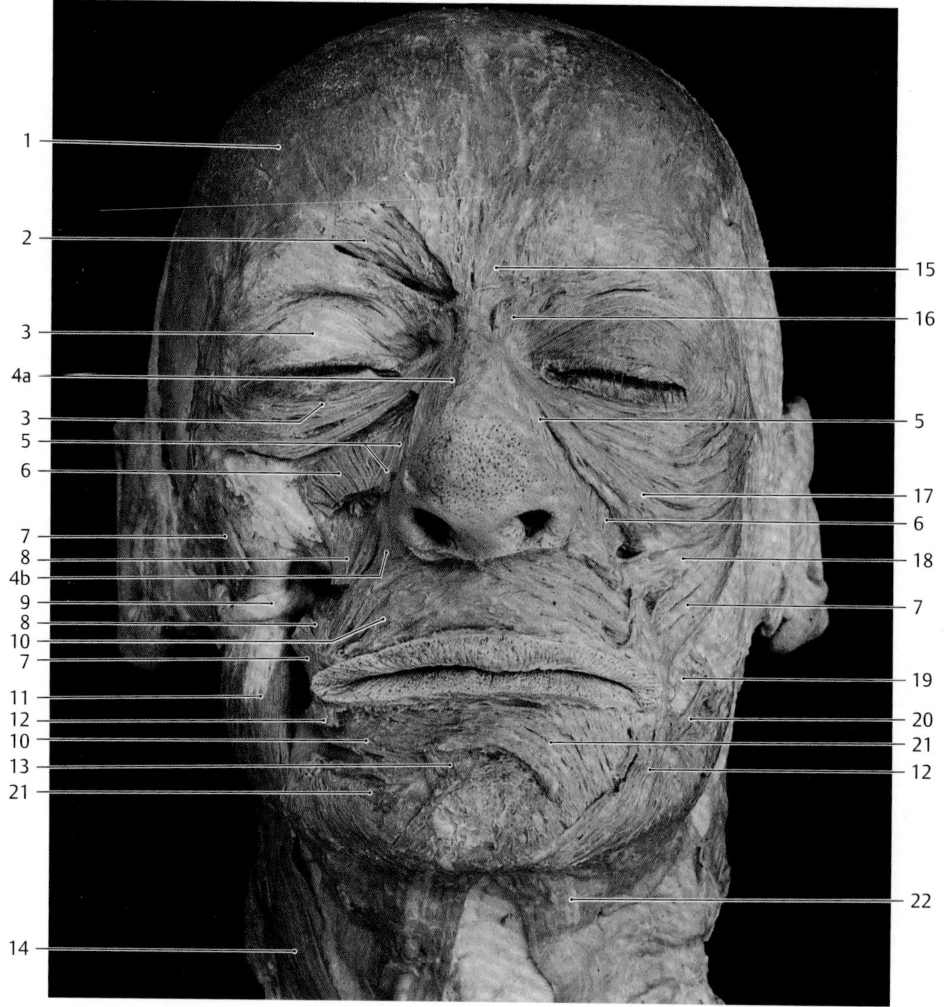


1 Frontal belly of occipitofrontalis muscle
2 Corrugator supercilii muscle
3 Palpebral part of orbicularis oculi muscle
4a Transverse part of nasalis muscle
4b Alar part of nasalis muscle
5 Levator labii superioris alaeque nasi muscle
6 Levator labii superioris muscle
7 Zygomaticus major muscle
8 Levator anguli oris muscle
9 Parotid duct
10 Orbicularis oris muscle
11 Masseter muscle
12 Depressor anguli oris muscle
13 Mentalis muscle
14 Sternocleidomastoid muscle
15 Procerus muscle
16 Depressor supercilii muscle
17 Orbital part of orbicularis oculi muscle
18 Zygomaticus minor muscle
19 Buccinator muscle
20 Risorius muscle
21 Depressor labii inferioris muscle
22 Platysma muscle
23 Galea aponeurotica
24 Temporoparietalis muscle
25 Occipital belly of occipitofrontalis muscle
26 Parotid gland with fascia
27 Temporal fascia
28 Orbicularis oculi muscle
29 Parotid duct and masseter muscle

**Fig. 8.105 Facial muscles** (anterior aspect). Left side = superficial layer; right side = deeper layer.

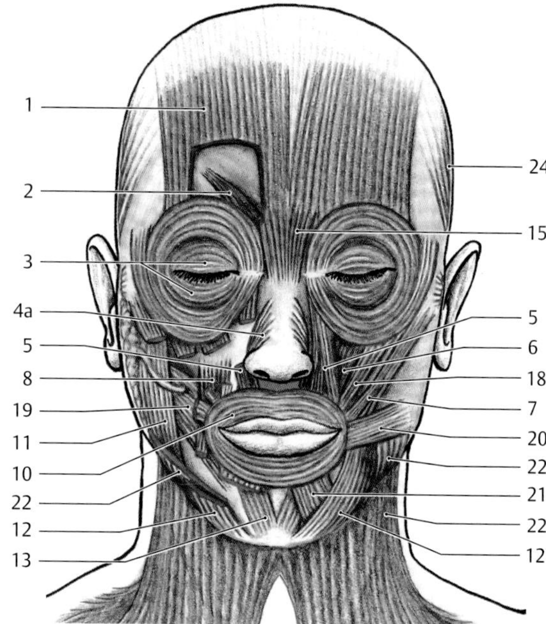


**Fig. 8.106 Facial muscles** (anterior aspect). Left side = superficial layer; right side = deeper layer.

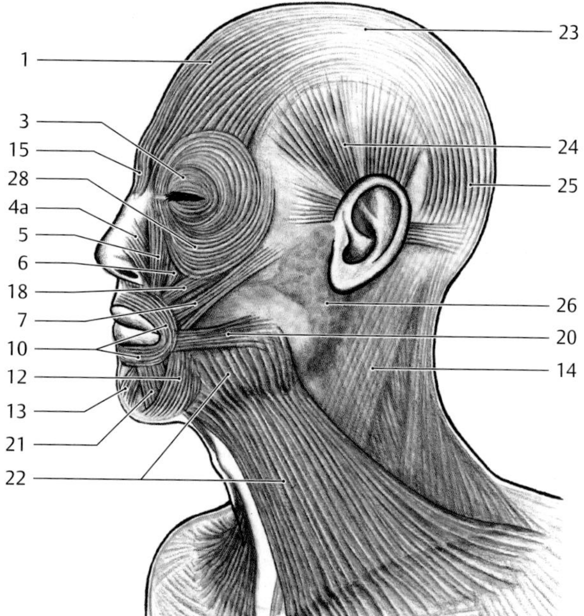


**Fig. 8.107 Facial muscles** (lateral aspect). Sphincter-like muscles surround the orifices of the head. Radially arranged muscles work as their antagonists.

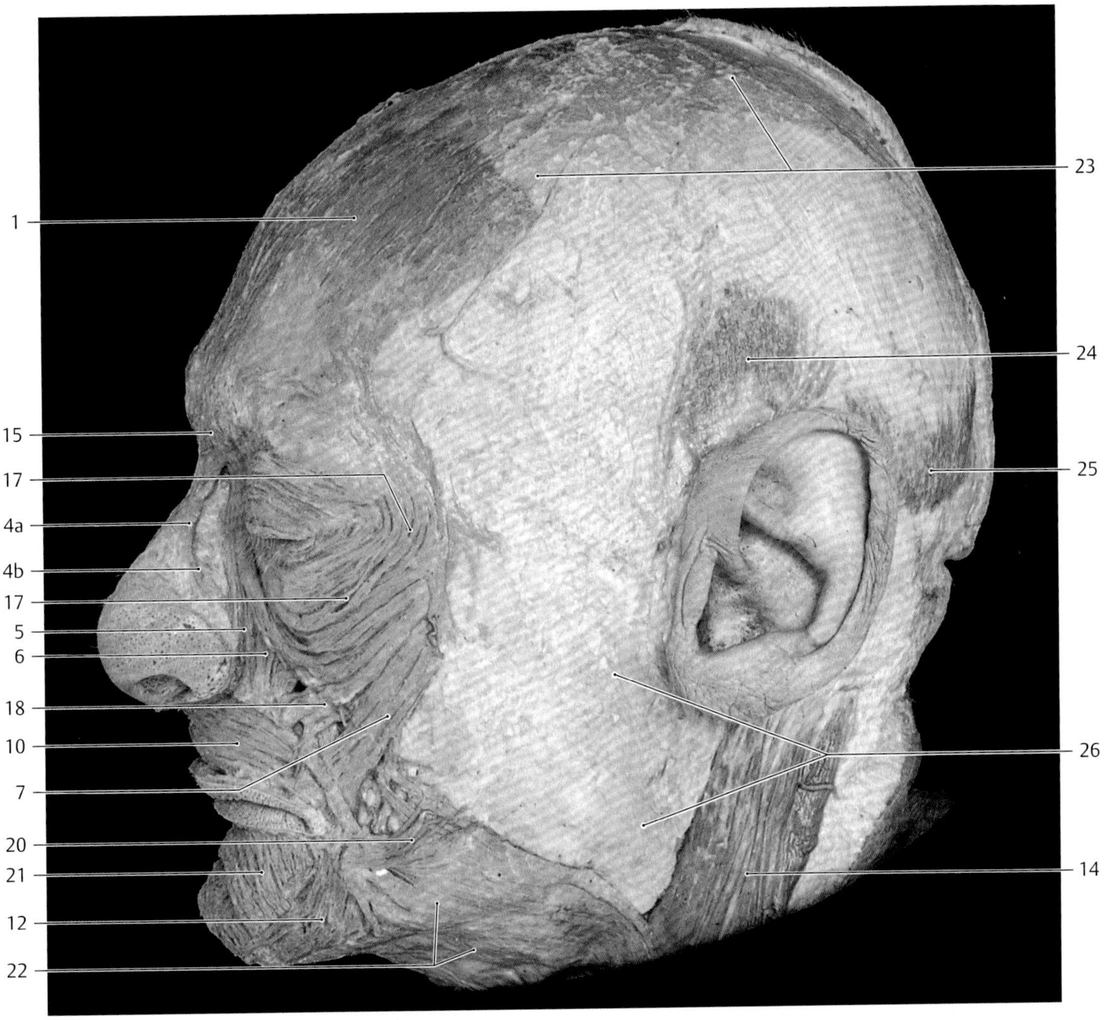

Fig. 8.108 **Facial muscles** (lateral aspect).

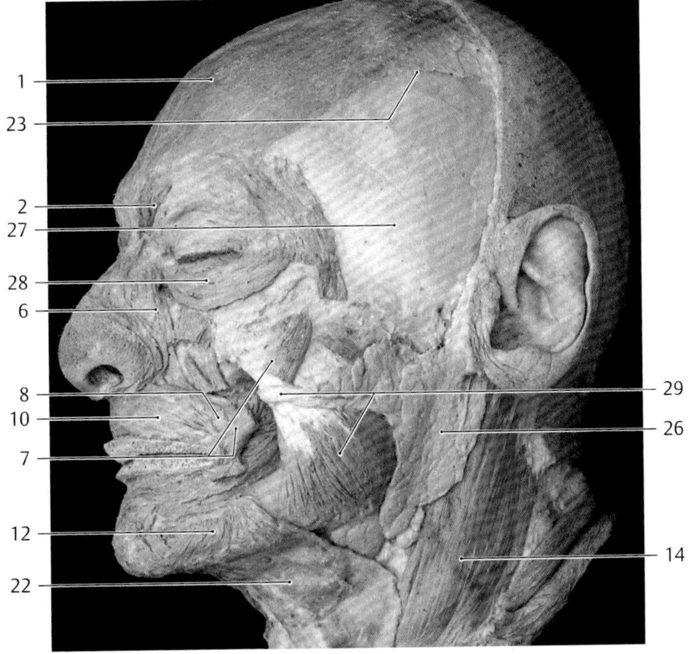


Fig. 8.109 **Facial muscles and parotid gland** (lateral aspect).

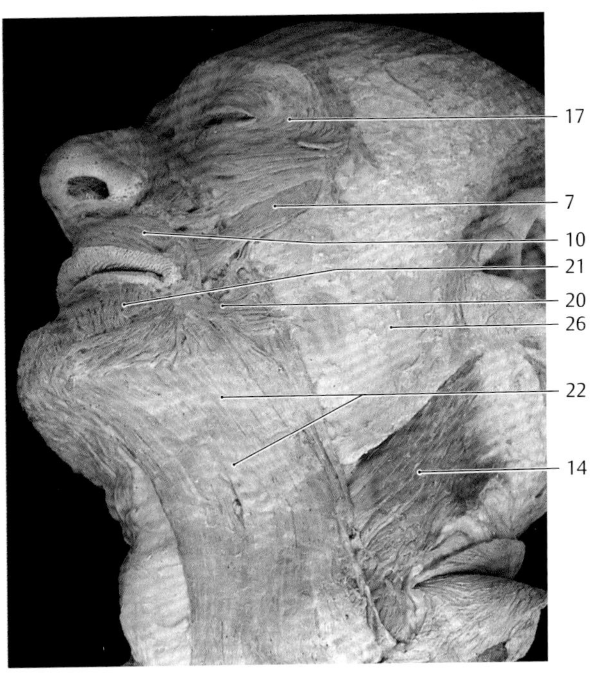


Fig. 8.110 **Platysma muscle** (oblique-lateral aspect). The superficial lamina of the cervical fascia has been partly removed.

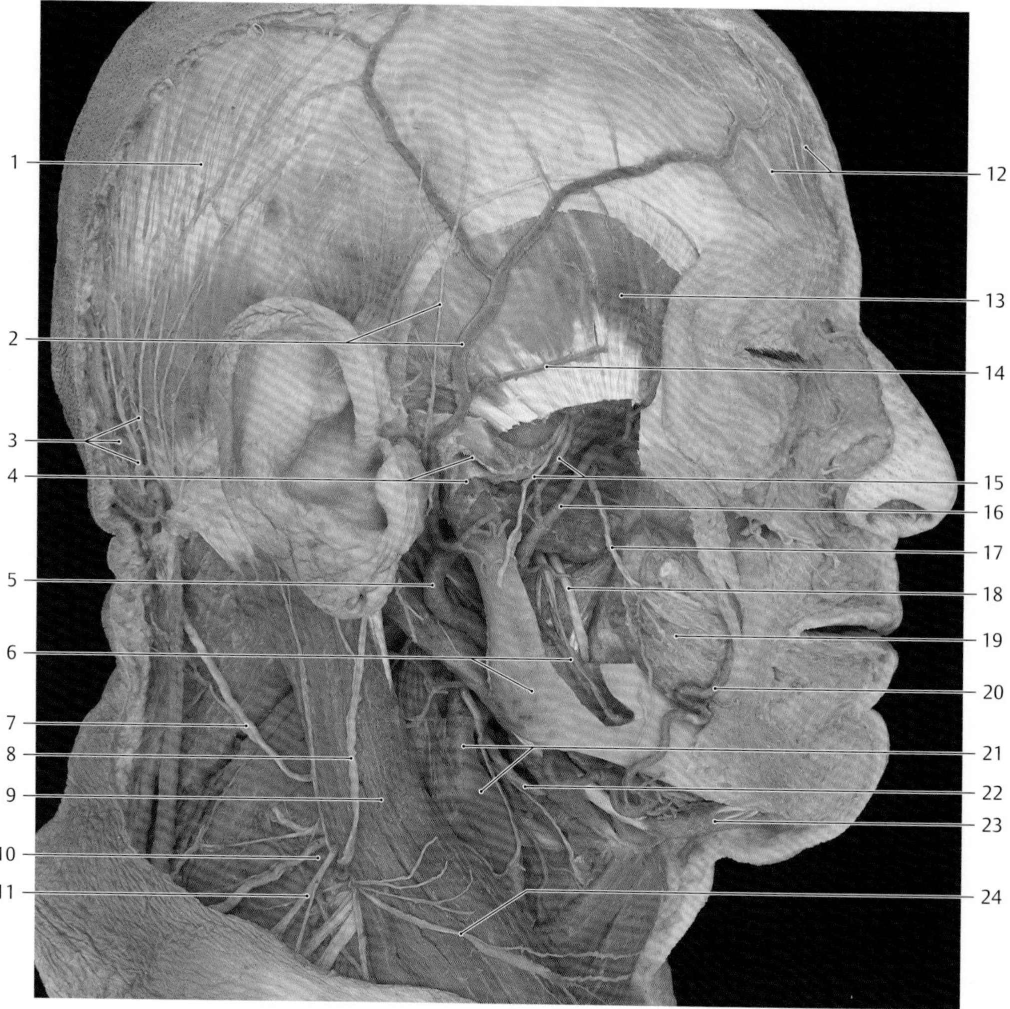


1 Galea aponeurotica
2 Superficial temporal artery and auriculotemporal nerve
3 Occipital artery and greater occipital nerve (C2)
4 Temporomandibular joint (opened)
5 External carotid artery
6 Mandible and inferior mandibular artery and nerve
7 Accessory nerve (var.)
8 Great auricular nerve
9 Sternocleidomastoid muscle
10 Punctum nervosum
11 Supraclavicular nerves
12 Supra-orbital nerves
13 Temporal muscle
14 Transverse facial artery
15 Masseteric nerve and deep temporal branch of maxillary artery
16 Maxillary artery
17 Buccal nerve
18 Lingual nerve
19 Buccinator muscle
20 Facial artery
21 External carotid artery and sinus caroticus
22 Hypoglossal nerve
23 Digastric muscle
24 Transverse cervical nerves

Fig. 8.111 **Dissection of maxillary artery** (lateral aspect). The ramus mandibulae has been partly removed and the canalis mandibulae has been opened.

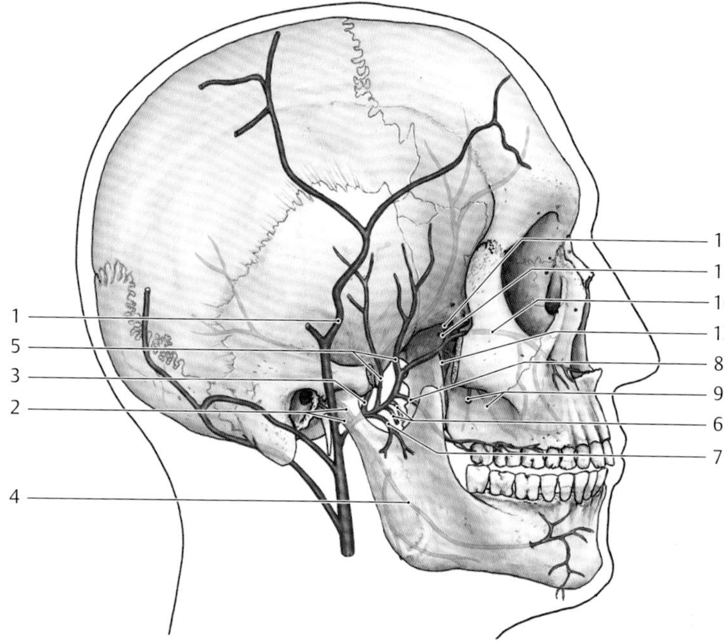


1 Superficial temporal artery

**Branches of the first part**
2 Deep auricular artery and anterior tympanic artery
3 Middle meningeal artery
4 Inferior alveolar artery

**Branches of the second part**
5 Deep temporal branches
6 Pterygoid branches
7 Masseteric artery
8 Buccal artery

**Branches of the third part**
9 Posterior superior alveolar artery
10 Infra-orbital artery
11 Sphenopalatine artery and branches to the nasal cavity
12 Descending palatine artery
13 Artery of the pterygoid canal

Fig. 8.112 **Main branches of maxillary artery** (lateral aspect).

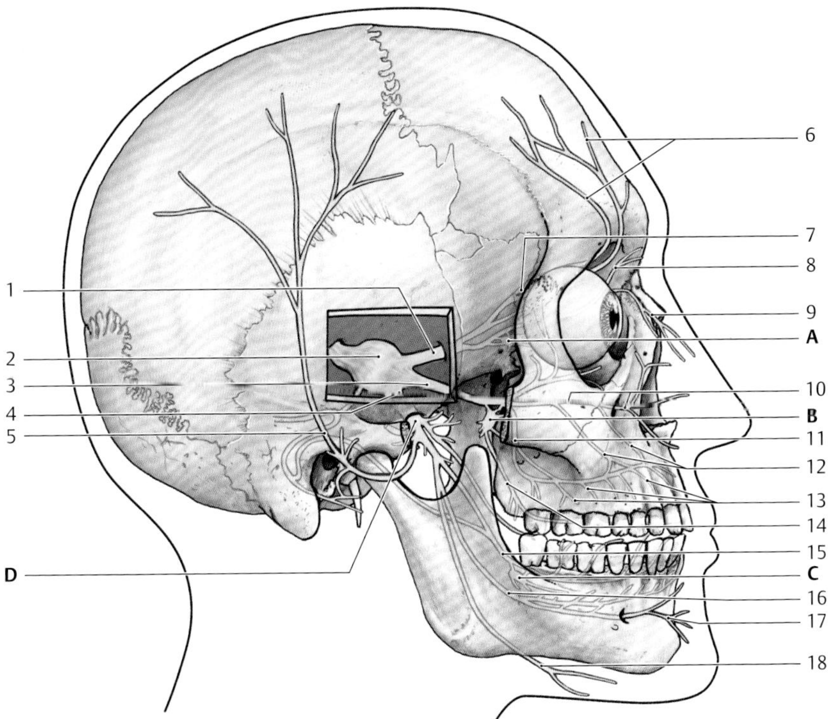


**Trigeminal nerve**
1 Ophthalmic nerve (CN $V_1$)
2 Trigeminal ganglion
3 Maxillary nerve (CN $V_2$)
4 Mandibular nerve (CN $V_3$)
5 Auriculotemporal nerve
6 Lateral and medial branch of supra-orbital nerve
7 Frontal nerve
8 Nasociliary nerve
9 External nasal branch
10 Infra-orbital nerve
11 Posterior superior alveolar nerve
12 Anterior and middle superior alveolar nerves
13 Superior dental plexus
14 Greater palatine nerve
15 Lingual nerve
16 Inferior alveolar nerve
17 Mental nerve
18 Mylohyoid nerve

A = Ciliary ganglion
B = Pterygopalatine ganglion
C = Submandibular ganglion
D = Otic ganglion

Fig. 8.113 **Trigeminal nerve (CN V) and its major branches.** Letters indicate the position of the three autonomic ganglia that are related to the three major divisions of the trigeminal nerve.

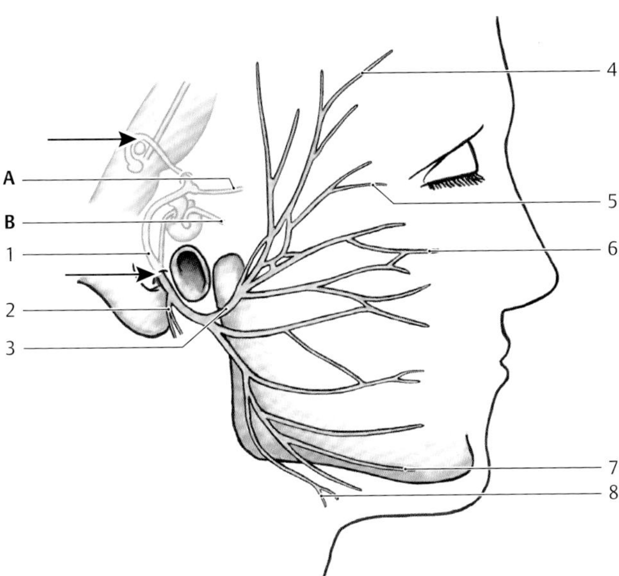


Fig. 8.114 **Facial nerve (CN VII) and its branches.** Letters indicate the autonomic branches. Upper arrow = internal geniculum of the facial nerve; lower arrow = stylomastoid foramen.

**Facial nerve (CN VII)**
1 Posterior auricular nerve
2 Styloid branch, digastric branch
3 Parotid plexus
4 Temporal branch
5 Zygomatic branch
6 Buccal branch
7 Marginal mandibular branch
8 Cervical branch

A = Greater petrosal nerve
B = Chorda tympani

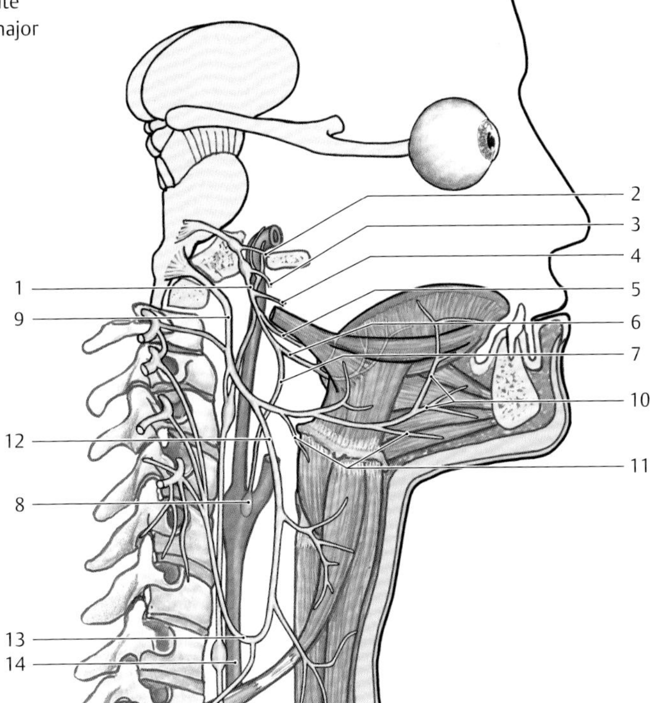


Fig. 8.115 **Glossopharyngeal (CN IX) and hypoglossal (CN XII) nerves and their branches.**

1 **Glossopharyngeal nerve (CN IX)**
2 Tympanic nerve
3 Stylopharyngeal branch
4 Pharyngeal branch
5 Tonsillar branch
6 Lingual branch
7 Carotid sinus branch
8 Carotid body
9 **Hypoglossal nerve (CN XII)**
10 Lingual branch
11 Geniohyoid and thyrohyoid branch
12 Superior root of ansa cervicalis
13 Ansa cervicalis
14 Common carotid artery

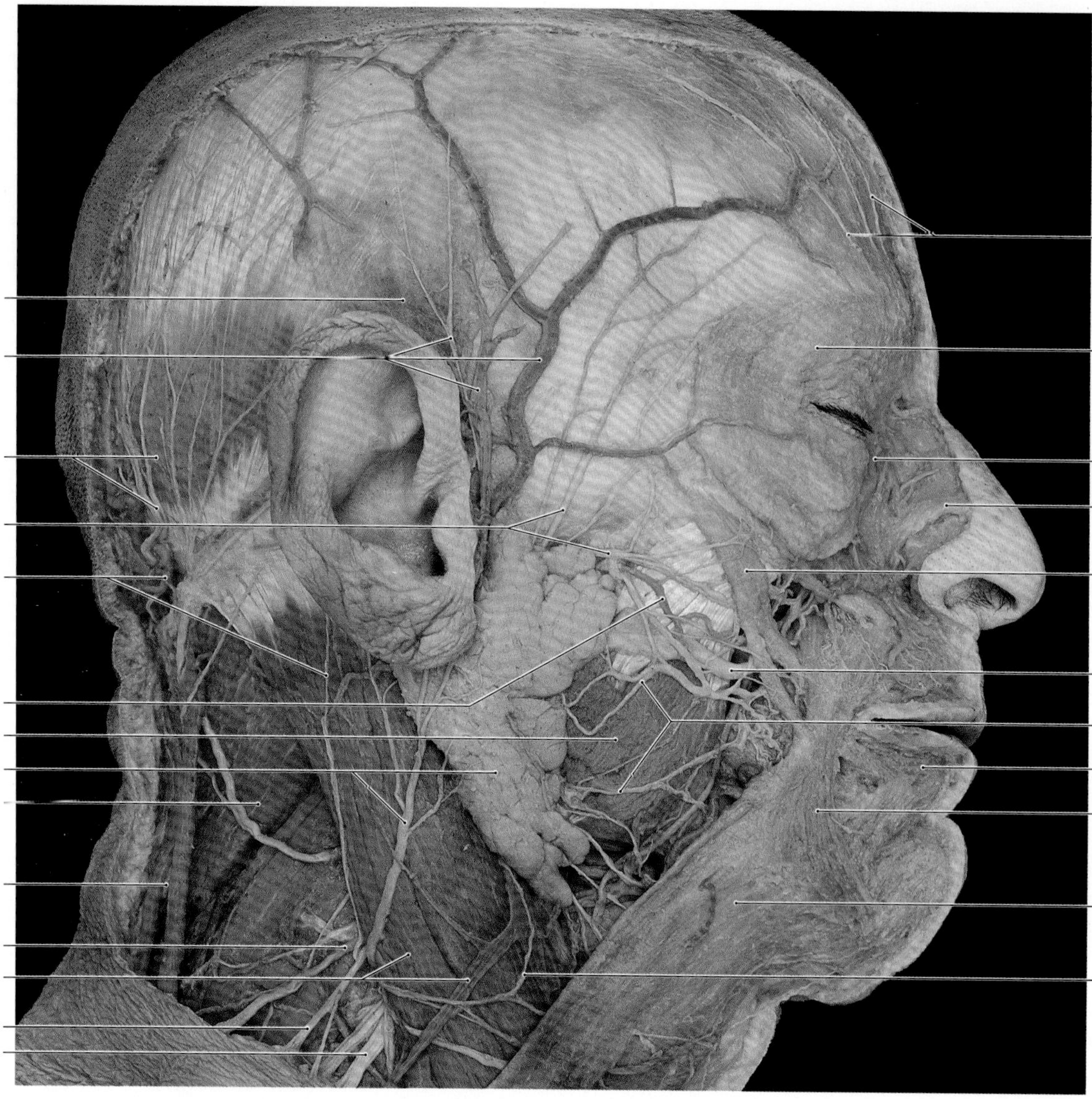

**Fig. 8.116 Superficial dissection of lateral region of the face.** Peripheral distribution of facial nerve (CN VII).

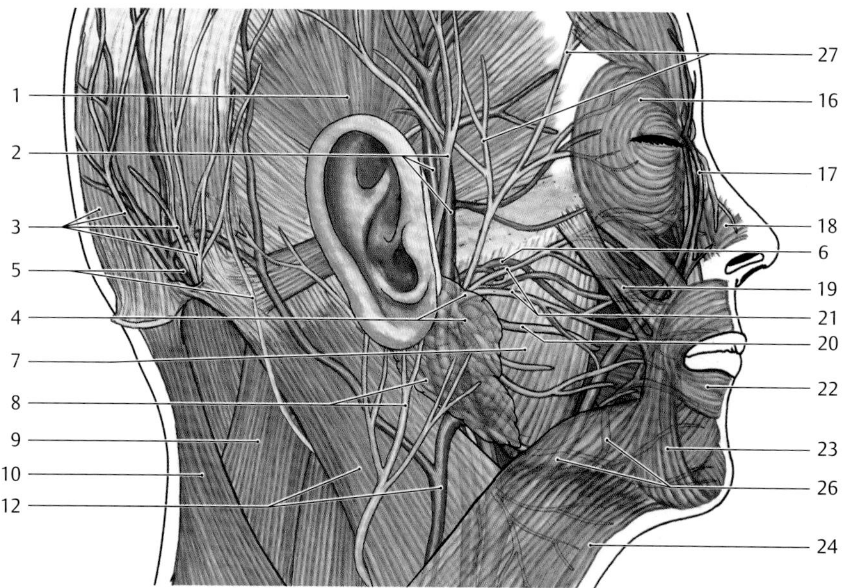


**Fig. 8.117 Superficial region of the face.** Note the facial plexus within the parotid gland (lateral aspect).

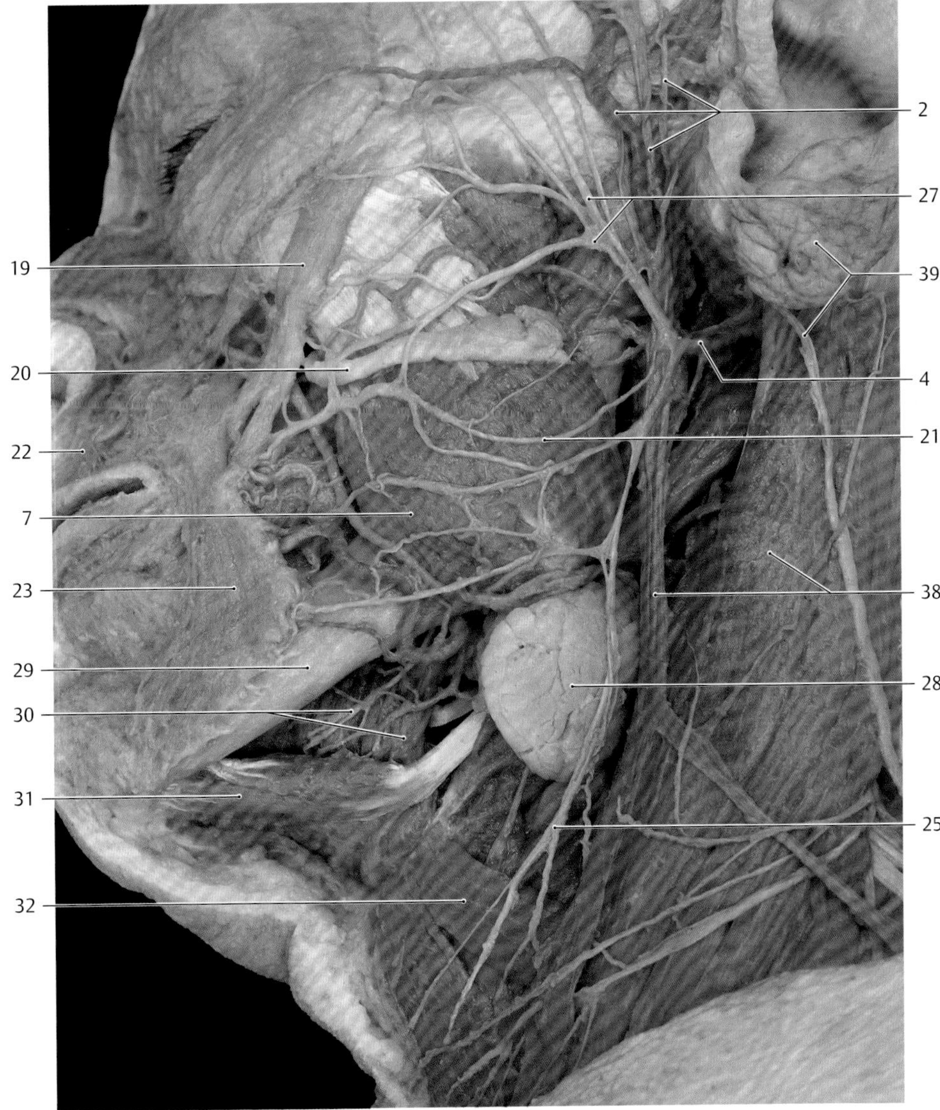


Fig. 8.118 **Retromandibular and submandibular regions** (lateral aspect). The parotid gland has been removed.

1 Temporoparietalis muscle
2 Superficial temporal artery and vein, and auriculotemporal nerve
3 Occipital belly of occipitofrontalis muscle and greater occipital nerve (C2)
4 Facial nerve (CN VII)
5 Lesser occipital nerve and occipital artery
6 Transverse facial artery
7 Masseter muscle
8 Parotid gland and great auricular nerve
9 Splenius capitis muscle
10 Trapezius muscle
11 Punctum nervosum, point of distribution of cutaneous nerves of cervical plexus
12 Sternocleidomastoid muscle and external jugular vein
13 Supraclavicular nerves
14 Brachial plexus
15 Supra-orbital nerves
16 Orbicularis oculi muscle
17 Angular artery (terminal branch of facial artery)
18 Nasalis muscle
19 Zygomaticus major muscle
20 Parotid duct
21 Zygomatic and buccal branches of facial nerve
22 Orbicularis oris muscle
23 Depressor anguli oris muscle
24 Platysma muscle
25 Cervical branch of facial nerve (anastomosing with transverse cervical nerve of cervical plexus)
26 Facial artery and vein
27 Temporal branches of facial nerve
28 Submandibular gland
29 Mandible
30 Mylohyoid muscle and nerve
31 Anterior belly of digastric muscle
32 Omohyoid muscle
33 Greater petrosal nerve
34 Geniculate ganglion
35 Chorda tympani
36 Posterior auricular nerve
37 Stylomastoid foramen
38 Sternocleidomastoid muscle and retromandibular vein
39 Lobule of auricle and great auricular nerve

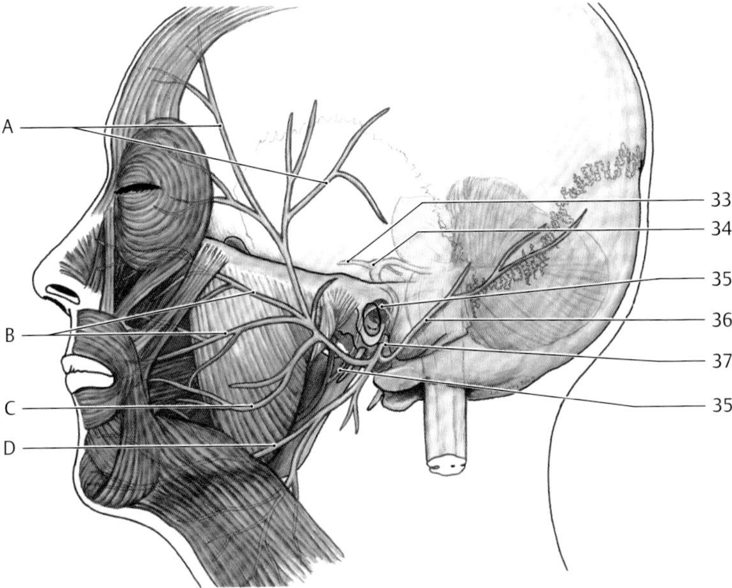


Fig. 8.119 **Main branches of facial nerve** (lateral aspect). A = temporal branches; B = zygomatic branches; C = buccal branches; D = marginal mandibular branch.

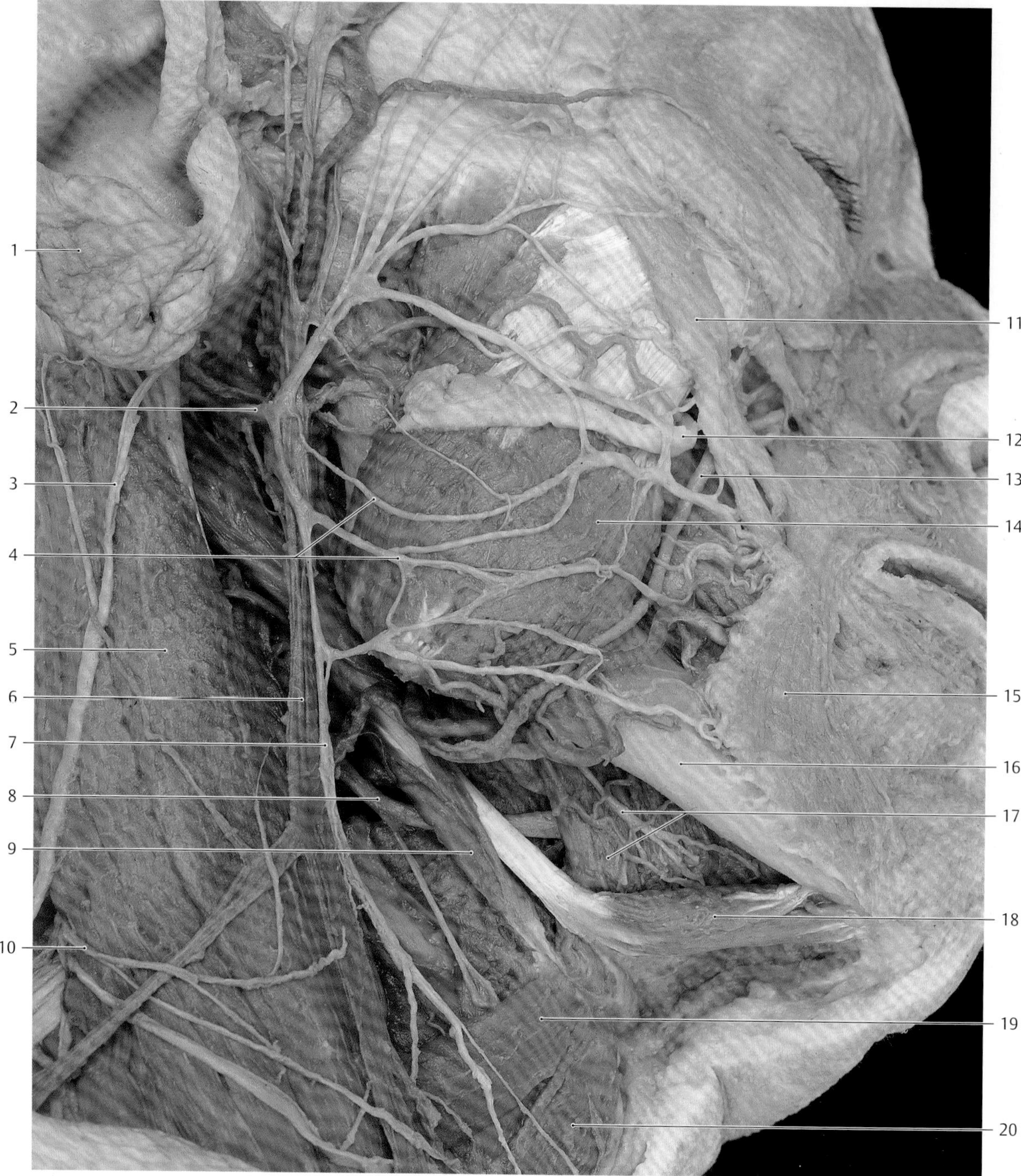


Fig. 8.120 **Retromandibular and submandibular regions** (lateral aspect). The parotid gland and the submandibular gland have been removed. The parotid plexus (4) is formed by anastomosis of the temporal, zygomatic, buccal, marginal mandibular, and cervical branches of the facial nerve, arising in the parotid gland.

1 Lobule of auricle
2 Facial nerve (CN VII)
3 Great auricular nerve
4 Parotid plexus
5 Sternocleidomastoid muscle
6 Retromandibular vein
7 Cervical branch of facial nerve
8 Hypoglossal nerve (CN XII)
9 Stylohyoid muscle
10 Transverse cervical nerve
11 Zygomaticus major muscle
12 Parotid duct
13 Facial artery
14 Masseter muscle
15 Depressor anguli oris muscle
16 Mandible
17 Mylohyoid muscle and nerve
18 Anterior belly of digastric muscle
19 Omohyoid muscle
20 Sternohyoid muscle

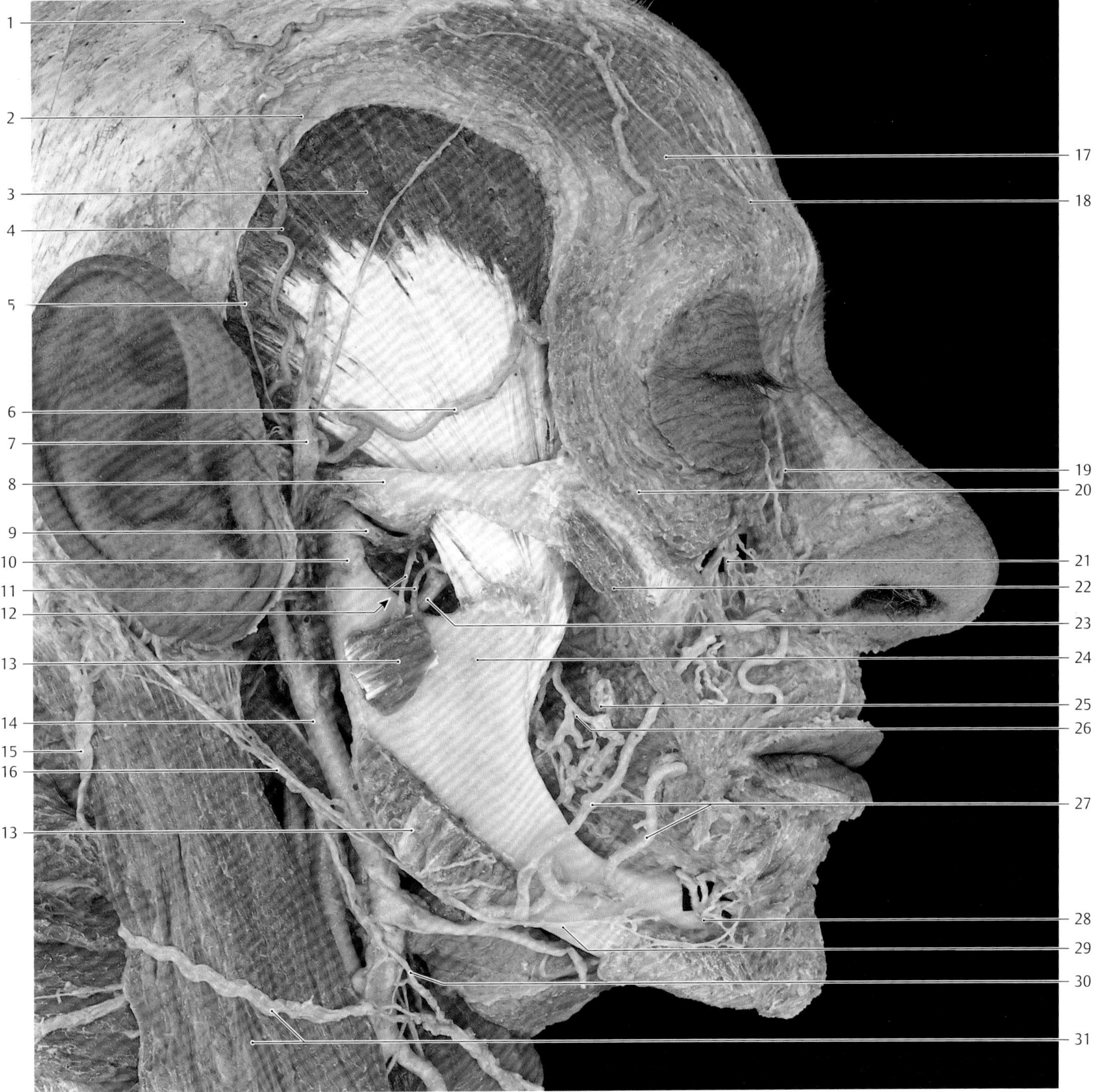


Fig. 8.121 **Superficial dissection of lateral region of the face.** Masseter muscle and temporal fascia have been partly removed to display the masseteric artery and nerve.

1 Galea aponeurotica
2 Temporal fascia
3 Temporal muscle
4 Parietal branch of superficial temporal artery
5 Auriculotemporal nerve
6 Frontal branch of superficial temporal artery
7 Superficial temporal vein
8 Zygomatic arch
9 Articular disc of temporomandibular joint
10 Head of mandible
11 Masseteric artery and nerve
12 Mandibular notch
13 Masseter muscle (divided)
14 External carotid artery
15 Great auricular nerve
16 Facial nerve (reflected)
17 Frontal belly of occipitofrontalis muscle
18 Medial branch of supra-orbital nerve
19 Angular artery
20 Orbicularis oculi muscle
21 Infra-orbital nerve
22 Zygomaticus major muscle
23 Maxillary artery
24 Coronoid process
25 Parotid duct (divided)
26 Buccal nerve
27 Facial artery and vein
28 Mental nerve
29 Mandibular branch of facial nerve
30 Cervical branch of facial nerve
31 Transverse cervical nerve (communicating branch with facial nerve) and sternocleidomastoid muscle

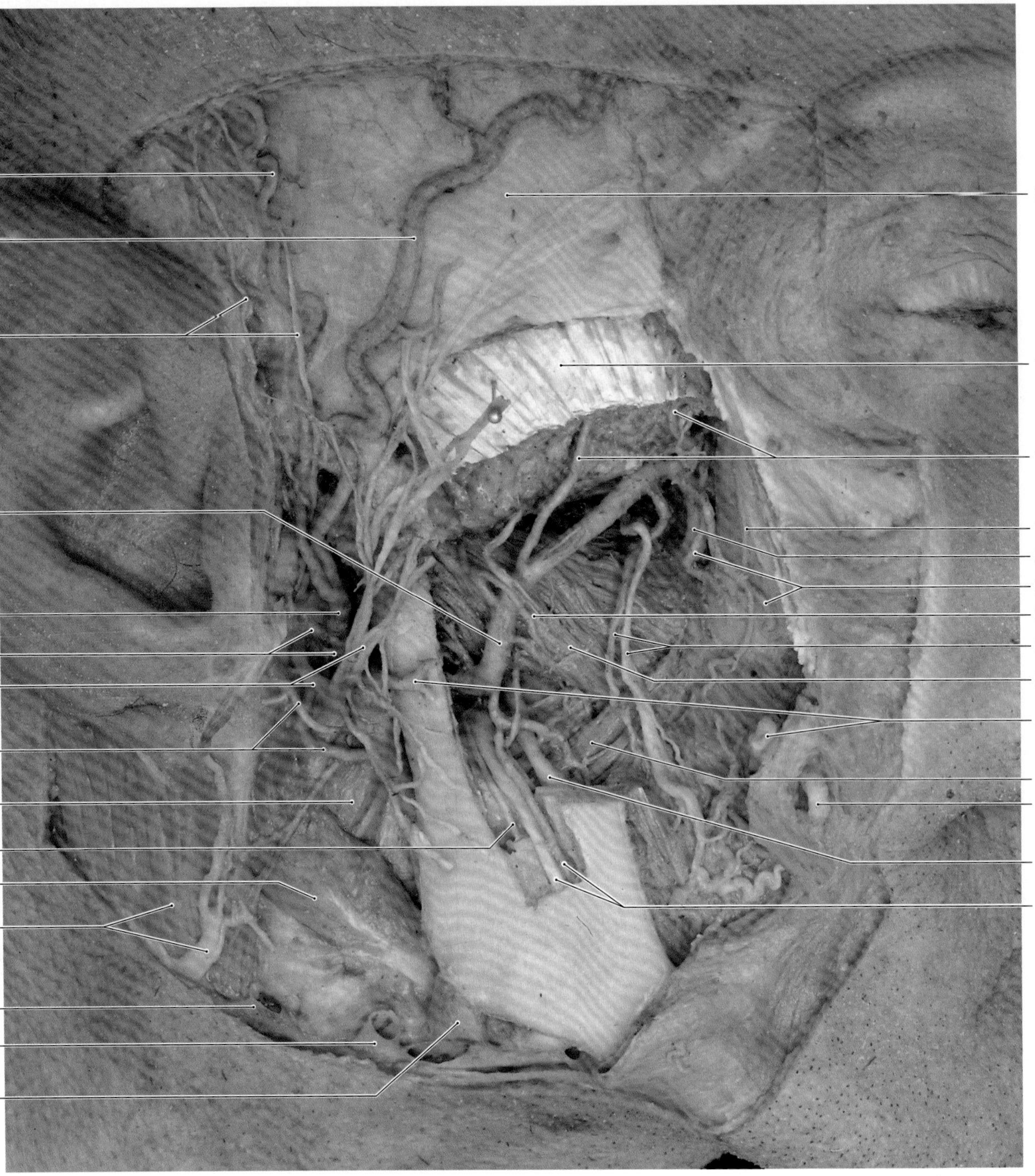

**Fig. 8.122 Deep dissection of facial and retromandibular regions.** The coronoid process together with the insertions of temporal muscle have been removed to display the maxillary artery. The upper part of the mandibular canal has been opened.

1 Parietal branch of superficial temporal artery
2 Frontal branch of superficial temporal artery
3 Auriculotemporal nerve
4 Maxillary artery
5 Superficial temporal artery
6 Communicating branches between facial and auriculotemporal nerves
7 Facial nerve
8 Posterior auricular artery and anterior auricular branch of superficial temporal artery
9 Internal jugular vein
10 Mylohyoid nerve
11 Posterior belly of digastric muscle
12 Great auricular nerve and sternocleidomastoid muscle
13 External jugular vein
14 Retromandibular vein
15 Submandibular gland
16 Temporal fascia
17 Temporal tendon
18 Deep temporal arteries
19 Posterior superior alveolar nerve
20 Sphenopalatine artery
21 Posterior superior alveolar arteries
22 Masseteric artery and nerve
23 Buccal nerve and artery
24 Lateral pterygoid
25 Transverse facial artery and parotid duct (divided)
26 Medial pterygoid muscle
27 Facial artery
28 Lingual nerve
29 Inferior alveolar artery and nerve (mandibular canal opened)

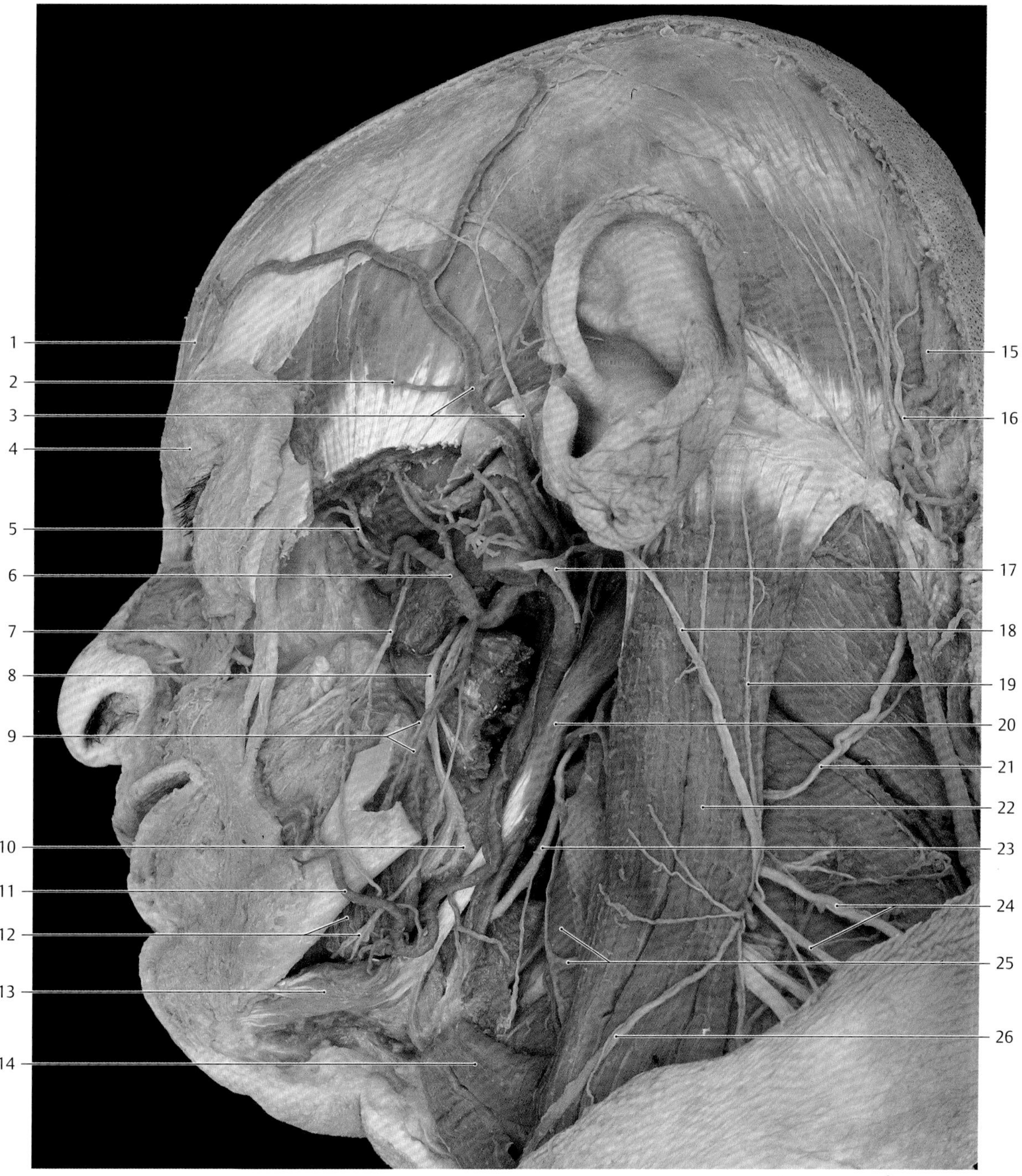


Fig. 8.123 **Dissection of peripharyngeal and retromandibular regions** (oblique-lateral aspect). The mandible has been partly removed.

1 Supra-orbital nerve (medial branch)
2 Temporal muscle
3 Superficial temporal artery and auriculotemporal nerve
4 Orbicularis oculi muscle
5 Anterior deep temporal artery
6 Maxillary artery
7 Buccal nerve
8 Lingual nerve
9 Inferior alveolar nerve and artery
10 Submandibular ganglion
11 Facial artery
12 Mylohyoid muscle and nerve
13 Anterior belly of digastric muscle
14 Omohyoid muscle
15 Occipital artery
16 Greater occipital nerve (C2)
17 Facial nerve (cut) (CN VII)
18 Great auricular nerve
19 Lesser occipital nerve
20 Posterior belly of digastric muscle
21 Accessory nerve (var.)
22 Sternocleidomastoid muscle
23 Hypoglossal nerve (CN XII)
24 Supraclavicular nerves (lateral and intermedial branches)
25 Internal jugular vein and ansa cervicalis
26 Anterior supraclavicular nerve

**Fig. 8.124 Deep dissection of facial and retromandibular regions.** The mandible and pterygoid muscles have been removed and the temporal muscle has been fenestrated.

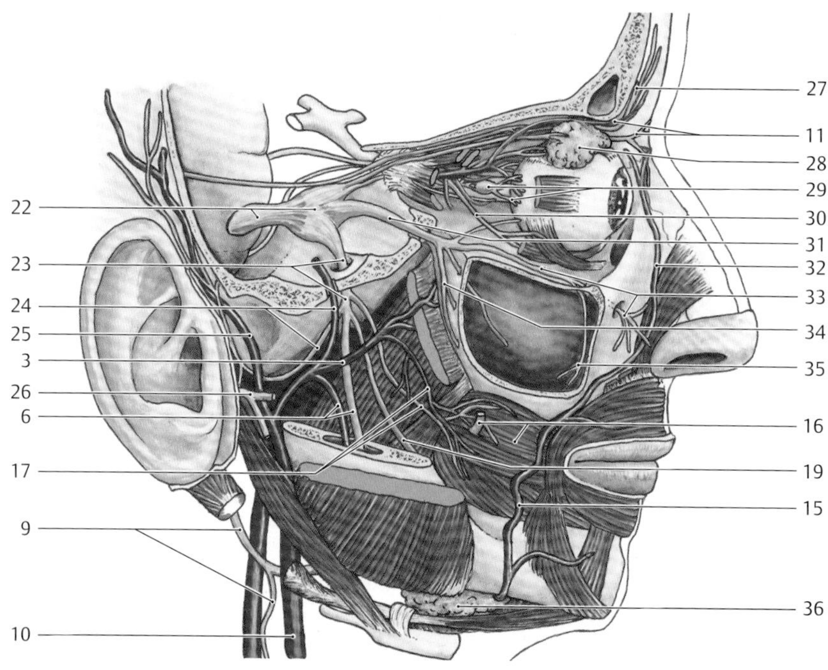


**Fig. 8.125 Deep region of the face with arteries and nerves,** particularly the dissection of the maxillary artery and trigeminal nerve.

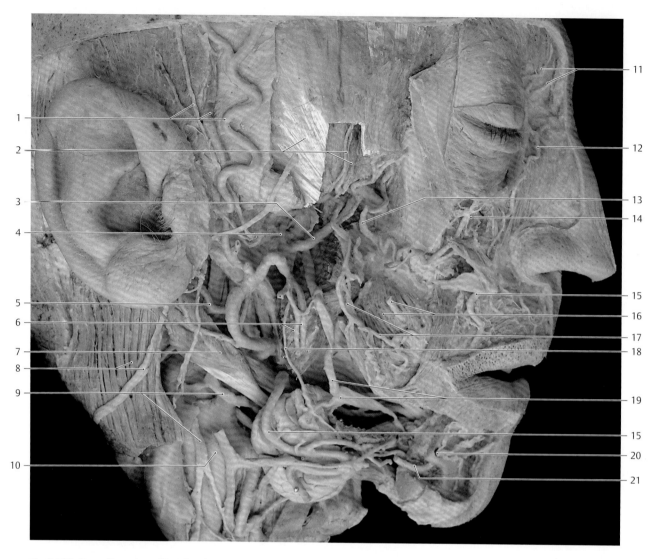

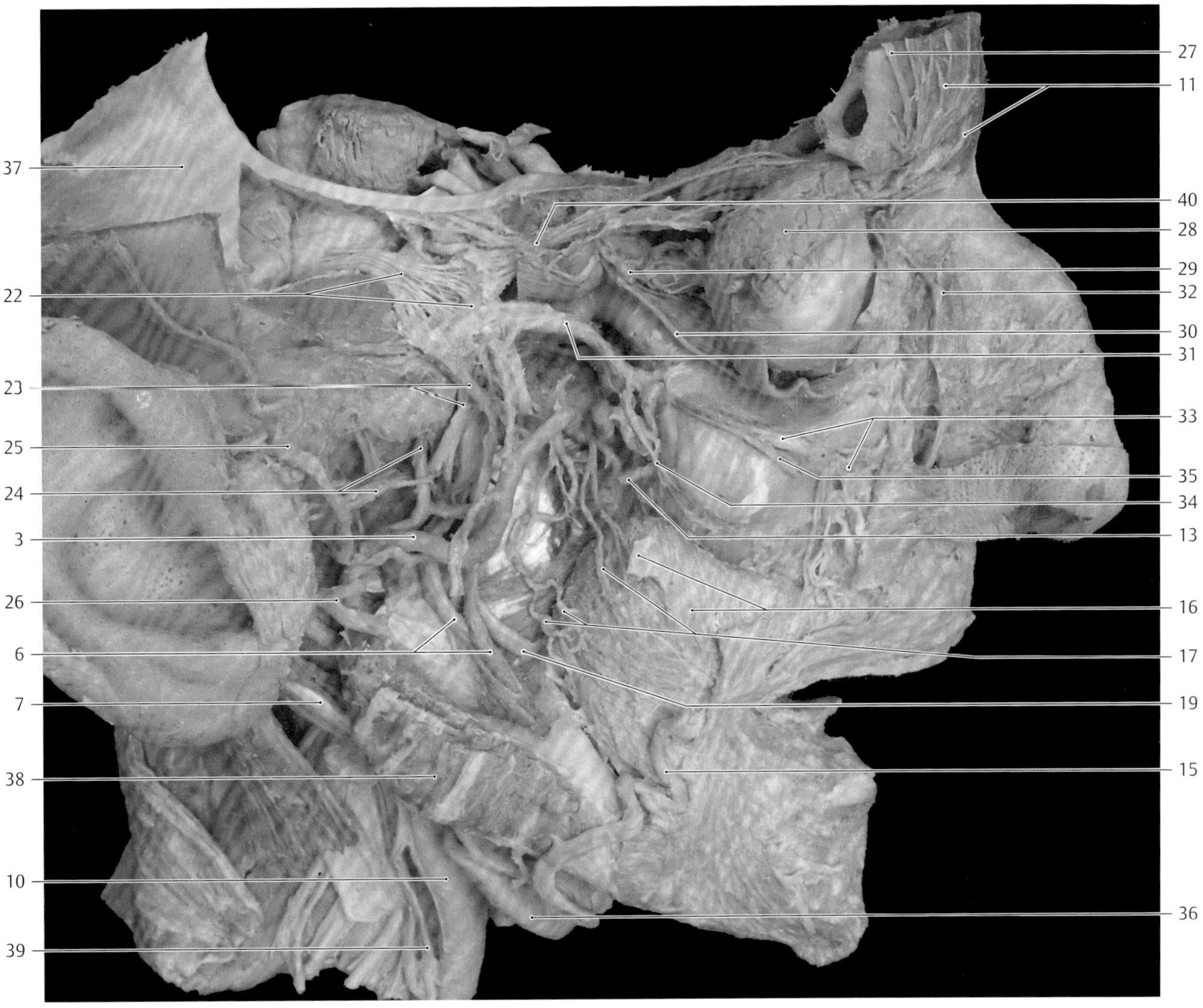


Fig. 8.126 **Deep dissection of the infratemporal region.** The mandible and the lateral wall of the orbit have been removed. The main branches of the trigeminal nerve and its ganglion are displayed.

1 Superficial temporal artery and vein and auriculotemporal nerve
2 Tendon of temporal muscle, deep temporal nerves and artery
3 Maxillary artery
4 Middle meningeal artery
5 Occipital artery
6 Inferior alveolar artery and nerve
7 Posterior belly of digastric muscle
8 Great auricular nerve and sterno-cleidomastoid muscle
9 Hypoglossal nerve and superior root of ansa cervicalis
10 External carotid artery
11 Supratrochlear nerve and medial branch of supra-orbital artery
12 Angular artery
13 Posterior superior alveolar artery
14 Infra-orbital nerve
15 Facial artery
16 Parotid duct (divided) and buccinator muscle
17 Buccal artery and nerve
18 Mylohyoid nerve
19 Lingual nerve and submandibular ganglion
20 Mental nerve and foramen
21 Inferior alveolar nerve
22 Trigeminal nerve and ganglion
23 Mandibular nerve (CN $V_3$)
24 Auriculotemporal nerve and middle meningeal artery
25 Superficial temporal artery
26 Facial nerve
27 Lateral branch of supra-orbital nerve
28 Lacrimal gland
29 Ciliary ganglion and short ciliary nerves
30 Inferior branch of oculomotor nerve
31 Maxillary nerve (CN $V_2$)
32 Angular artery
33 Infra-orbital nerve
34 Posterior superior alveolar nerve
35 Anterior superior alveolar nerve
36 Submandibular gland
37 Cerebellar tentorium
38 Masseter muscle
39 Superior root of ansa cervicalis
40 Ophthalmic nerve (CN $V_1$)

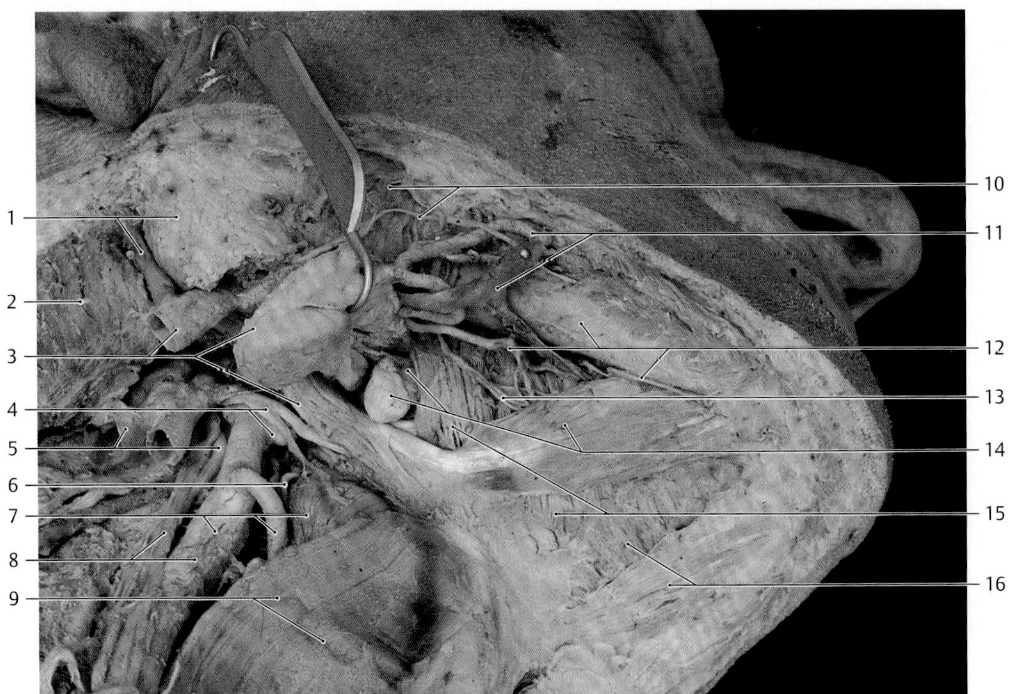


**Fig. 8.127 Submandibular triangle,** superficial dissection (inferior aspect of right side). The submandibular gland has been reflected.

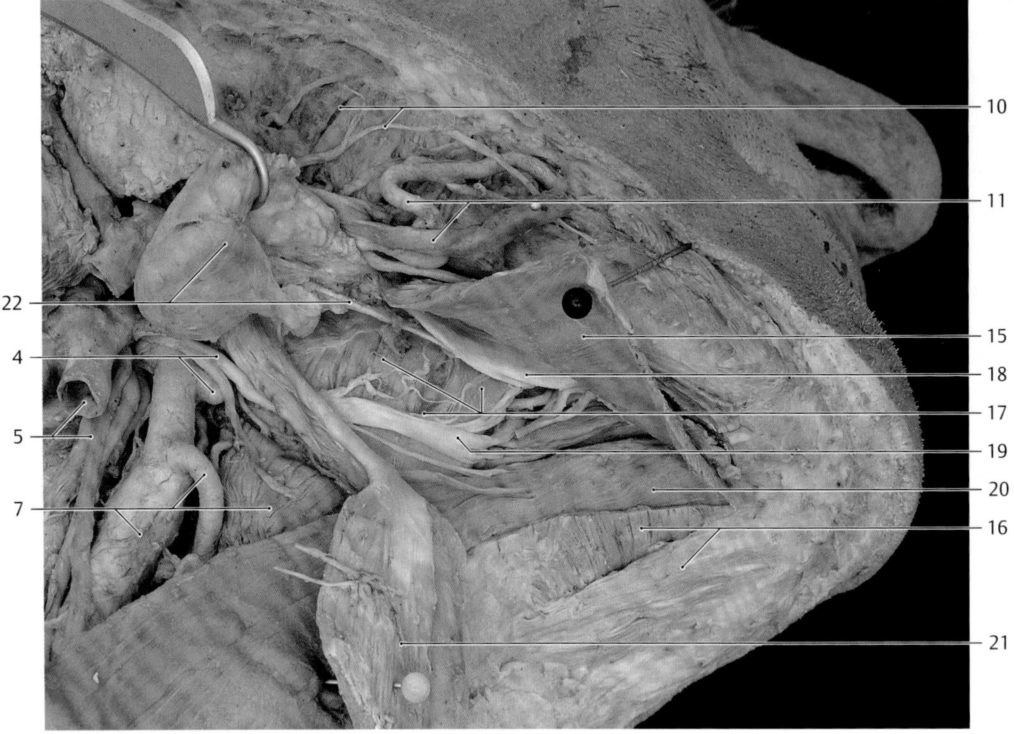


**Fig. 8.128 Submandibular triangle,** deep dissection (inferior aspect of right side). The mylohyoid muscle has been severed and reflected to display the lingual and hypoglossal nerves.

1 Parotid gland and retromandibular vein
2 Sternocleidomastoid muscle
3 Retromandibular vein, submandibular gland, and stylohyoid muscle
4 Hypoglossal nerve and lingual artery
5 Vagus nerve and internal jugular vein
6 Superior laryngeal artery
7 External carotid artery, thyrohyoid muscle, and superior thyroid artery
8 Common carotid artery and superior root of ansa cervicalis
9 Omohyoid and sternohyoid muscles
10 Masseter muscle and marginal mandibular branch of facial nerve
11 Facial artery and vein
12 Mandible and submental artery and vein
13 Mylohyoid nerve
14 Submandibular duct, sublingual gland, and anterior belly of digastric muscle
15 Mylohyoid muscle
16 Mylohyoid muscle and anterior belly of left digastric muscle
17 Hyoglossus muscle and lingual artery
18 Lingual nerve
19 Hypoglossal nerve
20 Geniohyoid muscle
21 Anterior belly of right digastric muscle
22 Submandibular gland and duct

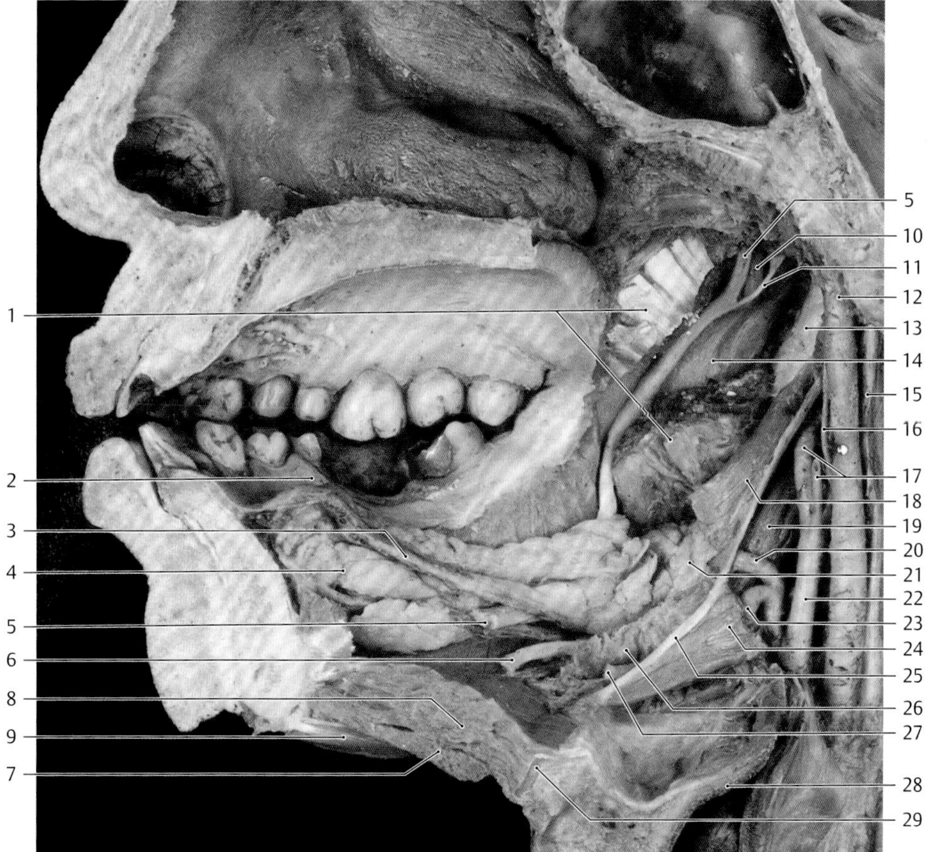


Fig. 8.129 **Oral cavity** (internal aspect). The tongue and pharyngeal wall has been removed.

1 Medial pterygoid muscle
2 Sublingual papilla
3 Submandibular duct
4 Sublingual gland
5 Lingual nerve
6 Hypoglossal nerve
7 Mylohyoid muscle
8 Geniohyoid muscle
9 Anterior belly of digastric muscle
10 Inferior alveolar nerve
11 Chorda tympani
12 Internal carotid artery
13 Parotid gland
14 Sphenomandibular ligament
15 Vagus nerve
16 Glossopharyngeal nerve
17 Superficial temporal artery and ascending pharyngeal artery
18 Styloglossus muscle
19 Posterior belly of digastric muscle
20 Facial artery
21 Submandibular gland
22 External carotid artery
23 Lingual artery
24 Middle pharyngeal constrictor muscle
25 Stylohyoid ligament
26 Hyoglossus muscle
27 Deep lingual artery
28 Epiglottis
29 Hyoid bone
30 Buccinator muscle
31 Tongue
32 Mandible (divided)
33 Parotid duct
34 Masseter muscle
35 Right and left sublingual caruncle
36 Left sublingual caruncle

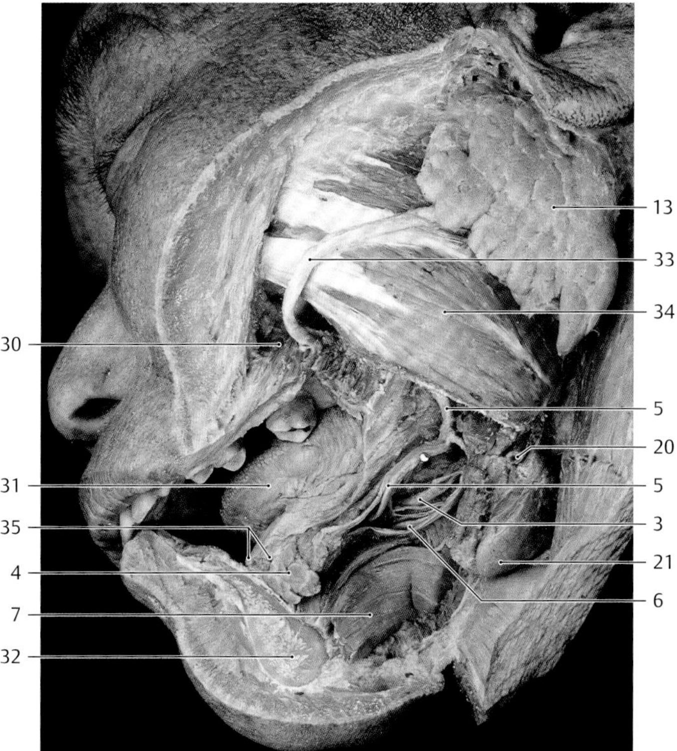


Fig. 8.130 **Dissection of the major salivary glands** (infero-lateral aspect). The left mandible and buccinator muscle have been partly removed to view the oral cavity.

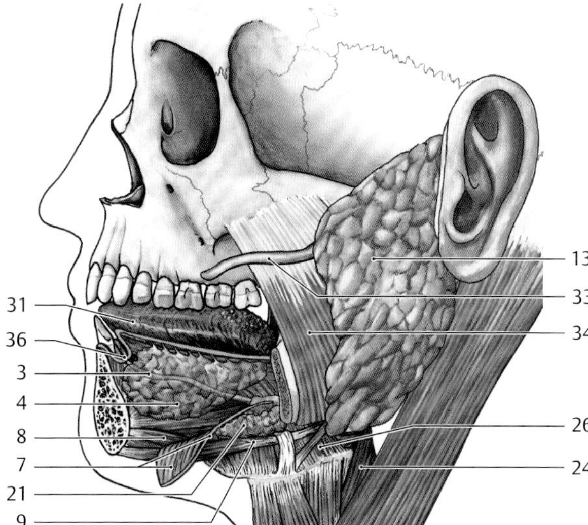


Fig. 8.131 **Location of the major salivary glands** in relation to the oral cavity (lateral aspect).

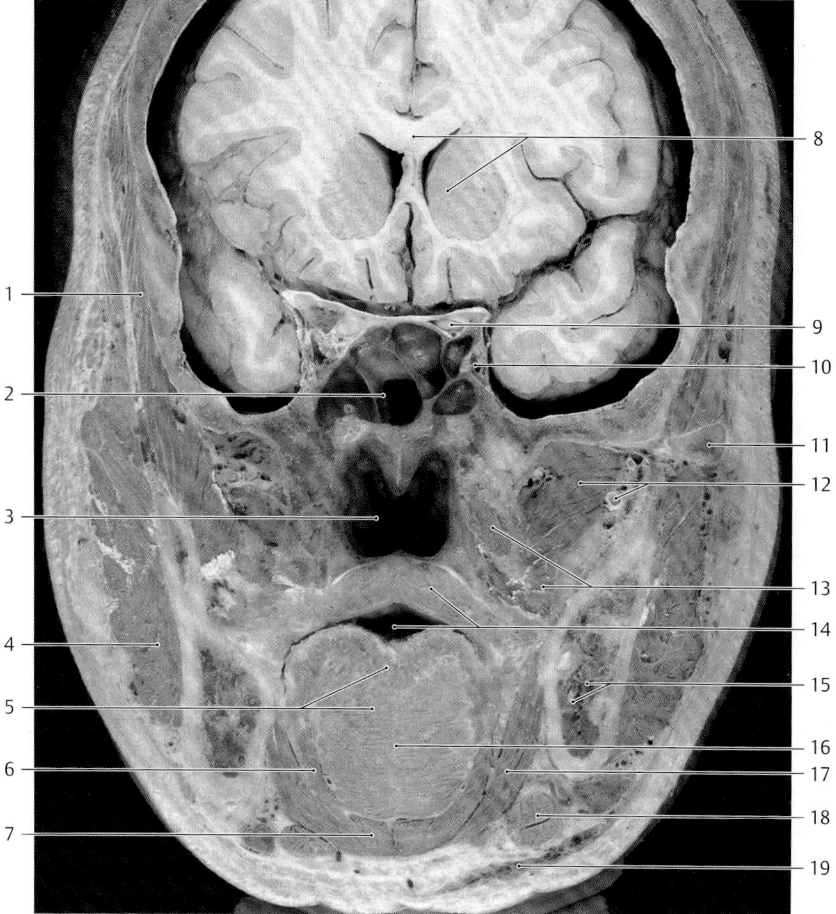


Fig. 8.132 **Coronal section through cranial, nasal, and oral cavities** at the level of sphenoidal sinus.

1 Temporal muscle
2 Sphenoidal sinus
3 Nasopharynx
4 Masseter muscle
5 Superior longitudinal, transverse, and vertical muscles of tongue
6 Hyoglossus muscle
7 Geniohyoid muscle
8 Corpus callosum (caudate nucleus)
9 Optic nerve
10 Cavernous sinus
11 Zygomatic arch
12 Cross section of lateral pterygoid muscle and maxillary artery
13 Section of medial pterygoid muscle
14 Soft palate
15 Mandible and inferior alveolar nerve
16 Septum of the tongue
17 Mylohyoid muscle
18 Submandibular gland
19 Platysma muscle
20 Foramen magnum, vertebral artery, and spinal cord
21 Internal carotid artery
22 Head of mandible
23 Styloid process
24 Inferior alveolar nerve
25 Lingual nerve and chorda tympani nerve
26 Medial pterygoid muscle
27 Uvula
28 Anterior belly of digastric muscle (cut)
29 Condyle of occipital bone
30 Mastoid process
31 Lateral pterygoid muscle
32 Auditory tube and levator veli palatini muscle
33 Tensor veli palatini muscle
34 Nasal septum
35 Mandible
36 Spinal medulla
37 Depressor labii inferioris muscle
38 Mentalis muscle
39 Genioglossus muscle

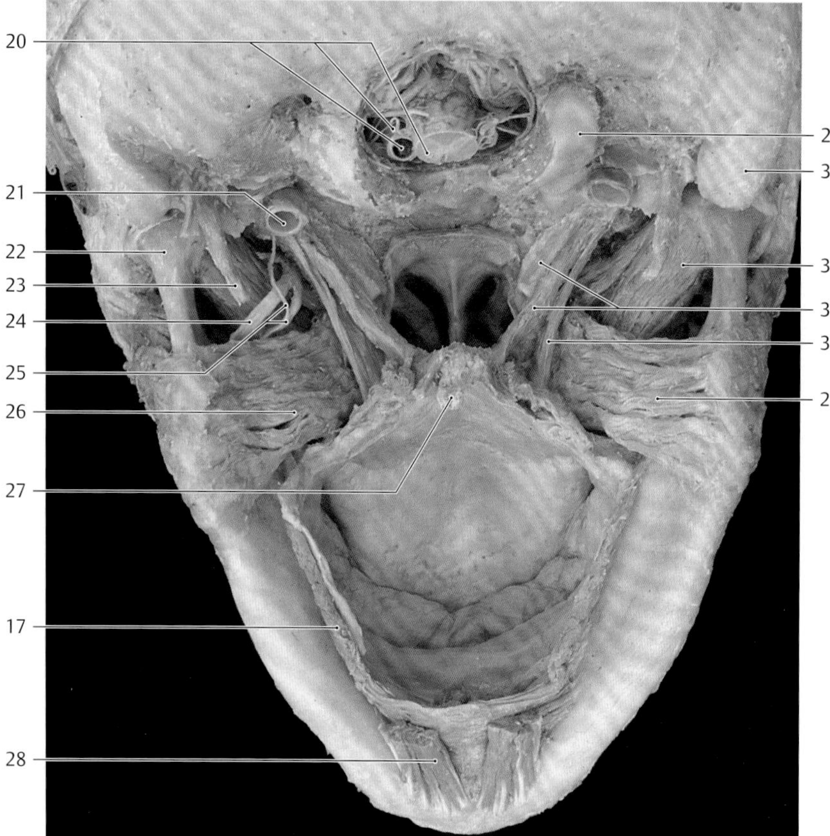


Fig. 8.133 **Pterygoid and palatine muscles** (posterior aspect).

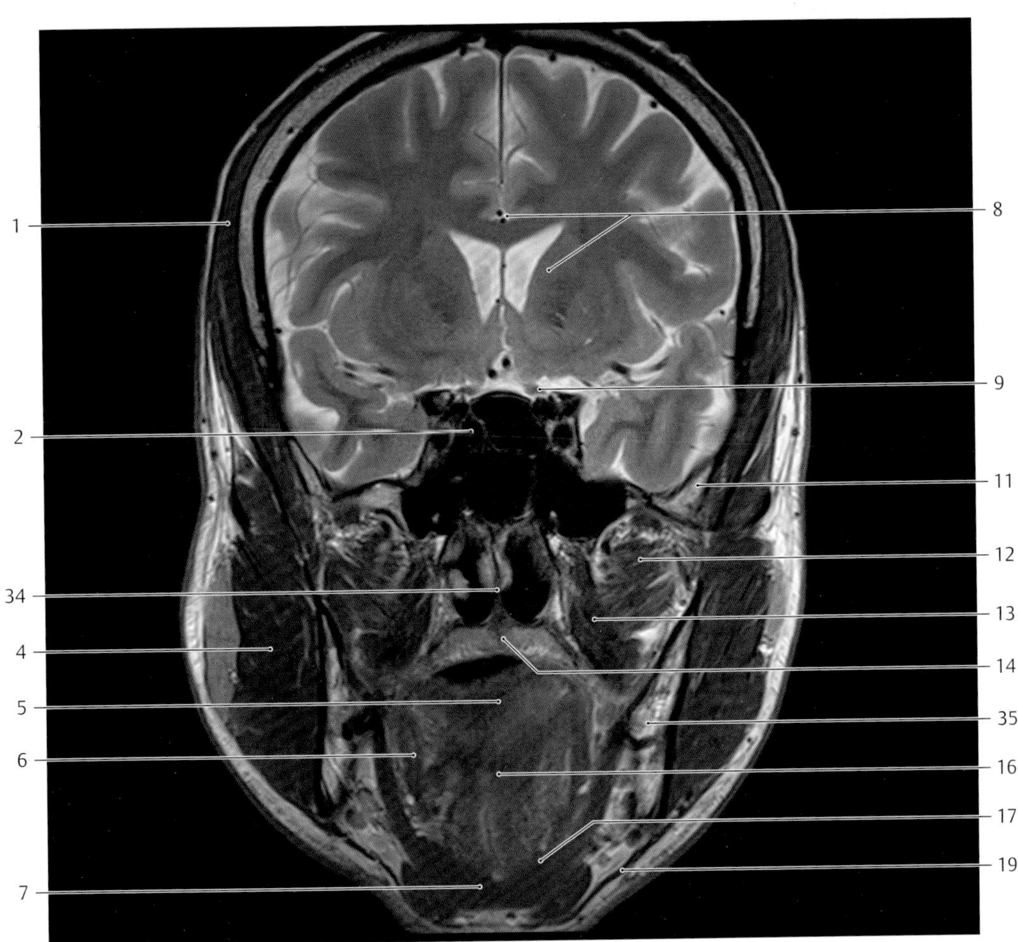


Fig. 8.134 **Frontal section through the cavities of the head** at the level of sphenoidal sinus (MRI scan). (Courtesy of Prof. Uder, Institute of Radiology, University Hospital Erlangen, Germany.)

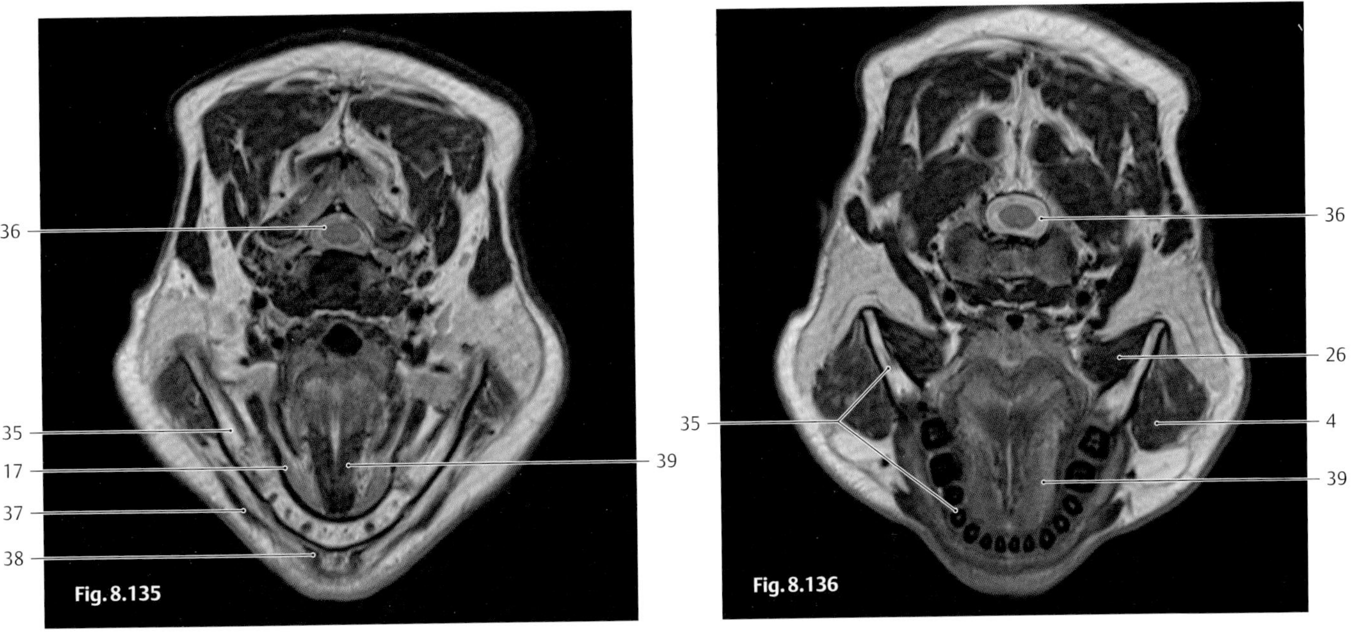


Fig. 8.135 and 8.136 **Horizontal sections** (obliquely at the course of the mandible) **through the oral cavity at different levels** (MRI scans). Note that the section in Figure 8.136 is more cranially situated than the section in Figure 8.135. (Courtesy of Prof. Uder, Institute of Radiology, University Hospital Erlangen, Germany.)

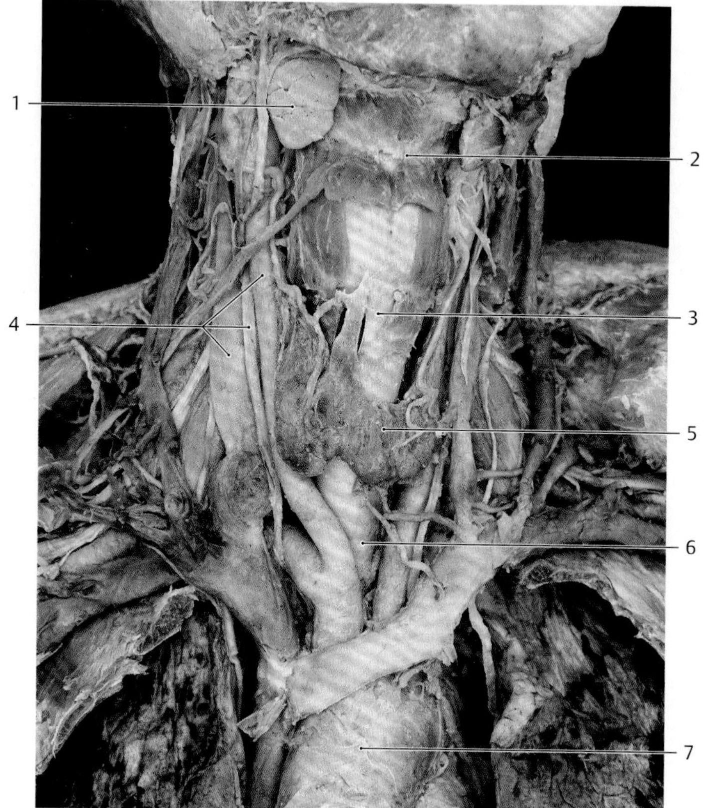


1 Submandibular gland
2 Hyoid bone
3 Larynx (thyroid cartilage)
4 Nerves and vessels of the neck (carotid artery, internal jugular vein, and vagus nerve)
5 Thyroid gland
6 Trachea
7 Aortic arch

**Fig. 8.137 Regional anatomy of the neck** (anterior aspect). The anteriorly located muscles and the thoracic wall have been removed.

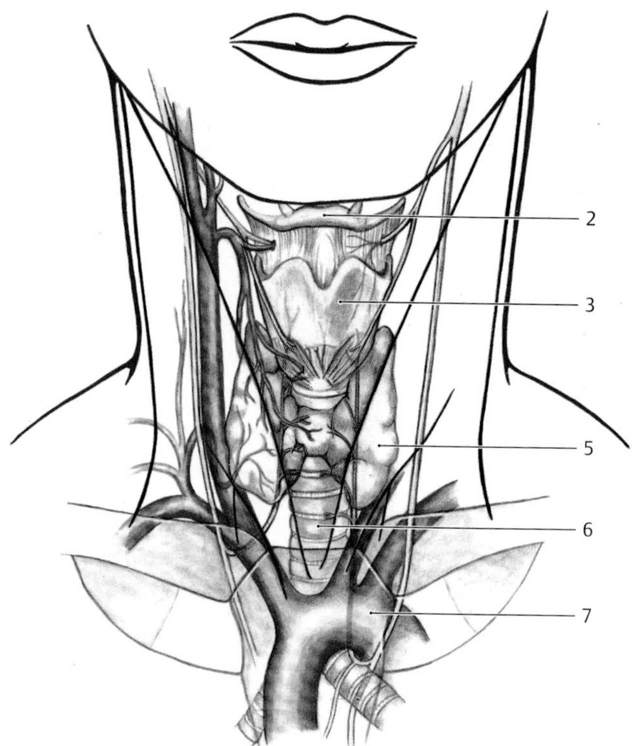


**Fig. 8.138 Organs of the neck** (anterior aspect). The main arterial trunks are indicated in red.

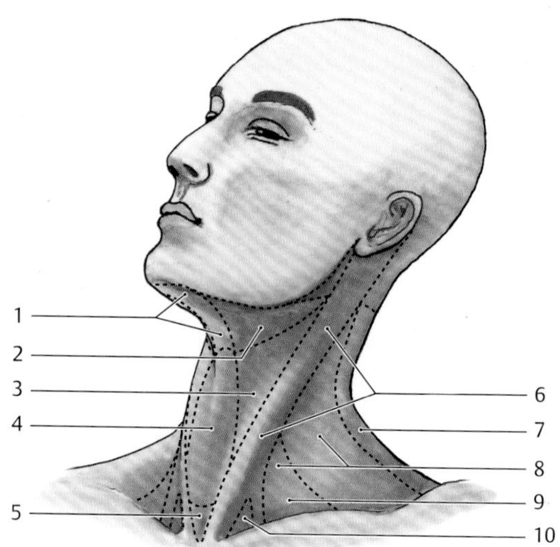


1 Submental triangle
2 Submandibular triangle
3 Carotid triangle
4 Muscular triangle
} Anterior cervical region
5 Jugular fossa
6 Sternocleidomastoid region
7 Posterior cervical region
8 Lateral cervical region
9 Greater supraclavicular fossa (supraclavicular triangle)
10 Lesser supraclavicular fossa

**Fig. 8.139 Regions and triangles of the neck** (oblique-lateral aspect).

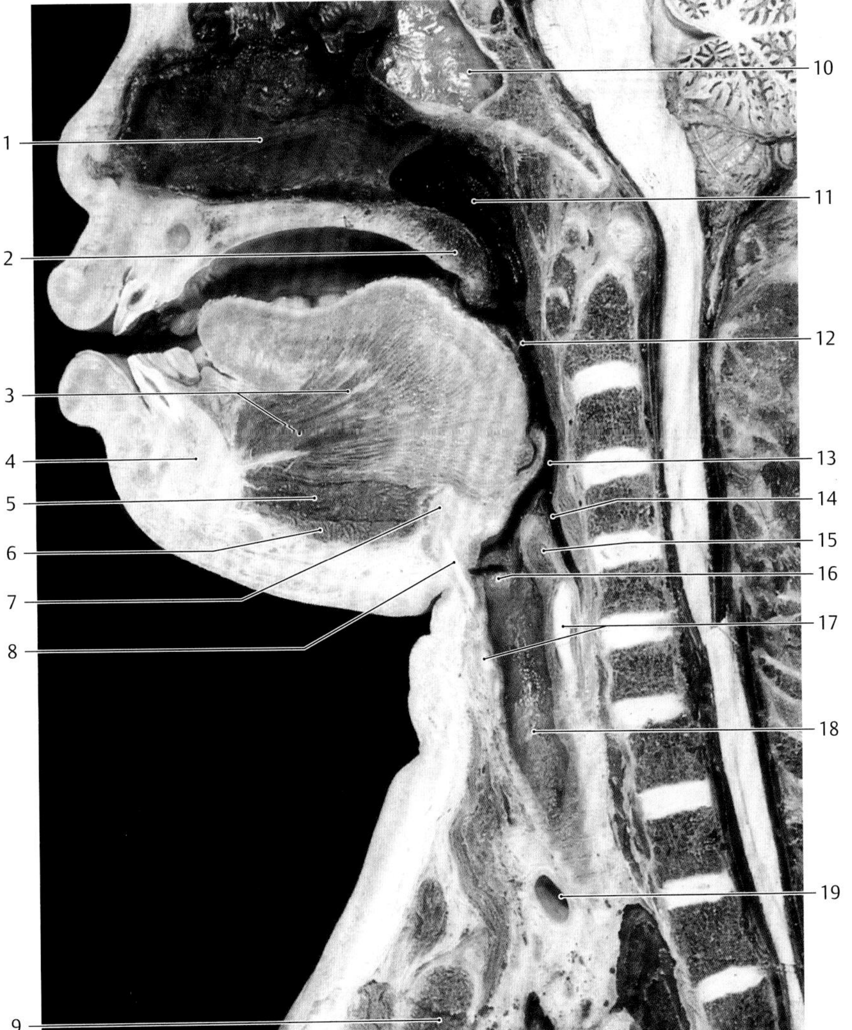


**Fig. 8.140 Median section through adult head and neck.** Note the low position of the adult larynx compared to that of the neonate in Figure 8.141 below.

1 Nasal septum
2 Uvula
3 Genioglossus muscle
4 Mandible
5 Geniohyoid muscle
6 Mylohyoid muscle
7 Hyoid bone
8 Thyroid cartilage
9 Manubrium sterni
10 Sphenoidal sinus
11 Nasopharynx
12 Oropharynx
13 Epiglottis
14 Laryngopharynx
15 Arytenoid muscle
16 Vocal fold
17 Cricoid cartilage
18 Trachea
19 Left brachiocephalic vein
20 Thymus
21 Esophagus

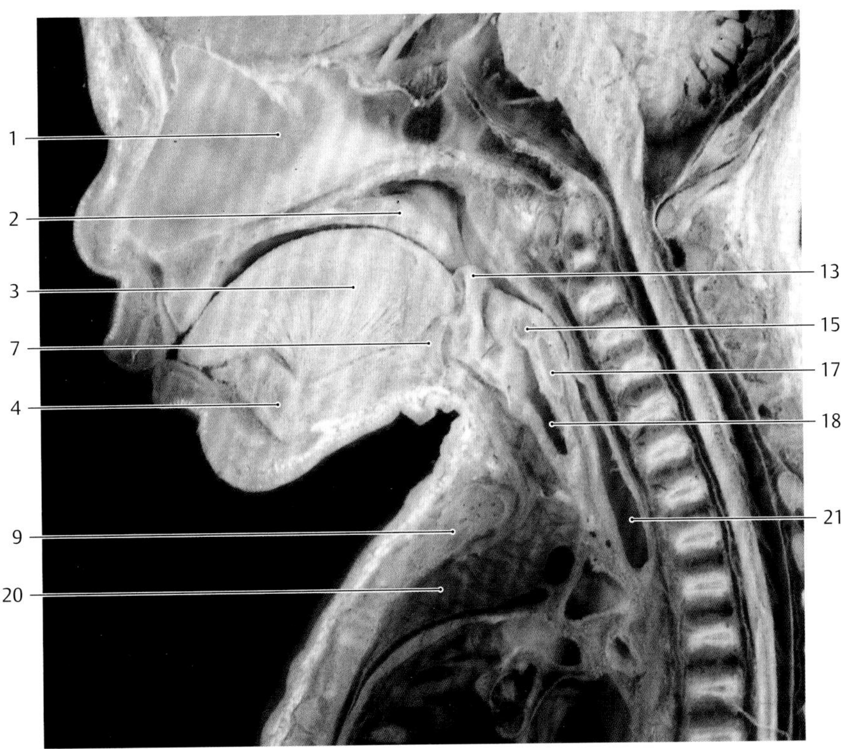


**Fig. 8.141 Median section through neonate head and neck.** Note the high position of the larynx permitting the epiglottis to nearly reach the uvula compared to that of the adult in Figure 8.140 above.

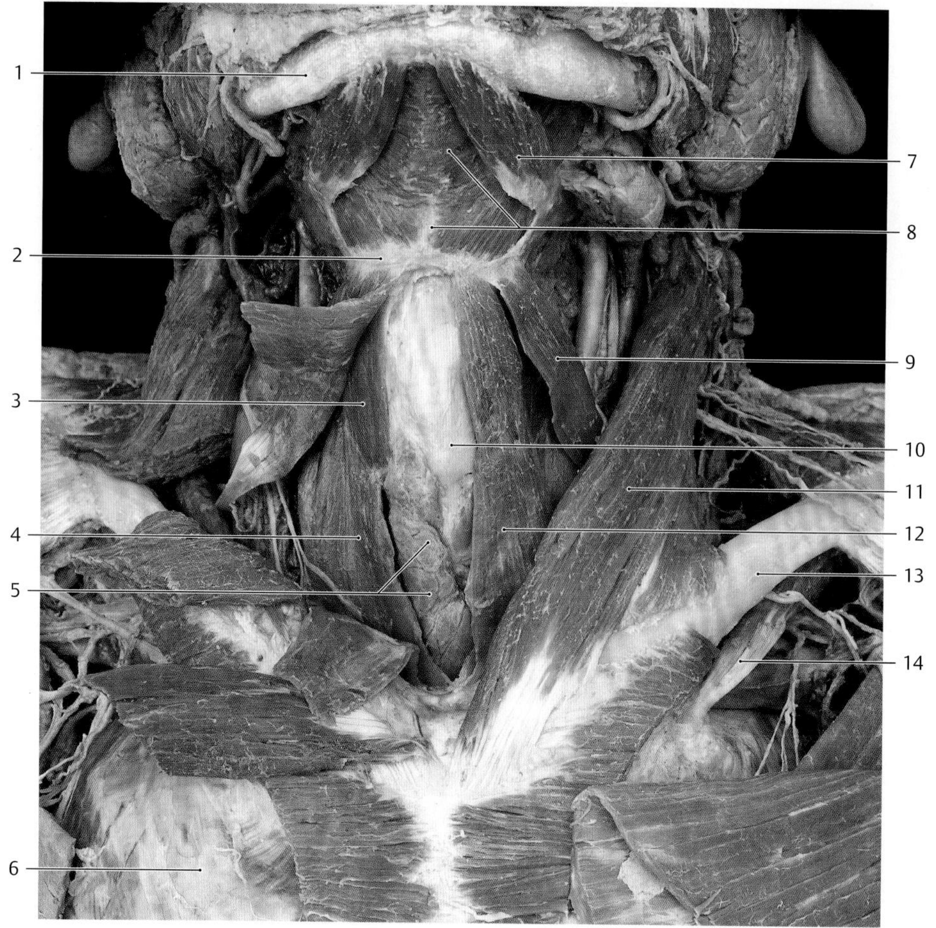


1 Mandible
2 Hyoid bone
3 Thyrohyoid muscle
4 Sternothyroid muscle
5 Thyroid gland
6 Second rib
7 Anterior belly of digastric muscle
8 Mylohyoid muscle (and mylohyoid raphe)
9 Omohyoid muscle
10 Thyroid cartilage
11 Sternocleidomastoid muscle
12 Sternohyoid muscle
13 Clavicle
14 Subclavius muscle
15 Posterior belly of digastric muscle
16 Stylohyoid muscle
17 Scalene muscles
18 Trapezius muscle
19 First rib
20 Scapula
21 Trachea
22 Manubrium sterni

Fig. 8.142 **Muscles of the neck** (anterior aspect). The sternocleidomastoid and sternohyoid muscles on the right have been divided and reflected.

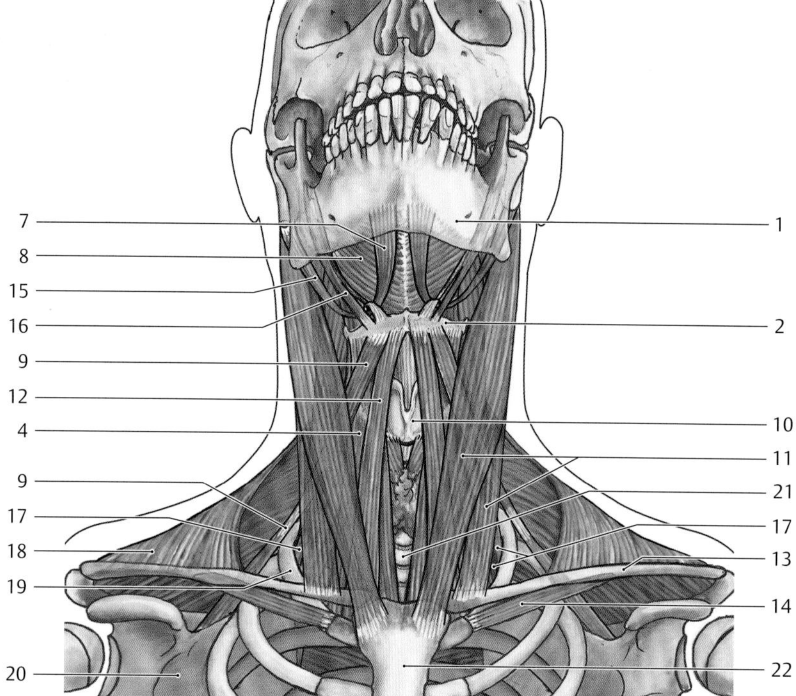


Fig. 8.143 **Muscles of the neck** (anterior aspect).

The muscles of the neck are complex and highly sophisticated. There are two major groups of muscles to be distinguished according to their functional aspects. One group is made up of muscles connecting the head to the hyoid bone and the larynx. The second category of muscles links the head and the ribcage.

The sternocleidomastoid muscle represents the border between the anterior and posterior cervical triangle.

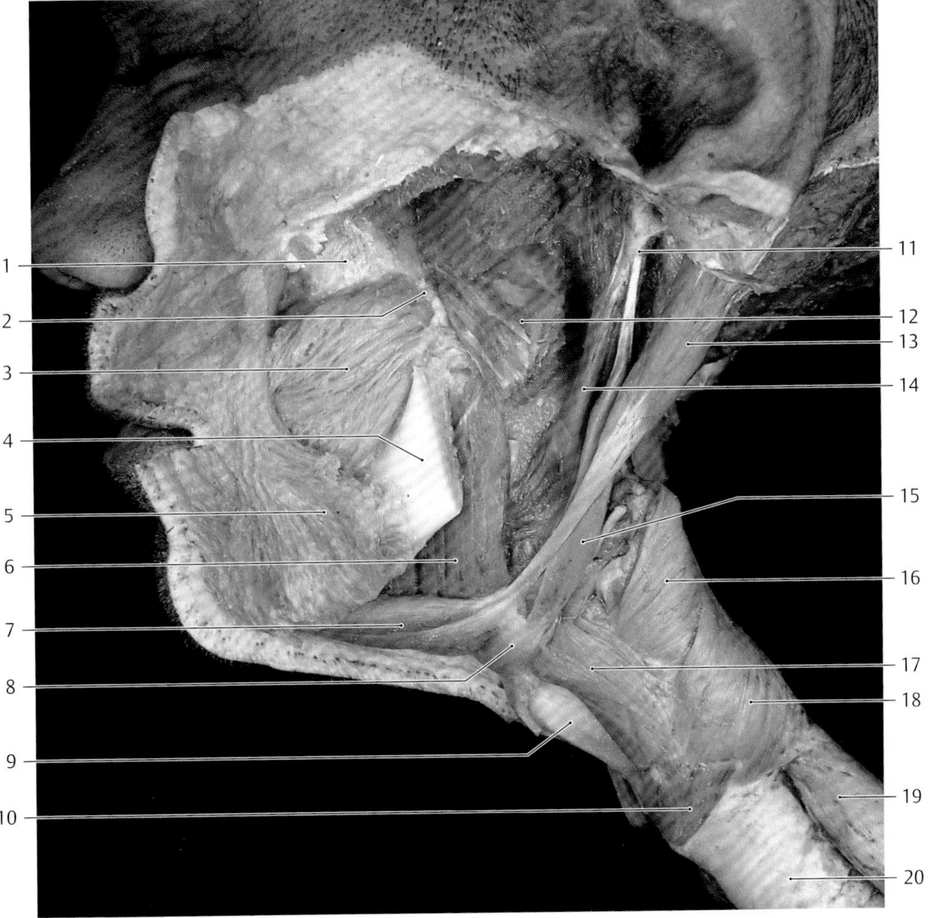


Fig. 8.144 **Dissection of pharynx, supra-, and infrahyoid muscles** (lateral aspect). The mandible has been partly removed.

1 Maxilla
2 Pterygomandibular raphe
3 Buccinator muscle
4 Mandible (divided)
5 Depressor anguli oris muscle
6 Mylohyoid muscle
7 Anterior belly of digastric muscle
8 Hyoid bone
9 Thyroid cartilage
10 Cricothyroid muscle
11 Styloid process
12 Medial pterygoid muscle (divided)
13 Posterior belly of digastric muscle
14 Styloglossus muscle
15 Stylohyoid muscle
16 Thyropharyngeal part of inferior constrictor muscle of pharynx
17 Thyrohyoid muscle
18 Cricopharyngeal part of inferior constrictor muscle of pharynx
19 Esophagus
20 Trachea
21 First molar of maxilla
22 Tongue
23 Inferior longitudinal muscle of tongue
24 Genioglossus muscle
25 Superior constrictor muscle of pharynx
26 Hypoglossal nerve
27 Hyoglossus muscle
28 Superior laryngeal nerve and superior laryngeal artery

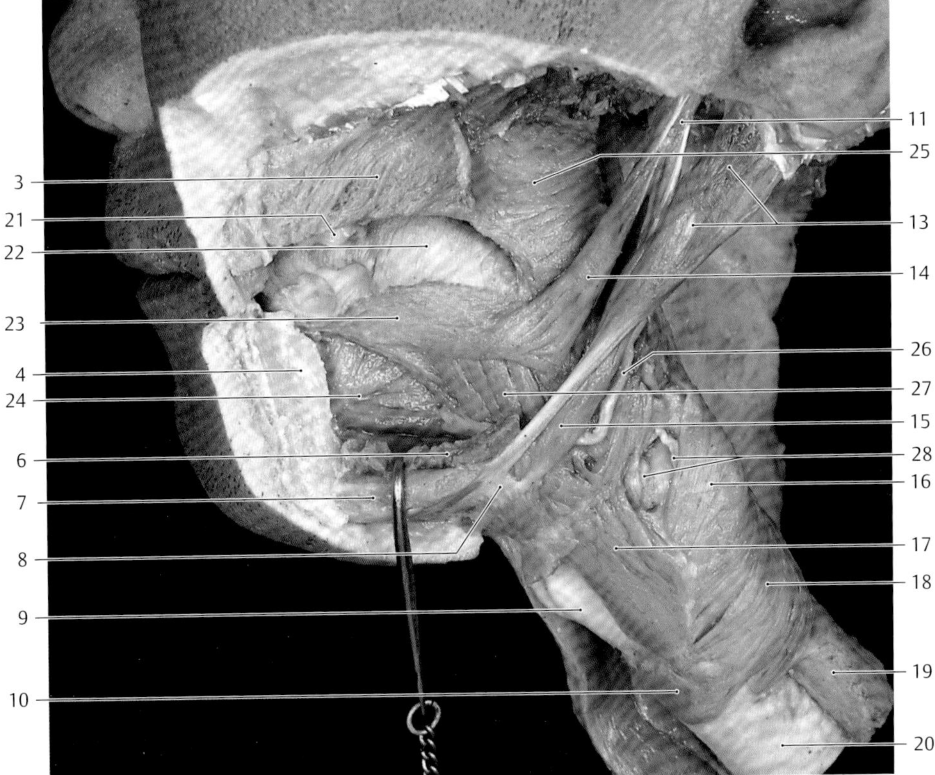


Fig. 8.145 **Dissection of pharynx, supra-, and infrahyoid muscles** (lateral aspect). The oral cavity has been opened.

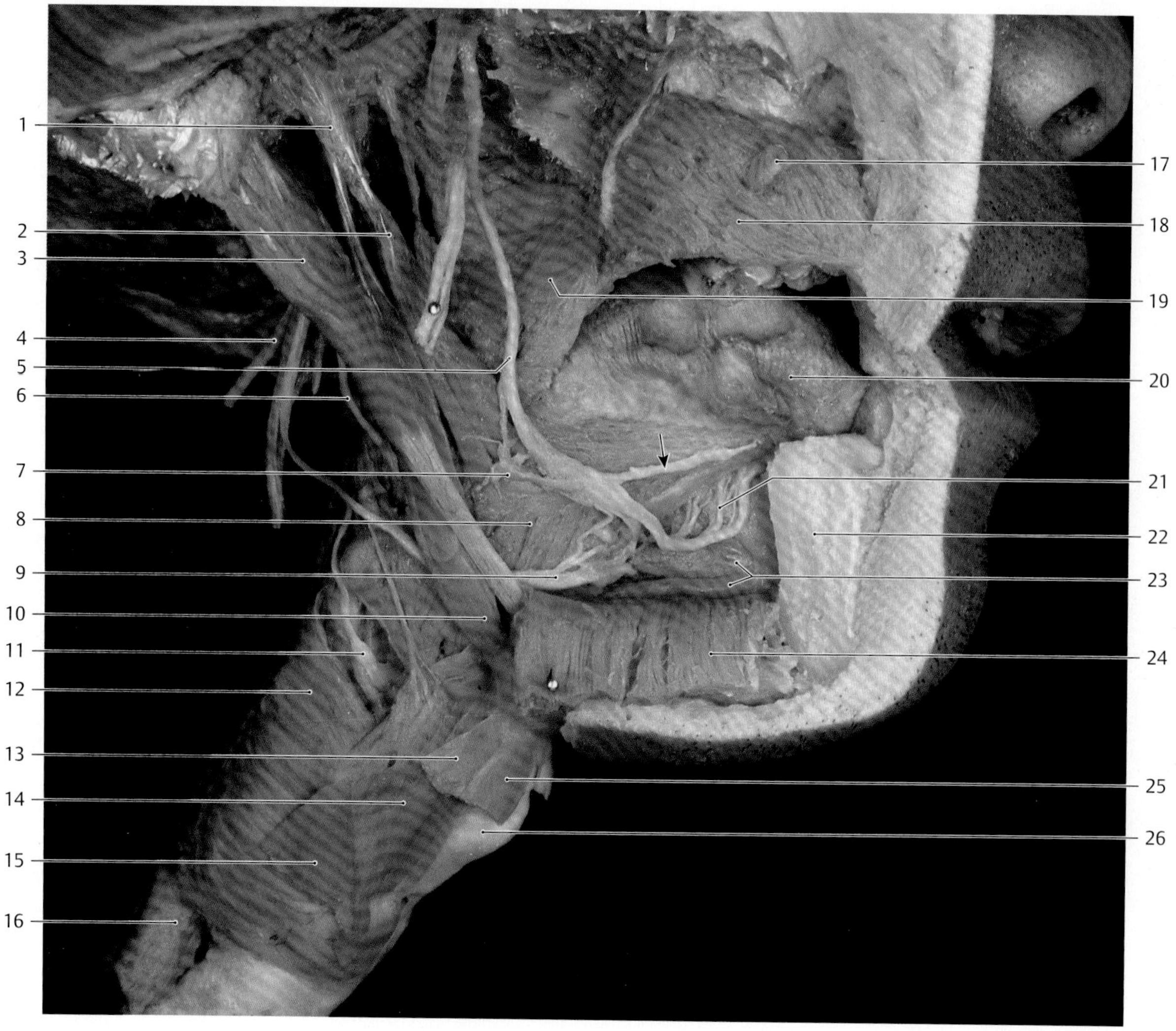

**Fig. 8.146 Parapharyngeal and sublingual regions.** Innervation of the tongue. The lateral part of the face and the mandible have been removed and the oral cavity opened. Arrow = submandibular duct.

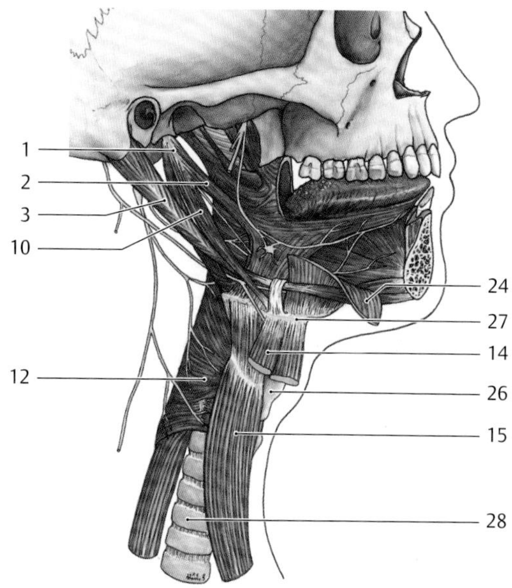


**Fig. 8.147 Supra- and infrahyoid muscles and pharynx.**

1 Styloid process
2 Styloglossus muscle
3 Posterior belly of digastric muscle
4 Vagus nerve (CN X)
5 Lingual nerve (CN $V_3$)
6 Glossopharyngeal nerve (CN IX)
7 Submandibular ganglion
8 Hyoglossus muscle
9 Hypoglossal nerve (CN XII)
10 Stylohyoid muscle
11 Internal branch of superior laryngeal nerve (branch of vagus nerve, not visible)
12 Middle constrictor muscle of pharynx
13 Omohyoid muscle (divided)
14 Thyrohyoid muscle
15 Sternothyroid muscle
16 Esophagus
17 Parotid duct (divided)
18 Buccinator muscle
19 Superior constrictor muscle of pharynx
20 Tongue
21 Terminal branches of lingual nerve
22 Mandible (divided)
23 Genioglossus and geniohyoid muscles
24 Mylohyoid muscle (divided and reflected)
25 Sternohyoid muscle (divided)
26 Thyroid cartilage
27 Hyoid bone
28 Trachea

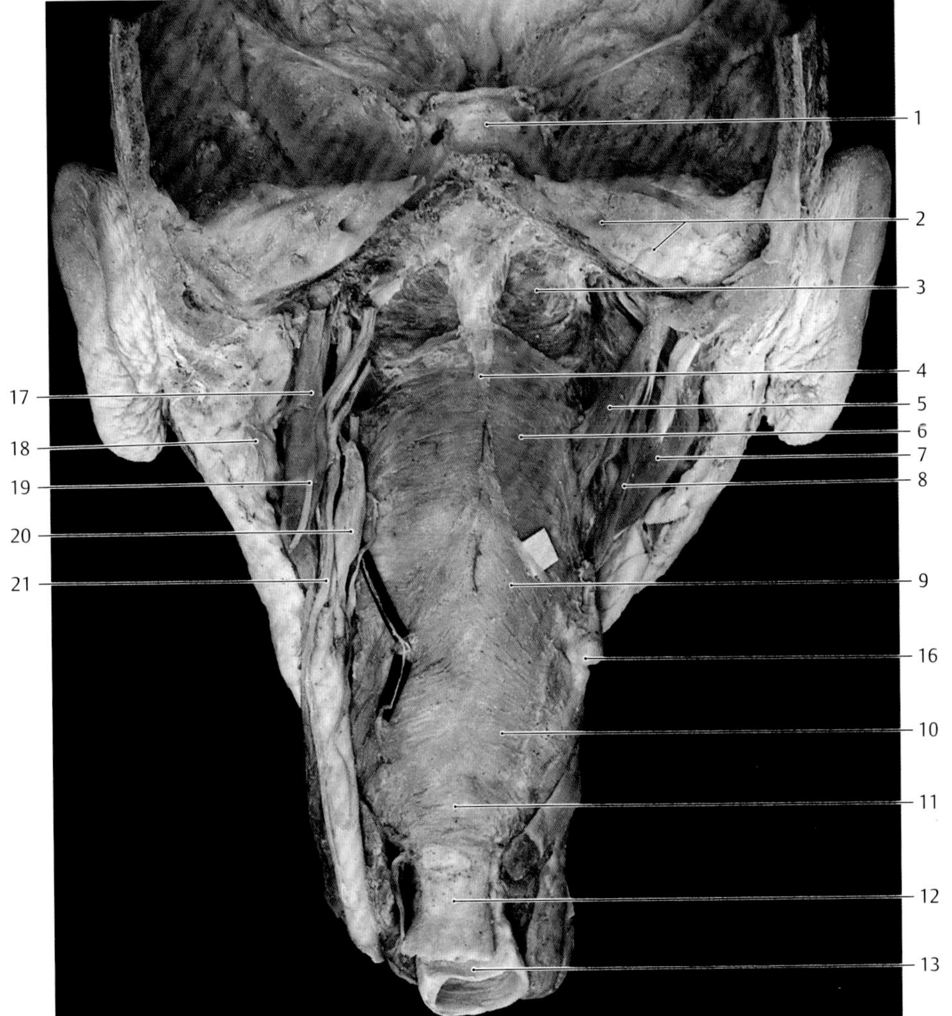


Fig. 8.148 **Muscles of the pharynx** (posterior aspect).

1 Sella turcica
2 Internal acoustic meatus and petrous part of temporal bone
3 Pharyngobasilar fascia
4 Fibrous raphe of pharynx
5 Stylopharyngeal muscle
6 Superior constrictor muscle of pharynx
7 Posterior belly of digastric muscle
8 Stylohyoid muscle
9 Middle constrictor muscle of pharynx
10 Inferior constrictor muscle of pharynx
11 Muscle-free area (Killian's triangle)
12 Esophagus
13 Trachea
14 Thyroid and parathyroid glands
15 Medial pterygoid muscle
16 Greater horn of hyoid bone
17 Internal jugular vein
18 Parotid gland
19 Accessory nerve
20 Superior cervical ganglion of sympathetic trunk
21 Vagus nerve
22 Laimer's triangle (area prone to developing diverticula)
23 Orbicularis oculi muscle
24 Nasalis muscle
25 Levator labii superioris and levator labii alaeque nasi muscles
26 Levator anguli oris muscle
27 Orbicularis oris muscle
28 Buccinator muscle
29 Depressor labii inferioris muscle
30 Hyoglossus muscle
31 Thyrohyoid muscle
32 Thyroid cartilage
33 Cricothyroid muscle
34 Pterygomandibular raphe
35 Tensor veli palatini muscle
36 Levator veli palatini muscle
37 Depressor anguli oris muscle
38 Mentalis muscle
39 Styloglossus muscle

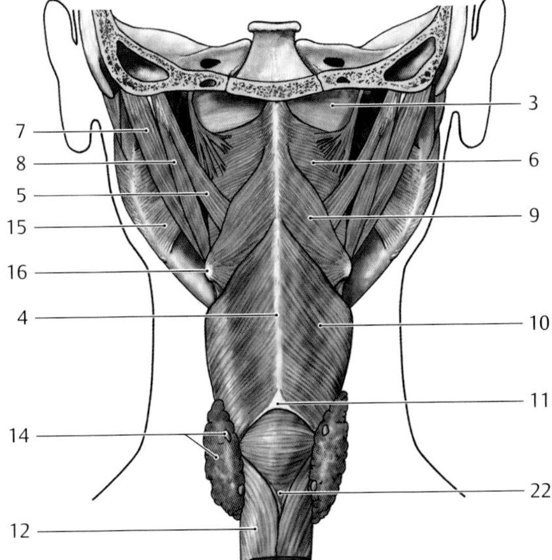


Fig. 8.149 **Muscles of the pharynx** (posterior aspect).

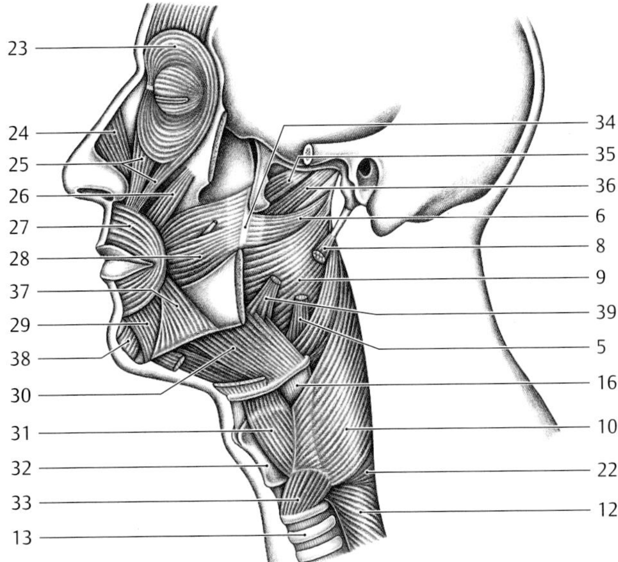


Fig. 8.150 **Muscles of the pharynx** (lateral aspect).

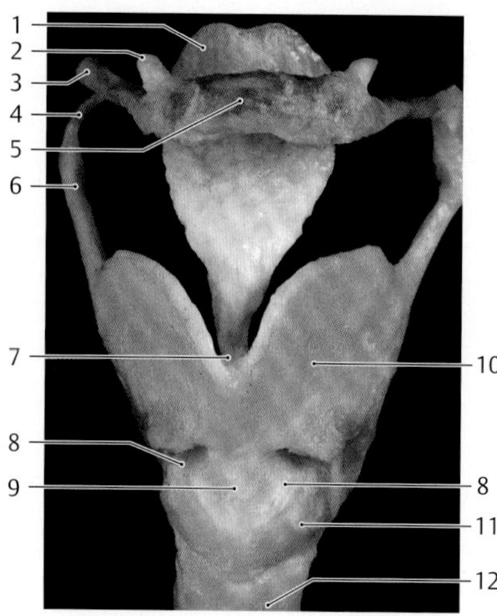

Fig. 8.151 **Cartilages of the larynx with the hyoid bone** (anterior aspect).

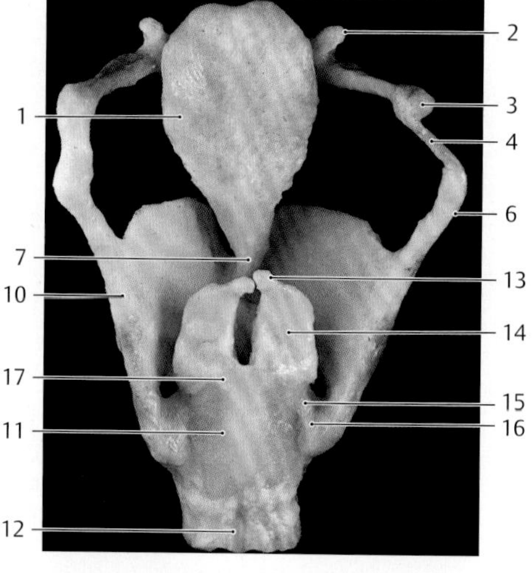
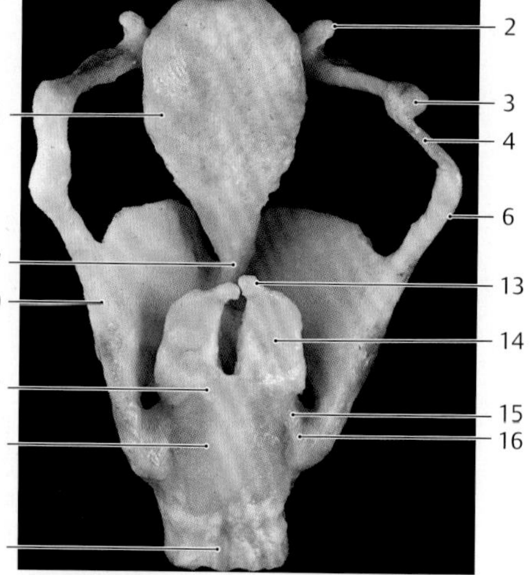
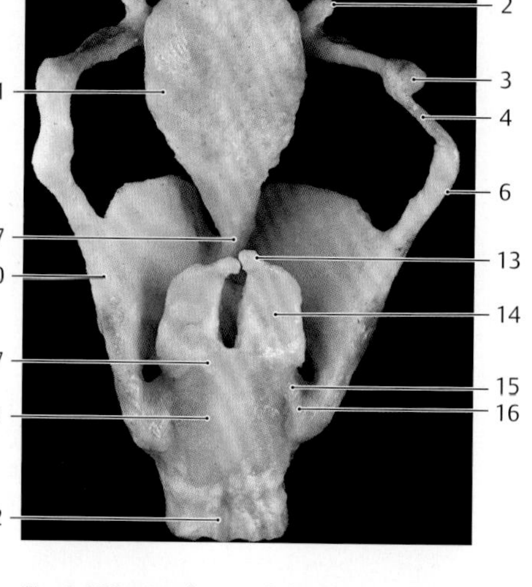

Fig. 8.152 **Cartilages of the larynx with the hyoid bone** (posterior aspect).

1 Epiglottis
2 Lesser cornu } of hyoid bone
3 Greater cornu } of hyoid bone
4 Lateral thyrohyoid ligament
5 Body of hyoid bone
6 Superior cornu of thyroid cartilage
7 Thyro-epiglottic ligament
8 Conus elasticus
9 Cricothyroid ligament
10 Thyroid cartilage
11 Cricoid cartilage
12 Trachea
13 Corniculate cartilage
14 Arytenoid cartilage
15 Posterior crico-arytenoid ligament
16 Cricothyroid joint
17 Crico-arytenoid joint

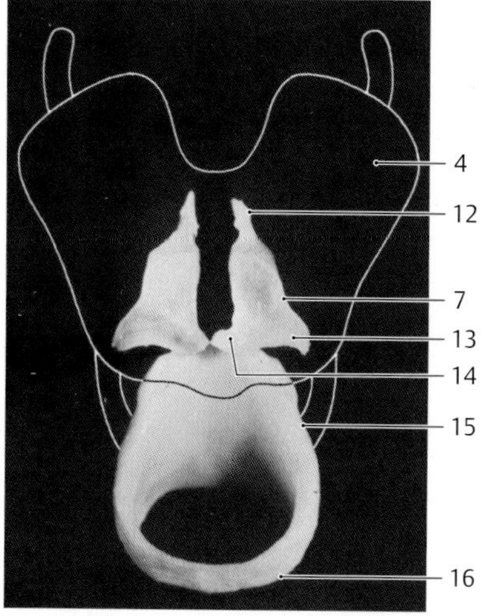

Fig. 8.153 **Cartilages of the larynx** (anterior aspect). Thyroid cartilage is indicated by the outline.

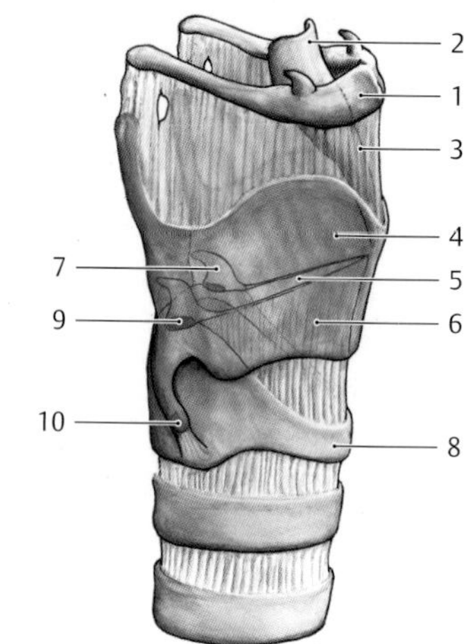

Fig. 8.154 **Cartilages and ligaments of the larynx** (lateral aspect).

1 Hyoid bone
2 Epiglottis
3 Thyrohyoid membrane
4 Thyroid cartilage
5 Vocal ligament
6 Conus elasticus
7 Arytenoid cartilage
8 Cricoid cartilage
9 Crico-arytenoid joint
10 Cricothyroid joint
11 Tracheal cartilages
12 Corniculate cartilage
13 Muscular process } of arytenoid cartilage
14 Vocal process } of arytenoid cartilage
15 Lamina of cricoid cartilage
16 Arch of cricoid cartilage

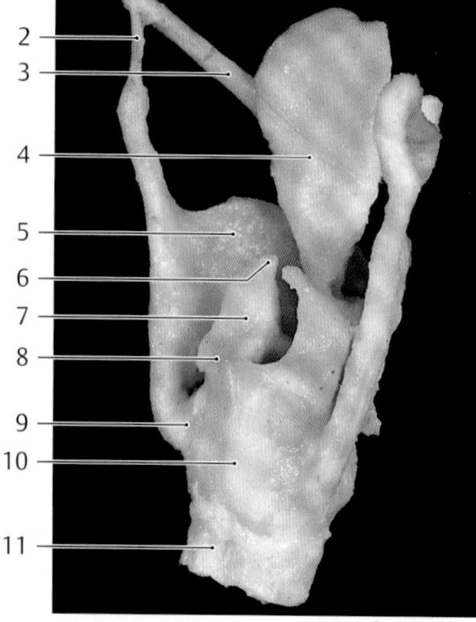

Fig. 8.155 **Cartilages of the larynx** (obliqueposterior aspect).

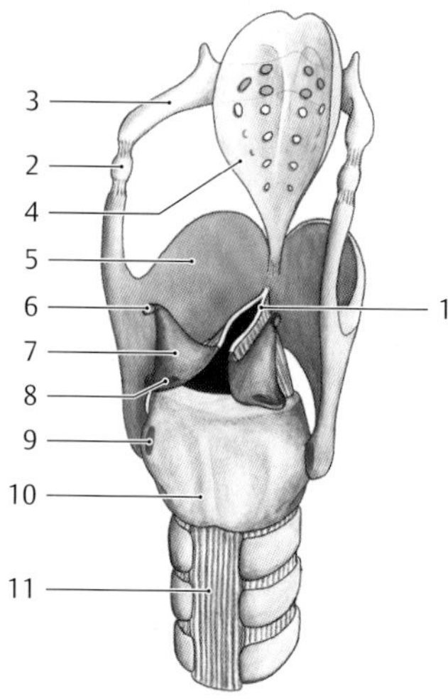

Fig. 8.156 **Cartilages of the larynx** (oblique-posterior aspect).

1 Vocal ligament
2 Lateral thyrohyoid ligament
3 Greater cornu of hyoid bone
4 Epiglottis
5 Thyroid cartilage
6 Corniculate cartilage
7 Arytenoid cartilage
8 Crico-arytenoid joint
9 Cricothyroid joint
10 Cricoid cartilage
11 Trachea

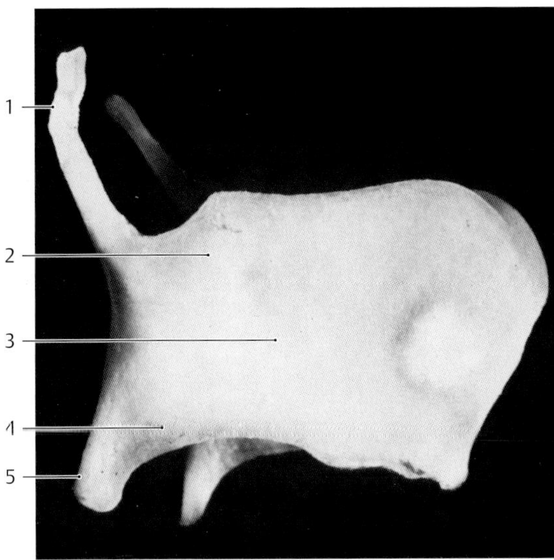


Fig. 8.157 **Thyroid cartilage** (lateral aspect).

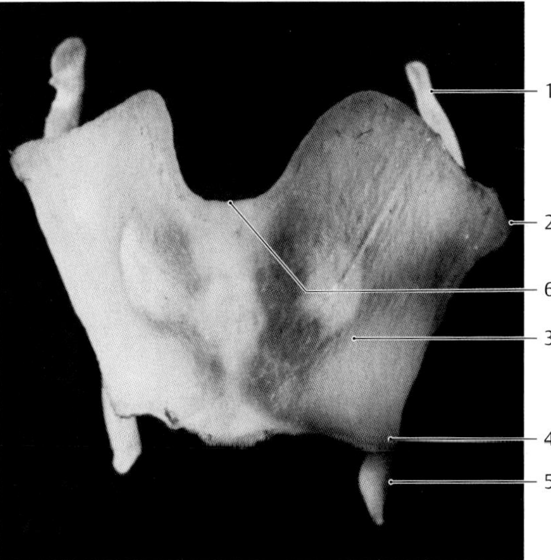


Fig. 8.158 **Thyroid cartilage** (anterior aspect).

1 Superior cornu
2 Superior thyroid tubercle
3 Lamina of thyroid cartilage
4 Inferior thyroid tubercle
5 Inferior cornu
6 Superior thyroid notch

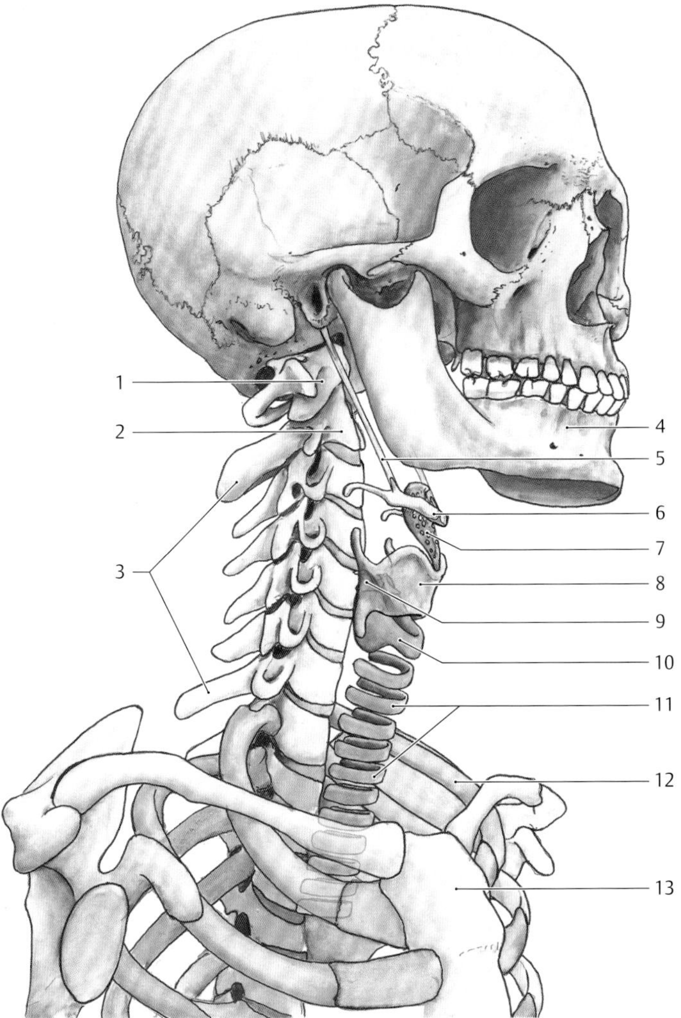


1 Atlas
2 Axis
3 Cervical vertebrae (C2–C7)
4 Mandible
5 Stylohyoid ligament
6 Hyoid bone
7 Epiglottis
8 Thyroid cartilage
9 Arytenoid cartilage
10 Cricoid cartilage
11 Tracheal cartilages
12 First rib
13 Manubrium of sternum

Fig. 8.159 **Position of the larynx and hyoid bone** in the neck (oblique-lateral aspect).

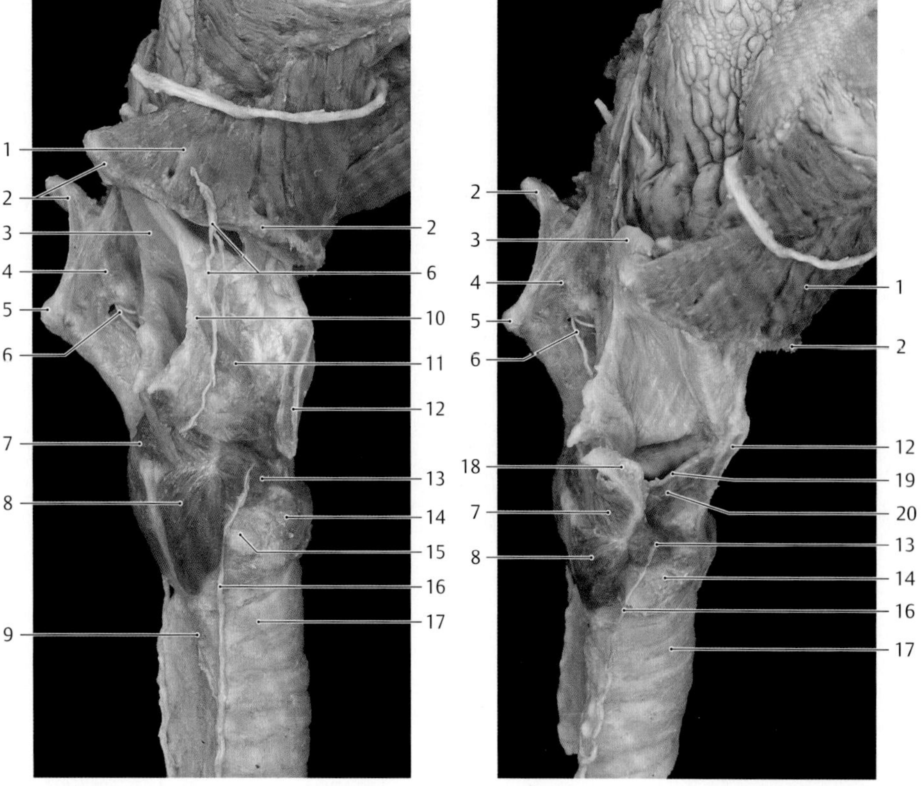


**Fig. 8.160 Laryngeal muscles** (lateral aspect). The thyroid cartilage and thyro-arytenoid muscle have been partly removed.

**Fig. 8.161 Laryngeal muscles** (lateral aspect). Dissection of the vocal ligament. Half of the thyroid cartilage has been removed.

1 Hyoglossus muscle
2 Hyoid bone
3 Epiglottis
4 Thyrohyoid membrane
5 Superior cornu of thyroid cartilage
6 Superior laryngeal nerve
7 Transverse arytenoid muscle
8 Posterior crico-arytenoid muscle
9 Transverse muscle of trachea
10 Ary-epiglottic fold
11 Thyro-epiglottic muscle
12 Thyroid cartilage
13 Lateral crico-arytenoid muscle
14 Cricoid cartilage
15 Articular facet for thyroid cartilage
16 Inferior laryngeal nerve (branch of recurrent nerve)
17 Trachea
18 Arytenoid cartilage
19 Vocal ligament
20 Vocalis muscle (part of thyro-arytenoid muscle)
21 Thyrohyoideus muscle
22 Cricothyroid muscle
23 Root of tongue
24 Cuneiform tubercle
25 Corniculate tubercle
26 Ary-epiglottic muscle

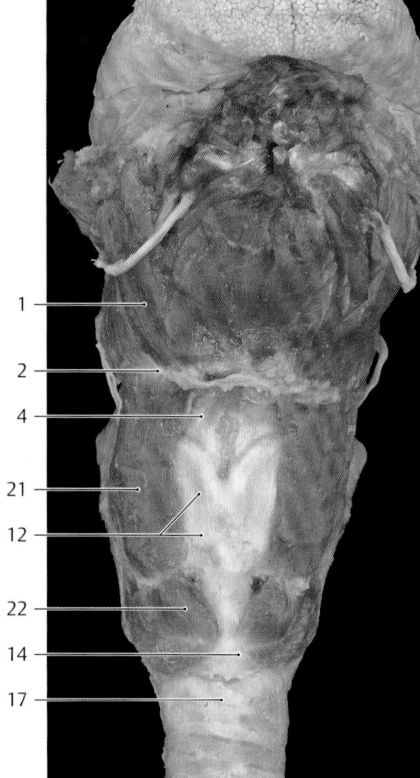


**Fig. 8.162 Laryngeal muscles and larynx** (anterior aspect).

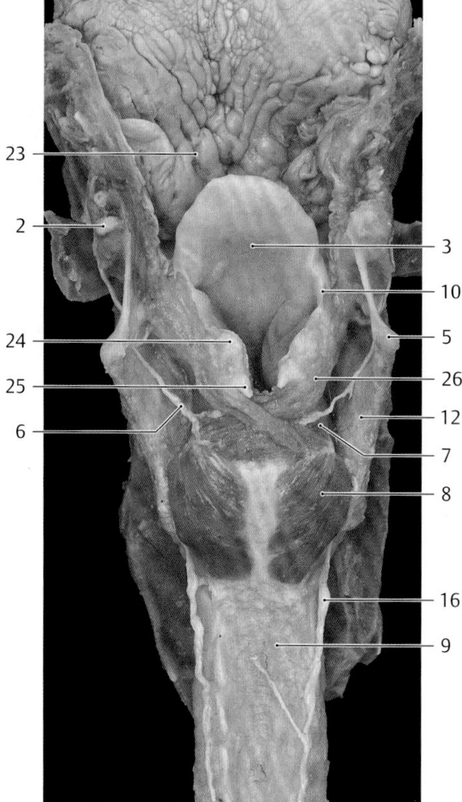


**Fig. 8.163 Laryngeal muscles and larynx** (posterior aspect).

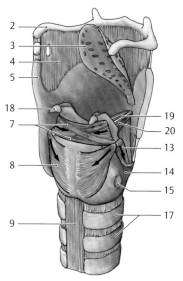

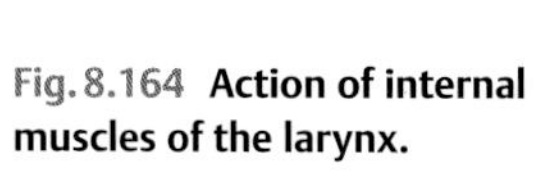


**Fig. 8.164 Action of internal muscles of the larynx.**

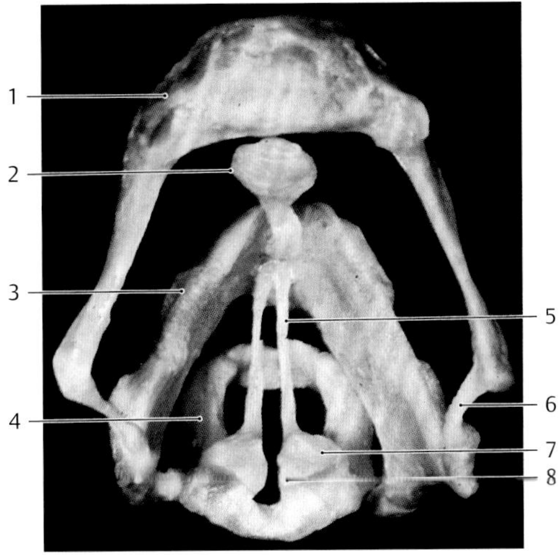


Fig. 8.165 **Laryngeal cartilages and vocal ligaments** (superior aspect).

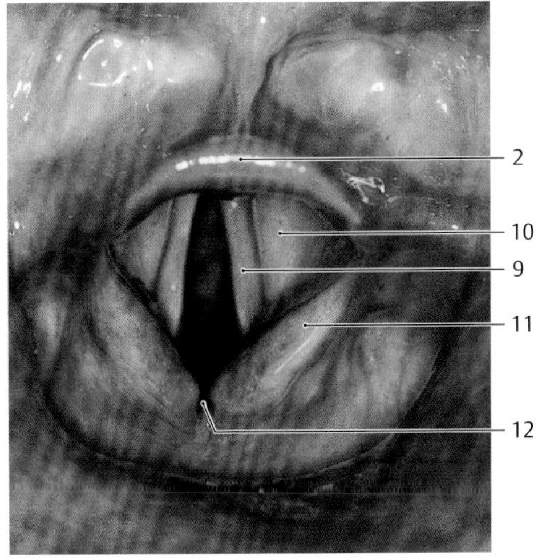


Fig. 8.166 **Glottis in vivo** (superior aspect).

1 Hyoid bone
2 Epiglottis
3 Thyroid cartilage
4 Cricoid cartilage
5 Vocal ligament
6 Thyrohyoid ligament
7 Arytenoid cartilage
8 Corniculate cartilage
9 Vocal fold
10 Vestibular fold
11 Ary-epiglottic fold
12 Interarytenoid notch
13 Mandible
14 Anterior belly of digastric muscle
15 Mylohyoid muscle
16 Pyramidal lobe of thyroid gland
17 Sternohyoid and sternothyroid muscles
18 Common carotid artery
19 Internal jugular vein
20 Rima glottidis
21 Sternocleidomastoid muscle
22 Transverse arytenoid muscle
23 Pharynx and inferior constrictor muscle
24 Ventricle of larynx
25 Vocalis muscle
26 Trachea
27 Superior cornu of thyroid cartilage
28 Root of tongue (lingual tonsil)
29 Piriform recess
30 Vocalis muscle
31 Lateral crico-arytenoid muscle
32 Thyroid gland

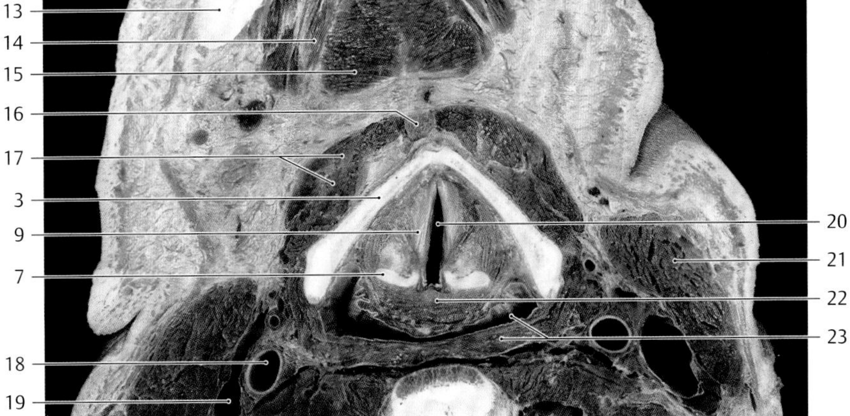


Fig. 8.167 **Horizontal section through the larynx** at the level of the vocal folds (superior aspect).

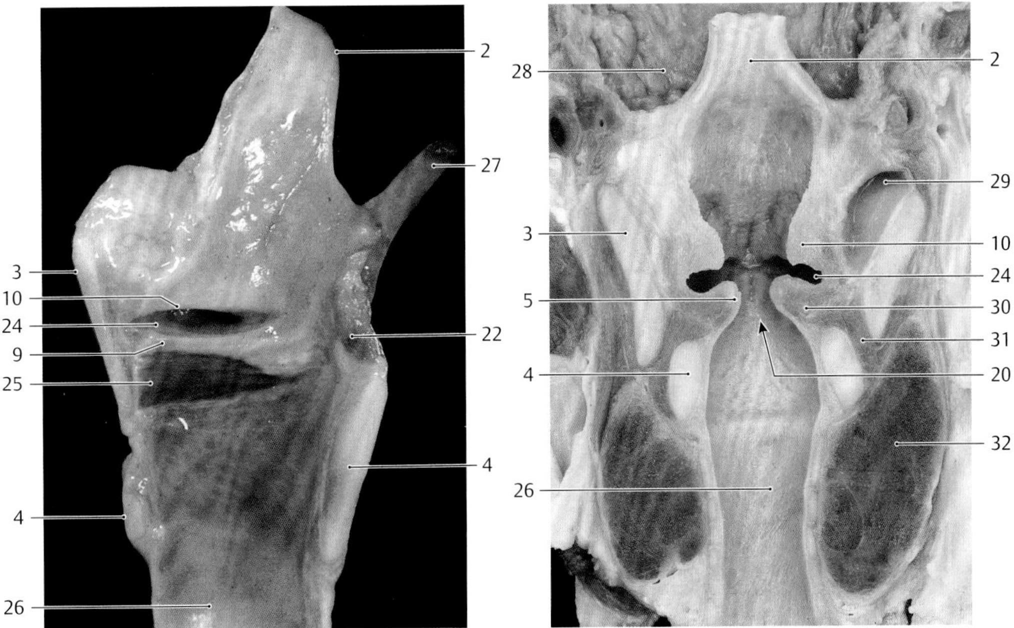


Fig. 8.168 **Sagittal section through larynx and trachea.**

Fig. 8.169 **Coronal section through larynx and trachea.**

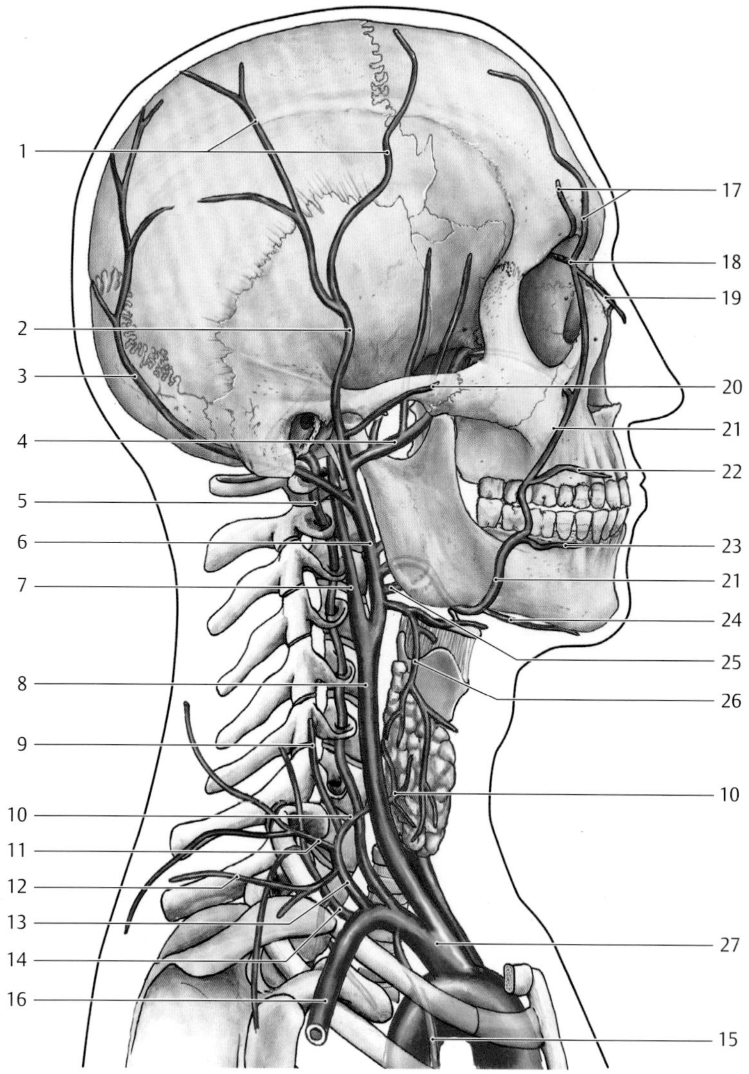

1 Frontal and parietal branches of superficial temporal artery
2 Superficial temporal artery
3 Occipital artery
4 Maxillary artery
5 Vertebral artery
6 External carotid artery
7 Internal carotid artery
8 Common carotid artery (divided)
9 Ascending cervical artery
10 Inferior thyroid artery
11 Transverse cervical artery with two branches (superficial cervical artery and descending scapular artery)
12 Suprascapular artery

(9–12: Thyro-cervical trunk)

13 Thyrocervical trunk
14 Costocervical trunk with two branches (deep cervical artery and supreme intercostal artery)
15 Internal thoracic artery
16 Axillary artery
17 Supra-orbital and supra-trochlear arteries
18 Angular artery
19 Dorsal nasal artery
20 Transverse facial artery
21 Facial artery
22 Superior labial artery
23 Inferior labial artery
24 Submental artery
25 Lingual artery
26 Superior thyroid artery
27 Brachiocephalic trunk

Fig. 8.170 **Arteries of head and neck** (lateral aspect). Diagram of the main branches of the external carotid and subclavian arteries.

▸ **Labels for Figure 8.171 (next page):**

1 Galea aponeurotica
2 Frontal branch } of superficial temporal artery
3 Parietal branch } of superficial temporal artery
4 Superior auricular muscle
5 Superficial temporal artery and vein
6 Middle temporal artery
7 Auriculotemporal nerve
8 Branches of facial nerve
9 Facial nerve
10 External carotid artery within the retromandibular fossa
11 Posterior belly of digastric muscle
12 Sternocleidomastoid artery
13 Sympathetic trunk and superior cervical ganglion
14 Sternocleidomastoid muscle (divided and reflected)
15 Clavicle (divided)
16 Transverse cervical artery
17 Ascending cervical artery and phrenic nerve
18 Anterior scalene muscle
19 Suprascapular artery
20 Dorsal scapular artery
21 Brachial plexus and axillary artery
22 Thoraco-acromial artery
23 Lateral thoracic artery
24 Median nerve (displaced) and pectoralis minor muscle (reflected)
25 Frontal belly of occipitofrontalis muscle
26 Orbital part of orbicularis oculi muscle
27 Angular artery and vein
28 Facial artery
29 Superior labial artery
30 Zygomaticus major muscle
31 Inferior labial artery
32 Parotid duct
33 Buccal fat pad
34 Maxillary artery
35 Masseter muscle
36 Facial artery and mandible
37 Submental artery
38 Anterior belly of digastric muscle
39 Hyoid bone
40 Internal carotid artery
41 External carotid artery
42 Superior laryngeal artery
43 Superior thyroid artery
44 Common carotid artery
45 Thyroid ansa of sympathetic trunk and inferior thyroid artery
46 Thyroid gland (right lobe)
47 Vertebral artery
48 Thyrocervical trunk
49 Vagus nerve
50 Ansa subclavia of sympathetic trunk
51 Brachiocephalic trunk
52 Superior vena cava (divided)
53 Aortic arch

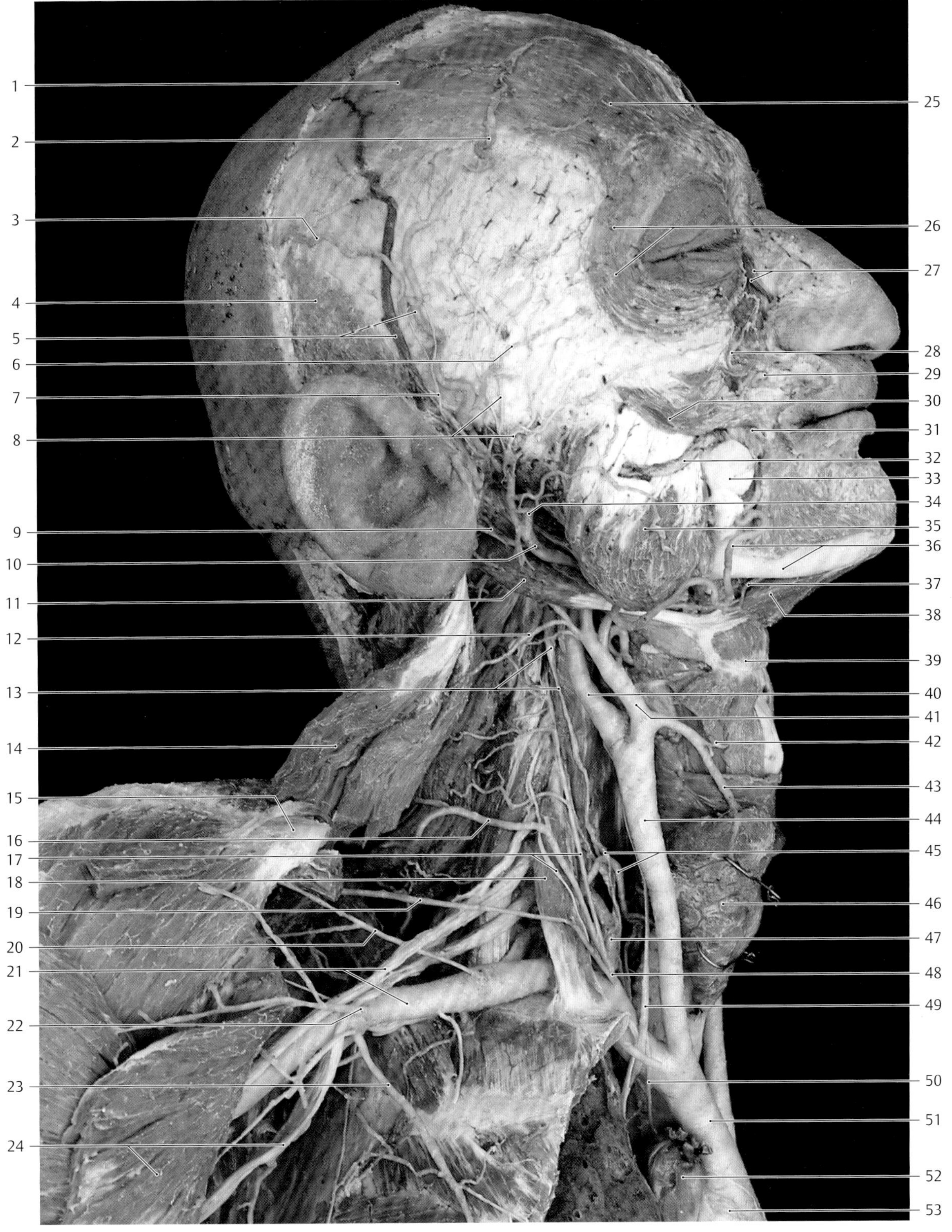


Fig. 8.171 **Main branches of head and neck arteries** (lateral aspect). The anterior thoracic wall and clavicle have been partly removed and the pectoralis muscles have been reflected to display the subclavian and axillary arteries.

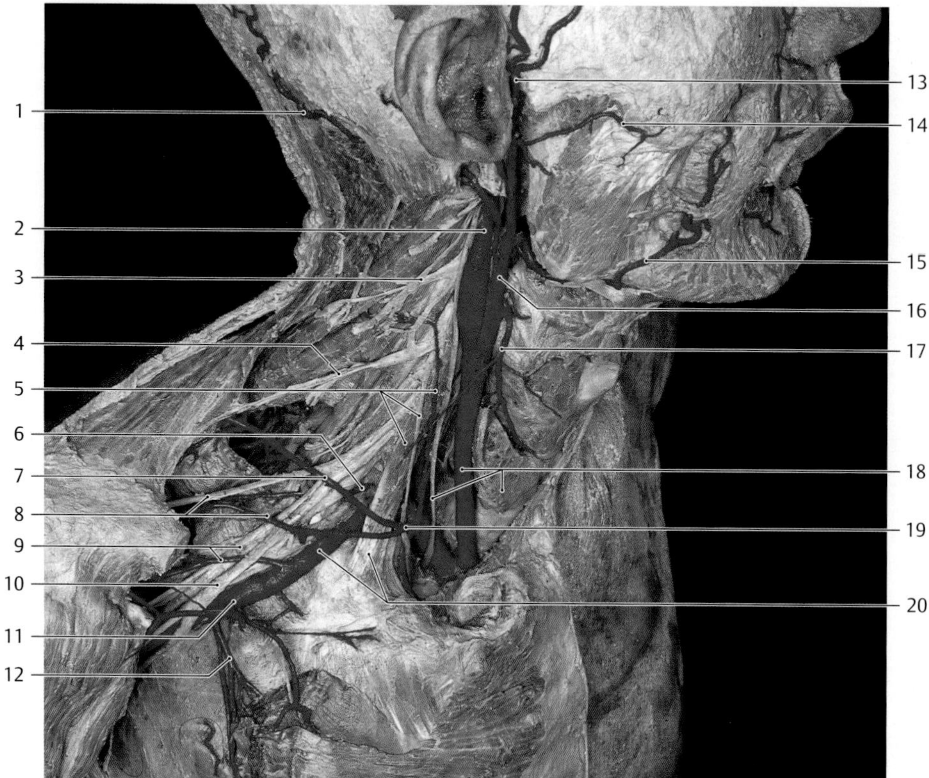


Fig. 8.172 **Arteries of head and neck** (antero-lateral aspect). The clavicle, sternocleidomastoid muscle, and veins have been partly removed. Arteries have been colored red.

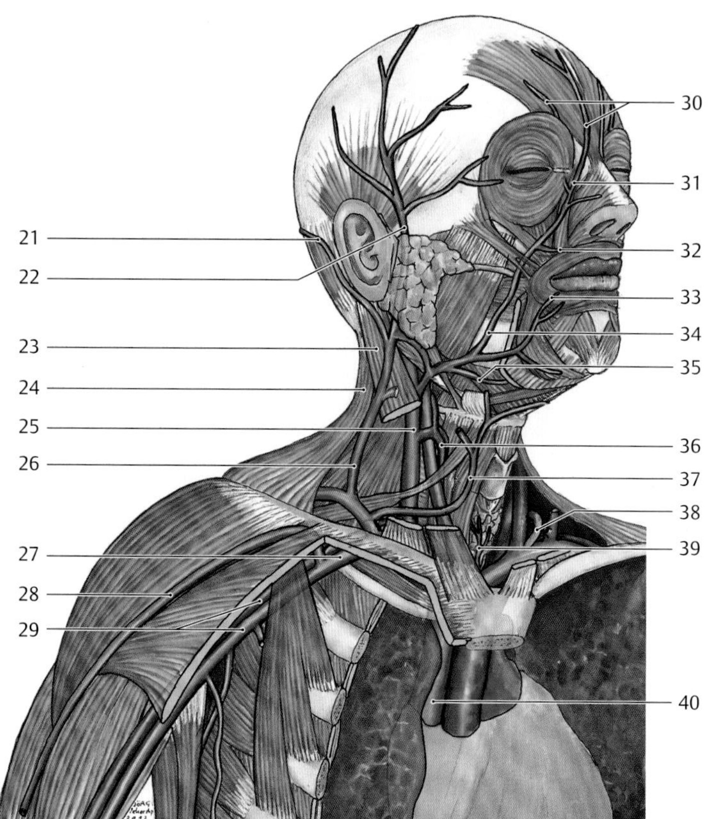


Fig. 8.173 **Veins of head, neck, and shoulder** (anterior aspect). The sternocleidomastoid muscle and anterior thoracic wall have been partly removed. Note the venous connection with the superior vena cava.

1 Occipital branch of occipital artery
2 Internal carotid artery
3 Cervical plexus
4 Supraclavicular nerve
5 Phrenic nerve and ascending cervical artery on anterior scalene muscle
6 Transverse cervical artery
7 Superficial cervical artery
8 Suprascapular artery and nerve
9 Brachial plexus and transverse cervical artery
10 Lateral cord of brachial plexus
11 Thoraco-acromial artery
12 Lateral thoracic artery
13 Superficial temporal artery
14 Transverse facial artery
15 Facial artery
16 External carotid artery
17 Superior thyroid artery
18 Common carotid artery, vagus nerve, and thyroid gland
19 Thyrocervical trunk
20 Subclavian artery and anterior scalene muscle
21 Occipital vein
22 Superficial temporal vein
23 Sternocleidomastoid muscle
24 Trapezius muscle
25 Internal jugular vein
26 External jugular vein
27 Subclavian vein
28 Cephalic vein
29 Axillary vein and artery
30 Supra-orbital veins
31 Angular vein
32 Superior labial vein
33 Inferior labial vein
34 Facial vein
35 Submental vein
36 Superior thyroid vein
37 Anterior jugular vein
38 Thoracic duct
39 Inferior thyroid vein
40 Superior vena cava
41 Parotid gland and facial nerve
42 Great auricular nerve
43 External jugular vein
44 Brachial plexus
45 Cephalic vein within the delto-pectoral triangle
46 Right brachiocephalic vein
47 Superior vena cava
48 Right lung (reflected)
49 Superficial temporal artery and vein
50 Facial artery and vein
51 Cervical branch of facial nerve and submandibular gland
52 Internal jugular vein, common carotid artery, and omohyoid muscle
53 Anterior jugular vein and thyroid gland
54 Jugular venous arch
55 Left brachiocephalic vein
56 Pericardium of heart (location of right atrium)

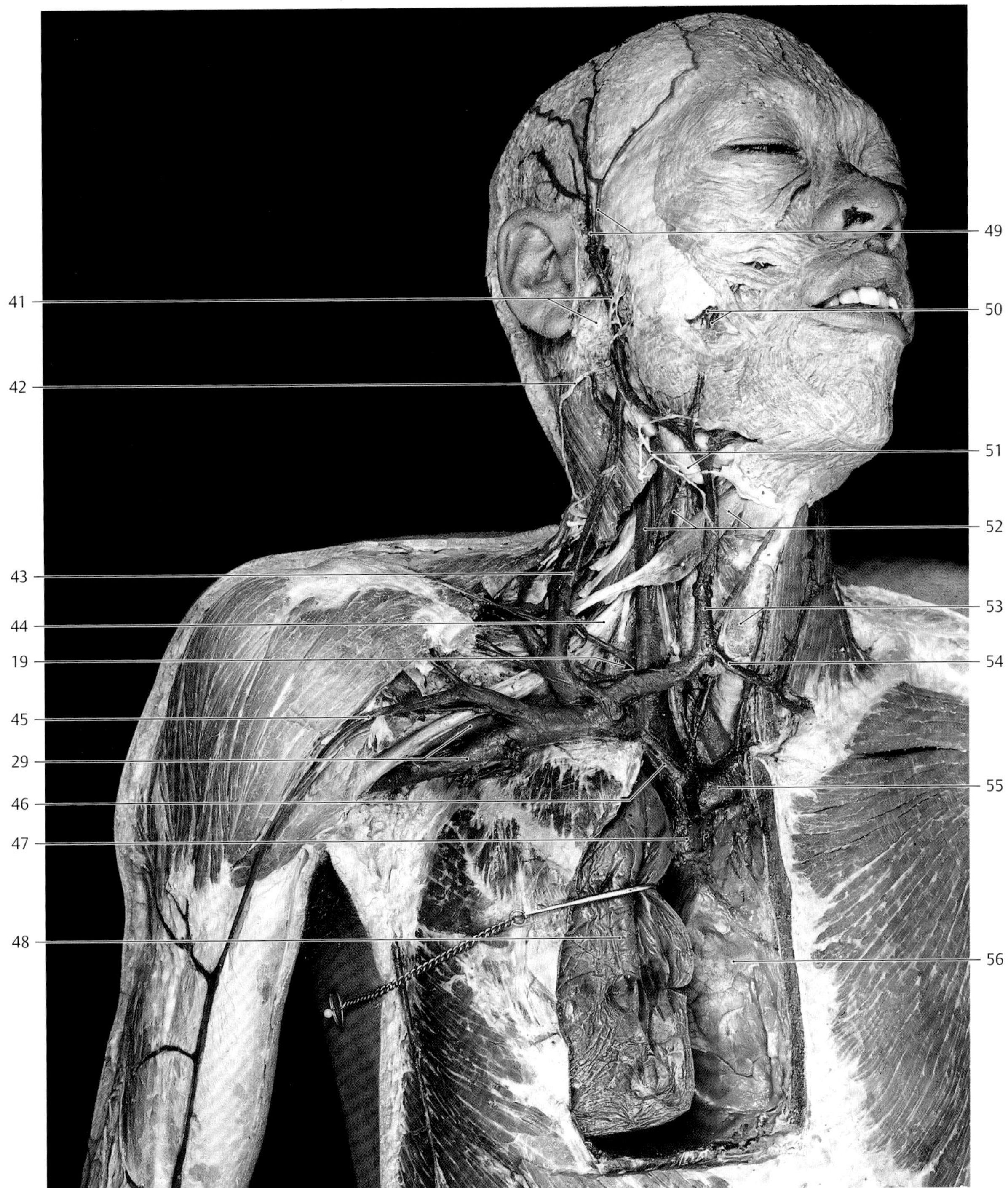


**Fig. 8.174 Veins of head, neck, and shoulder** (anterior aspect). Part of the thoracic wall, clavicle, and sternocleidomastoid muscle have been removed. Blue = veins; red = arteries.

The **internal jugular vein** is the continuation of the sigmoid sinus, which drains most of the venous blood from the brain together with the external cerebrospinal fluid. By joining the subclavian vein, it forms the right brachiocephalic vein, which continues on the right side directly into the superior vena cava. The common way to introduce the lead from a pacemaker device into the heart is by way of the cephalic vein. On the left side, the thoracic duct joins the internal jugular vein at the point where the subclavian vein and the internal jugular vein form the left brachiocephalic vein. Note that the subclavian vein lies in front of the anterior scalene muscle, whereas the subclavian artery and the brachial plexus lie posterior to that muscle. The **cephalic vein** joins the axillary vein by passing into the deltopectoral triangle. **The subclavian vein** is strongly fixed to the first rib, so it can be punctured with a needle at that point (underneath the sternal end of the clavicle) to introduce a catheter (subclavian line).

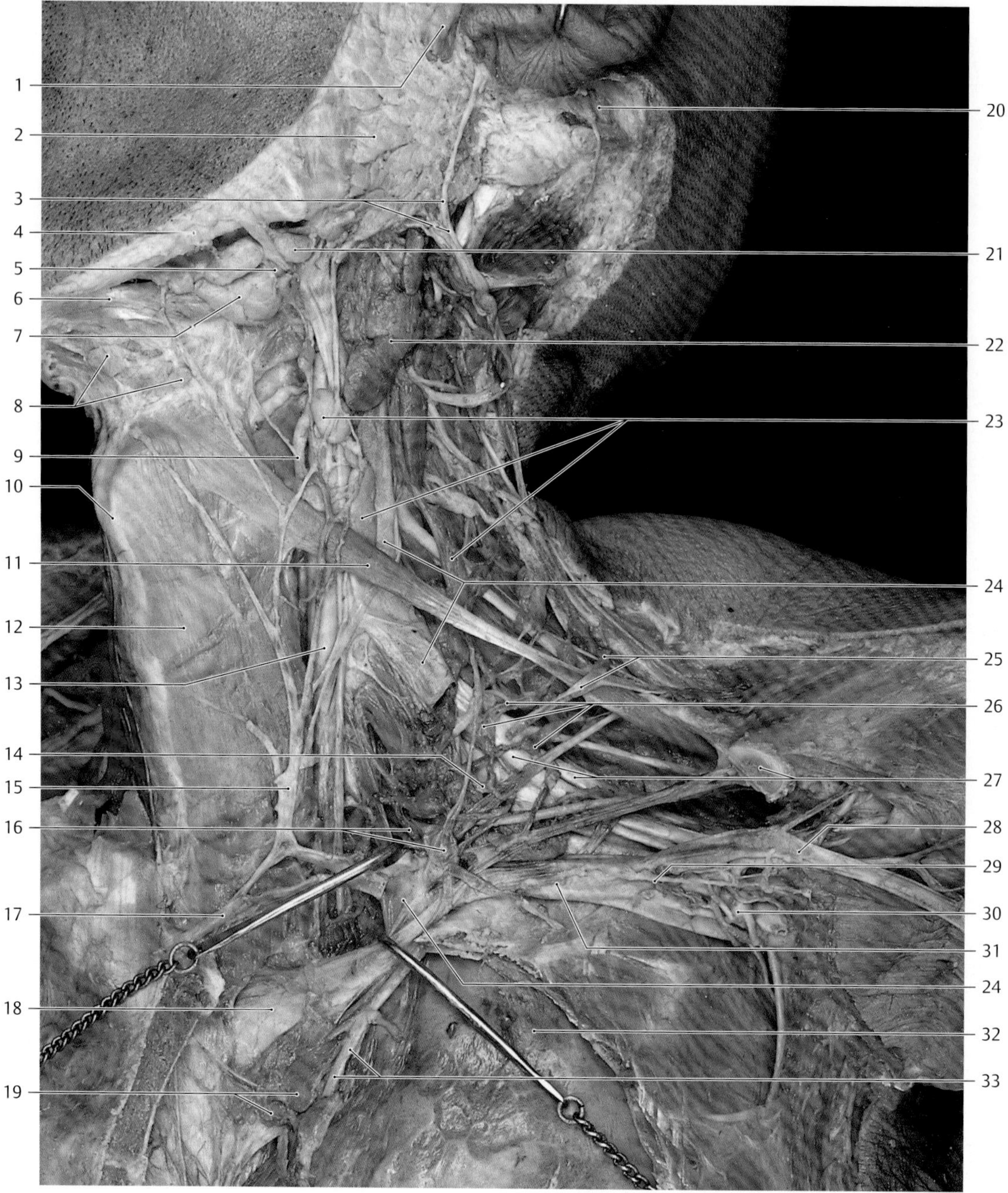


Fig. 8.175 **Lymph nodes and lymph vessels of the neck,** left side (oblique-lateral aspect). The sternocleidomastoid muscle and the left half of the thoracic wall have been removed. The lower part of the internal jugular vein has been cut and laterally displaced to show the thoracic duct.

1 Superficial parotid lymph node
2 Parotid gland
3 Great auricular nerve
4 Mandible
5 Facial vein
6 Anterior belly of digastric muscle
7 Submandibular gland
8 Submental lymph nodes
9 Superior thyroid artery
10 Thyroid cartilage
11 Omohyoid muscle
12 Sternohyoid muscle
13 Common carotid artery
14 Supraclavicular lymph nodes
15 Anterior jugular vein
16 Thoracic duct and internal jugular vein
17 Jugular venous arch
18 Left brachiocephalic vein
19 Superior mediastinal lymph nodes
20 Retro-auricular lymph nodes
21 Submandibular nodes
22 Superficial cervical lymph nodes
23 Jugulodigastric lymph nodes and jugular trunk
24 Internal jugular vein
25 External jugular vein
26 Jugulo-omohyoid lymph nodes
27 Brachial plexus
28 Cephalic vein
29 Subclavian trunk
30 Infraclavicular lymph nodes
31 Subclavian vein
32 Lung
33 Internal thoracic artery and vein

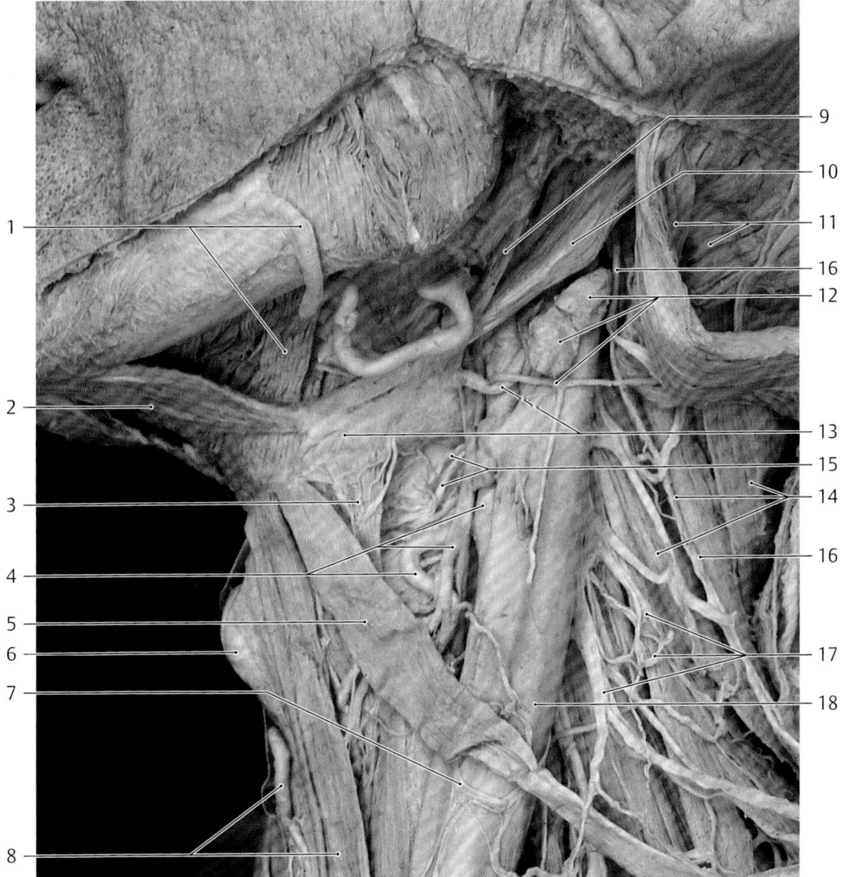


Fig. 8.176 **Carotid triangle,** left side (lateral aspect). The sternocleidomastoid muscle has been reflected.

1 Mylohyoid muscle and facial artery
2 Anterior belly of digastric muscle
3 Thyrohyoid muscle
4 External carotid artery, superior thyroid artery, and vein
5 Omohyoid muscle
6 Thyroid cartilage
7 Ansa cervicalis
8 Sternohyoid muscle and superior thyroid artery
9 Stylohyoid muscle
10 Posterior belly of digastric muscle
11 Sternocleidomastoid muscle (reflected)
12 Superior cervical lymph nodes and sternocleidomastoid artery
13 Hyoid bone and hypoglossal nerve (CN XII)
14 Splenius capitis and levator scapulae muscles
15 Superior laryngeal artery and internal branch of superior laryngeal nerve
16 Accessory nerve
17 Cervical plexus
18 Internal jugular vein
19 Facial vein
20 Submandibular lymph nodes
21 Submental lymph nodes
22 Thoracic duct
23 Retro-auricular lymph nodes
24 Occipital lymph nodes
25 Parotid lymph nodes
26 Jugulodigastric lymph node
27 Deep cervical lymph nodes
28 External jugular vein
29 Jugulo-omohyoid lymph node
30 Jugular trunk
31 Subclavian trunk
32 Infraclavicular lymph nodes

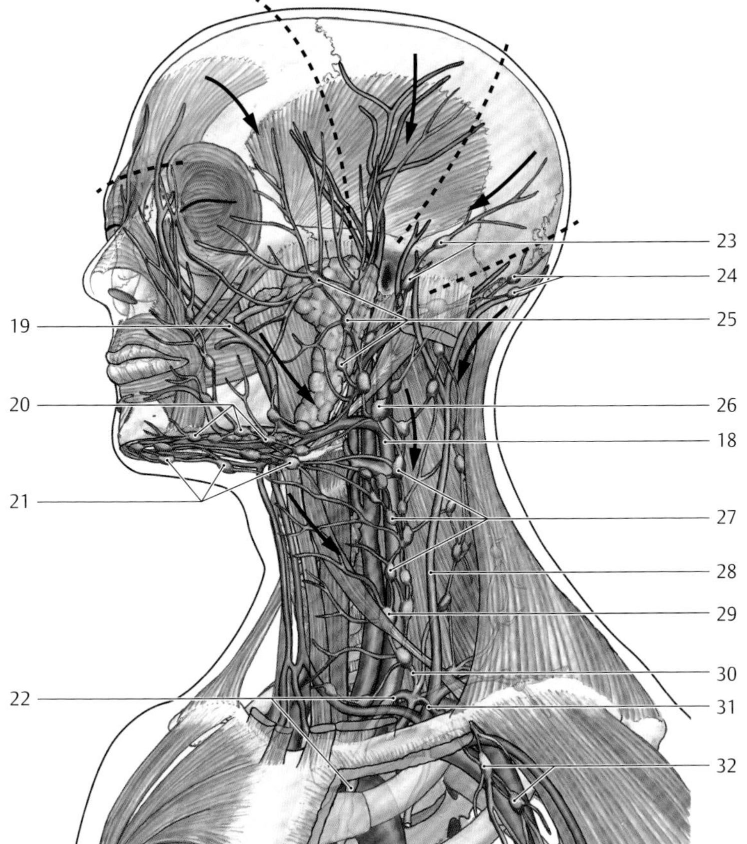


Fig. 8.177 **Lymph nodes and veins of head and neck** (oblique-lateral aspect). Dotted lines = border between irrigation areas; arrows = direction of lymph flow.

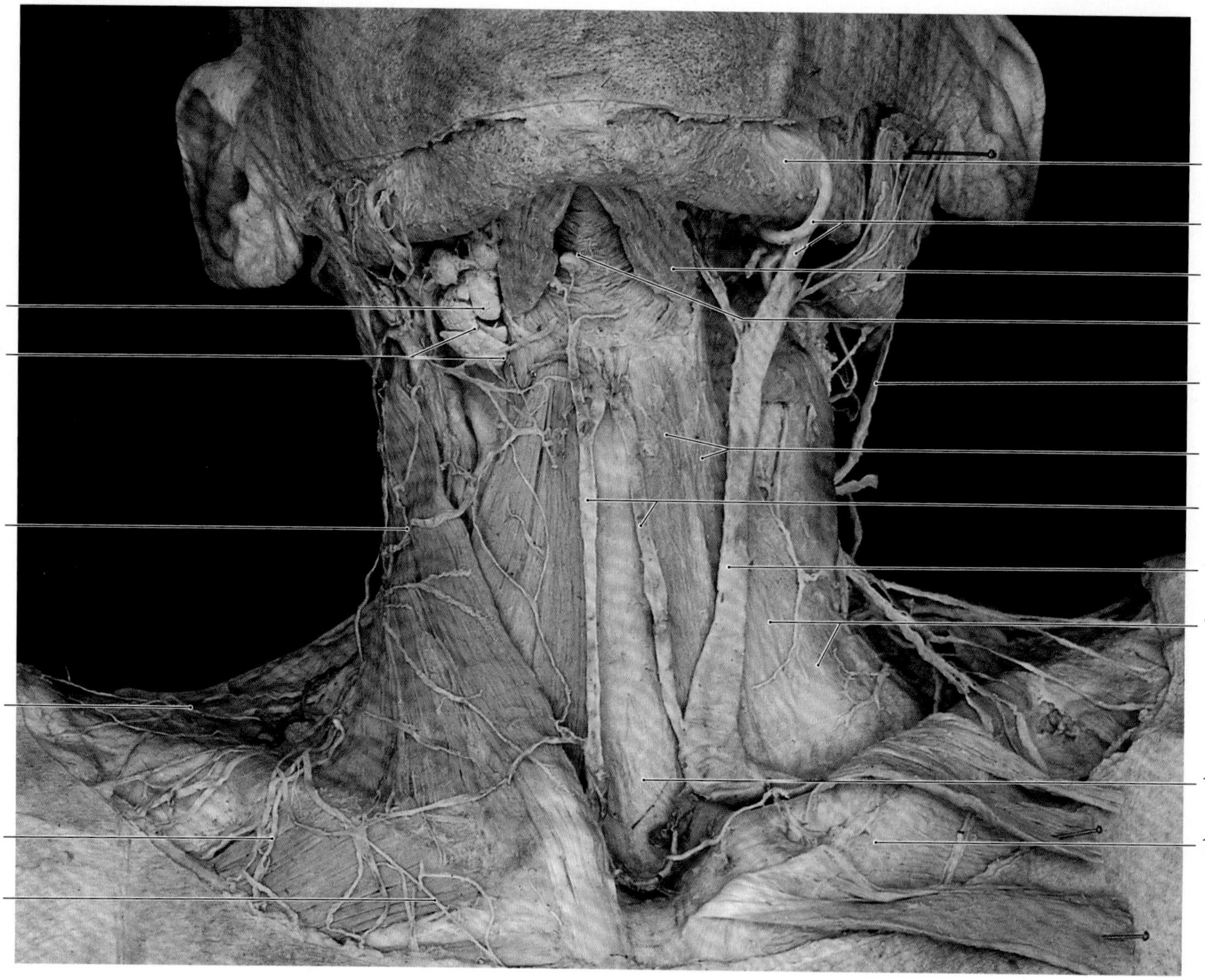

Fig. 8.178 **Anterior region of the neck** (superficial layer). The superficial fascia has been removed.

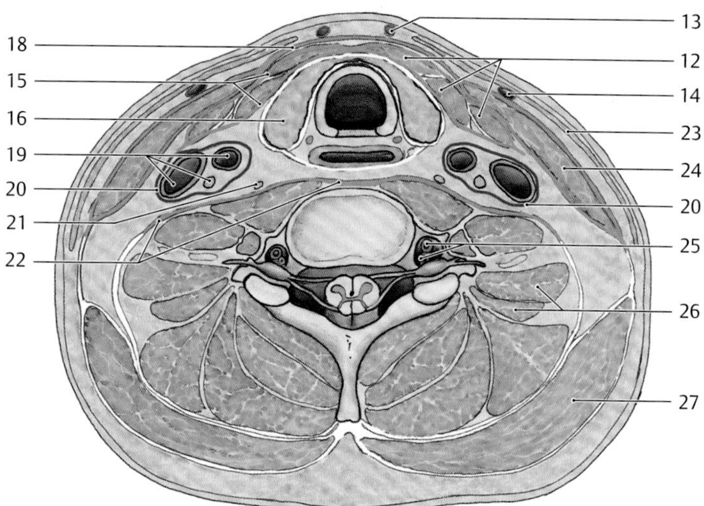


Fig. 8.179 **Cross section through the neck** at the level of the thyroid gland. Notice the position of the three laminae of cervical fascia (colored blue).

1 Submandibular gland
2 Cervical branch of facial nerve
3 Transverse cervical nerve *
4 Lateral supraclavicular nerves *
5 Middle supraclavicular nerves *
6 Medial supraclavicular nerves *
7 Great auricular nerve *
8 Mandible
9 Facial artery and vein
10 Anterior belly of digastric muscle
11 Mylohyoid muscle
12 Infrahyoid muscles (sternohyoid, sternothyroid, and omohyoid muscles)
13 Anterior jugular veins
14 External jugular vein
15 Pretracheal lamina of cervical fascia
16 Thyroid gland
17 Clavicle
18 Superficial lamina of cervical fascia
19 Carotid sheath with common carotid artery, internal jugular vein, and vagus nerve
20 Carotid sheath
21 Cervical part of sympathetic trunk
22 Prevertebral lamina of cervical fascia
23 Platysma muscle
24 Sternocleidomastoid muscle
25 Vertebral artery and vein
26 Scalene muscles
27 Trapezius muscle

* Cutaneous branches of cervical plexus

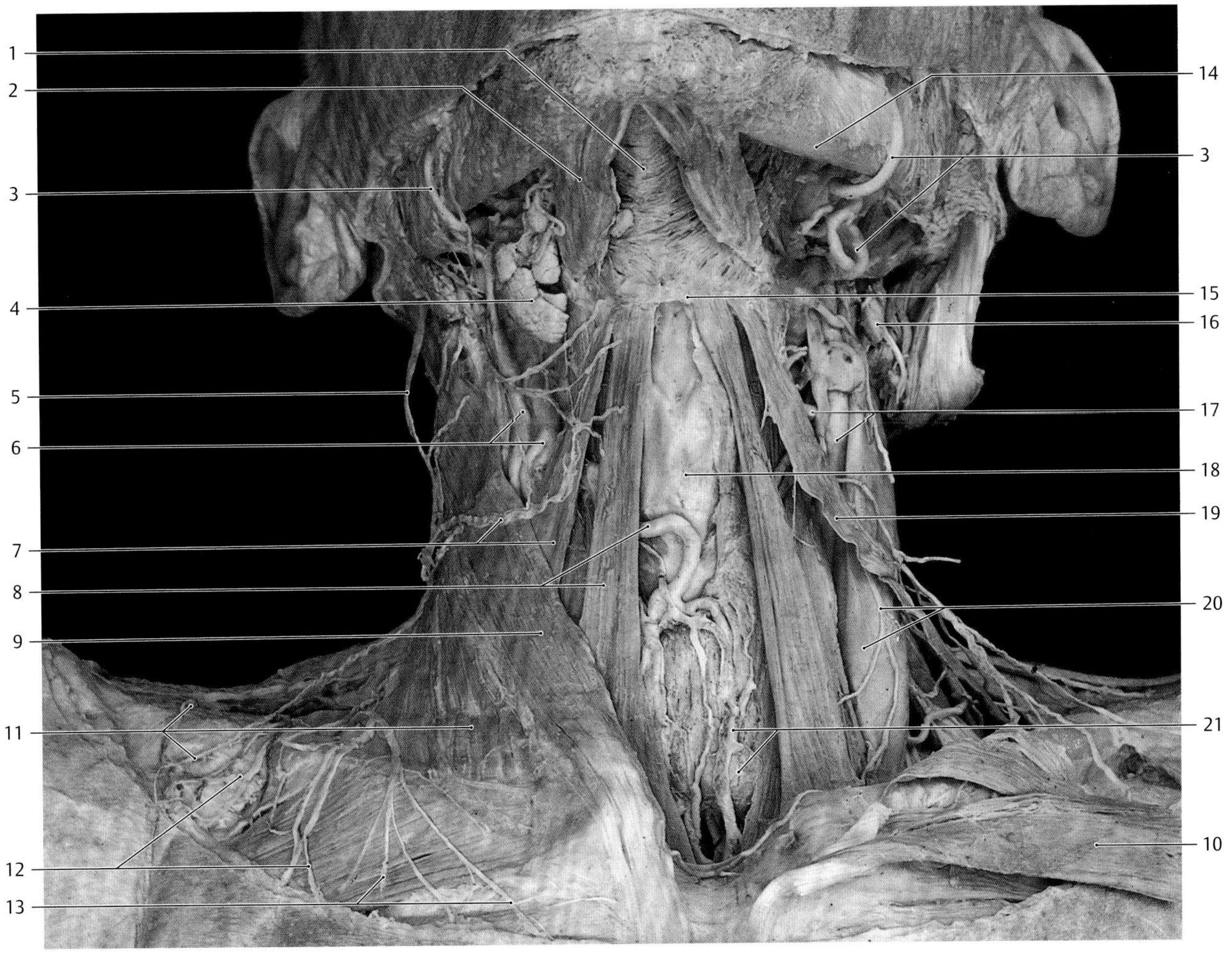

**Fig. 8.180 Anterior region of the neck** with anterior triangle (superficial layer [right side]; deeper layer [left side]). The pretracheal lamina of the cervical fascia and left sternocleidomastoid muscle have been removed.

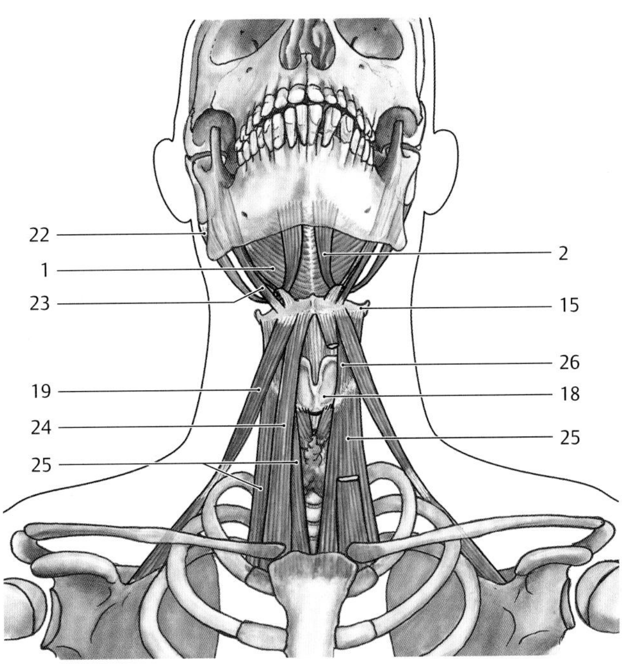


**Fig. 8.181 Supra- and infrahyoid muscles** (anterior aspect).

1 Mylohyoid muscle
2 Anterior belly of digastric muscle
3 Facial artery
4 Submandibular gland
5 Great auricular nerve
6 Internal jugular vein and common carotid artery
7 Transverse cervical nerve and omohyoid muscle
8 Sternohyoid muscle and superior thyroid artery
9 Sternocleidomastoid muscle (sternal head)
10 Left sternocleidomastoid muscle (reflected)
11 Sternocleidomastoid muscle (clavicular head) and lateral supraclavicular nerves
12 Middle supraclavicular nerves
13 Medial supraclavicular nerves
14 Mandible
15 Hyoid bone
16 Superficial cervical lymph nodes
17 Left superior thyroid artery and external carotid artery
18 Thyroid cartilage
19 Superior belly of omohyoid muscle
20 Internal jugular vein and branches of ansa cervicalis
21 Thyroid gland and unpaired inferior thyroid vein
22 Posterior belly of digastric muscle
23 Stylohyoid muscle
24 Sternohyoid muscle
25 Sternothyroid muscle
26 Thyrohyoid muscle

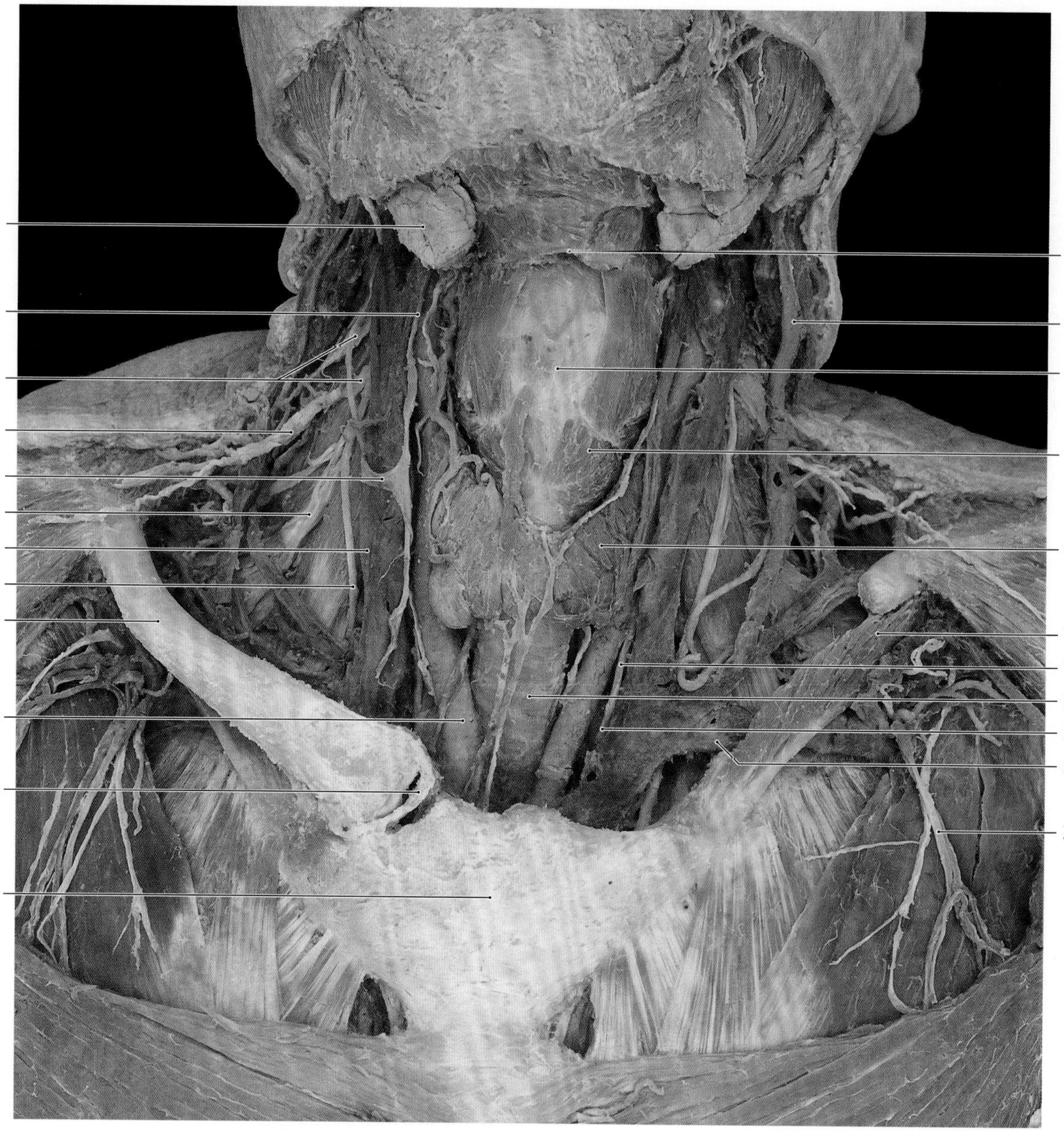

**Fig. 8.182 Anterior region of the neck** (deeper layer). The sternocleidomastoid muscles and left clavicle have been removed. The thyroid gland in relation to the trachea, larynx, and vessels of the neck is shown.

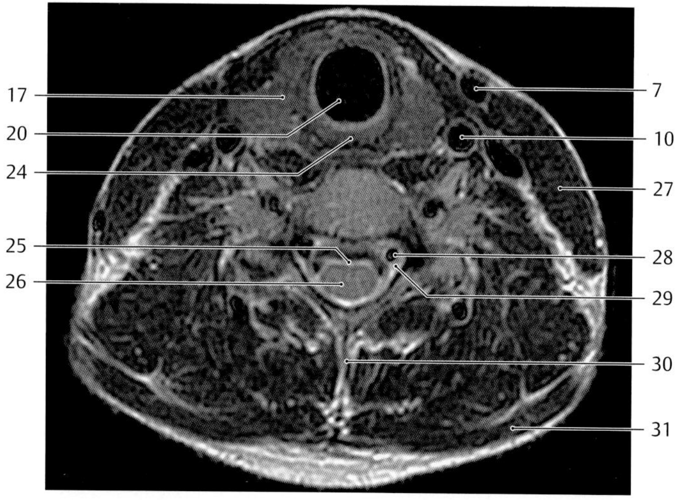


**Fig. 8.183 Cross section through the neck** at the level of the thyroid gland (MRI scan). (Courtesy of Prof. Uder, Institute of Radiology, University Hospital Erlangen, Germany.)

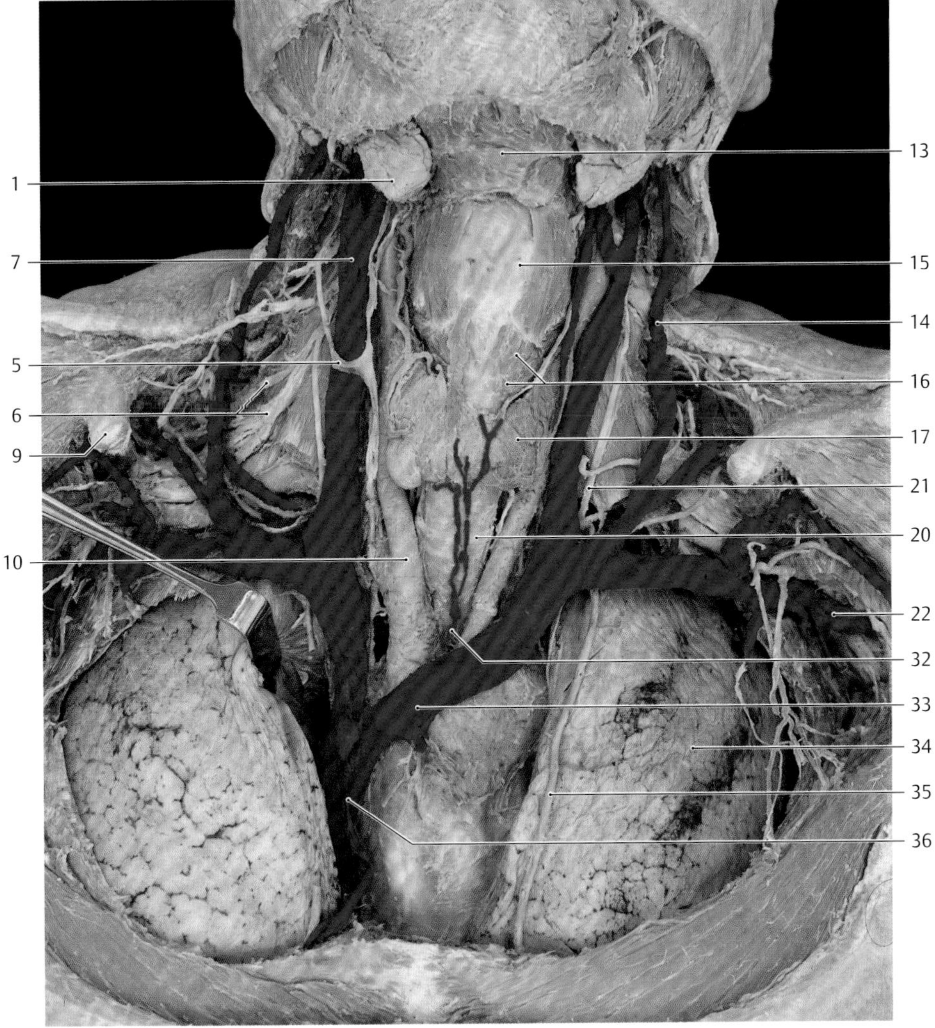


Fig. 8.184 **Anterior region of the neck** and thoracic cavity (deeper layer). Both clavicles, sternum, and ribs have been removed. The main veins have been colored blue.

1 Submandibular gland
2 Cervical branch of facial nerve (CN VII)
3 Cervical plexus
4 Middle supraclavicular nerves
5 Ansa cervicalis
6 Brachial plexus
7 Internal jugular vein
8 Phrenic nerve
9 Clavicle
10 Common carotid artery
11 Sternoclavicular joint with articular disc
12 Manubrium of sternum
13 Hyoid bone
14 External jugular vein
15 Thyroid cartilage
16 Cricothyroid muscle
17 Thyroid gland
18 Subclavius muscle
19 Recurrent laryngeal nerve
20 Trachea
21 Vagus nerve (CN X)
22 Subclavian vein
23 Middle pectoral nerve
24 Esophagus
25 Body of cervical vertebra
26 Spinal cord
27 Sternocleidomastoid muscle
28 Vertebral artery
29 Transverse process of cervical vertebra
30 Spinous process of cervical vertebra
31 Trapezius muscle
32 Inferior thyroid vein
33 Left brachiocephalic vein
34 Superior lobe of left lung
35 Internal thoracic artery
36 Superior vena cava
37 Superior thyroid artery
38 Inferior thyroid artery
39 Thyrocervical trunk
40 Subclavian artery
41 Aortic arch

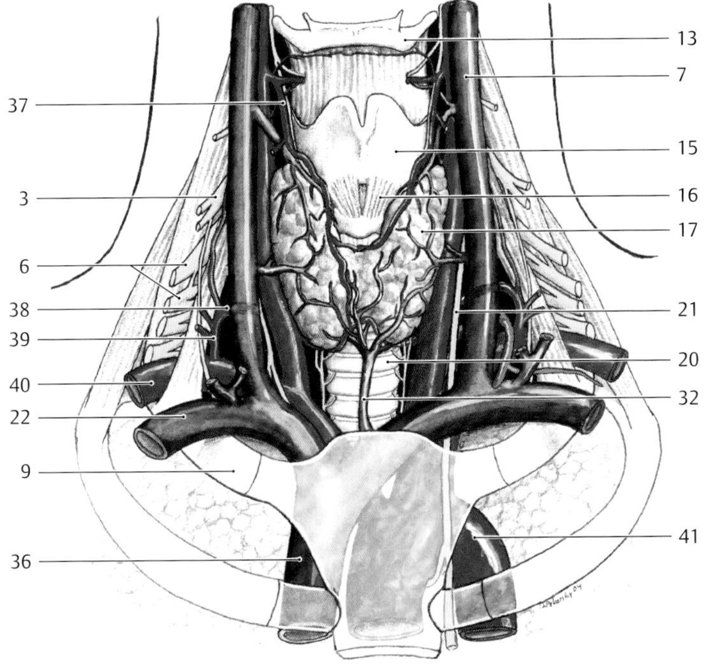


Fig. 8.185 **Anterior region of the neck.** Regional anatomy of the thyroid gland with related blood vessels.

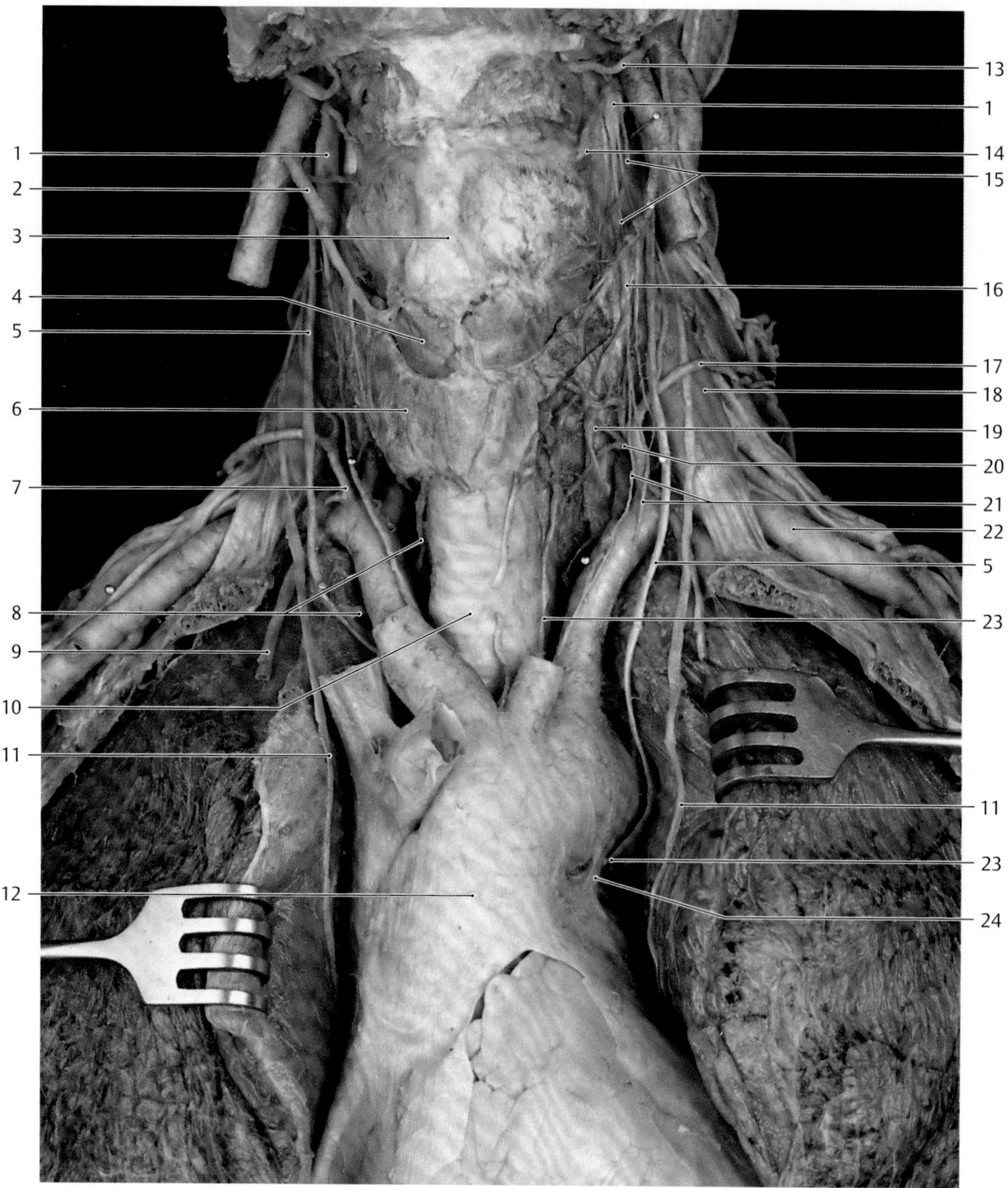


**Fig. 8.186 Larynx and thoracic organs** (anterior aspect). Dissection of vagus and recurrent laryngeal nerves.

1 Superior cervical ganglion
2 Superior thyroid artery
3 Thyroid cartilage
4 Cricothyroid muscle
5 Vagus nerve (CN X)
6 Thyroid gland
7 Thyrocervical trunk
8 Right recurrent laryngeal nerve
9 Internal thoracic artery
10 Trachea
11 Phrenic nerve
12 Aortic arch
13 Hypoglossal nerve (CN XII)
14 Internal branch of superior laryngeal nerve
15 External branch of superior laryngeal nerve
16 Sympathetic trunk
17 Transverse cervical artery
18 Anterior scalene muscle
19 Middle cervical ganglion
20 Inferior thyroid artery
21 Inferior cervical cardiac nerves (branches of sympathetic trunk)
22 Left subclavian artery
23 Left recurrent laryngeal nerve
24 Ligamentum arteriosum
25 Tongue
26 Inferior constrictor muscle of pharynx
27 Left common carotid artery
28 Glossopharyngeal nerve (CN IX)
29 Superior laryngeal nerve
30 Epiglottis
31 Posterior crico-arytenoid muscle and cricoid cartilage
32 Recurrent laryngeal nerve
33 Middle and posterior scalene muscles
34 Longus capitis muscle
35 Right subclavian artery
36 Brachiocephalic trunk
37 Hyoid bone
38 Thyrohyoid membrane
39 Second rib

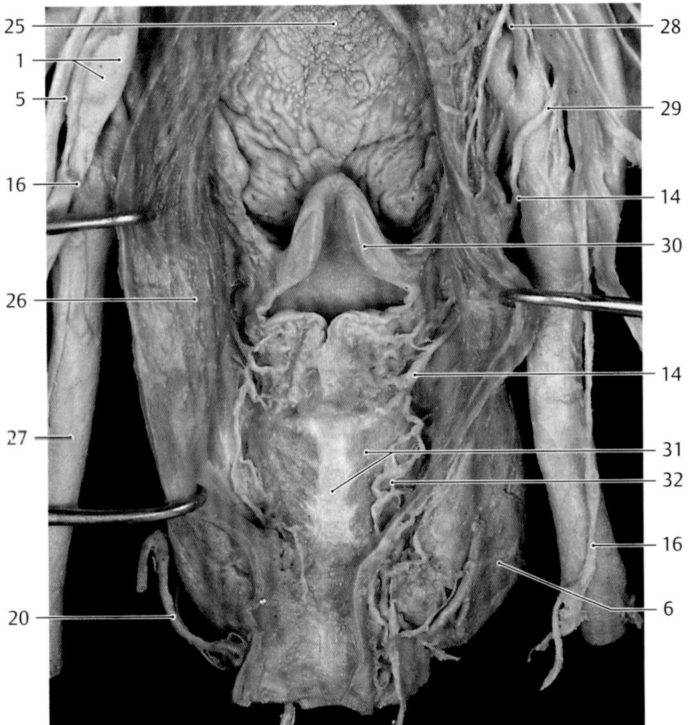


Fig. 8.187 **Innervation of the larynx** (posterior aspect). Dissection of the superior and inferior laryngeal nerves. The pharynx has been opened.

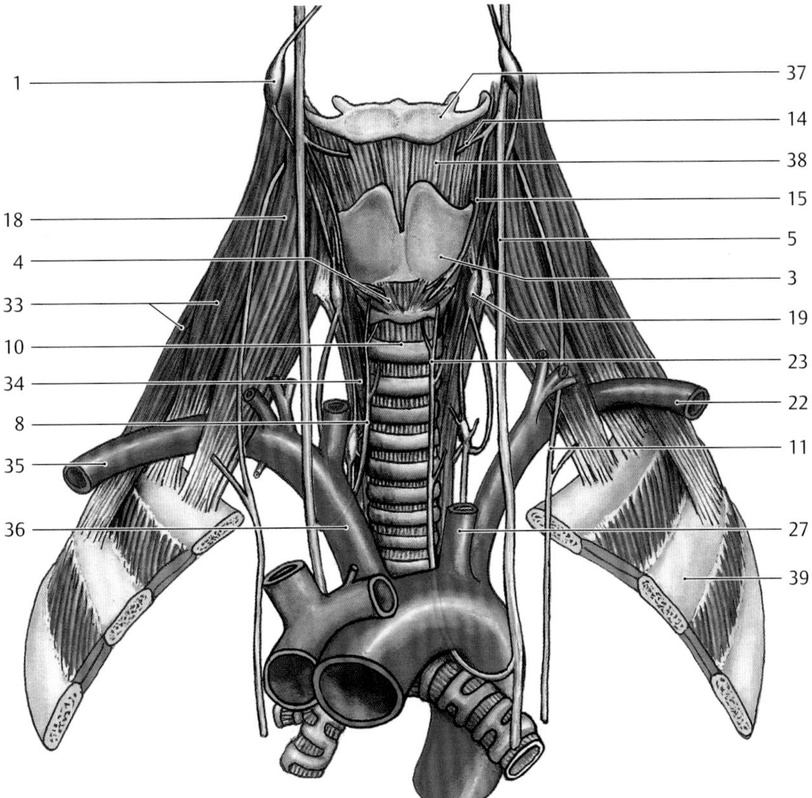


Fig. 8.188 **Innervation of the larynx.**

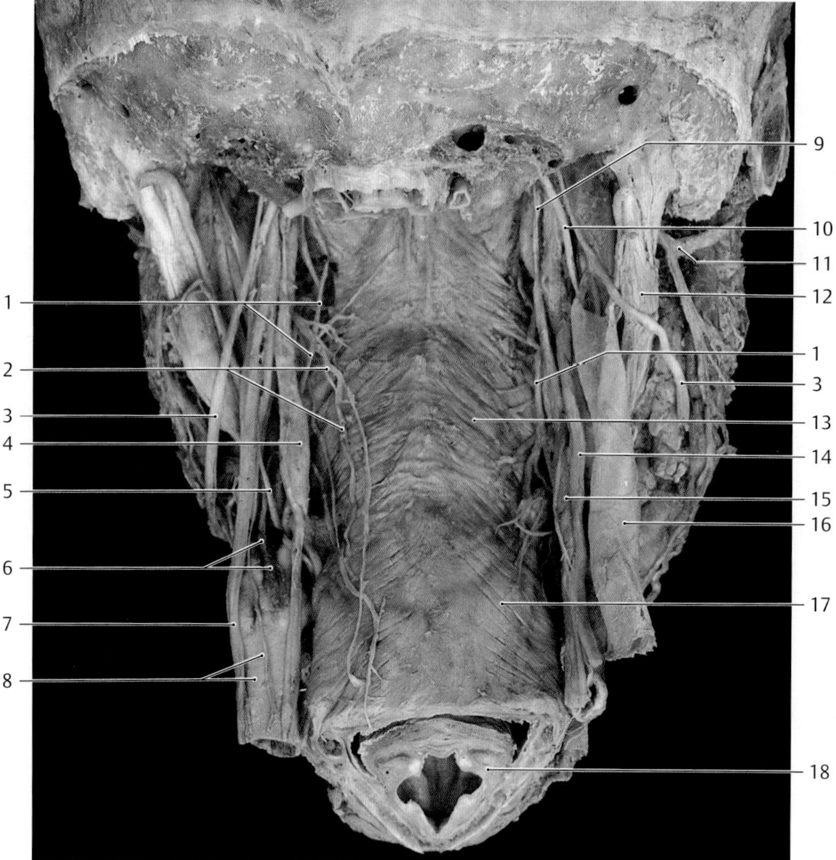


Fig. 8.189 **Pharynx with parapharyngeal nerves and vessels** (posterior aspect).

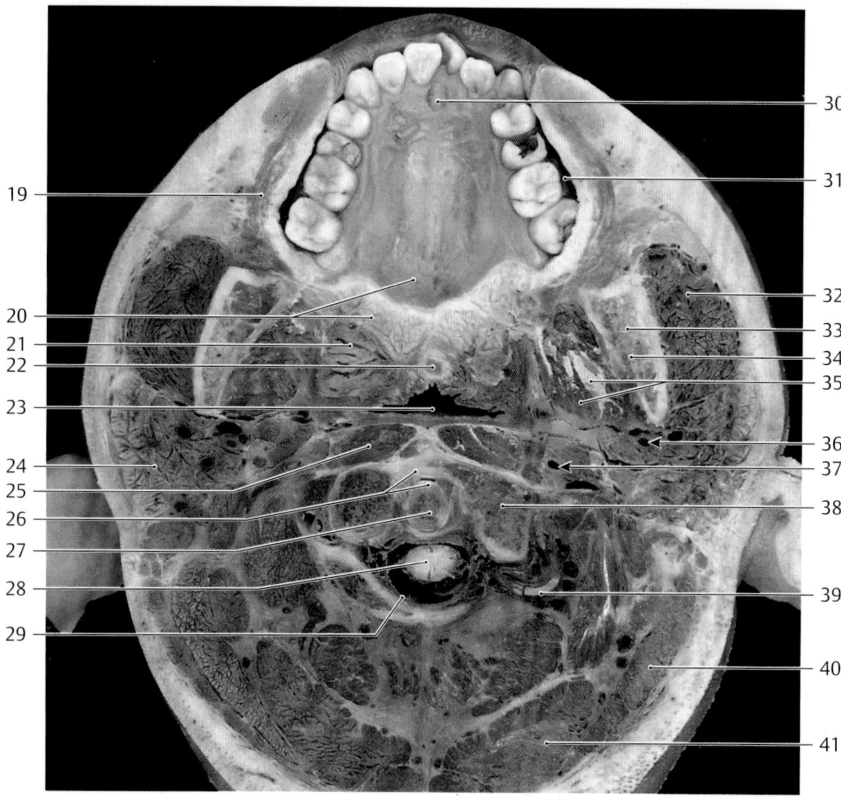


Fig. 8.190 **Cross section through head and neck** at the level of the atlas (inferior aspect).

1 Ascending pharyngeal artery
2 Pharyngeal plexus
3 Accessory nerve
4 Superior cervical ganglion of sympathetic trunk
5 Superior laryngeal nerve
6 Carotid body and carotid sinus nerve
7 Left vagus nerve
8 Common carotid artery and cardiac branch of vagus nerve
9 Glossopharyngeal nerve
10 Hypoglossal nerve
11 Facial nerve
12 Posterior belly of digastric muscle
13 Middle constrictor muscle of pharynx
14 Right vagus nerve
15 Sympathetic trunk
16 Internal jugular vein
17 Inferior constrictor muscle of pharynx
18 Larynx
19 Buccinator muscle
20 Soft palate and palatine glands
21 Palatine tonsil
22 Uvula of palate
23 Pharynx (oral part)
24 Parotid gland
25 Longus capitis muscle
26 Median atlanto-axial joint and anterior arch of atlas
27 Dens of axis
28 Spinal cord
29 Dura mater
30 Incisive papilla
31 Oral vestibule
32 Masseter muscle
33 Mandible
34 Mandibular canal with vessels and nerve
35 Medial pterygoid muscle
36 External carotid artery
37 Internal carotid artery
38 Atlas
39 Vertebral artery
40 Splenius capitis muscle
41 Semispinalis capitis muscle

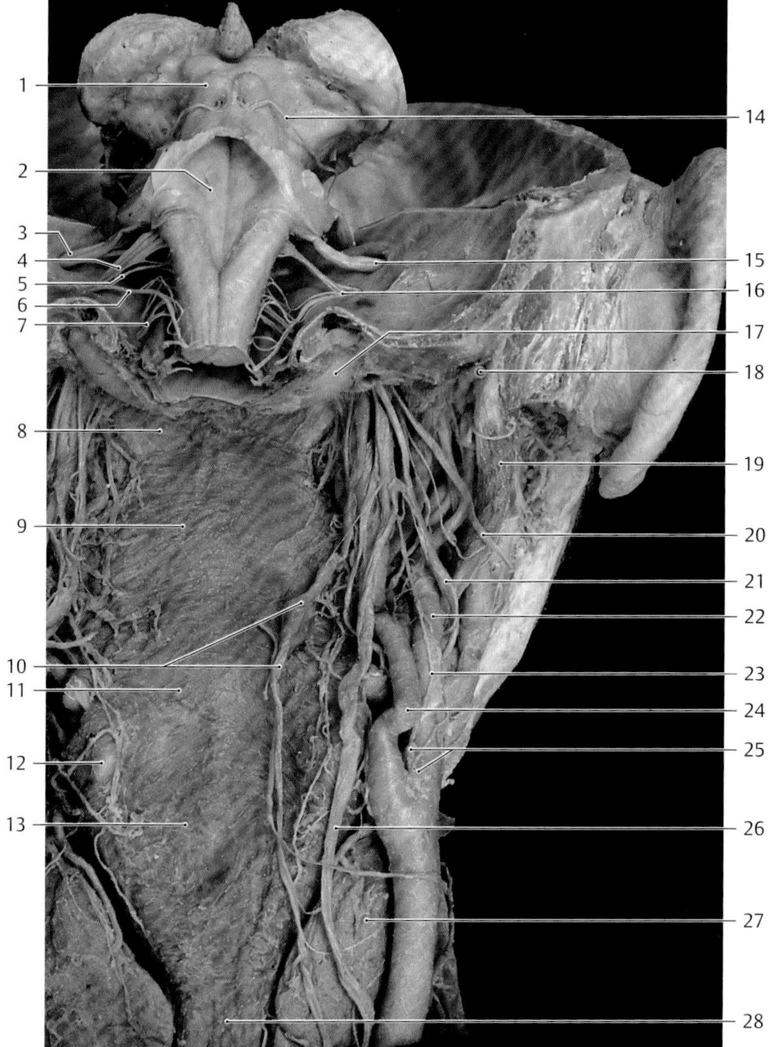


Fig. 8.191 **Pharynx and parapharyngeal nerves in connection with the brainstem** (posterior aspect).

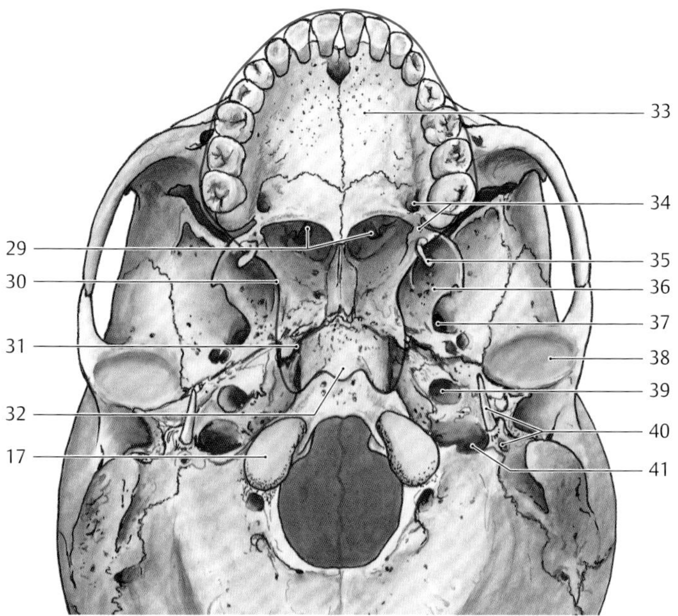


1 Inferior colliculus of midbrain
2 Facial colliculus in floor of rhomboid fossa
3 Vestibulocochlear and facial nerves
4 Glossopharyngeal nerve
5 Vagus nerve
6 Accessory nerve
7 Hypoglossal nerve
8 Pharyngobasilar fascia
9 Superior constrictor muscle of pharynx
10 Sympathetic trunk and superior cervical ganglion (medially displaced)
11 Middle constrictor muscle of pharynx
12 Greater cornu of hyoid bone
13 Inferior constrictor muscle of pharynx
14 Trochlear nerve
15 Internal acoustic meatus with facial and vestibulocochlear nerves
16 Jugular foramen with glossopharyngeal, vagus, and assessory nerves
17 Occipital condyle
18 Occipital artery
19 Posterior belly of digastric muscle
20 Accessory nerve (extracranial part)
21 Hypoglossal nerve (extracranial part)
22 External carotid artery
23 Carotid sinus nerve
24 Internal carotid artery
25 Carotid sinus and carotid body
26 Vagus nerve
27 Thyroid gland
28 Esophagus
29 Choanae
30 Medial pterygoid plate
31 Foramen lacerum
32 Pharyngeal tubercle
33 Hard palate
34 Greater and lesser palatine foramen
35 Pterygoid hamulus
36 Lateral pterygoid plate
37 Foramen ovale
38 Mandibular fossa
39 Carotid canal
40 Styloid process and stylomastoid foramen
41 Jugular foramen

Fig. 8.192 **Base of the skull** (inferior aspect). Red line = outline of superior constrictor muscle in continuation with buccinator and orbicularis oris muscles.

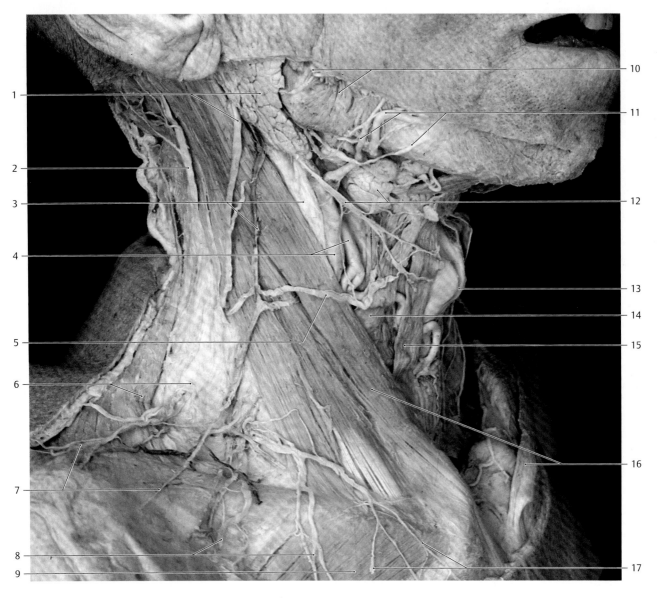

**Fig. 8.193 Lateral region of the neck** with posterior and carotid triangles (superficial layer).

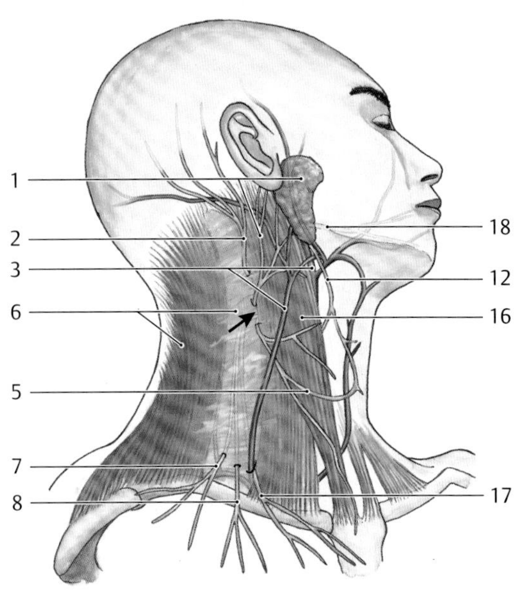


1 Parotid gland and great auricular nerve
2 Lesser occipital nerve
3 Internal and external jugular veins
4 Retromandibular vein and external carotid artery
5 Transverse cervical nerve with communicating branch to cervical branch of facial nerve
6 Trapezius muscle and superficial lamina of cervical fascia
7 Lateral supraclavicular nerves
8 Intermediate supraclavicular nerves
9 Pectoralis major muscle
10 Buccal branch of facial nerve and masseter muscle
11 Facial artery and vein and mandibular branch of facial nerve
12 Cervical branch of facial nerve and submandibular gland (gland only in Fig. 8.193)
13 Thyroid cartilage
14 Omohyoid muscle
15 Sternohyoid muscle
16 Sternocleidomastoid muscle
17 Medial supraclavicular nerves
18 Mandibular branch of facial nerve

**Fig. 8.194 Cutaneous branches of cervical plexus** (lateral region). Arrow = Erb's point.

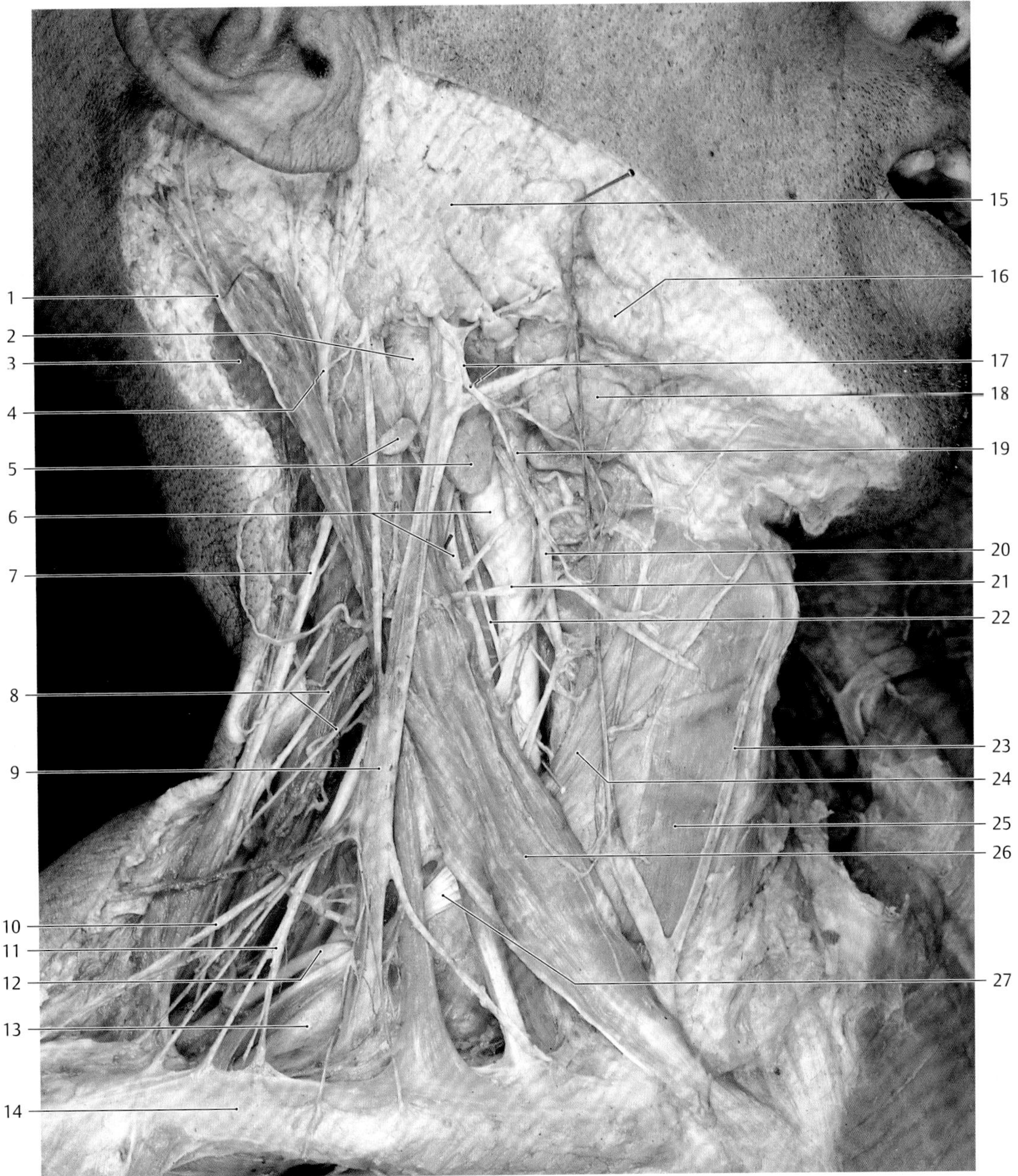


**Fig. 8.195 Lateral region of the neck** with posterior and carotid triangles (superficial layer). The superficial lamina of cervical fascia has been removed to display the cutaneous branches of the cervical plexus and subcutaneous veins.

1 Lesser occipital nerve
2 Internal jugular vein
3 Splenius capitis muscle
4 Great auricular nerve
5 Submandibular nodes
6 Internal carotid artery and vagus nerve
7 Accessory nerve
8 Muscular branches of cervical plexus
9 External jugular vein
10 Posterior supraclavicular nerves
11 Middle supraclavicular nerves
12 Suprascapular artery
13 Pretracheal lamina of fascia of neck
14 Clavicle
15 Parotid gland
16 Mandible
17 Cervical branch of facial nerve
18 Submandibular gland
19 External carotid artery
20 Superior thyroid artery
21 Transverse cervical nerve
22 Superior root of ansa cervicalis
23 Anterior jugular vein
24 Omohyoid muscle
25 Sternohyoid muscle
26 Sternocleidomastoid muscle
27 Intermediate tendon of omohyoid muscle

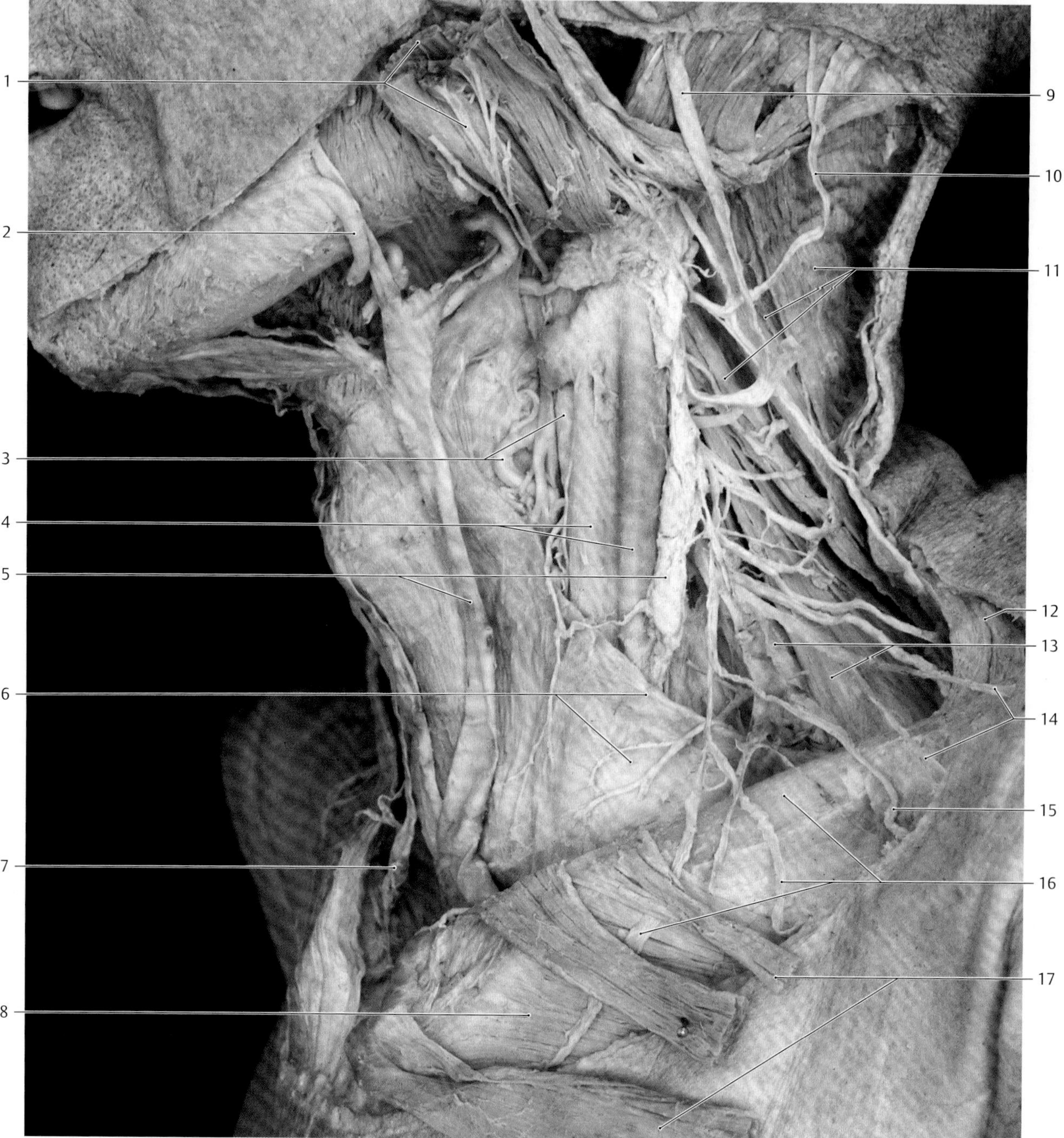


**Fig. 8.196 Lateral region of the neck** (deeper layer). The sternocleidomastoid muscle has been cut and reflected to display the pretracheal lamina of the cervical fascia.

1 Sternocleidomastoid muscle (reflected) and branch of accessory nerve
2 Facial artery
3 External carotid artery and superior thyroid artery
4 Internal jugular vein
5 Deep cervical lymph nodes and external jugular vein
6 Omohyoid muscle and pretracheal lamina of cervical fascia
7 Anterior jugular vein
8 Pectoralis major muscle
9 Great auricular nerve
10 Lesser occipital nerve
11 Splenius capitis and levator scapulae muscles
12 Trapezius muscle
13 Middle scalene muscle and brachial plexus
14 Lateral supraclavicular nerves
15 Intermediate supraclavicular nerve
16 Clavicle and medial supraclavicular nerves
17 Sternocleidomastoid muscle (reflected)

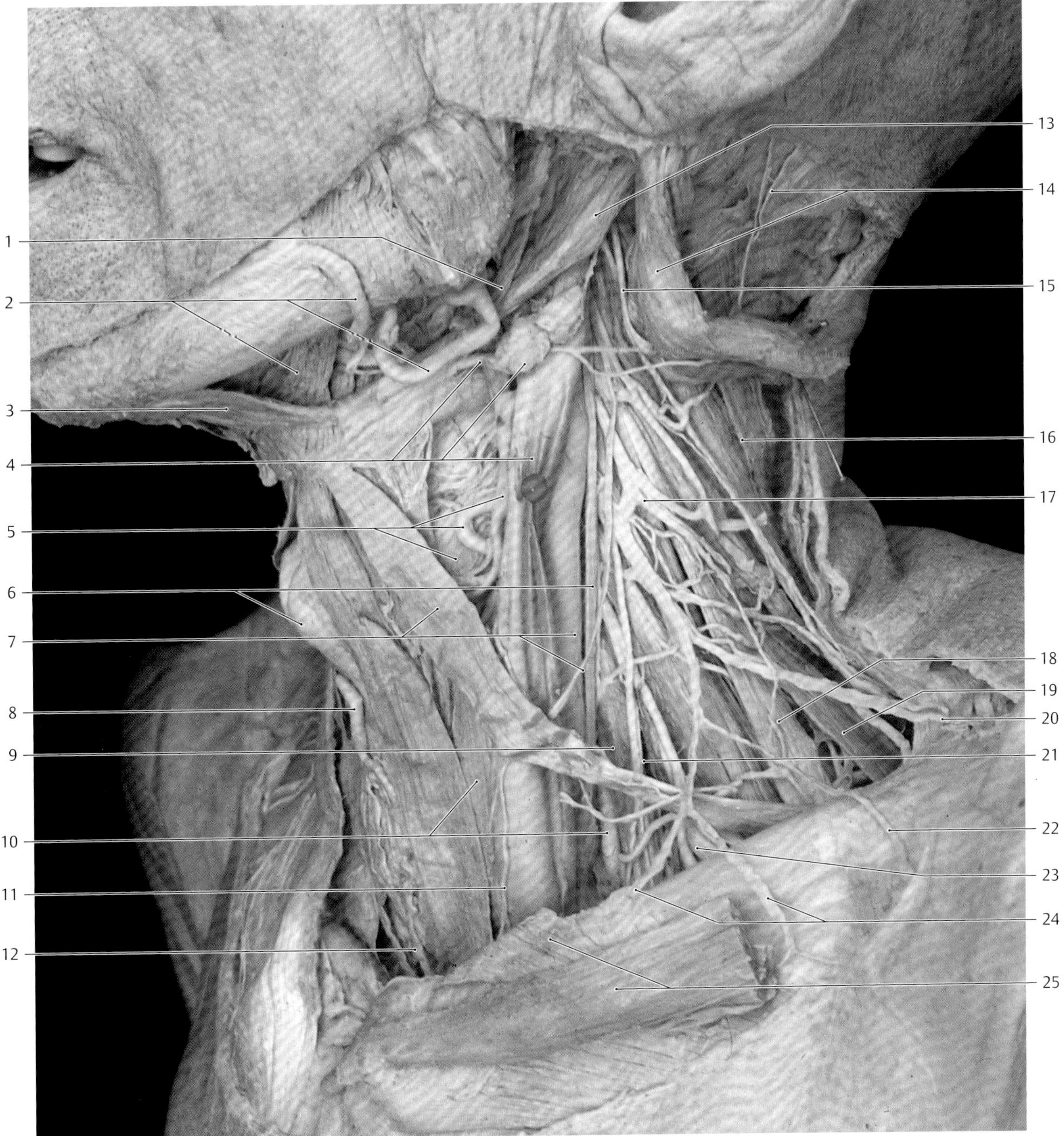


**Fig. 8.197 Lateral region of the neck** (deeper layer). The internal jugular vein has been reflected to expose the carotid artery and vagus nerve.

1 Stylohyoid muscle
2 Facial artery and mylohyoid muscle
3 Anterior belly of digastric muscle
4 Internal jugular vein, hypoglossal nerve, and superficial cervical lymph nodes
5 Superior thyroid artery and vein and inferior pharyngeal constrictor muscle
6 Thyroid cartilage and vagus nerve
7 Ansa cervicalis, omohyoid muscle, and common carotid artery
8 Right superior thyroid artery
9 Anterior scalene muscle
10 Sternothyroid muscle and inferior thyroid artery
11 Muscular branches of ansa cervicalis to the infrahyoid muscles
12 Inferior thyroid vein
13 Posterior belly of digastric muscle
14 Sternocleidomastoid muscle and lesser occipital nerve
15 Accessory nerve
16 Splenius capitis muscle
17 Cervical plexus
18 Posterior scalene muscle
19 Levator scapulae muscle
20 Lateral supraclavicular nerves
21 Phrenic nerve
22 Intermediate supraclavicular nerve
23 Brachial plexus
24 Medial supraclavicular nerves
25 Sternocleidomastoid muscle

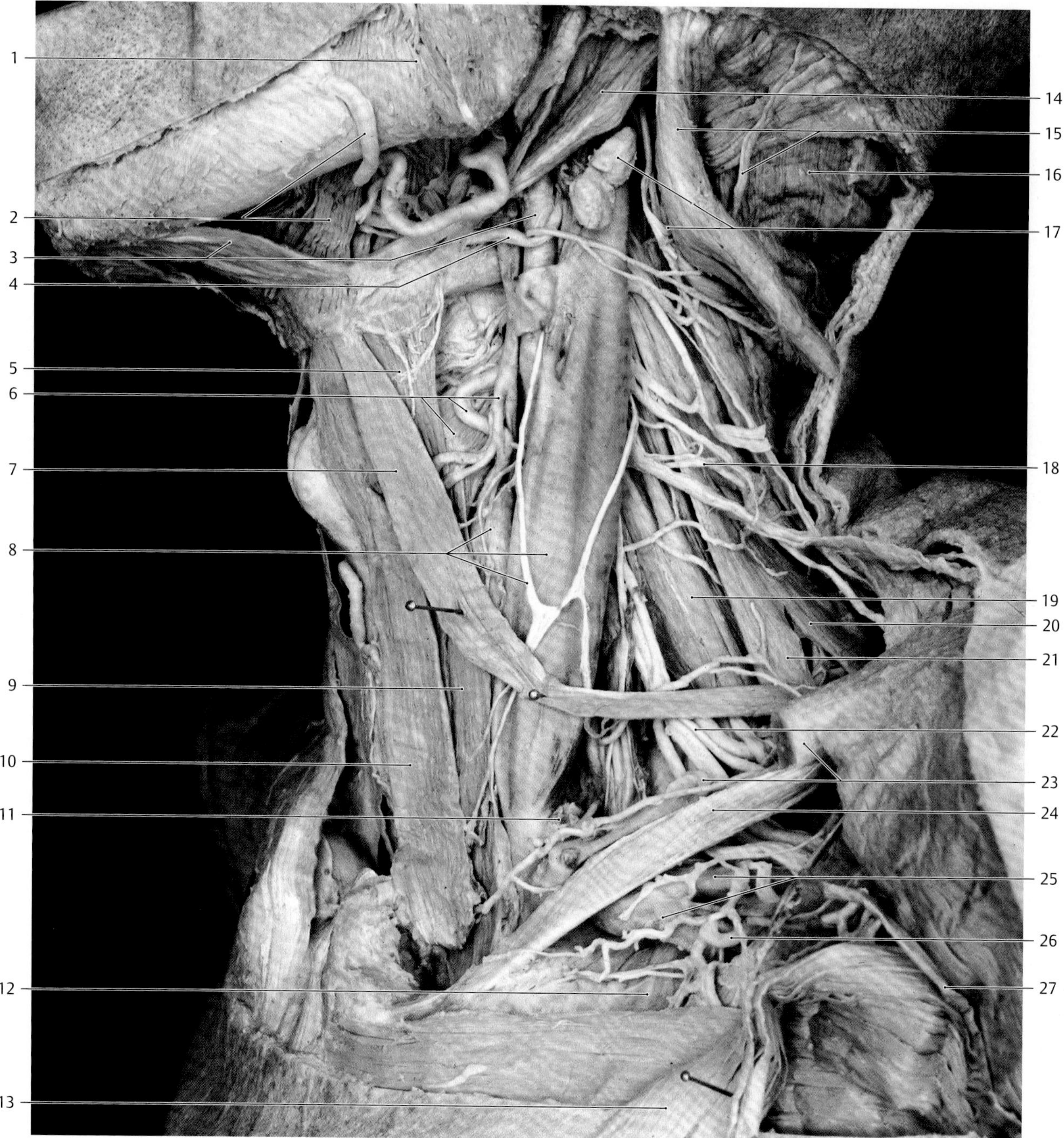


**Fig. 8.198 Lateral region of the neck** with ansa cervicalis (deeper layer). The cervical fascia and the clavicle have been partly removed. The ansa cervicalis and infrahyoid muscles are displayed.

1 Masseter muscle
2 Mylohyoid muscle and facial artery
3 External carotid artery and anterior belly of digastric muscle
4 Hypoglossal nerve
5 Thyrohyoid muscle
6 Superior thyroid artery and vein and inferior pharyngeal constrictor muscle
7 Superior belly of omohyoid muscle
8 Ansa cervicalis, thyroid gland, and internal jugular vein
9 Sternothyroid muscle
10 Sternohyoid muscle
11 Thoracic duct
12 Pectoralis minor muscle
13 Pectoralis major muscle
14 Posterior belly of digastric muscle
15 Sternocleidomastoid muscle and lesser occipital nerve
16 Splenius capitis muscle
17 Superficial cervical lymph nodes and accessory nerve
18 Cervical plexus
19 Middle scalene muscle
20 Levator scapulae muscle
21 Posterior scalene muscle
22 Brachial plexus
23 Transverse cervical artery and clavicle
24 Subclavius muscle
25 Subclavian artery and vein
26 Thoraco-acromial artery
27 Cephalic vein

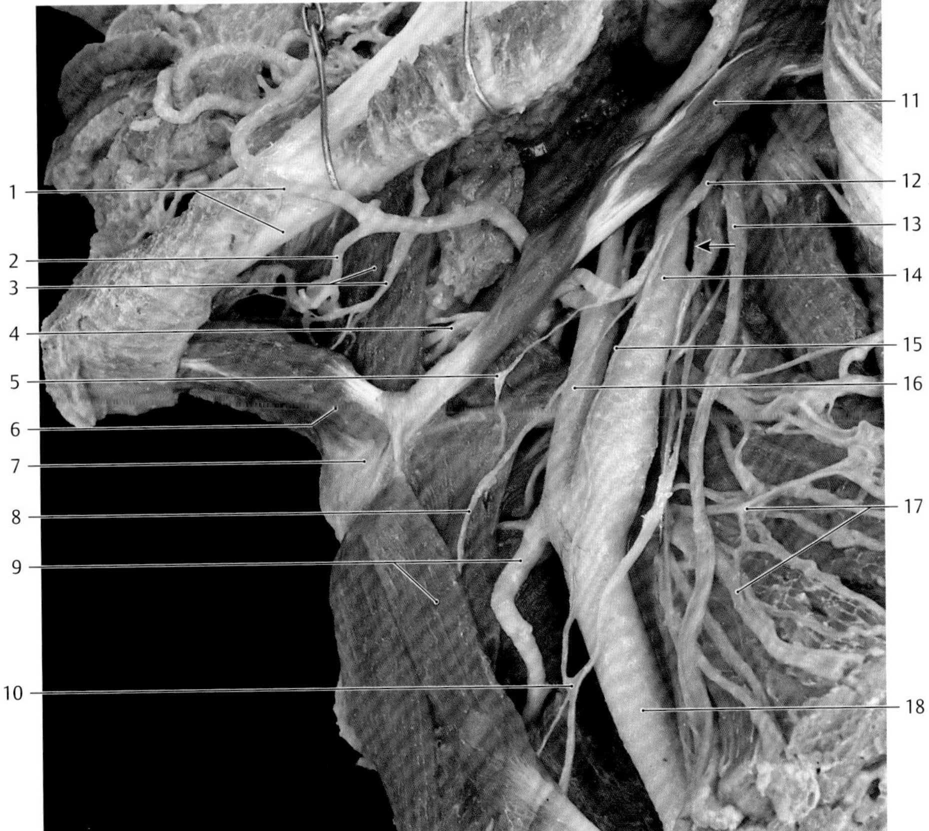


Fig. 8.199 **Lateral region of the neck and submandibular region** with hypoglossal nerve (CN XII). The mandible has been slightly elevated. Arrow = superior cervical ganglion.

1 Facial artery and mandible
2 Submental artery
3 Mylohyoid muscle and nerve
4 Hypoglossal nerve (lingual branches)
5 Thyrohyoid branch of hypoglossal nerve (CN XII)
6 Anterior belly of digastric muscle
7 Hyoid bone
8 Omohyoid branch of hypoglossal nerve (CN XII)
9 Omohyoid muscle and superior thyroid artery
10 Ansa cervicalis
11 Posterior belly of digastric muscle
12 Hypoglossal nerve (CN XII)
13 Vagus nerve (CN X)
14 Internal carotid artery
15 Superior root of ansa cervicalis
16 External carotid artery
17 Cervical plexus
18 Common carotid artery
19 Facial artery and vein
20 Omohyoid muscle
21 Internal jugular vein
22 Sternohyoid and sternothyroid muscles
23 Clavicle
24 Superficial temporal artery and vein
25 Occipital artery
26 Supraclavicular nerves (C3 and C4)
27 Spinal processes of cervical vertebrae (C4 and C5)
28 Scapula

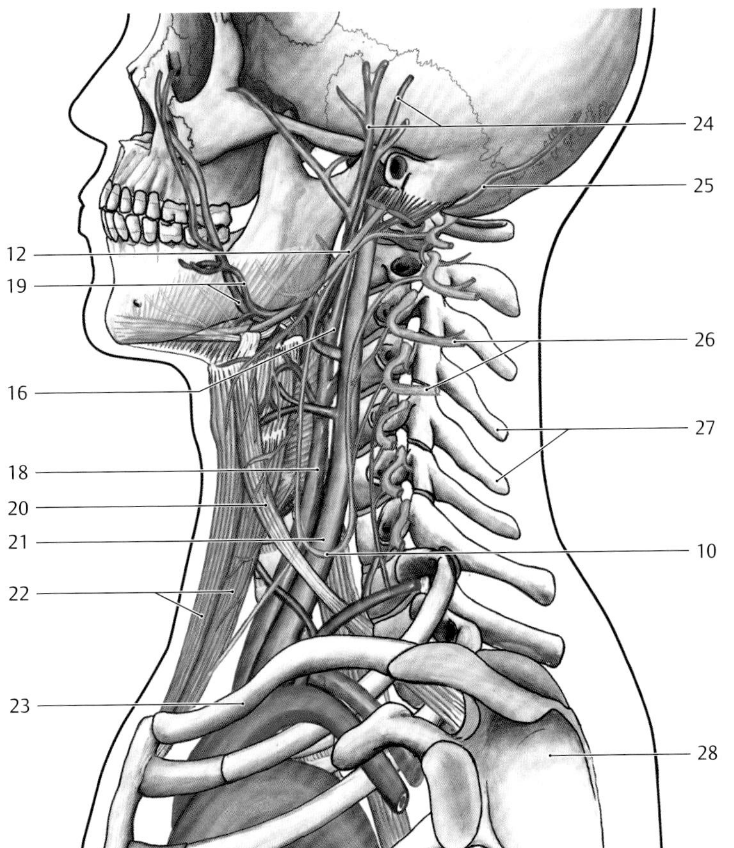


Fig. 8.200 **Nerves and vessels of the neck** (lateral aspect). The ansa cervicalis with its connection to the spinal nerves is depicted.

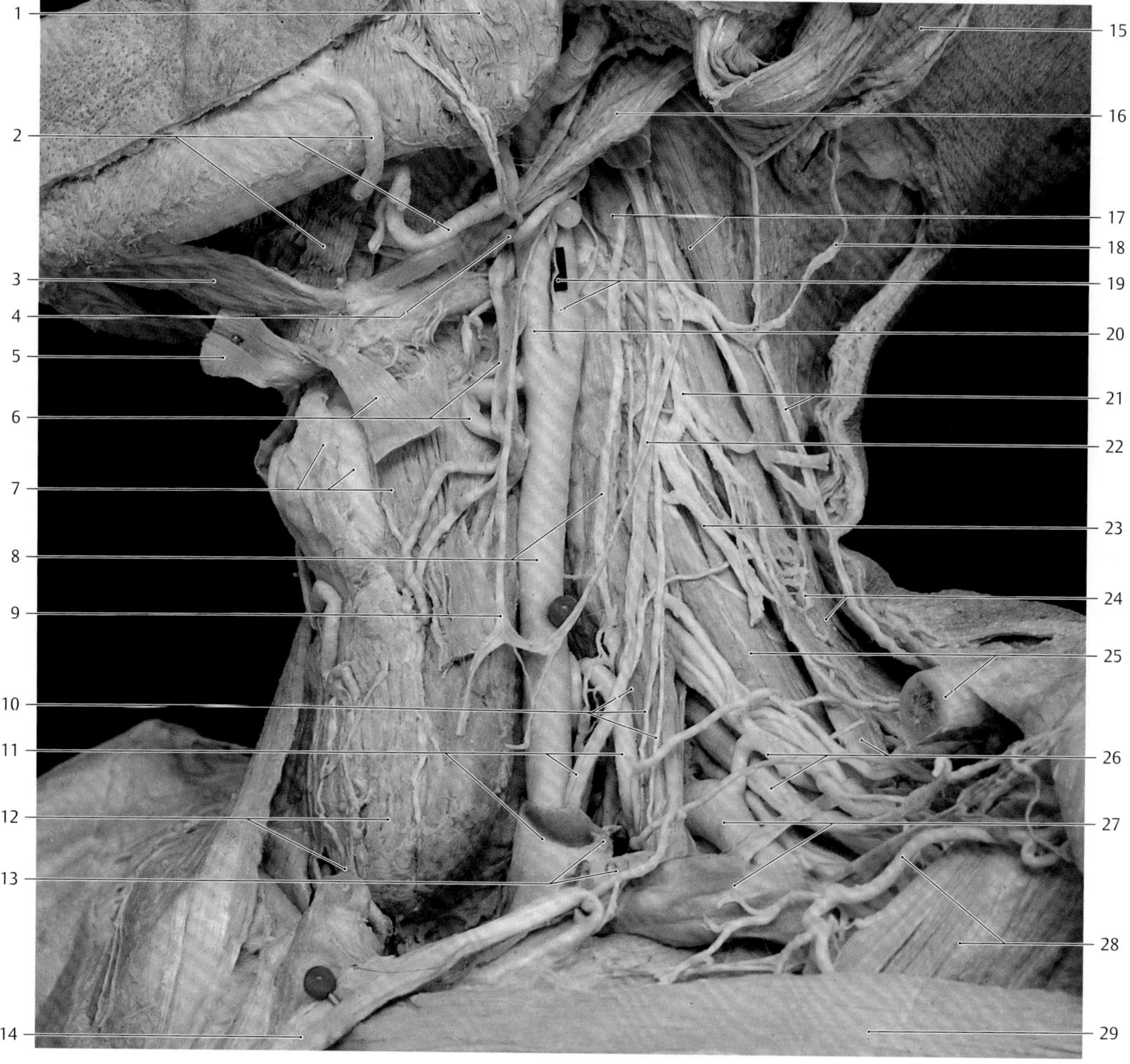


**Fig. 8.201 Lateral region of the neck** (deeper layer). The clavicle partly has been removed to show the gap between the scalene muscles. Internal jugular vein removed.

1 Masseter muscle
2 Mylohyoid muscle and facial artery
3 Anterior belly of digastric muscle
4 Hypoglossal nerve
5 Sternohyoid muscle
6 Omohyoid muscle, superior thyroid artery and vein
7 Sternothyroid muscle, thyroid cartilage, and pyramidal lobe of thyroid gland
8 Common carotid artery and sympathetic trunk
9 Deep ansa cervicalis
10 Phrenic nerve, ascending cervical artery, and anterior scalene muscle
11 Inferior thyroid artery, vagus nerve, and internal jugular vein (cut)
12 Thyroid gland and unpaired inferior thyroid venous plexus
13 Thoracic duct and left subclavian trunk
14 Subclavius muscle (reflected)
15 Sternocleidomastoid muscle (reflected)
16 Posterior belly of digastric muscle
17 Superior cervical ganglion and splenius muscle
18 Lesser occipital nerve
19 Internal carotid artery and branch of the glossopharyngeal nerve to the carotid body (marked black)
20 External carotid artery
21 Cervical plexus and accessory nerve (CN XI)
22 Inferior root of ansa cervicalis
23 Supraclavicular nerve
24 Levator scapulae muscle
25 Middle scalene muscle and clavicle
26 Transverse cervical artery, brachial plexus, and posterior scalene muscle
27 Subclavian artery and vein
28 Thoraco-acromial artery and pectoralis minor muscle
29 Pectoralis major muscle

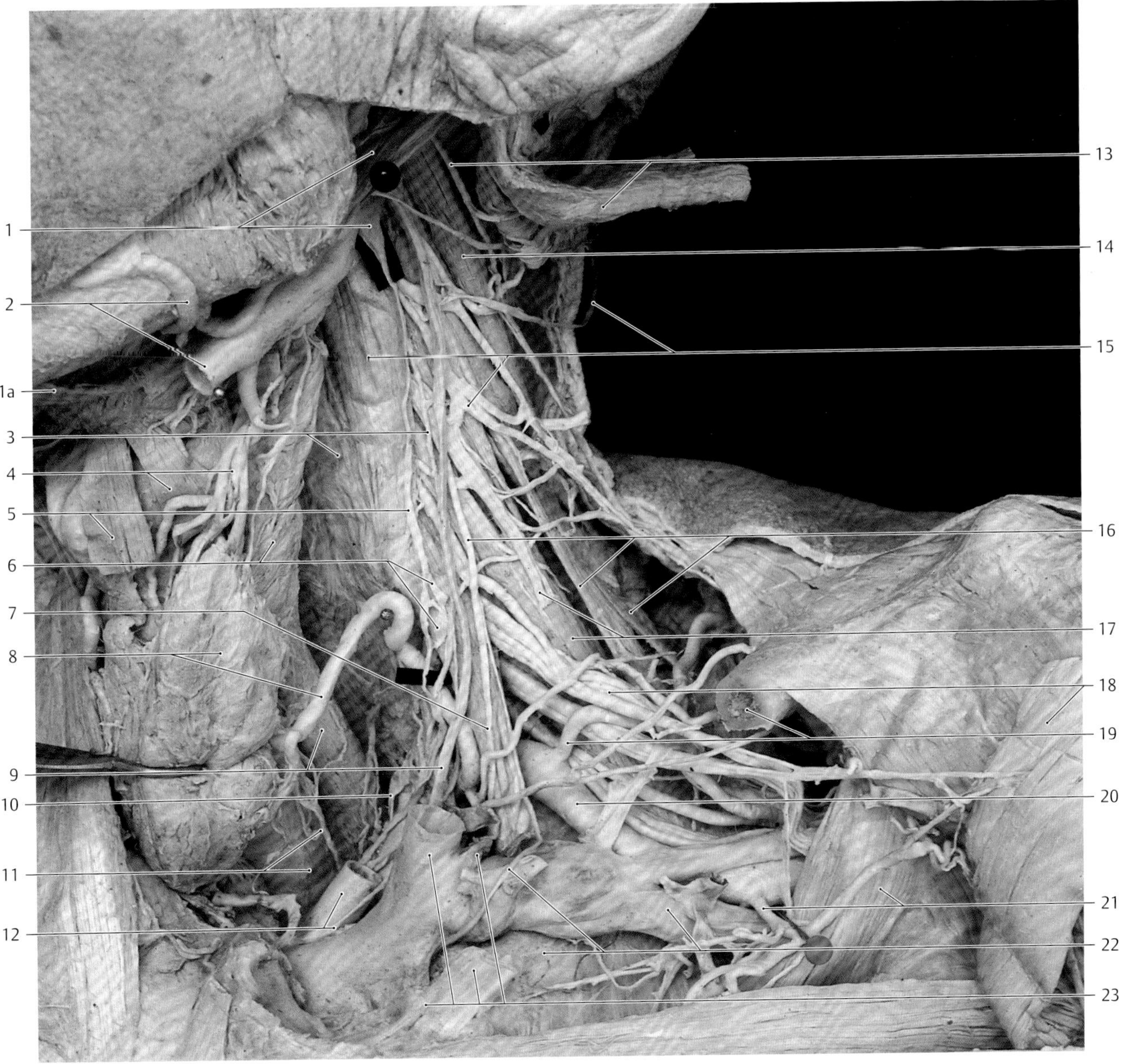


Fig. 8.202 **Lateral region of the neck** (deep layer). The thyroid gland has been reflected to expose the esophagus and the recurrent laryngeal nerve.

1 Superior cervical ganglion of sympathetic trunk and posterior belly of digastric muscle
1a Anterior belly of digastric muscle
2 Facial artery and common carotid artery (reflected anteriorly)
3 Ascending cervical artery and longus colli muscle
4 Omohyoid muscle and superior thyroid artery
5 Sympathetic trunk and sternohyoid muscle
6 Middle cervical ganglion and inferior pharyngeal constrictor muscle
7 Anterior scalene muscle and phrenic nerve
8 Thyroid gland and inferior thyroid artery
9 Vagus nerve and esophagus
10 Stellate ganglion
11 Recurrent laryngeal nerve and trachea
12 Common carotid artery and cervical cardiac branch of vagus nerve
13 Sternocleidomastoid muscle and accessory nerve
14 Splenius capitis muscle
15 Lesser occipital nerve, longus capitis muscle, and cervical plexus
16 Phrenic nerve, posterior scalene muscle, and levator scapulae muscle
17 Supraclavicular nerves and middle scalene muscle
18 Brachial plexus and pectoralis major muscle (clavicular head)
19 Transverse cervical artery and clavicle
20 Subclavian artery
21 Thoraco-acromial artery and pectoralis minor muscle
22 First rib, accessory phrenic nerve, and subclavian vein
23 Internal jugular vein, thoracic duct, and subclavius muscle

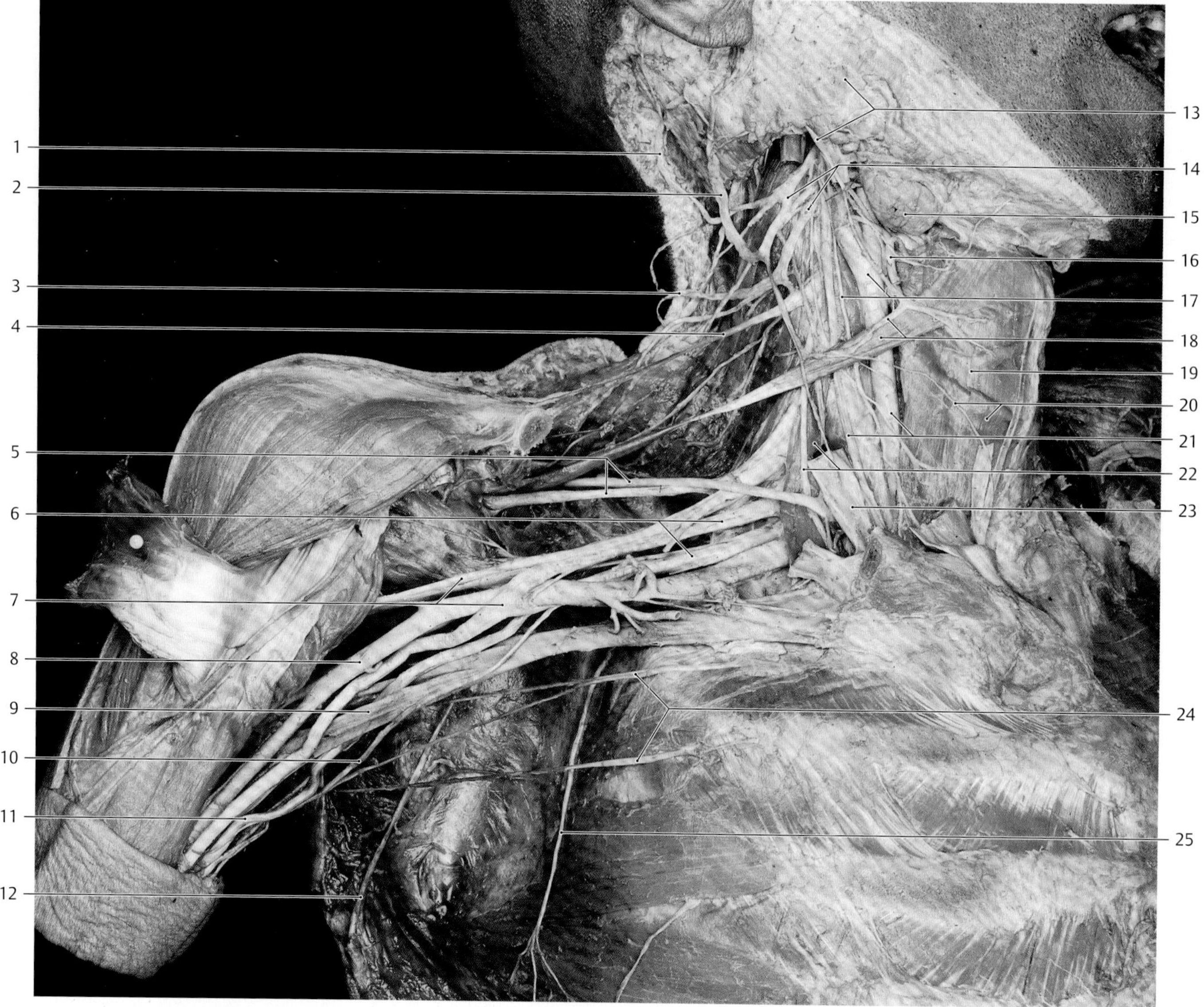


**Fig. 8.203 Cervical and brachial plexuses and their relation to blood vessels.** Note the location and content of the scalene triangle. The sternocleidomastoid muscle and clavicle have been removed and the internal jugular vein has been divided to display the roots of the cervical and brachial plexuses.

1 Lesser occipital nerve
2 Great auricular nerve
3 Cutaneous branches of cervical plexus
4 Supraclavicular nerve
5 Suprascapular nerve and artery
6 Brachial plexus
7 Median nerve (with two roots) and musculocutaneous nerve
8 Axillary artery
9 Axillary vein
10 Medial brachial cutaneous nerve
11 Ulnar nerve
12 Thoracodorsal nerve
13 Parotid gland and facial nerve (cervical branch)
14 Cervical plexus
15 Submandibular gland
16 Superior thyroid artery
17 Common carotid artery dividing in internal and external carotid artery and superior root of ansa cervicalis
18 Omohyoid muscle and cervical branch of facial nerve joining the transverse cervical nerve (C2, C3)
19 Sternohyoid muscle
20 Transverse cervical nerve and sternothyroid muscle
21 Common carotid artery and vagus nerve
22 Phrenic nerve and anterior scalene muscle
23 Internal jugular vein
24 Intercostobrachial nerves
25 Long thoracic nerve

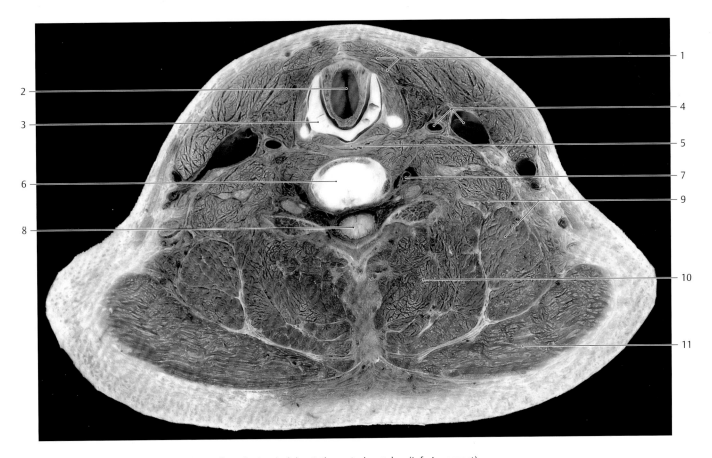

Fig. 8.204 **Axial section through the neck** at the level of the sixth cervical vertebra (inferior aspect).

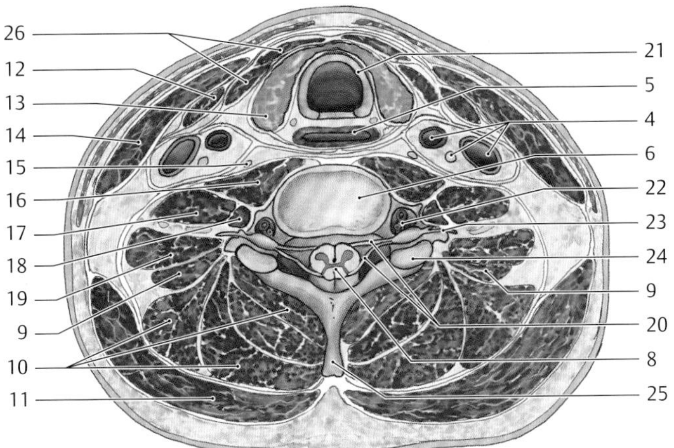


Fig. 8.205 **Organization of the neck** (axial section at the level of the thyroid gland).

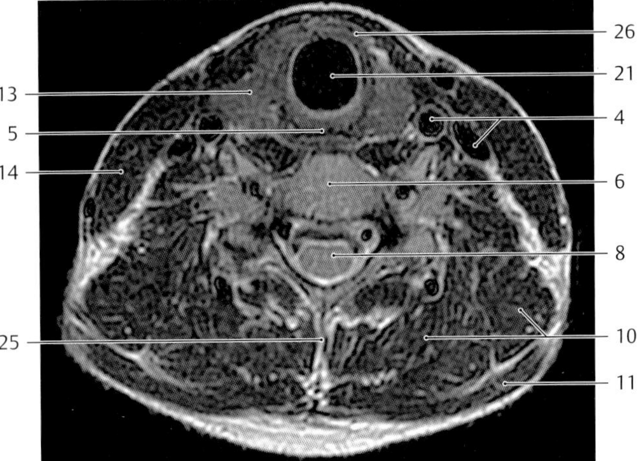


Fig. 8.206 **Axial section through the neck** at the level of the sixth cervical vertebra (MRI scan). (Courtesy of Prof. Uder, Institute of Radiology, University Hospital Erlangen, Germany.)

1 Sternohyoid and thyrohyoid muscles
2 Larynx
3 Cricoid cartilage
4 Internal jugular vein, common carotid artery, and vagus nerve (CN X)
5 Esophagus
6 Body of cervical vertebra
7 Vertebral artery
8 Spinal cord
9 Posterior scalene muscle
10 Deep muscles of the neck
11 Trapezius muscle
12 Omohyoid muscle
13 Thyroid gland
14 Sternocleidomastoid muscle
15 Sympathetic trunk
16 Longus colli muscle
17 Anterior scalene muscle
18 Longissimus capitis muscle
19 Middle scalene muscle
20 Ventral and dorsal root of cervical spinal nerve
21 Trachea
22 Vertebral artery and vein, and foramen transversarium
23 Cervical spinal nerve
24 Superior facet of articular process
25 Spinous process
26 Sternohyoid and sternothyroid muscles

# 9 Brain and Sensory Organs

Head, Neck, and Brain

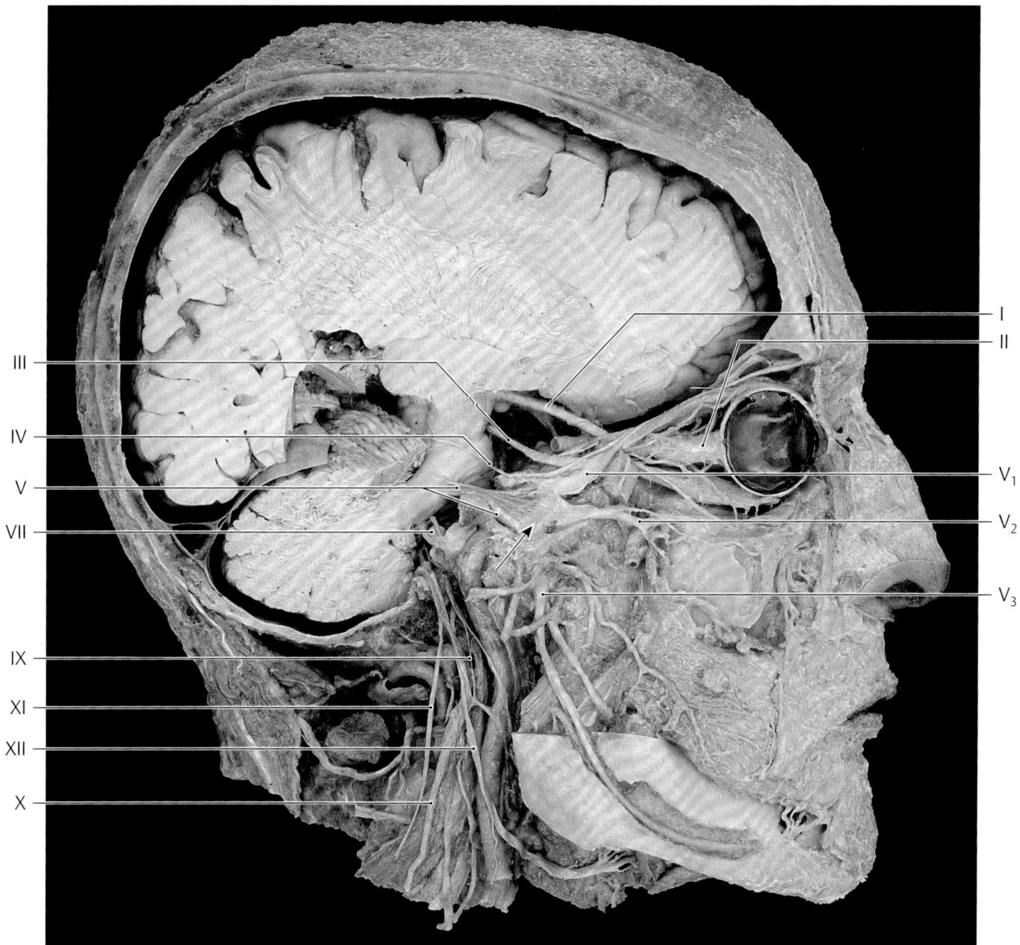


Fig. 9.1 **Dissection of the cranial nerves** (lateral aspect). The cranial nerves are numbered I–XII. The brain, brainstem, and cerebellum have been partly removed. Arrow = trigeminal ganglion.

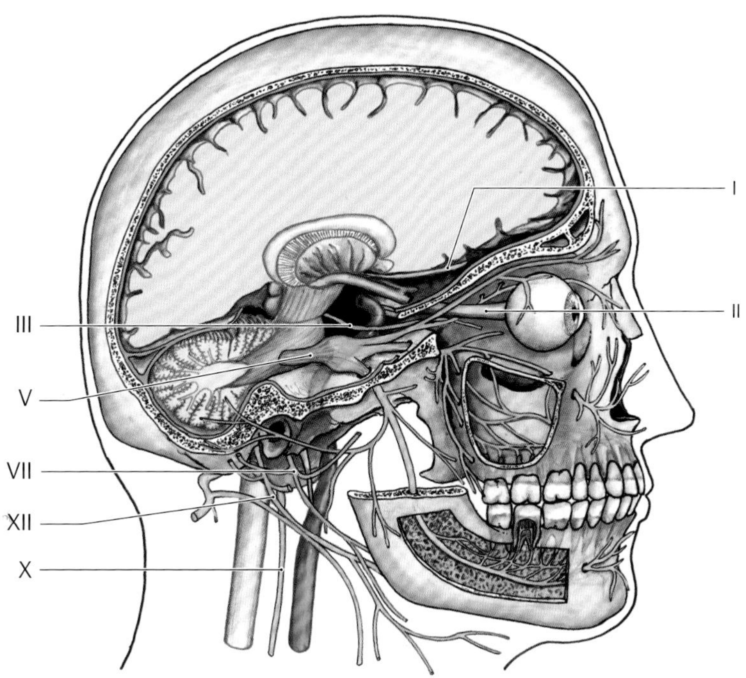


Fig. 9.2 **Schematic drawing of the cranial nerves I–XII** (lateral aspect).

**Cranial nerves and their innervation areas**

- I = Olfactory nerve (to the olfactory mucosa of the nasal cavity)
- II = Optic nerve (to the retina)
- III = Oculomotor nerve (to the extra-ocular muscles)
- IV = Trochlear nerve (to the superior oblique muscle)
- V = Trigeminal nerve (for sensitive innervation and innervation of the muscles of mastication)
- $V_1$ = Ophthalmic nerve (to the orbit)
- $V_2$ = Maxillary nerve (to the upper jaw and to the teeth)
- $V_3$ = Mandibular nerve (to the lower jaw, to the teeth, and to the muscles of mastication)
- VI = Abducent nerve (to the lateral rectus muscle)
- VII = Facial nerve (to the facial muscles)
- VIII = Vestibulocochlear nerve (to the auditory and vestibulary apparatus)
- IX = Glossopharyngeal nerve (to the taste buds)
- X = Vagus nerve (to the pharynx, the larynx, and to the digestive tract)
- XI = Accessory nerve (to the trapezius and sternocleidomastoid muscles)
- XII = Hypoglossal nerve (to the tongue and to the suprahyoid muscles)

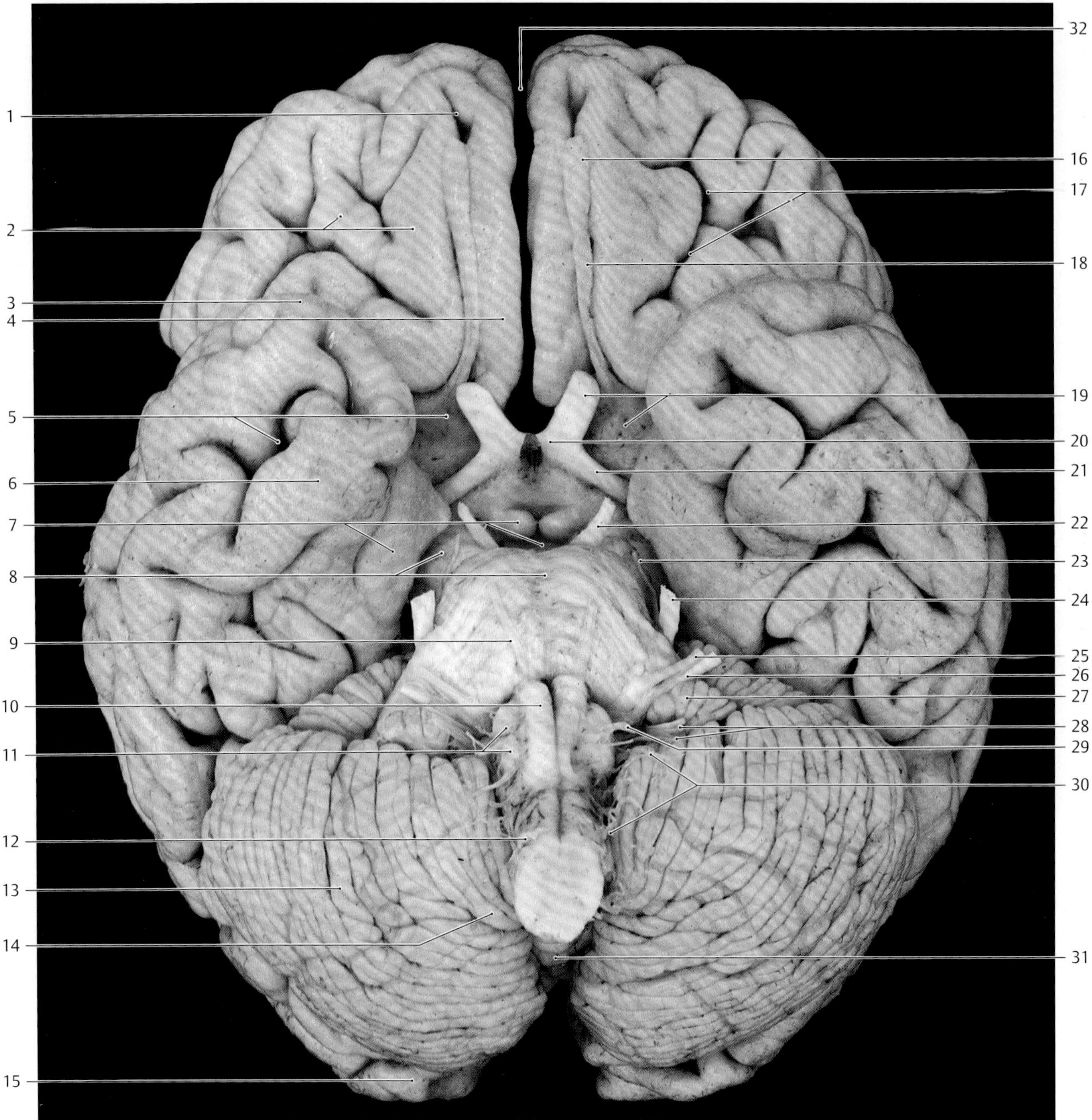


Fig. 9.3 **Brain with cranial nerves** (inferior aspect). Meninges removed.

1 Olfactory sulcus (termination)
2 Orbital gyri
3 Temporal lobe
4 Straight gyrus
5 Olfactory trigone and inferior temporal sulcus
6 Medial occipitotemporal gyrus
7 Parahippocampal gyrus, mamillary body, and interpeduncular fossa
8 Pons and cerebral peduncle
9 Abducent nerve (CN VI)
10 Pyramid
11 Inferior olive
12 Cervical spinal nerves
13 Cerebellum
14 Tonsil of cerebellum
15 Occipital lobe (posterior pole)
16 Olfactory bulb
17 Orbital sulci of frontal lobe
18 Olfactory tract
19 Optic nerve (CN II) and anterior perforated substance
20 Optic chiasma
21 Optic tract
22 Oculomotor nerve (CN III)
23 Trochlear nerve (CN IV)
24 Trigeminal nerve (CN V)
25 Facial nerve (CN VII)
26 Vestibulocochlear nerve (CN VIII)
27 Flocculus of cerebellum
28 Glossopharyngeal nerve (CN IX) and vagus nerve (CN X)
29 Hypoglossal nerve (CN XII)
30 Accessory nerve (CN XI)
31 Vermis of cerebellum
32 Longitudinal fissure

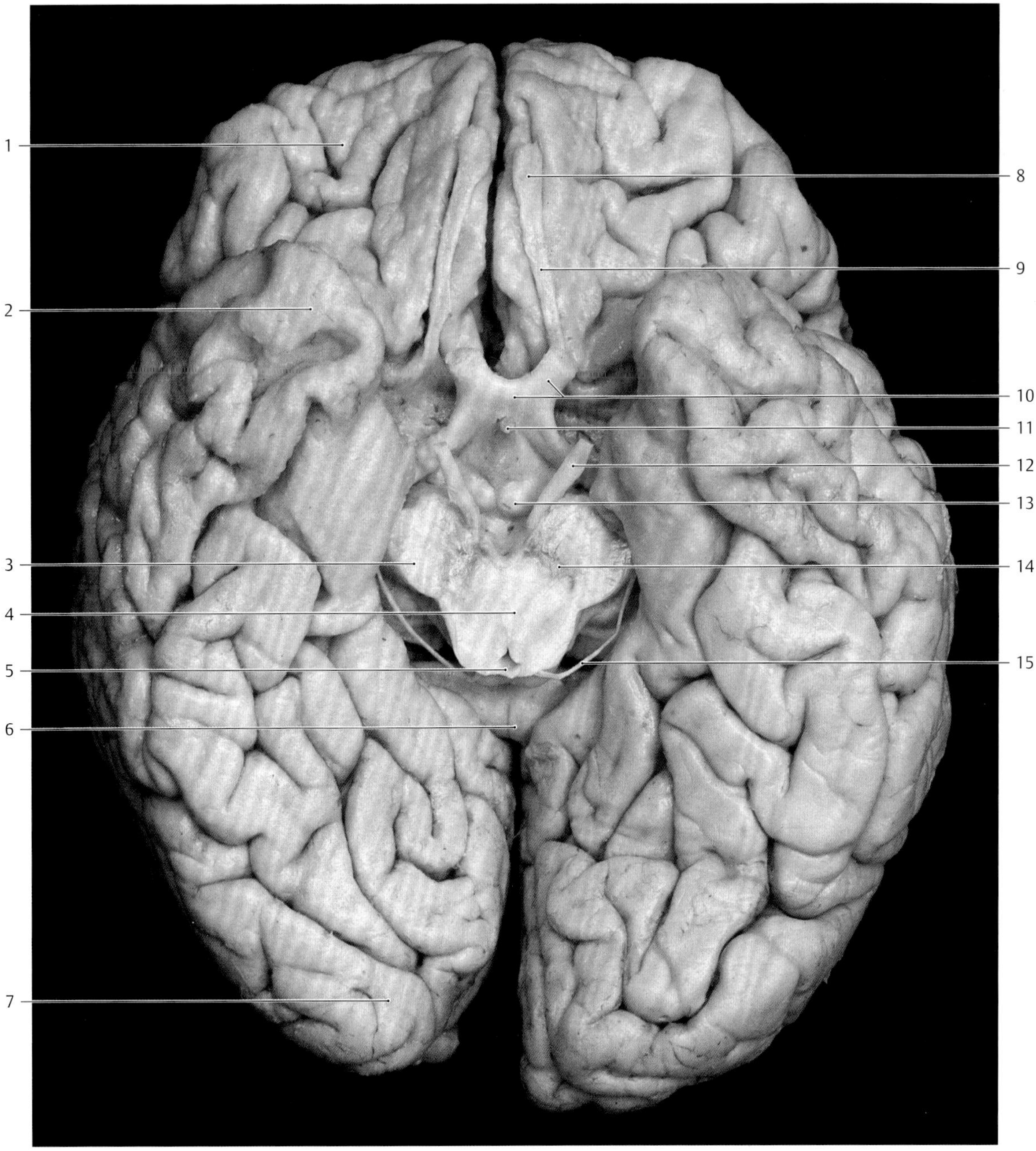


Fig. 9.4 **Brain with cranial nerves** (inferior aspect). Midbrain divided.

1 Frontal lobe
2 Temporal lobe
3 Pedunculus cerebri
4 Midbrain (divided)
5 Cerebral aqueduct
6 Splenium of corpus callosum
7 Occipital lobe
8 Olfactory bulb
9 Olfactory tract
10 Optic nerve and optic chiasma
11 Infundibulum
12 Oculomotor nerve (CN III)
13 Mamillary body
14 Substantia nigra
15 Trochlear nerve (CN IV)

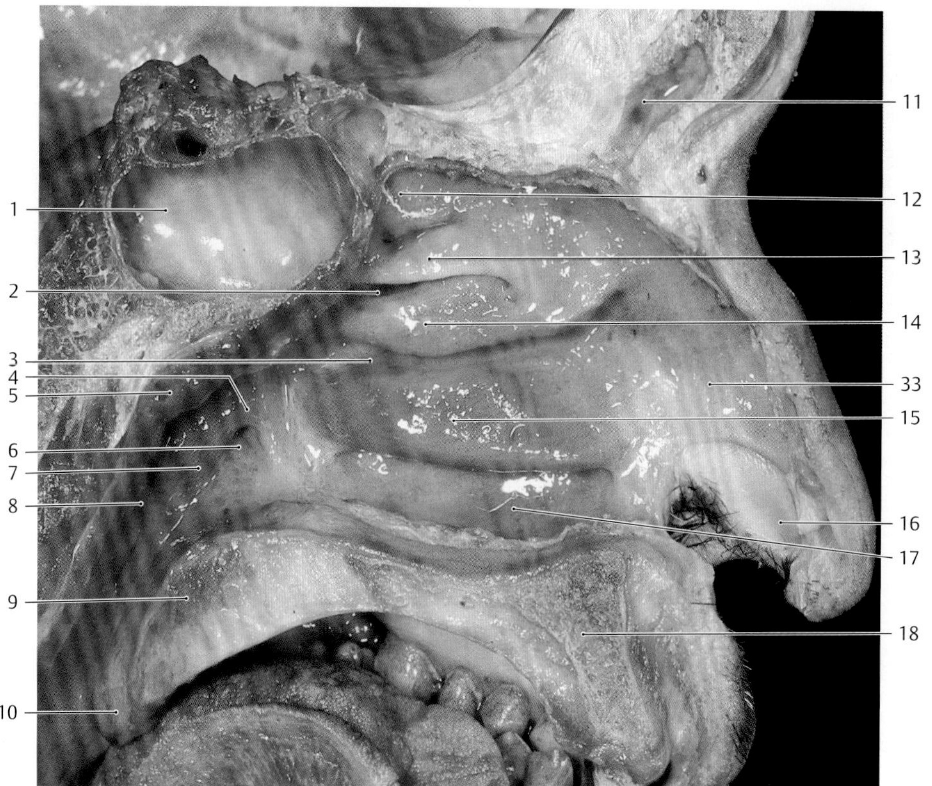


Fig. 9.5 **Lateral wall of the nasal cavity.** Septum removed.

1 Sphenoidal sinus
2 Superior meatus
3 Middle meatus
4 Tubal elevation
5 Pharyngeal tonsil
6 Pharyngeal orifice of auditory tube
7 Salpingopharyngeal fold
8 Pharyngeal recess
9 Soft palate
10 Uvula
11 Frontal sinus
12 Spheno-ethmoidal recess
13 Superior nasal concha
14 Middle nasal concha
15 Inferior nasal concha
16 Vestibule
17 Inferior meatus
18 Hard palate
19 Grooves for the middle meningeal artery and parietal bone (yellow)
20 Maxillary hiatus
21 Perpendicular process of palatine bone
22 Openings of ethmoidal air cells
23 Nasofrontal duct
24 Medial pterygoid plate (red)
25 Horizontal plate of palatine process
26 Ethmoidal air cells
27 Maxillary sinus
28 Nasal septum
29 Pterygoid hamulus
30 Nasal bone (white)
31 Frontal process of maxilla (violet)
32 Palatine process of maxilla (violet)
33 Nasal atrium

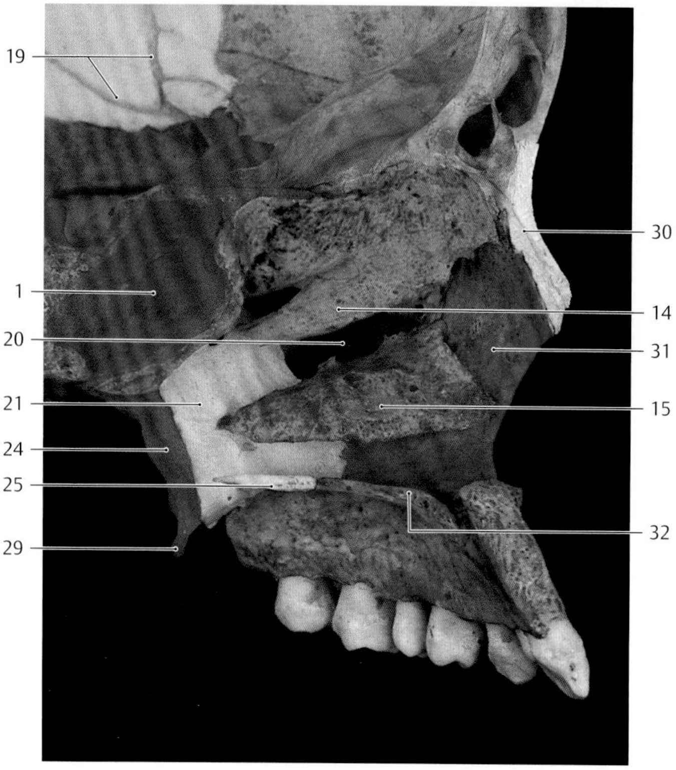

Fig. 9.6 **Bones of the left nasal cavity** (medial aspect).

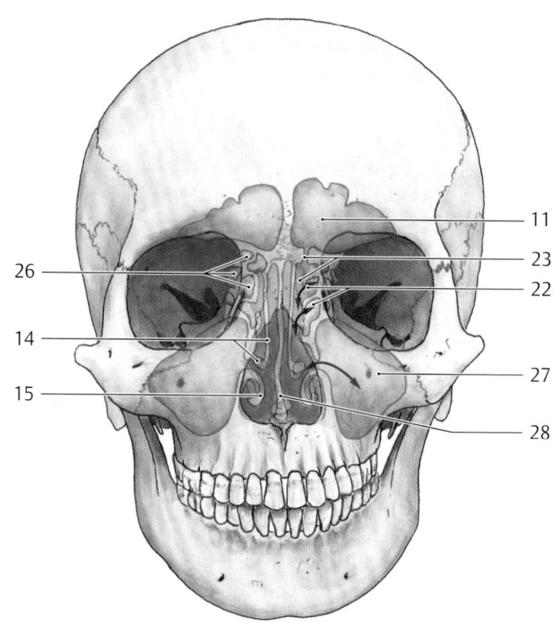


Fig. 9.7 **Paranasal sinuses and their connections with the nasal cavity.** Arrows = Openings.

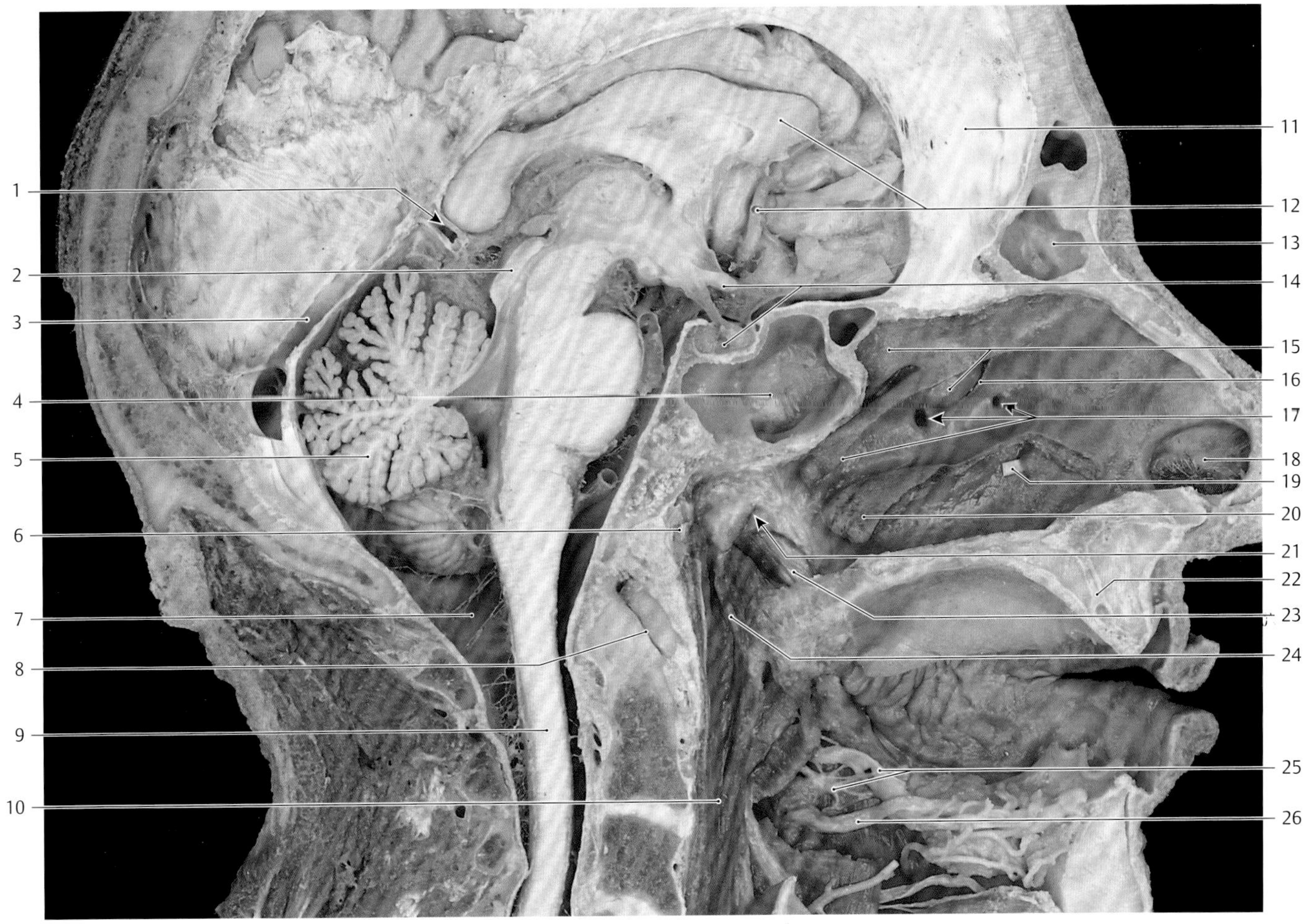

**Fig. 9.8 Median section through the head with nasal and oral cavities.** The middle and inferior nasal conchae have been partly removed to show the openings of the paranasal sinuses.

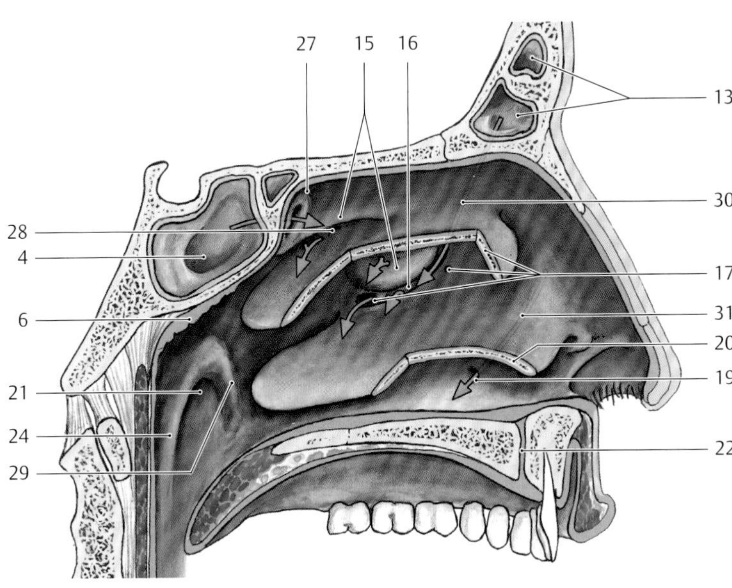


**Fig. 9.9 Lateral wall of the nasal cavity.** Arrows = Openings.

1 Great cerebral vein (Galen's vein)
2 Tectum of midbrain
3 Straight sinus
4 Sphenoidal sinus
5 Cerebellum
6 Pharyngeal tonsil
7 Cerebellomedullary cistern
8 Median atlanto-axial joint
9 Spinal cord
10 Oral part of pharynx
11 Falx cerebri
12 Corpus callosum and anterior cerebral artery
13 Frontal sinus
14 Optic chiasm and pituitary gland
15 Superior nasal concha and ethmoidal bulla
16 Semilunar hiatus
17 Accessory openings to maxillary sinus and cut edge of middle nasal concha
18 Vestibule
19 Opening of nasolacrimal duct
20 Inferior nasal concha (cut)
21 Opening of auditory tube
22 Incisive canal
23 Levator veli palatini muscle
24 Salpingopharyngeal fold
25 Lingual nerve and submandibular ganglion
26 Submandibular duct
27 Spheno-ethmoidal recess
28 Superior nasal meatus
29 Salpingopalatine fold
30 Nasofrontal duct
31 Nasolacrimal duct

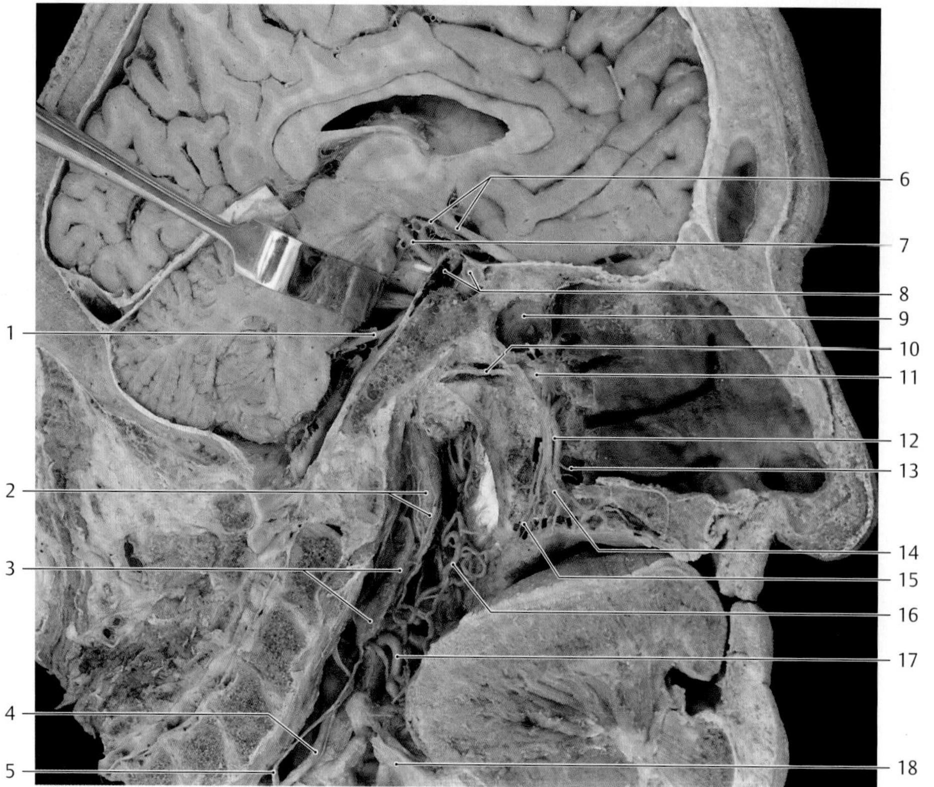


**Fig. 9.10 Nerves of the lateral wall of nasal cavity** (sagittal section through the head). The mucous membranes have been partly removed and the pterygoid canal opened.

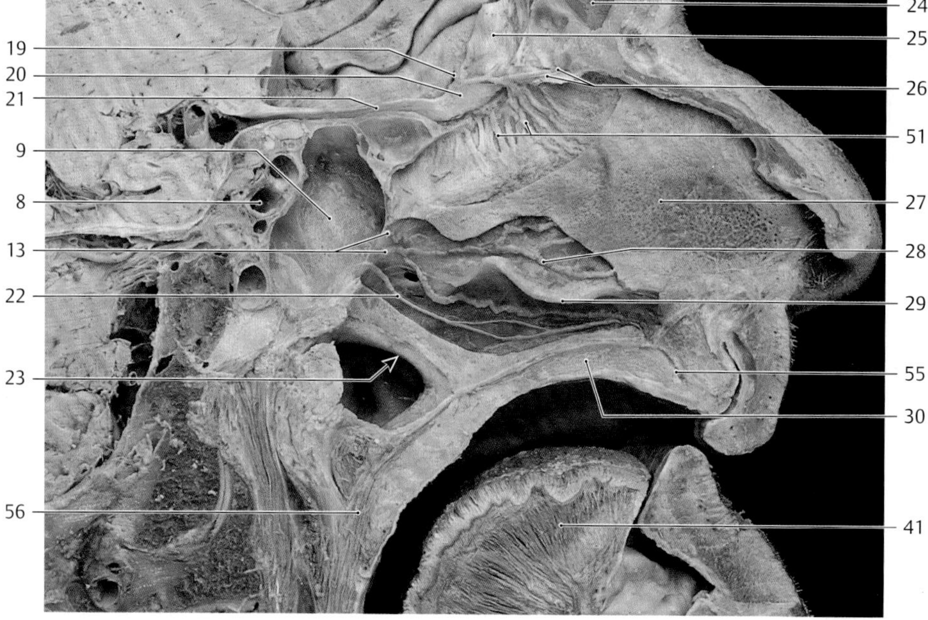


**Fig. 9.11 Nasal septum.** Dissection of nerves and vessels.

1 Facial nerve
2 Internal carotid artery and internal carotid plexus
3 Superior cervical ganglion
4 Vagus nerve (CN X)
5 Sympathetic trunk
6 Optic nerve (CN II) and ophthalmic artery
7 Oculomotor nerve (CN III)
8 Internal carotid artery and cavernous sinus
9 Sphenoidal sinus
10 Nerve of the pterygoid canal
11 Pterygopalatine ganglion
12 Descending palatine artery
13 Lateral inferior posterior nasal branches and lateral posterior nasal and septal arteries
14 Greater palatine nerves and artery
15 Lesser palatine nerves and arteries
16 Branches of ascending pharyngeal artery
17 Lingual artery
18 Epiglottis
19 Anterior ethmoidal artery
20 Olfactory bulb
21 Olfactory tract
22 Nasopalatine nerve
23 Choanae
24 Frontal sinus
25 Crista galli
26 Anterior ethmoidal artery and nerve, and nasal branch of anterior ethmoidal artery
27 Nasal septum
28 Septal artery
29 Crest of nasal septum
30 Hard palate
31 Cerebellar tentorium
32 Trochlear nerve (CN IV)
33 Trigeminal nerve (CN V) with motor root
34 Internal carotid plexus
35 Lingual nerve with chorda tympani
36 Medial pterygoid muscle and medial pterygoid plate
37 Inferior alveolar nerve
38 Sympathetic trunk
39 Greater petrosal nerve
40 Palatine nerves
41 Tongue
42 Olfactory bulb
43 Ophthalmic nerve (CN $V_1$)
44 Trigeminal ganglion
45 Maxillary nerve (CN $V_2$)
46 Mandibular nerve (CN $V_3$)
47 Deep petrosal nerve
48 Medial pterygoid muscle
49 Tensor veli palatine muscle
50 Greater palatine nerve
51 Olfactory nerves
52 Internal and medial nasal branches of anterior ethmoidal nerve
53 Lateral superior posterior nasal branches
54 Lateral inferior posterior nasal branches
55 Incisive canal with nasopalatine nerve
56 Uvula

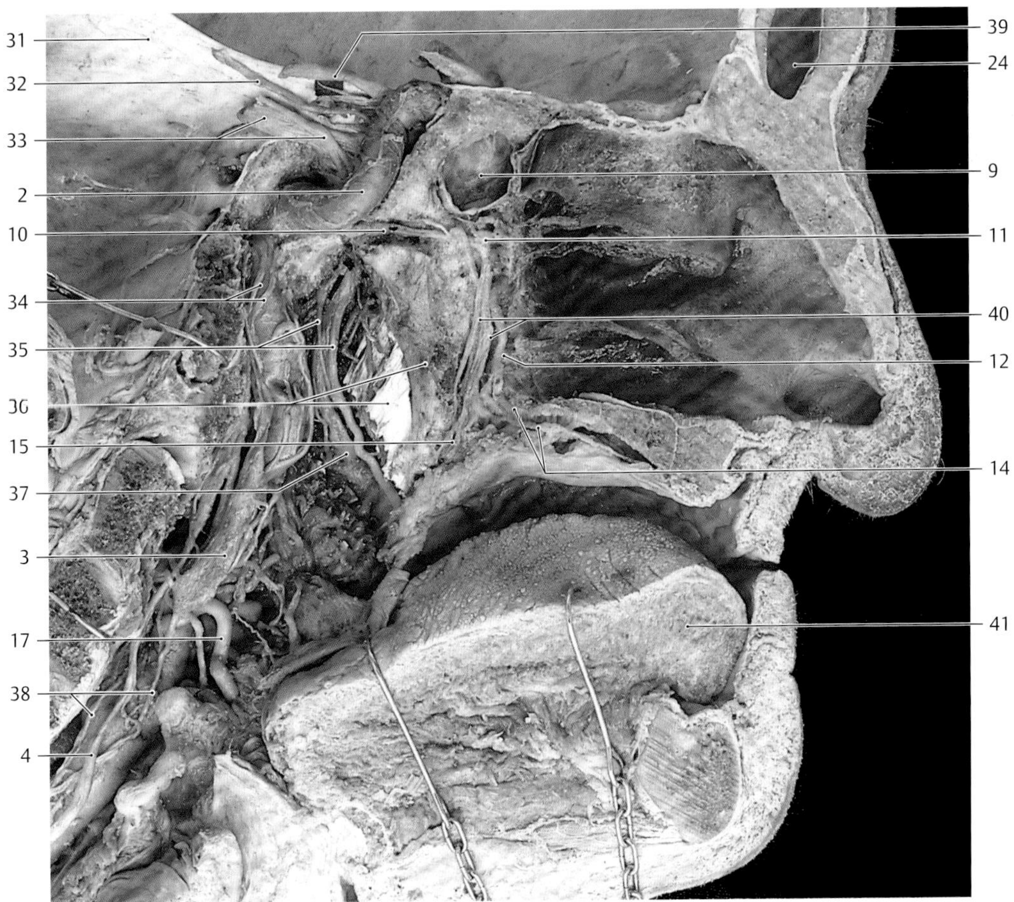


Fig. 9.12 **Nerves of the lateral wall of the nasal cavity** (sagittal section through the head). The carotid canal has been opened and the mucous membranes of the pharynx and nasal cavity partly removed.

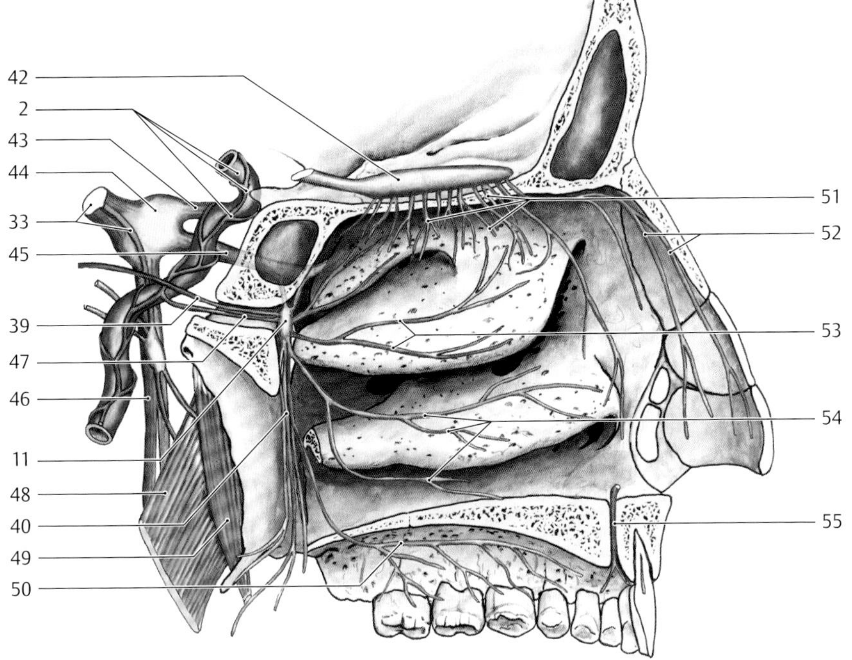


Fig. 9.13 **Nerves of the lateral wall of the nasal cavity** (sagittal section).

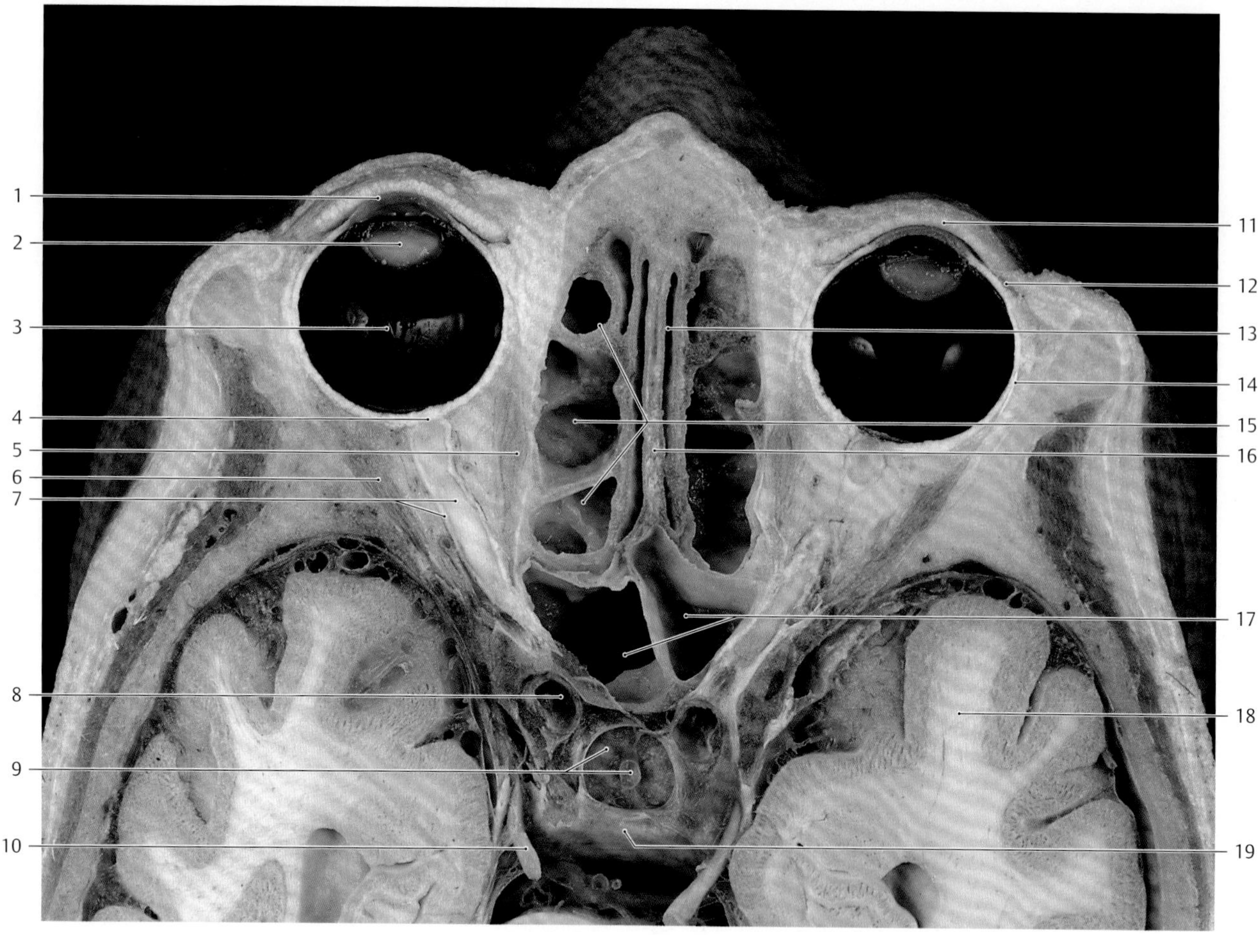

**Fig. 9.14 Horizontal section through the nasal cavity, the orbits, and temporal lobes of the brain** at the level of the pituitary gland.

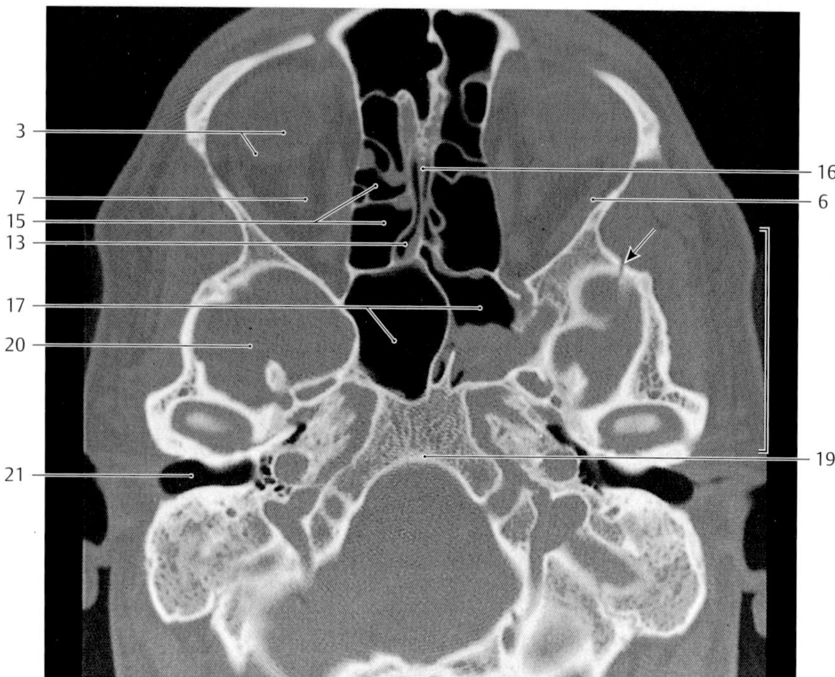


**Fig. 9.15 Horizontal section through the nasal cavity, the orbits, and temporal lobes of the brain** (CT scan). Bar = 2cm; arrow = fracture. (Courtesy of Prof. Uder, Institute of Radiology, University Hospital Erlangen, Germany.)

1 Cornea
2 Lens
3 Vitreous body (eyeball)
4 Head of optic nerve
5 Medial rectus muscle
6 Lateral rectus muscle
7 Optic nerve with dural sheath
8 Internal carotid artery
9 Pituitary gland and infundibulum
10 Oculomotor nerve
11 Superior tarsal plate of eyelid
12 Fornix of conjunctiva
13 Nasal cavity
14 Sclera
15 Ethmoidal sinus
16 Nasal septum
17 Sphenoidal sinus
18 Temporal lobe
19 Clivus
20 Middle cranial fossa
21 External acoustic meatus
22 Superior sagittal sinus
23 Falx cerebri
24 Superior rectus and levator palpebrae superioris muscles

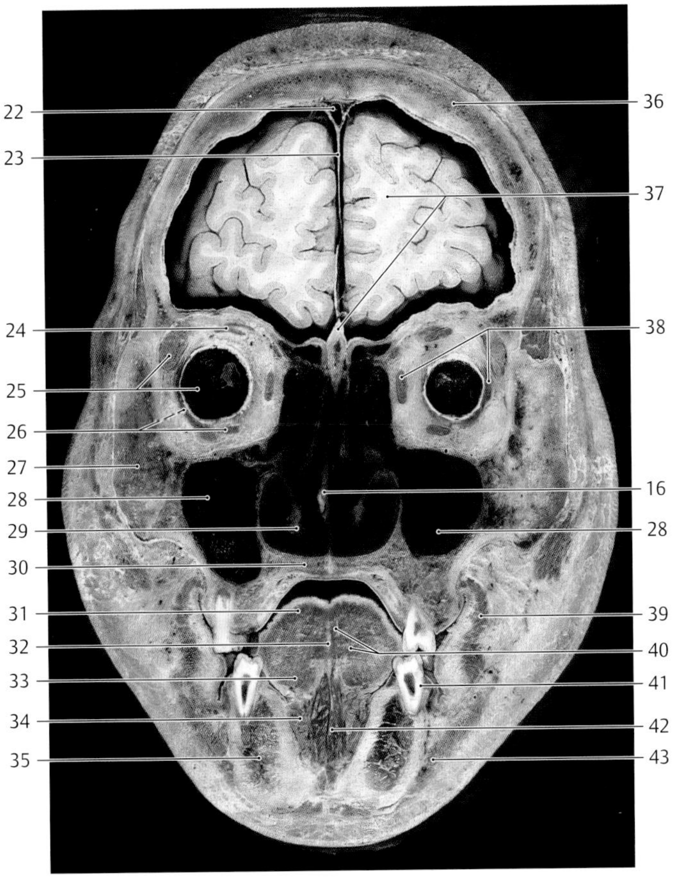

Fig. 9.16 **Coronal section through the head** at the level of the second premolar of the mandible.

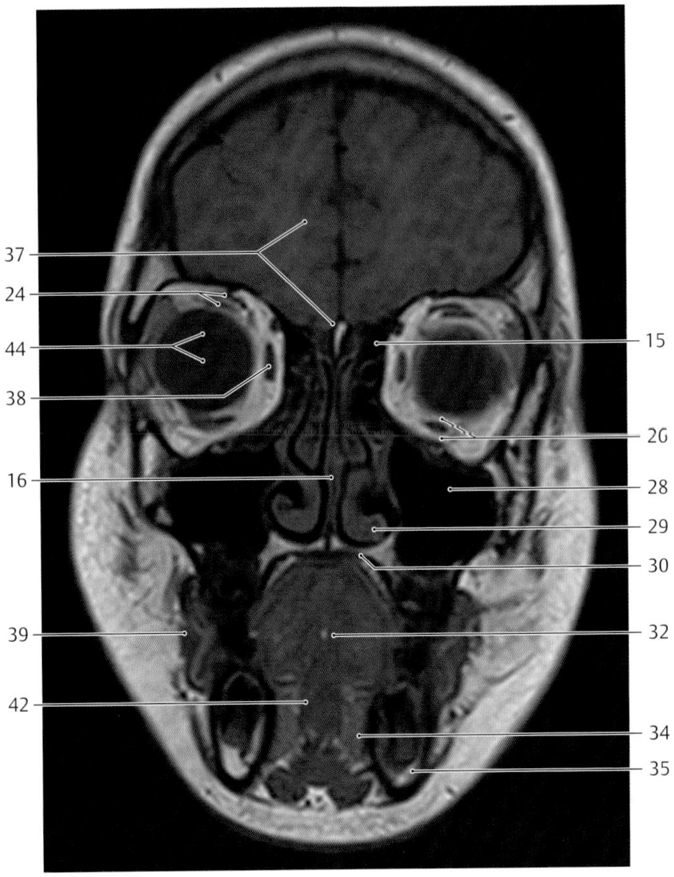

Fig. 9.17 **Coronal section through the head** (MRI scan). Note the position of the head cavities. (Courtesy of Prof. Uder, Institute of Radiology, University Hospital Erlangen, Germany.)

25 Eyeball and lacrimal gland
26 Inferior rectus and inferior oblique muscles
27 Zygomatic bone
28 Maxillary sinus
29 Inferior nasal concha
30 Hard palate
31 Superior longitudinal muscle of tongue
32 Lingual septum
33 Inferior longitudinal muscle of tongue
34 Sublingual gland
35 Mandible
36 Calvaria
37 Frontal lobe of brain and crista galli
38 Lateral and medial rectus muscles
39 Buccinator muscle
40 Vertical and transverse muscles of tongue
41 Second premolar of the mandible
42 Genioglossus muscle
43 Platysma muscle
44 Orbit and optic nerve (CN II)
45 Hyoid bone
46 Mylohyoid muscle
47 Submandibular gland

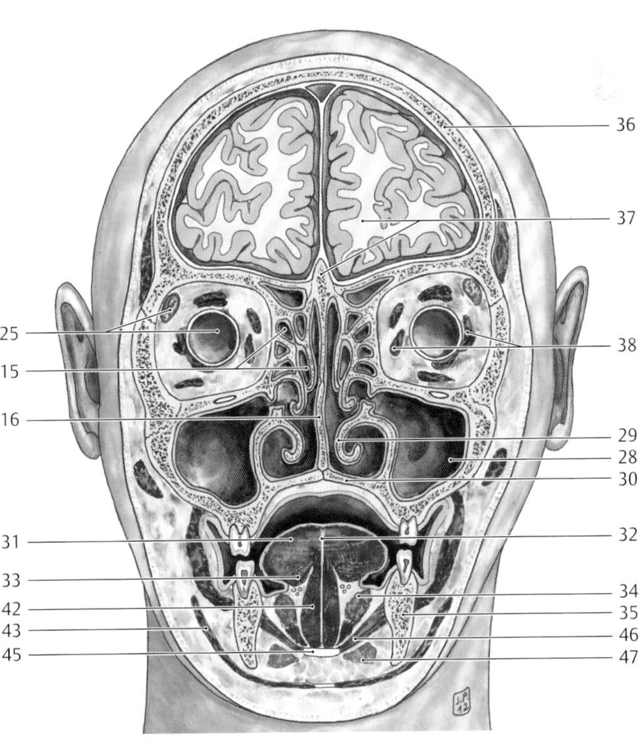


Fig. 9.18 **Coronal section through the head** at the level of the second premolar of the mandible.

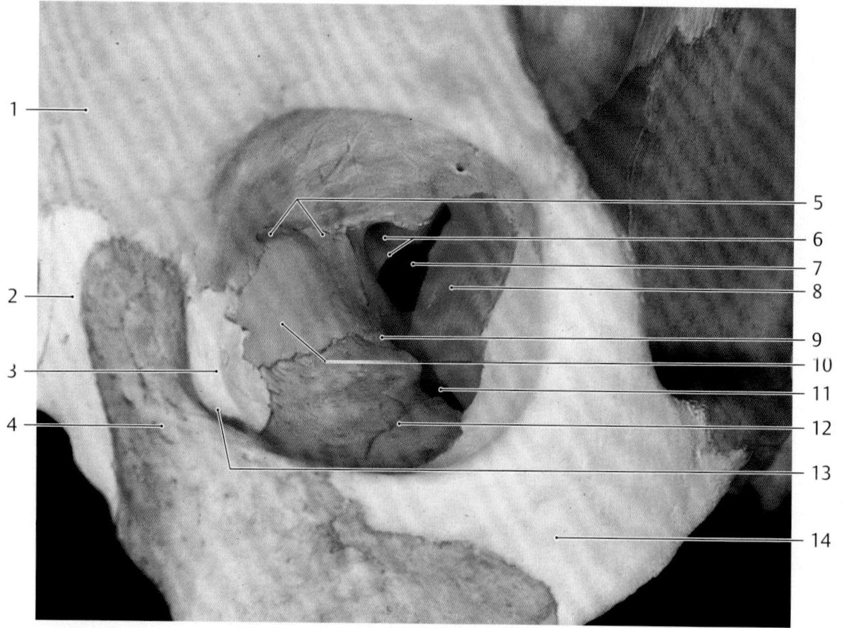


**Fig. 9.19 Bones of the left orbit** (indicated by different colors).

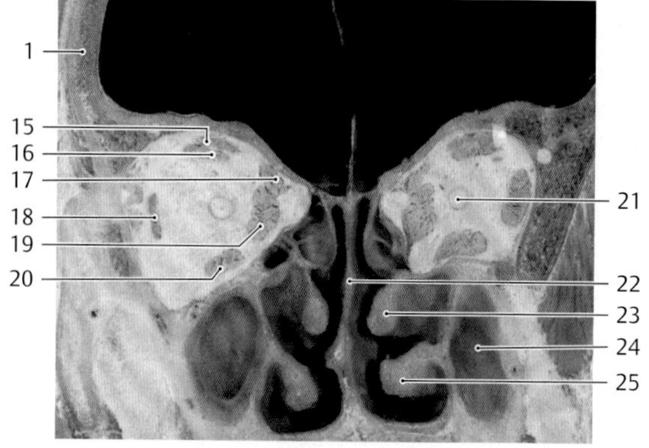


**Fig. 9.20 Frontal section through the posterior part of the orbit.**

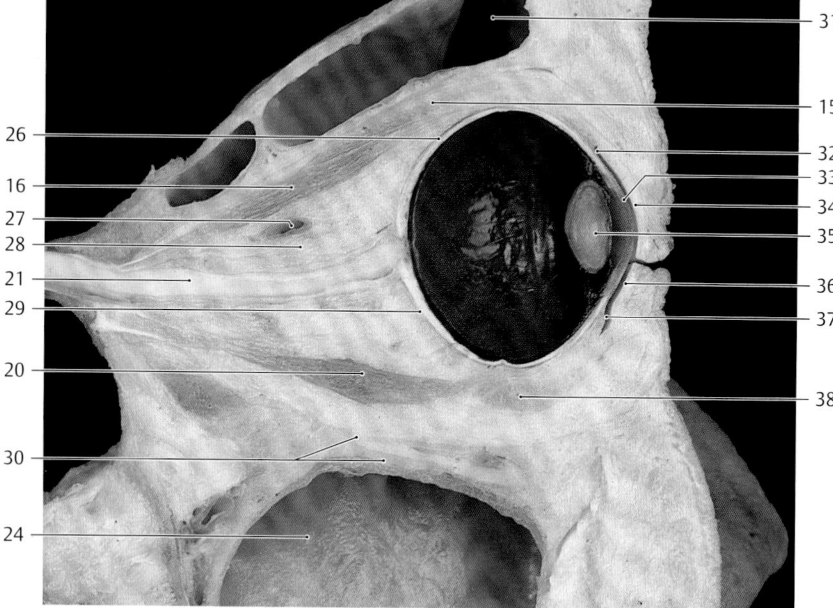


**Fig. 9.21 Sagittal section through the orbit and eyeball.**

1 Frontal bone
2 Nasal bone
3 Lacrimal bone
4 Maxilla (frontal process)
5 Ethmoidal foramina
6 Lesser wing of sphenoid bone and optic canal
7 Superior orbital fissure
8 Greater wing of sphenoid bone
9 Orbital process of palatine bone
10 Orbital plate of ethmoid bone
11 Inferior orbital fissure
12 Infra-orbital sulcus
13 Nasolacrimal canal
14 Zygomatic bone
15 Levator palpebrae superioris muscle
16 Superior rectus muscle
17 Superior oblique muscle
18 Lateral rectus muscle
19 Medial rectus muscle
20 Inferior rectus muscle
21 Optic nerve (CN II)
22 Nasal septum
23 Middle nasal concha
24 Maxillary sinus
25 Inferior nasal concha
26 Sclera
27 Ophthalmic artery
28 Orbital fatty tissue
29 Tenon's space
30 Periorbita and maxilla
31 Frontal sinus
32 Superior conjunctival fornix
33 Cornea
34 Superior tarsal plate
35 Lens
36 Inferior tarsal plate
37 Inferior conjunctival fornix
38 Inferior oblique muscle

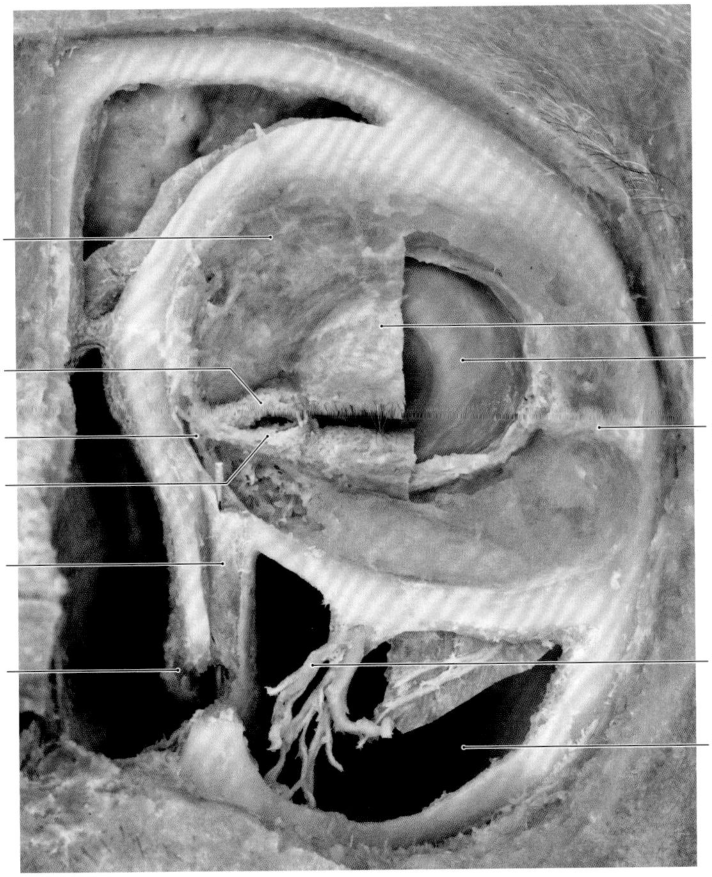

**Fig. 9.22 Eyelids and lacrimal apparatus of the left eye** (anterior aspect). Parts of the eyelids have been removed to reveal the underlying eyeball. The maxillary sinus has been opened.

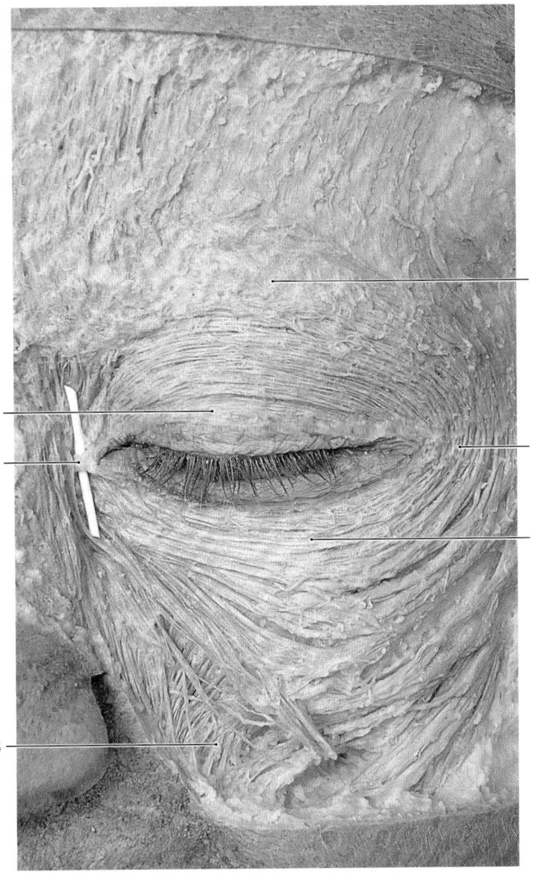

**Fig. 9.23 Facial muscles of the left eye** (anterior aspect). The orbicularis oculi muscle and its connection to the superior labial muscles are shown. Note the medial palpebral ligament (probe).

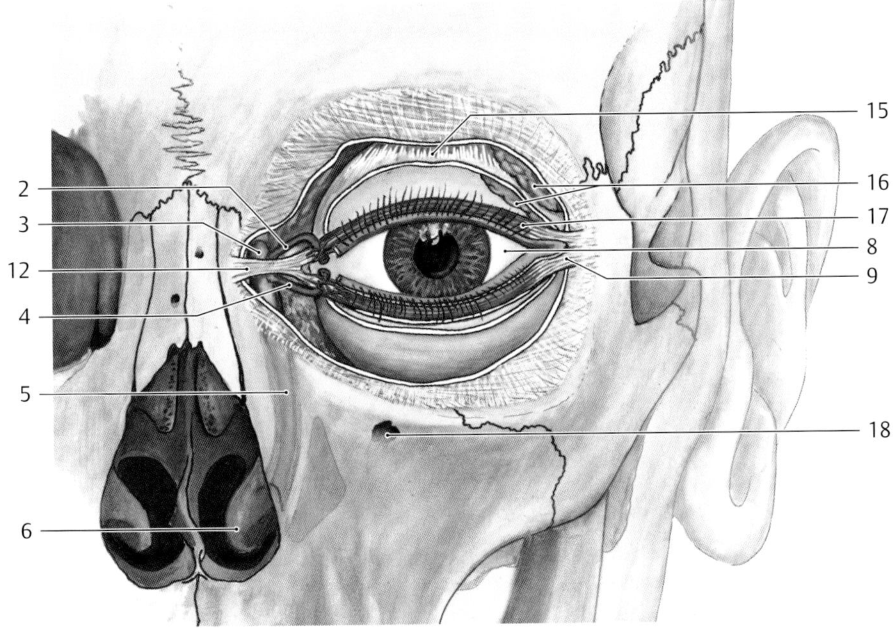


**Fig. 9.24 Lacrimal apparatus of the left eye** (anterior aspect). Red = Palpebral portion of the orbicularis oculi muscle.

1 Orbicularis oculi muscle
2 Superior lacrimal canaliculus
3 Lacrimal sac
4 Inferior lacrimal canaliculus
5 Nasolacrimal duct
6 Inferior nasal concha
7 Upper eyelid
8 Eyeball
9 Lateral palpebral ligament
10 Infra-orbital artery and nerve
11 Maxillary sinus
12 Medial palpebral ligament
13 Levator labii superioris muscle
14 Frontal belly of occipitofrontalis muscle
15 Aponeurosis of levator palpebrae superioris muscle
16 Lacrimal gland
17 Palpebral portion of orbicularis oculi muscle
18 Infra-orbital foramen

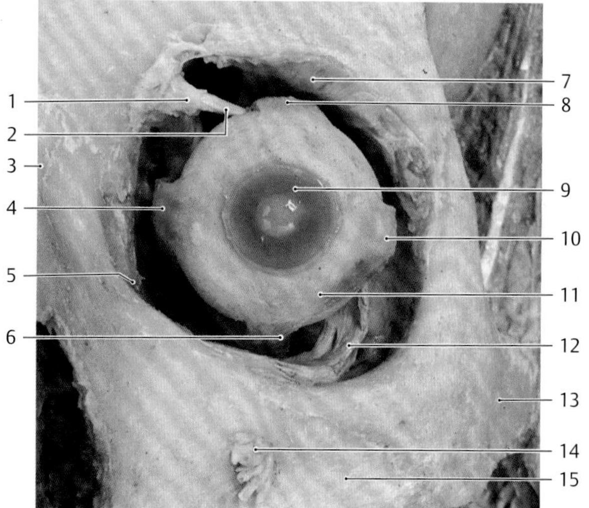


Fig. 9.25 **Left orbit with eyeball and extra-ocular muscles (anterior aspect).** The eyelids, conjunctiva, and lacrimal apparatus have been removed.

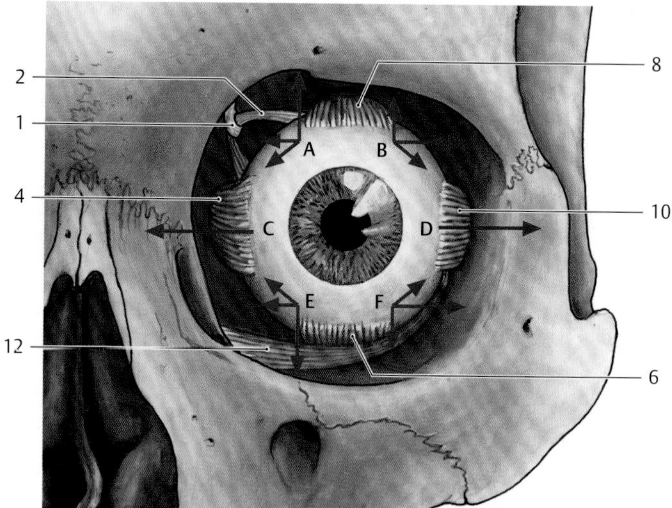


Fig. 9.26 **Action of the extra-ocular muscles** (anterior aspect).

A = Superior rectus muscle
B = Inferior oblique muscle
C = Medial rectus muscle
D = Lateral rectus muscle
E = Inferior rectus muscle
F = Superior oblique muscle

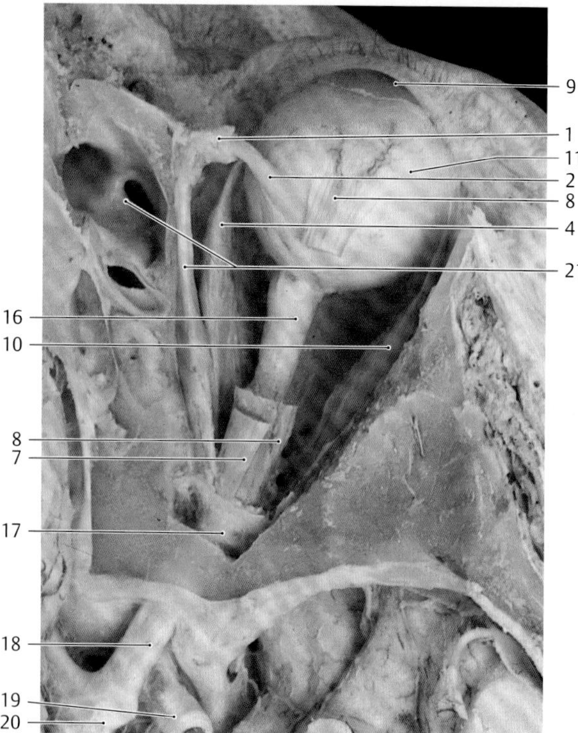


Fig. 9.27 **Right orbit with eyeball and extra-ocular muscles** (from above). The roof of the orbit has been removed, and the superior rectus muscle and the levator palpebrae superioris muscle have been severed.

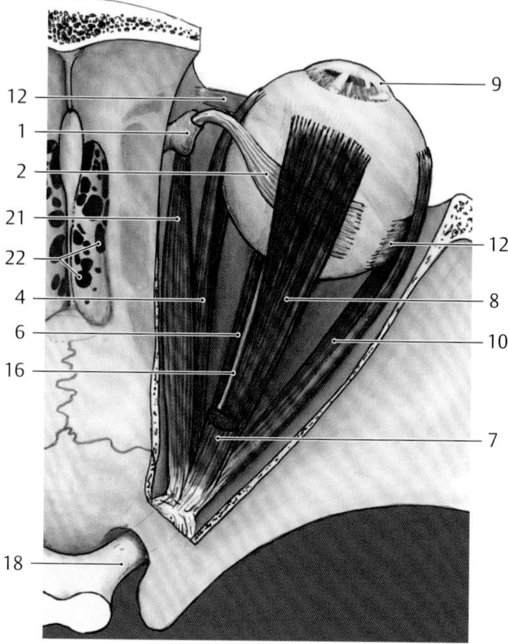


Fig. 9.28 **Right orbit with eyeball and extra-ocular muscles** (from above). The levator palpebrae superioris muscle has been severed.

1 Trochlea
2 Tendon of superior oblique muscle
3 Nasal bone
4 Medial rectus muscle
5 Nasolacrimal duct
6 Inferior rectus muscle
7 Levator palpebrae superioris muscle
8 Superior rectus muscle
9 Cornea
10 Lateral rectus muscle
11 Sclera
12 Inferior oblique muscle
13 Zygomatic bone
14 Infra-orbital nerves
15 Maxilla
16 Optic nerve (CN II) (extracranial part)
17 Common annular tendon
18 Optic nerve (intracranial part)
19 Internal carotid artery
20 Optic chiasma
21 Superior oblique muscle
22 Ethmoidal cells

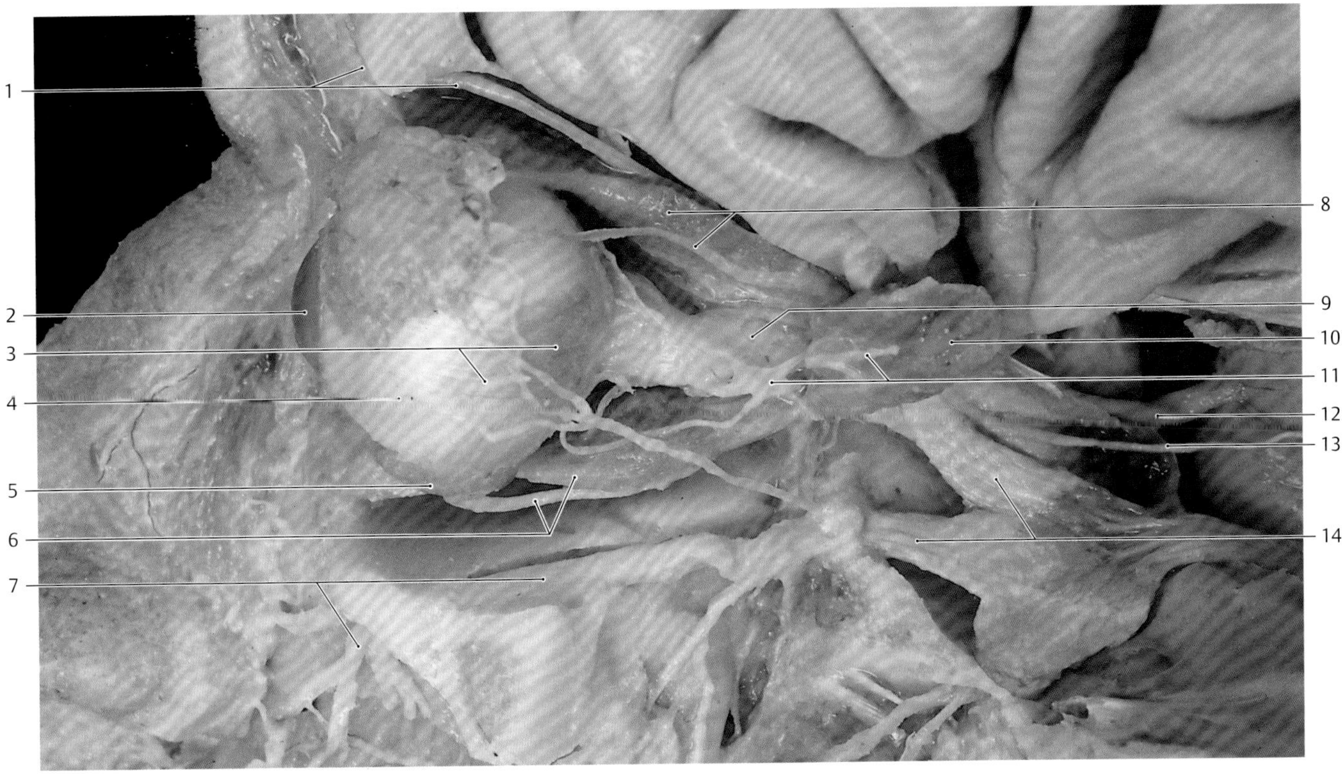


Fig. 9.29 **Extra-ocular muscles and their nerves** (lateral aspect of the left eye). The lateral rectus muscle has been divided and reflected.

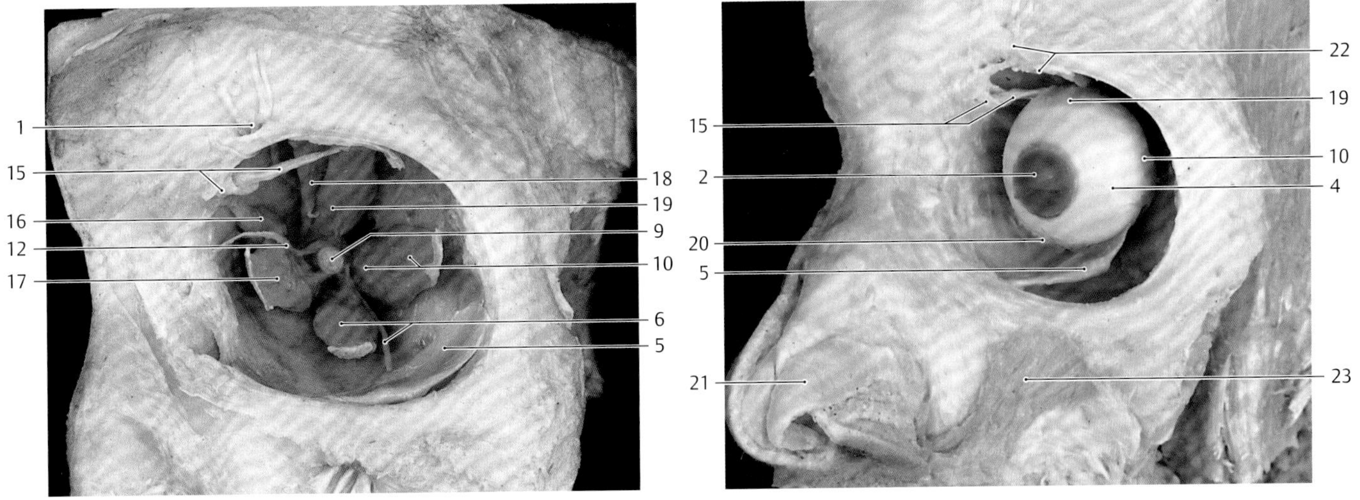


Fig. 9.30 **Left orbit with extra-ocular muscles** (anterior aspect). The eyeball has been removed.

Fig. 9.31 **Extra-ocular muscles** (antero-lateral aspect). The fatty tissue of the orbit has been removed.

1 Supra-orbital nerve
2 Cornea
3 Insertion of lateral rectus muscle
4 Eyeball (sclera)
5 Inferior oblique muscle
6 Inferior rectus muscle and inferior branch of oculomotor nerve
7 Infra-orbital nerve
8 Superior rectus muscle and lacrimal nerve
9 Optic nerve (CN II)
10 Lateral rectus muscle
11 Ciliary ganglion and abducens nerve (CN VI)
12 Oculomotor nerve (CN III)
13 Trochlear nerve (CN IV)
14 Ophthalmic nerve (CN $V_1$) and maxillary nerve (CN $V_2$)
15 Trochlea and tendon of superior oblique muscle
16 Superior oblique muscle
17 Medial rectus muscle
18 Levator palpebrae superioris muscle
19 Superior rectus muscle
20 Inferior rectus muscle
21 Greater alar cartilage
22 Supra-orbital nerve and levator palpebrae superioris muscle
23 Levator labii superioris muscle

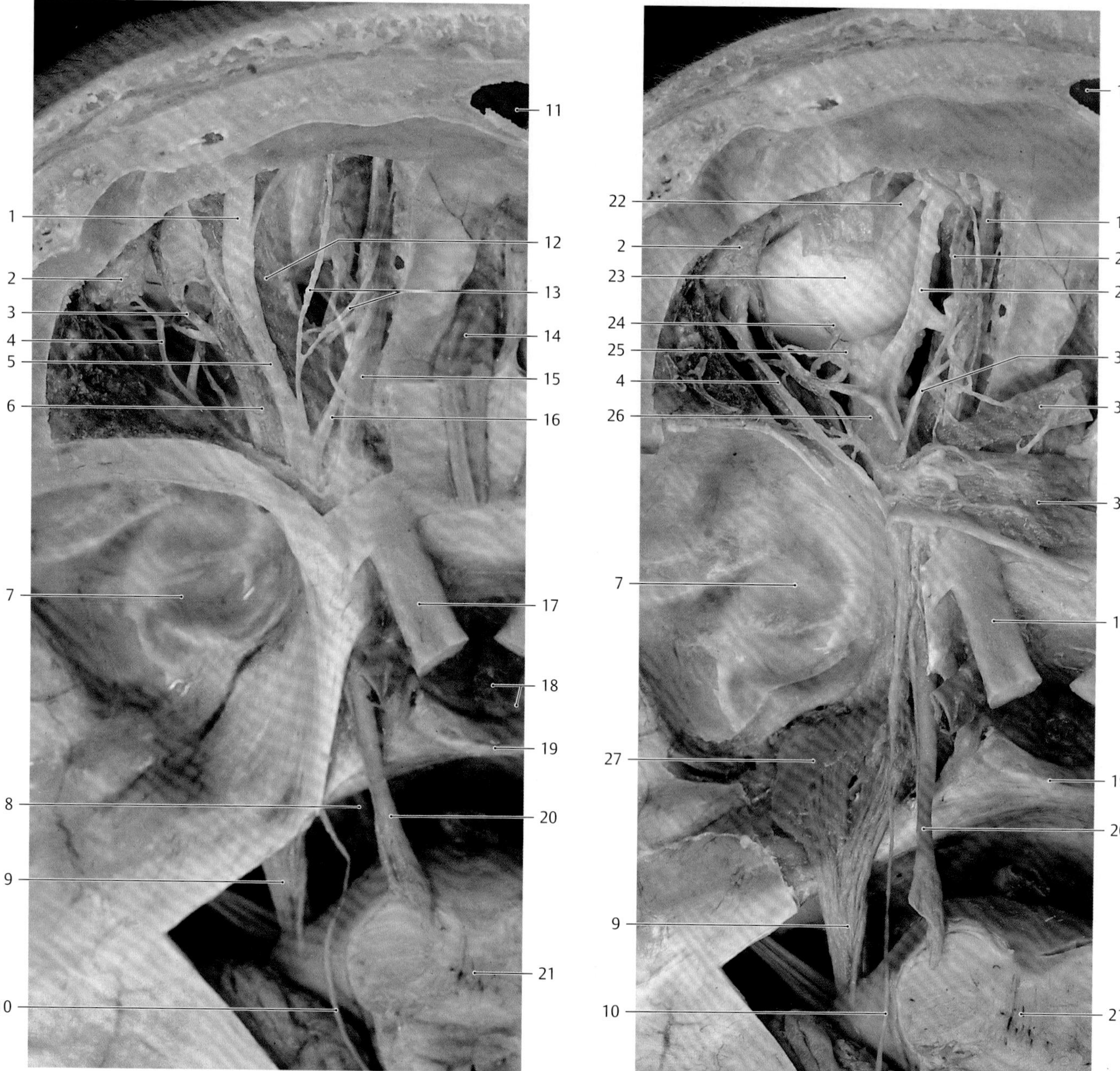


**Fig. 9.32 Superficial layer of the left orbit** (superior aspect). The roof of the orbit and a portion of the left tentorium have been removed.

**Fig. 9.33 Middle layer of the left orbit** (superior aspect). The roof of the orbit has been removed and the superior extra-ocular muscles have been divided and reflected.

1 Lateral branch of frontal nerve
2 Lacrimal gland
3 Lacrimal vein
4 Lacrimal nerve
5 Frontal nerve
6 Superior rectus
7 Middle cranial fossa
8 Abducent nerve (CN VI)
9 Trigeminal nerve (CN V)
10 Trochlear nerve (CN IV) (intracranial part)
11 Frontal sinus
12 Levator palpebrae superioris muscle
13 Branches of supratrochlear nerve
14 Olfactory bulb
15 Superior oblique muscle
16 Trochlear nerve (CN IV) (intra-orbital part)
17 Optic nerve (CN II) (intracranial part)
18 Pituitary gland and infundibulum
19 Dorsum sellae
20 Oculomotor nerve (CN III)
21 Midbrain
22 Tendon of superior oblique muscle
23 Eyeball
24 Vena vorticosa
25 Short ciliary nerves
26 Optic nerve (CN II) (extracranial part)
27 Trigeminal ganglion
28 Ophthalmic artery
29 Superior ophthalmic vein

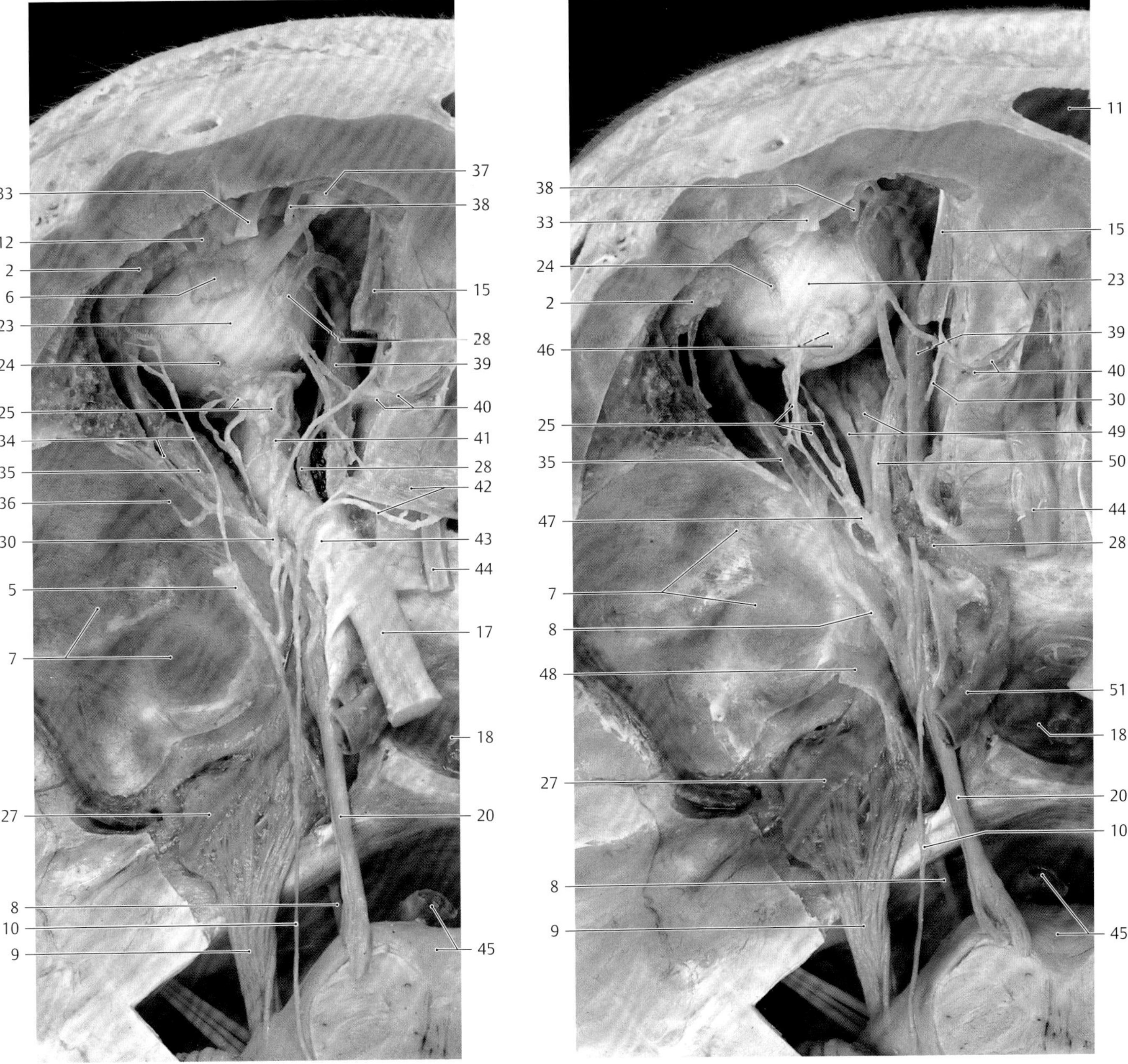


**Fig. 9.34 Middle layer of the left orbit** (superior aspect). The roof of the orbit and the superior extra-ocular muscles have been removed.

**Fig. 9.35 Deeper layer of the left orbit** (superior aspect). The optic nerve has been removed.

30 Nasociliary nerve (CN $V_1$)
31 Levator palpebrae superioris muscle (reflected)
32 Superior rectus muscle (reflected)
33 Lateral branch of supra-orbital nerve
34 Lacrimal nerve and artery
35 Lateral rectus muscle
36 Meningolacrimal artery (anastomosing with middle meningeal artery)
37 Trochlea
38 Medial branch of supra-orbital nerve
39 Medial rectus muscle
40 Anterior ethmoidal artery and nerve
41 Long ciliary nerve
42 Superior oblique muscle and trochlear nerve
43 Common tendinous ring
44 Olfactory tract
45 Basilar artery and pons
46 Optic nerve (external sheath of optic nerve, divided)
47 Ciliary ganglion
48 Ophthalmic nerve (divided, reflected)
49 Inferior branch of oculomotor nerve and inferior rectus muscle
50 Superior branch of oculomotor nerve
51 Internal carotid artery

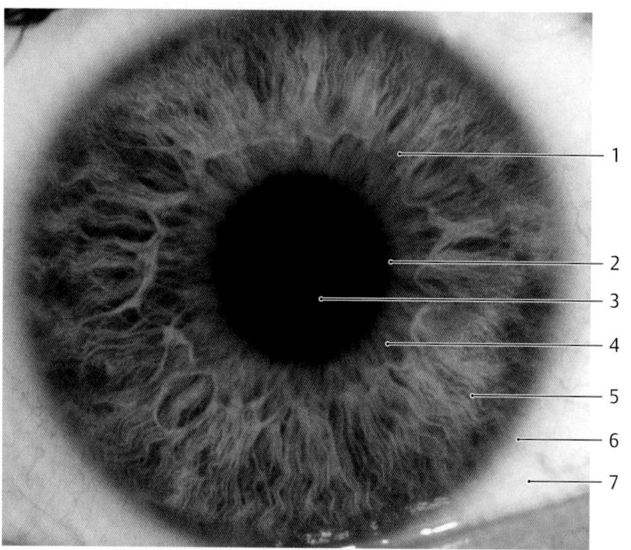


Fig. 9.36 **Anterior segment of the human eye.** Note the colored iris and the location of the lens behind the iris.

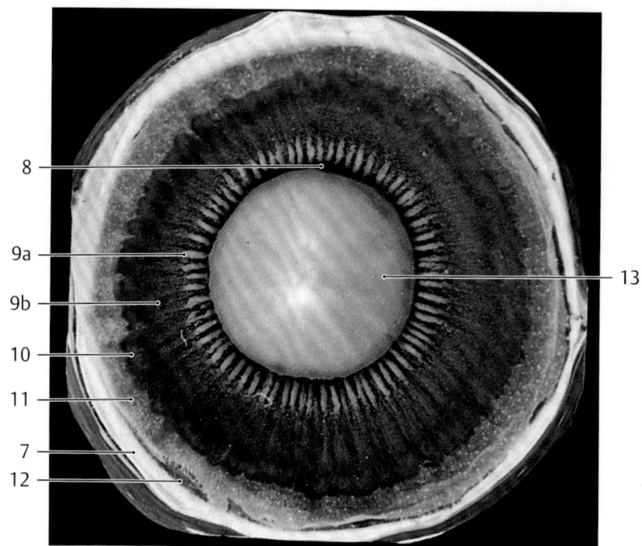


Fig. 9.37 **Anterior segment of the eyeball** (posterior aspect).

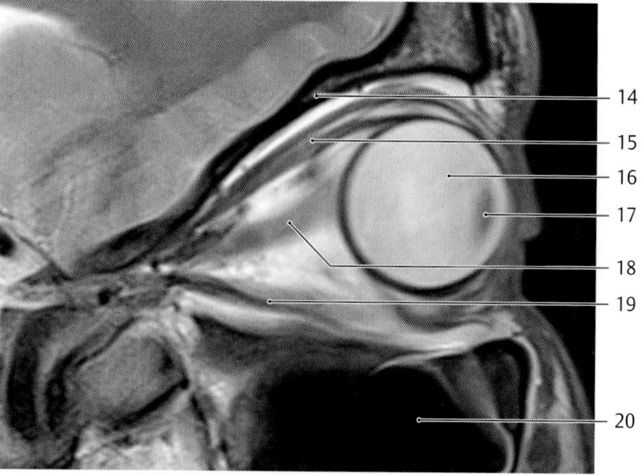


Fig. 9.38 **Sagittal section through the orbit and eyeball** (MRI scan). (Courtesy of Prof. Uder, Institute of Radiology, University Hospital Erlangen, Germany.)

1 Fold of iris
2 Pupillary margin of iris
3 Anterior surface of the lens
4 Inner border of iris
5 Outer border of iris
6 Corneal limbus
7 Sclera
8 Zonular fibers
9 Ciliary body
(a) Ciliary processes (pars plicata)
(b) Ciliary ring (pars plana)
10 Ora serrata
11 Retina
12 Choroid
13 Posterior surface of the lens
14 Orbital bone
15 Superior rectus muscle
16 Vitreous body
17 Lens
18 Optic nerve (CN II)
19 Inferior rectus muscle
20 Maxillary sinus
21 Supratrochlear artery
22 Supra-orbital artery
23 Anterior ciliary artery
24 Dorsal nasal artery
25 Iridial arteries
26 Posterior and anterior ethmoidal arteries
27 Long and short posterior ciliary arteries
28 Optic nerve (CN II) and ophthalmic artery
29 Central retinal artery
30 Fovea centralis and macula lutea
31 Retinal arteries

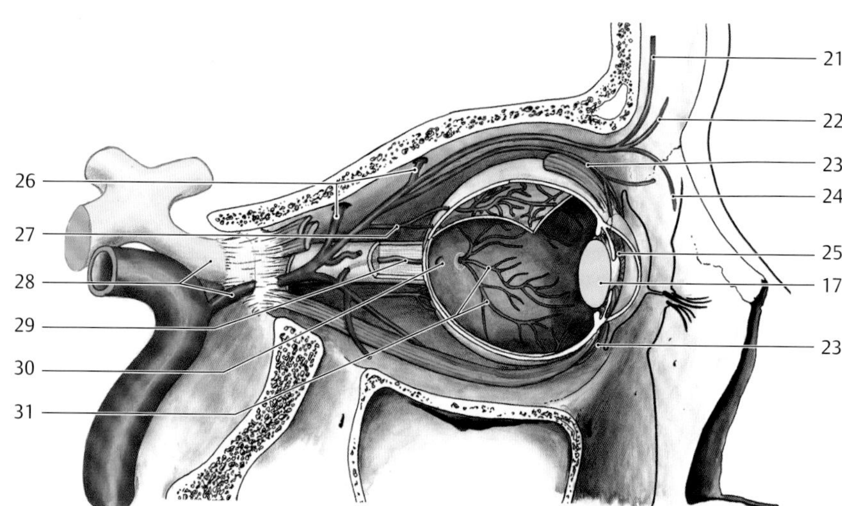


Fig. 9.39 **Orbit with eyeball, optic nerve, and vessels of the eye.** The ophthalmic artery and its branches are shown.

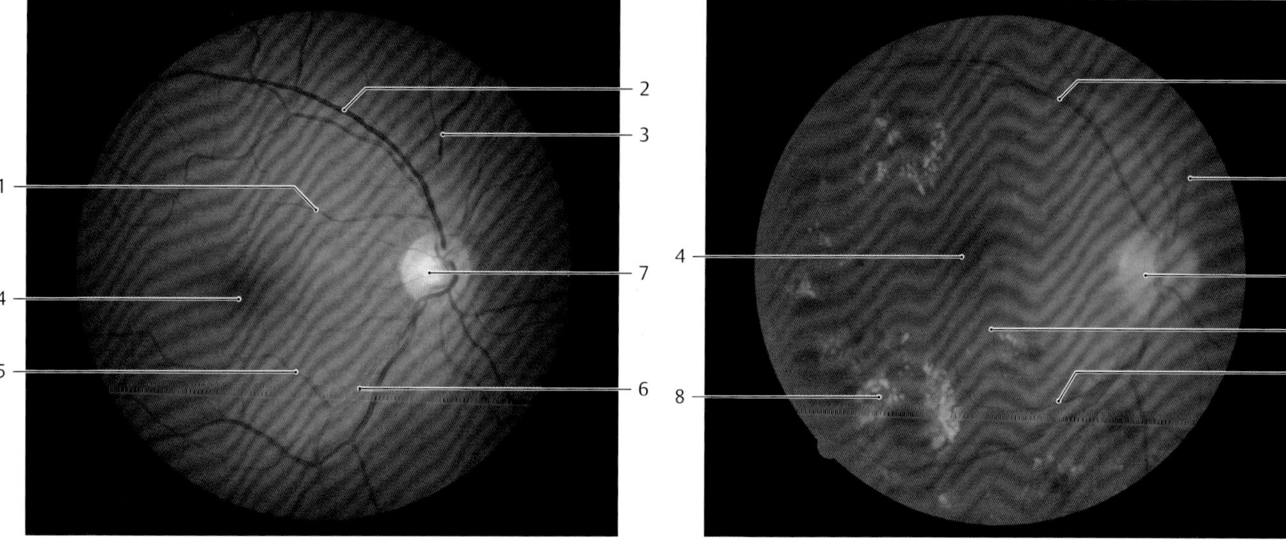


**Fig. 9.40 Fundus of a normal right eye.** Notice, the arteries are smaller and lighter than the veins. (Courtesy of Prof. Mardin, Department of Ophthalmology, University of Erlangen, Germany.)

**Fig. 9.41 Fundus of an eye with diabetic retinopathy.** The retinal veins are compressed and signs of retinal degeneration, seen here as white patches (cotton wool spots), are visible. (Courtesy of Prof. Mardin, Department of Ophthalmology, University of Erlangen, Germany.)

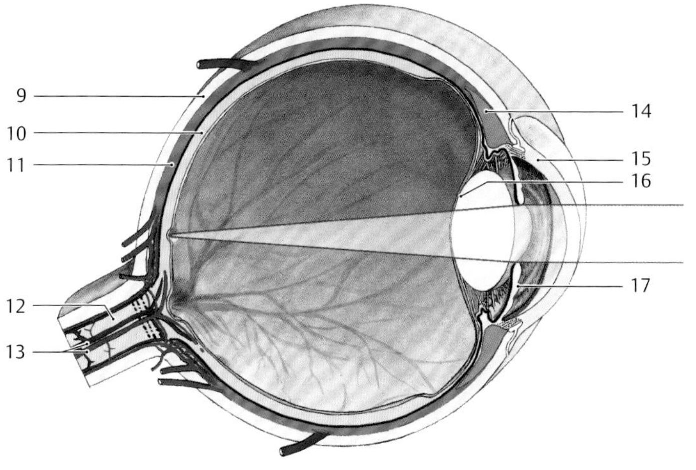


**Fig. 9.42 Organization of the eyeball** (sagittal section). Red lines = projection of the light on the fovea centralis.

1 Superior macular artery
2 Superior temporal artery and vein of retina
3 Medial artery and vein of retina
4 Fovea centralis and macula lutea
5 Inferior macular artery
6 Inferior temporal artery and vein of retina
7 Optic disc
8 Cotton-wool spots
9 Sclera
10 Retina
11 Choroid
12 Optic nerve (CN II)
13 Central retinal artery and vein
14 Ciliary muscle
15 Cornea
16 Posterior surface of lens
17 Iris
18 Internal limiting membrane
19 Branches of the central retinal artery
20 Nerve fiber layer
21 Ganglion cell layer
22 Inner plexiform layer
23 Inner nuclear layer
24 Outer plexiform layer
25 Outer nuclear layer
26 External limiting membrane
27 Outer and inner segments of photoreceptors
28 Retinal pigment epithelium
29 Macular edema

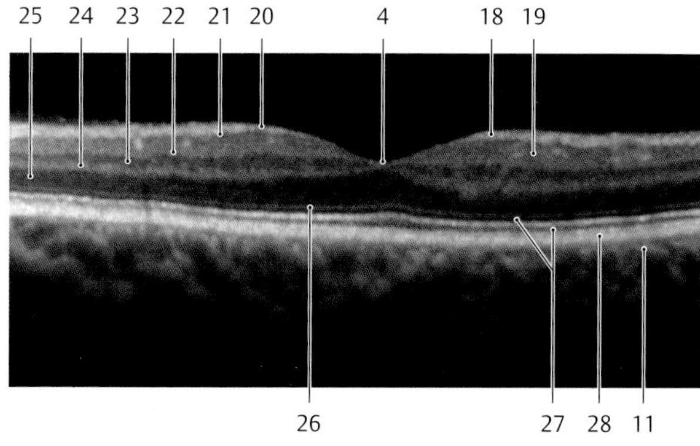


**Fig. 9.43 Section through the fovea centralis and the central retina of a normal eye** (OCT scan). (Courtesy of Prof. Mardin, Department of Ophthalmology, University of Erlangen, Germany.)

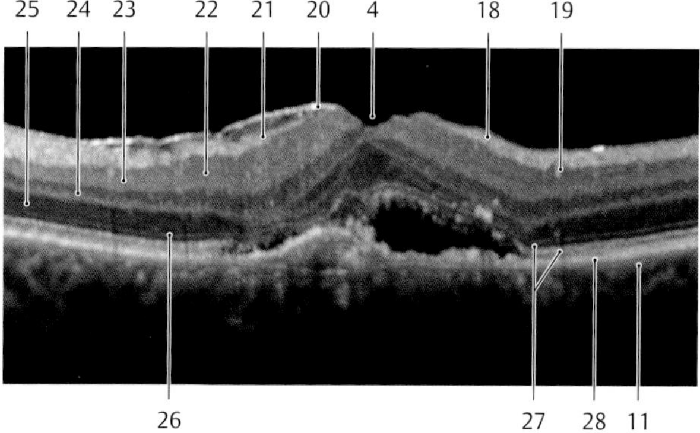


**Fig. 9.44 Section through the fovea centralis of an eye with macular degeneration.** Macular edema has formed between the retinal pigment epithelium and the adjacent photoreceptor cells (OCT scan). (Courtesy of Prof. Mardin, Department of Ophthalmology, University of Erlangen, Germany.)

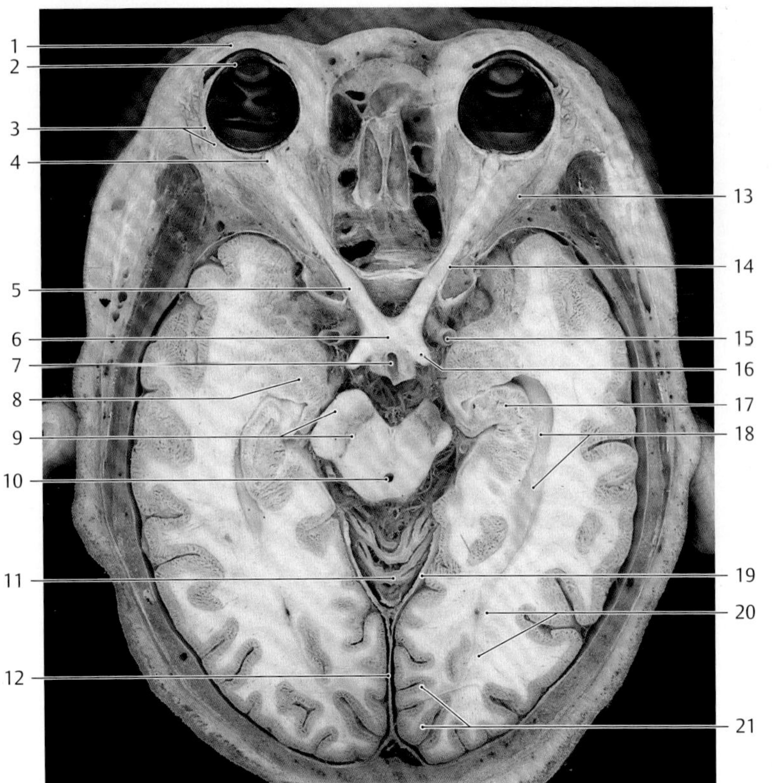


**Fig. 9.45 Horizontal section through the head** at the level of optic chiasma and striate cortex (superior aspect). Note the relationship of the hypothalamic infundibulum to the optic chiasma.

1 Upper lid
2 Cornea
3 Eyeball (sclera, retina)
4 Head of optic nerve
5 Optic nerve
6 Optic chiasma
7 Infundibular recess of hypothalamus
8 Amygdaloid body
9 Substantia nigra and crus cerebri
10 Cerebral aqueduct
11 Vermis of cerebellum
12 Falx cerebri
13 Lateral rectus muscle
14 Optic canal
15 Internal carotid artery
16 Optic tract
17 Hippocampus
18 Inferior horn of lateral ventricle
19 Cerebellar tentorium
20 Optic radiation of Gratiolet
21 Visual cortex (area calcarina, striate cortex)
22 Lens
23 Eyeball
24 Medial rectus muscle
25 Cerebral peduncle
26 Ethmoidal cells
27 Optic nerve (CN II) with dura sheath
28 Temporal muscle
29 Oculomotor nerve (CN III) and pituitary gland (hypophysis)
30 Midbrain
31 Occipital lobe
32 Long and short ciliary nerves
33 Ciliary ganglion
34 Oculomotor nerve (CN III) within the cavernous sinus
35 Accessory oculomotor nuclei
36 Colliculi of midbrain
37 Corpus callosum
38 Visual field
39 Retina
40 Lateral geniculate body

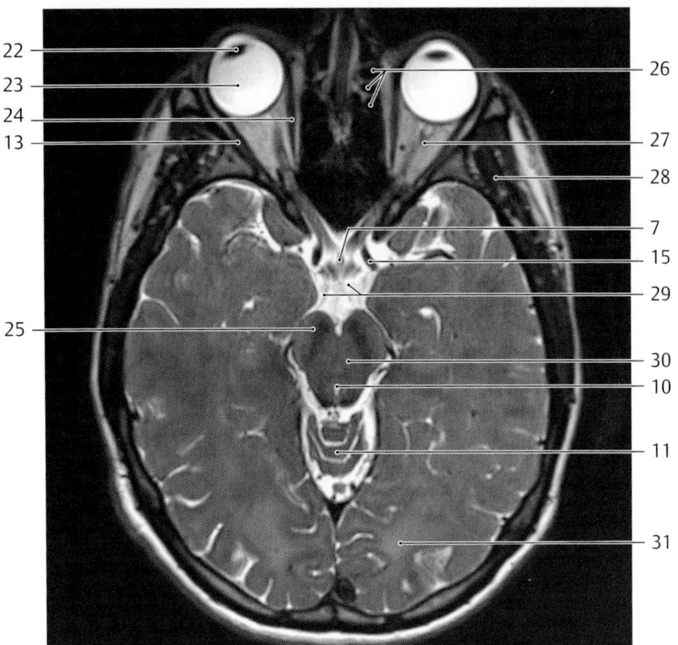


**Fig. 9.46 Horizontal section through the head** at the level of the sella turcica (MRI scan). (Courtesy of Prof. Uder, Institute of Radiology, University Hospital Erlangen, Germany.)

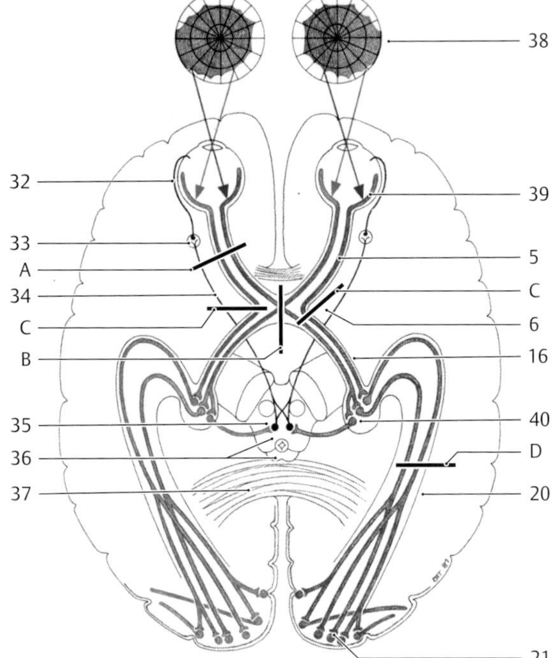


**Fig. 9.47 Diagram of the visual pathway and path of the light reflex.**

In **binocular vision** the visual field (38) is projected upon portions of both retinae (blue and red in the drawing). In the chiasma the fibers from the two retinal portions are combined to form the left optic tract. The fibers of the two eyes remain separated from each other throughout the entire visual pathway up to their final termination in the visual cortex (21). **Injuries on the optic pathway** produce visual defects whose nature depends on the location of the injury. Destruction of one optic nerve (A) produces **blindness in the corresponding eye** with loss of pupillary light reflex. If **lesions of the chiasma** destroy the crossing fibers of the nasal portions of the retina (B), both temporal fields of vision are lost **(bitemporal hemianopsia)**. If both lateral angles of the chiasma are compressed (C), the nondecussating fibers from the temporal retinae are affected, resulting in loss of nasal visual fields **(binasal hemianopsia)**. Lesions posterior to the chiasma (D) (i.e., optic tract, lateral geniculate body, optic radiation, or visual cortex) result in a loss of the entire opposite field of vision **(homonymous hemianopsia)**.

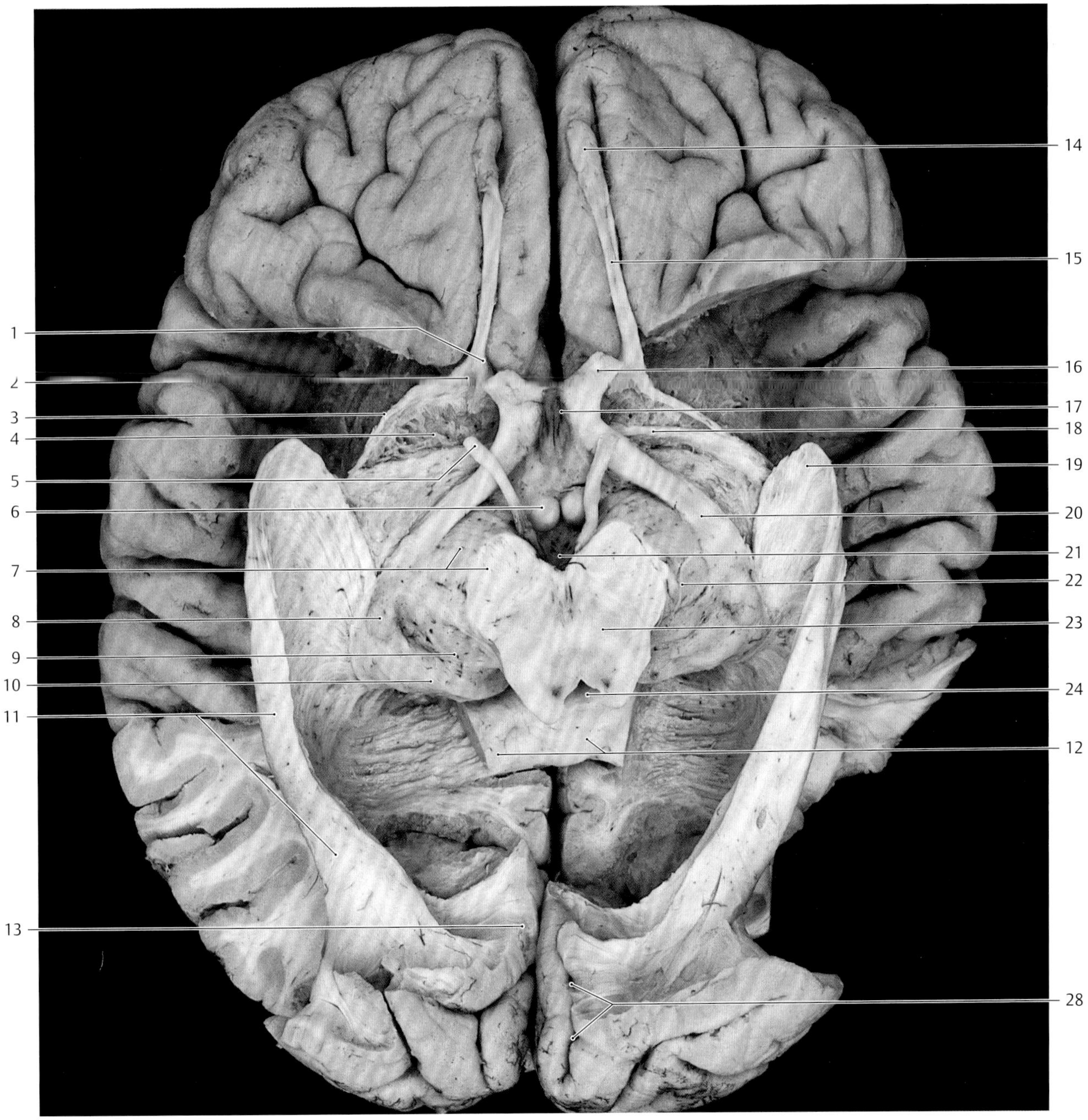

Fig. 9.48 **Dissection of the visual pathway** (inferior aspect). The midbrain has been divided. Frontal pole at the top.

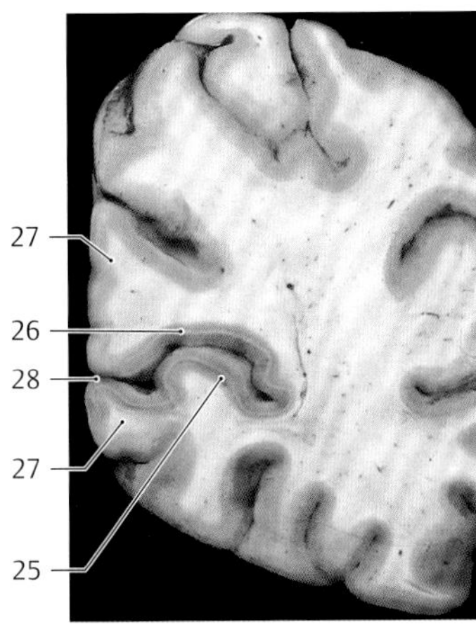


Fig. 9.49 **Frontal section of the striate cortex** at the level of the striate area in the occipital lobe.

1 Medial olfactory stria
2 Olfactory trigone
3 Lateral olfactory stria
4 Anterior perforated substance
5 Oculomotor nerve (CN III)
6 Mamillary body
7 Cerebral peduncle
8 Lateral geniculate body
9 Medial geniculate body
10 Pulvinar of thalamus
11 Optic radiation
12 Splenium of the corpus callosum (commissural fibers)
13 Cuneus
14 Olfactory bulb
15 Olfactory tract
16 Optic nerve (CN II)
17 Infundibulum
18 Anterior commissure
19 Genu of optic radiation
20 Optic tract
21 Interpeduncular fossa and posterior perforated substance
22 Trochlear nerve (CN IV)
23 Substantia nigra
24 Cerebral aqueduct
25 Visual cortex
26 Line of Gennari
27 Gyrus of striate cortex
28 Calcarine sulcus

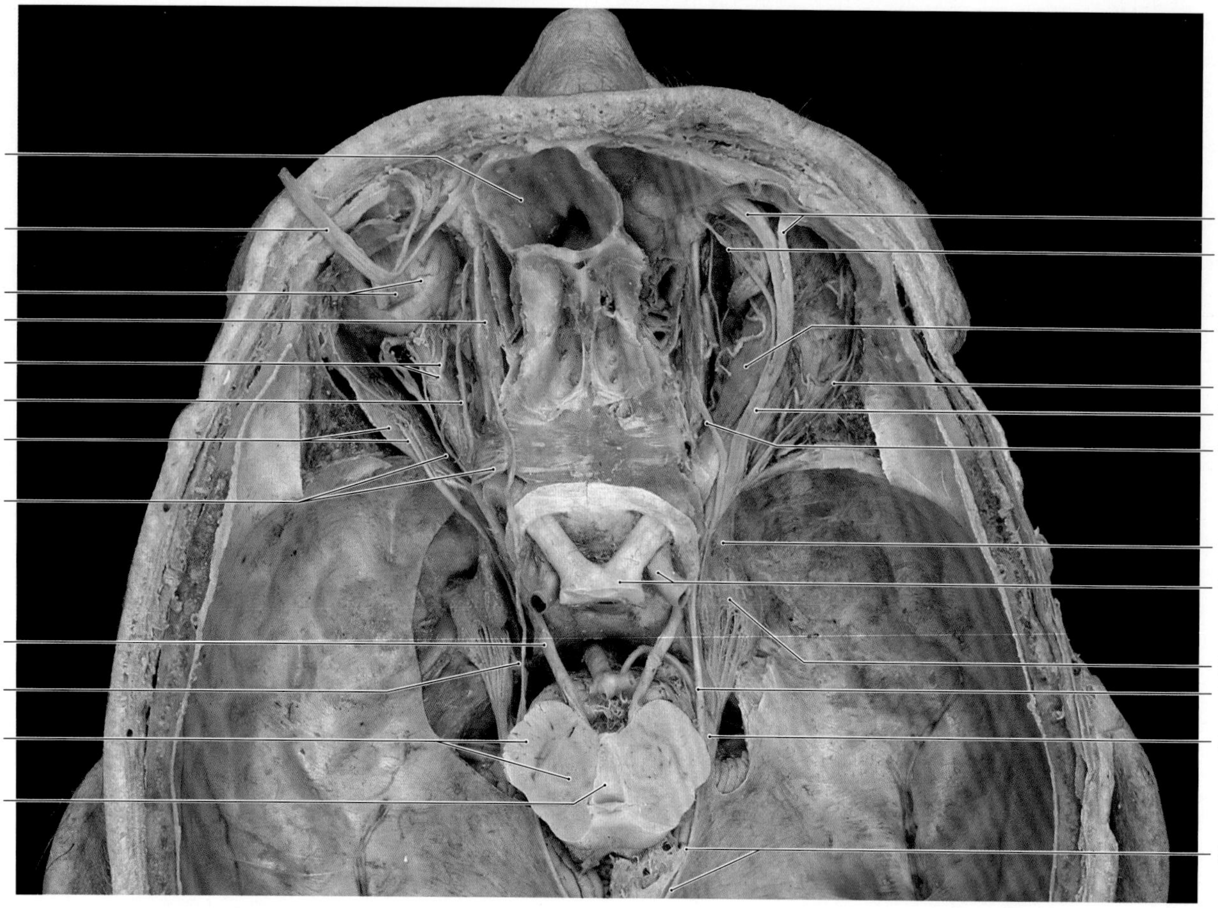

**Fig. 9.50 Cranial nerves of the orbit** (superficial layer [right side] and middle layer of the orbit [left side], superior aspect). The superior rectus muscle and frontal nerve have been divided and reflected and the tentorium and dura mater partly removed.

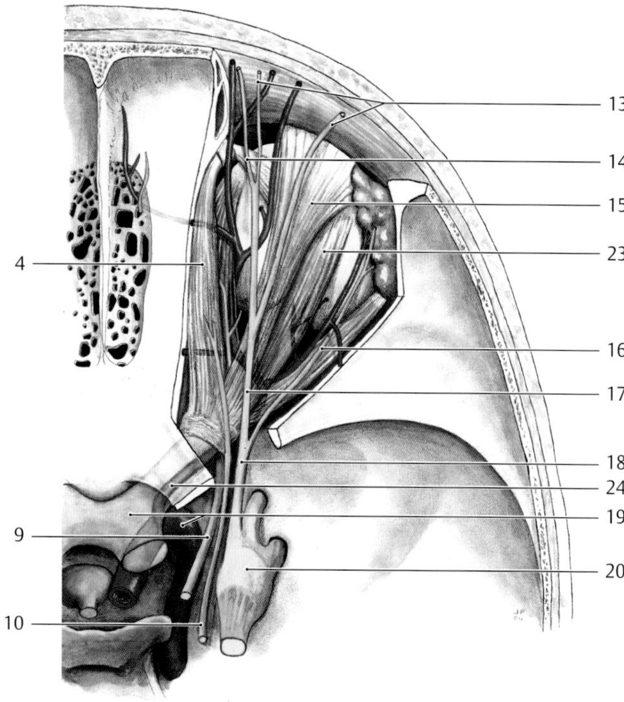


**Fig. 9.51 Cranial nerves within the orbit (superior aspect).**

1 Frontal sinus (enlarged)
2 Frontal nerve (divided and reflected)
3 Superior rectus muscle (divided) and eyeball
4 Superior oblique muscle
5 Short ciliary nerves and optic nerve (CN II)
6 Nasociliary nerve
7 Abducent nerve (CN VI) and lateral rectus muscle
8 Ciliary ganglion and superior rectus muscle (reflected)
9 Oculomotor nerve (CN III)
10 Trochlear nerve (CN IV)
11 Crus cerebri and midbrain
12 Inferior wall of the third ventricle connected with cerebral aqueduct
13 Lateral and medial branches of supra-orbital nerve
14 Supratrochlear nerve
15 Superior levator palpebrae muscle
16 Lacrimal nerve
17 Frontal nerve
18 Ophthalmic nerve (CN $V_1$)
19 Optic chiasma and internal carotid artery
20 Trigeminal ganglion
21 Trigeminal nerve (CN V)
22 Tentorial notch
23 Superior rectus muscle
24 Ophthalmic artery

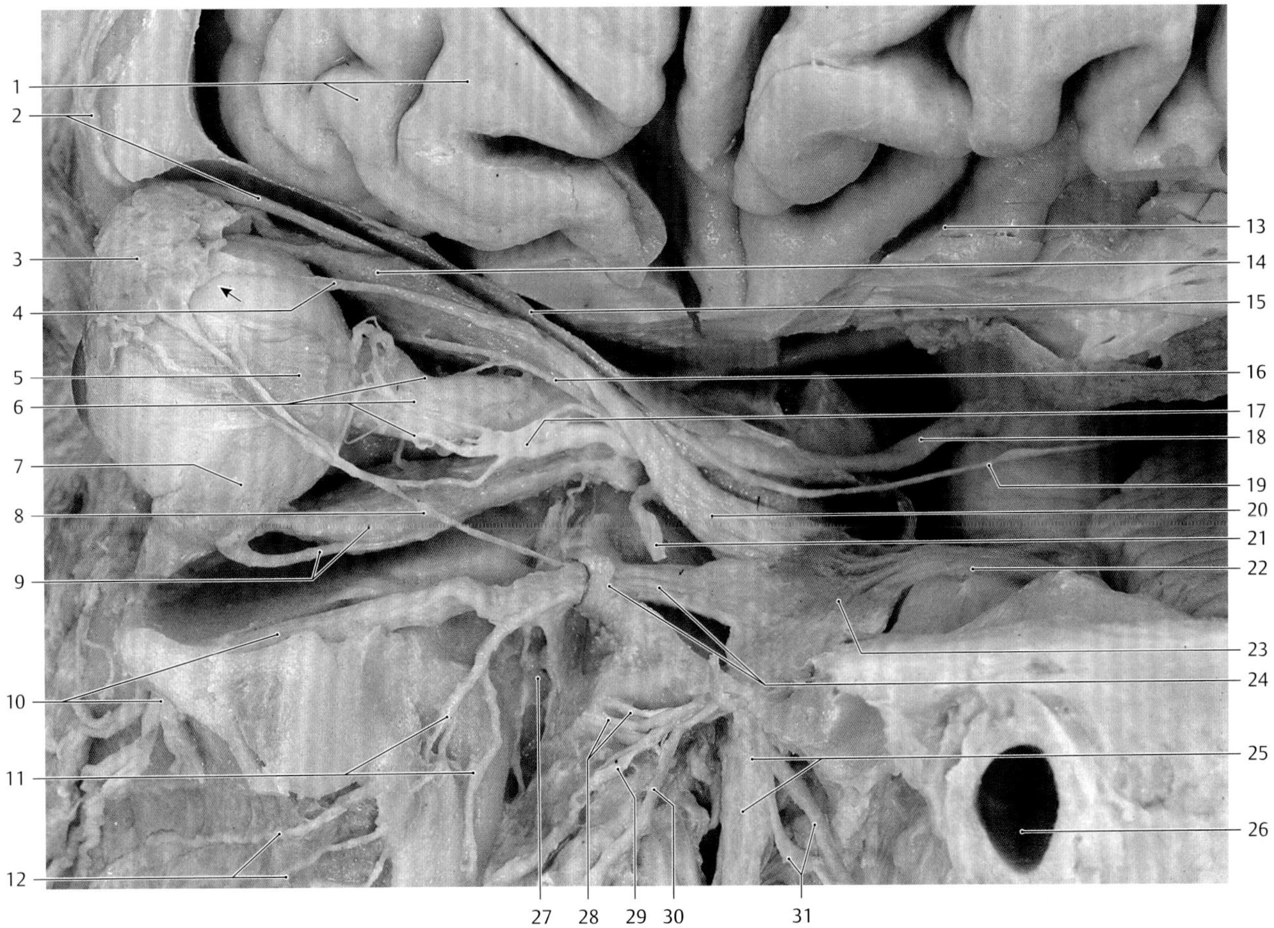

Fig. 9.52 **Cranial nerves of the orbit and pterygopalatine fossa** (left orbit, lateral aspect). **Dissection of optic (CN II), oculomotor (CN III), trochlear (CN IV), ophthalmic (CN $V_1$), and abducent (CN VI) nerves.** Arrow = zygomaticolacrimal anastomosis.

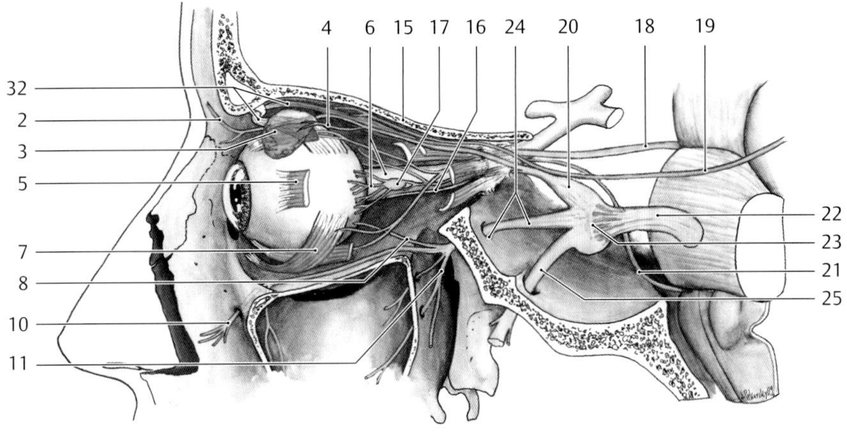


Fig. 9.53 **Cranial nerves innervating extra-ocular muscles** (lateral aspect).

1 Frontal lobe
2 Supra-orbital nerve
3 Lacrimal gland
4 Lacrimal nerve
5 Lateral rectus muscle (divided)
6 Optic nerve (CN II) and short ciliary nerves
7 Inferior oblique muscle
8 Zygomatic nerve
9 Inferior branch of oculomotor nerve (CN III) and inferior rectus muscle
10 Infra-orbital nerve
11 Posterior superior alveolar nerves
12 Branches of superior alveolar plexus adjacent to mucous membrane of maxillary sinus
13 Central sulcus of insula
14 Superior rectus muscle
15 Periorbita (roof of orbit)
16 Nasociliary nerve
17 Ciliary ganglion
18 Oculomotor nerve (CN III)
19 Trochlear nerve (CN IV)
20 Ophthalmic nerve (CN $V_1$)
21 Abducent nerve (CN VI) (divided)
22 Trigeminal nerve (CN V)
23 Trigeminal ganglion
24 Maxillary nerve (CN $V_2$) and foramen rotundum
25 Mandibular nerve (CN $V_3$)
26 External acoustic meatus
27 Pterygopalatine nerves
28 Deep temporal nerves
29 Buccal nerve
30 Masseteric nerve
31 Auriculotemporal nerve
32 Trochlea and superior oblique muscle

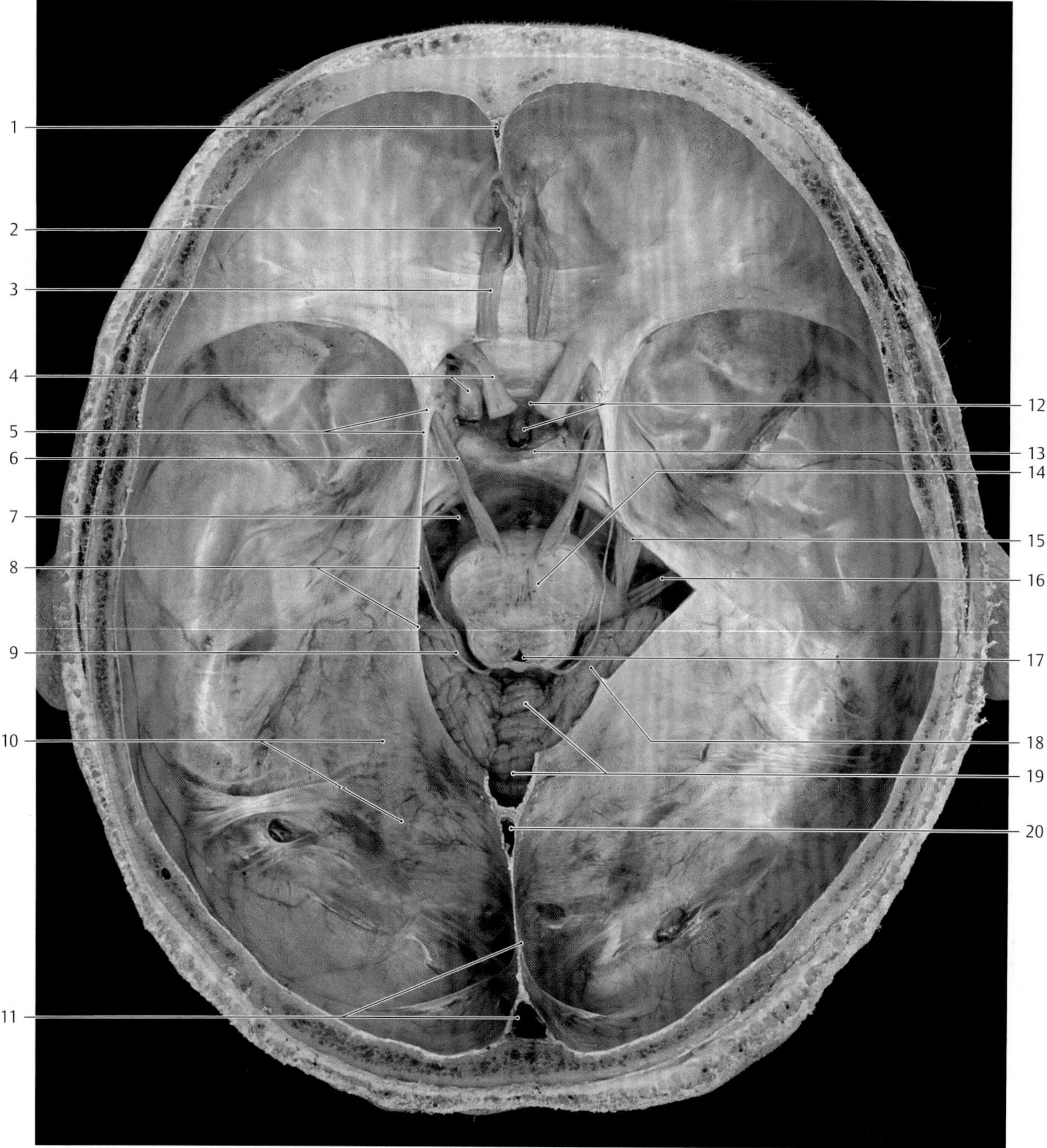


**Fig. 9.54 Base of the skull with cranial nerves** (internal aspect). Both cerebral hemispheres and upper part of the brainstem have been removed. Incision on the right cerebellar tentorium to display the cranial nerves of the infratentorial space.

1 Superior sagittal sinus with falx cerebri
2 Olfactory bulb
3 Olfactory tract
4 Optic nerve and internal carotid artery
5 Anterior clinoid process and anterior attachment of cerebellar tentorium
6 Oculomotor nerve (CN III)
7 Abducent nerve (CN VI)
8 Tentorial notch (incisura tentorii)
9 Trochlear nerve (CN IV)
10 Cerebellar tentorium
11 Falx cerebri and confluence of sinuses
12 Hypophysial fossa, infundibulum, and diaphragma sellae
13 Dorsum sellae
14 Midbrain (divided)
15 Trigeminal nerve (CN V)
16 Facial nerve (CN VII), nervus intermedius, and vestibulocochlear nerve (CN VIII)
17 Cerebral aqueduct
18 Right hemisphere of cerebellum
19 Vermis of cerebellum
20 Straight sinus

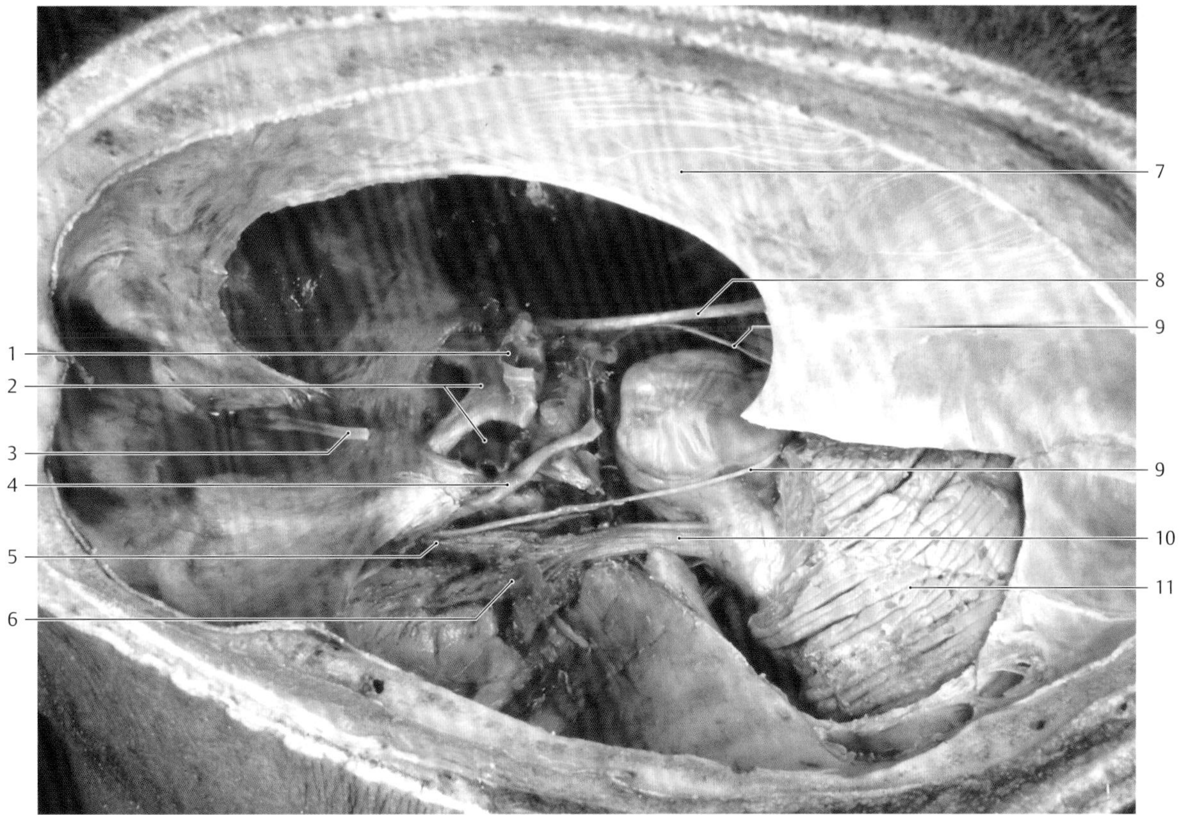


Fig. 9.55 **Base of the skull with cranial nerves.** The brainstem was divided and the tentorium fenestrated. Both hemispheres have been removed.

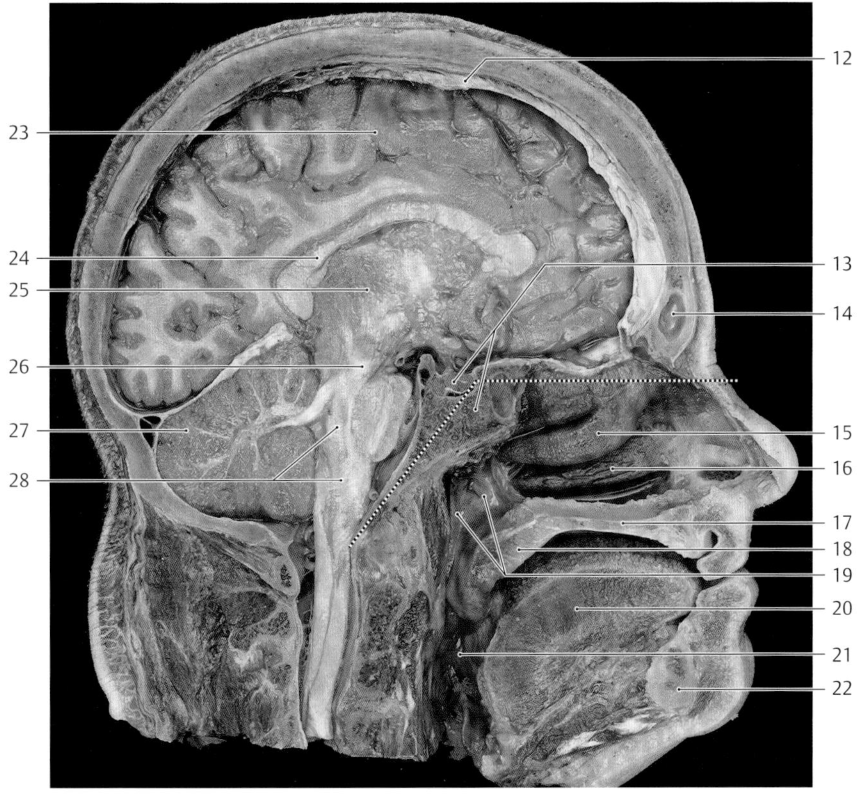


Fig. 9.56 **Median sagittal section through the head.** The palate separates the nasal and oral cavities. The base of the skull forms an angle of about 150° at the sella turcica (dotted line).

1 Infundibulum
2 Optic chiasma and internal carotid artery
3 Olfactory tract
4 Oculomotor nerve (CN III)
5 Ophthalmic nerve (CN $V_1$)
6 Trigeminal ganglion
7 Falx cerebri
8 Tentorial notch
9 Trochlear nerve (CN IV)
10 Trigeminal nerve (CN V)
11 Cerebellum
12 Dura mater
13 Hypophysis within hypophysial fossa
14 Frontal sinus
15 Middle nasal concha
16 Inferior nasal concha
17 Hard palate
18 Soft palate
19 Pharynx with auditory tube
20 Tongue
21 Pharynx with palatine tonsil
22 Mandible
23 Cerebrum (telencephalon)
24 Corpus callosum
25 Thalamus
26 Midbrain (mesencephalon) with cranial nerve nuclei III and IV
27 Cerebellum
28 Hindbrain (rhombencephalon)

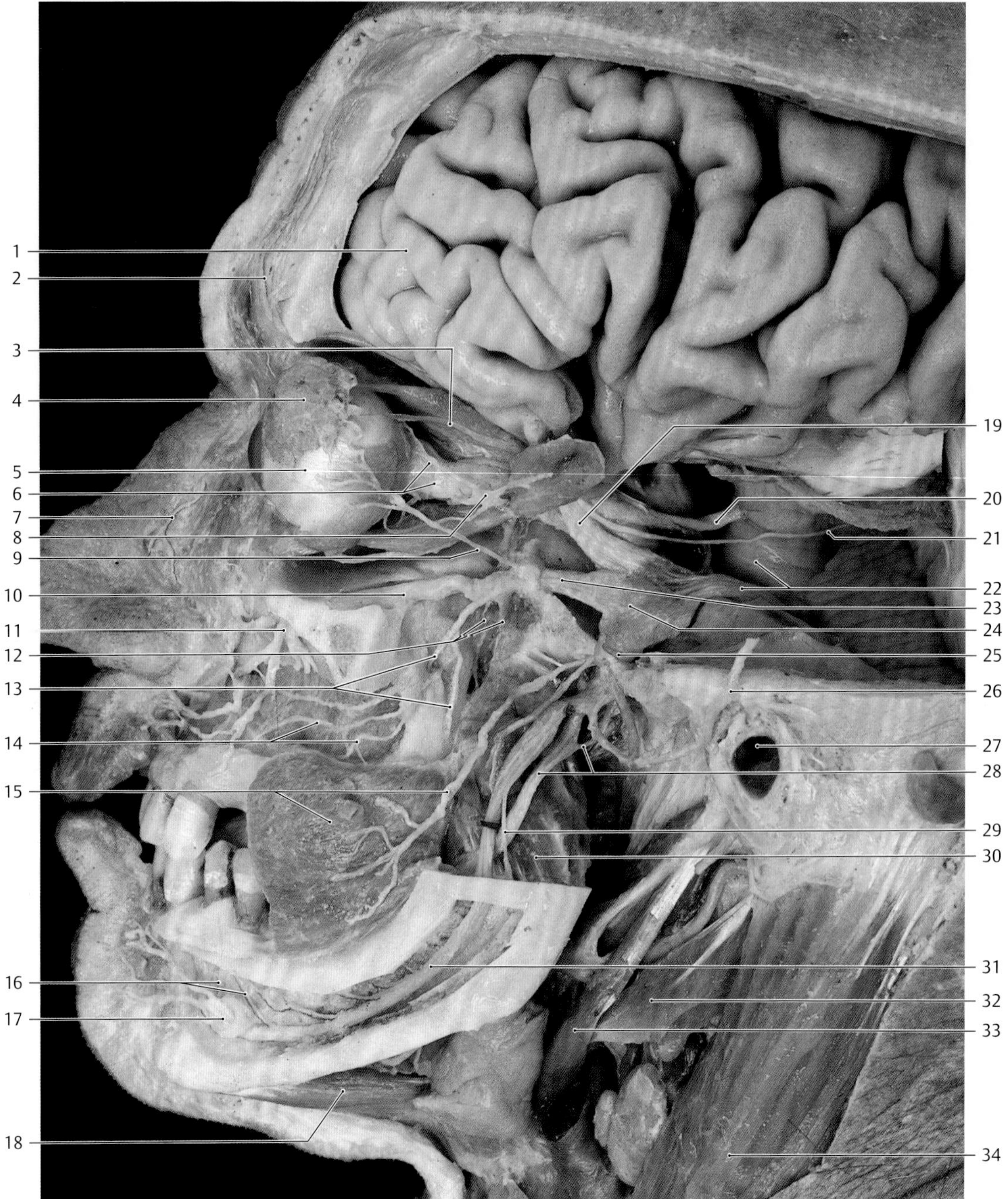


**Fig. 9.57 Dissection of the trigeminal nerve (CN V) in its entirety.** The lateral wall of the cranial cavity, lateral wall of the orbit, zygomatic arch, and ramus of the mandible have been removed and the mandibular canal opened.

1 Frontal lobe of cerebrum
2 Supra-orbital nerve
3 Lacrimal nerve
4 Lacrimal gland
5 Eyeball
6 Optic nerve and short ciliary nerves
7 External nasal branch of anterior ethmoidal nerve
8 Ciliary ganglion
9 Zygomatic nerve
10 Infra-orbital nerve
11 Infra-orbital foramen and terminal branches of infra-orbital nerve
12 Pterygopalatine ganglion and pterygopalatine nerves
13 Posterior superior alveolar nerves
14 Superior dental plexus
15 Buccinator muscle and buccal nerve
16 Inferior dental plexus
17 Mental foramen and mental nerve
18 Anterior belly of digastric muscle
19 Ophthalmic nerve (CN $V_1$)
20 Oculomotor nerve (CN III)
21 Trochlear nerve (CN IV)
22 Trigeminal nerve (CN V) and pons
23 Maxillary nerve (CN $V_2$)
24 Trigeminal ganglion
25 Mandibular nerve (CN $V_3$)
26 Auriculotemporal nerve
27 External acoustic meatus (divided)
28 Lingual nerve and chorda tympani
29 Mylohyoid nerve
30 Medial pterygoid muscle
31 Inferior alveolar nerve
32 Posterior belly of digastric muscle
33 Stylohyoid muscle
34 Sternocleidomastoid muscle

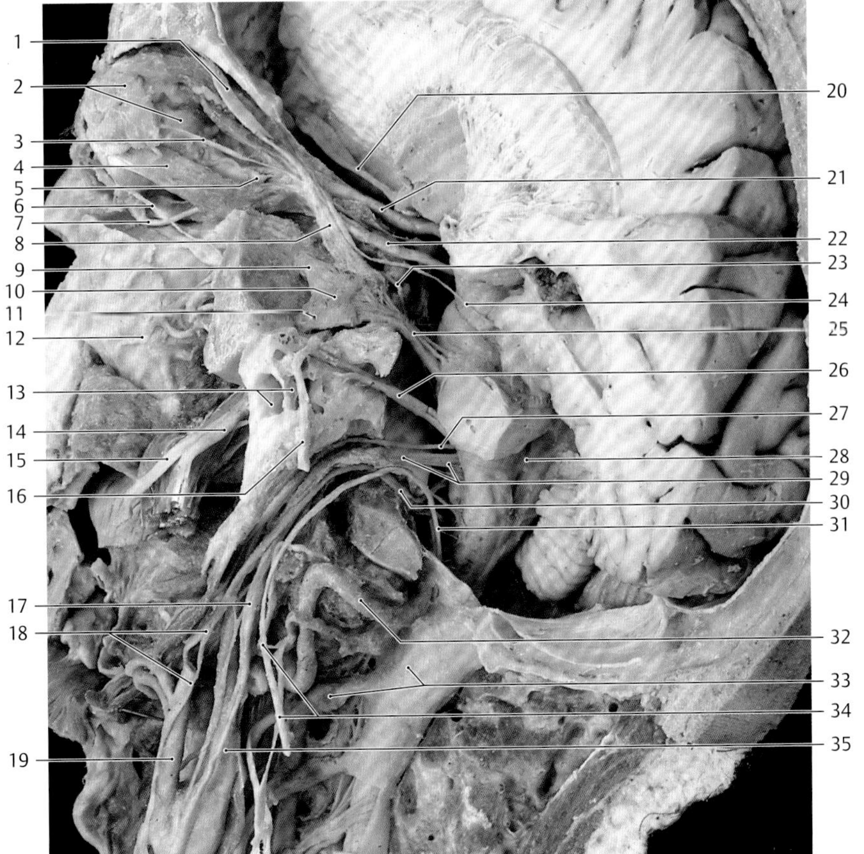


**Fig. 9.58 Cranial nerves in connection with the brainstem** (lateral superior aspect, left side). The left half of the brain and the head have been partly removed. Notice the location of the trigeminal ganglion.

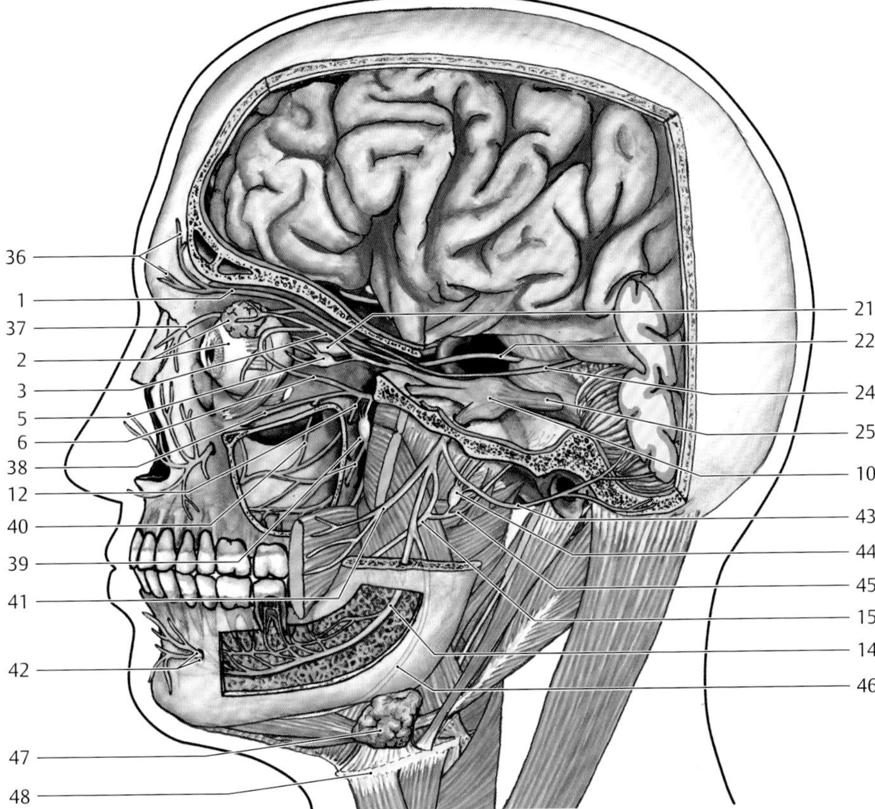


**Fig. 9.59 Main branches of trigeminal nerve** (see corresponding Fig. 9.57 on previous page).

1 Frontal nerve
2 Lacrimal gland and eyeball
3 Lacrimal nerve
4 Lateral rectus muscle
5 Ciliary ganglion lateral to optic nerve
6 Zygomatic nerve
7 Inferior branch of oculomotor nerve
8 Ophthalmic nerve (CN $V_1$)
9 Maxillary nerve (CN $V_2$)
10 Trigeminal ganglion
11 Mandibular nerve (CN $V_3$)
12 Posterior superior alveolar nerves
13 Tympanic cavity, external acoustic meatus, and tympanic membrane
14 Inferior alveolar nerve
15 Lingual nerve
16 Facial nerve (CN VII)
17 Vagus nerve (CN X)
18 Hypoglossal nerve (CN XII) and superior root of ansa cervicalis
19 External carotid artery
20 Olfactory tract (CN I)
21 Optic nerve (CN II) (intracranial part)
22 Oculomotor nerve (CN III)
23 Abducent nerve (CN VI)
24 Trochlear nerve (CN IV)
25 Trigeminal nerve (CN V)
26 Vestibulocochlear nerve (CN VIII) and facial nerve (CN VII)
27 Glossopharyngeal nerve (CN IX) (leaving brainstem)
28 Rhomboid fossa
29 Vagus nerve (CN X) (leaving brainstem)
30 Hypoglossal nerve (CN XII) (leaving medulla oblongata)
31 Accessory nerve (CN XI) (ascending from foramen magnum)
32 Vertebral artery
33 Spinal ganglion and dura mater of spinal cord
34 Accessory nerve (CN XI)
35 Internal carotid artery
36 Lateral and medial branch of supra-orbital nerve
37 Infratrochlear nerve
38 Infra-orbital nerve
39 Pterygopalatine ganglion and pterygopalatine nerves
40 Middle superior alveolar nerves (entering superior dental plexus)
41 Buccal nerve
42 Mental nerve and mental foramen
43 Auriculotemporal nerve
44 Otic ganglion
45 Chorda tympani
46 Mylohyoid nerve
47 Submandibular gland
48 Hyoid bone

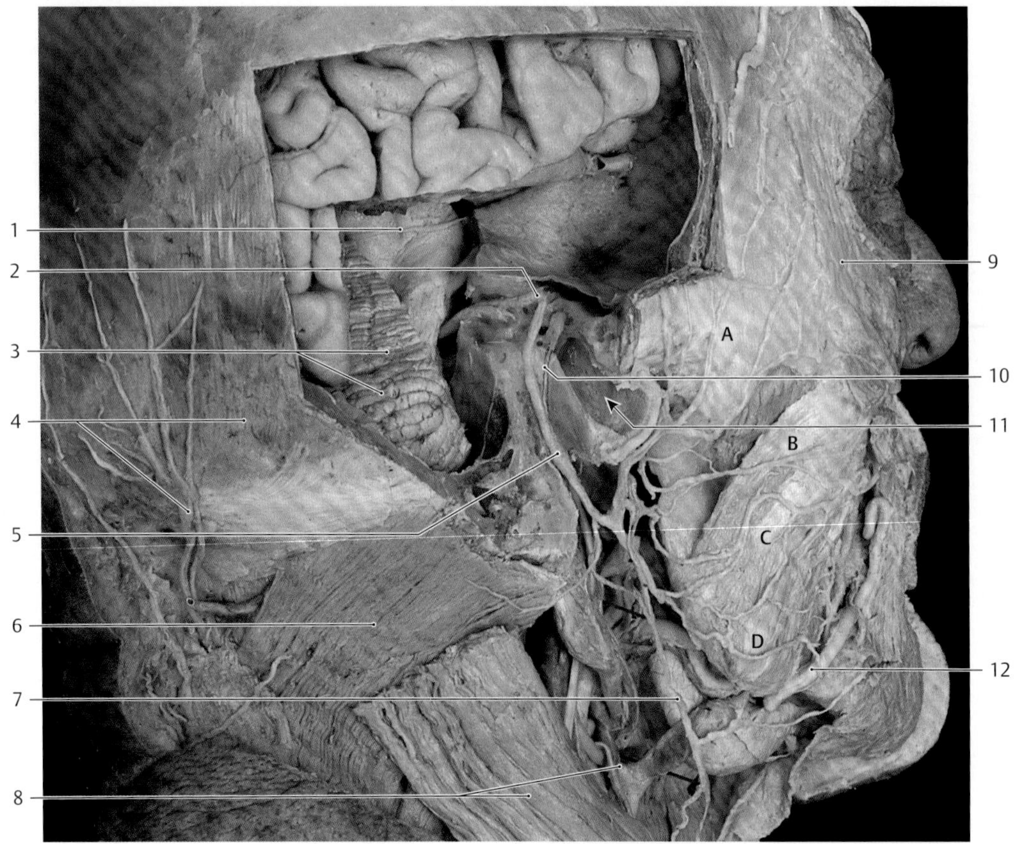


Fig. 9.60 **Dissection of the facial nerve (CN VII) in its entirety.** The cranial cavity has been fenestrated and the temporal lobe partly removed. The facial canal and tympanic cavity have been opened and the posterior wall of the external acoustic meatus removed.

**Branches of the facial nerve**
A = Temporal branch
B = Zygomatic branches
C = Buccal branches
D = Marginal mandibular branch

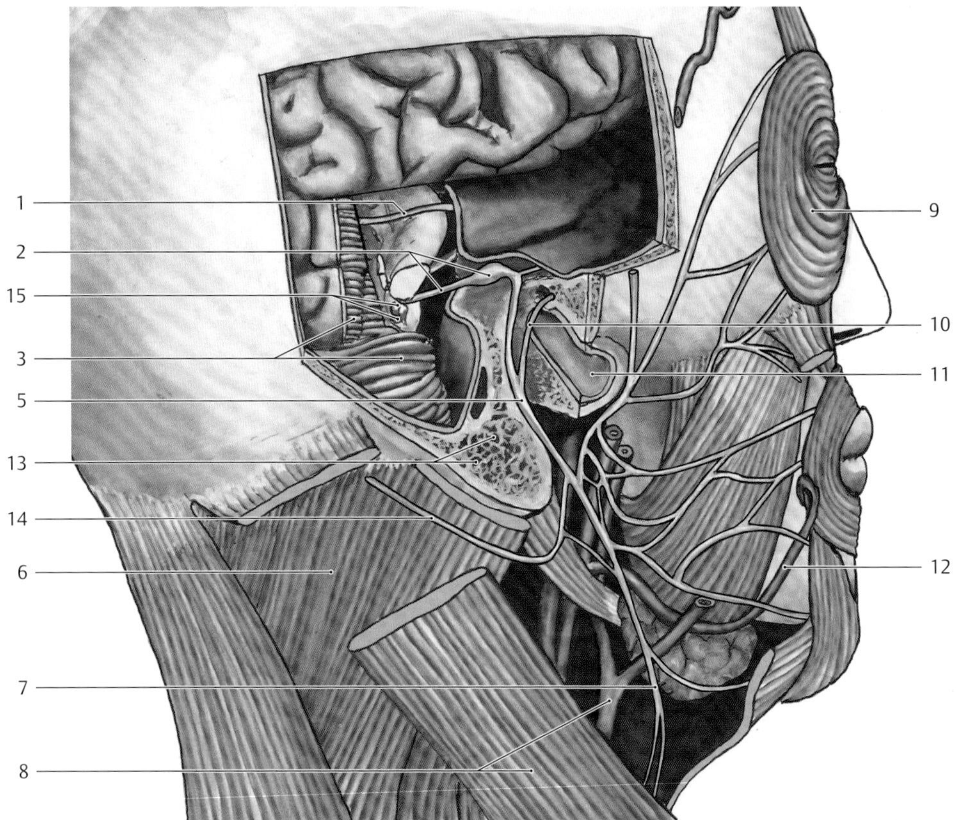


1 Trochlear nerve (CN IV)
2 Facial nerve (CN VII) with geniculate ganglion
3 Cerebellum (right hemisphere)
4 Occipital belly of occipito-frontalis muscle and greater occipital nerve
5 Facial nerve (CN VII) at stylomastoid foramen
6 Splenius capitis muscle
7 Cervical branch of facial nerve (CN VII)
8 Sternocleidomastoid muscle and retro-mandibular vein
9 Orbicularis oculi muscle
10 Chorda tympani
11 External acoustic meatus
12 Facial artery
13 Mastoid air cells
14 Posterior auricular nerve
15 Nucleus and genu of facial nerve

Fig. 9.61 **Facial nerve** (see corresponding Fig. 9.60 above).

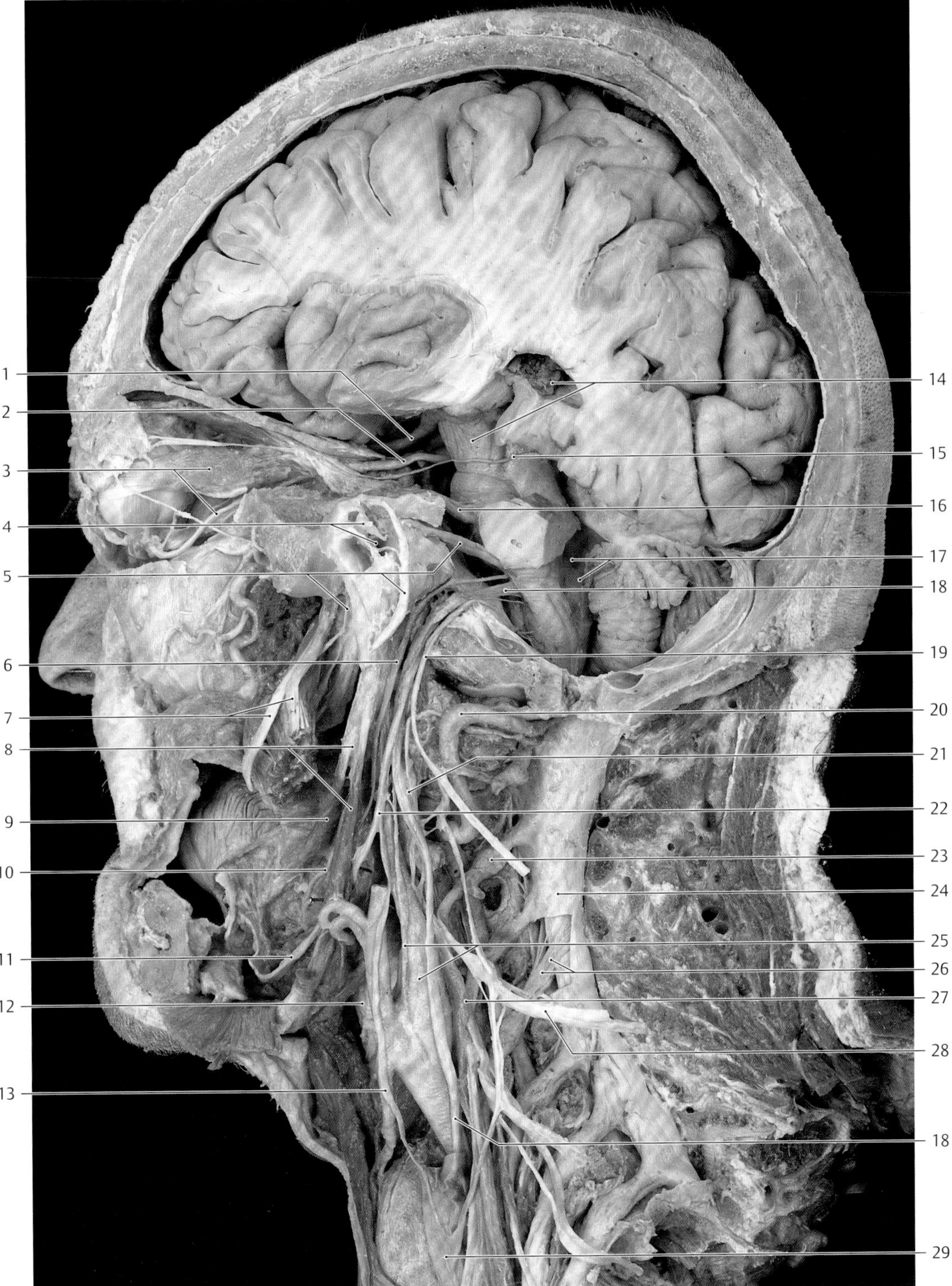


**Fig. 9.62 Cranial nerves in connection with the brainstem** (oblique-lateral aspect). Lateral portion of the skull, brain, neck and facial structures and the lateral wall of the orbit and oral cavity have been removed. The tympanic cavity has been opened. The mandible has been divided and the muscles of mastication have been removed.

1 Optic tract
2 Oculomotor nerve (CN III)
3 Lateral rectus muscle and inferior branch of oculomotor nerve
4 Malleus and chorda tympani
5 Chorda tympani, facial nerve (CN VII), and vestibulocochlear nerve (CN VIII)
6 Glossopharyngeal nerve (CN XI)
7 Lingual nerve and inferior alveolar nerve
8 Styloid process and stylohyoid muscle
9 Styloglossus muscle
10 Lingual branches of glossopharyngeal nerve
11 Lingual branch of hypoglossal nerve
12 External carotid artery
13 Superior root of ansa cervicalis (branch of hypoglossal nerve, derived from C1)
14 Lateral ventricle with choroid plexus and cerebral peduncle
15 Trochlear nerve (CN IV)
16 Trigeminal nerve (CN V)
17 Fourth ventricle and rhomboid fossa
18 Vagus nerve (CN X)
19 Accessory nerve (CN XI)
20 Vertebral artery
21 Superior cervical ganglion
22 Hypoglossal nerve (CN XII)
23 Spinal ganglion with dural sheath
24 Dura mater of spinal cord
25 Internal carotid artery and carotid sinus branch of glossopharyngeal nerve
26 Dorsal roots of spinal nerve
27 Sympathetic trunk
28 Branch of cervical plexus (ventral primary ramus of third cervical spinal nerve)
29 Ansa cervicalis

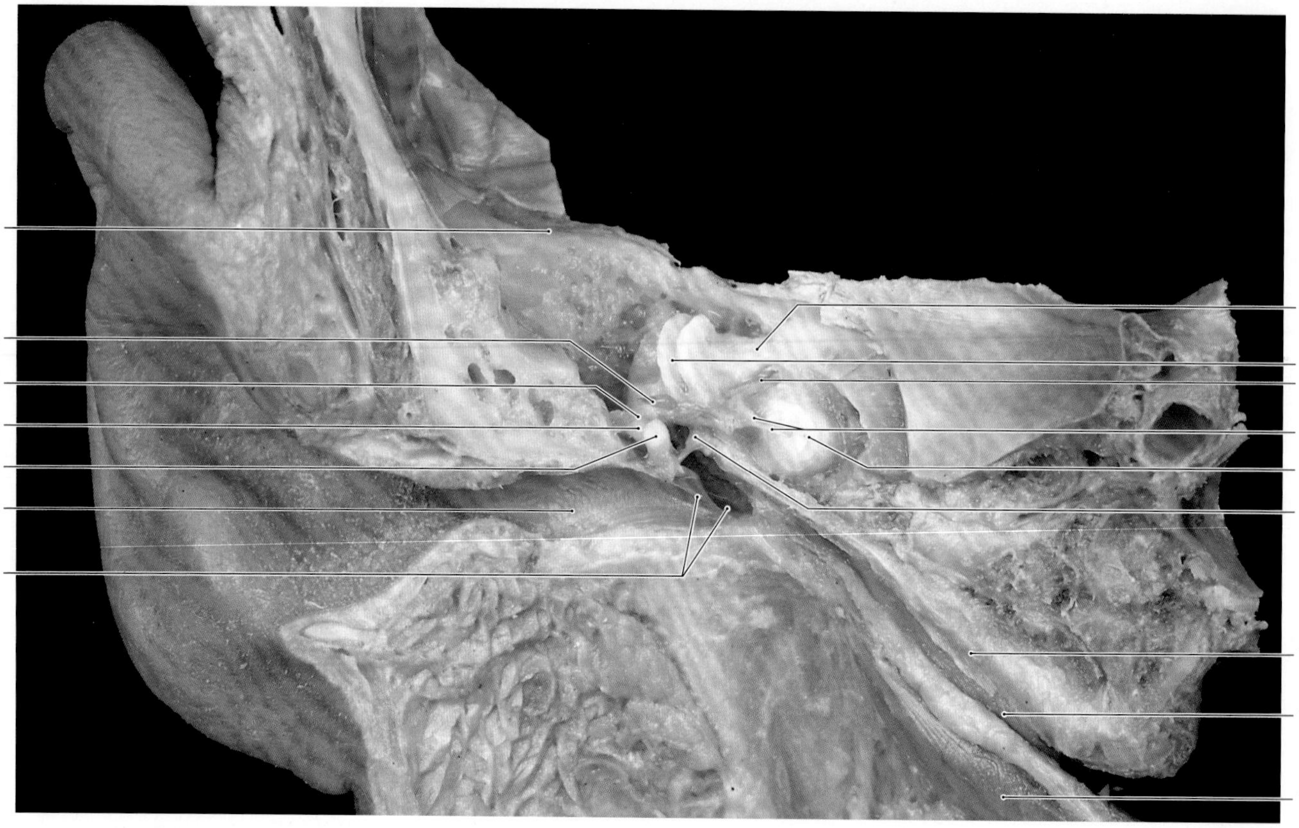

**Fig. 9.63 Longitudinal section through the right outer, middle, and inner ear** (anterior aspect). The cochlea and semicircular canals have been further dissected.

1 Roof of tympanic cavity
2 Lateral osseous semicircular canal
3 Facial nerve
4 Incus
5 Malleus
6 External acoustic meatus
7 Tympanic cavity and tympanic membrane
8 Vestibulocochlear nerve
9 Anterior osseous semicircular canal
10 Geniculate ganglion and greater petrosal nerve
11 Cochlea
12 Stapes
13 Tensor tympani muscle
14 Auditory tube
15 Levator veli palatini muscle
16 Styloid process

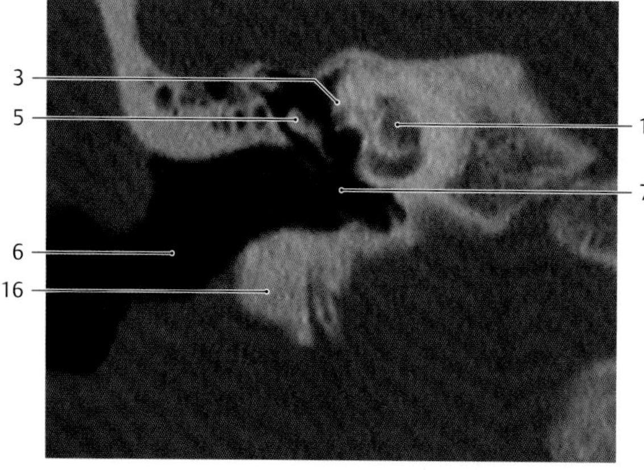


**Fig. 9.64 Auditory and Vestibular Apparatus** (MRI scan, see corresponding Fig. 9.67). (Courtesy of Prof. Uder, Institute of Radiology, University Hospital Erlangen, Germany.)

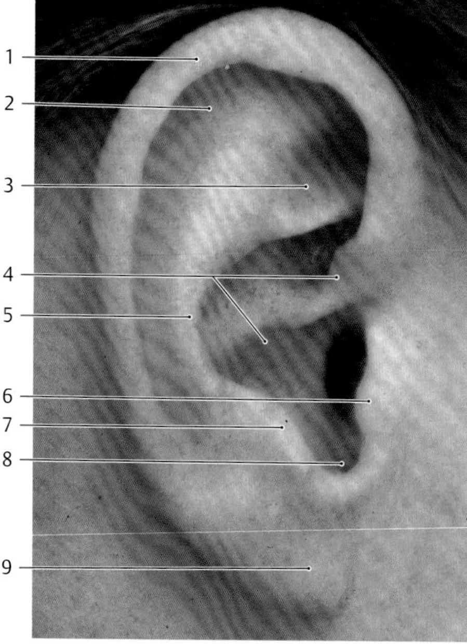


1 Helix
2 Scaphoid fossa
3 Triangular fossa
4 Concha
5 Antihelix
6 Tragus
7 Antitragus
8 Intertragic notch
9 Lobule

**Fig. 9.65 Right auricle** (lateral aspect).

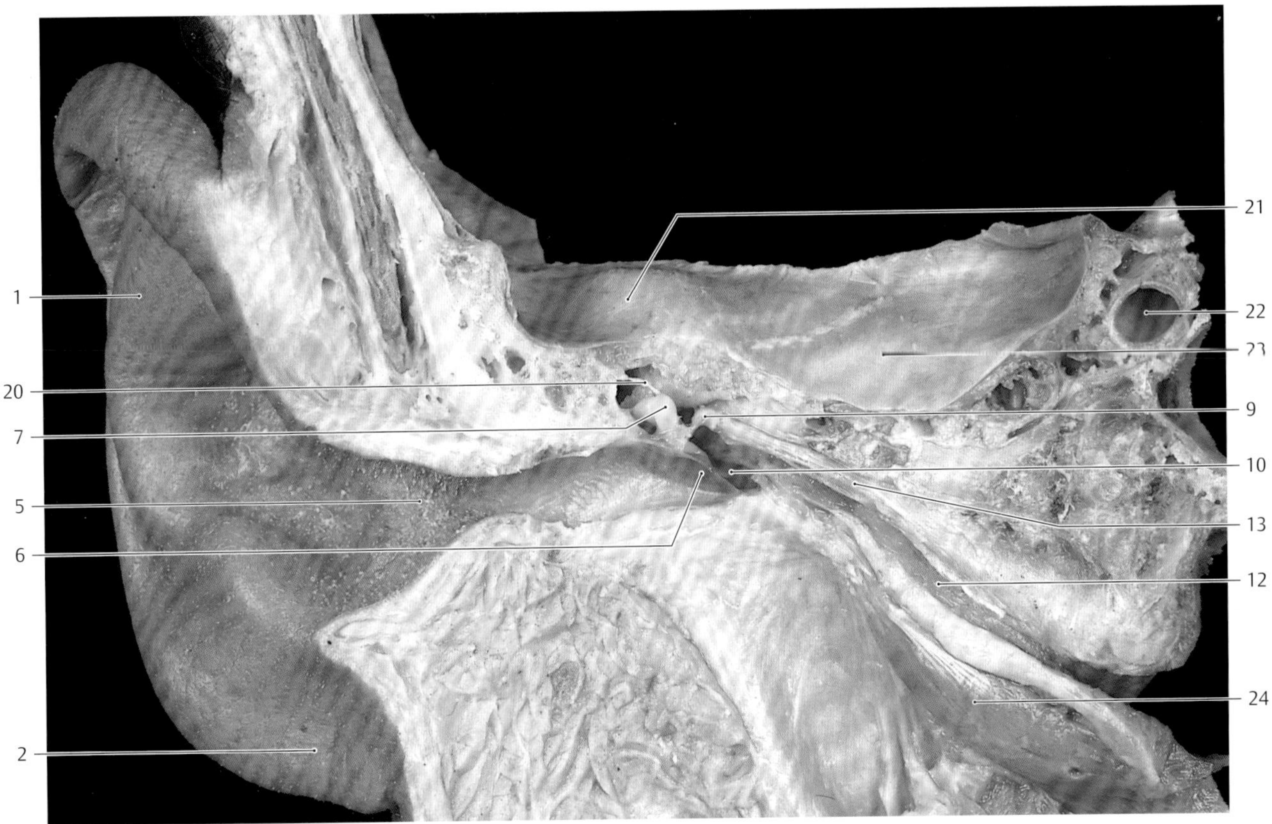


Fig. 9.66 **Longitudinal section through the right outer, middle, and inner ear** (anterior aspect).

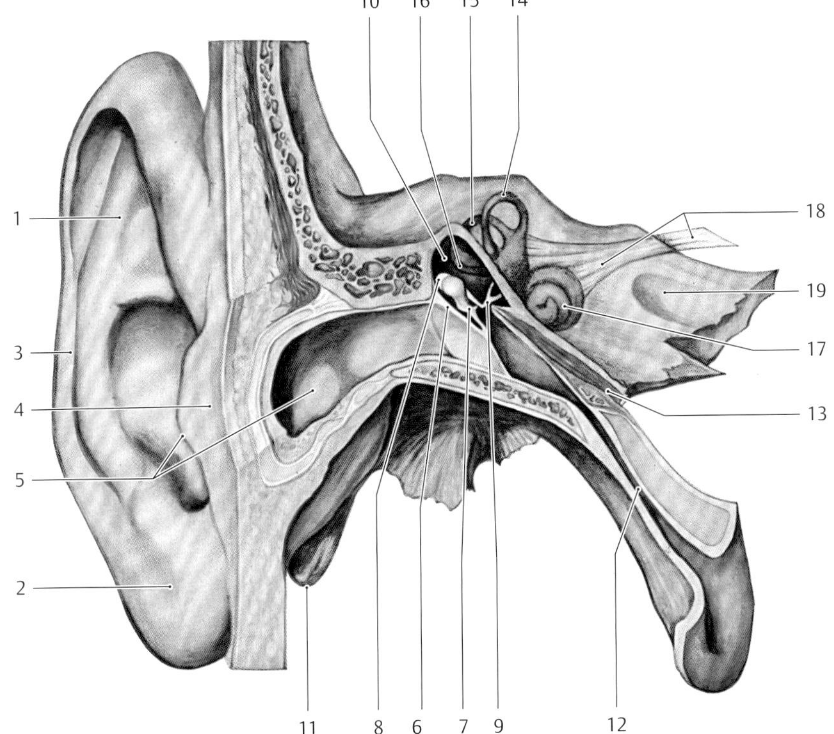


Fig. 9.67 **Right auditory and vestibular apparatus** (anterior aspect).
(See corresponding Fig. 9.64.)

**Outer ear**

1 Auricle
2 Lobule of auricle
3 Helix
4 Tragus
5 External acoustic meatus

**Middle ear**

6 Tympanic membrane
7 Malleus
8 Incus
9 Stapes
10 Tympanic cavity
11 Mastoid process
12 Auditory tube
13 Tensor tympani muscle

**Inner ear**

14 Anterior semicircular duct
15 Posterior semicircular duct
16 Lateral semicircular duct
17 Cochlea
18 Vestibulocochlear nerve (CN VIII)
19 Petrous part of the temporal bone

**Additional structures**

20 Superior ligament of malleus
21 Arcuate eminence
22 Internal carotid artery
23 Anterior surface of pyramid with dura mater
24 Levator veli palatini muscle

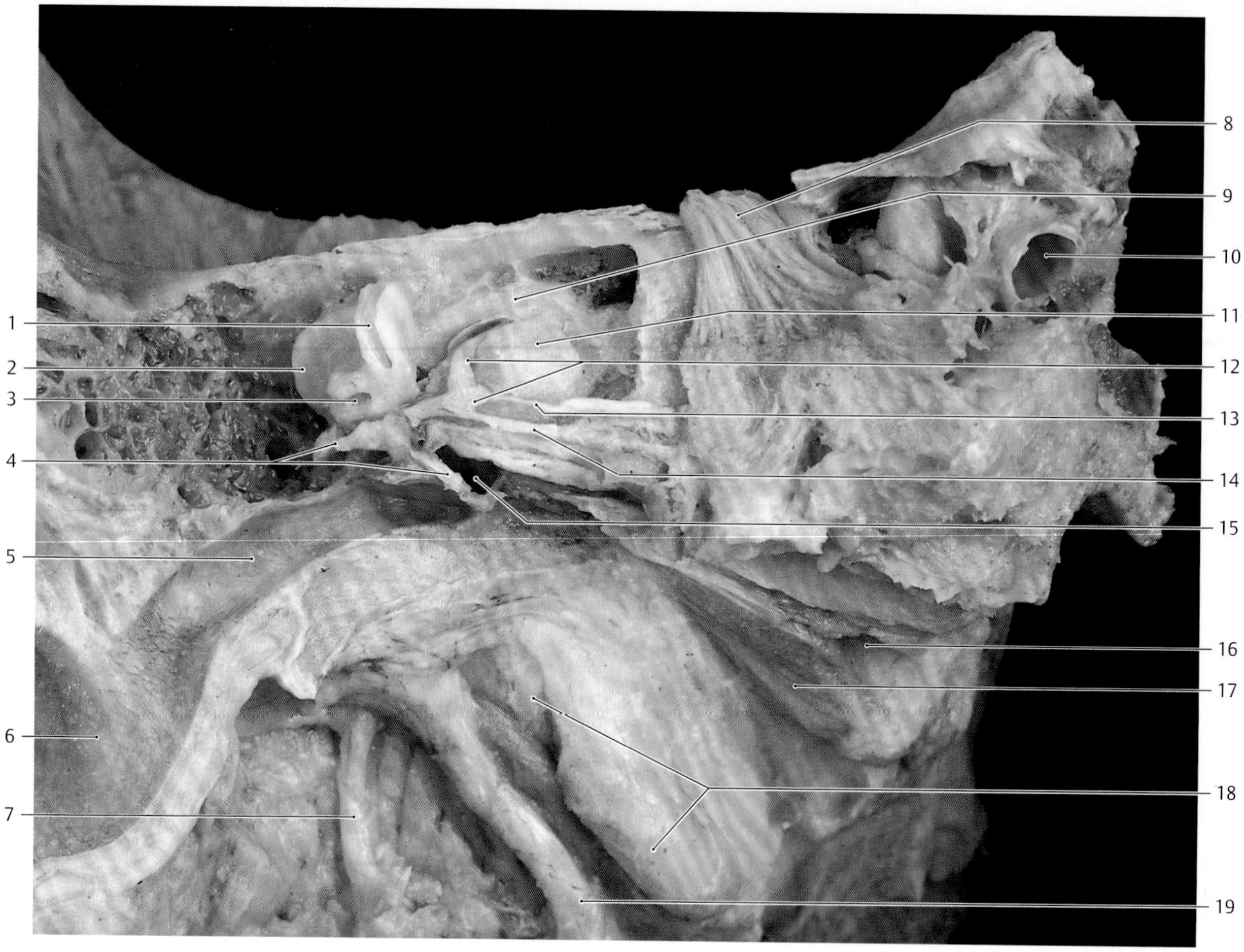

**Fig. 9.68 Longitudinal section through the outer, middle, and inner ear** (anterior aspect). Deeper dissection to display the facial nerve and lesser and greater petrosal nerves.

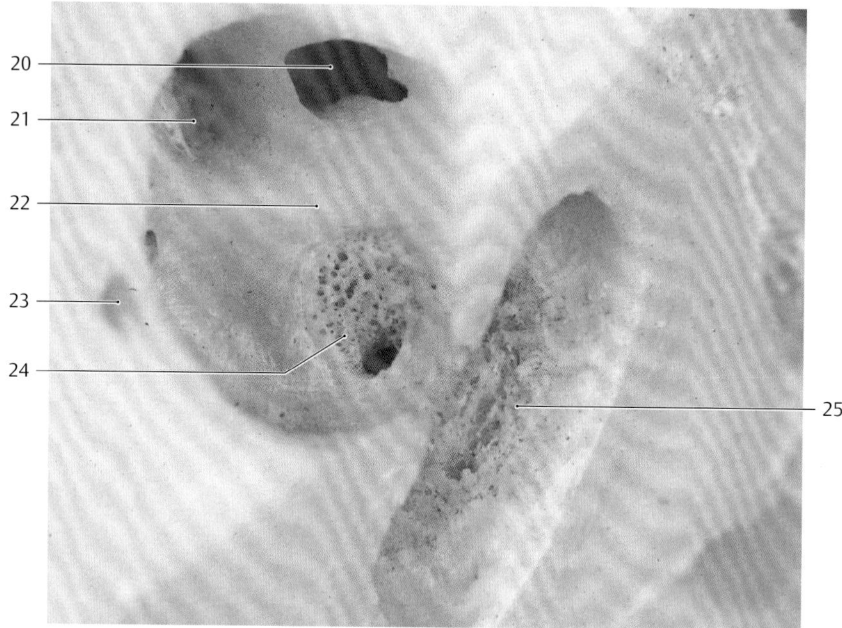


**Fig. 9.69 Internal acoustic meatus,** left side. The bone has been partly removed to show the bottom of the meatus.

1 Anterior osseous semicircular canal (opened)
2 Posterior osseous semicircular canal
3 Lateral osseous semicircular canal (opened)
4 Facial nerve and chorda tympani
5 External acoustic meatus
6 Auricle
7 Facial nerve
8 Trigeminal nerve
9 Bony base of internal acoustic meatus
10 Internal carotid artery within cavernous sinus
11 Cochlea
12 Facial nerve with geniculate ganglion
13 Greater petrosal nerve
14 Lesser petrosal nerve
15 Tympanic cavity
16 Auditory tube
17 Levator veli palatini muscle
18 Internal carotid artery and internal jugular vein
19 Styloid process
20 Area of facial nerve
21 Superior vestibular area
22 Transverse crest
23 Foramen singulare
24 Foraminous spiral tract (outlet of cochlear part of vestibulocochlear nerve)
25 Base of cochlea

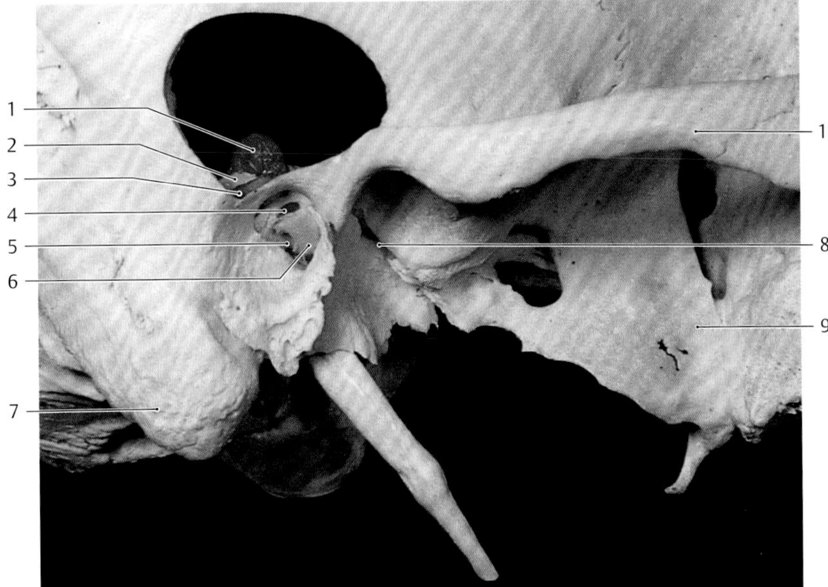


Fig. 9.70 **Right temporal bone** (lateral aspect). The petrosquamous portion has been partly removed to display the semicircular canals.

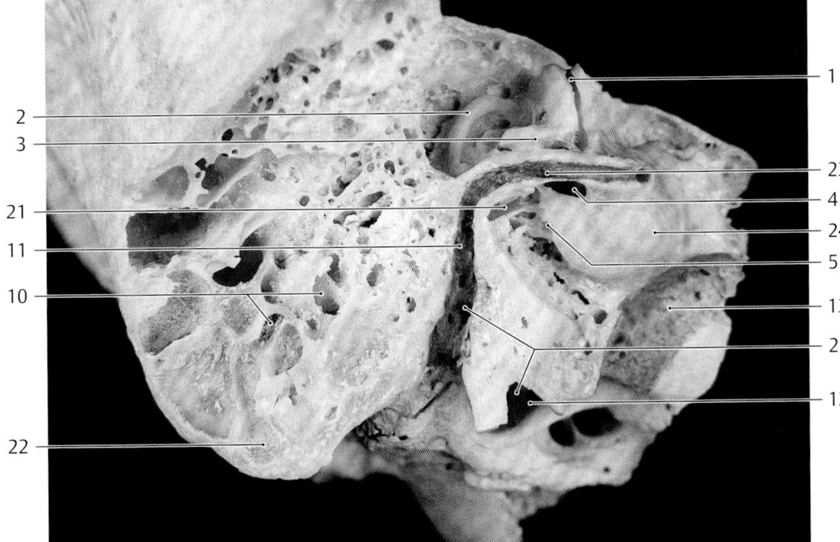


Fig. 9.71 **Right temporal bone** (lateral aspect). The mastoid air cells and facial canal have been opened and the three semicircular canals dissected.

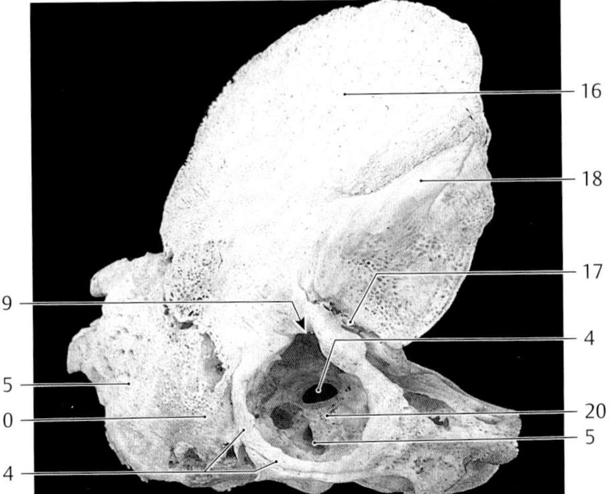


Fig. 9.72 **Right temporal bone of the newborn** (lateral aspect).

1 Anterior semicircular canal (red)
2 Posterior semicircular canal (yellow)
3 Lateral or horizontal semicircular canal (green)
4 Fenestra vestibuli
5 Fenestra cochleae
6 Tympanic cavity
7 Mastoid process
8 Petrotympanic fissure (red probe: chorda tympani)
9 Lateral pterygoid plate
10 Mastoid air cells
11 Facial canal (blue)
12 Foramen ovale
13 Carotid canal (red)
14 Tympanic ring
15 Petromastoid part of temporal bone
16 Squamous part of temporal bone
17 Squamomastoid suture
18 Zygomatic process of temporal bone
19 Incisure of tympanic ring
20 Promontory
21 Canaliculus chordae tympani (green probe)
22 Mastoid process
23 Canaliculus for stapedius nerve (red)
24 Cochlea
25 Canaliculus mastoideus (red probe)

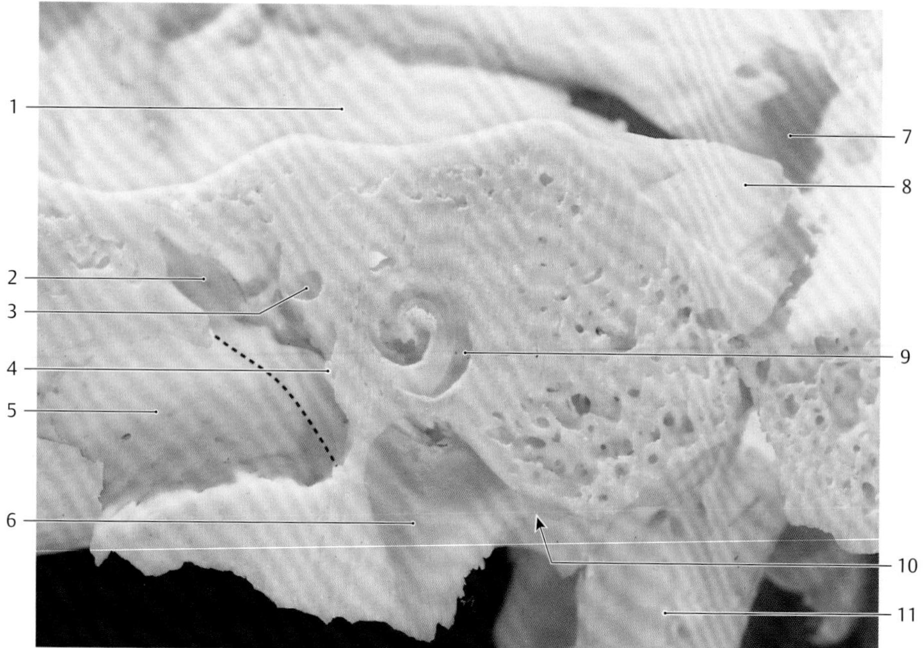


Fig. 9.73 **Frontal section through the petrous part of the left temporal bone** at the level of the cochlea (posterior aspect). Dotted line = Position of the tympanic membrane.

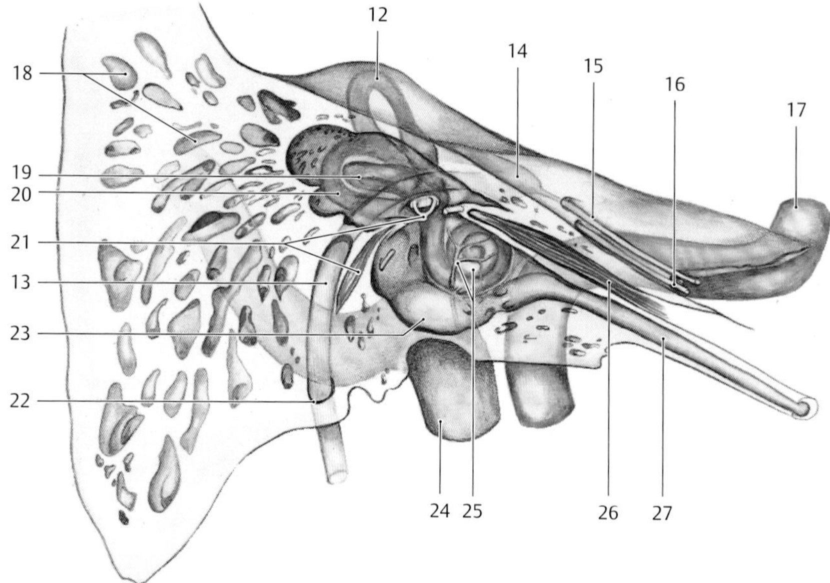


Fig. 9.74 **Medial wall of the tympanic cavity** and its relation to neighboring structures of the inner ear, facial nerve, and blood vessels. Frontal section through the right temporal bone (anterior aspect).

1 Anterior surface of the pyramid
2 Mastoid antrum
3 Lateral semicircular canal
4 Cochleariform process
5 External acoustic meatus
6 Jugular fossa
7 Foramen lacerum
8 Apex of petrous part
9 Position of cochlea (modiolus with crista spiralis ossea)
10 Carotid canal
11 Pterygoid process
12 Anterior semicircular duct
13 Facial nerve
14 Geniculate ganglion
15 Greater petrosal nerve
16 Lesser petrosal nerve
17 Internal carotid artery
18 Mastoid air cells
19 Lateral semicircular duct
20 Posterior semicircular duct
21 Stapes with stapedius muscle
22 Stylomastoid foramen
23 Inferior recess of tympanic cavity (hypotympanum)
24 Internal jugular vein
25 Promontory with tympanic plexus (position of cochlea)
26 Tensor muscle of tympanum
27 Auditory tube

The medial wall of the tympanic cavity is directly adjacent to the inner ear. The promontory of the tympanic cavity is formed by a bulge of the basal turn of the cochlea. The facial nerve (CN VII, see p. 468) travels between the lateral semicircular duct (which also comes in close proximity to the middle ear) and the base of the stapes (which is enclosed by the oval window) in an arc to the stylomastoid foramen. At this point, the facial nerve is particularly at risk as the middle ear mucosa is very close to it. An equally clinically important regional relationship affects the sigmoid sinus in its transition to the internal jugular vein. The venous sinus curves slightly inward at the base of the tympanic cavity. The mucosa of the middle ear is directly connected to the nasal mucosa in the area of the nasopharynx via the pharyngotympanic tube (Eustachian tube).

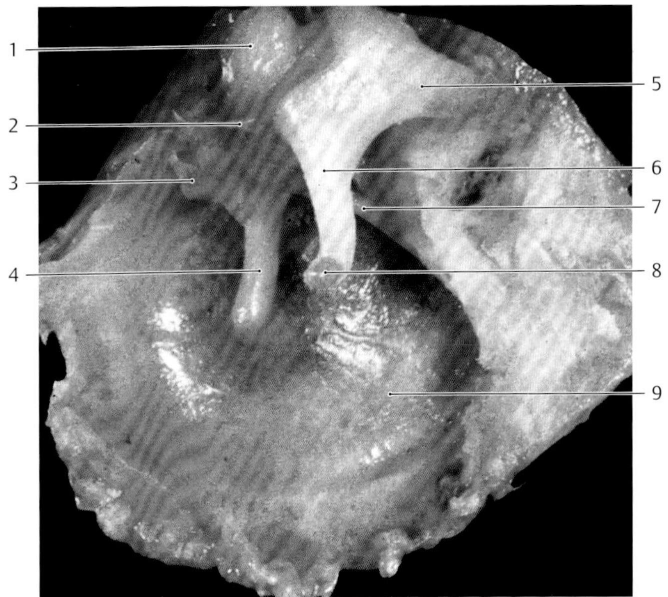

1 Head of malleus
2 Anterior ligament of malleus
3 Tendon of tensor tympani muscle
4 Handle of malleus
5 Short crus of incus
6 Long crus of incus
7 Chorda tympani
8 Lenticular process
9 Tympanic membrane

Fig. 9.75 **Tympanic membrane with malleus and incus** (internal aspect, right side).

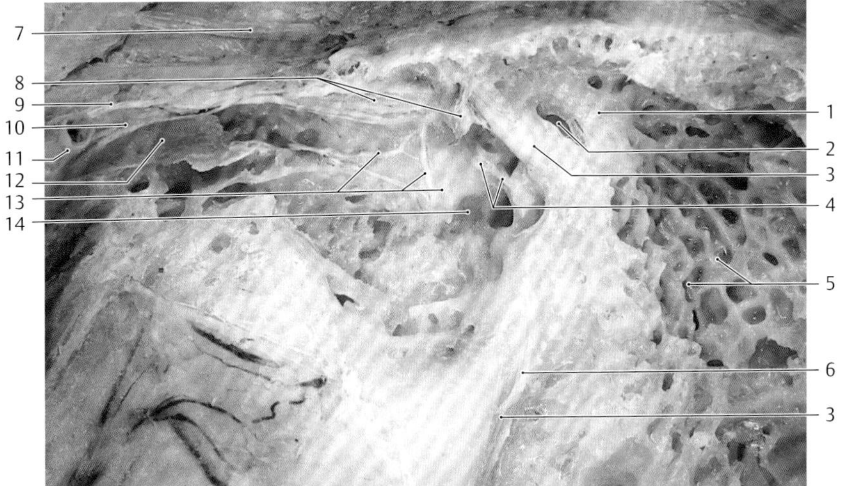

1 Tympanic antrum
2 Lateral semicircular canal (opened)
3 Facial canal
4 Stapes with tendon of stapedius
5 Mastoid air cells
6 Chorda tympani (intracranial part)
7 Greater petrosal nerve
8 Tensor tympani muscle (processus cochleariformis)
9 Lesser petrosal nerve
10 Anterior tympanic artery
11 Middle meningeal artery
12 Auditory tube
13 Promontory with tympanic plexus
14 Fenestra cochleae

Fig. 9.76 **Tympanic cavity, medial wall** (left side). External acoustic meatus and lateral wall of tympanic cavity together with incus. The malleus and tympanic membrane have been removed and the mastoid air cells opened.

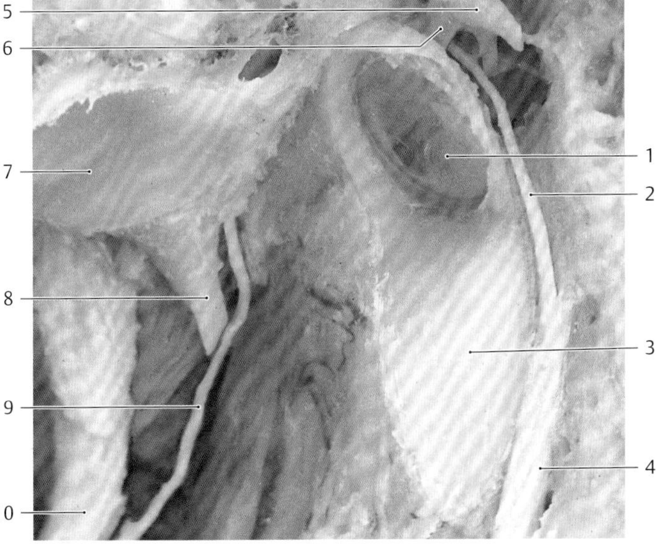

1 Tympanic membrane
2 Chorda tympani (intracranial part)
3 Floor of the external acoustic meatus
4 Facial nerve and facial canal
5 Incus
6 Head of malleus
7 Mandibular fossa
8 Spine of sphenoid
9 Chorda tympani (extracranial part)
10 Styloid process

Fig. 9.77 **Tympanic membrane** (lateral aspect, left side). External acoustic meatus and facial canal have been opened to expose the chorda tympani (approx. ×1.5).

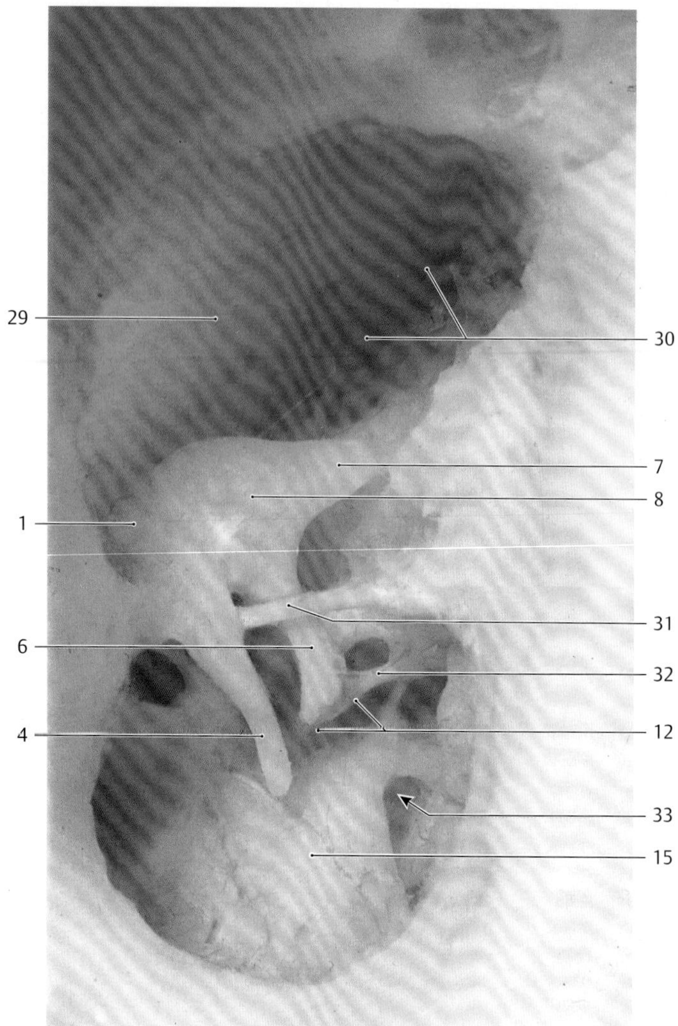


**Fig. 9.78 Tympanic cavity with malleus, incus, and stapes** (lateral aspect, left side). Tympanic membrane removed, mastoid antrum opened.

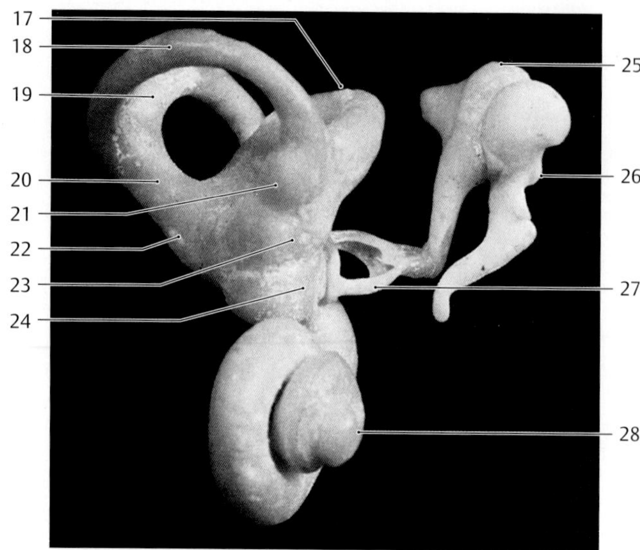


**Fig. 9.79 Chain of auditory ossicles** in connection with the inner ear (antero-lateral aspect, left side).

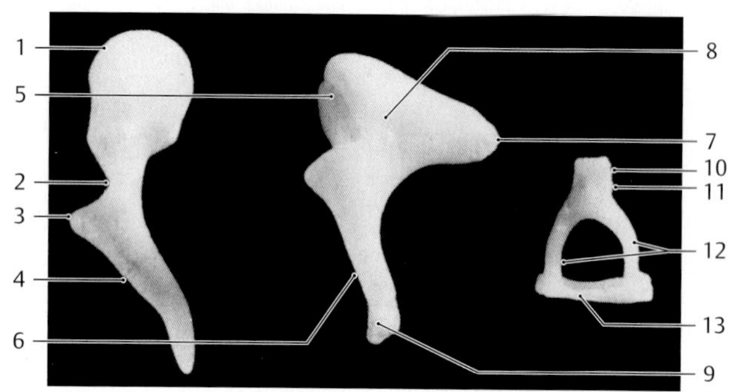


**Fig. 9.80 Auditory ossicles** (isolated).

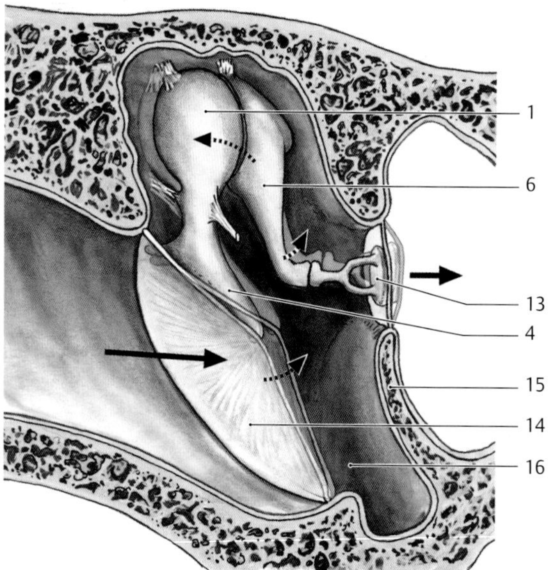


**Fig. 9.81 Position and movements of the auditory ossicles during transmission of sound waves.**

**Malleus**
1 Head
2 Neck
3 Lateral process
4 Handle

**Incus**
5 Articular facet for malleus
6 Long crus
7 Short crus
8 Body
9 Lenticular process

**Stapes**
10 Head
11 Neck
12 Anterior and posterior crura
13 Base

**Walls of tympanic cavity**
14 Tympanic membrane
15 Promontory
16 Hypotympanic recess of tympanic cavity

**Auditory ossicles and internal ear (labyrinth)**
17 Lateral semicircular duct
18 Anterior semicircular duct
19 Posterior semicircular duct
20 Common crus
21 Ampulla
22 Beginning of endolymphatic duct
23 Utricular prominence
24 Saccular prominence
25 Incus
26 Malleus
27 Stapes
28 Cochlea

**Tympanic cavity**
29 Epitympanic recess
30 Mastoid antrum
31 Chorda tympani
32 Tendon of stapedius muscle
33 Round window (fenestra cochleae)

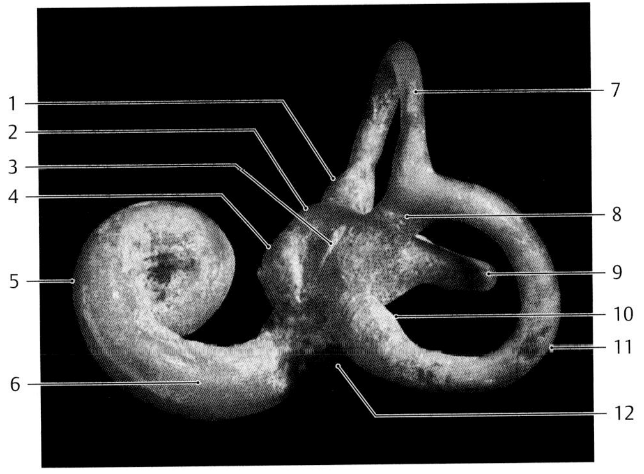


Fig. 9.82 **Cast of the right labyrinth** (postero-medial aspect).

1 Ampulla (anterior semicircular canal)
2 Elliptical recess
3 Aqueduct of the vestibule
4 Spherical recess
5 Cochlea
6 Base of cochlea
7 Anterior semicircular canal
8 Crus commune or common limb
9 Lateral semicircular canal
10 Posterior bony ampulla
11 Posterior semicircular canal (posterior canal)
12 Fenestra cochleae
13 Bony ampulla
14 Fenestra vestibuli
15 Cupula of cochlea
16 External acoustic meatus
17 Mastoid air cells
18 Tympanic cavity and fenestra cochleae (probe)
19 External acoustic meatus
20 Facial canal
21 Base of cochlea and musculotubal canal
22 Malleus and incus
23 Stapes
24 Tympanic membrane
25 Tympanic cavity
26 Aqueduct of cochlea
27 Endolymphatic sac
28 Endolymphatic duct
29 Macula of utricle
30 Macula of saccule

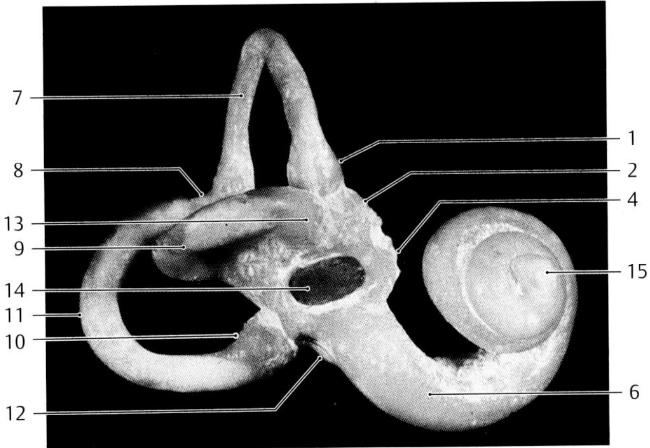


Fig. 9.83 **Cast of the right labyrinth** (lateral aspect).

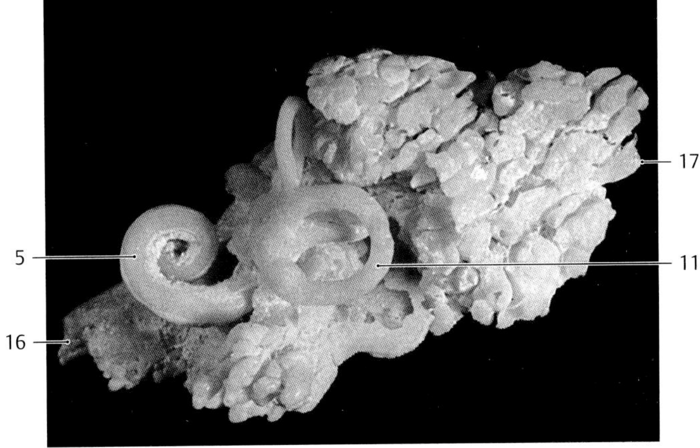


Fig. 9.84 **Cast of the labyrinth and mastoid cells** (posterior aspect). Life size.

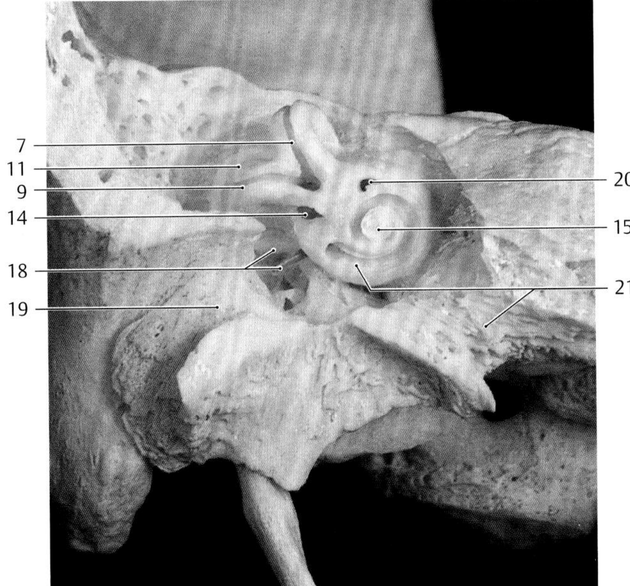


Fig. 9.85 **Dissection of bony labyrinth in situ.** Semicircular canals and cochlear duct have been opened.

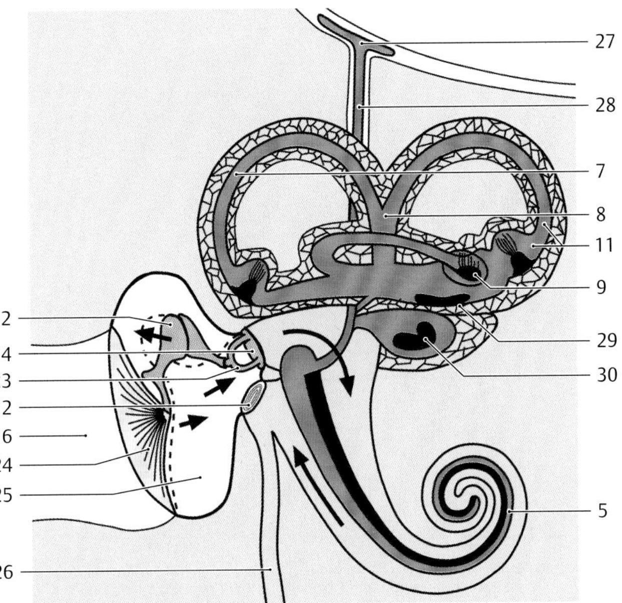


Fig. 9.86 **Auditory and vestibular apparatus.** Arrows = direction of sound waves; blue = perilymphatic ducts.

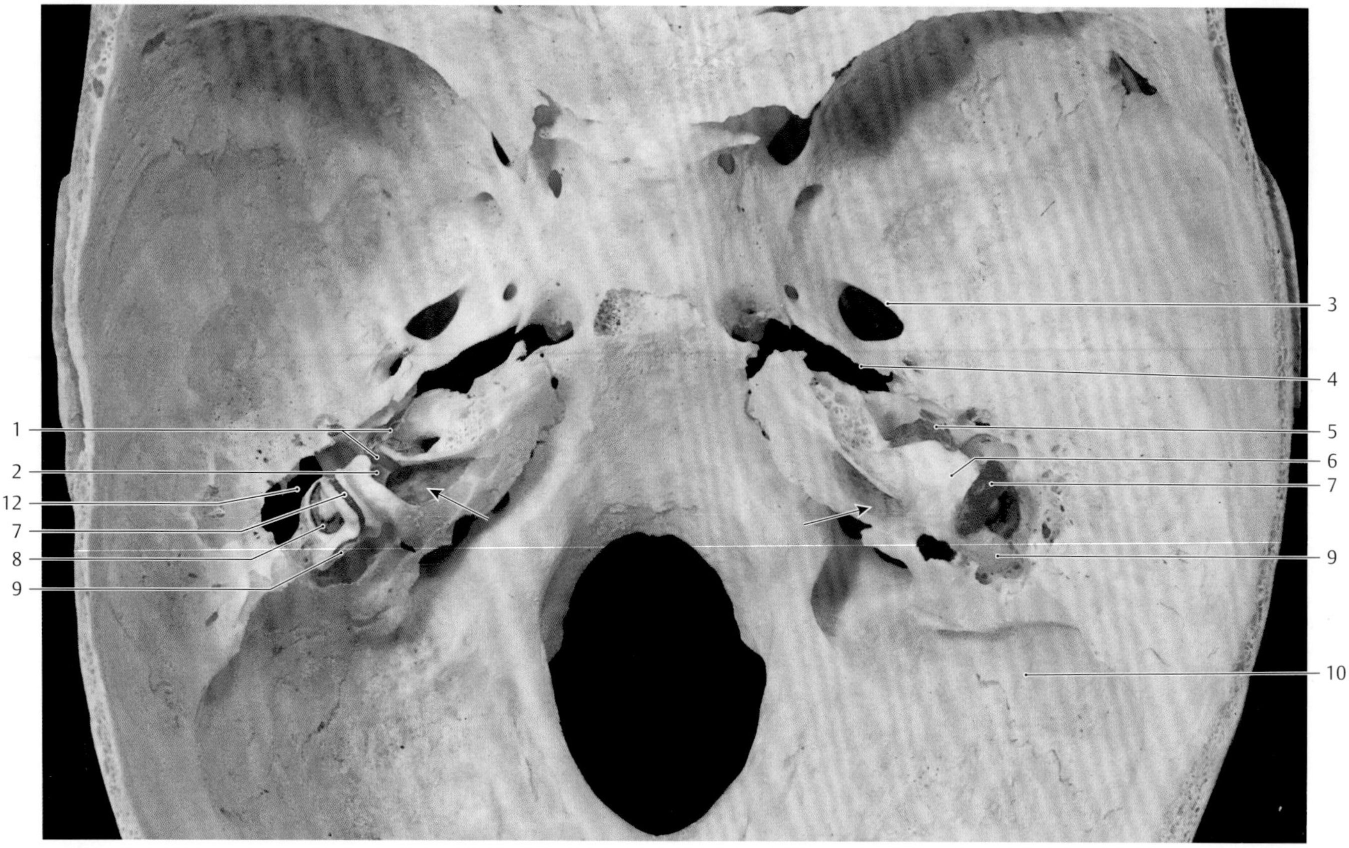

Fig. 9.87 **Bony labyrinth, petrous part of the temporal bone** (from above). Left = semicircular canals opened; right = semicircular canals closed; arrows = internal acoustic meatus.

1 Facial canal and semicanal of auditory tube
2 Superior vestibular area
3 Foramen ovale
4 Foramen lacerum
5 Cochlea
6 Vestibule
7 Anterior semicircular canal
8 Lateral semicircular canal
9 Posterior semicircular canal
10 Groove for sigmoid sinus
11 Sigmoid sinus
12 Tympanic cavity
13 Auditory tube
14 Mastoid air cells
15 Facial, vestibulocochlear, and intermediate nerves
16 Temporal fossa
17 Fenestra vestibuli
18 Promontory
19 Zygomatic process
20 Fenestra cochleae
21 Mastoid process

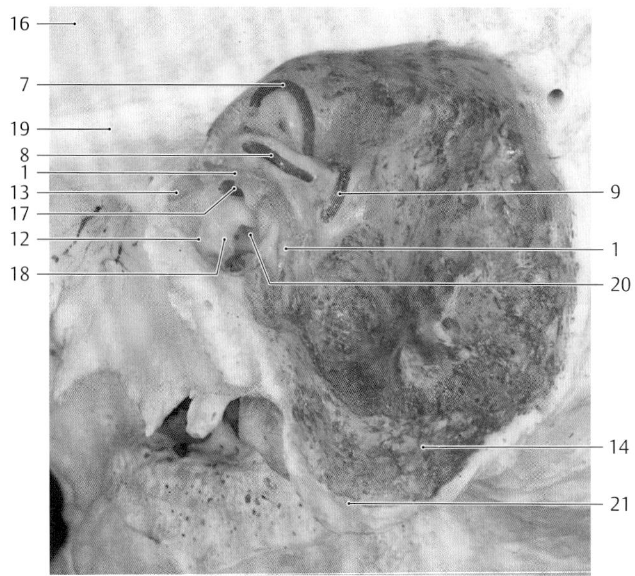


Fig. 9.88 **Bony labyrinth** (left lateral aspect). The temporal and tympanic bones have been partly removed and the semicircular canals opened.

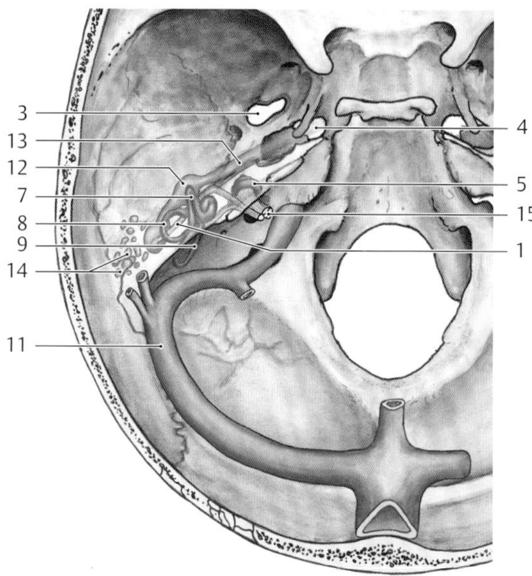


Fig. 9.89 **Internal ear** (from above). Diagram showing the position of the membranous labyrinth and the tympanic cavity.

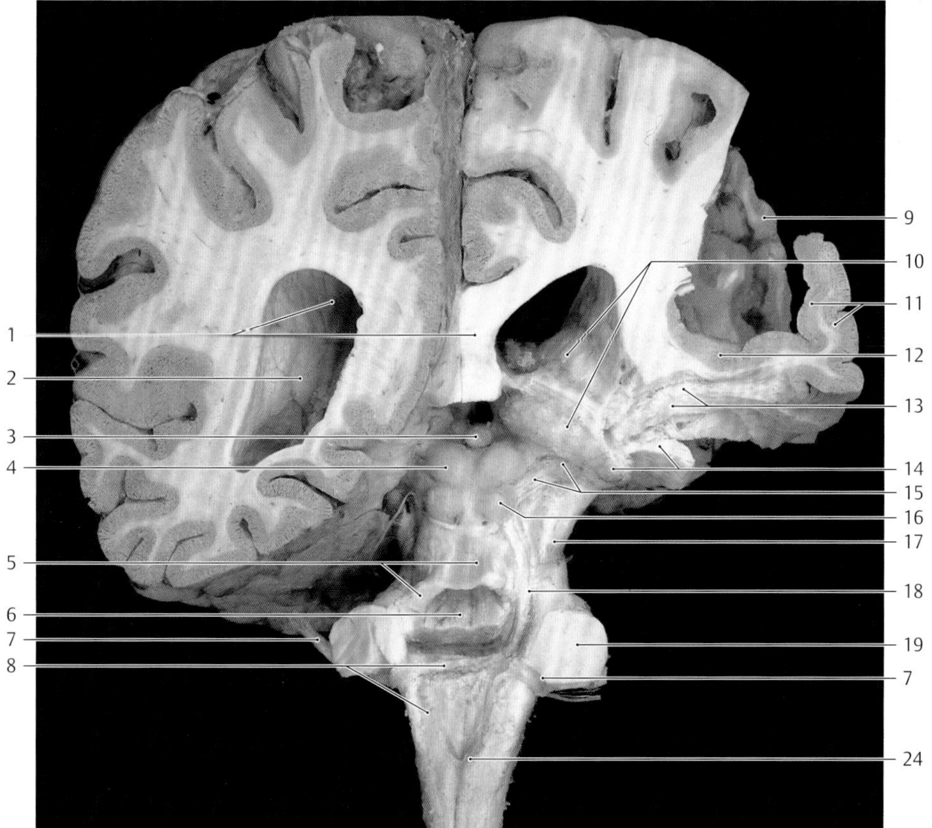


Fig. 9.90 **Dissection of the brainstem showing the auditory pathway** (posterior aspect). The cerebellum and posterior part of the two hemispheres have been removed.

1 Left lateral ventricle and corpus callosum
2 Thalamus
3 Pineal gland (epiphysis)
4 Superior colliculus
5 Superior medullary velum and superior cerebellar peduncle
6 Rhomboid fossa
7 Vestibulocochlear nerve (CN VIII)
8 Dorsal acoustic striae and inferior cerebellar peduncle
9 Insular lobe
10 Caudate nucleus and thalamus
11 Temporal lobe (superior temporal gyrus) (area of acoustic centers)
12 Transverse temporal gyri of Heschl (area of primary acoustic centers)
13 Acoustic radiation of internal capsule
14 Lateral geniculate body and optic radiation (cut)
15 Medial geniculate body and brachium of inferior colliculus
16 Inferior colliculus
17 Cerebral peduncle
18 Lateral lemniscus
19 Middle cerebellar peduncle
20 Dorsal (posterior) cochlear nucleus
21 Ventral (anterior) cochlear nucleus
22 Inferior olive with olivocochlear tract of Rasmussen (red)
23 Ganglion spirale
24 Obex
25 Frontal lobe
26 Temporal lobe
27 Middle temporal gyrus (area of tertiary acoustic centers)
28 Trapezoid body

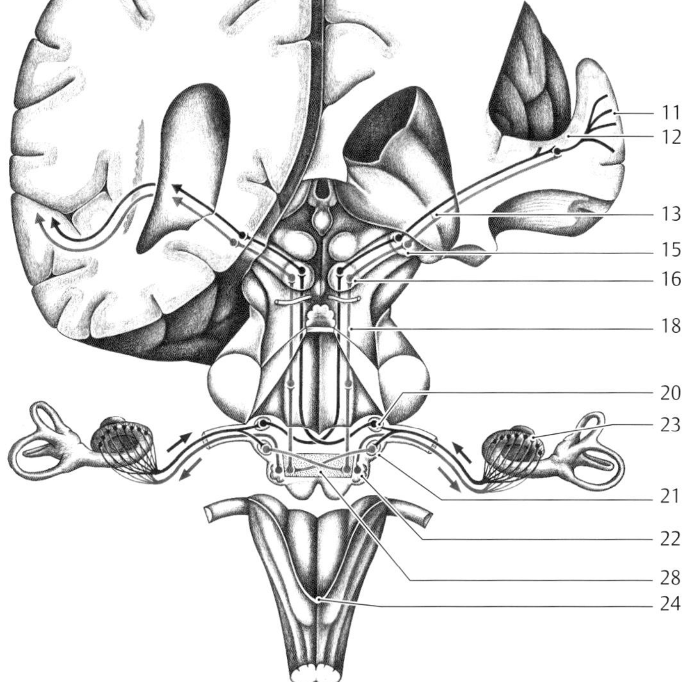


Fig. 9.91 **Auditory pathway** (see corresponding Fig. 9.90 above). Red = descending (efferent) pathway (olivocochlear tract of Rasmussen); green and blue = ascending (afferent) pathways.

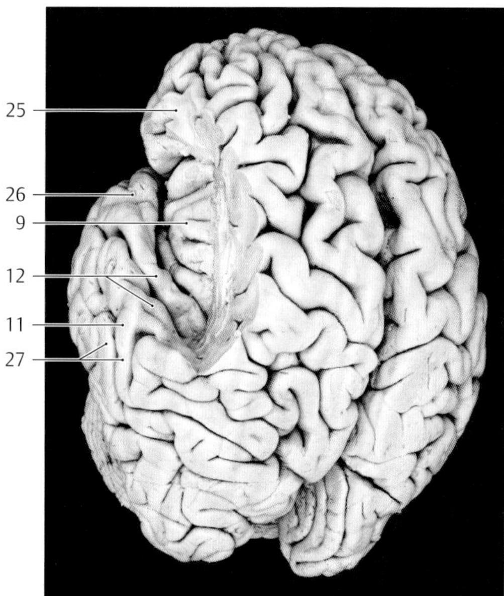


Fig. 9.92 **Auditory areas in the left hemisphere** (superolateral aspect). Parts of the frontal and parietal lobes have been removed.

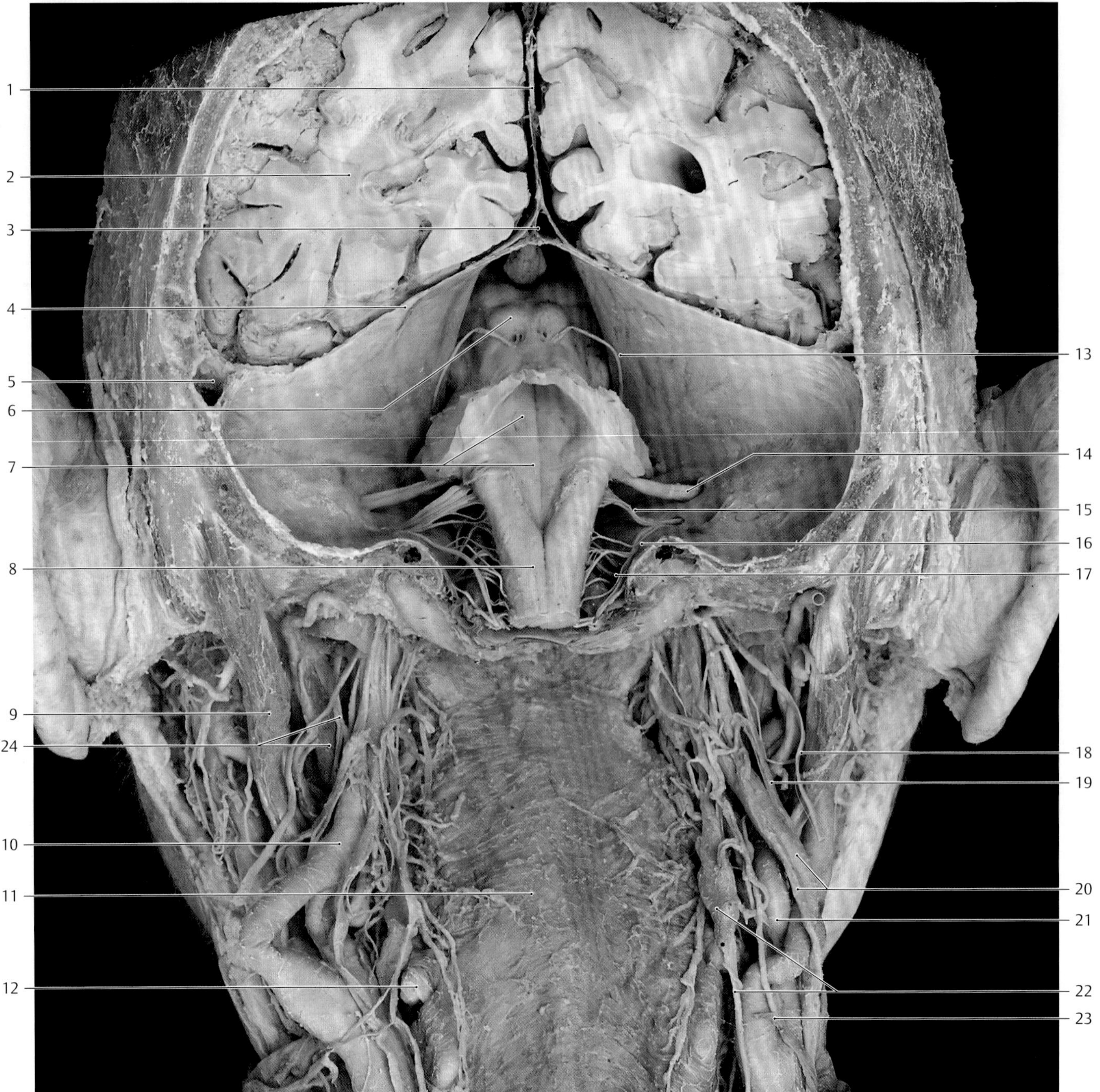


Fig. 9.93 **Brainstem and pharynx with cranial nerves** (posterior aspect). **Dissection of trochlear (CN IV), facial (CN VII), vestibulocochlear (CN VIII), glossopharyngeal (CN IX), vagus (CN X), accessory (CN XI), and hypoglossal (CN XII) nerves.** The cranial cavity has been opened and the cerebellum removed.

1 Falx cerebri
2 Occipital lobe
3 Straight sinus
4 Cerebellar tentorium
5 Transverse sinus
6 Inferior colliculus of midbrain
7 Rhomboid fossa
8 Medulla oblongata
9 Posterior belly of digastric muscle
10 Internal carotid artery
11 Pharynx (middle constrictor muscle)
12 Hyoid bone (greater horn)
13 Trochlear nerve (CN IV)
14 Facial nerve (CN VII) and vestibulocochlear nerve (CN VIII)
15 Glossopharyngeal nerve (CN IX) and vagus nerve (CN X)
16 Accessory nerve (intracranial portion) (CN XI)
17 Hypoglossal nerve (intracranial portion) (CN XII)
18 Accessory nerve (CN XI)
19 Hypoglossal nerve (CN XII)
20 Vagus nerve (CN X) and internal carotid artery
21 External carotid artery
22 Sympathetic trunk and superior cervical ganglion
23 Ansa cervicalis (superior root of hypoglossal nerve)
24 Glossopharyngeal nerve (CN IX) and stylopharyngeus muscle

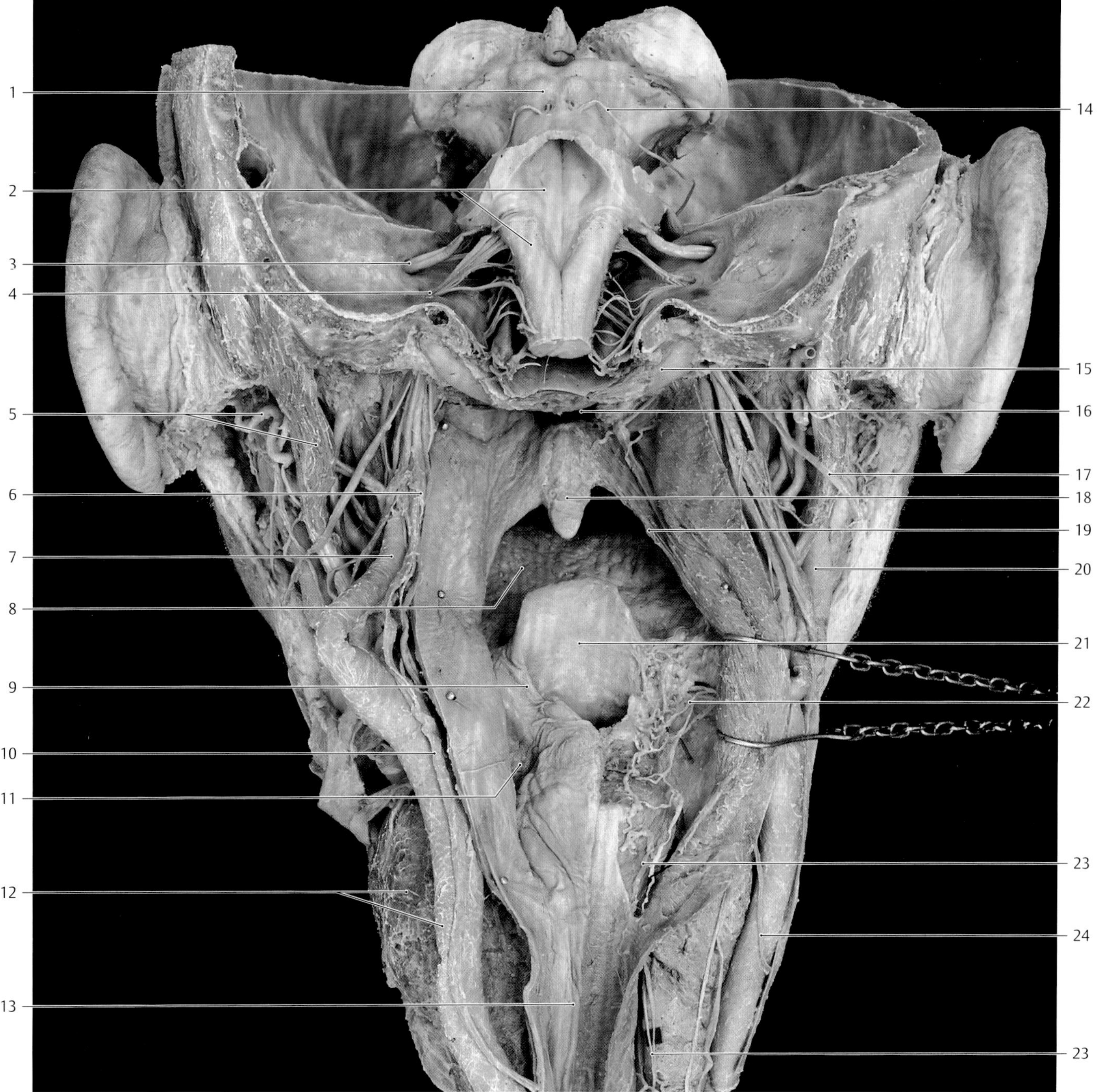


Fig. 9.94 **Larynx and oral cavity (posterior aspect).** Dissection of trochlear (CN IV), facial (CN VII), vestibulocochlear (CN VIII), glossopharyngeal (CN IX), vagus (CN X), and accessory (CN XI) nerves. The mucous membrane on the right half of the pharynx has been removed.

1 Midbrain (inferior colliculus)
2 Rhomboid fossa and medulla oblongata
3 Vestibulocochlear and facial nerve (CN VII)
4 Glossopharyngeal (CN IX), vagus (CN X), and accessory nerves (CN XI)
5 Occipital artery and posterior belly of digastric muscle
6 Superior cervical ganglion
7 Internal carotid artery
8 Oral cavity (tongue)
9 Ary-epiglottic fold
10 Vagus nerve (CN X)
11 Piriform recess
12 Thyroid gland and common carotid artery
13 Esophagus
14 Trochlear nerve (CN IV)
15 Occipital condyle
16 Nasal cavity (choana)
17 Accessory nerve (CN XI)
18 Uvula and soft palate
19 Palatopharyngeus muscle
20 External carotid artery
21 Epiglottis
22 Internal branch of superior laryngeal nerve
23 Inferior laryngeal nerve
24 Ansa cervicalis

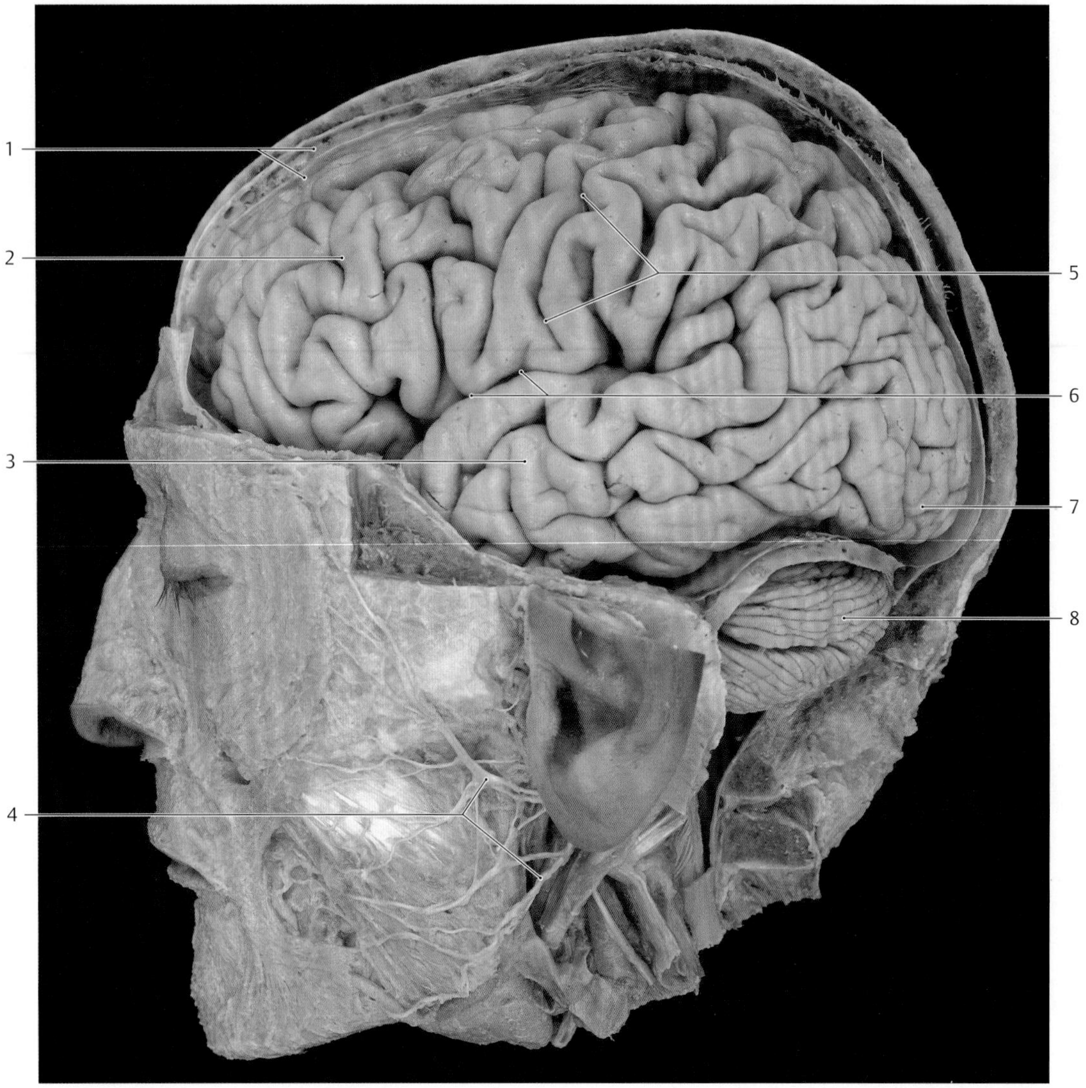

**Fig. 9.95 Dissection of the head to show the brain with pia mater and arachnoid in situ** (lateral aspect).

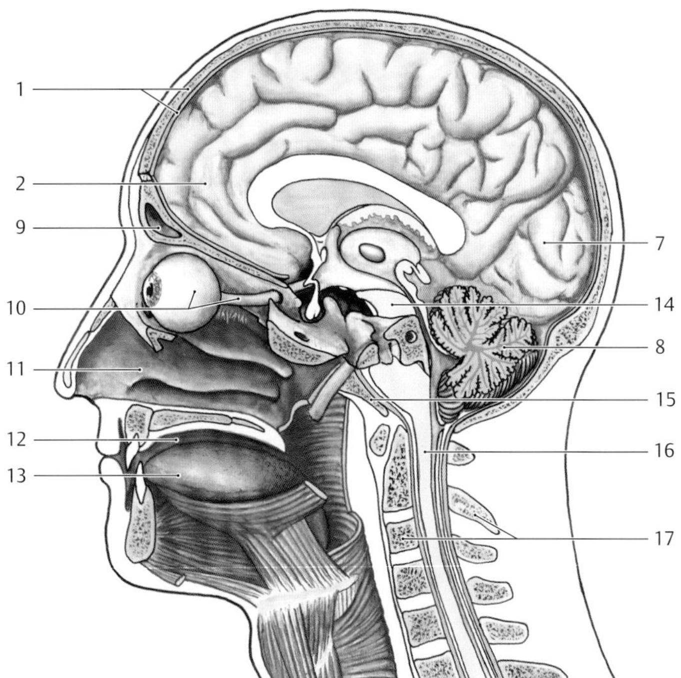


1 Vertex of the skull and dura mater
2 Frontal lobe
3 Temporal lobe
4 Facial nerve (CN VII)
5 Central sulcus
6 Lateral sulcus
7 Occipital lobe
8 Cerebellum
9 Frontal sinus
10 Eye and optic nerve (CN II)
11 Nasal cavity
12 Oral cavity
13 Tongue
14 Brainstem
15 Base of skull
16 Spinal cord
17 Vertebral column

**Fig. 9.96 Sagittal section through the head with brain and sensory organs.** The eye with the optic nerve is located within the orbit and the labyrinth organ within the petrous bone.

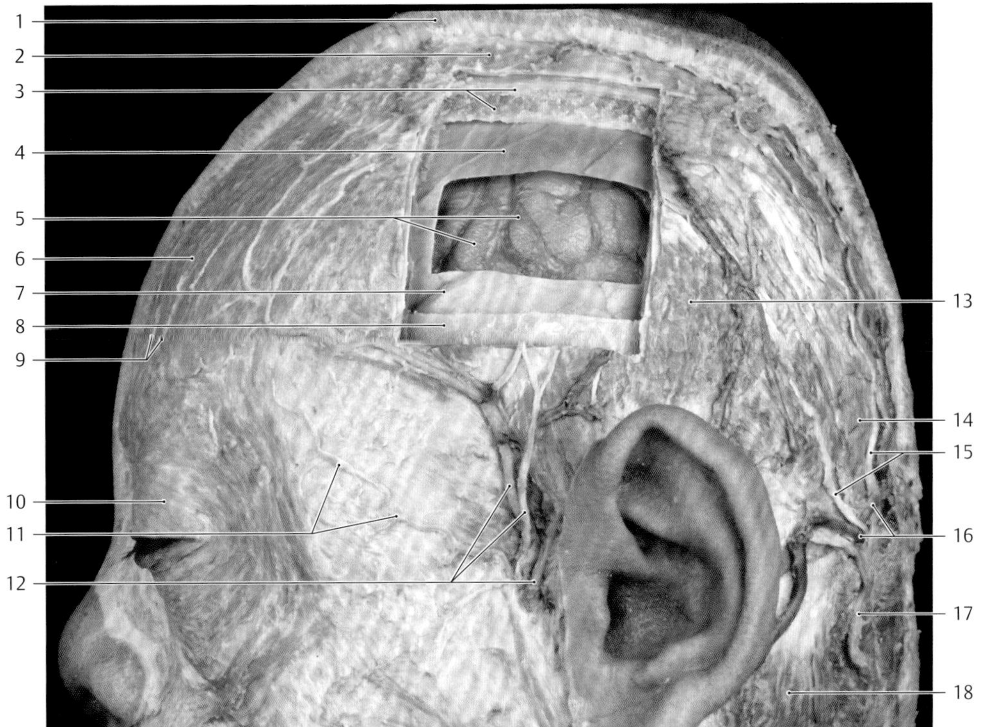


Fig. 9.97 **Lateral aspect of the head. Scalp, vertex of the skull, and meninges** are demonstrated by a series of window-like openings.

1 Skin
2 Galea aponeurotica
3 Skull diploe
4 Dura mater
5 Arachnoid and pia mater with cerebral vessels
6 Frontal belly of occipito-frontalis muscle
7 Branch of middle meningeal artery
8 Pericranium (periosteum)
9 Lateral and medial branches of supra-orbital nerve
10 Orbicularis oculi muscle
11 Zygomatico-orbital artery
12 Auriculotemporal nerve and superficial temporal artery and vein
13 Superior auricular muscle
14 Occipital belly of occipito-frontalis muscle
15 Occipital nerve
16 Occipital artery and vein
17 Greater occipital nerve
18 Sternocleidomastoid muscle
19 Frontal lobe
20 Chiasmatic cistern
21 Interpeduncular cistern
22 Arachnoid granulations
23 Subarachnoid space
24 Superior sagittal sinus
25 Inferior sagittal sinus
26 Corpus callosum
27 Straight sinus
28 Confluence of sinuses
29 Cerebellum
30 Cerebellomedullar cistern
31 Cerebral cortex

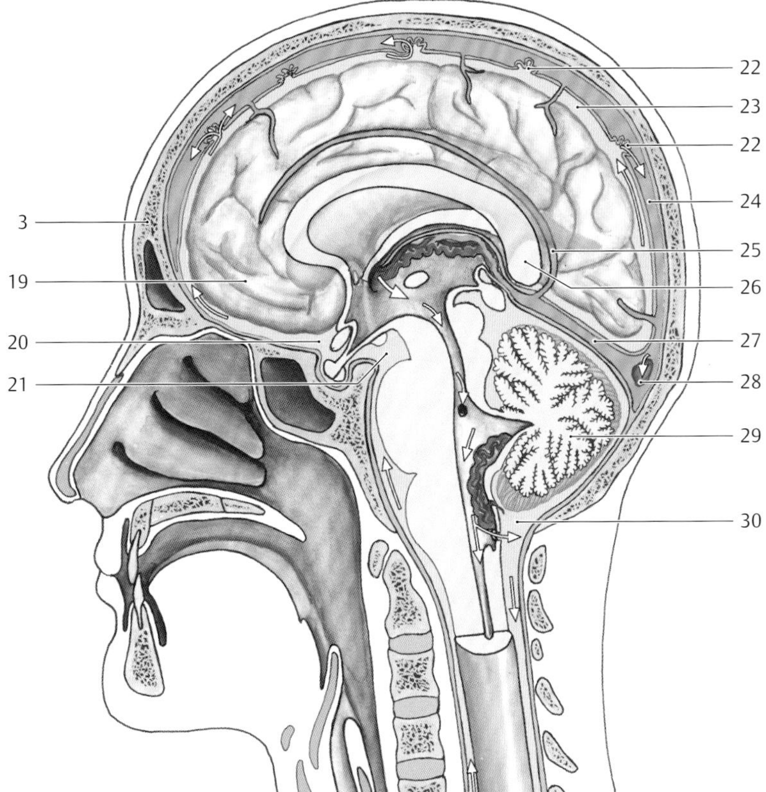


Fig. 9.98 **Subarachnoid cisterns of the brain** (midsagittal section). Green = cisterns; blue = dural sinus and ventricles; red = choroid plexus of third and fourth ventricles; arrows = flow of cerebrospinal fluid.

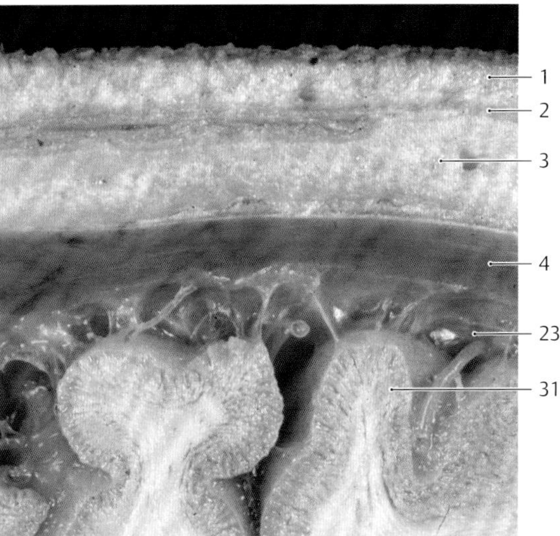


Fig. 9.99 **Cross section of the scalp and the meninges.** The subarachnoid space (23) is shown.

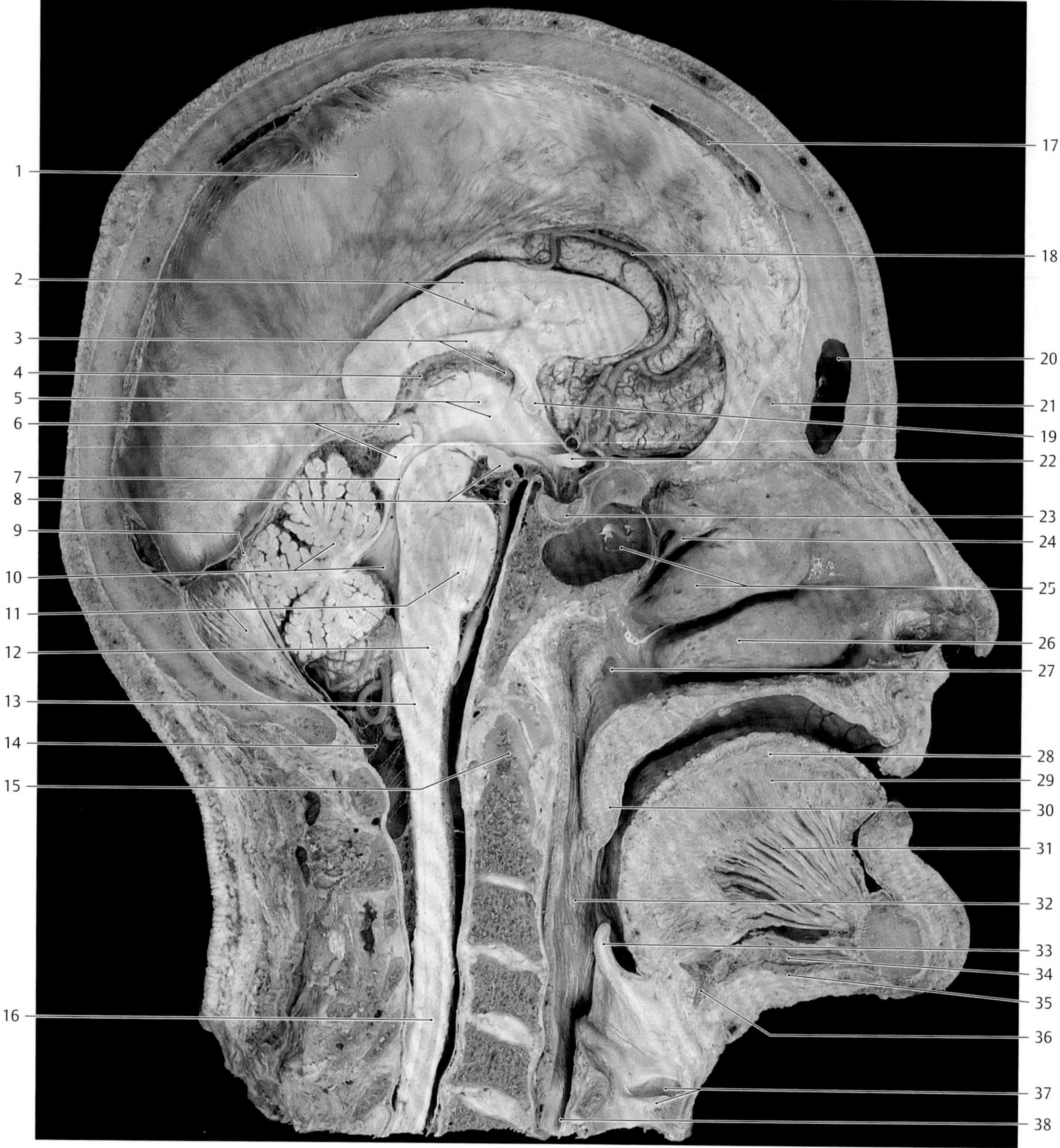


**Fig. 9.100 Median sagittal section through the head and neck.**

1 Falx cerebri
2 Corpus callosum and septum pellucidum
3 Interventricular foramen and fornix
4 Choroid plexus of third ventricle and internal cerebral vein
5 Third ventricle and interthalamic adhesion
6 Pineal body and colliculi of the midbrain
7 Cerebral aqueduct
8 Mamillary body and basilar artery
9 Straight sinus
10 Fourth ventricle and cerebellum
11 Pons and falx cerebelli
12 Medulla oblongata
13 Central canal
14 Cerebellomedullary cistern
15 Dens of the axis (odontoid process)
16 Spinal cord
17 Superior sagittal sinus
18 Anterior cerebral artery
19 Anterior commissure
20 Frontal sinus
21 Crista galli
22 Optic chiasma
23 Pituitary gland (hypophysis)
24 Superior nasal concha
25 Middle nasal concha and sphenoid sinus
26 Inferior nasal concha
27 Pharyngeal opening of auditory tube
28 Superior longitudinal muscle of tongue
29 Vertical muscle of the tongue
30 Uvula
31 Genioglossus muscle
32 Pharynx
33 Epiglottis
34 Geniohyoid muscle
35 Mylohyoid muscle
36 Hyoid bone
37 Vocal fold and sinus of larynx
38 Esophagus

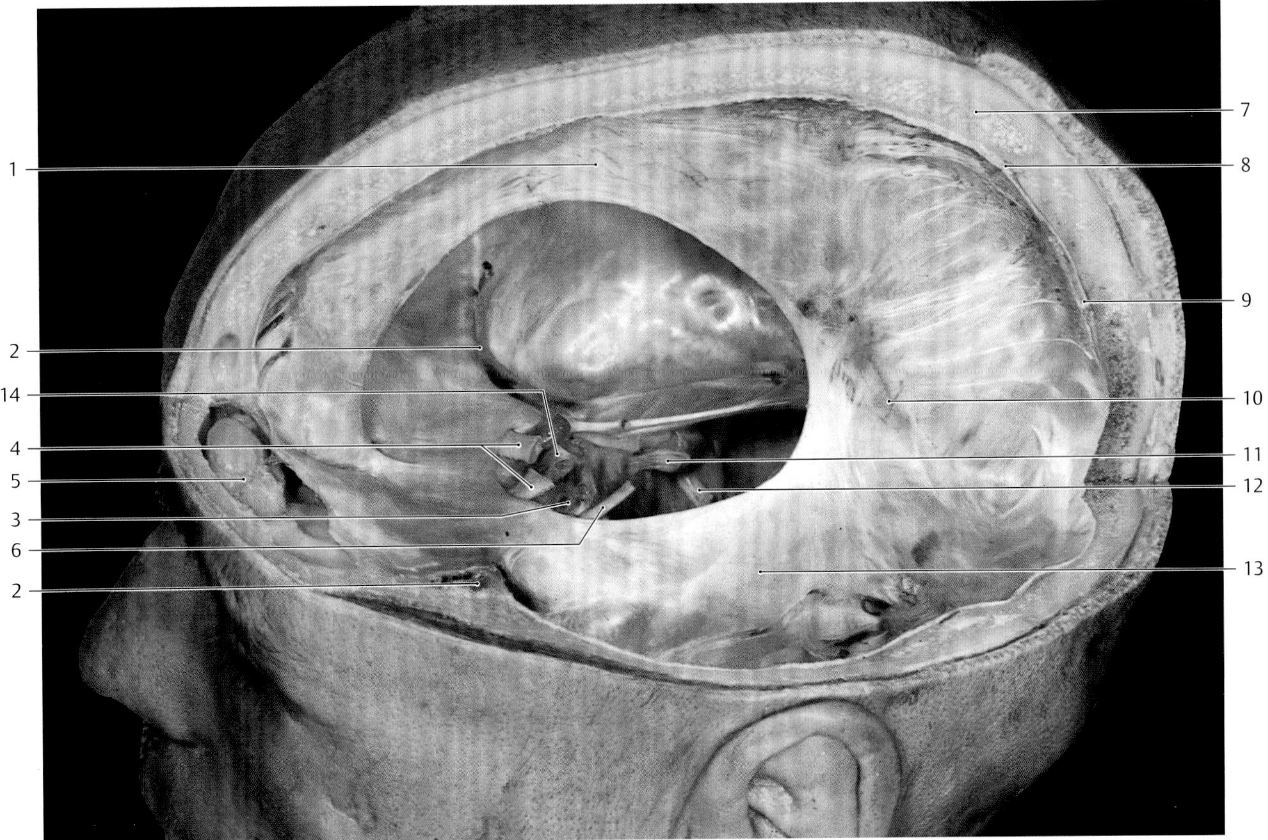


Fig. 9.101 **Dura mater and venous sinuses of the dura mater** (oblique-lateral aspect). The brain has been removed.

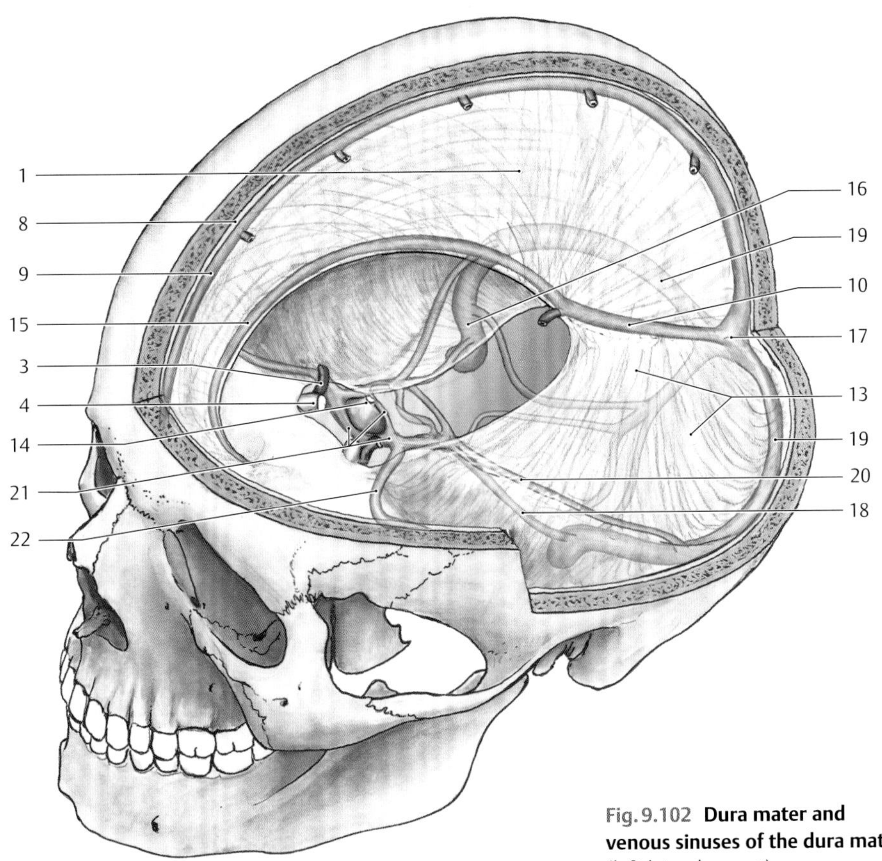


1 Falx cerebri
2 Position of middle meningeal artery and vein
3 Internal carotid artery
4 Optic nerve (CN II)
5 Frontal sinus
6 Oculomotor nerve (CN III)
7 Diploë
8 Dura mater
9 Superior sagittal sinus
10 Straight sinus
11 Trigeminal nerve (CN V)
12 Facial and vestibulocochlear nerve (CN VII and CN VIII)
13 Cerebellar tentorium
14 Pituitary gland (hypophysis)
15 Inferior sagittal sinus
16 Sigmoid sinus
17 Confluence of sinuses
18 Inferior petrosal sinus
19 Transverse sinus
20 Superior petrosal sinus
21 Cavernous and intercavernous sinuses
22 Sphenoparietal sinus

Fig. 9.102 **Dura mater and venous sinuses of the dura mater** (left lateral aspect).

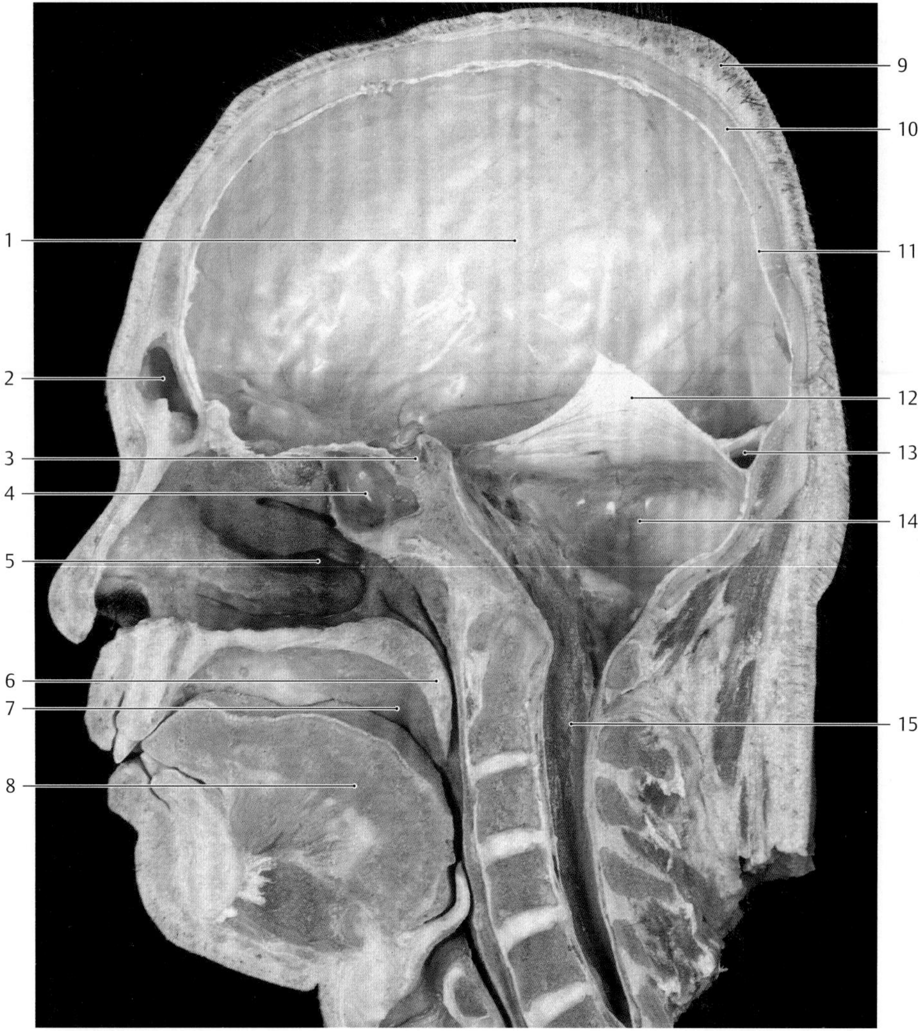


Fig. 9.103 **Median section through the head. Demonstration of dura mater covering the cranial cavity** (right half of the head). The brain and spinal cord have been removed.

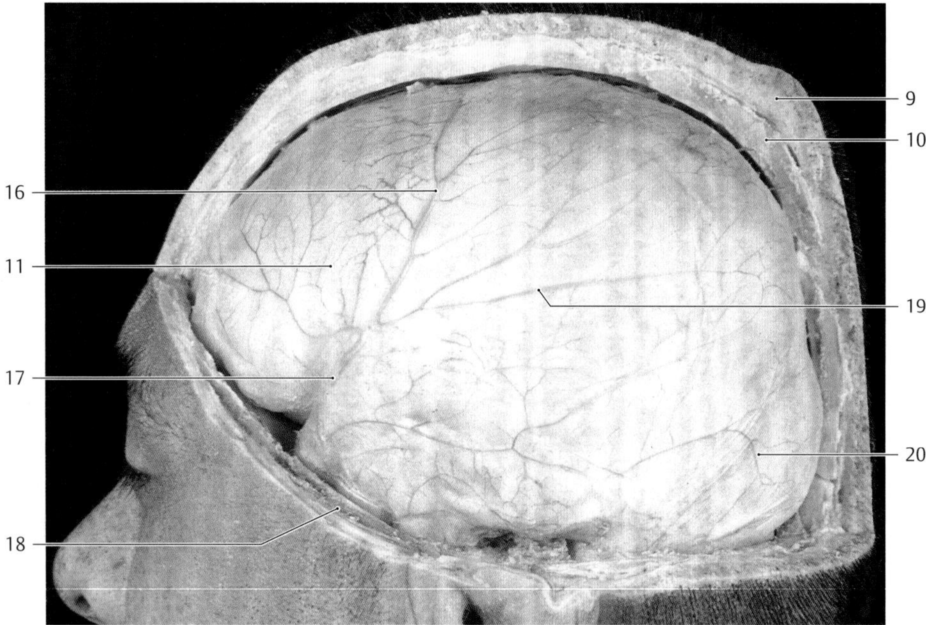


Fig. 9.104 **Dissection of dura mater and meningeal vessels.** The left half of the calvaria has been removed.

1 Cranial cavity with dura mater (right cerebral hemisphere has been removed)
2 Frontal sinus
3 Hypophysial fossa with pituitary gland
4 Sphenoidal sinus
5 Nasal cavity
6 Soft palate (uvula)
7 Oral cavity
8 Tongue
9 Skin
10 Calvaria
11 Dura mater
12 Cerebellar tentorium
13 Confluence of sinuses
14 Infratentorial space (cerebellum and part of the brainstem have been removed)
15 Vertebral canal
16 Frontal branch of middle meningeal artery and veins
17 Middle meningeal artery
18 Diploë
19 Parietal branch of middle meningeal artery and vein
20 Occipital pole of left hemisphere covered with dura mater

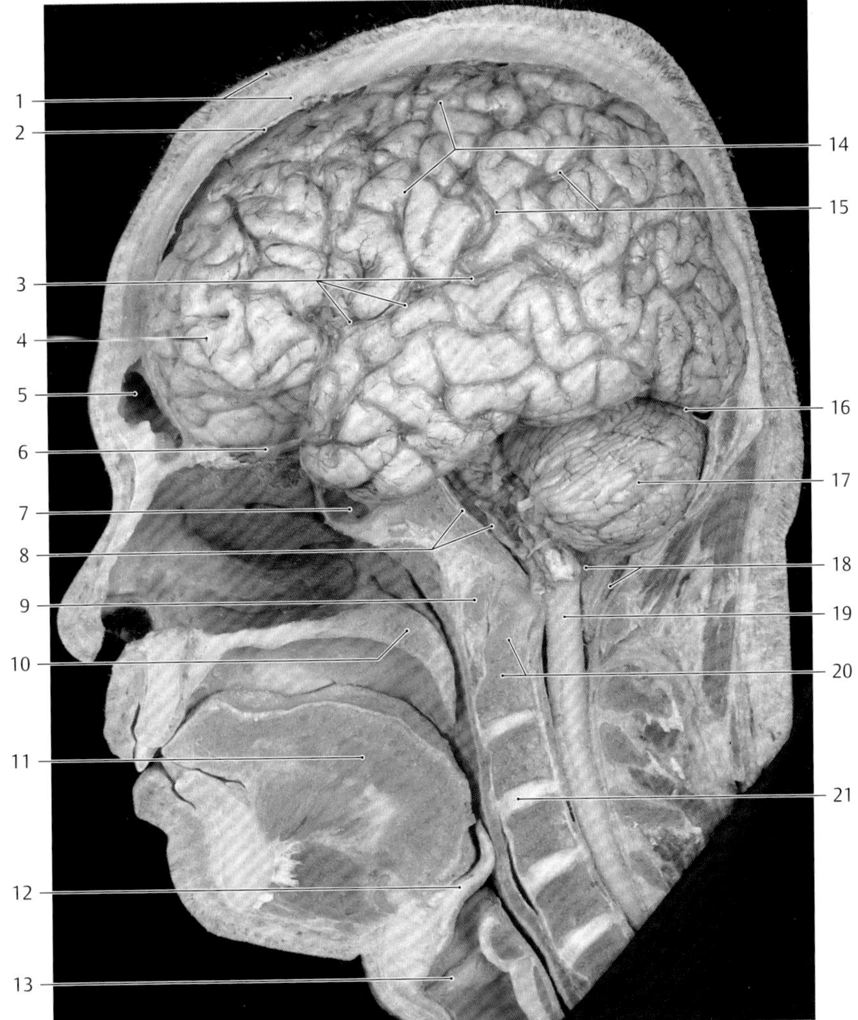


1 Calvaria and skin of the scalp
2 Dura mater (divided)
3 Position of lateral sulcus
4 Frontal lobe covered by arachnoid and pia mater
5 Frontal sinus
6 Olfactory bulb
7 Sphenoidal sinus
8 Dura mater on clivus and basilar artery
9 Atlas (anterior arch, divided)
10 Soft palate
11 Tongue
12 Epiglottis
13 Vocal fold
14 Position of central sulcus
15 Superior cerebral veins
16 Tentorium (divided)
17 Cerebellum
18 Cerebellomedullary cistern
19 Position of foramen magnum and spinal cord
20 Dens of axis
21 Intervertebral disc

Fig. 9.105 **Dissection of the brain with pia mater and arachnoid in situ.** The head has been cut in half except for the brain, which is shown in its entirety.

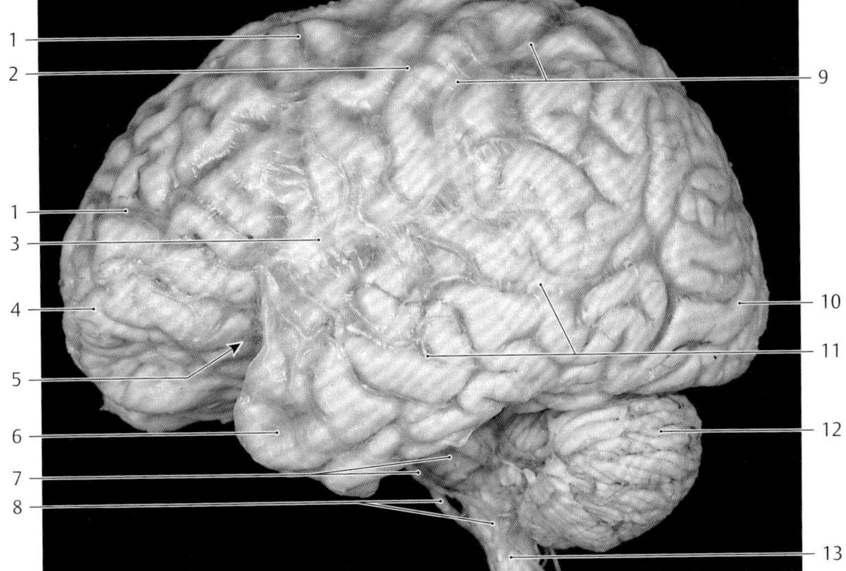


1 Superior cerebral veins
2 Position of central sulcus
3 Position of lateral sulcus and cistern of lateral cerebral fossa
4 Frontal pole
5 Lateral sulcus (arrow)
6 Temporal pole
7 Pons and basilar artery
8 Vertebral arteries
9 Superior anastomotic vein
10 Occipital pole
11 Inferior cerebral veins
12 Hemisphere of cerebellum
13 Medulla oblongata

Fig. 9.106 **Brain with pia mater and arachnoid.** Frontal pole to the left (lateral aspect).

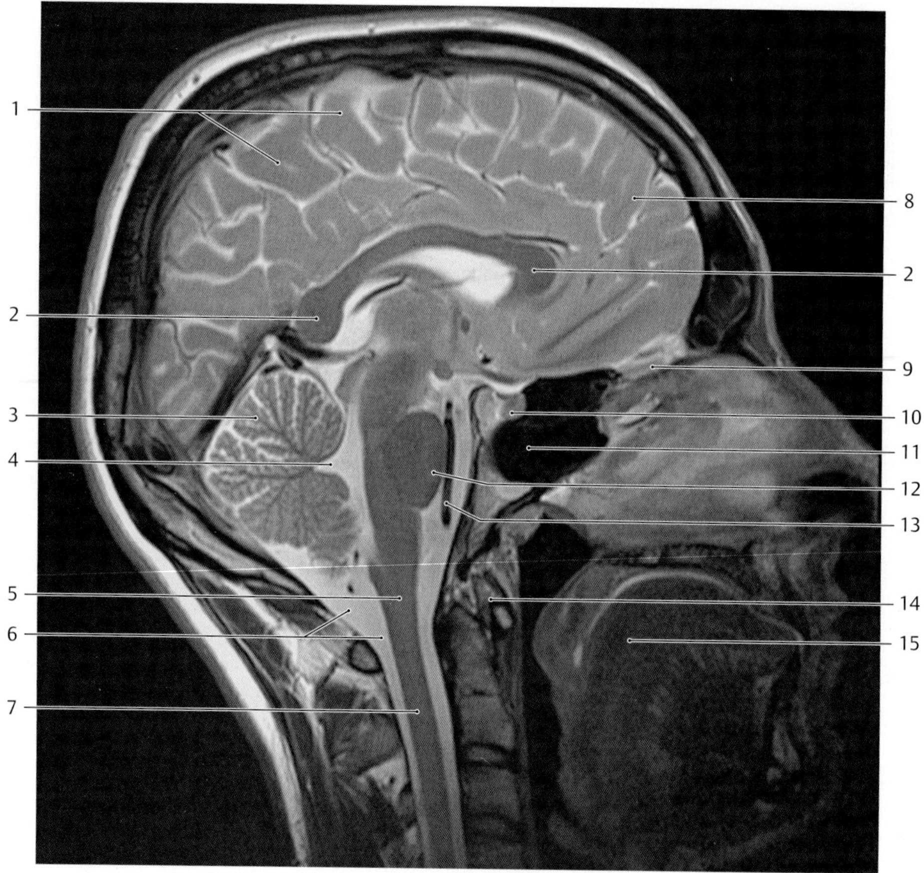


1 Parietal lobe
2 Corpus callosum
3 Cerebellum
4 Fourth ventricle
5 Medulla oblongata
6 Cerebellomedullar cistern
7 Spinal cord
8 Frontal lobe
9 Olfactory bulb
10 Hypophysial fossa (sella turcica) with pituitary gland
11 Sphenoid sinus
12 Pons
13 Basilar artery
14 Ligaments to the dens of axis
15 Tongue

Fig. 9.107 **Median section through the head** (MRI scan). (Courtesy of Prof. Uder, Institute of Radiology, University Hospital Erlangen, Germany.)

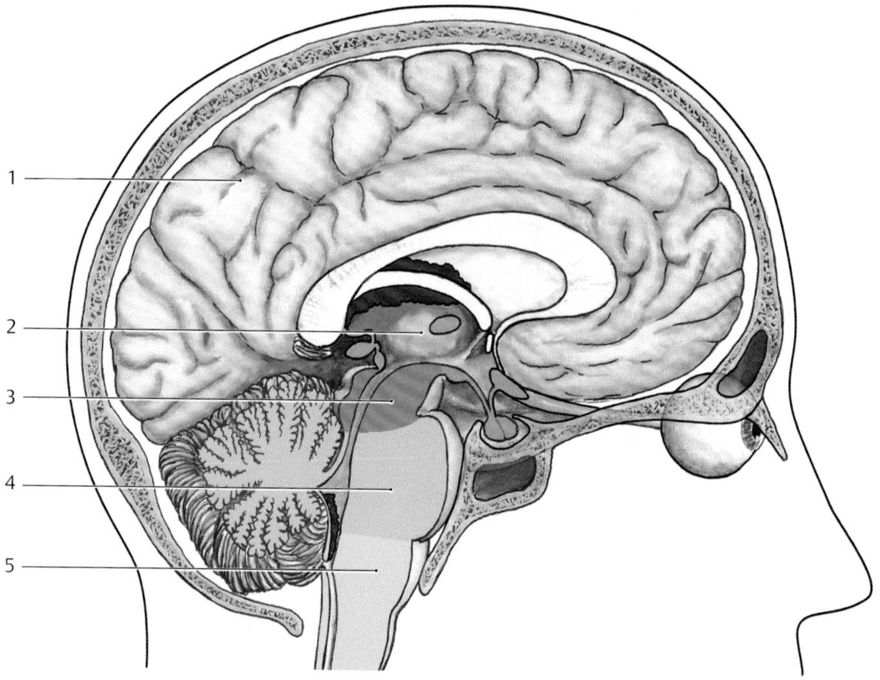

1 Telencephalon (yellow) with lateral ventricles
2 Diencephalon (orange) with third ventricle, optic nerve, and retina
3 Mesencephalon (blue) with cerebral aqueduct
4 Metencephalon (green) with fourth ventricle
5 Myelencephalon (yellow-green)

Fig. 9.108 **Median section through the head with colored highlighting of the brain divisions.** Red = choroid plexus.

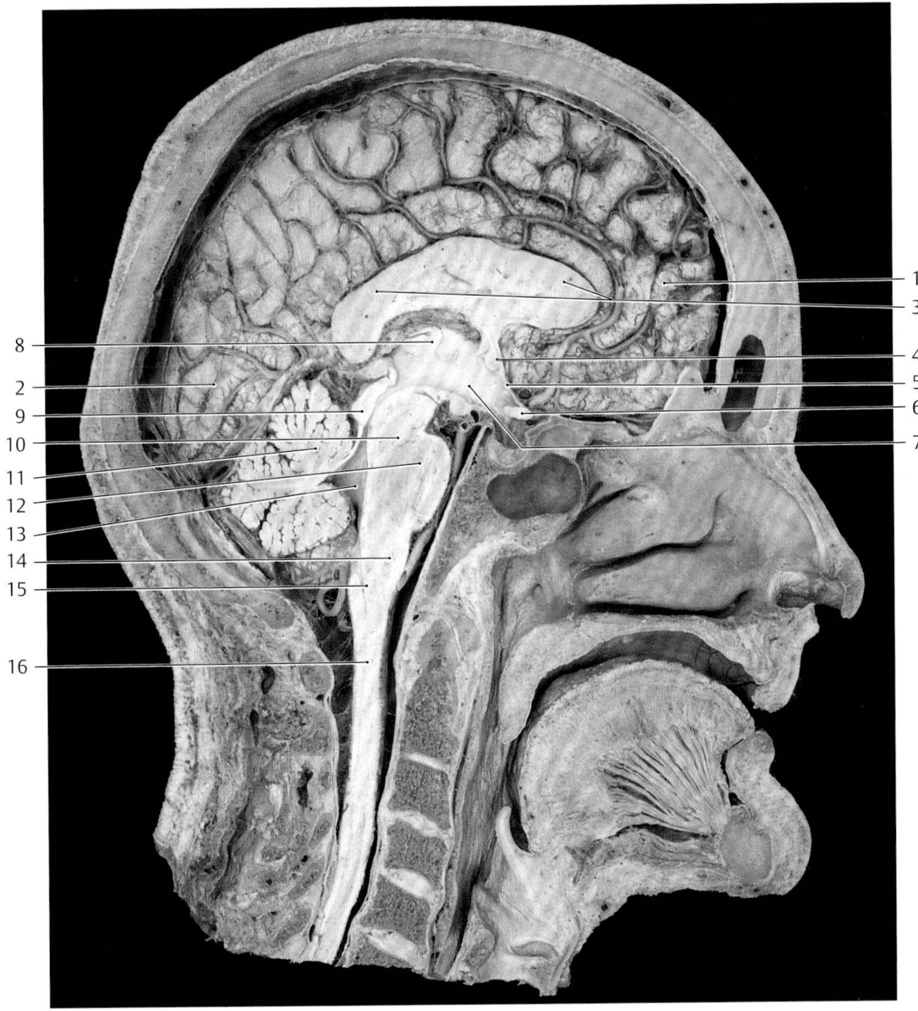


1 Frontal lobe of cerebrum
2 Occipital lobe of cerebrum
3 Corpus callosum
4 Anterior commissure
5 Lamina terminalis
6 Optic chiasma
7 Hypothalamus
8 Thalamus and third ventricle
9 Colliculi of the midbrain
10 Midbrain (inferior portion)
11 Cerebellum
12 Pons
13 Fourth ventricle
14 Medulla oblongata
15 Central canal
16 Spinal cord

Fig. 9.109 **Median section through the head.** Regions of the brain. The falx cerebri has been removed.

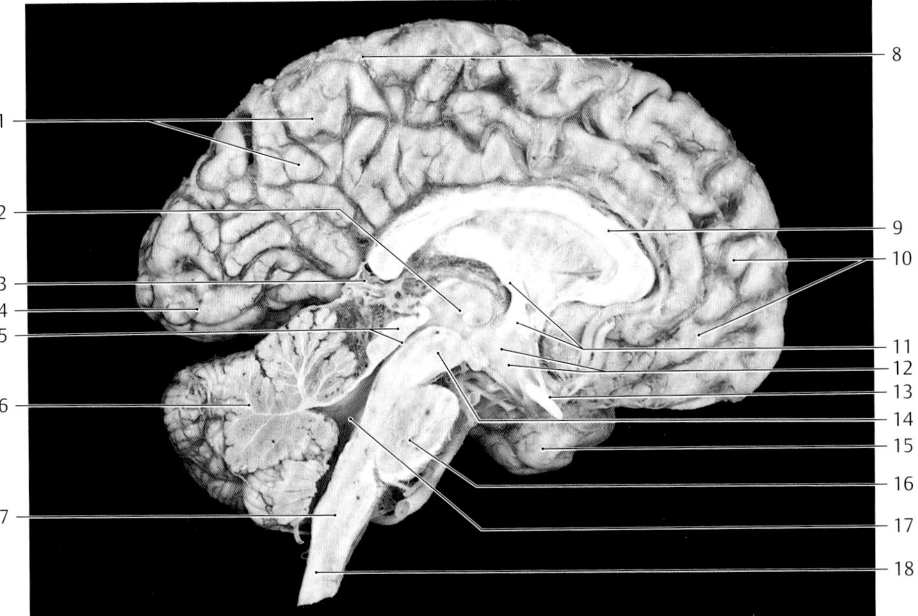


1 Parietal lobe
2 Thalamus and third ventricle
3 Great cerebral vein
4 Occipital lobe
5 Colliculi of the midbrain and cerebral aqueduct
6 Cerebellum
7 Medulla oblongata
8 Central sulcus
9 Corpus callosum
10 Frontal lobe
11 Fornix and anterior commissure
12 Hypothalamus
13 Optic chiasma
14 Midbrain
15 Temporal lobe
16 Pons
17 Fourth ventricle
18 Spinal cord

Fig. 9.110 **Median section through brain and brainstem.** Frontal pole to the right.

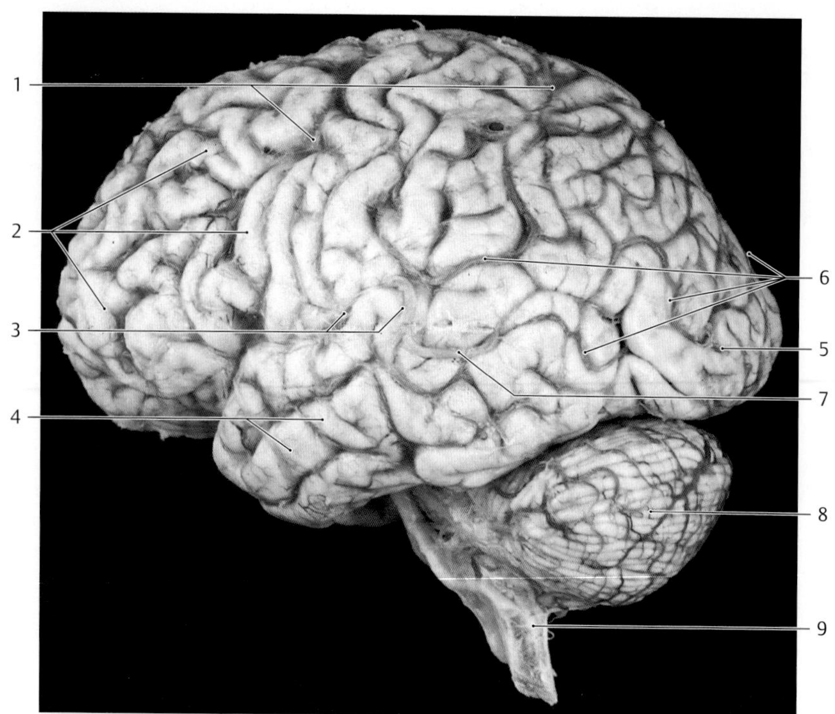


1 Superior cerebral veins and parietal lobe
2 Frontal lobe
3 Superficial middle cerebral vein and cistern of lateral cerebral fossa
4 Temporal lobe
5 Occipital lobe
6 Inferior cerebral veins and transverse occipital sulcus
7 Inferior anastomotic vein
8 Cerebellum
9 Medulla oblongata

Fig. 9.111 **Brain with pia mater and arachnoid** (lateral aspect). **Cerebral veins** (bluish). In the lateral sulcus the cistern of the lateral fossa is recognizable. Frontal lobe to the left.

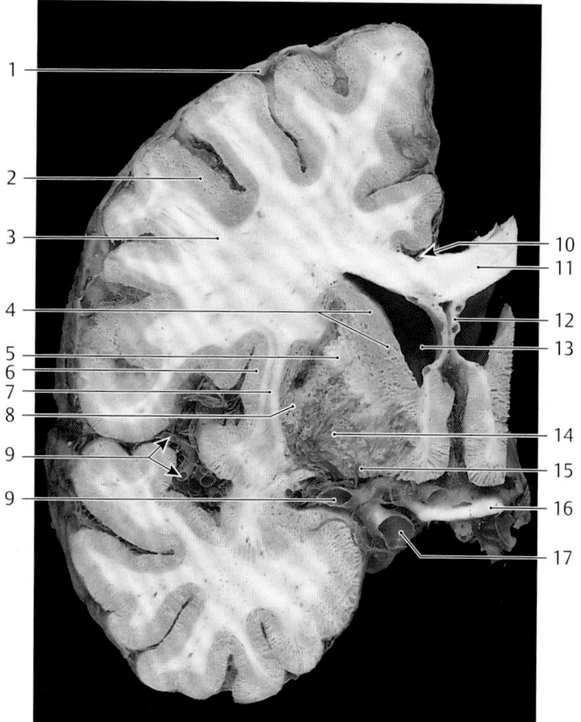


Fig. 9.112 **Coronal section through the right hemisphere,** showing arachnoid, pia mater, and the arterial blood supply (anterior aspect).

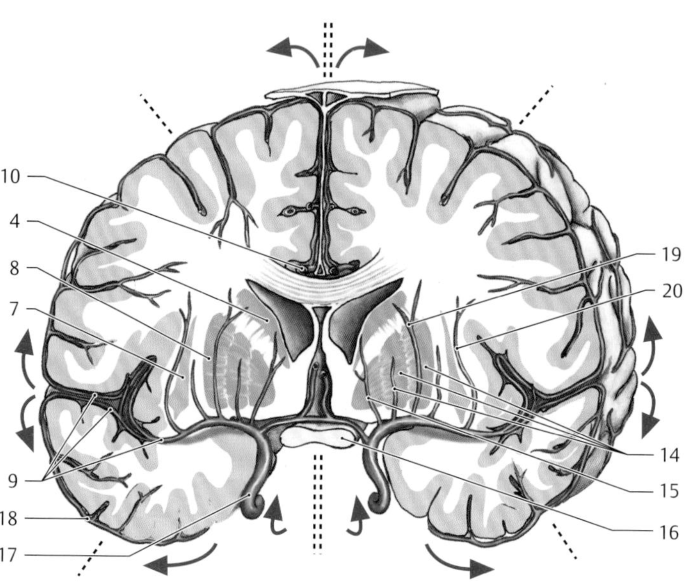


Fig. 9.113 **Arteries of the brain** (coronal section). Areas supplied by cortical and central arteries. Dotted lines = boundaries of arterial supply; arrows = direction of blood flow.

1 Arachnoid
2 Cortex
3 Frontal lobe (white matter)
4 Caudate nucleus
5 Internal capsule
6 Insular lobe
7 Claustrum
8 Putamen
9 Middle cerebral arteries
10 Anterior cerebral artery
11 Corpus callosum
12 Septum pellucidum
13 Lateral ventricle
14 Globus pallidus and pallidostriate artery
15 Thalamic artery
16 Optic chiasma
17 Internal carotid artery
18 Posterior cerebral artery
19 Posterior striate branch
20 Insular artery

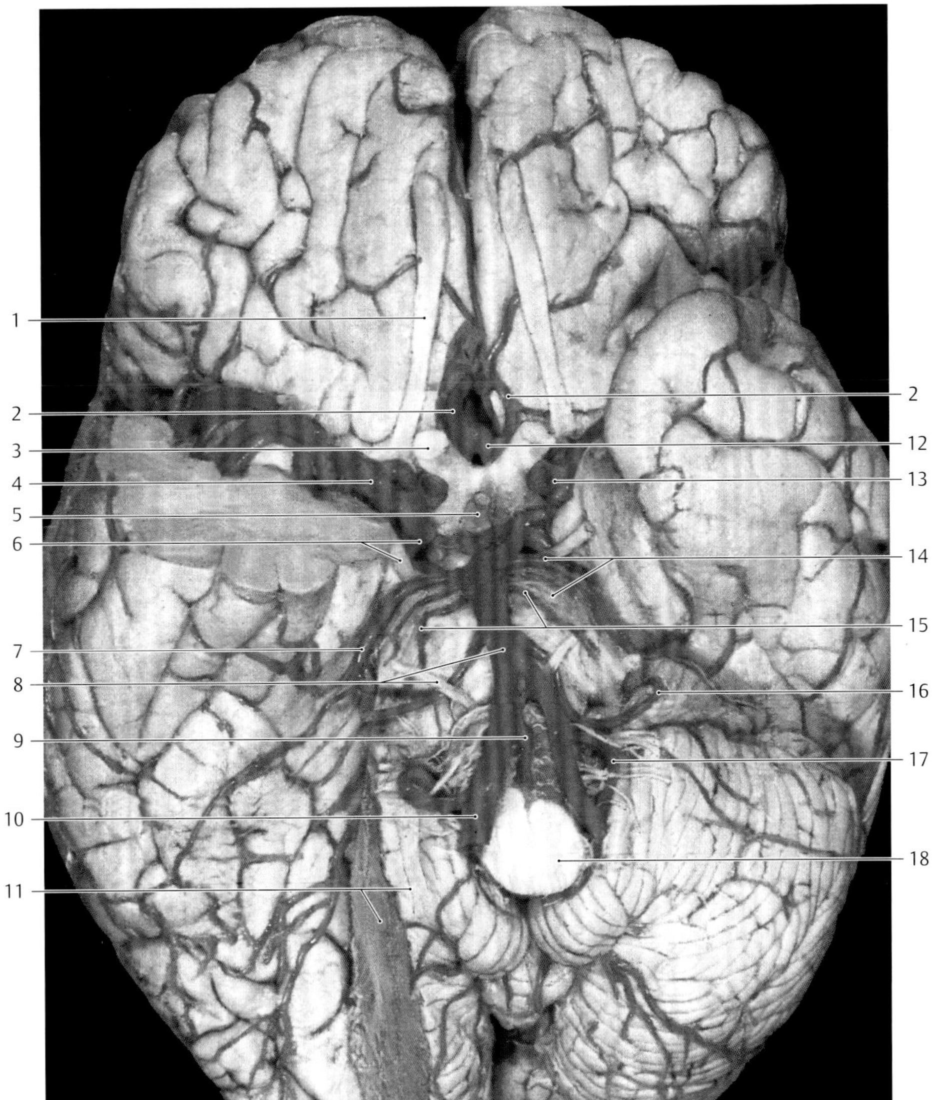


**Fig. 9.114 Arteries of the brain** (inferior aspect, frontal pole above). The right temporal lobe and cerebellum have been partly removed.

1 Olfactory tract
2 Anterior cerebral artery
3 Optic nerve (CN II)
4 Middle cerebral artery
5 Infundibulum
6 Oculomotor nerve (CN III) and posterior communicating artery
7 Posterior cerebral artery
8 Basilar artery and abducent nerve (CN VI)
9 Anterior spinal artery
10 Vertebral artery
11 Cerebellum
12 Anterior communicating artery
13 Internal carotid artery
14 Superior cerebellar artery and pons
15 Labyrinthine arteries
16 Inferior anterior cerebellar artery
17 Inferior posterior cerebellar artery
18 Medulla oblongata
19 Supratrochlear artery
20 Anterior ciliary arteries
21 Lacrimal artery
22 Posterior ciliary arteries
23 Ophthalmic artery with central retinal artery
24 Trigeminal nerve (CN V)
25 Facial nerve (CN VII) and vestibulocochlear nerve (CN VIII)
26 Glossopharyngeal nerve (CN IX), vagus nerve (CN X), and accessory nerve (CN XI)
27 Olfactory bulb
28 Posterior spinal artery

**Fig. 9.115 Arteries of the brain** (inferior aspect). The right temporal lobe and cerebellum have been partly removed. Note the arterial circle of Willis around the infundibulum.

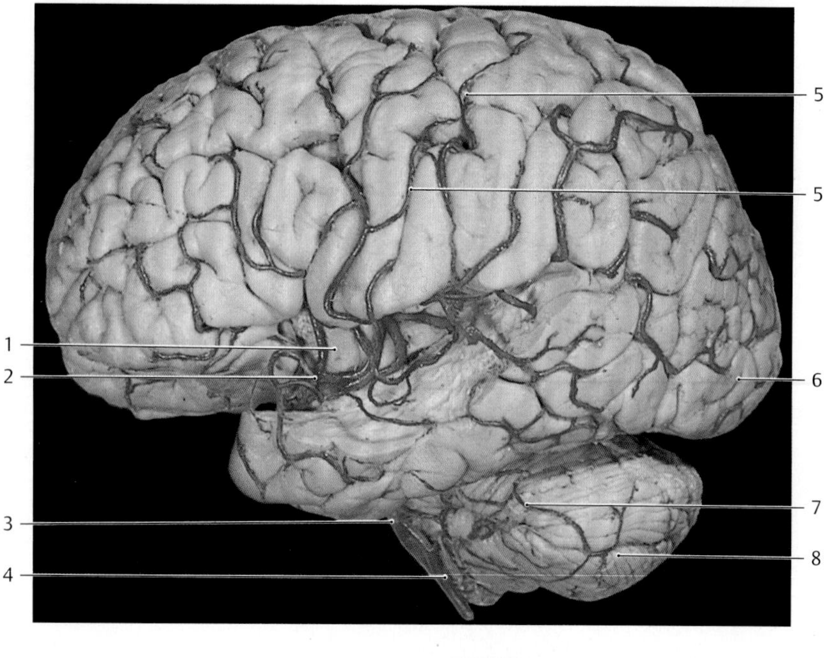


**Fig. 9.116 Arteries of the brain** (lateral aspect of the left hemisphere). The upper part of the temporal lobe has been removed to display the insula and cerebral arteries (injected with red resin).

1 Insula
2 Middle cerebral artery with two branches:
(a) Parietal branches
(b) Temporal branches
3 Basilar artery
4 Vertebral artery
5 Central sulcus
6 Occipital lobe
7 Superior cerebellar artery
8 Cerebellum
9 Anterior cerebral artery
10 Ethmoidal arteries
11 Ophthalmic artery
12 Internal carotid artery
13 Posterior communicating artery
14 Posterior cerebral artery
15 Anterior inferior cerebellar artery
16 Posterior inferior cerebellar artery

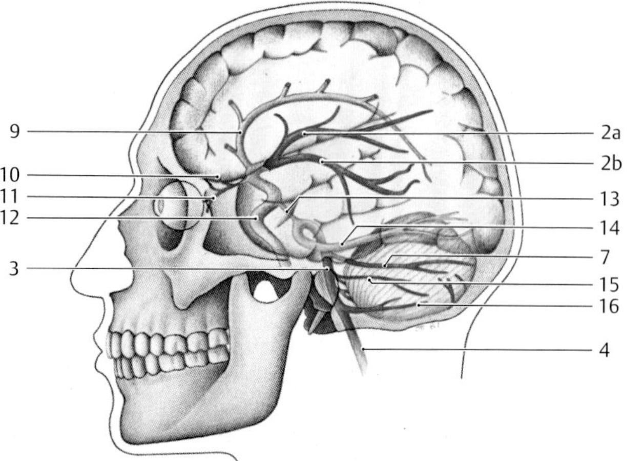


**Fig. 9.117 Arteries of the brain** (lateral aspect).

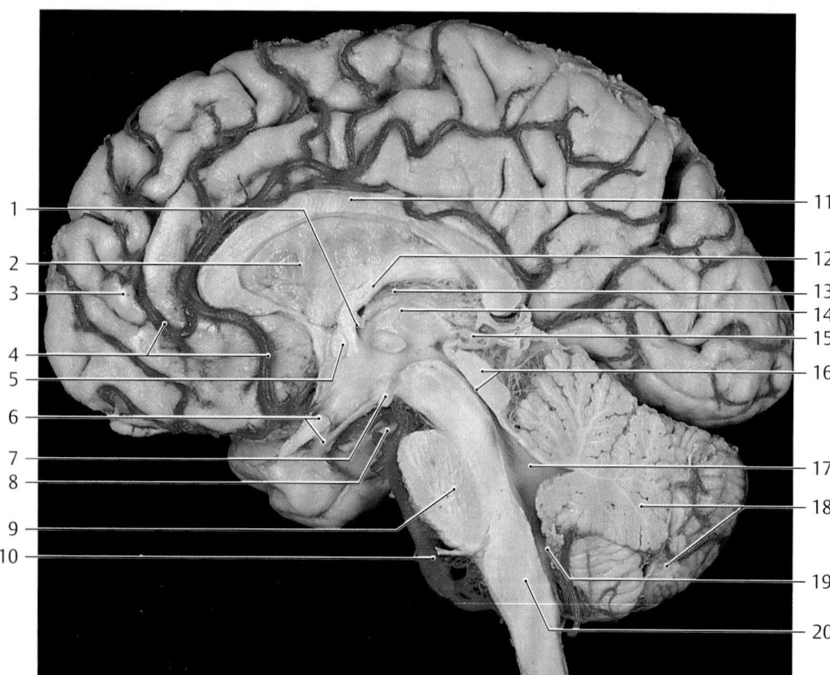


1 Interventricular foramen
2 Septum pellucidum
3 Frontal lobe
4 Anterior cerebral artery
5 Anterior commissure
6 Optic chiasma and infundibulum
7 Mamillary body
8 Oculomotor nerve (CN III)
9 Pons
10 Basilar artery
11 Corpus callosum
12 Fornix
13 Choroid plexus
14 Third ventricle
15 Pineal body
16 Tectum and cerebral aqueduct
17 Fourth ventricle
18 Cerebellum (arbor vitae, vermis)
19 Median aperture of Magendie
20 Medulla oblongata

**Fig. 9.118 Median section through the brain and brainstem.** Cerebral arteries have been injected with red resin.

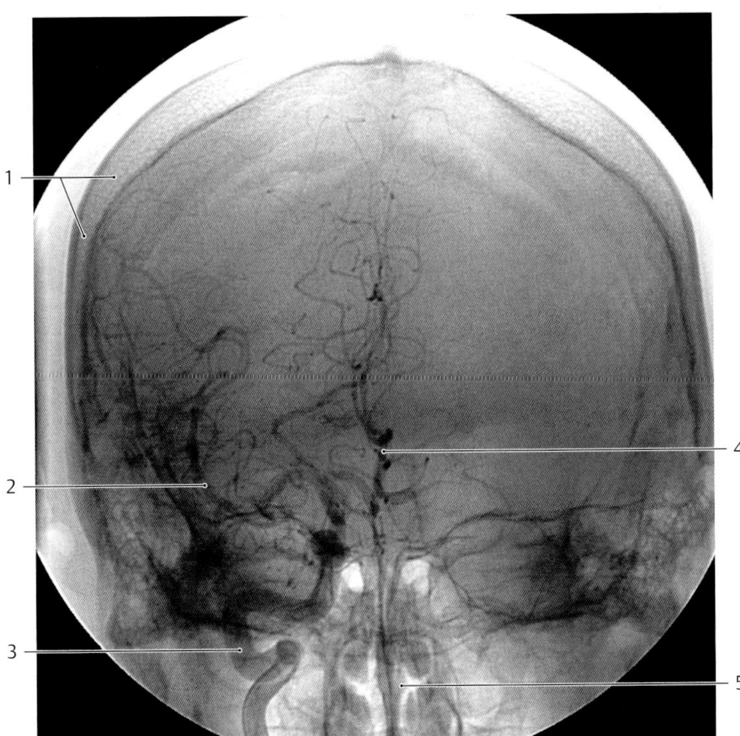


**Fig. 9.119 Arteriogram of the internal carotid artery** (anterior aspect, right side). (Courtesy of Dr. Wieners, Department of Radiology, Charité Universitätsmedizin, Berlin, Germany.)

1 Skull diploe
2 Middle cerebral artery
3 Internal carotid artery
4 Anterior cerebral artery
5 Nasal cavity
6 Arterial circle of Willis
7 Vertebral artery
8 Common carotid artery
9 Subclavian artery
10 Posterior communicating artery
11 Posterior cerebral artery
12 Basilar artery
13 Aortic arch

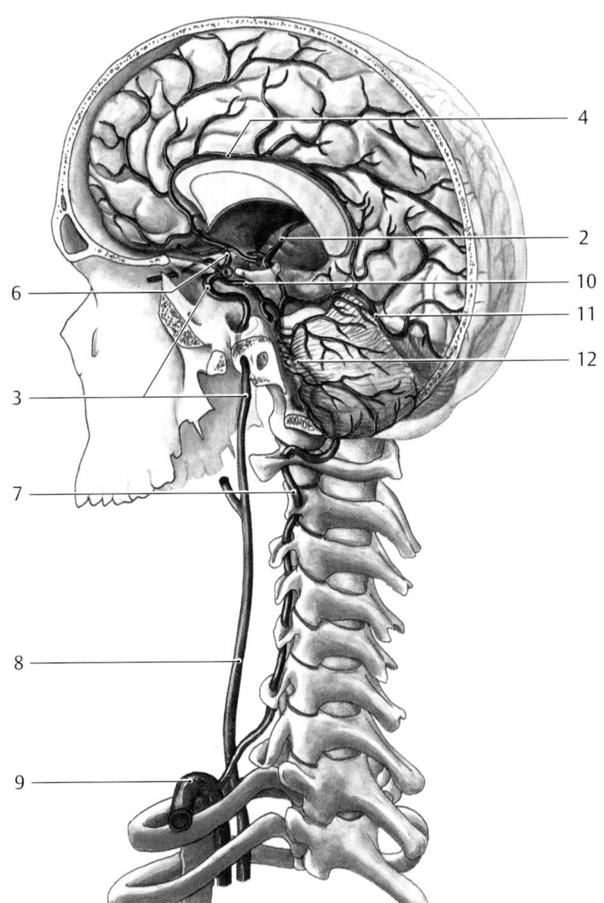


**Fig. 9.120 Arteries of the brain.** The left hemisphere and brainstem have been removed. Note the arterial circle of Willis around the sella turcica.

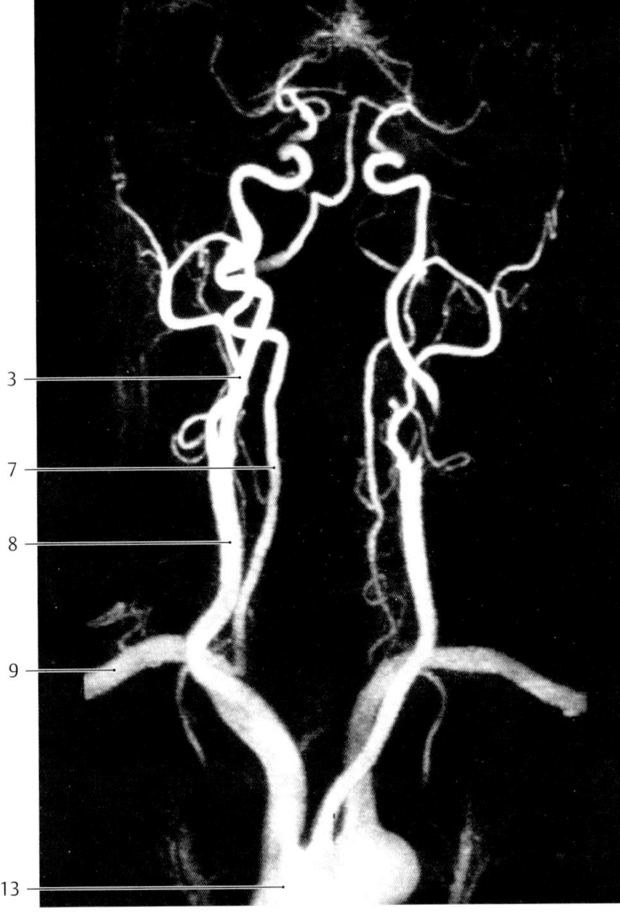


**Fig. 9.121 Main arteries for brain supply** (anterior aspect; MRI angiograph). (Courtesy of Prof. Uder, Institute of Radiology, University Hospital Erlangen, Germany.)

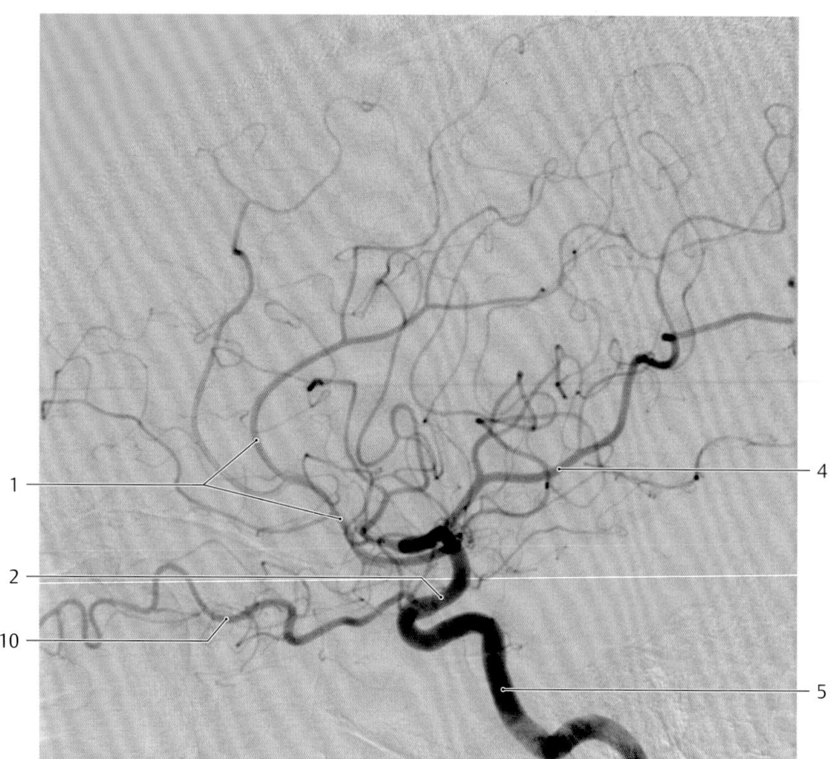


Fig. 9.122 **Arteriogram of the internal carotid artery** (lateral aspect). (Courtesy of Dr. Wieners, Department of Radiology, Charité Universitätsmedizin, Berlin, Germany.)

1 Anterior cerebral artery
2 Loop of the internal carotid artery
3 Middle cerebral artery
4 Posterior cerebral artery
5 Internal carotid artery
6 Superior cerebellar artery
7 Anterior inferior cerebellar artery
8 Posterior inferior cerebellar artery
9 Vertebral artery
10 Ophthalmic artery

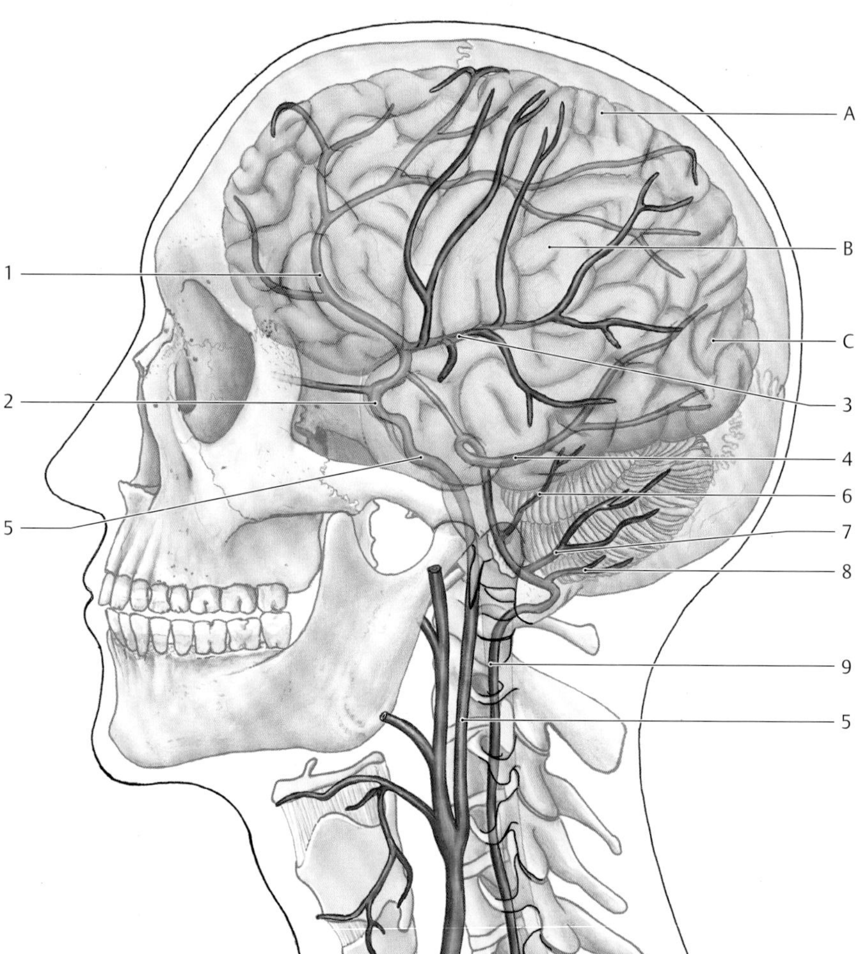


**Areas of blood supply of the brain** (cerebellum = light blue).
A = Anterior cerebral artery (upper and medial parts of the cortex) (orange)
B = Middle cerebral artery (lateral areas of the frontal, parietal, and temporal lobes) (white)
C = Posterior cerebral artery (occipital lobe and inferior parts of the temporal lobe) (blue)

Fig. 9.123 **Arteries of the brain** (lateral aspect). The areas supplied by the main arteries are indicated by different colors.

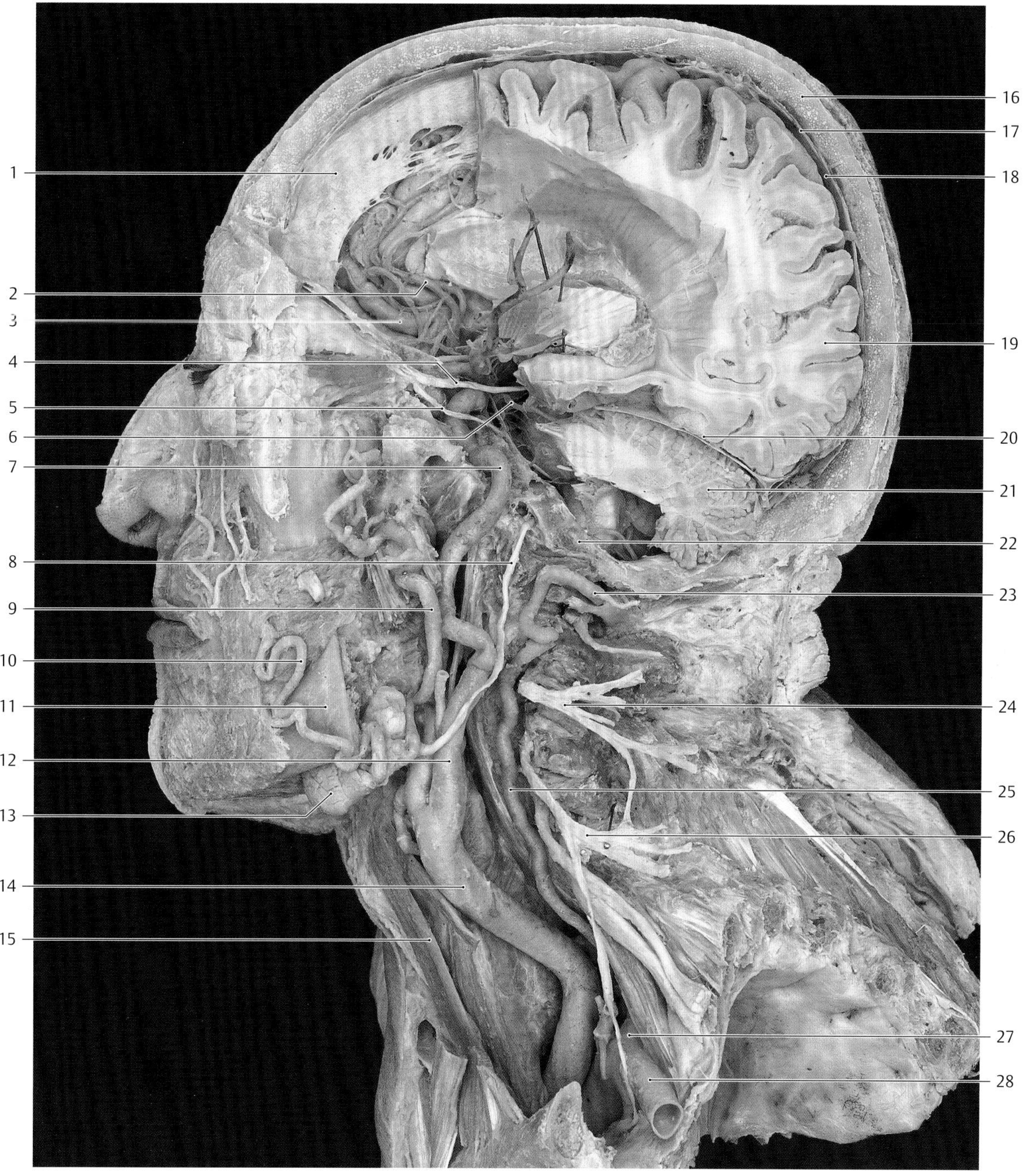


Fig. 9.124 **Dissection of the arteries of the brain and head** (lateral aspect). The superficial layers of facial region and left hemisphere and cerebellum have been partly removed.

1 Falx cerebri
2 Anterior cerebral artery
3 Frontal lobe
4 Oculomotor nerve (CN III)
5 Abducent nerve (CN VI)
6 Posterior cerebral artery
7 Internal carotid artery, entering sinus cavernosus
8 Hypoglossal nerve (CN XII)
9 Maxillary artery
10 Facial artery
11 Mandible
12 External carotid artery
13 Submandibular gland
14 Common carotid artery
15 Sternohyoid muscle
16 Calvaria
17 Dura mater
18 Subarachnoid space
19 Occipital lobe
20 Tentorium of cerebellum
21 Cerebellum
22 Base of skull
23 Vertebral artery (on the posterior arch of the atlas)
24 Cervical plexus
25 Vertebral artery (removed from the cervical vertebrae)
26 Brachial plexus
27 Vertebral artery (branching from the subclavian artery)
28 Subclavian artery

Fig. 9.125 **Dissection of the arterial circle of Willis at the base of the skull** (superior aspect). Calvaria and brain have been removed. Red = arteries; yellow = cranial nerves I–XII.

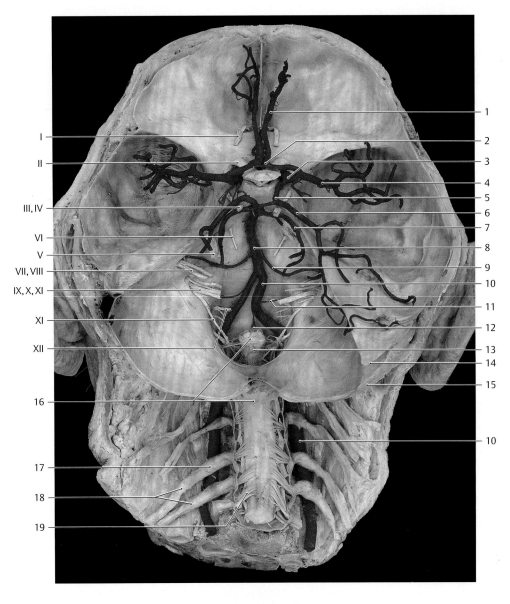

1 Anterior cerebral artery
2 Anterior communicating artery
3 Internal carotid artery
4 Medial cerebral artery
5 Posterior communicating artery
6 Posterior cerebral artery
7 Superior cerebellar artery
8 Basilar artery
9 Anterior inferior cerebellar artery with artery of the labyrinth
10 Vertebral artery
11 Posterior inferior cerebellar artery
12 Anterior spinal artery
13 Pia mater of spinal cord
14 Cerebellar tentorium
15 Dura mater of the cranial cavity
16 Spinal cord
17 Spinal ganglion
18 Spinal nerves (C3, C4)
19 Posterior root filaments (fila radicularia post.)
20 Ophthalmic artery (within the orbit)
21 Internal carotid artery (within carotid canal)

I = Olfactory tract
II = Optic nerve
III = Oculomotor nerve
IV = Trochlear nerve
V = Trigeminal nerve
VI = Abducent nerve
VII = Facial nerve
VIII = Vestibulocochlear nerve
IX = Glossopharyngeal nerve
X = Vagus nerve
XI = Accessory nerve
XII = Hypoglossal nerve

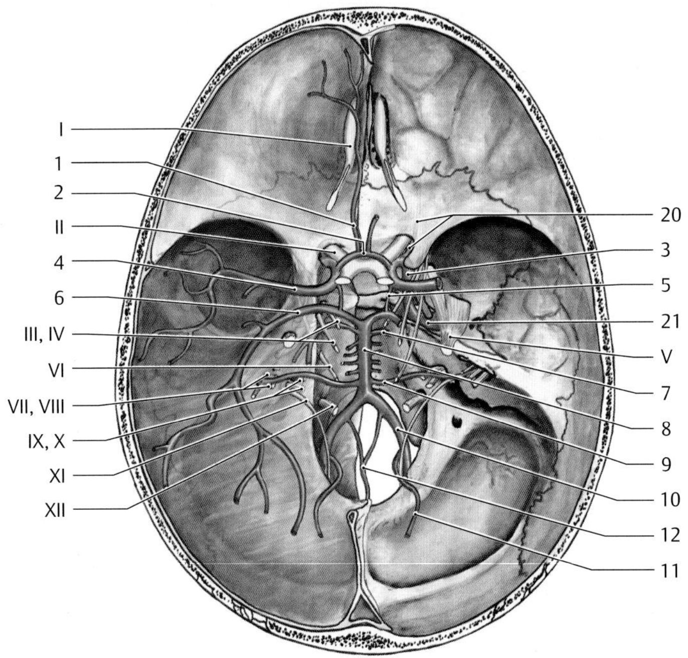


Fig. 9.126 **Arterial circle of Willis at the base of the skull** (superior aspect). Red = arteries; yellow = cranial nerves I–XII.

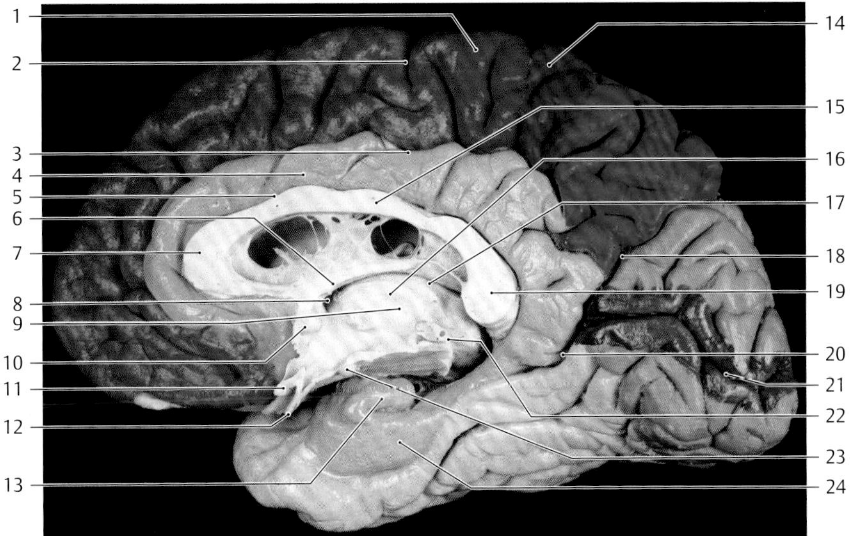


Fig. 9.127 **Brain, right hemisphere** (medial aspect). The midbrain has been divided and the cerebellum and inferior part of the brainstem removed. Frontal pole to the left.

| | | | |
|---|---|---|---|
| Red | = Frontal lobe | Dark blue | = Postcentral lobe |
| Blue | = Parietal lobe | Dark green | = Calcarine sulcus |
| Green | = Occipital lobe | Dark yellow | = Limbic cortex (cingulate and parahippocampal gyri) |
| Yellow | = Temporal lobe | | |
| Dark red | = Precentral lobe | | |

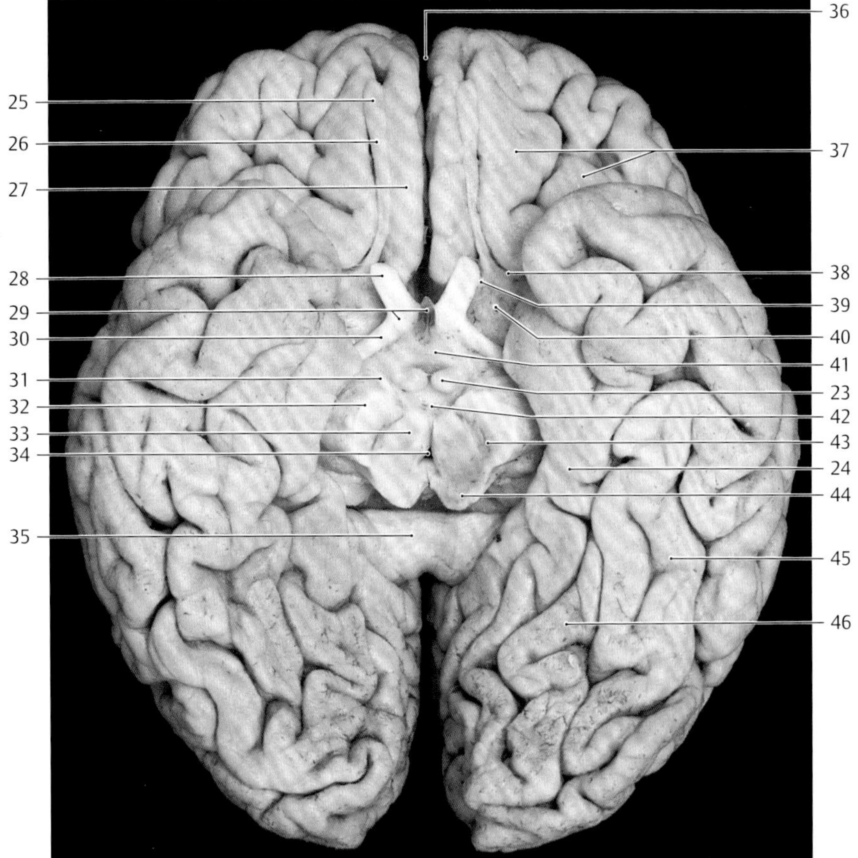


Fig. 9.128 **Brain** (inferior aspect). The midbrain has been divided and the cerebellum and inferior part of the brainstem removed. Frontal pole at the top.

1 Precentral gyrus
2 Precentral sulcus
3 Cingulate sulcus
4 Cingulate gyrus
5 Sulcus of corpus callosum
6 Fornix
7 Genu of corpus callosum
8 Interventricular foramen
9 Intermediate mass
10 Anterior commissure
11 Optic chiasma
12 Infundibulum
13 Uncus hippocampi
14 Postcentral gyrus
15 Body of corpus callosum
16 Third ventricle and thalamus
17 Stria medullaris
18 Parieto-occipital sulcus
19 Splenium of corpus callosum
20 Communication of calcarine and parieto-occipital sulcus
21 Calcarine sulcus
22 Pineal body
23 Mamillary body
24 Parahippocampal gyrus
25 Olfactory bulb
26 Olfactory tract
27 Gyrus rectus
28 Optic nerve
29 Infundibulum and optic chiasma
30 Optic tract
31 Oculomotor nerve
32 Pedunculus cerebri
33 Red nucleus
34 Cerebral aqueduct
35 Corpus callosum
36 Longitudinal fissure
37 Orbital gyri
38 Lateral root of olfactory tract
39 Medial root of olfactory tract
40 Olfactory tubercle and anterior perforated substance
41 Tuber cinereum
42 Interpeduncular fossa
43 Substantia nigra
44 Colliculi of the midbrain
45 Lateral occipitotemporal gyrus
46 Medial occipitotemporal gyrus

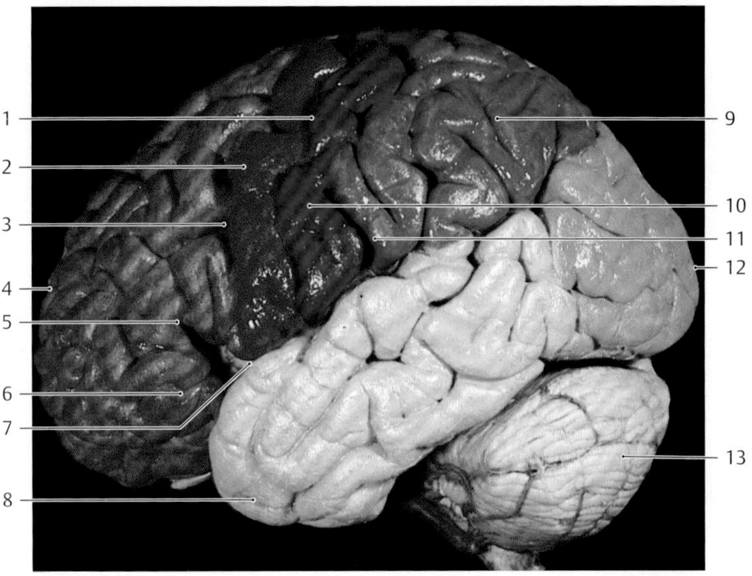


Fig. 9.129 **Brain, left hemisphere** (lateral aspect). Frontal pole to the left.

1 Central sulcus
2 Precentral gyrus
3 Precentral sulcus
4 Frontal lobe
5 Anterior ascending ramus } of lateral sulcus
6 Anterior horizontal ramus } of lateral sulcus
7 Lateral sulcus
8 Temporal lobe
9 Parietal lobe
10 Postcentral gyrus
11 Postcentral sulcus
12 Occipital lobe
13 Cerebellum
14 Superior frontal sulcus
15 Middle frontal gyrus
16 Lunate sulcus
17 Longitudinal fissure
18 Arachnoid granulations

| | | |
|---|---|---|
| Pink | = | Frontal lobe |
| Blue | = | Parietal lobe |
| Green | = | Occipital lobe |
| Yellow | = | Temporal lobe |
| Dark red | = | Precentral gyrus |
| Dark blue | = | Postcentral gyrus |

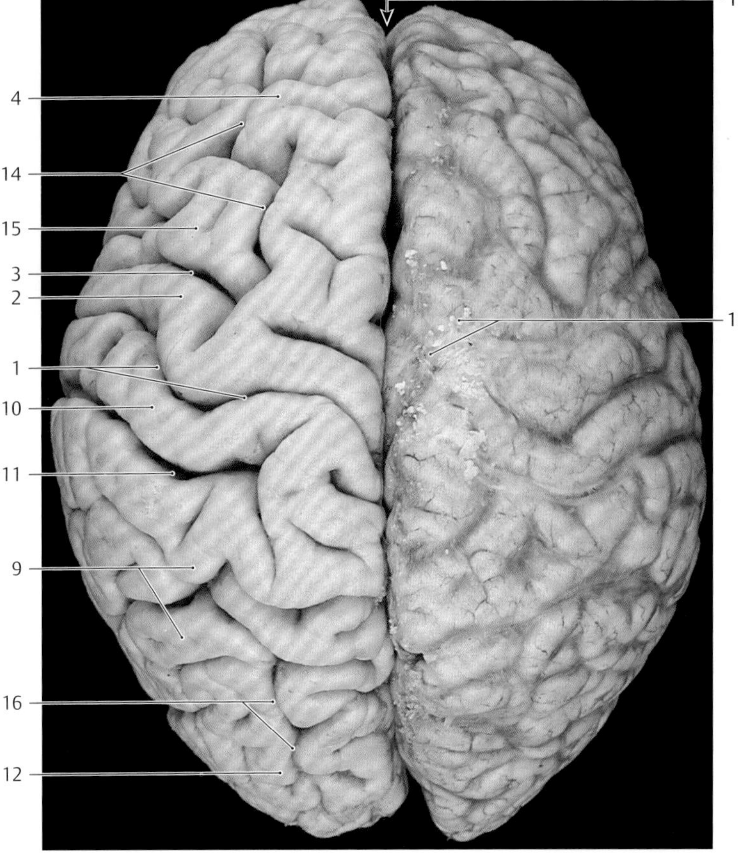


Fig. 9.130 **Brain** (superior aspect). Right hemisphere with arachnoid and pia mater.

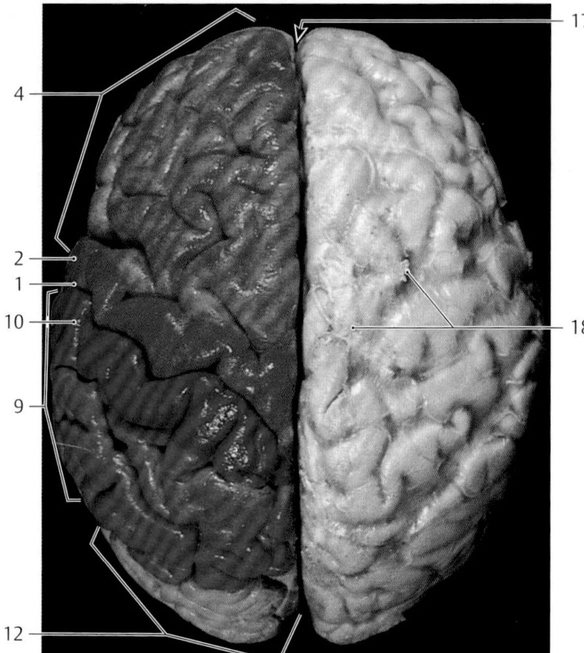


Fig. 9.131 **Brain** (superior aspect). Lobes of the left hemisphere indicated by color; right hemisphere is covered with arachnoid and pia mater.

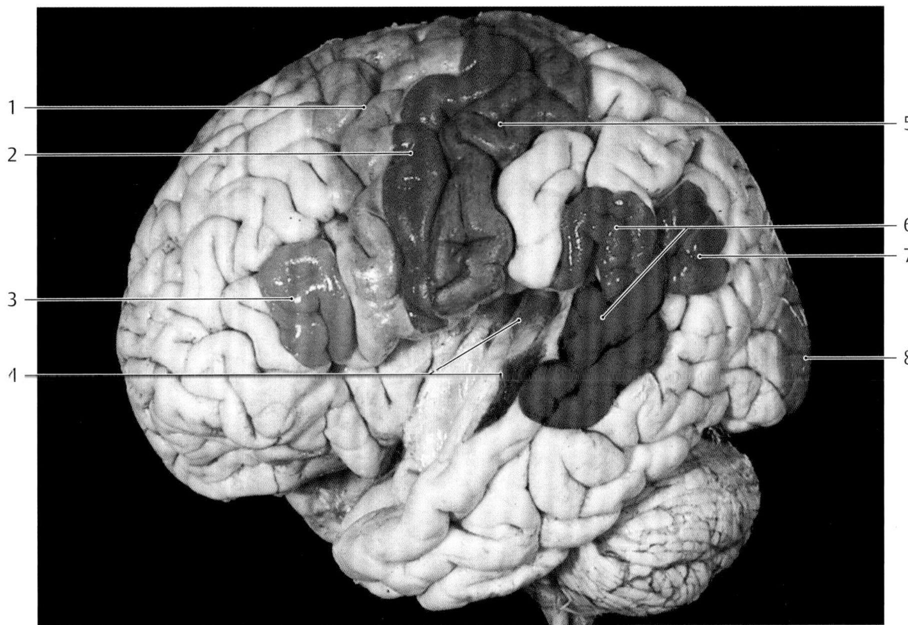


1 Premotor area
2 Somatomotor area
3 Motor speech area of Broca
4 Acoustic area (red: high tone, dark green: low tone)
5 Somatosensory area
6 Sensory speech area of Wernicke
7 Reading comprehension area
8 Visuosensory area

Fig. 9.132 **Brain, left hemisphere** (lateral aspect). **Main cortical areas** are colored. The lateral sulcus has been opened to display the insula and the inner surface of the temporal lobe.

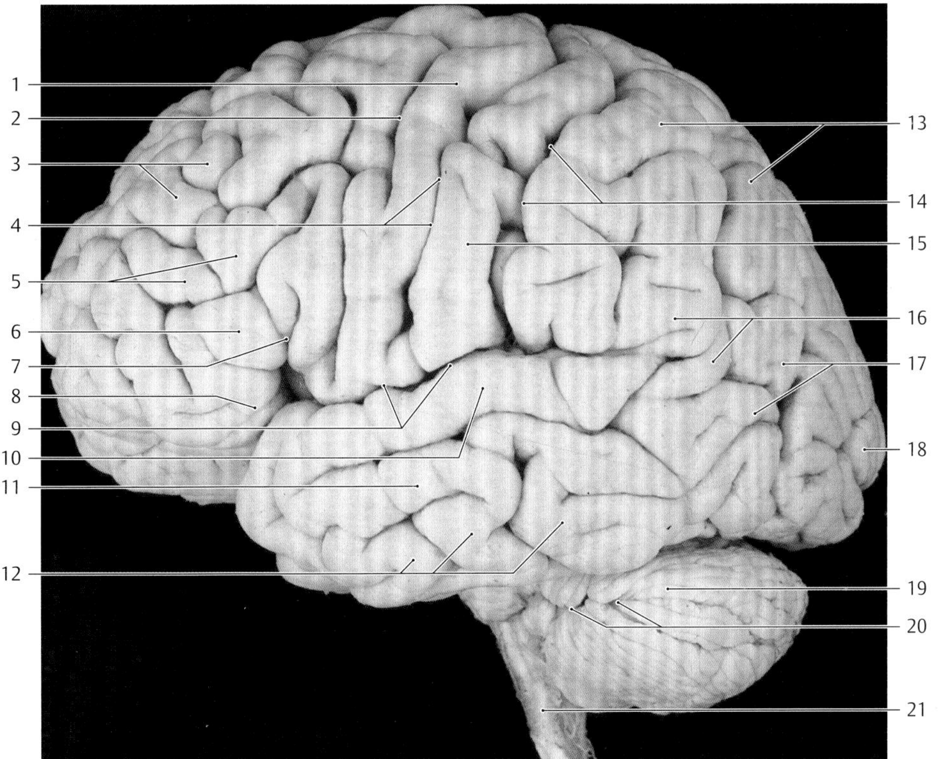


1 Precentral gyrus
2 Precentral sulcus
3 Superior frontal gyrus
4 Central sulcus
5 Middle frontal gyrus
6 Inferior frontal gyrus
7 Ascending ramus } of lateral sulcus
8 Horizontal ramus } of lateral sulcus
9 Posterior ramus } of lateral sulcus
10 Superior temporal gyrus
11 Middle temporal gyrus
12 Inferior temporal gyrus
13 Parietal lobe
14 Postcentral sulcus
15 Postcentral gyrus
16 Supramarginal gyrus
17 Angular gyrus
18 Occipital lobe
19 Cerebellum
20 Horizontal fissure of cerebellum
21 Medulla oblongata

Fig. 9.133 **Brain, left hemisphere** (lateral aspect). Frontal pole to the left.

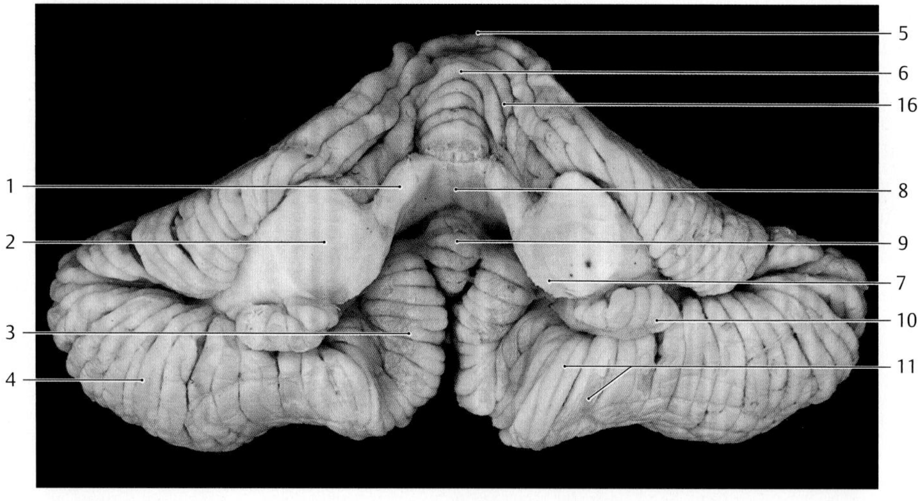


Fig. 9.134 **Cerebellum** (infero-anterior aspect). The cerebellar peduncles have been severed.

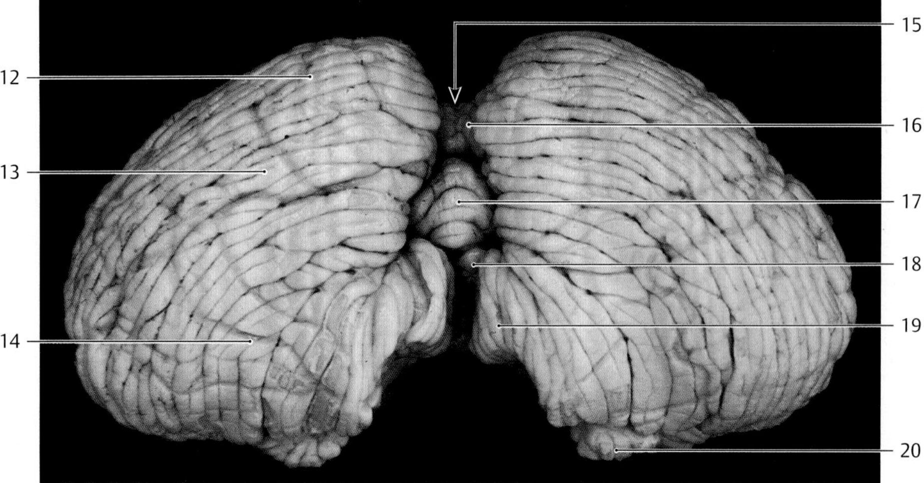


Fig. 9.135 **Cerebellum** (infero-posterior aspect).

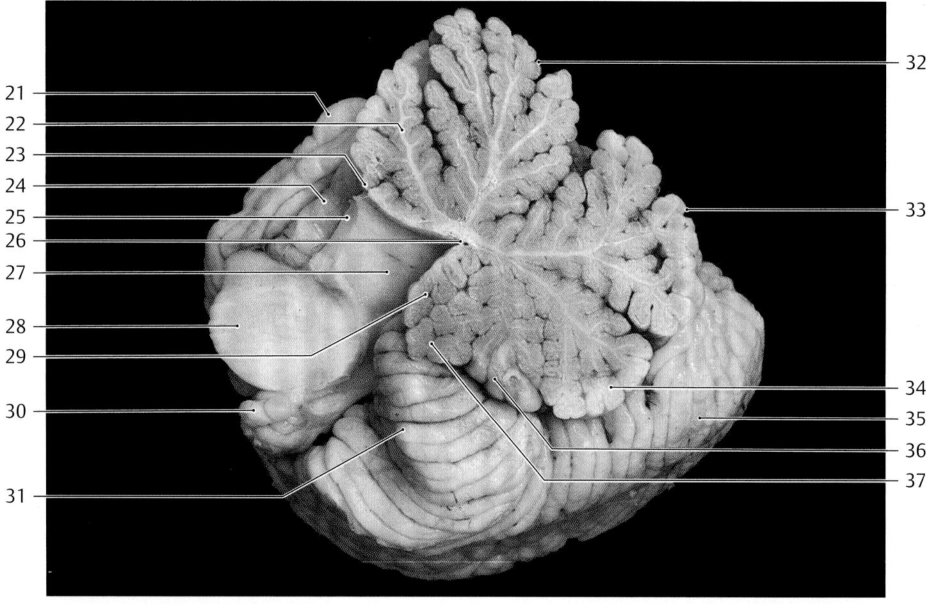


Fig. 9.136 **Median section through the cerebellum.** Right cerebellar hemisphere and right half of vermis.

1 Superior cerebellar peduncle
2 Middle cerebellar peduncle
3 Cerebellar tonsil
4 Inferior semilunar lobule
5 Vermis
6 Central lobule of vermis
7 Inferior cerebellar peduncle
8 Superior medullary velum
9 Nodule of vermis
10 Flocculus of cerebellum
11 Biventral lobule
12 Left cerebellar hemisphere
13 Inferior semilunar lobule
14 Biventral lobule
15 Vermis of cerebellum
16 Tuber of vermis
17 Pyramid of vermis
18 Uvula of vermis
19 Tonsil of cerebellum
20 Flocculus of cerebellum
21 Right cerebellar hemisphere
22 Vermis (central lobule)
23 Cerebellar lingula
24 Ala of central lobule
25 Superior cerebellar peduncle
26 Fastigium
27 Fourth ventricle
28 Middle cerebellar peduncle
29 Nodule of vermis
30 Flocculus of cerebellum
31 Cerebellar tonsil
32 Culmen of vermis
33 Declive of vermis
34 Tuber of vermis
35 Inferior semilunar lobule
36 Pyramid of vermis (cut)
37 Uvula of vermis

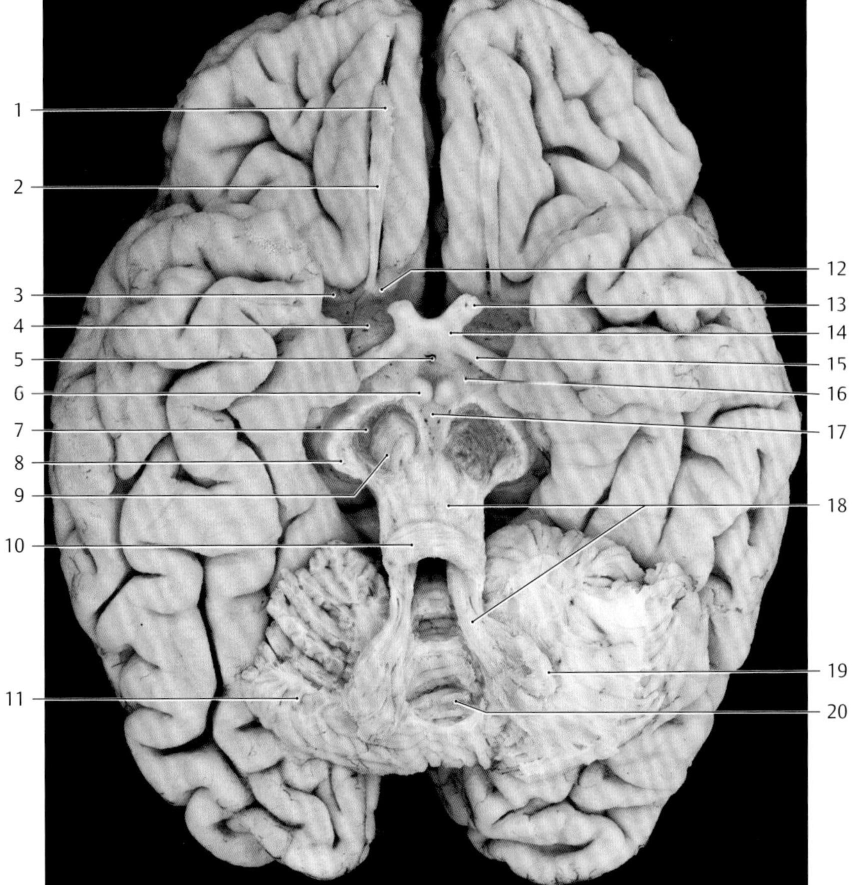


Fig. 9.137 **Brain and cerebellum** (inferior aspect). Parts of the cerebellum have been removed to display the dentate nucleus and the main pathway to the midbrain (cerebellorubral tract).

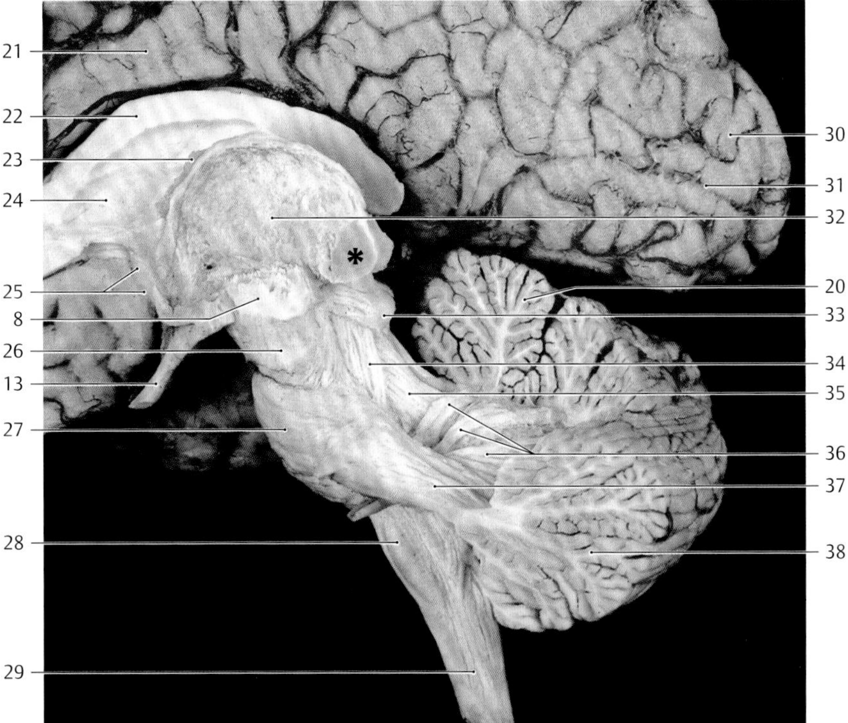


1 Olfactory bulb
2 Olfactory tract
3 Lateral olfactory stria
4 Anterior perforated substance
5 Infundibulum (divided)
6 Mamillary body
7 Substantia nigra
8 Cerebral peduncle (cut)
9 Red nucleus
10 Decussation of superior cerebellar peduncle
11 Cerebellar hemisphere
12 Medial olfactory stria
13 Optic nerve
14 Optic chiasma
15 Optic tract
16 Posterior perforated substance
17 Interpeduncular fossa
18 Superior cerebellar peduncle and cerebellorubral tract
19 Dentate nucleus
20 Vermis of cerebellum
21 Cingulate gyrus
22 Corpus callosum
23 Stria terminalis
24 Septum pellucidum
25 Columna fornicis
26 Cerebral peduncle at midbrain level
27 Pons
28 Inferior olive
29 Medulla oblongata with lateral pyramidal tract
30 Occipital lobe
31 Calcarine sulcus
32 Thalamus
33 Inferior colliculus with brachium
34 Medial lemniscus
35 Superior cerebellar peduncle
36 Inferior cerebellar peduncle
37 Middle cerebellar peduncle
38 Cerebellar hemisphere

Fig. 9.138 **Dissection of the cerebellar peduncles and their connection with midbrain and diencephalon.** A small part of the pulvinar thalami (*) has been cut to show the inferior brachium.

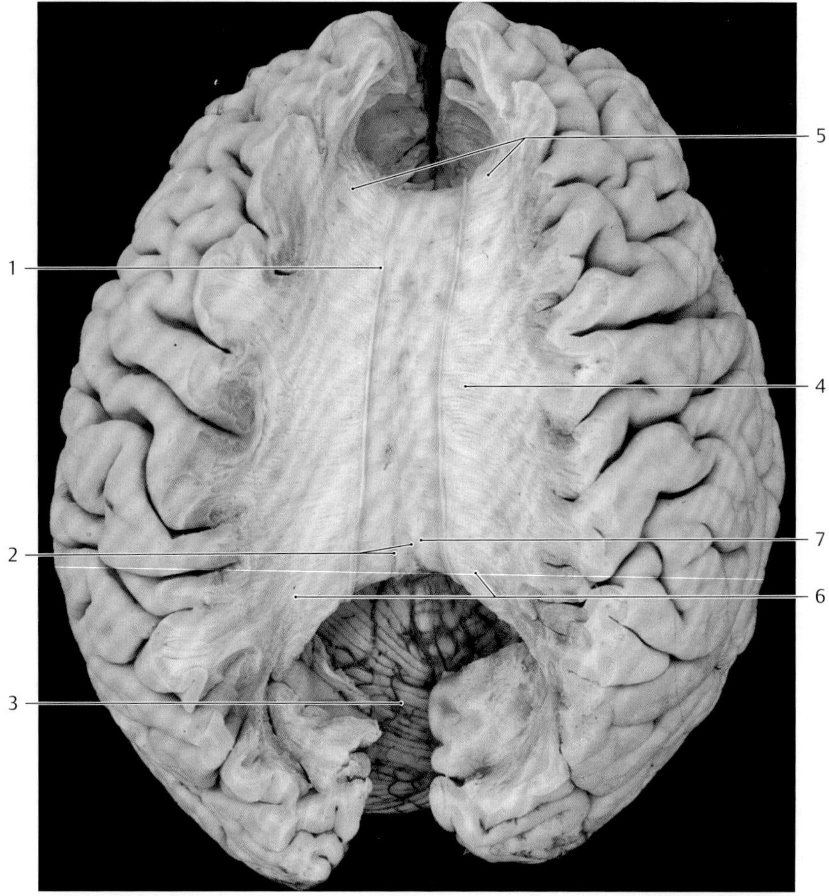


1 Lateral longitudinal stria of indusium griseum
2 Medial longitudinal stria of indusium griseum
3 Cerebellum
4 Radiating fibers of the corpus callosum
5 Forceps minor of corpus callosum
6 Forceps major of corpus callosum
7 Splenium of corpus callosum

**Fig. 9.139 Dissection of the brain I.** The fiber system of the corpus callosum has been displayed by removing the cortex lying above it. Frontal pole at the top.

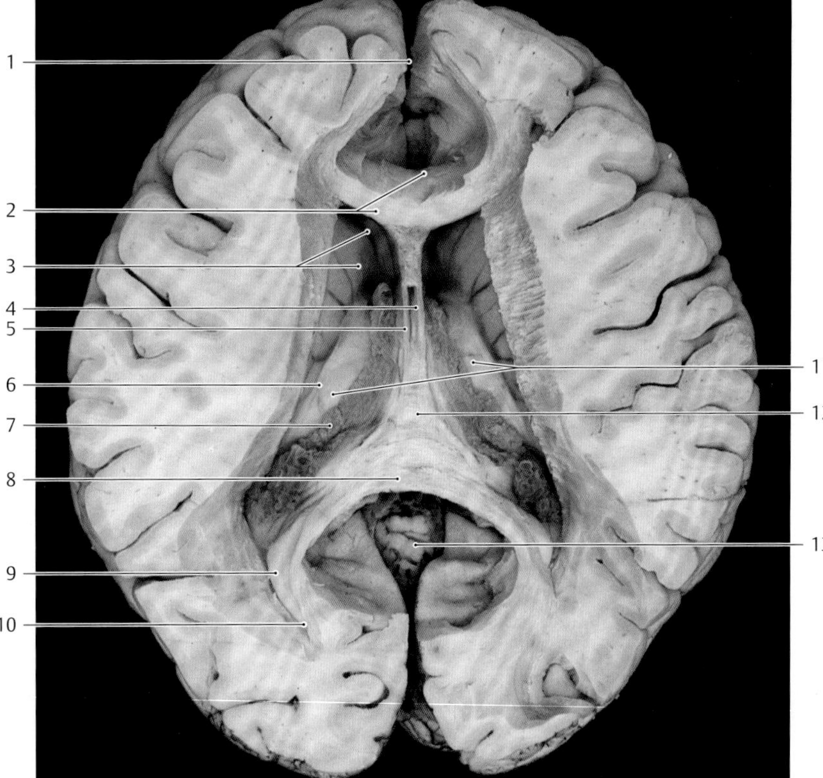


1 Longitudinal cerebral fissure
2 Genu of corpus callosum
3 Head of caudate nucleus and anterior horn of lateral ventricle
4 Cavum of septum pellucidum
5 Septum pellucidum
6 Stria terminalis
7 Choroid plexus of lateral ventricle
8 Splenium of corpus callosum
9 Calcar avis
10 Posterior horn of lateral ventricle
11 Thalamus (lamina affixa)
12 Commissure of fornix
13 Vermis of cerebellum

**Fig. 9.140 Dissection of the brain II.** The lateral ventricles and subcortical nuclei of the brain have been dissected and the corpus callosum has been partly removed. Frontal pole at the top.

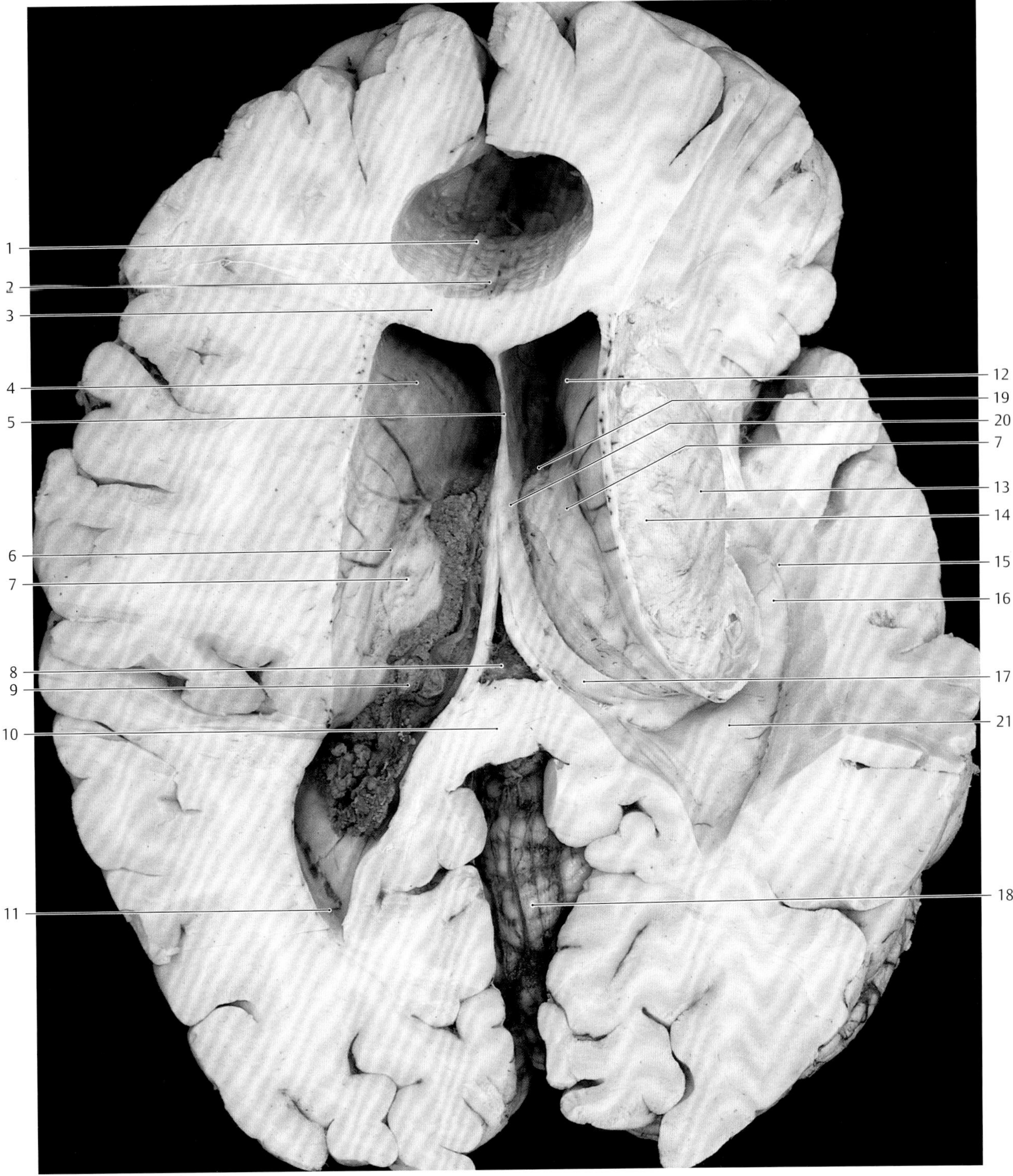


Fig. 9.141 **Dissection of the brain III** (superior aspect of lateral ventricle and subcortical nuclei of the brain). The corpus callosum has been partly removed. On the right side, the entire lateral ventricle has been opened and the insula with claustrum and the extreme and external capsules have been removed, exposing the lentiform nucleus and the internal capsule.

1 Lateral longitudinal stria
2 Medial longitudinal stria
3 Genu of corpus callosum
4 Head of caudate nucleus
5 Septum pellucidum
6 Stria terminalis
7 Thalamus (lamina affixa)
8 Choroid plexus of third ventricle
9 Choroid plexus of lateral ventricle
10 Splenium of corpus callosum
11 Posterior horn of lateral ventricle
12 Anterior horn of lateral ventricle (head of caudate nucleus)
13 Putamen of lentiform nucleus
14 Internal capsule
15 Inferior horn of lateral ventricle
16 Pes hippocampi
17 Crus of fornix
18 Vermis of cerebellum with arachnoid and pia mater
19 Interventricular foramen
20 Right column of fornix
21 Collateral eminence

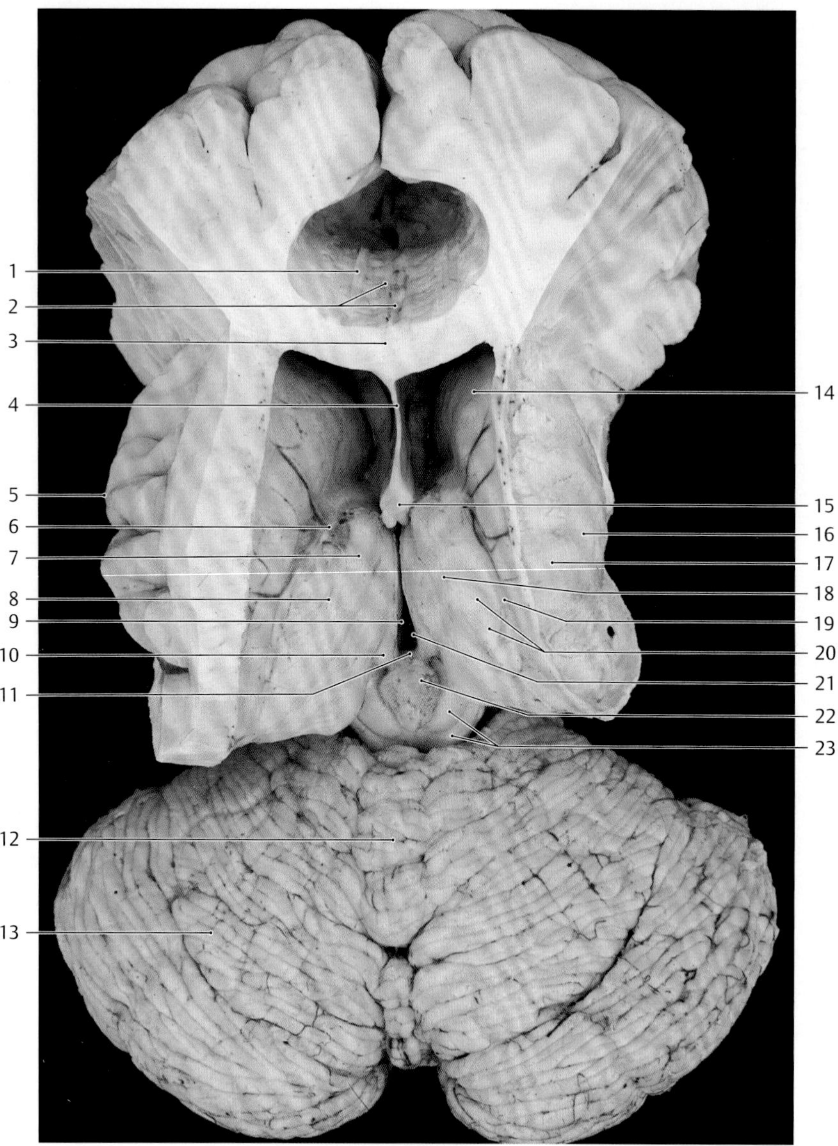


**Fig. 9.142 Dissection of the brain IVa** (superior aspect). The temporal lobe, fornix, and posterior corpus callosum have been removed (which can be seen in Fig. 9.143 below). Frontal pole at the top.

1 Lateral longitudinal stria
2 Medial longitudinal stria
3 Corpus callosum
4 Septum pellucidum
5 Insular gyri
6 Thalamostriate vein
7 Anterior tubercle of thalamus
8 Thalamus
9 Stria medullaris of thalamus
10 Habenular trigone
11 Habenular commissure
12 Vermis of cerebellum
13 Left hemisphere of cerebellum
14 Head of caudate nucleus
15 Columns of fornix
16 Putamen of lentiform nucleus
17 Internal capsule
18 Taenia of choroid plexus
19 Stria terminalis and thalamostriate vein
20 Lamina affixa
21 Third ventricle
22 Pineal body
23 Superior and inferior colliculi of midbrain

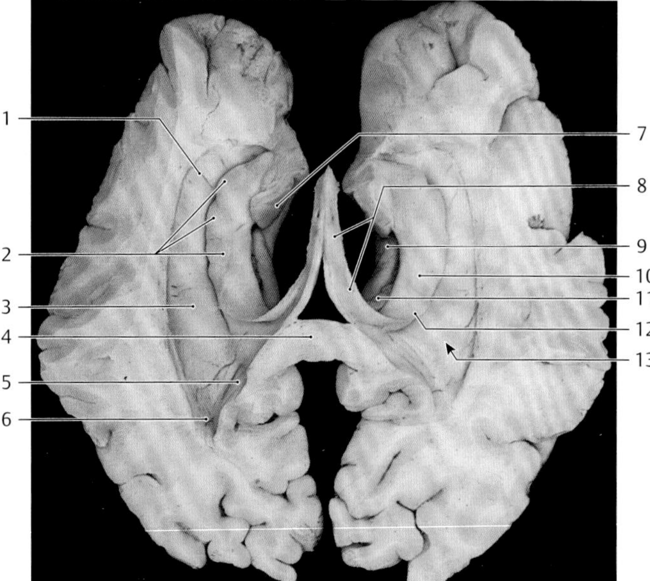


1 Inferior horn of lateral ventricle
2 Hippocampal digitations
3 Collateral eminence
4 Splenium of corpus callosum
5 Calcar avis
6 Posterior horn of lateral ventricle
7 Uncus of parahippocampal gyrus
8 Body and crus of fornix
9 Parahippocampal gyrus
10 Pes hippocampi
11 Dentate gyrus
12 Hippocampal fimbria
13 Lateral ventricle

**Fig. 9.143 Dissection of the brain IVb.** Depicted is the portion of the brain removed from the specimen above: temporal lobe and limbic system. Columns of fornix are cut (superior aspect).

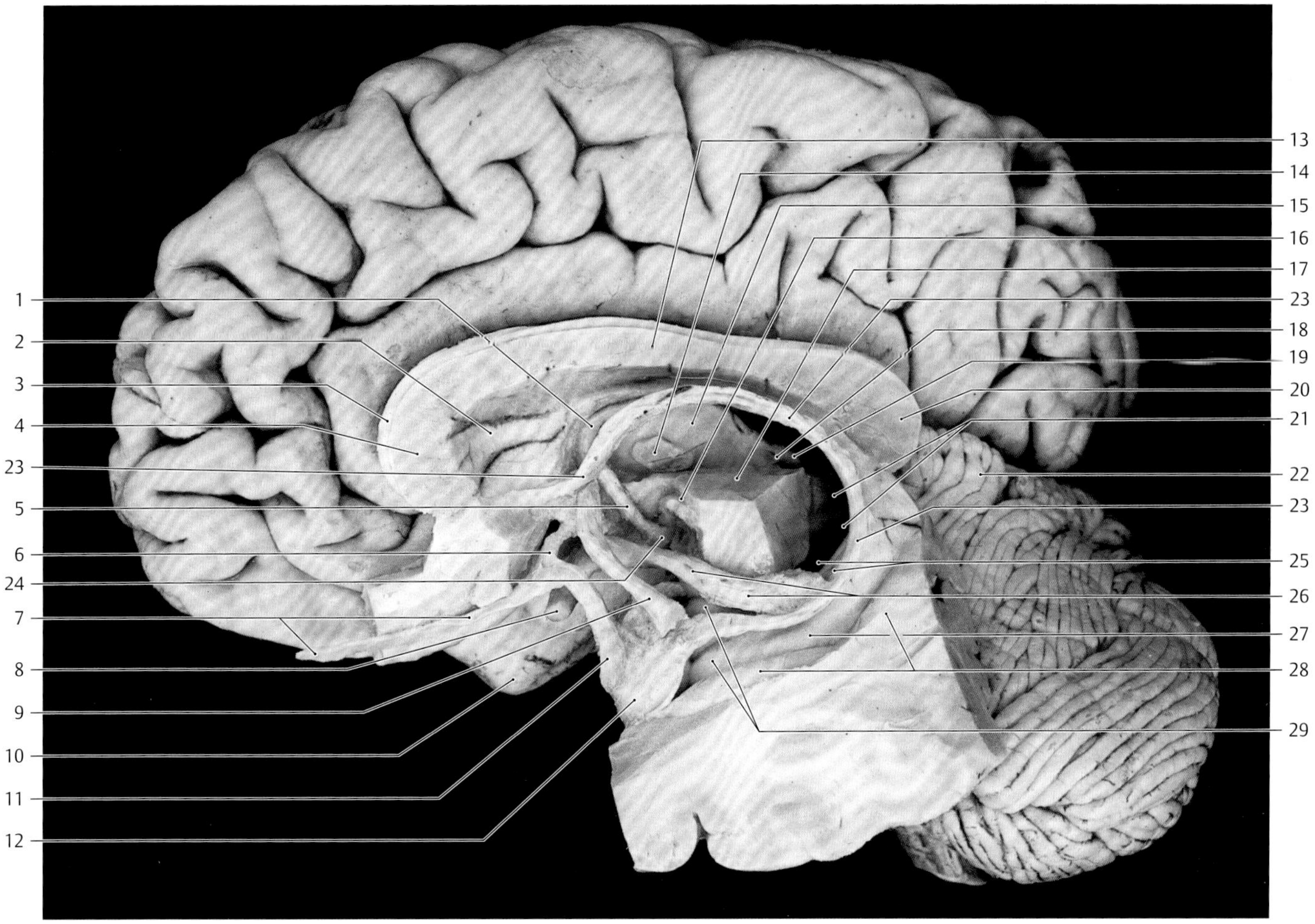

**Fig. 9.144 Dissection of the limbic system** (left side, lateral aspect). The corpus callosum has been cut at the median plane. The left thalamus and the left hemisphere have been partly removed.

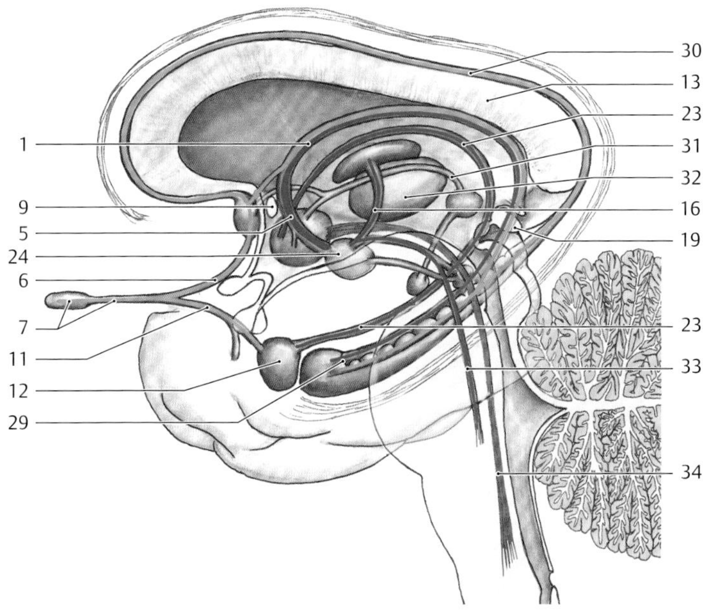


**Fig. 9.145 Main pathways of limbic and olfactory system.** Blue = afferent pathways; red = efferent pathways.

1 Body of fornix
2 Septum pellucidum
3 Lateral longitudinal stria
4 Genu of corpus callosum
5 Column of fornix
6 Medial olfactory stria
7 Olfactory bulb and olfactory tract
8 Optic nerve
9 Anterior commissure (left half)
10 Right temporal lobe
11 Lateral olfactory stria
12 Amygdala
13 Body of corpus callosum
14 Interthalamic adhesion
15 Third ventricle and right thalamus
16 Mammillothalamic fasciculus
17 Part of the thalamus
18 Habenular commissure
19 Pineal body
20 Splenium of corpus callosum
21 Colliculi of midbrain
22 Vermis of cerebellum
23 Stria terminalis
24 Mamillary body
25 Fimbria of hippocampus and pes hippocampi
26 Left optic tract and lateral geniculate body
27 Lateral ventricle and parahippocampal gyrus
28 Collateral eminence
29 Hippocampal digitations
30 Supracallosal gyrus (longitudinal stria)
31 Stria medullaris of thalamus
32 Dorsomedial nucleus of thalamus
33 Mammillotegmental fasciculus
34 Dorsal longitudinal fasciculus (Schütz)

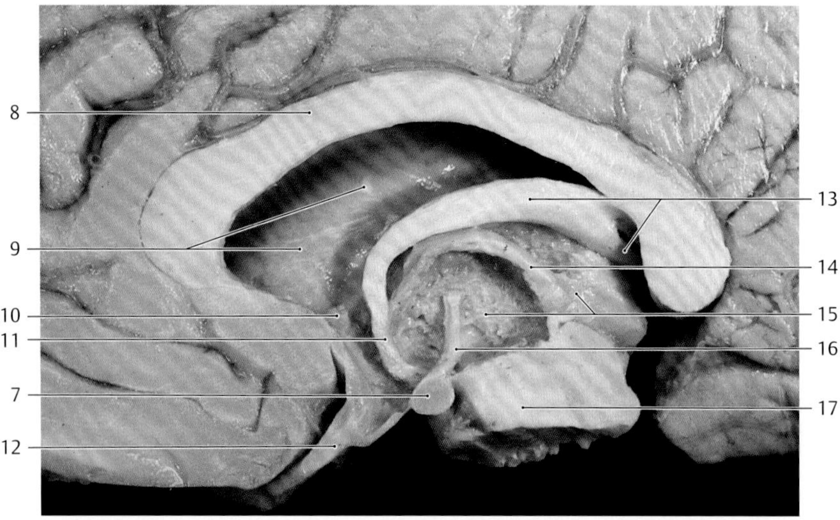


Fig. 9.146 **Median section through the diencephalon.** Medial part of the thalamus and septum pellucidum have been removed to show the fornix and mammillothalamic fasciculus.

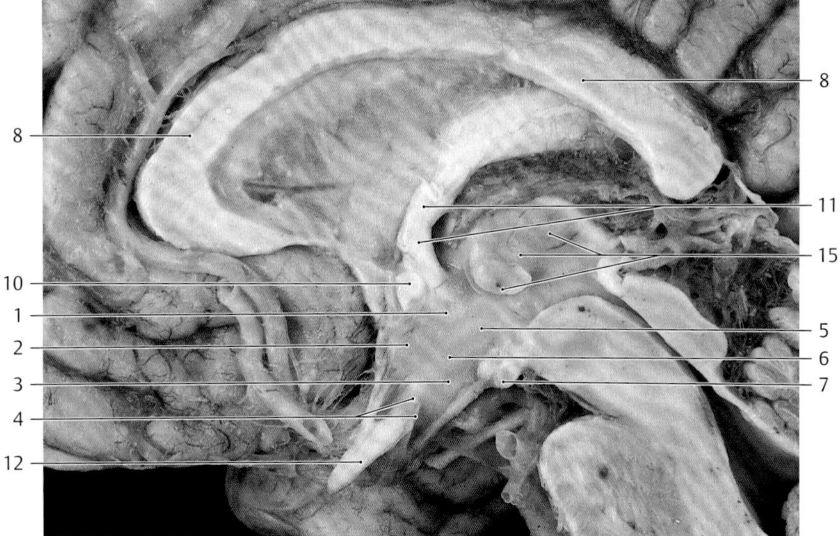


Fig. 9.147 **Median section through diencephalon and midbrain. Location of the hypothalamic nuclei.**

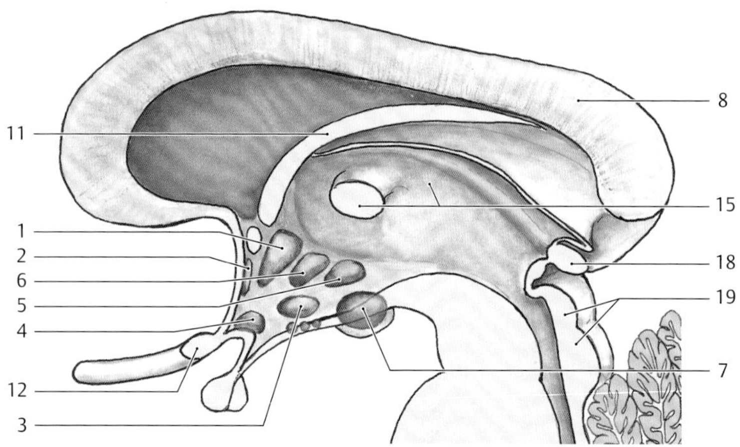


Fig. 9.148 **Location of the main hypothalamic nuclei.**

1 Paraventricular nucleus
2 Pre-optic nucleus
3 Ventromedial nucleus
4 Supra-optic nucleus
5 Posterior nucleus
6 Dorsomedial nucleus
(1–6: Hypothalamic nuclei)
7 Mamillary body
8 Corpus callosum
9 Lateral ventricle (showing caudate nucleus)
10 Anterior commissure
11 Column of fornix
12 Optic chiasma
13 Crus of fornix
14 Stria medullaris of thalamus
15 Thalamus and interthalamic adhesion
16 Mammillothalamic fasciculus of Vicq d'Azyr
17 Cerebral peduncle
18 Pineal body
19 Tectum of midbrain

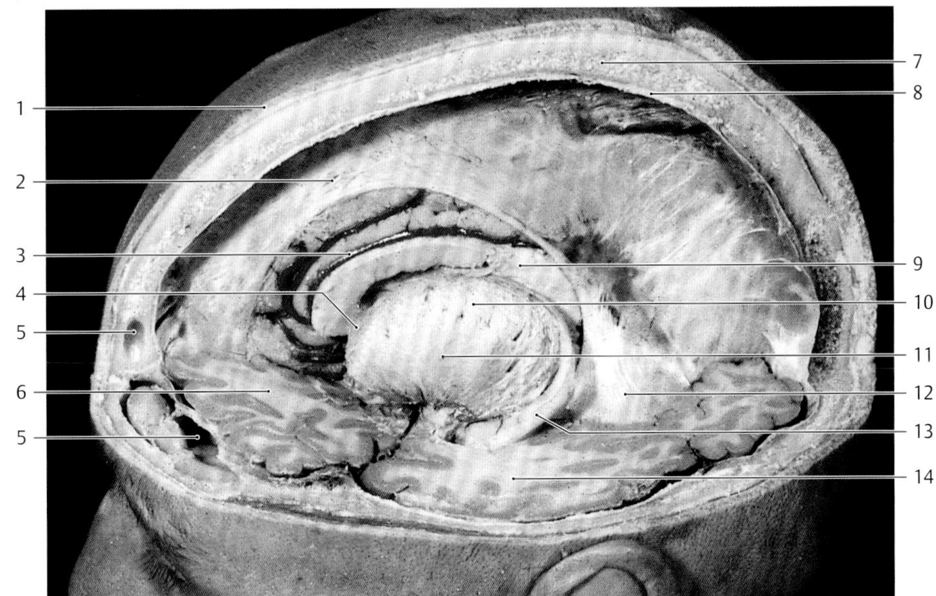


1 Skin of scalp
2 Falx cerebri
3 Anterior cerebral artery
4 Caudate nucleus
5 Frontal sinus
6 Frontal lobe
7 Diploë of the skull
8 Dura mater
9 Corpus callosum
10 Internal capsule
11 Lentiform nucleus (putamen)
12 Cerebellar tentorium
13 Hippocampus
14 Temporal lobe of the left hemisphere

Fig. 9.149 **Dissection of brainstem in situ.** The left hemisphere has been partly removed.

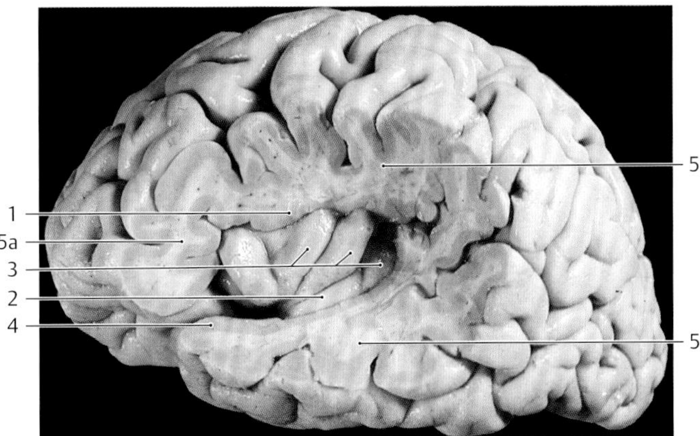


Fig. 9.150 **Insula (Reili),** left hemisphere. The opercula of the frontal, parietal, and temporal lobes have been removed to display the insular gyri.

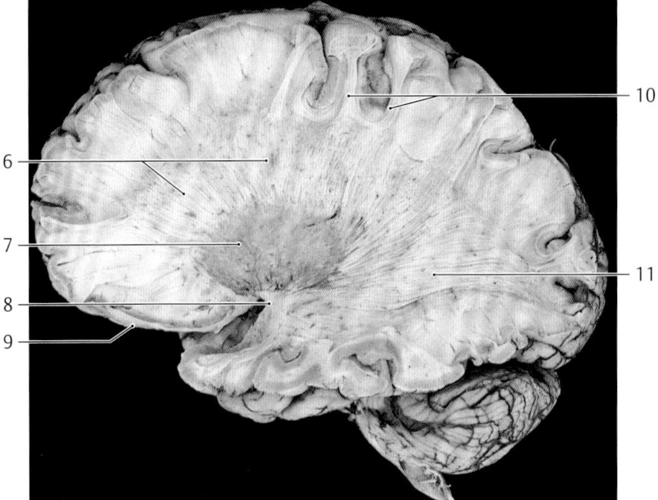


Fig. 9.151 **Corona radiata,** left hemisphere. Frontal pole to the left.

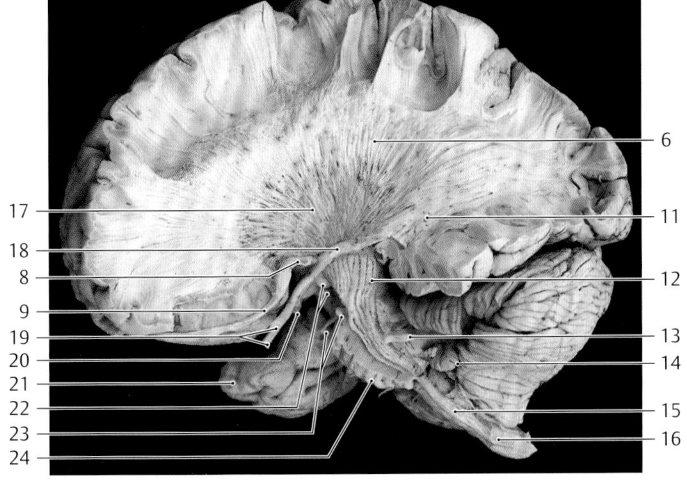


Fig. 9.152 **Corona radiata and internal capsule,** left hemisphere. The lentiform nucleus has been removed. Frontal pole to the left.

1 Circular sulcus of insula
2 Long gyrus of insula
3 Short gyri of insula
4 Limen insulae
5 Opercula (cut)
(a) Frontal operculum
(b) Frontoparietal operculum
(c) Temporal operculum
6 Corona radiata
7 Lentiform nucleus
8 Anterior commissure
9 Olfactory tract
10 Cerebral arcuate fibers
11 Optic radiation
12 Cerebral peduncle
13 Trigeminal nerve (CN V)
14 Flocculus of cerebellum
15 Pyramidal tract
16 Decussation of pyramidal tract
17 Internal capsule
18 Optic tract
19 Optic nerve (CN II)
20 Infundibulum
21 Temporal lobe (right side)
22 Mamillary bodies
23 Oculomotor nerve (CN III)
24 Transverse fibers of pons

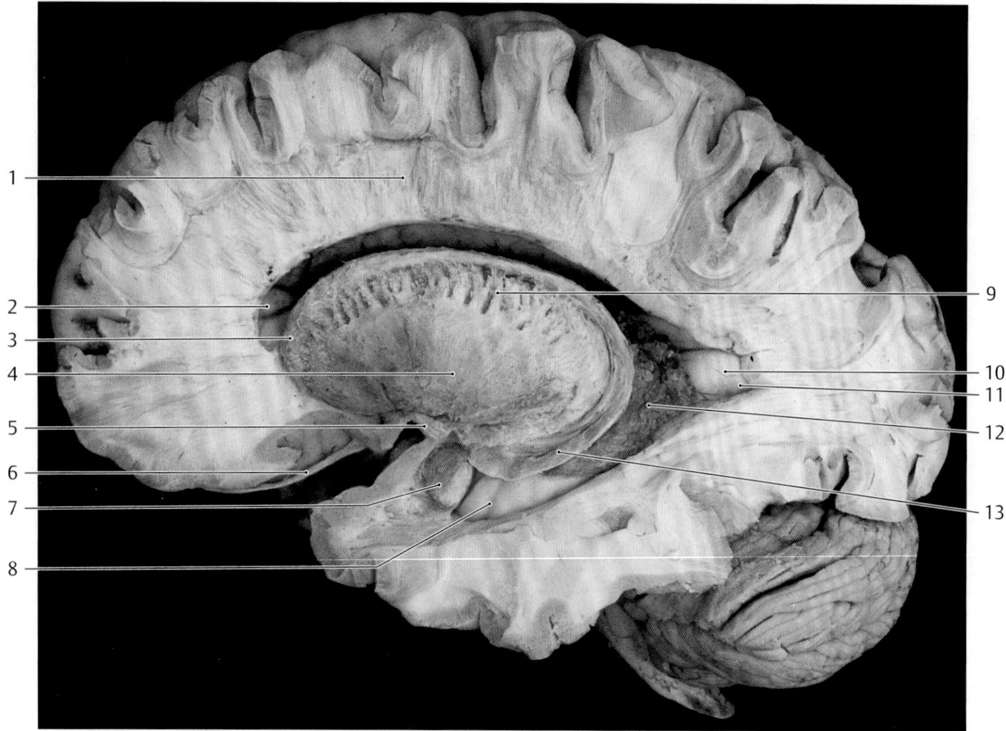


Fig. 9.153 **Dissection of the subcortical nuclei and internal capsule,** left hemisphere (lateral aspect). The lateral ventricle has been opened and the insular gyri and claustrum have been removed, revealing the lentiform nucleus and the internal capsule. Frontal pole to the left.

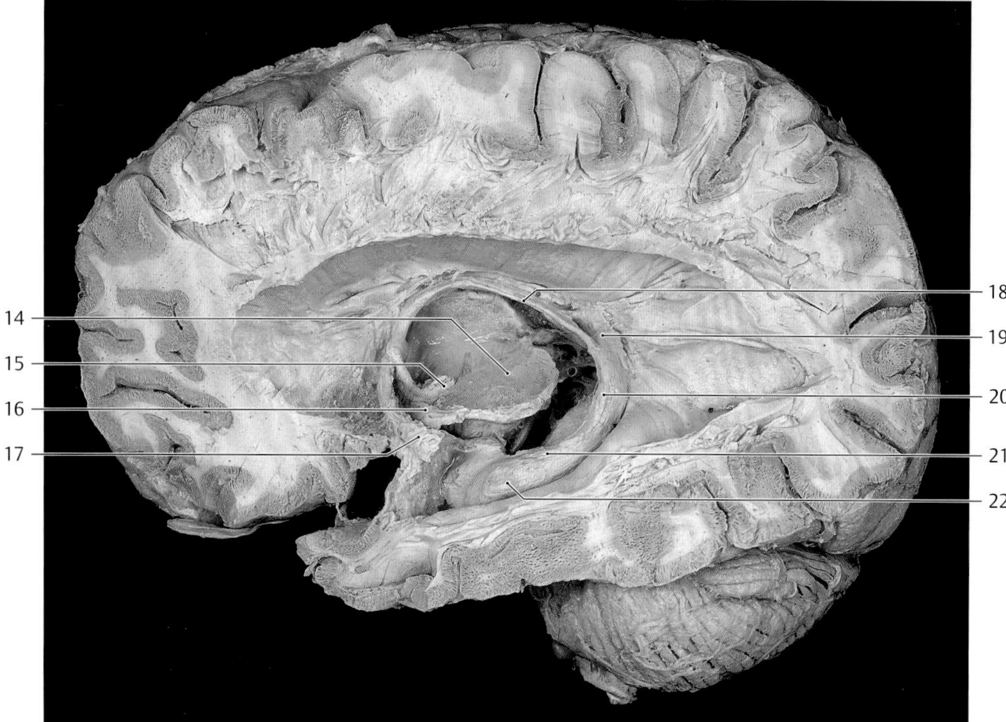


Fig. 9.154 **Dissection of the limbic system and fornix,** left hemisphere (lateral aspect). Frontal pole to the left.

1 Corona radiata
2 Anterior horn of lateral ventricle
3 Head of caudate nucleus
4 Putamen
5 Anterior commissure
6 Olfactory tract
7 Amygdala
8 Hippocampal digitations
9 Internal capsule
10 Calcar avis
11 Posterior horn of lateral ventricle
12 Choroid plexus of lateral ventricle
13 Caudal extremity of caudate nucleus
14 Pulvinar of thalamus
15 Mamillary body
16 Optic tract
17 Anterior commissure
18 Fornix
19 Longitudinal stria
20 Dentate gyrus
21 Hippocampal fimbria
22 Pes hippocampi

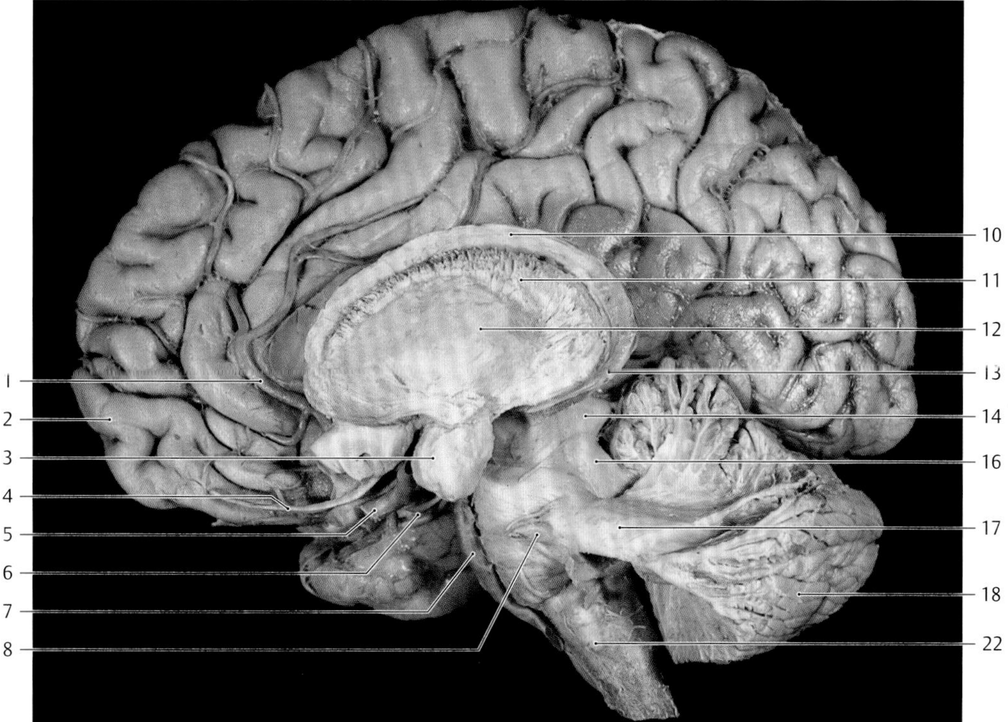


Fig. 9.155 **Dissection of the brainstem and cerebellum** (lateral aspect). The connections of the brainstem with the cerebellum have been dissected. The amygdala of the left hemisphere is shown. The corpus callosum has been partly removed. Frontal pole to the left.

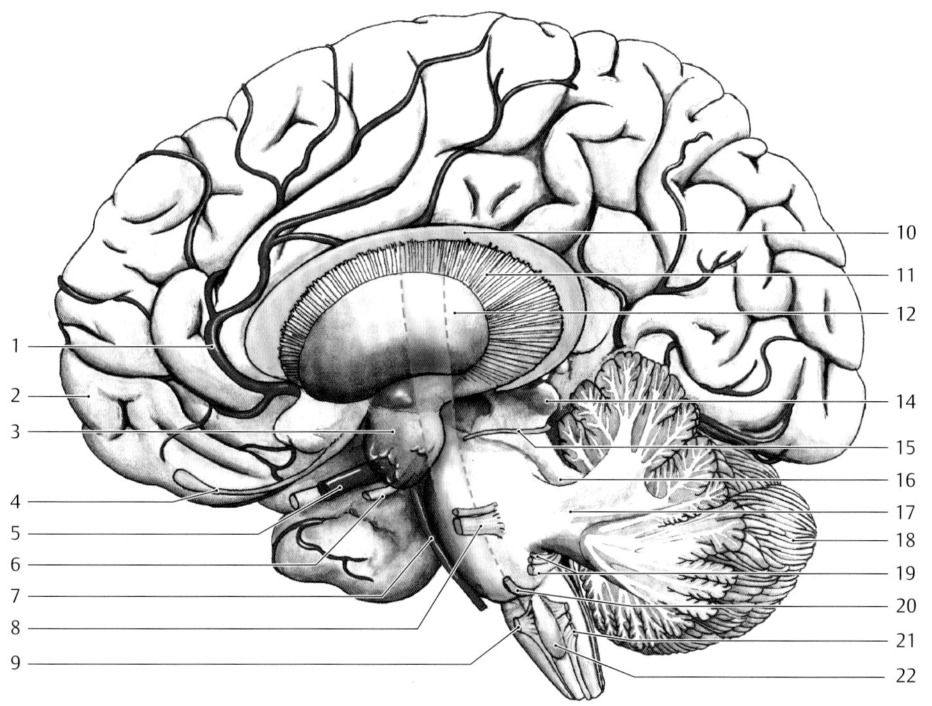


Fig. 9.156 **Schematic drawing of the dissected brainstem and cerebellum** (lateral aspect; see Fig. 9.155 above). Red = course of the pyramidal tracts; yellow = cranial nerves.

1 Anterior cerebral artery
2 Frontal lobe
3 Amygdala (amygdaloid body)
4 Olfactory tract
5 Internal carotid artery
6 Oculomotor nerve (CN III)
7 Basilar artery
8 Trigeminal nerve (CN V)
9 Hypoglossal nerve (CN XII)
10 Caudate nucleus
11 Internal capsule
12 Lentiform nucleus
13 Caudal extremity of caudate nucleus
14 Inferior colliculus of midbrain
15 Trochlear nerve (CN IV)
16 Superior cerebellar peduncle
17 Middle cerebellar peduncle
18 Cerebellum
19 Facial nerve (CN VII) and vestibulocochlear nerve (CN VIII)
20 Abducent nerve (CN VI)
21 Glossopharyngeal nerve (CN IX), vagus nerve (CN X), and accessory nerve (CN XI)
22 Inferior olive

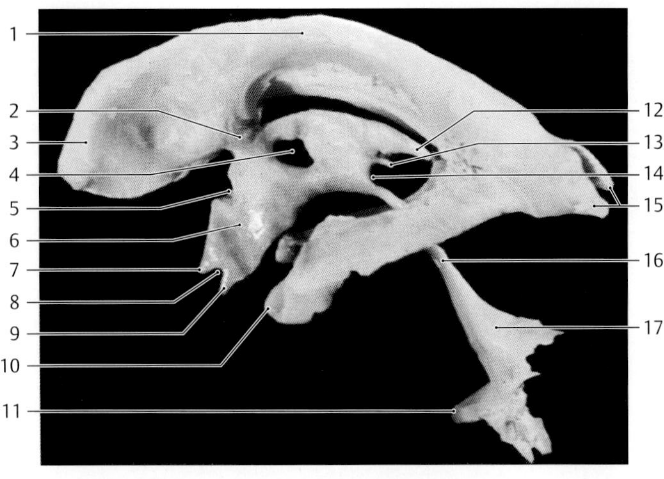


1 Central part of the lateral ventricle
2 Interventricular foramen of Monro
3 Anterior horn of the lateral ventricle
4 Site of interthalamic adhesion
5 Notch for anterior commissure
6 Third ventricle
7 Optic recess
8 Notch for optic chiasma
9 Infundibular recess
10 Inferior horn of lateral ventricle with indentation of amygdaloid body
11 Lateral recess and lateral aperture of Luschka
12 Suprapineal recess
13 Pineal recess
14 Notch for posterior commissure
15 Posterior horn of lateral ventricle
16 Cerebral aqueduct
17 Fourth ventricle
18 Median aperture of Magendie

**Fig. 9.157 Cast of ventricular cavities of the brain** (lateral aspect). Frontal pole to the left.

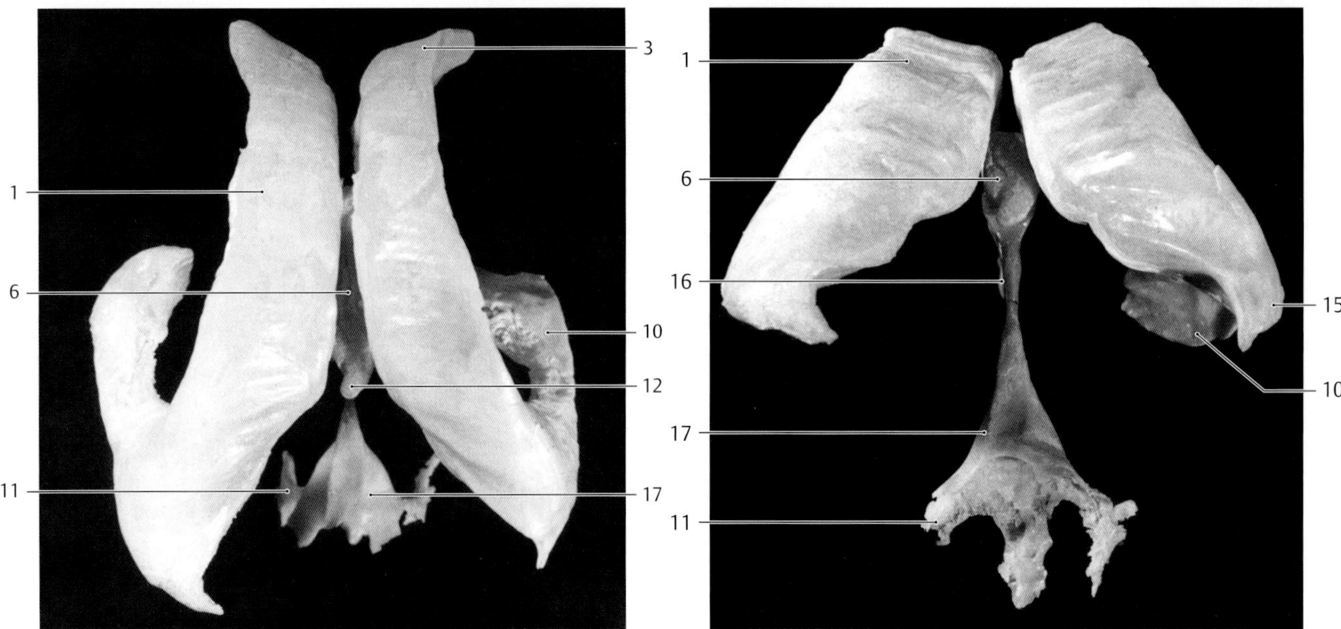


**Fig. 9.158 Cast of ventricular cavities of the brain** (superior aspect). Frontal pole at the top.

**Fig. 9.159 Cast of ventricular cavities of the brain and cerebral aqueduct** (posterior aspect). Posterior horns of the lateral ventricles (15) are shown. Fourth ventricle (17) from below.

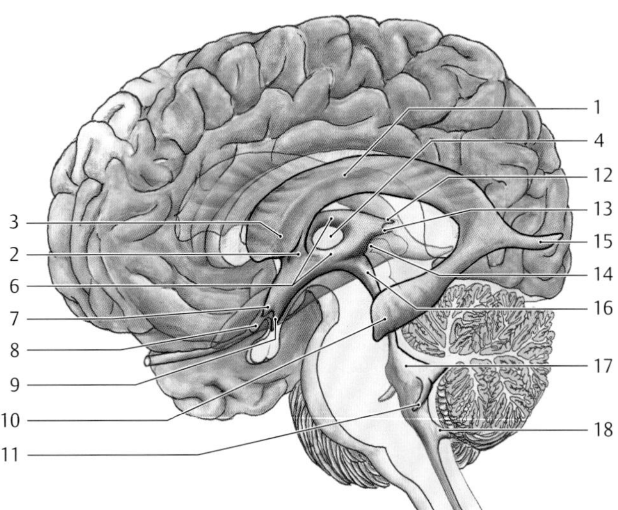


**Fig. 9.160 Position of ventricular cavities.**

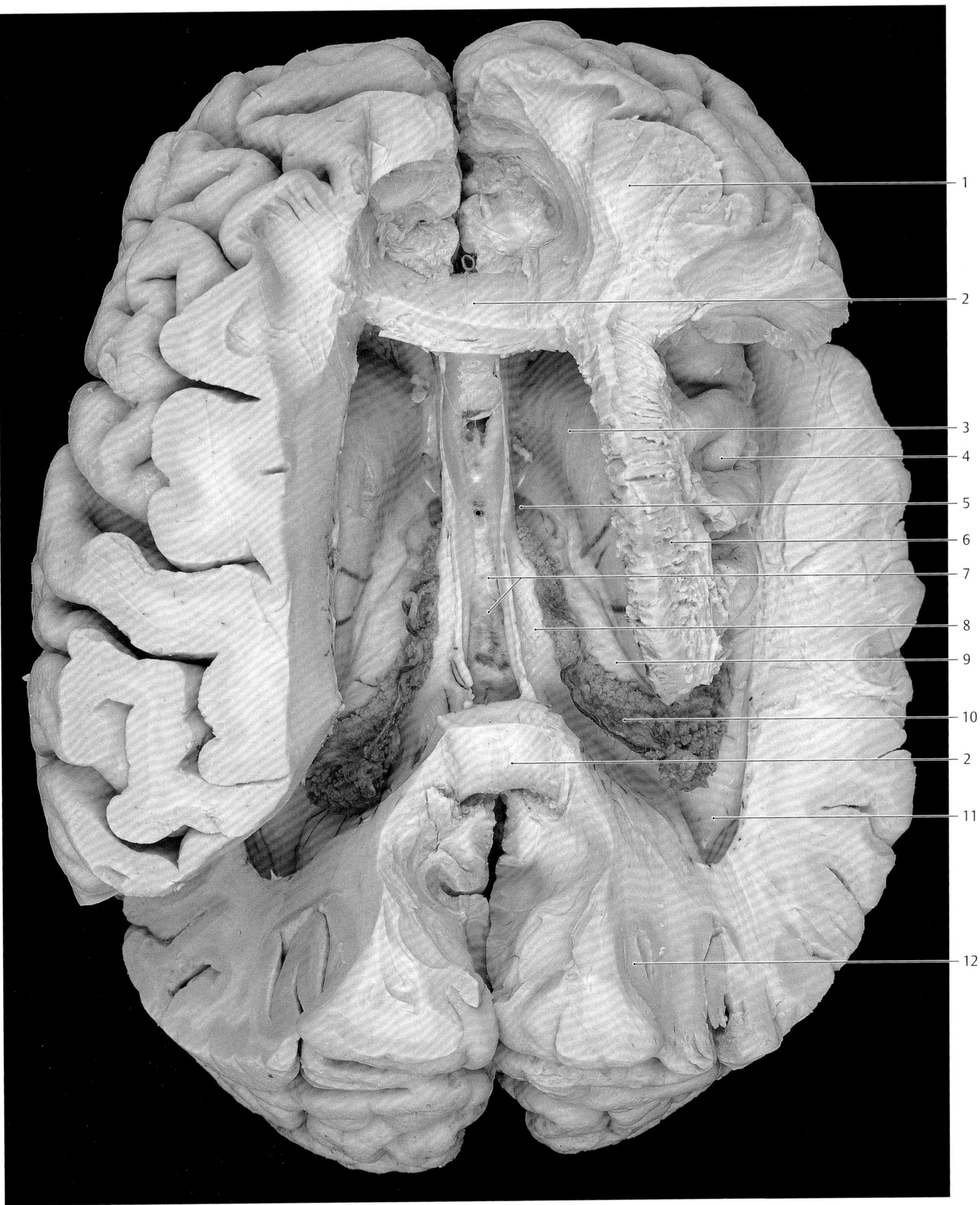


Fig. 9.161 **Dissection of the brain** (superior aspect of the lateral ventricle and of the subcortical nuclei of the brain). The corpus callosum has been partly removed. Fornix and choroid plexus of the left lateral ventricle are shown.

1 Frontal lobe of brain
2 Corpus callosum
3 Caudate nucleus (head)
4 Insular cortex
5 Interventricular foramen
6 Internal capsule
7 Choroid plexus of third ventricle
8 Body of fornix
9 Thalamus
10 Choroid plexus
11 Lateral ventricle (occipital horn)
12 Occipital lobe of brain

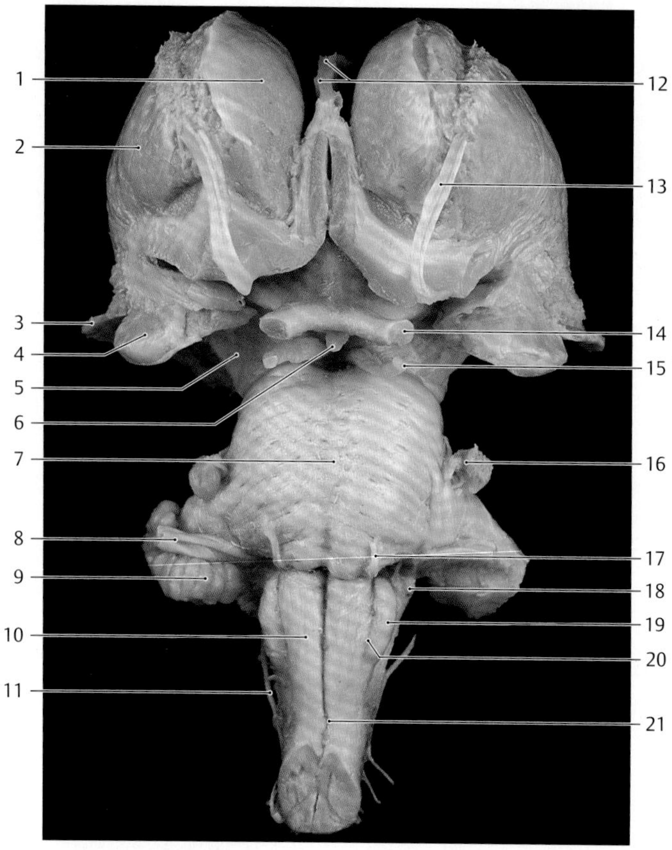

**Fig. 9.162 Brainstem** (anterior aspect). The cerebrum has been removed.

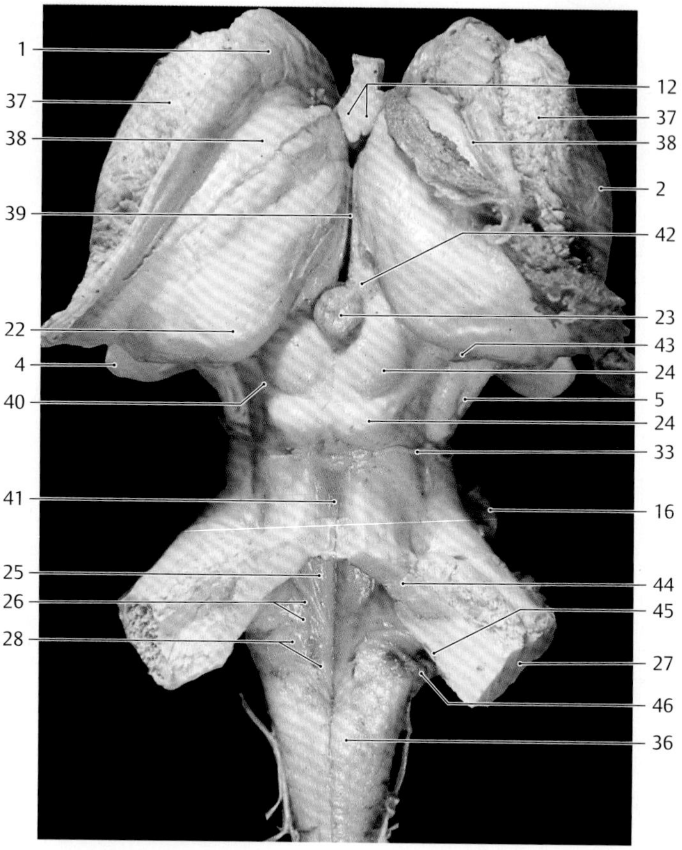

**Fig. 9.163 Brainstem** (posterior aspect). The cerebrum has been removed.

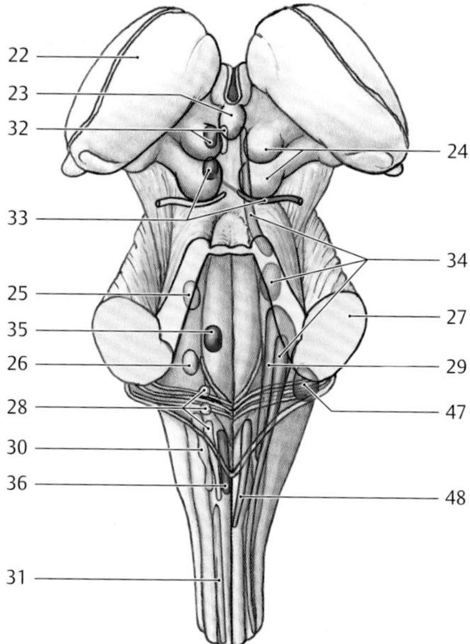


**Fig. 9.164 Brainstem** (posterior aspect). **Location of cranial nerve nuclei.** The somatic motor and visceral motor nuclei (derivations of the basal plate of the spinal cord) lie in two rows next to the median line in the rhomboid fossa (orange, yellow). The somatic efferent nuclei areas of CN III, IV, VI, and XII are located further medially (orange). The somatic sensory and visceral sensory nuclei (derivations of the wing plate) join laterally (green, blue). The purely sensory nuclei of CN VIII are located most laterally (blue).

1 Caudate nucleus
2 Lentiform nucleus
3 Caudal extremity of caudate nucleus
4 Amygdaloid body
5 Cerebral peduncle
6 Infundibulum
7 Pons
8 Facial and vestibulocochlear nerves (CN VII, CN VIII)
9 Cerebellar flocculus
10 Medulla oblongata
11 Accessory nerve (CN XI)
12 Fornix and column of fornix
13 Olfactory tract
14 Optic nerve (CN II)
15 Oculomotor nerve (CN III)
16 Trigeminal nerve (CN V)
17 Abducent nerve (CN VI)
18 Glossopharyngeal and vagus nerves (CN IX, CN X)
19 Inferior olive
20 Hypoglossal nerve (CN XII)
21 Decussation of the pyramids
22 Thalamus
23 Epiphysis
24 Tectum of midbrain (superior and inferior colliculus)
25 Motor nucleus of trigeminal nerve (CN V)
26 Facial nucleus (CN VII)
27 Middle cerebellar peduncle
28 Visceral nucleus of glossopharyngeal and vagus nerves (CN IX and CN X), salivatory nucleus
29 Vestibular nucleus (CN VIII)
30 Ambiguus nucleus (CN IX, CN X, CN XI)
31 Spinal nucleus of accessory nerve (CN XI)
32 Motor nucleus of oculomotor nerve (CN III)
33 Trochlear nucleus and nerve (CN IV)
34 Sensory nucleus of trigeminal nerve (CN V)
35 Abducent nucleus (CN VI)
36 Hypoglossal nucleus (CN XII)
37 Internal capsule
38 Lamina affixa
39 Third ventricle
40 Brachium of inferior colliculus
41 Superior medullary velum
42 Habenular trigone
43 Medial geniculate body
44 Superior cerebellar peduncle
45 Inferior cerebellar peduncle
46 Choroid plexus of fourth ventricle
47 Cochlear nuclei
48 Nucleus of solitary tract

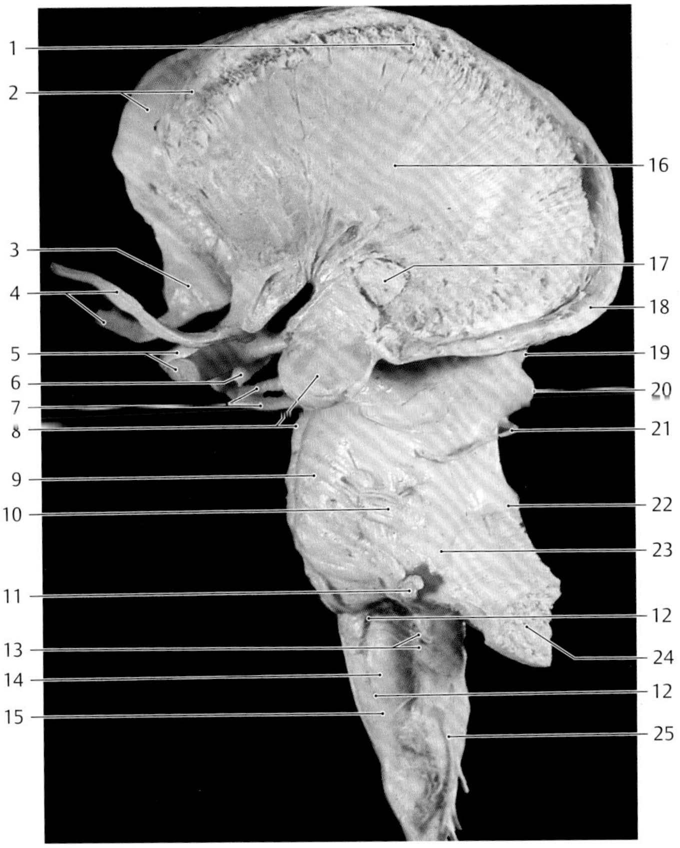

**Fig. 9.165 Brainstem** (left lateral aspect). The cerebellar peduncles have been severed and the cerebellum and cerebral cortex have been removed.

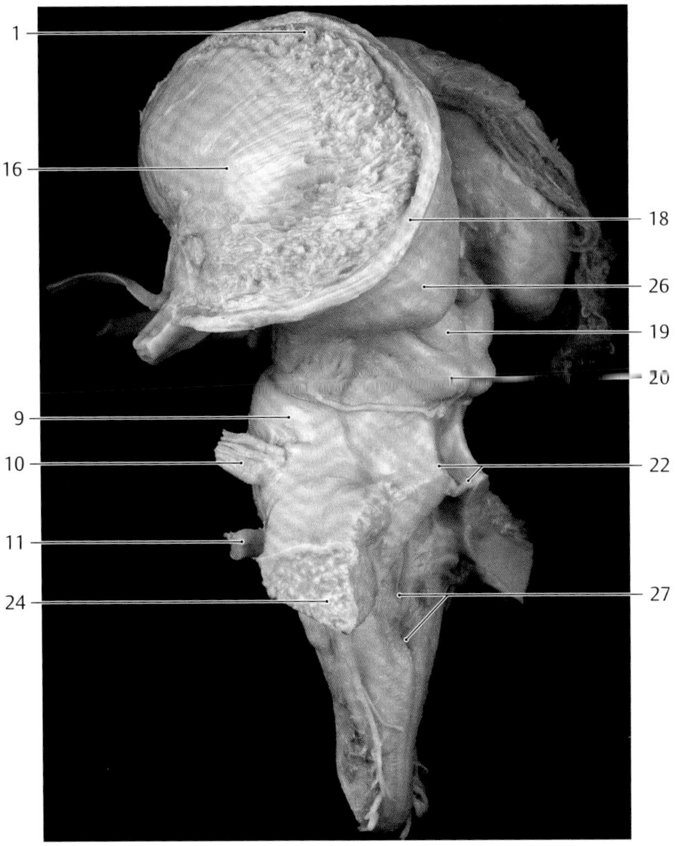

**Fig. 9.166 Brainstem** (dorso-lateral aspect). The cerebellum has been removed.

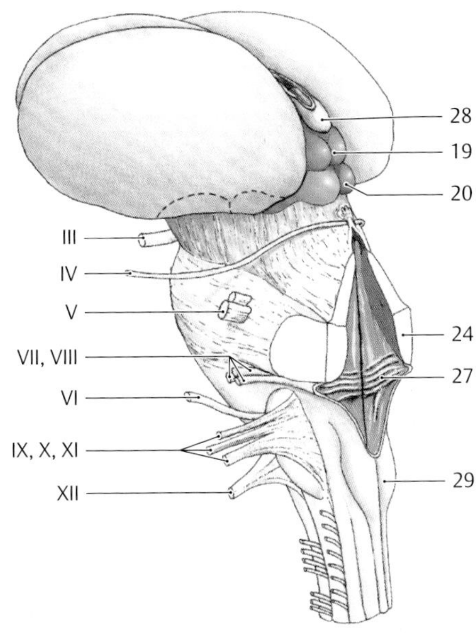


**Fig. 9.167 Brainstem** (lateral aspect). Note the location of the cranial nerves III–XII.

1 Internal capsule
2 Head of the caudate nucleus
3 Olfactory trigone
4 Olfactory tracts
5 Optic nerves (CN II)
6 Infundibulum
7 Oculomotor nerve (CN III)
8 Amygdaloid body
9 Pons
10 Trigeminal nerve (CN V)
11 Facial and vestibulo-cochlear nerves (CN VII, CN VIII)
12 Hypoglossal nerve (CN XII)
13 Glossopharyngeal and vagus nerves (CN IX, CN X)
14 Inferior olive
15 Medulla oblongata
16 Lentiform nucleus
17 Anterior commissure
18 Tail of caudate nucleus
19 Superior colliculus
20 Inferior colliculus
21 Trochlear nerve (CN IV)
22 Superior cerebellar peduncle
23 Inferior cerebellar peduncle
24 Middle cerebellar peduncle
25 Accessory nerve (CN XI)
26 Pulvinar of thalamus
27 Striae medullares and rhomboid fossa
28 Pineal body
29 Clava

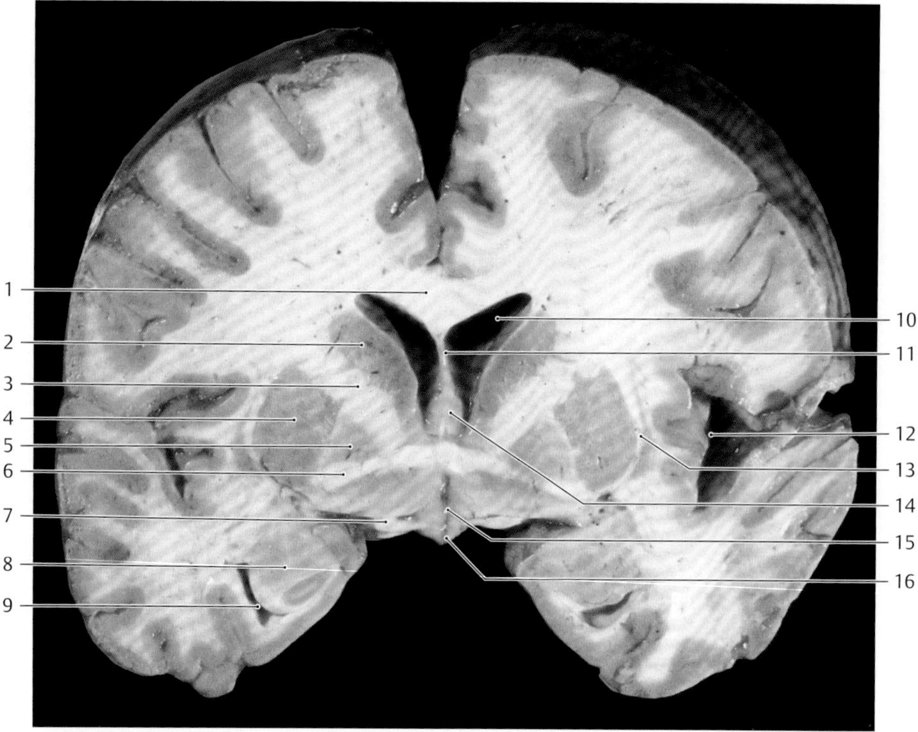


**Fig. 9.168 Coronal section through the brain** at the level of the anterior commissure. Section 1.

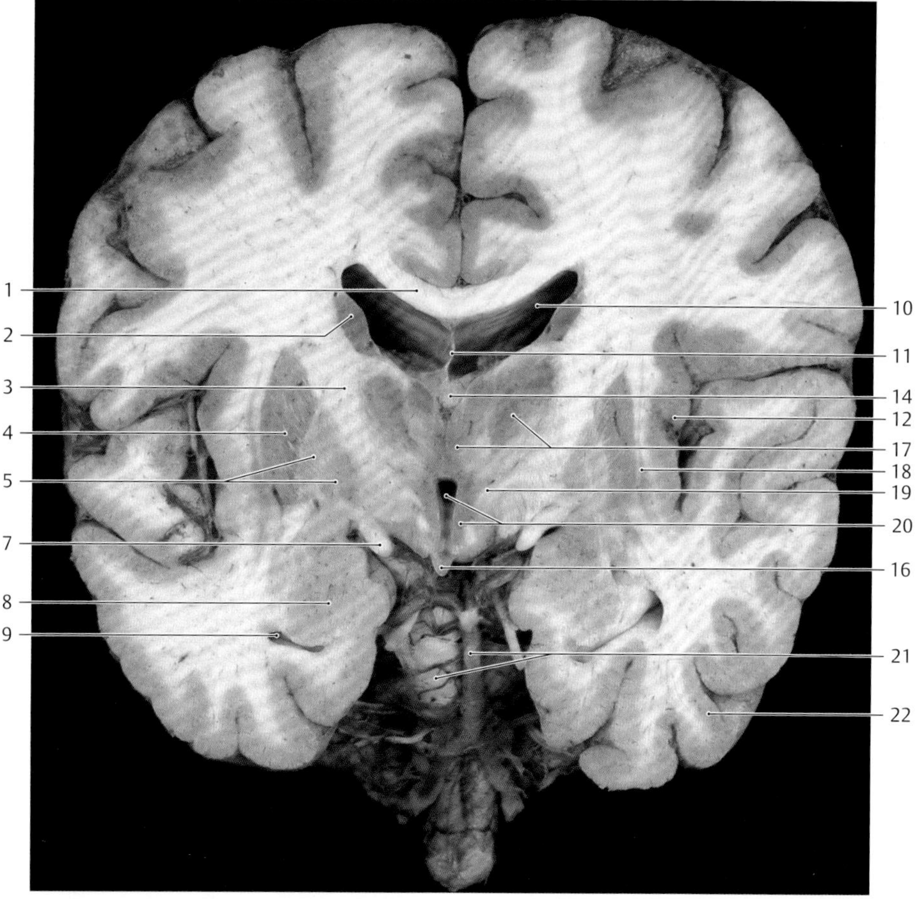


**Fig. 9.169 Coronal section through the brain** at the level of the third ventricle and the interthalamic adhesion. Section 2.

1 Corpus callosum
2 Head of caudate nucleus
3 Internal capsule
4 Putamen
5 Globus pallidus
6 Anterior commissure
7 Optic tract
8 Amygdaloid body
9 Inferior horn of lateral ventricle
10 Lateral ventricle
11 Septum pellucidum
12 Lobus insularis (insula)
13 External capsule
14 Column of fornix
15 Optic recess
16 Infundibulum
17 Thalamus
18 Claustrum
19 Lenticular ansa
20 Third ventricle and hypothalamus
21 Basilar artery and pons
22 Cortex of temporal lobe
23 Inferior colliculus
24 Superior colliculus
25 Cerebral aqueduct
26 Red nucleus
27 Substantia nigra
28 Cerebral peduncle
29 Trochlear nerve (CN IV)
30 Gray matter
31 Nucleus of oculomotor nerve
32 Fibers of oculomotor nerve (CN III)
33 Vermis of cerebellum
34 Fourth ventricle
35 Reticular formation
36 Pons and transverse pontine fibers
37 Emboliform nucleus
38 Dentate nucleus
39 Middle cerebellar peduncle
40 Choroid plexus
41 Hypoglossal nucleus at rhomboid fossa
42 Medial longitudinal fasciculus
43 Trigeminal nerve (CN V)
44 Inferior olivary nucleus
45 Corticospinal fibers and arcuate fibers
46 Fourth ventricle with choroid plexus
47 Vestibular nuclei
48 Nucleus and tractus solitarius
49 Inferior cerebellar peduncle (restiform body)
50 Reticular formation
51 Medial lemniscus
52 Cuneate nucleus of Burdach
53 Central canal
54 Pyramidal tract
55 Flocculus of cerebellum
56 Cerebellar hemisphere with pia mater
57 “Arbor vitae” of cerebellum
58 Nucleus gracilis of Goll
59 Lateral recess of choroid plexus of fourth ventricle
60 Posterior inferior cerebellar artery
61 Choroid plexus of lateral ventricle

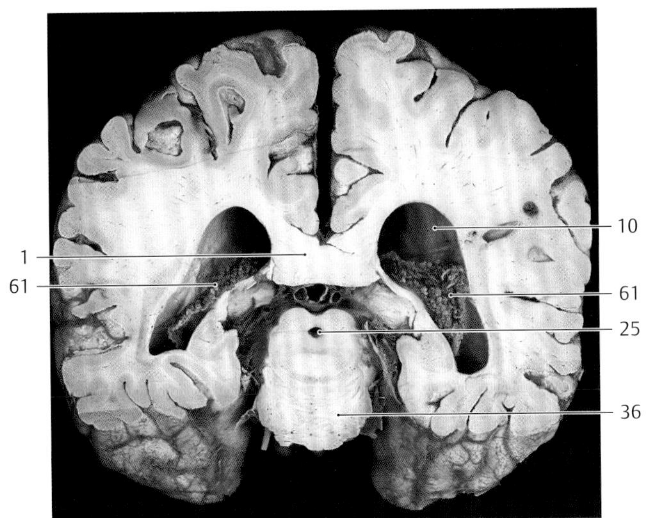


Fig. 9.170 **Coronal section through the brain** at the level of the inferior colliculus (posterior aspect). Section 3.

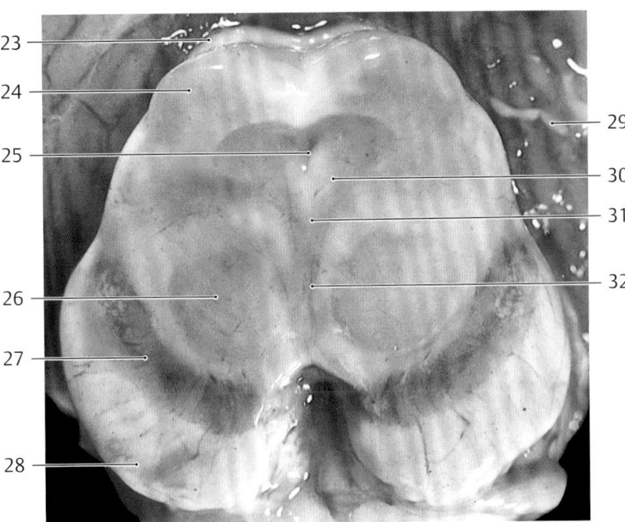


Fig. 9.171 **Cross section through the midbrain** (mesencephalon) at the level of the superior colliculus (superior aspect). Section 4.

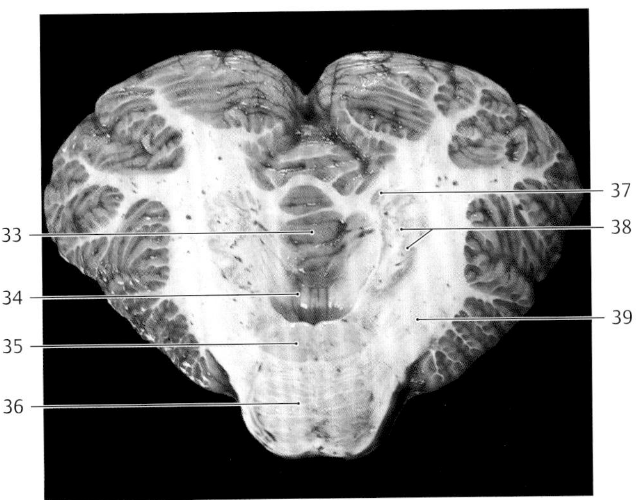


Fig. 9.172 **Cross section through the rhombencephalon** at the level of the pons (inferior aspect). Section 5.

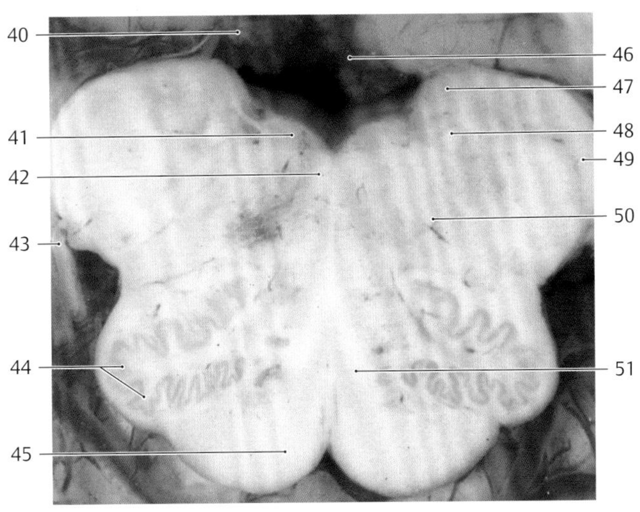


Fig. 9.173 **Cross section through the rhombencephalon** at the level of the olive (inferior aspect). Section 6.

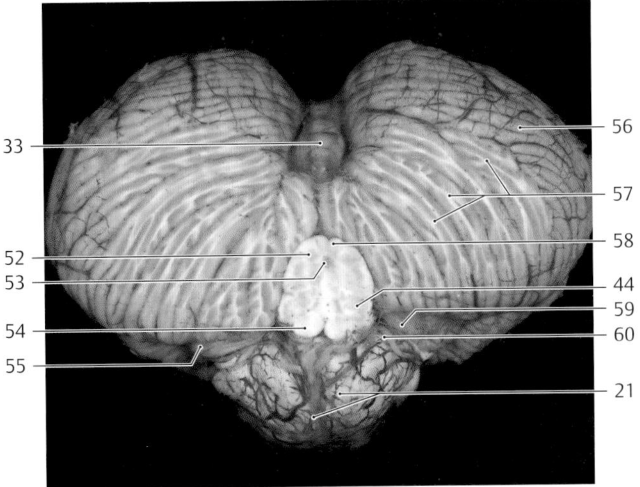


Fig. 9.174 **Cross section through medulla oblongata and cerebellum** (inferior aspect). Section 7.

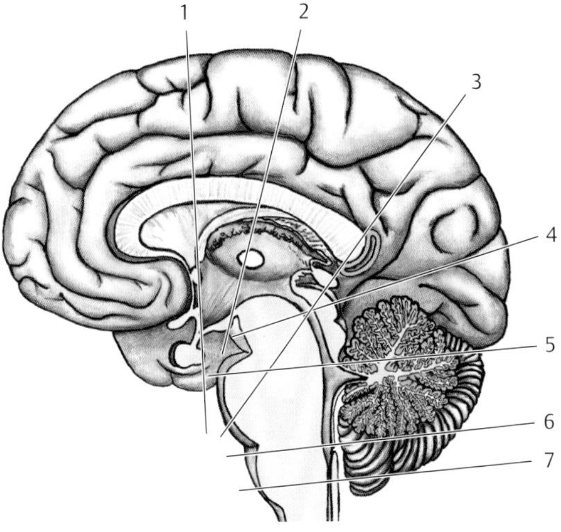


Fig. 9.175 **Right half of the brain.** Levels of the sections are indicated.

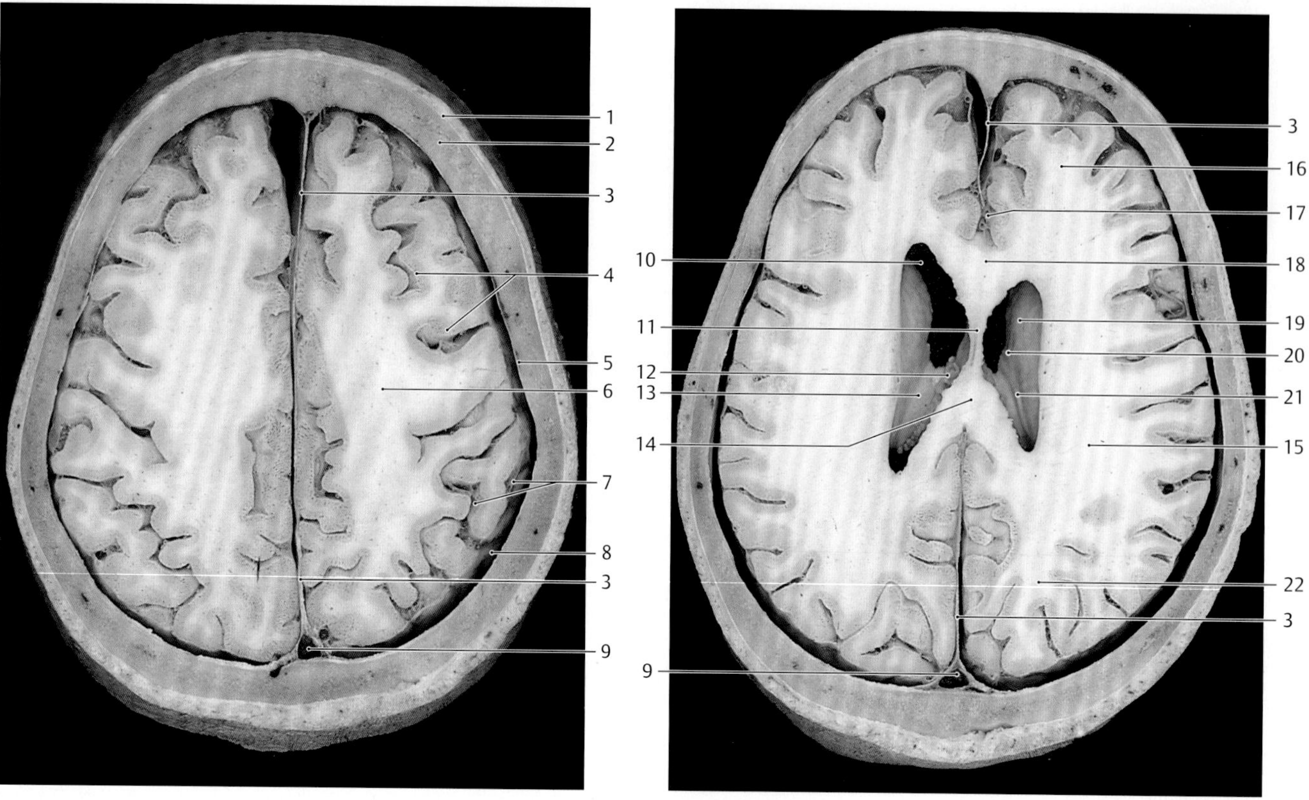


**Fig. 9.176 Horizontal section through the head and brain.** Section 1.

**Fig. 9.177 Horizontal section through the head and brain.** Section 2.

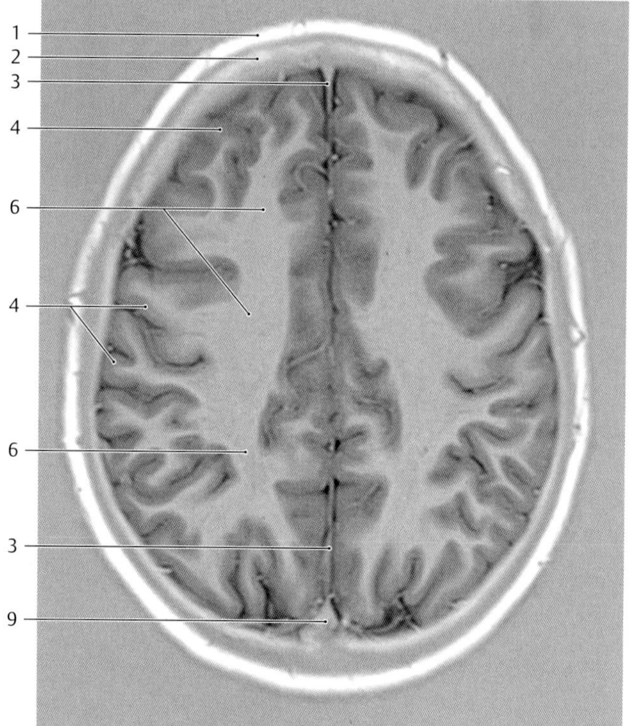


**Fig. 9.178 Horizontal section through the head and brain** at the level of section 1 (MRI scan). (Courtesy of Prof. Uder, Institute of Radiology, University Hospital Erlangen, Germany.)

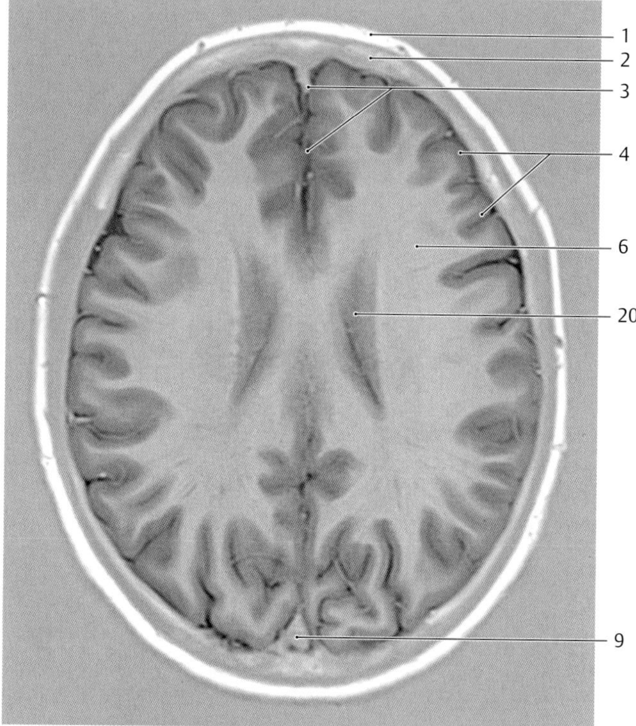


**Fig. 9.179 Horizontal section through the head and brain** at the level of section 2 (MRI scan). (Courtesy of Prof. Uder, Institute of Radiology, University Hospital Erlangen, Germany.)

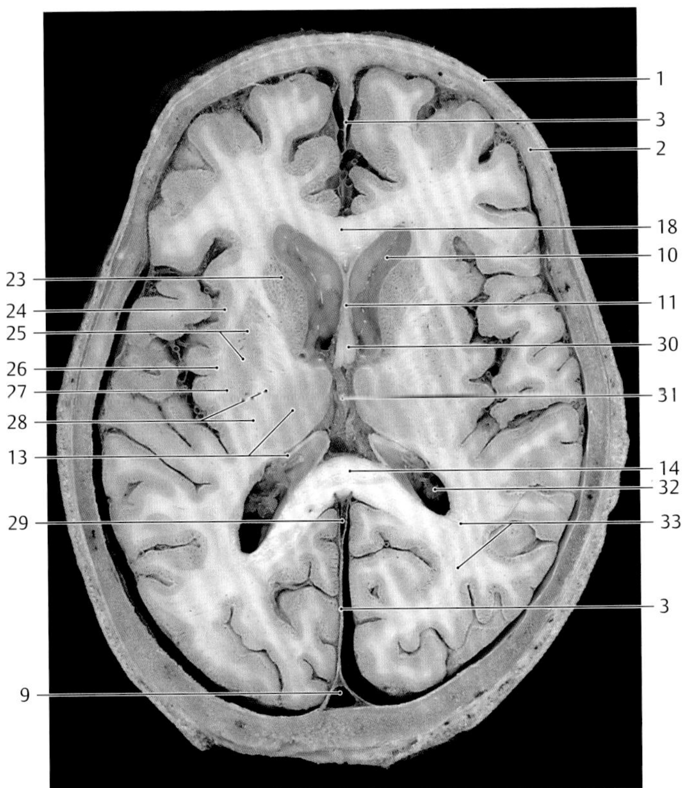


Fig. 9.180 **Horizontal section through the head and brain** at the level of third ventricle of internal capsule and neighboring nuclei. Section 3.

1 Skin of scalp
2 Calvaria (diploe of the skull)
3 Falx cerebri
4 Gray matter of brain (cortex)
5 Dura mater
6 White matter of brain
7 Arachnoid and pia mater with vessles
8 Subdural space (slightly expanded due to shrinkage of the brain)
9 Superior sagittal sinus
10 Anterior horn of lateral ventricle
11 Septum pellucidum
12 Choroid plexus
13 Thalamus
14 Splenium of corpus callosum
15 Parietal lobe
16 Frontal lobe
17 Anterior cerebral artery
18 Genu of corpus callosum
19 Caudate nucleus
20 Central part of lateral ventricle
21 Stria terminalis
22 Occipital lobe
23 Caudate nucleus
24 Lobus insularis (insula)
25 Putamen
26 Claustrum
27 External capsule
28 Internal capsule
29 Inferior sagittal sinus
30 Column of fornix
31 Choroid plexus of third ventricle
32 Entrance to inferior horn of lateral ventricle with choroid plexus
33 Optic radiation
34 Third ventricle

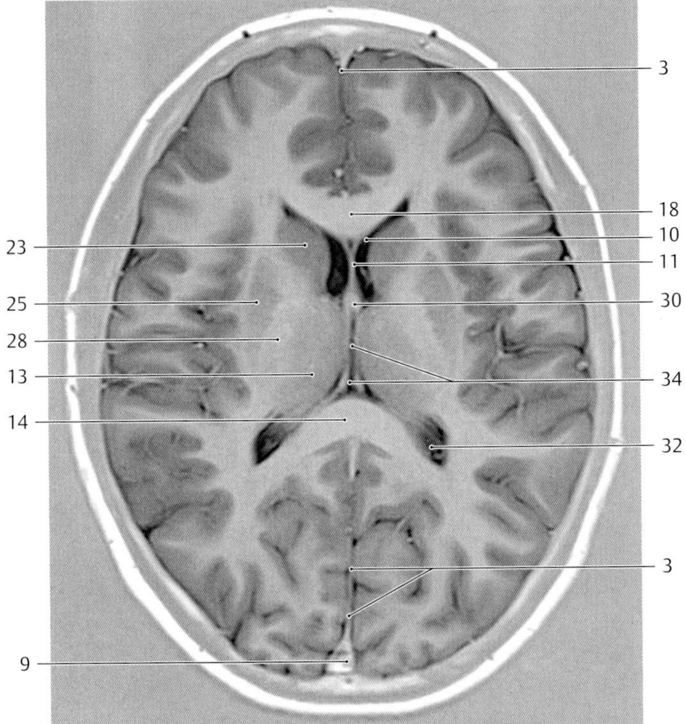


Fig. 9.181 **Horizontal section through the head and brain** at the level of section 3 (MRI scan). (Courtesy of Prof. Uder, Institute of Radiology, University Hospital Erlangen, Germany.)

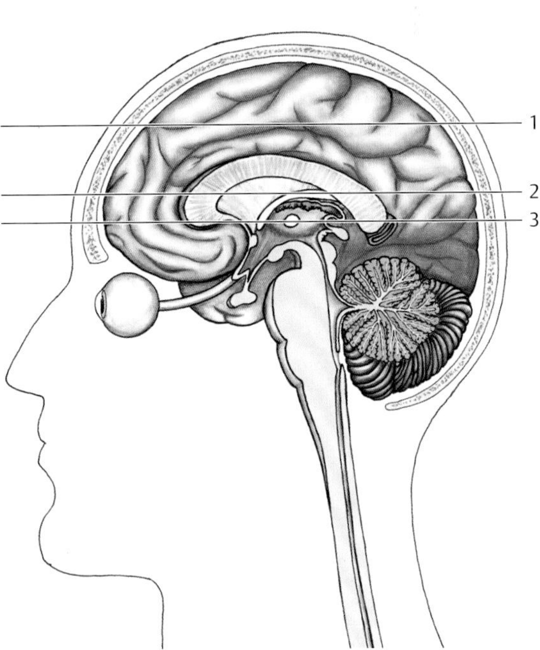


Fig. 9.182 **Sagittal section through the head and brain.** Levels of the sections are indicated.

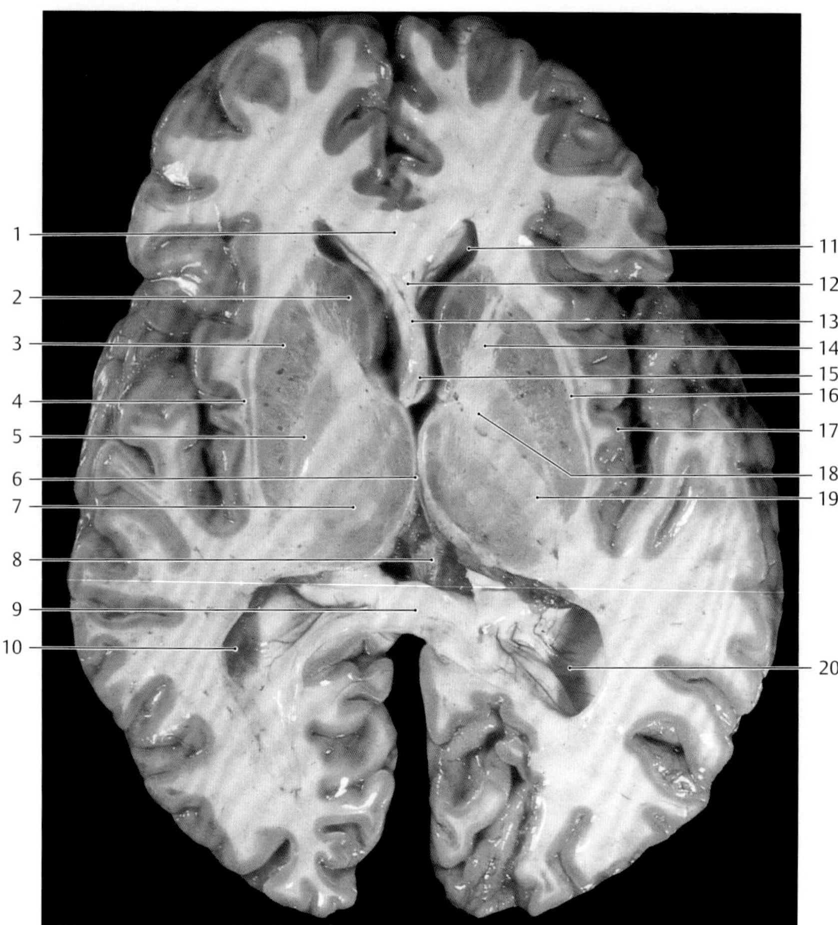


Fig. 9.183 **Horizontal section through the brain,** showing the subcortical nuclei and internal capsule. Section 1.

1 Genu of corpus callosum
2 Head of caudate nucleus
3 Putamen
4 Claustrum
5 Globus pallidus
6 Third ventricle
7 Thalamus
8 Pineal body
9 Splenium of corpus callosum
10 Choroid plexus of the lateral ventricle
11 Anterior horn of lateral ventricle
12 Cavity of septum pellucidum
13 Septum pellucidum
14 Anterior limb of internal capsule
15 Column of fornix
16 External capsule
17 Lobus insularis (insula)
18 Genu of internal capsule
19 Posterior limb of internal capsule
20 Posterior horn of lateral ventricle
21 Anterior commissure
22 Optic radiation
23 Falx cerebri
24 Maxillary sinus
25 Position of auditory tube
26 Tympanic cavity
27 External acoustic meatus
28 Medulla oblongata
29 Fourth ventricle
30 Cerebellum (left hemisphere)
31 Temporomandibular joint
32 Tympanic membrane
33 Base of cochlea
34 Mastoid air cells
35 Sigmoid sinus
36 Vermis of cerebellum
37 Intermediate mass

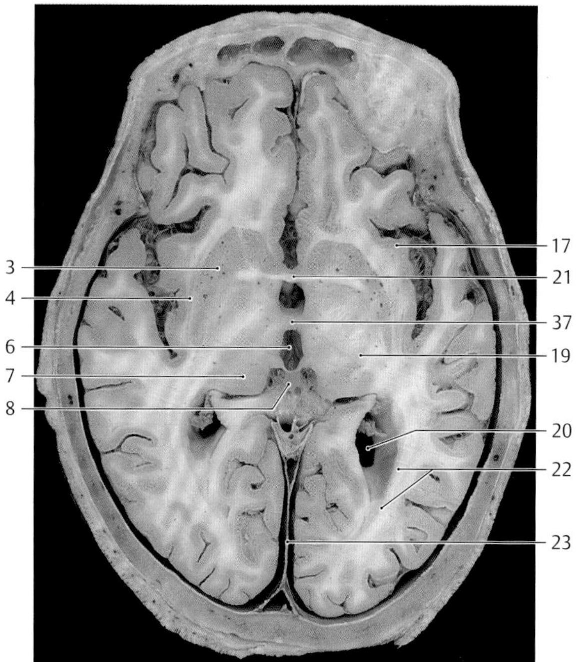


Fig. 9.184 **Horizontal section through the head and brain.** Section 2.

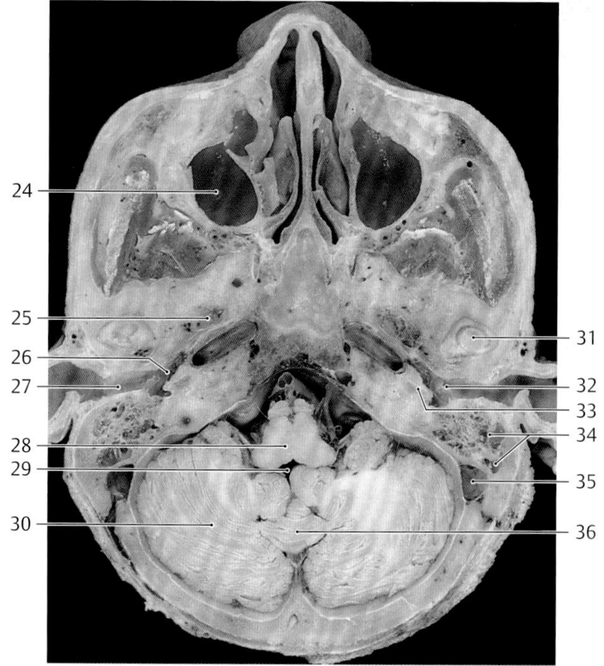


Fig. 9.185 **Horizontal section through the head and brain.** Section 4.

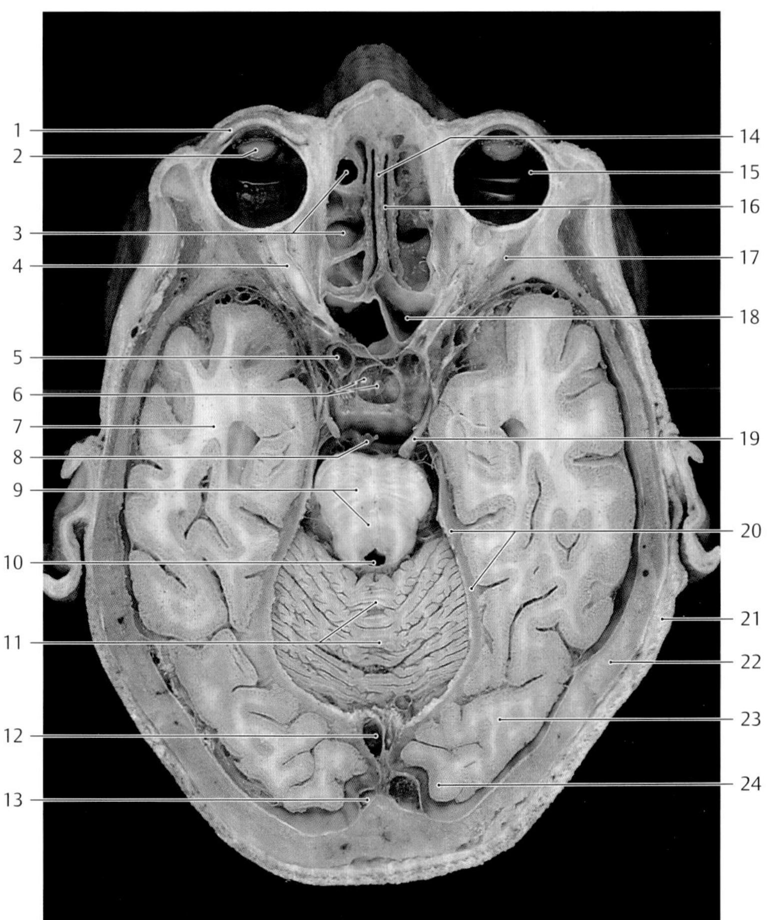


1 Upper lid (tarsal plate)
2 Lens
3 Ethmoidal sinus
4 Optic nerve (CN II)
5 Internal carotid artery
6 Infundibulum and pituitary gland
7 Temporal lobe
8 Basilar artery
9 Pons (cross section of brainstem)
10 Cerebral aqueduct (beginning of fourth ventricle)
11 Vermis of cerebellum
12 Straight sinus
13 Transverse sinus
14 Nasal septum
15 Eyeball (sclera)
16 Nasal cavity
17 Lateral rectus muscle
18 Sphenoidal sinus
19 Oculomotor nerve (CN III)
20 Cerebellar tentorium
21 Skin of scalp
22 Calvaria (diploe of the skull)
23 Occipital lobe
24 Striate cortex (visual cortex)

Fig. 9.186 **Horizontal section through the head and brain.** Section 3.

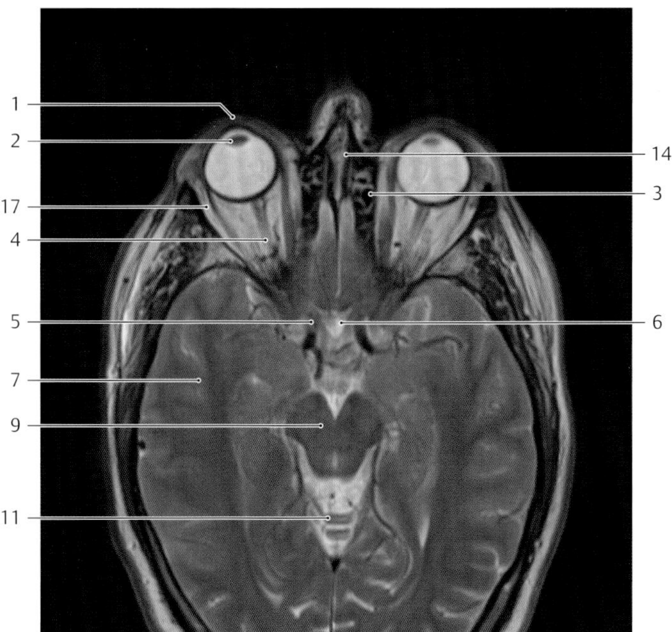


Fig. 9.187 **Cerebral peduncles.** Cross section through the brainstem with the cerebral aqueduct (MRI scan). (Courtesy of Prof. Uder, Institute of Radiology, University Hospital Erlangen, Germany.)

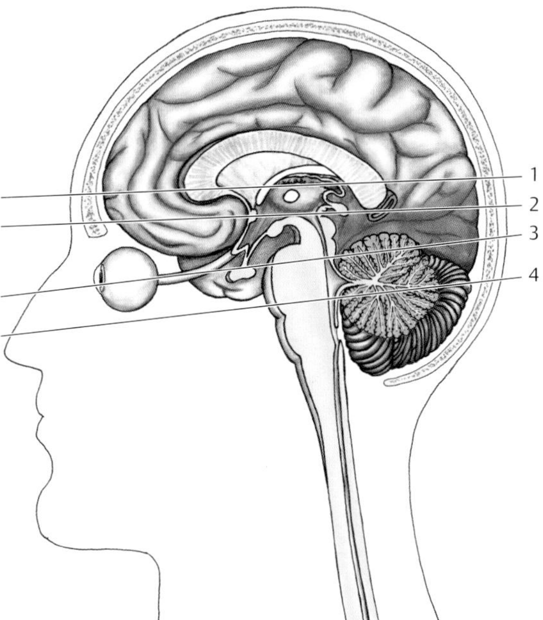


Fig. 9.188 **Sagittal section through the head and brain.** Levels of the sections are indicated.

# Appendix
# Additional Resources

## Arteries of Trunk, Chest and Abdominal Wall

See also Pages: 16–17 / 42 / 43–45 / 243–244 / 249 / 155 / 259 / 310

Aortic arch
- **brachiocephalic trunk** (divides into **right common carotid artery** [for right half of head and neck] and **right subclavian artery** [for right shoulder and arm])
- **left common carotid artery** (for left half of head and neck)
- **left subclavian artery** (for left shoulder and arm)

Vertebral artery
(through foramina transversaria of cervical spine and foramen occip. to brain; confluence of basilar artery)

Int. thoracic artery
(next to sternum to diaphragm and anterior abdominal wall)
- **ant. intercostal arteries** (to intercostal musculature)
- **med. mammary branches** (to mammary gland)
- **musculophrenic artery** (to diaphragm)
- **sup. epigastric artery** (to the anterior muscles of abdominal wall)

Thyrocervical trunk
- **inf. thyroid artery** (for the thyroid gland and esophagus)
- **ascending cervical artery** (for scalene muscles and the prevertebral cervical muscles)
- **transverse cervical artery** (to the superficial dorsal muscles)
- **suprascapular artery** (to the scapula muscles; anastomoses with circumflex scapular artery)
- **doral scapular artery** (autonomous branch of transverse cervical artery)

Costocervical trunk
- **deep cervical artery** (to neck muscles)
- **supreme intercostal artery** (to 1st and 2nd intercostal space)

Aorta (thoracic part)
- **post. intercostal arteries** (to 3rd to 12th intercostal spaces; anastomose with ant. intercostal arteries)
- **bronchial branches** (to bronchi and lung)
- **esophageal branches** (to esophagus)
- **pericardiac branches** (to pericardium)
- **sup. phrenic arteries** (to diaphragm)
- **subcostal artery** (intercostal artery beneath 12th rib)

Aorta (abdominal part)
- **inf. phrenic artery** (to diaphragm, branch to adrenal gland [sup. suprarenal artery])
- **middle suprarenal artery** (to adrenal gland)

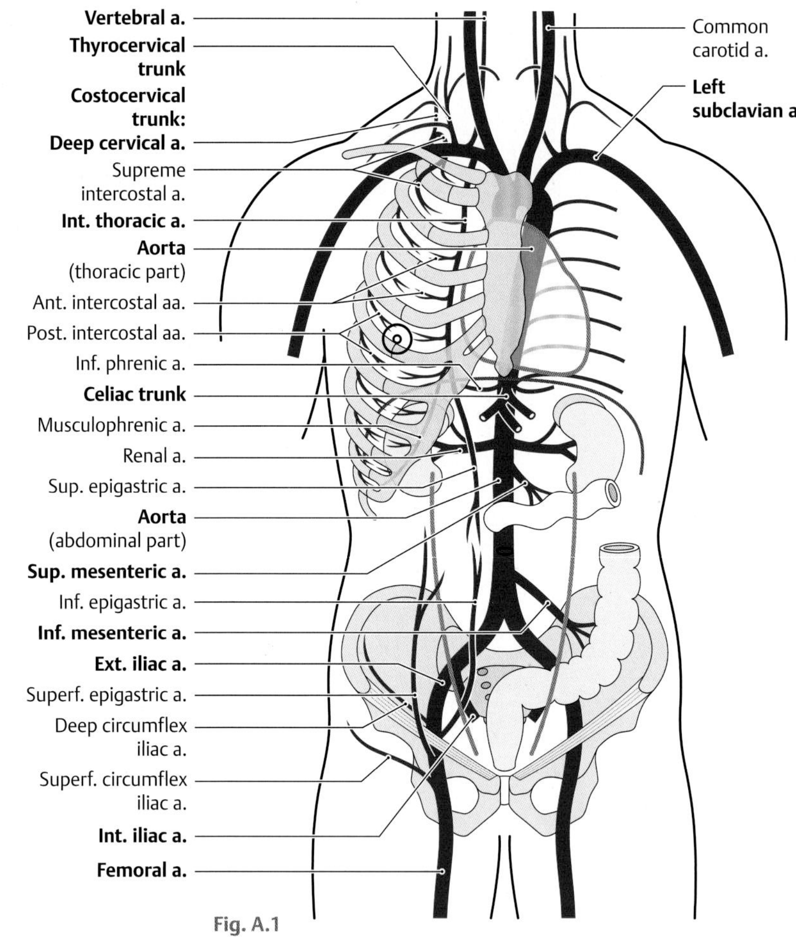


Fig. A.1

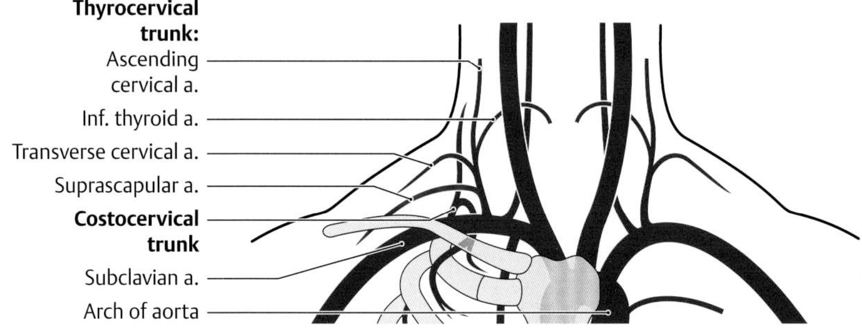


Fig. A.2

- **lumbar arteries** (4 segmental arteries; to core muscles and spinal cord)
- **renal artery** (to kidney)

Celiac trunk (see p. 523)
Sup. mesenteric artery (see p. 523)
Inf. mesenteric artery (see p. 523)
Ext. iliac artery
- **Inf. epigastric artery** (to anterior abdominal muscles; anastomoses with sup. epigastric artery)
- **Deep circumflex iliac artery** (to abdominal wall at pelvic edge)

Femoral artery (see p. 544)
- **superf. epigastric artery** (to anterior abdominal wall)
- **superf. circumflex iliac artery** (to abdominal wall of groin region)

Clinical

**Intercostal arteries:**
run at lower edge of ribs; puncture of pleura can be carried out at upper edge of the ribs.

**Sup. and inf. epigastric arteries:**
form a collateral cycle above abdominal wall, which can be clinically relevant.

## Arteries of the Abdominal Organs

See also Pages: 259 / 279–283 / 290/ 291–295 / 305–306 / 310 / 312–313

**Epigastrium**
**Celiac trunk** (Tripus Halleri) has 3 branches: **left gastric artery** runs to the front of the stomach; **common hepatic artery**, right of the median plane (dashed line), supplies organs positioned on the right (liver, head of pancreas, duodenum, etc.); and the **splenic artery**, supplies organs positioned on the left (spleen, fundus of stomach, pancreas, etc.).

**Hypogastrium**
**Sup. mesenteric artery** right of the diagonal marked line (root of mesentery), supplies all parts of the intestine until left colic flexure. The **inf. mesenteric artery** supplies all parts of the intestine lying left from marked line (descending colon until rectum).

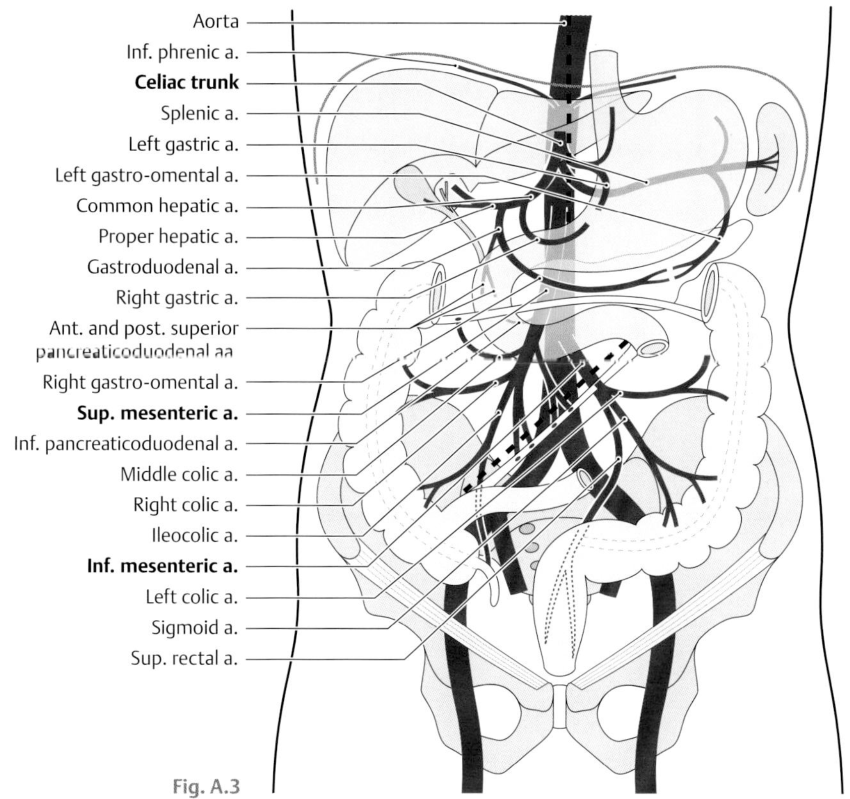


Fig. A.3

**Aorta**
(transition from thoracic part into abdominal part)
- **inf. phrenic artery** (to bottom of diaphragm)

**Celiac trunk**
(with 3 main branches to organs of the epigastrium [stomach, spleen, liver and first part of duodenum])
- **splenic artery** (to spleen; branches to fundus of stomach [short gastric branches] and to the greater curvature of the stomach and the greater omentum [left gastro-omental artery])
- **left gastric artery** (to lesser curvature of stomach)
- **common hepatic artery** (branches to liver, stomach and upper duodenum; continues into **proper hepatic artery** [to the liver] with branches to gallbladder [**cystic artery**])
  - **gastroduodenal artery** (behind pylorus; branches to the stomach and duodenum)
  - **right gastric artery** (to lesser curvature of stomach; anastomoses with left gastric artery)
  - **ant. and post. sup. pancreaticoduodenal arteries** (to duodenum and head of pancreas)
  - **right gastro-omental artery** (anastomoses with left gastro-omental artery at greater curvature of stomach; supplies stomach and greater omentum)

**Sup. mesenteric artery**
(crosses horizontal part of duodenum; numerous branches to duodenum, jejunum and ileum and garland of colon until left colic flexure)
- **inf. pancreaticoduodenal artery** (to duodenum and head of pancreas; anastomoses with ant. and post. sup. pancreaticoduodenal arteries)
- **middle colic artery** (in transverse mesocolon to transverse colon)
- **right colic artery** (to ascending colon)
- **ileocolic artery** (to cecum, ileum and vermiform appendix [appendicular artery])
- **inf. mesenteric artery** (provides descending colon, sigmoid colon and rectum)
- **left colic artery** (runs retroperitoneal to descending colon; anastomoses with middle colic artery [riolan-anastomosis])
- **sigmoid arteries** (a number of branches to sigmoid colon)
- **sup. rectal artery** (right and left branches supply rectum up to the anal valves)

Clinical

**Splenic artery:**
branches of artery of spleen are functional final branches, so partial resections of spleen are possible.

**Pancreaticoduodenal artery:**
tight locality with duodenum; carcinoma of head of pancreas can cause erosion of the arteries which can lead to life-threatening bleedings.

**Riolan-anastomosis:**
connection between middle colic artery and left colic artery in region of left colic flexure; this collateral cycle can be clinically relevant if resection of colon is needed.

## Veins of the Torso, Chest and Abdominal Wall

See also Pages: 44–45 / 242–243 / 246–247 / 252–253 / 256–257 / 310 / 312

Clinical

**Sup. vena cava:**
access to right atrium of the heart (for example with cardiac catheter).
**Inf. vena cava:**
obstruction can lead to development of collateral circulation with epigastric veins, vertebral venous plexus and ascending lumbar veins.
**Azygos vein** and **hemiazygos vein:**
obstruction of portal vein can lead to collateral circulation to superior vena cava.
**Testicular vein:**
an obstruction of the drainage of the left side leads more often to varicoceles than of the right side (left: confluence in renal vein and fewer venous valves).

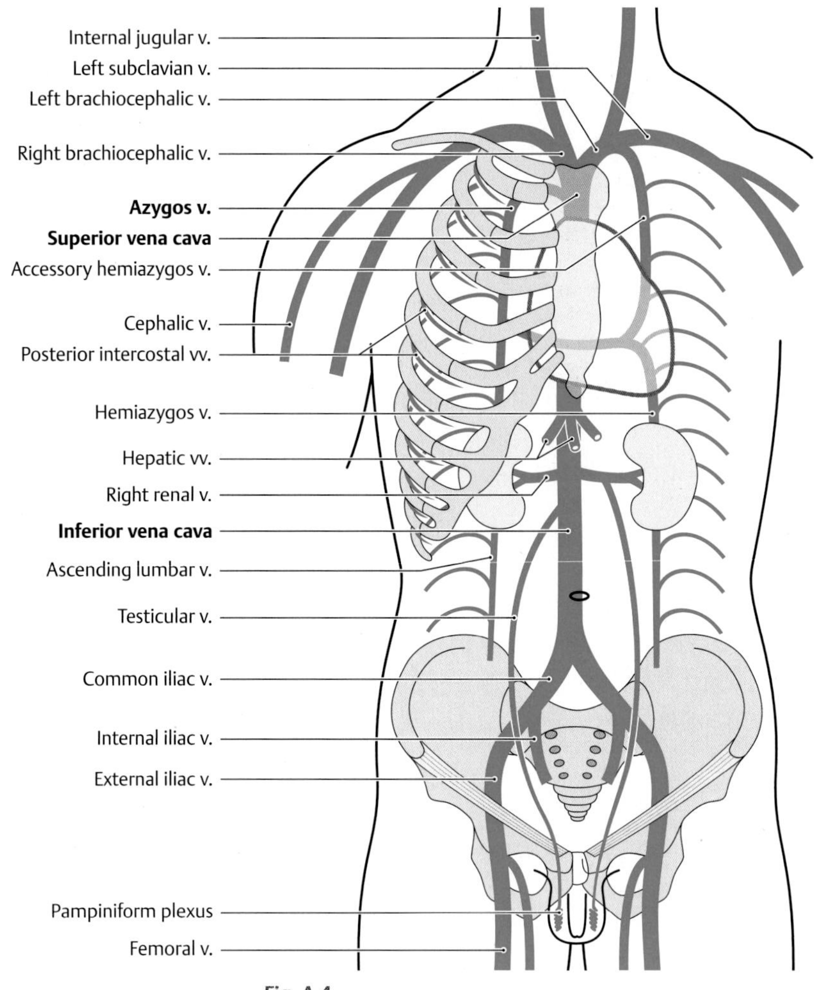


Fig. A.4

**Sup. vena cava**
(from confluence of both **brachiocephalic veins**; drainage from head and arm and from dorsal torso wall, [**azygos vein**])
**Inf. vena cava**
(from confluence of both **common iliac veins**; drainage of blood from the liver [**hepatic veins**]; kidneys [**renal veins**] and from the pelvic organs [**int. iliac veins**]) and legs [**femoral veins**])

**Azygos vein**
(receives blood from **posterior intercostal veins, lumbar veins, hemiazygos vein** and **accessory hemiazygos vein** [drainage from the entire posterior torso wall])

Note:
The **testicular veins** or **ovarian veins** flow on the left side into the renal vein and on the right side into the inferior vena cava.

## Veins of the Abdominal Organs: Portal Venous System

See also Pages: 278–280 / 305 / 312

The regions of the anastomosis between the vena cava and portal venous system (portocaval anastomosis, red circles) are marked with a, b and c.

Clinical

**Portal vein:**
obstruction or disease of the liver (e.g. liver cirrhosis) leads to collateral circulation

a) through veins of the esophagus to azygos vein and sup. vena cava,
b) through sup. epigastric veins to sup. vena cava and inf. epigastric veins to femoral vein or ext. iliac vein (head of Medusa),
c) through middle and inf. rectal veins to int. iliac vein and inf. vena cava.

**Rectal veins:**
venous drainage from kidneys and pelvic organs (retroperitoneal space); do not belong to the portal venous system.

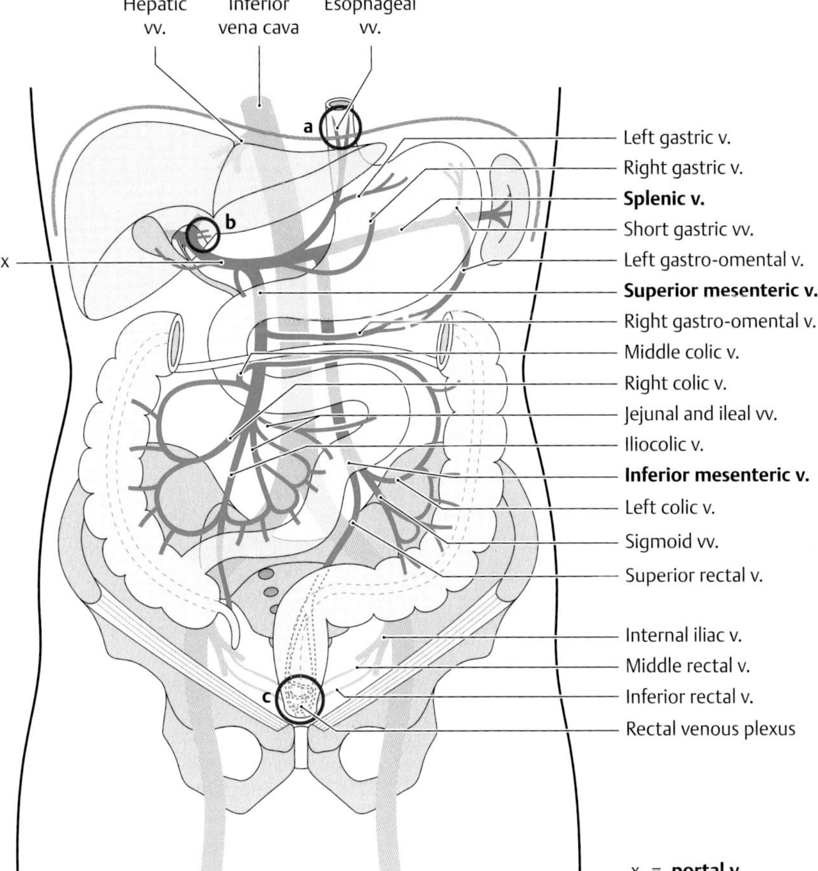


Fig. A.5

**Portal vein**
(collecting vessel for venous blood of all abdominal organs [stomach, spleen, duodenum, pancreas, jejunum, ileum and colon]; three anastomosis regions for drainage region of venae cavae [portocaval anastomoses]):

a = esophageal veins (connections to azygos veins)
b = periumbilical veins (connections to the azygos veins)
c = rectal venous plexus (connections to the int. iliac veins)

- **esophageal veins** (from esophagus to azygos vein [anastomoses with gastric veins])
- **left and right gastric veins** (accompanying veins of arteries with same name on lesser curvature of the stomach)

**Splenic vein**
(vein for spleen to portal vein)

- **short gastric veins** (branches from splenic vein; from fundus of stomach)
- **left gastro-omental vein** (at greater curvature of the stomach to splenic vein)

**Sup. mesenteric vein**
(collection vessel of veins from distal duodenum, jejunum, ileum and colon until left colic flexure; crosses duodenum and forms the portal vein behind the head of the pancreas together with **splenic artery**)

- **right gastro-omental vein** (at greater curvature of the stomach; anastomoses with left gastro-omental vein)
- **middle colic vein** (drains from transverse colon)
- **right colic vein** (drains from ascending colon)
- **jejunal veins** and **ileal veins** (in the mesentery of jejunum and ileum)
- **iliocolic veins** (of cecum, ileum and vermiform appendix [**appendicular vein**])

**Inf. mesenteric vein**
(retroperitoneal drainage of descending colon, sigmoid colon and rectum; confluence of splenic vein)

- **left colic vein** (of descending colon)
- **sigmoid veins** (veins of the sigmoid colon that run in the mesentery)
- **sup. rectal vein** (unpaired branch of the superior rectum; anastomoses with middle and inferior rectal veins of the internal iliac veins to **rectal venous plexus**)

## Arteries of the Pelvis of the Female

See also Pages: 338–340 / 344

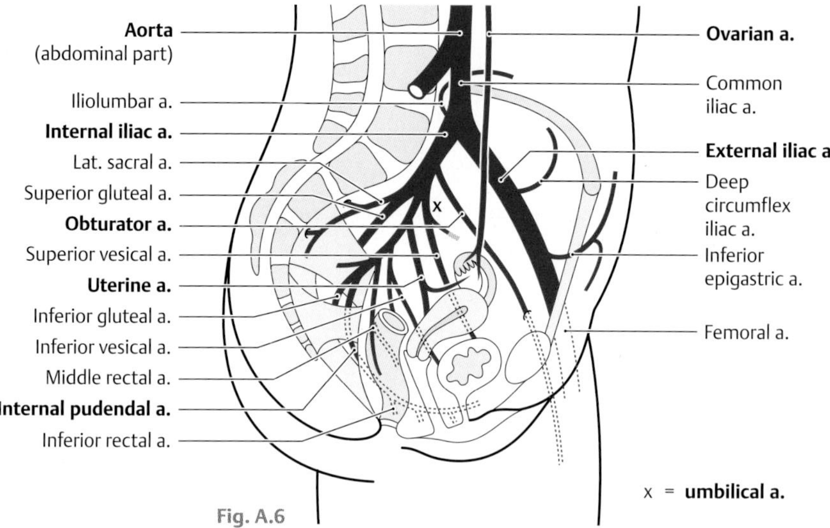

Fig. A.6

**Aorta** (abdominal part) (divides into ext. and int. iliac artery in front of fourth lumbar vertebra [aortic bifurcation])
**Ext. iliac artery** (continues as femoral artery after passage of the inguinal ligament)
- **deep circumflex iliac artery** (to the abdominal wall; along the iliac crest)
- **inf. epigastric artery** (runs in lat. umbilical fold upward to the abdominal wall)

**Ovarian artery** (separation of the aorta at L2; runs in the suspensory ligament of ovary to the ovary; anastomoses with ovarian branch of uterine artery)
**Int. iliac artery**
with **parietal branches:**
- **iliolumbar artery** (along iliac crest; anastomoses with deep circumflex iliac artery)
- **lat. sacral artery** (to sacrum and spinal canal)
- **sup. gluteal artery** (through greater sciatic foramen [suprapiriform foramen] gluteus medius and minimus muscle)
- **obturator artery** (through obturator canal to the adductor muscles; with **pubic branch** [internally to abdominal wall; anastomoses with inf. epigastric artery] and **acetabular branch** [in the ligament of head of femur for the head of the hip joint])
- **inf. gluteal artery** (through greater sciatic foramen [infrapiriform foramen] to gluteus maximus muscle)
- **int. pudendal artery** (through infrapiriform foramen and lesser sciatic foramen to anal and genital region) with
  - **inf. rectal artery** (to anus, rectum)
  - **perineal artery** (to perineum; forms post. labial arteries)
  - **artery of bulb of vestibule** (to bulb of vestible)
  - **urethral artery** (to corpus spongiosum urethrae)
  - **deep artery of clitoris** } final branches
  - **dorsal artery of clitoris** } for clitoris

and **viceral branches:**
- **umbilical artery** (with sup. vesical artery [to the bladder] and to the med. umbilical ligament [residuum of umbilical artery])
- **uterine artery** (for uterus and proximal vagina; with ovarian branch to ovary)
- **inf. vesical artery** (for base of bladder and vagina)
- **middle rectal artery** (for pelvic diaphragm and rectum)

## Veins of the Pelvis of the Female

See also Pages: 339–340

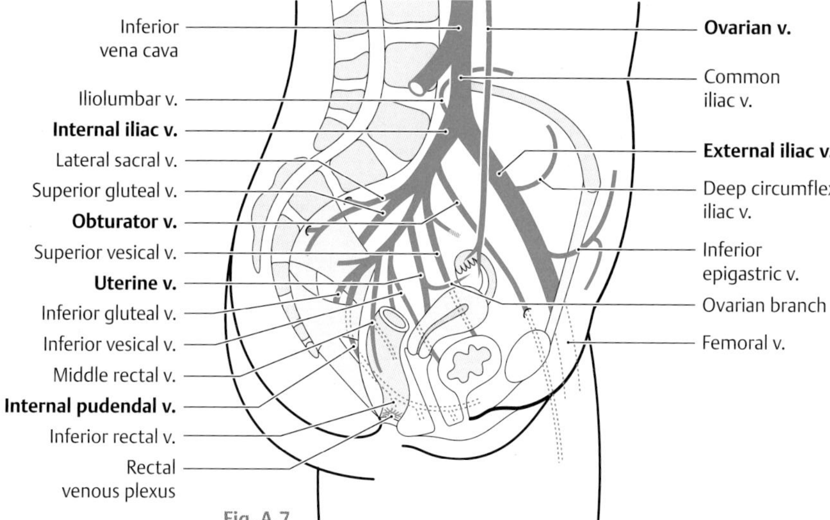

Fig. A.7

The veins of the female pelvis run together with the arteries of the same name and form mostly parallel vessels, which can arise from vast vascular networks (plexus).
**Ovarian vein**
(flows into the abdominal aorta on the right side and to the left renal vein on the left side; anastomoses with veins of uterine tube and uterus)
**Ext. iliac vein**
(continuation of femoral vein; intake of veins of the anterior abdominal wall [inf. epigastical vein] and of the iliac crest [deep circumflex iliac vein])
**Int. iliac vein**
with **parietal branches:**
- **iliolumbar vein** (of iliac crest)
- **lat. sacral vein** (of sacrum and spinal canal)
- **sup.** and **inf. gluteal veins** (of the gluteal muscles)
- **obturator vein** (of the adductor muscles)
- **int. pudendal vein** (with inf. rectal vein [rectal venous plexus]; perineal vein [of the perineal region and the labia], of the vein of bulb of vestibule and urethral vein [of urethra and bulb of vestibule] and of the veins of clitoris [of the clitoris])

and **visceral branches:**
- **middle rectal vein** (of rectum)
- **umbilical vein** (with sup. vesical vein and median umbilical ligament)
- **inf. vesical vein** (of the base of the bladder and vagina)
- **uterine vein** (runs in the parametrium [broad ligament of uterus] and forms connections with veins of the uterine tube and the ovaries)

## Arteries of the Pelvis of the Male

See also Pages: 310 / 312–313 / 324–329 / 332



Fig. A.8

**Testicular artery**
(separates from the aorta at L2; with ductus deferens through the inguinal canal to testicles and epididymis)
**Ext. iliac artery**
(continuation into femoral artery)
- **deep circumflex iliac artery** (anastomoses with iliolumbar artery at iliac crest)
- **inf. epigastric artery** (to the external abdominal wall; with **pubic branch** [anastomoses with obturator artery] and **cremasteric artery** [for spermatic cord and scrotum])

**Int. iliac artery**
with **parietal branches:**
- **iliolumbar artery**
(along iliac crest to the iliopsoas muscle and spinal canal; anastomoses with deep circumflex iliac artery)
- **lat. scrotal artery**
(to sacrum and spinal canal)
- **sup. gluteal artery**
(through suprapirifom foramen to gluteus medius and minimus muscle)
- **obturator artery**
(through the obturator canal to the adductor muscles; with **pubic branch** [internally to abdominal wall; anastomoses with inf. epigastric artery] and **acetabular branch** [in ligament of head of femur for the head of the hip joint])
- **inf. gluteal artery** (through infrapirifom foramen to gluteus maximus muscle)
- **int. pudendal artery** (through infrapiriform foramen and lesser sciatic foramen to anal and genital region) with **inf. rectal artery** [to anus and rectum])
  - **perineal artery** (to perineum; forms post. scrotal arteries)
  - **artery of bulb of penis** (to bulb of penis)
  - **urethral artery**
  (corpus spongiosum urethrae)
  - **dorsal artery of penis** (to glans penis)
  - **deep arteries of penis**
  (to erectile tissue of the penis)

and **visceral branches:**
- **middle rectal artery**
(for pelvic diaphragm, rectum, prostate and seminal vesicles)
- **umbilical artery**
  - **sup. vesical artery** (to the bladder)
  - **median umbilical ligament**
  (remnant of umbilical artery)
- **inf. vesical artery**
(to base of bladder, prostate)
- **artery of ductus deferens**
(for spermatic duct, seminal vesicle and spermatic cord)

## Veins of the Pelvis of the Male

See also Pages: 310 / 312 / 328–329 / 332

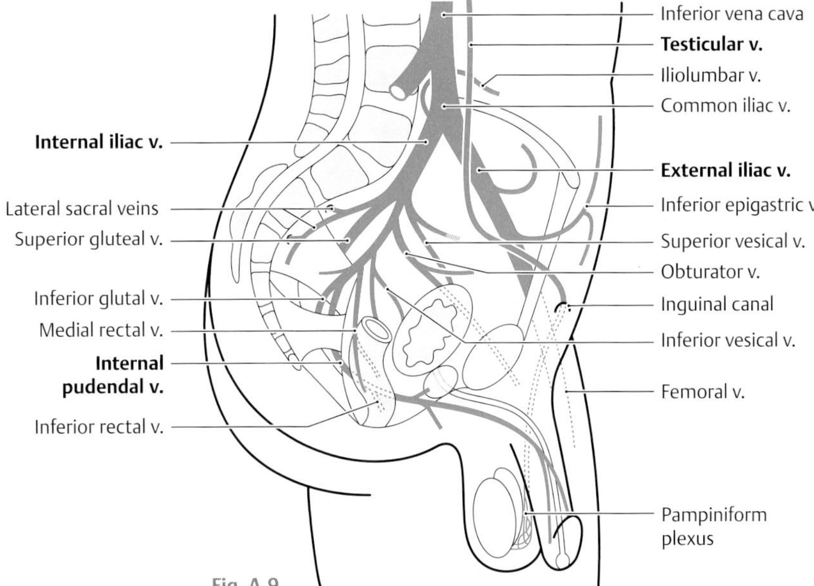


Fig. A.9

The veins accompany arteries of the same name, and often form double, interconnected venous cords and plexus attached to nearby organs.
**Ext. iliac vein**
(continues into femoral vein; before branching off into the inf. epigastric vein and deep circumflex iliac vein)
**Int. iliac vein**
(collects veins of lateral pelvic wall)
with **parietal branches:**
iliolumbar vein; lat. sacral veins, sup. and inf. gluteal veins (to pelvic wall, gluteal region and spinal canal) and
**Int. pudendal vein**
(of pelvic floor and genitalia)
and **visceral branches:**
(run from bladder [sup. and inf. vesical veins] and from rectum [middle and inf. rectal vein])

**Testicular vein**
(from pampiniform plexus; runs with ductus deferens through inguinal canal; confluence on right side in inf. vena cava, on left side in left renal vein)

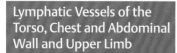

## Lymphatic Vessels of the Torso, Chest and Abdominal Wall and Upper Limb

See also Pages: 17 / 243–244 / 422–423 / 266 / 310-311 / 124–125

Clinical

**Supraclavicular lymph nodes** (Virchow nodes): often enlarged by metastasis of tumors of stomach or liver.

**Central axillary lymph nodes:** often primarily invaded by metastasis of tumor of the breast; in case of lymphadenectomy due to suspicion of a tumor, at least ten axillary lymph nodes need to be examined. Tumors of the breast can also metastasize into parasternal and supraclavicular lymph nodes.

**Regional groups of lymph nodes:** can provide information about the localization of the primary tumor (lymphatic metastasis).

**Lymphangitis:** inflammation of lymphatic vessels can be apparent as local swelling or red strips on the skin.

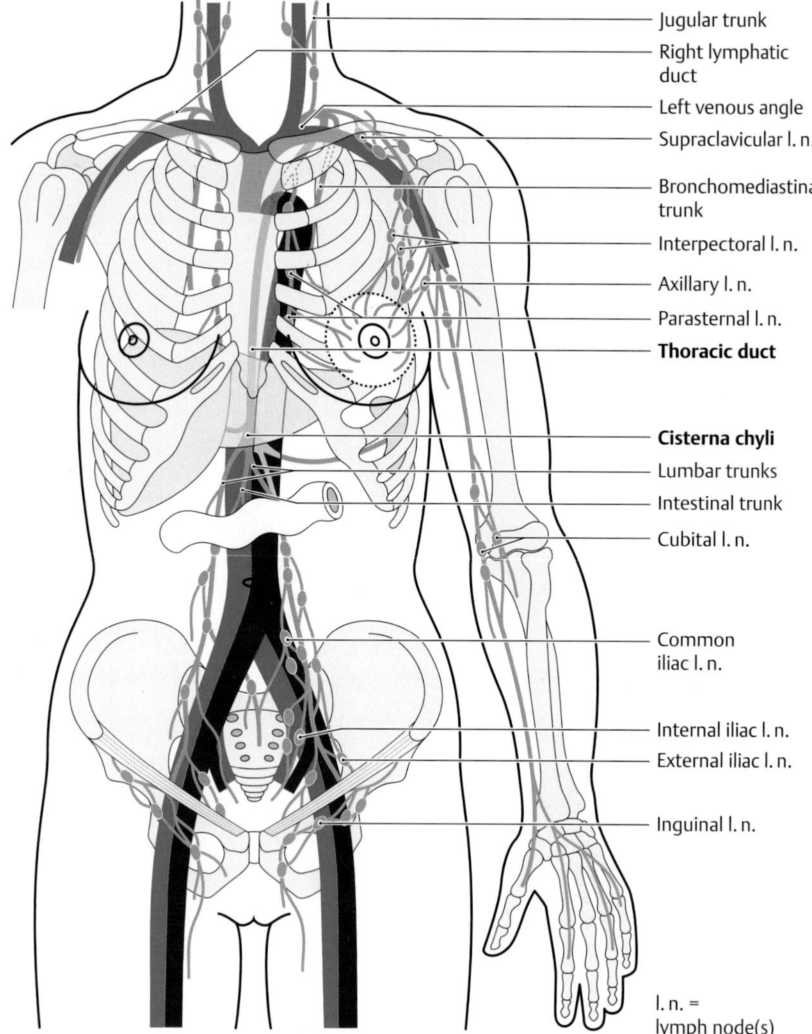


Fig. A.10

**Right lymphatic duct**
(lymphatic pathways of the right head and neck region [right jugular trunk], of the right arm [right subclavian trunk] and of the right upper half of the thorax, chest wall, breast and the anterior mediastinum [right broncho-mediastinal trunk]; confluence of right venous angle)
**Thoracic duct**
(confluence of left venous angle; receives lymph from left jugular trunk [lymphatic pathways of the left head and neck region] and of left subclavian trunk [of the left arm]); receives lymph from
**Left bronchomediastinal trunk**
(lymphatic pathways of left upper half of thorax, superior mediastinum, pericardium, trachea and bronchi, [tracheobronchial lymph nodes], chest wall and breast [parasternal and paramammary lymph nodes])
**Axillary lymphatic plexus**
(lymphatic pathways of the anterior chest wall [interpectoral, parasternal and intercostal lymph nodes] of the breast [paramammary lymph nodes] and of the arm [brachial, cubital, infraclavicular and deltopectoral lymph nodes])
**Cisterna chyli**
(receives lymph from
- **intestinal trunks** – lymphatic pathways of abdominal organs [visceral lymph nodes] and
- **lumbar trunks**
[paired], lymphatic pathways of the pelvic organs and lower limb; transition into thoracic duct)

## Muscles of the Antero-lateral Abdominal Wall

See also Pages: 36–41 / 44 / 46 / 48

**Intercostal and abdominal muscles, anterior head muscles**

The external and internal oblique muscles–connected by the rectus sheath–form an obliquly running tension band that crosses in the anterior abdominal wall (dotted lines).

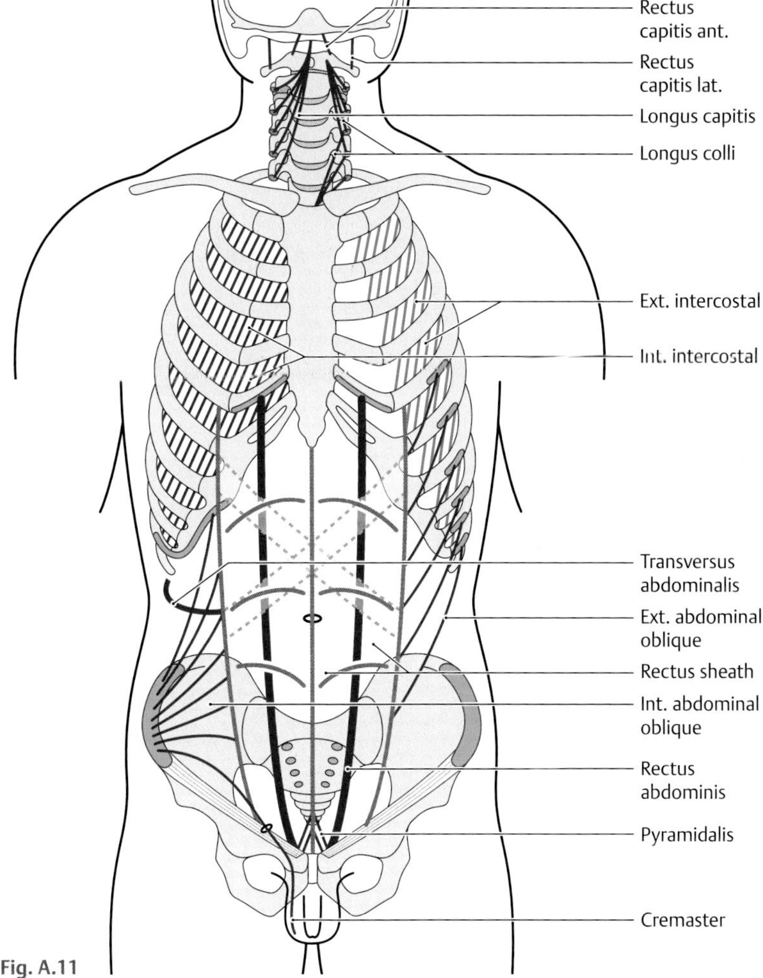


Fig. A.11

| Muscles | Origin | Insertion | Function | Innervation |
|---|---|---|---|---|
| **Rectus capitis anterior** | Atlas | Occipital bone | Anterior flexion of the head | Cervical plexus (C1, C2) |
| **Rectus capitis lateralis** | Transverse process of atlas | Occipital bone | Lateral flexion of the head | Cervical plexus (C1, C2) |
| **Longus capitis** | Transverse processes of C2–C6 | Occipital bone | Flexion of the cervical spine, anterior flexion of the head | Cervical plexus (C1, C2) |
| **Longus colli** | Body of vertebra C2–C7, T1–T3 | Body of vertebra and transverse process C2–T3 | Flexion of the cervical spine | Cervical plexus (C1–C8) |
| **External intercostal** | Lower border of ribs | Upper border of ribs | Inspiration | Anterior branches of the spinal nerves |
| **Internal intercostal** | Upper border of ribs | Upper border of ribs | Expiration | Anterior branches of the spinal branches |
| **Transversus abdominis** | 6th to 12th rib, iliac crest | Rectus sheath | Tension of the abdominal wall, abdominal press | Intercostal nn. (T6–T12), iliohypogastric n., ilioinguinal n. |
| **External abdominal oblique** | 5th to 12th rib | Iliac crest, inguinal ligament | As rectus abdominis and rotation of the trunk to the opposite side | Intercostal nn. (T5–T12), iliohypogastric n., ilioinguinal n. |
| **Internal abdominal oblique** (with cremaster) | Iliac crest, inguinal ligament | Costal arch, rectus sheath | As external abdominal oblique, rotation of the trunk to the same side (elevation of the testicles) | As external abdominal oblique (cremaster through genital branch of genitofemoral n.) |
| **Rectus abdominis** | Sternum, 5th to 7th rib | Pubic bone, symphysis | Anterior flexion of the trunk, elevation of the pelvis, abdominal press | Intercostal n. (T6–T12) |
| **Pyramidalis** | Pubic bone | Linea alba | Tension of the rectus sheath and linea alba | Intercostal n. (T12) |

## Muscles of the Posterior Abdominal Wall (I)

See also Pages: 56–59/62–64/60/80

**Superficial muscles of the back and posterior muscles of the head**

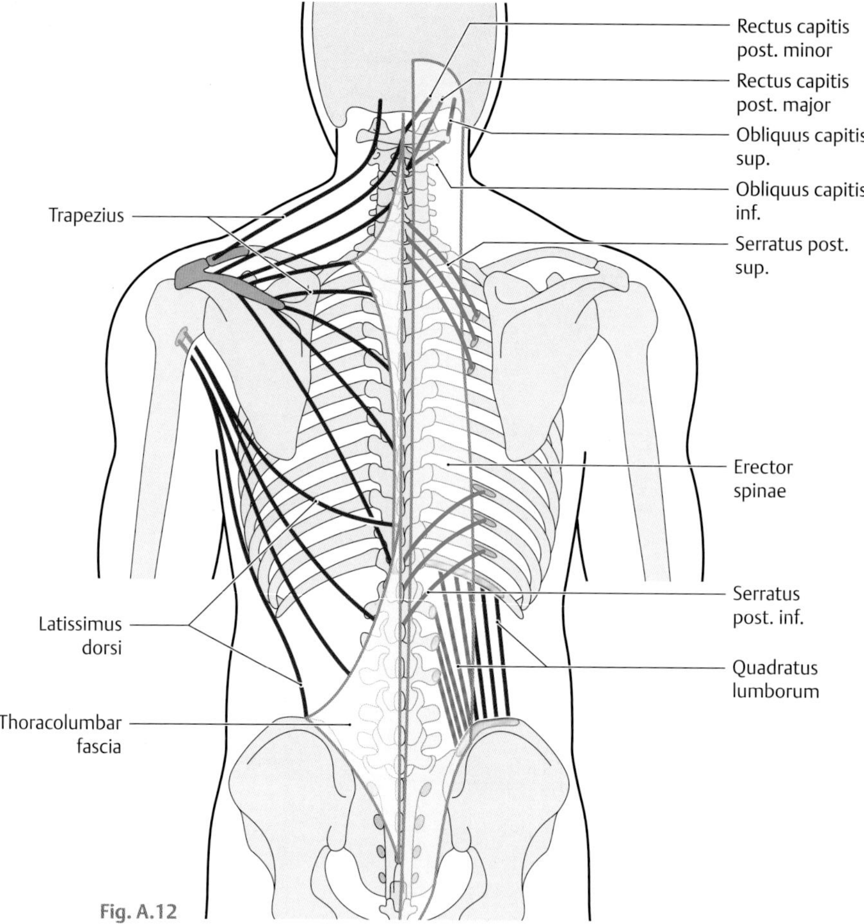


Fig. A.12

## Muscles of the Posterior Abdominal Wall (II)

See also Pages: 56–59 / 96

**Intrinsic back muscles, erector spinae muscles**
(*lateral and medial tract*)

1 = Rectus capitis posterior minor muscle
2 = Rectus capitis posterior major muscle
3 = Obliquus capitis superior muscle
4 = Obliquus capitis inferior muscle
(see table p. 532)

The levatores costarum breves and longi muscles run in the chest region from the transverse processes to the ribs.

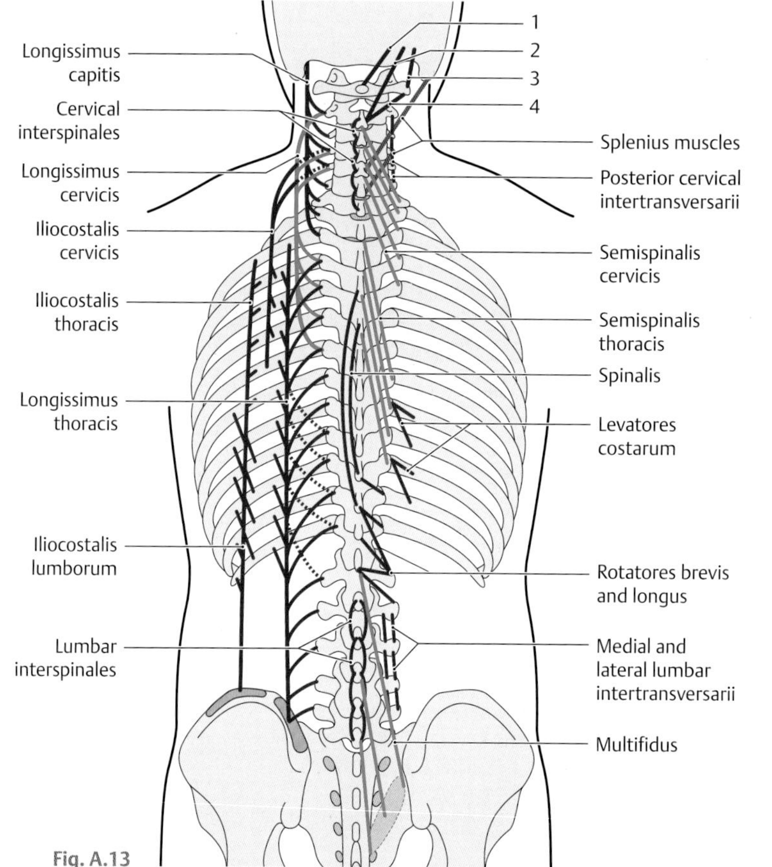


Fig. A.13

| Muscles | Origin | Insertion | Function | Innervation |
|---|---|---|---|---|
| **Muscles of the neck** | | | | |
| **Rectus capitis posterior minor** | Posterior tubercle of atlas | Occipital bone | Retroversion of the head | Suboccipital n. (C1) |
| **Rectus capitis posterior major** | Spinous process of axis | Occipital bone | Retroversion and lateral flexion of the head | Suboccipital n. (C1) |
| **Obliquus capitis superior** | Transverse process of atlas | Occipital bone | Retroversion and lateral flexion of the head | Suboccipital n. (C1) |
| **Obliquus capitis inferior** | Spinous process of axis | Transverse process of atlas | Rotation of the head | Suboccipital n. (C1) |
| **Muscles of the back** | | | | |
| **Trapezius**<br>• **descending part**<br>• **transverse part**<br>• **ascending part** | Ext. occipital protuberance, superior nuchal line, spinous processes of all cervical and thoracic vertebra | Clavicle,<br>acromion,<br>spine of scapula | Posterior elevation of the head and cervical spine, superior and inferior elevation of the shoulder girdle, rotation of the scapula | Accessory n. (CN XI), branches of cervical plexus |
| **Serratus posterior superior** | Spinous processes of C5–C7, T1 and T2 | 3rd to 5th rib | Tension of erector spinae, inspiration | Anterior branches of the spinal nerves |
| **Serratus posterior inferior** | Spinous processes of T11, T12, and L1–L3, thoraco-lumbar fascia | 9th to 12th rib | Tension of erector spinae, expiration | Anterior branches of the spinal nerves |
| **Quadratus lumborum** | Iliac crest | 12th rib, transverse process (L1–L4) | Lowering of the ribs, lateral flexion of the trunk | Subcostal n., lumbar plexus |
| **Latissimus dorsi** | Spinous processes of T6–L5, iliac crest, 9th to 12th rib, thoracolumbar fascia | Humerus (crest of lesser tubercle) | Adduction, internal rotation, retroversion of the arms | Thoracodorsal n. (brachial plexus) |

| Muscles | Origin | Insertion | Function | Innervation |
|---|---|---|---|---|
| **Erector spinae, lateral and intermediate column** | | | | |
| **Iliocostalis**<br>• **cervicis**<br>• **thoracis**<br>• **lumborum** | 3rd to 6th rib<br>7th to 12th rib<br>Iliac crest, sacrum | Transverse processes, C3–C6<br>1st to 6th rib<br>6th to 12th rib | Lateral flexion and extension of the trunk | Segmentally from the post. branches of the spinal nerves |
| **Longissimus**<br>• **capitis**<br>• **cervicis**<br>• **thoracis** | Transverse processes, C3–C7, T1–T3<br>Transverse processes, T1–T6<br>Sacrum, iliac crest, spinous and transverse processes of T1–L5 | Mastoid process<br>Transverse processes, C2–C7<br>2nd to 12th rib<br>Transverse processes, T1–T12, costal processes, L1–L5 | Lateral flexion of the neck<br>Rotation of the head<br>extension and lateral flexion of the trunk | Segmentally from the posterior branches of the spinal nerves |
| **Erector spinae: medial column (spinalis system)** | | | | |
| **Interspinalis** | Paired between spinous processes of cervical and lumbar spine | | Extension and retroflexion of the spine | Posterior branches of the respective segments of the spinal nerves |
| **Spinalis** | Muscle arches between spinous processes of the thoracic vertebra (middle of 9th thoracic vertebra) | | | |
| **Erector spinae: medial column (transversospinalis system)** | | | | |
| **Rotatores breves and longi** | Transverse processes of the cervical, thoracic or lumbar vertebra | Spinous processes of the next or the next but one vertebra | Rotation and extension of the spine | Posterior branches of the respective segments of the spinal nerves |
| **Multifidus** | Iliac crest, sacrum, transverse processes of the lumbar and thoracic vertebra | Transverse processes of the lumbar and thoracic vertebra | Retroflexion of the trunk | |
| **Semispinalis**<br>• **capitis**<br>• **cervicis**<br>• **thoracis** | Transverse processes, C4–T5<br>Transverse processes, T1–T6<br>Transverse processes, T6–T12 | Occipital bone<br>Transverse processes, C2–C7<br>Transverse processes, C6–T6 | Retroflexion and rotation of the head<br>Extension and rotation of the spine | Posterior branches of the respective segments of the spinal nerves |
| **Erector spinae: medial column (intertransversarii system)** | | | | |
| **Intertrans-versarii** | Run between transverse processes of the vertebra | | Lateral flexion of the vertebra | Post. and ant. branches of the spinal nerves |

## Directions of the Main Systems of the Intrinsic Back Muscles

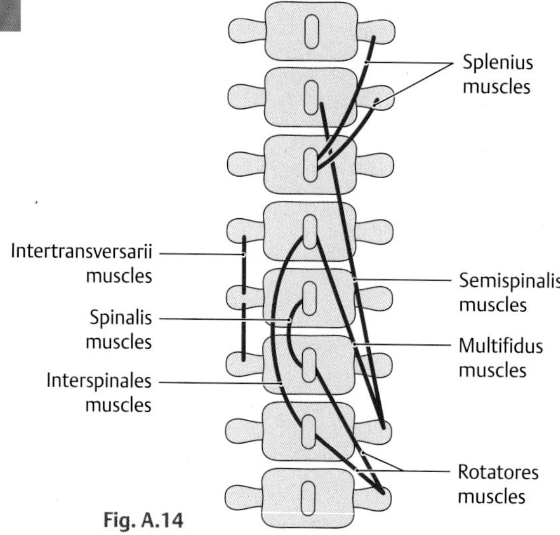


Fig. A.14

| Intrinsic back muscles (overview) | | |
|---|---|---|
| **Muscles of the neck** | Rectus capitis posterior minor<br>Rectus capitis posterior major<br>Obliquus capitis superior<br>Obliquus capitis inferior | between occipital bone, atlas and axis (posterior side) |
| | Rectus capitis anterior<br>Rectus capitis lateralis | between occipital bone and atlas (anterior side) |
| **Lateral tract** | | |
| | Iliocostalis (cervicis, thoracis, lumborum)<br>Longissimus (capitis, cervicis, thoracis) | between sacrum, iliac crest, ribs and spine (transverse processes) |
| **Medial tract** | | |
| | Interspinales<br>Spinalis | between spinous processes |
| | Rotatores (cervicis, thoracis, lumborum)<br>Multifidus<br>Semispinalis (capitis, cervicis, thoracis) | from transverse processes to the spinous processes and occipital bone |
| | Intertransversarii (posteriores and anteriores cervicis, thoracis, lateral and medial lumborum) | between the transverse processes |
| | Splenius capitis<br>Splenius cervicis | from spinous processes (C3–T6) to the transverse processes (C1–C3) and occipital bone |

## Innervation and Segmentation of the Posterior Wall of the Trunk

See also Pages: 54–55 / 60 / 62–64

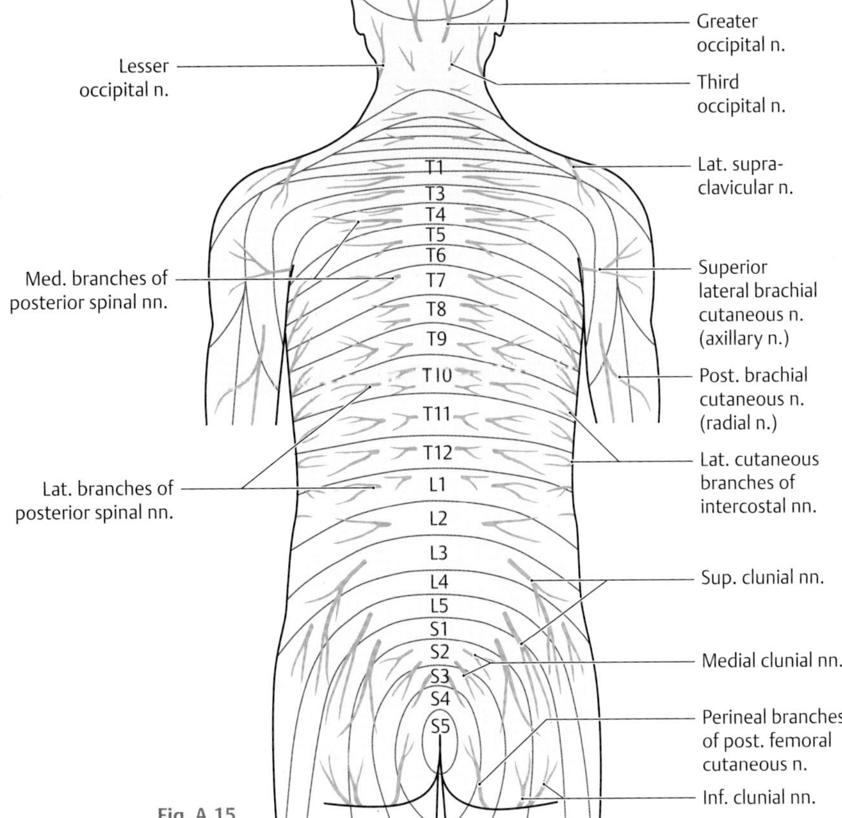


Fig. A.15

## Innervation and Segmentation of the Anterior Wall of the Trunk

See also Pages: 37 / 44–45 / 48

*Head's zones are marked in color.*

**Clinical**

Disease processes in different internal organs can lead to radiating pain in determined, firmly defined areas of the skin (Head's zones).

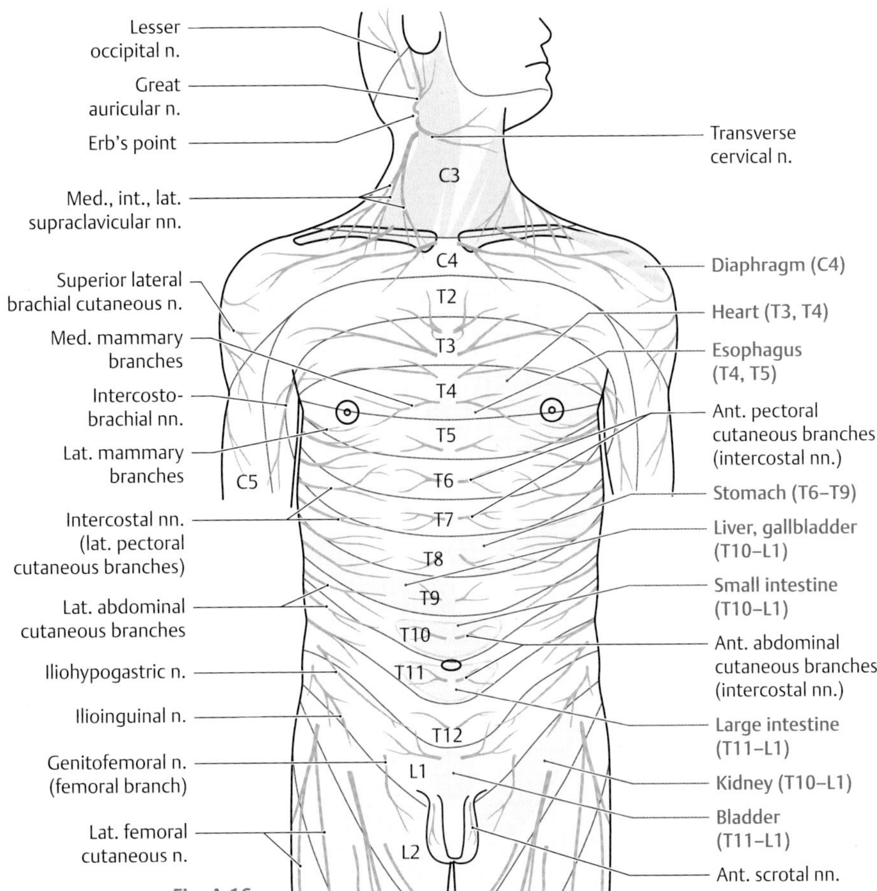


Fig. A.16

## Arteries of the Shoulder Girdle and Arm

See also Pages: 110–111 / 118–119 / 122 / 126 / 130–134 / 141 / 142–144

**Subclavian artery**
**Vertebral artery**
(through foramina transversaria of the cervical spine and foramen magnum to the brain; confluence of basilar artery)
**Int. thoracic artery**
(next to the sternum to the diaphragm and to the anterior abdominal wall)
- **pericardiophrenic artery; mediastinal branches, bronchial branches, sternal branches**
- **anterior intercostal branches**
- **medial mammary branches**
- **musculophrenic artery**
- **sup. epigastric artery**

**Costocervical trunk**
- **deep cervical artery** (to muscles of the neck)
- **supreme intercostal atery** (to 1st and 2nd intercostal space)

**Thyrocervical trunk**
- **ascending cervical artery** (for scalene muscles and prevertebral muscles of the neck)
- **inf. thyroid artery** (for thyroid gland and esophagus)
- **transverse cervical artery** (to the superficial muscles of the back)
- **suprascapular artery** (to the muscles of the scapular; anastomoses with circumflex scapular artery)
- **dorsal scapular artery** (independent deep branch of the transverse cervical artery)

**Axillary artery**
- **thoracoacromial artery** (deltopectorial triangle; with pectoral branches [to pectorales muscles], acromial branch [to acromial rete] and deltoid branch [to deltoid muscle])
- **sup. thoracic artery** (for subclavius muscle, pectoralis major muscle and spikes of seratus anterior muscle)
- **lat. thoracic artery** (to serratus ant. muscle and to the breast [lat. mammary branches])
- **arterior** and **posterior circumflex humeral artery** (anstomoses at the neck of humerus)

**Subscapular artery**
- **circumflex scapular artery** (for muscles of the scapular region)
- **thoracodorsal artery** (for latissimus dorsi muscle; teres major muscle and subscapular muscle)

**Brachial artery**
- **sup. and inf. ulnar collateral artery** (to cubital rete)
- **deep brachial artery** (in the groove for radial nerve to humerus)
  - **medial collateral artery**
  - **radial collateral artery** (to cubital rete)

**Radial artery**
- **radial recurrent artery**
- **palmar carpal branch** (palmar carpal rete)
- **superficial palmar branch** (to superficial palmar arch)
- **dorsal carpal branch** (to dorsal carpal rete)

**Ulnar artery**
- **ulnar recurrent artery**
- **common interosseous artery**
- **recurrent interosseous artery** (to cubital rete)
  - **post. interosseous artery** (to extensor muscles)
  - **ant. interosseous artery** (ventrally to interosseous membrane)
- **dorsal carpal branch** (to dorsal carpal rete)
- **palmar carpal branch** (to palmar carpal rete)
- **deep palmar branch** (to deep palmar arch)

**Superf. palmar arch**
- **common palmar digital arteries**
- **proper palmar digital arteries**

**Deep palmar arch**
- **princeps pollicis artery** (to thumb)
- **palmar metacarpal arteries**
- **radialis indicis artery** (to 2nd finger)

## Veins of the Shoulder Girdle and Arm

See also Pages: 112 / 116 / 120–121 / 132 / 135–136 / 140–141

**Subclavian vein**
(receives blood of the **internal** and **external jugular vein** of the neck as well as of the **internal thoracic vein** of the anterior chest wall and of the **pectoral veins** from the pectoralis muscles)
**Axillary vein** contains blood from the:
- **lateral thoracic vein** (on the serratus anterior muscle)
- **thoracodorsal vein** (on the lateral chest wall: receives blood from the **thoracoepigastric vein**, which anastomoses with the superficial epigastric vein [collateral circulation between superior and inferior vena cava])
- **cephalic vein** (comes from the side of the thumb of the back of the hand; connection with the basilic vein in the crook of the arm; confluence beneath the clavicle in the deltopectoral triangle into the axillary vein)

**Brachial vein**
contains blood from the:
- **basilic vein** (ulnar cutaneous vein; connection with the cephalic vein in the crook of the arm [median cubital vein])
- **radial vein** (accompanying vein of the radial artery)
- **ulnar vein** (accompanying vein of the ulnar artery)
- **deep venous palmar arch** (accompanying vein of the arterial anastomosis garland with the same name; connections with the metacarpal dorsal veins of the back of the hand and the veins of the palm and fingers [palmar metacarpal veins])
- **superficial venous plamar arch** (accompanying vein of the arterial anastomosis garland with the same name)

**Dorsal venous network of the hand**
(subcutaneous venous network on the back of the hand; drainage on the side of the thumb into the cephalic vein and ulnar into the basilic vein: receives blood from the **dorsal metacarpal veins** and the dorsal veins of the fingers)

Clinical

**Cephalic vein**
(on the right side):
possible access to the heart (e.g., with cardiac catheter).
**Median cubital vein**
(also median cephalic vein and median antebrachial vein):
used for intravenous injections and venipuncture.
**Palmar metacarpal veins**
(veins of the palm): in case of inflammation these veins can lead to swelling of the **back of the hand** (not of the palm).

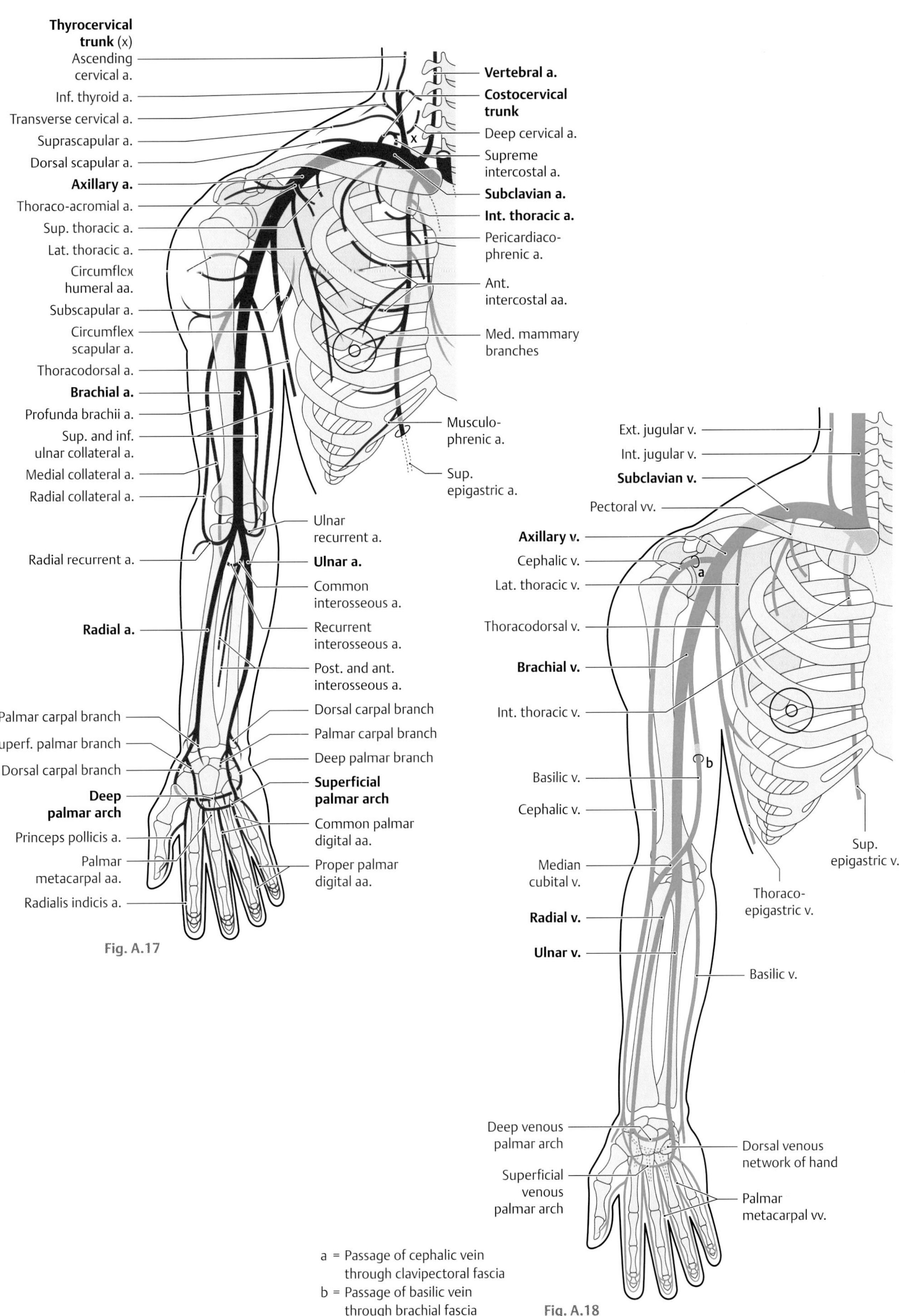
Thyrocervical trunk (x)
Ascending cervical a.
Inf. thyroid a.
Transverse cervical a.
Suprascapular a.
Dorsal scapular a.
Axillary a.
Thoraco-acromial a.
Sup. thoracic a.
Lat. thoracic a.
Circumflex humeral aa.
Subscapular a.
Circumflex scapular a.
Thoracodorsal a.
Brachial a.
Profunda brachii a.
Sup. and inf. ulnar collateral a.
Medial collateral a.
Radial collateral a.
Radial recurrent a.
Radial a.
Palmar carpal branch
Superf. palmar branch
Dorsal carpal branch
Deep palmar arch
Princeps pollicis a.
Palmar metacarpal aa.
Radialis indicis a.
Vertebral a.
Costocervical trunk
Deep cervical a.
Supreme intercostal a.
Subclavian a.
Int. thoracic a.
Pericardiacophrenic a.
Ant. intercostal aa.
Med. mammary branches
Musculophrenic a.
Sup. epigastric a.
Ulnar recurrent a.
Ulnar a.
Common interosseous a.
Recurrent interosseous a.
Post. and ant. interosseous a.
Dorsal carpal branch
Palmar carpal branch
Deep palmar branch
Superficial palmar arch
Common palmar digital aa.
Proper palmar digital aa.
x
Ext. jugular v.
Int. jugular v.
Subclavian v.
Pectoral vv.
Axillary v.
Cephalic v.
Lat. thoracic v.
Thoracodorsal v.
Brachial v.
Int. thoracic v.
Basilic v.
Cephalic v.
Median cubital v.
Radial v.
Ulnar v.
Basilic v.
Sup. epigastric v.
Thoraco-epigastric v.
a
b
Deep venous palmar arch
Superficial venous palmar arch
Dorsal venous network of hand
Palmar metacarpal vv.

Fig. A.17

a = Passage of cephalic vein through clavipectoral fascia
b = Passage of basilic vein through brachial fascia

Fig. A.18

## Brachial Plexus and Nerves of the Arm

See also Pages: 113 / 120–127 / 130–140 / 142–145

Brachial plexus (C5–T1)
- **suprascapular nerve** (through suprascapular notch to supra- and infraspinatus muscles)
- **dorsal scapular nerve** (for rhomboid muscles and levator scapulae muscle)
- **subclavian nerve** (for subclavius muscle)
- **middle** and **lat. pectoral nerves** (for pectoralis major and minor muscle)
- **subscapular nerves** (for subscapularis muscle and teres major muscle)
- **long thoracic nerve** (to serratus ant. muscle)
- **thoracodorsal nerve** (to latissimus dorsi muscle)

Lateral cord
- **lateral root of the fork of the median nerve**

Musculocutaneous nerve
- **muscular branches** (for biceps brachii muscle, coracobrachialis muscle)
- **lat. cutaneous nerve of forearm** (cutaneous branch to forearm)

Posterior cord

Axillary nerve
- **muscular branches** (for deltoid muscle and teres minor muscle)
- **lat. cutaneous nerve of the arm** (cutaneous branch to the shoulder)

Radial nerve
- **muscular branches** (for triceps brachii muscle, extensor carpi radialis muscles and brachioradialis muscle)
- **post. cutaneous nerve of the arm** (cutaneous branch to the dorsal side of the upper arm)
- **post. cutaneous nerve of the forearm** (cutaneous branch to the posterior side of the forearm)
- **deep branch** (for the extensors of the forearm, supinator muscle)
- **post. interosseous nerve of the forearm** (sensitive branch for wrist joint and periosteum)
- **superficial branch** (cutaneous branch for thumb and dorsal side of the hand, 2½ fingers [dorsal digital nerves])

Medial cord
- **lateral root of the fork of the median nerve**
- **medial cutaneous nerve of the arm** (cutaneous branch for the medial side of the upper arm)
- **intercostobrachial nerve** (anastomoses with intercostal nerves)
- **medial cutaneous nerve of the forearm** (cutaneous branch for the medial side of the forearm)

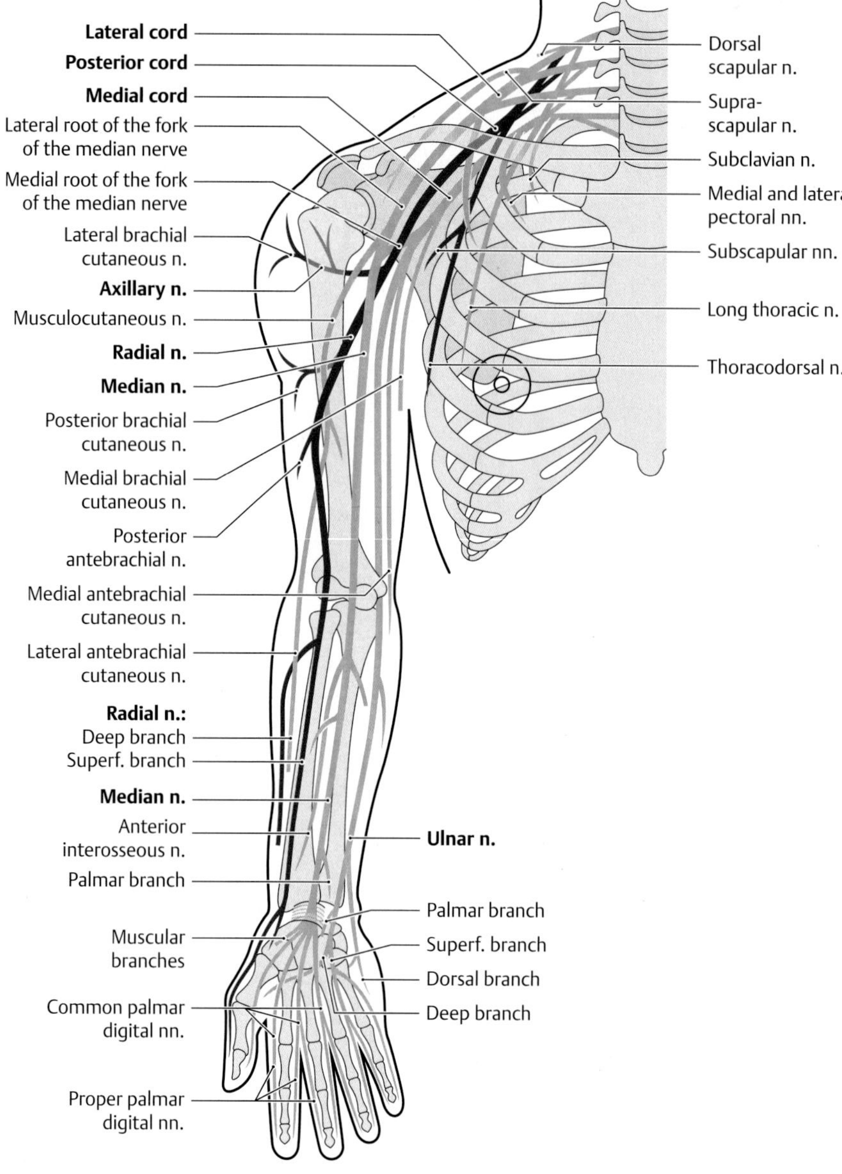


Fig. A.19

Median nerve
(no branches at the upper arm)
- **muscular branches** (for all flexors of the forearm, without the muscles that are provided by the ulnar nerve)
- **ant. interosseous nerve** (for pronator quadratus muscle)
- **palmar branch** (cutaneous branch to the palm)
- **muscular branches** (for muscles of the thenar eminence; exception: adductor pollicis muscle and deep head of flexor pollicis brevis muscle, lumbrical muscles I and II)
- **common palmar digital nerves**
- **proper palmar digital nerves**

} cutaneous branches for palmar side of 3½ radial fingers

Ulnar nerves
(no branches at the upper arm)
- **muscular branches** (for flexor carpi ulnaris muscle and the ulnar part of the flexor digitorum prof. muscle)
- **palmar branch** (cutaneous branch for forearm and hypothenar)
- **superficial branch** (cutaneous branch for palmar side of the 1½ ulnar fingers)
- **dorsal branch** (cutaneous branch for dorsal side of the 2½ ulnar fingers)
- **deep branch** (for all interosseal muscles, lumbrical muscles III and IV, adductor pollicis muscle, deep head of flexor pollicis brevis muscle and the muscles of the hypothenar)

## Vessels and Nerves of the Upper Limb

See also Pages: 110–113 / 118–127 / 130–131 / 142–143

*The veins are not shown, they run parallel with the arteries.*

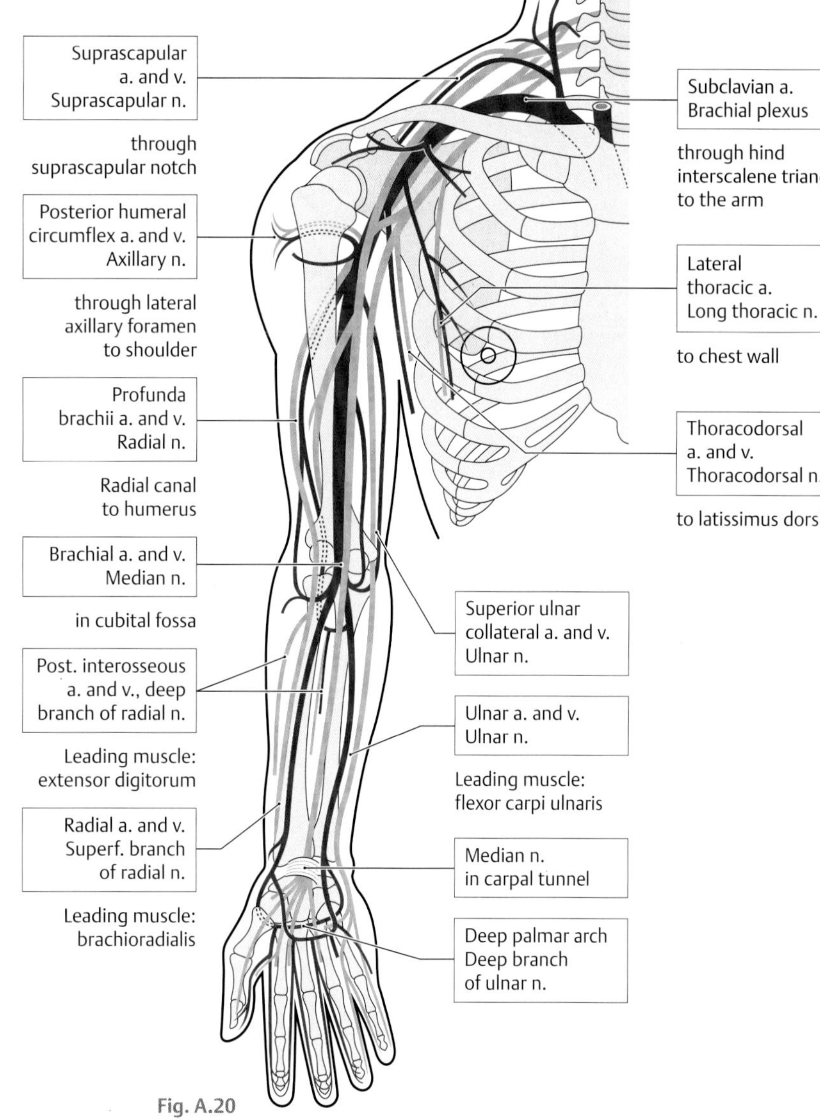


Fig. A.20

## Overview of the Main Muscle Functions of the Shoulder Girdle and Arm

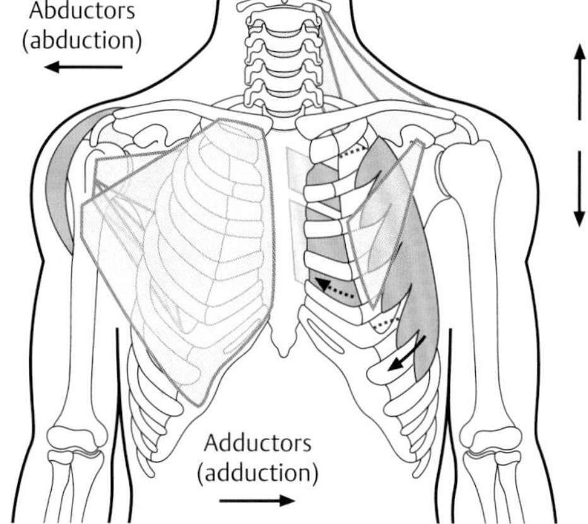


Fig. A.21

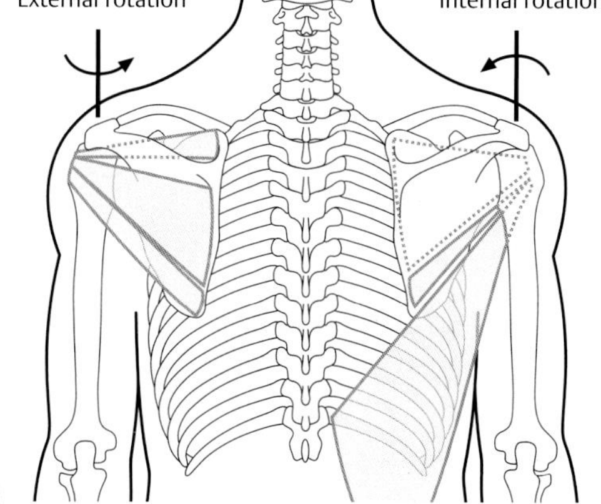


Fig. A.22

**Shoulder girdle:**

**Movement upward**
- levator scapulae
- trapezius

**Movement downward**
- pectoralis minor

**Anterior movement**
- serratus anterior

**Posterior movement**
- rhomboid major and minor

**Abduction of the arm**
- deltoid

**Adduction of the arm**
- pectoralis major
- teres major
- teres minor
- subscapularis

**Arm:**

**External rotation of the arm**
- infraspinatus
- teres minor
- deltoid

**Internal rotation of the arm**
- latissimus dorsi
- teres major
- subscapularis
- pectoralis major
- deltoid

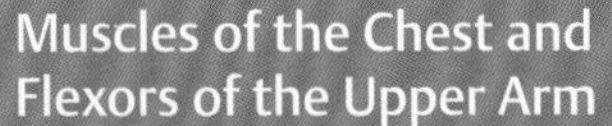

## Muscles of the Chest and Flexors of the Upper Arm

See also Pages: 35 / 47 / 98–101 / 120–121 / 126

*Anterior aspect.*

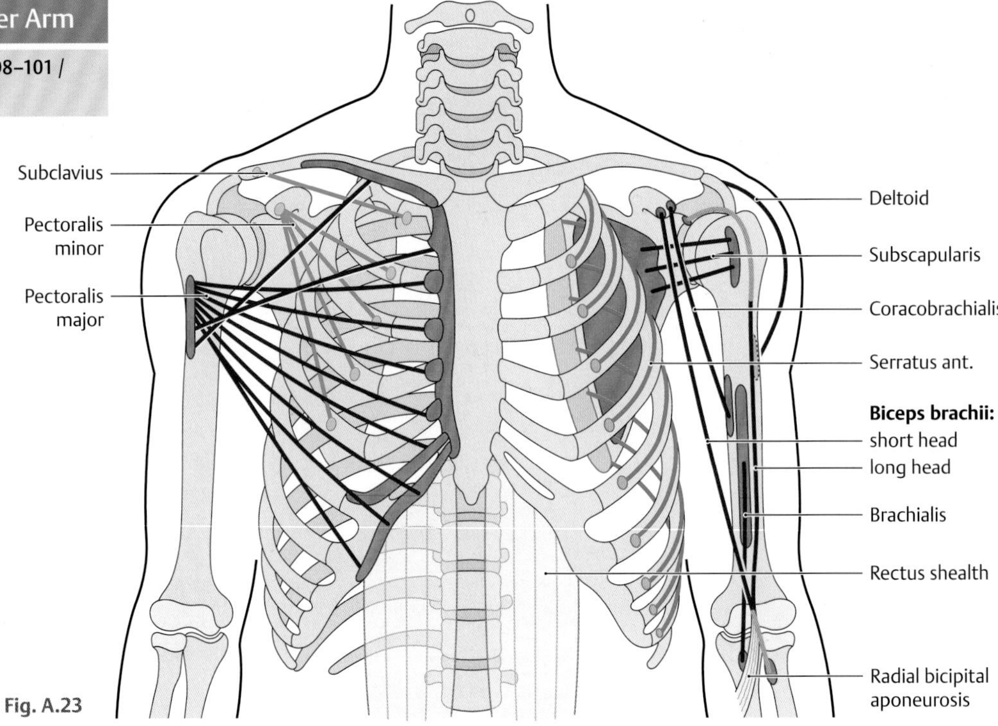


**Fig. A.23**

## Muscles of the Shoulder and Extensors of the Upper Arm

See also Pages: 72 / 96–97 / 117–118 / 122–123

*Posterior aspect.*

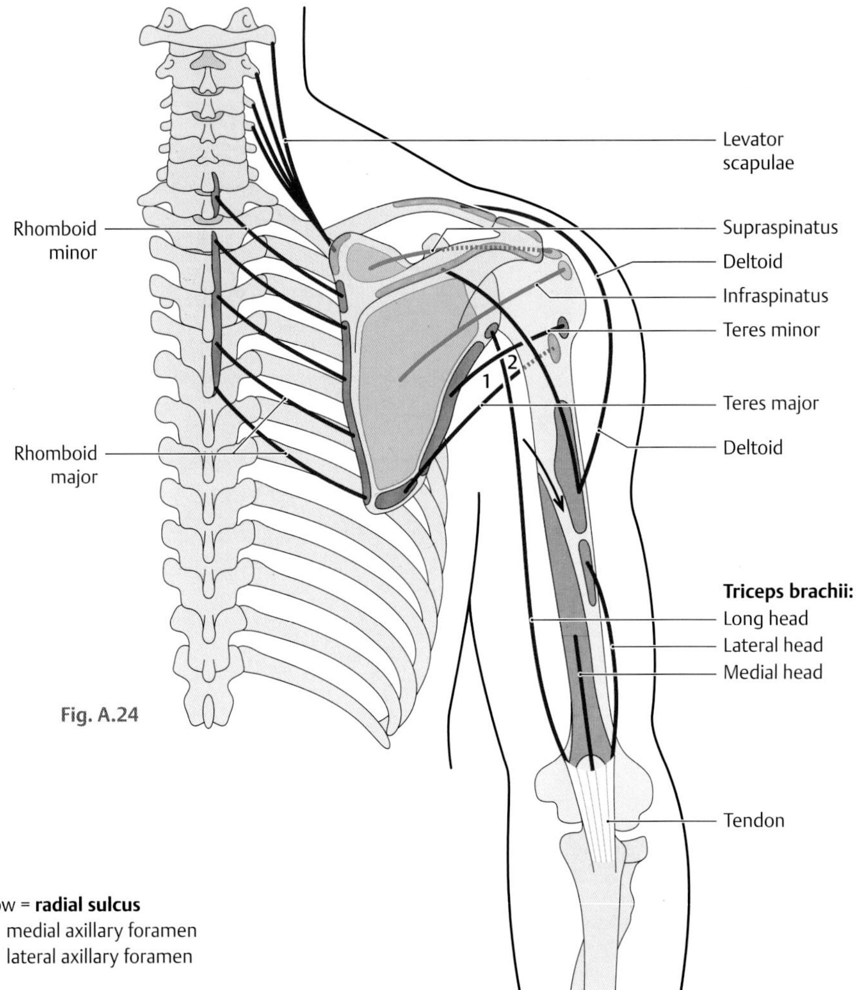


**Fig. A.24**

Arrow = **radial sulcus**
1 = medial axillary foramen
2 = lateral axillary foramen

| Muscles | Origin | Insertion | Function | Innervation |
|---|---|---|---|---|
| **Pectoralis major** | Clavicle, sternum, rectus sheath | Crest of greater tubercle of the humerus | Adduction, anteversion, internal rotation of the upper arm | Medial (C8, T1) and lateral (C5-C7) pectoral nn. |
| **Subclavius** | 1st rib | Clavicle | Fixation of the clavicle, tension of clavipectoral fascia | Subclavian n. (C5, C6) |
| **Pectoralis minor** | 2nd to 5th rib | Coracoid process of the scapula | Movement downward of the scapula, inspiration | Medial and lateral pectoral nn. (C8, T1) |
| **Deltoid**<br>• clavicular part<br>• acromial part<br>• spinal part | <br>Clavicle<br>Acromion<br>Spine of scapula | Humerus (deltoid tuberosity) | Ab- and adduction, internal and external rotation, ante- and retroversion of the arm | Axillary n. (C5, C6) |
| **Subscapularis** | Scapula, subscapular fossa | Lesser tubercle of the humerus | Internal rotation, adduction of the upper arm | Subscapular n. (C5, C6) |
| **Coracobrachialis** | Coracoid process of the scapula | Humerus | Adduction and internal rotation of the upper arm | Musculocutaneous n. (C6, C7) |
| **Serratus anterior** | 1st to 9th rib | Scapula (medial border) | Forward movement and rotation of the scapula, inspiration | Long thoracic n. (C5–C7) |
| **Biceps brachii** | Long head: supraglenoid tubercle of the scapula<br>Short head: coracoid process of the scapula | Radial tuberosity, aponeurosis of biceps brachii muscle to antebrachial fascia | In the joint of the shoulder: ab- and adduction, internal rotation, anteversion; in the joint of the elbow: flexion, supination | Musculocutaneous n. (C5–C7) |
| **Brachialis** | Humerus | Tuberosity of ulna | Flexion in the joint of the elbow | Musculocutaneous n. |

| Muscles | Origin | Insertion | Function | Innervation |
|---|---|---|---|---|
| **Levator scapulae** | Transverse processes C1–C4 | Superior angle of the scapula | Movement upward and rotation of the scapula | Dorsal scapular n. (C4–C5) |
| **Rhomboid minor** and **major** | Spinous processes C6, C7 (minor), spinous processes T1–T4 (major) | Medial border of the scapula | Medial and upward movement of the scapula | Dorsal scapular n. (C4, C5) |
| **Supraspinatus** | Supraspinous fossa of the scapula | Greater tubercle of the humerus | Abduction, external rotation of the upper arm | Suprascapular n. (C4–C6) |
| **Deltoid** | Clavicle, acromion, spine of scapula | Deltoid tuberosity | Takes part in all movements in the joint of the shoulder | Axillary n. (C5, C6) |
| **Infraspinatus** | Infraspinous fossa of the scapula | Greater tubercle of the humerus | Adduction, external rotation of the upper arm | Suprascapular n. (C4–C6) |
| **Teres minor** | Scapula | Greater tubercle of the humerus | Adduction, internal rotation of the upper arm | Axillary n. (C5, C6) |
| **Teres major** | Scapula | Crest of lesser tubercle | Adduction, internal rotation of the upper arm | Thoracodorsal n. (C6, C7) |
| **Triceps brachii** | Long head: infraglenoid tubercle of the scapula; medial and lateral head: humerus | Olecranon of the ulna | Extension in the joint of the elbow, long head: adduction and retroversion in the joint of the shoulder | Radial n., long head (C6–C8, T1), medial head (C7), lateral head (C6–C8) |

## Flexors of the Forearm and Hand

See also Pages: 102–105

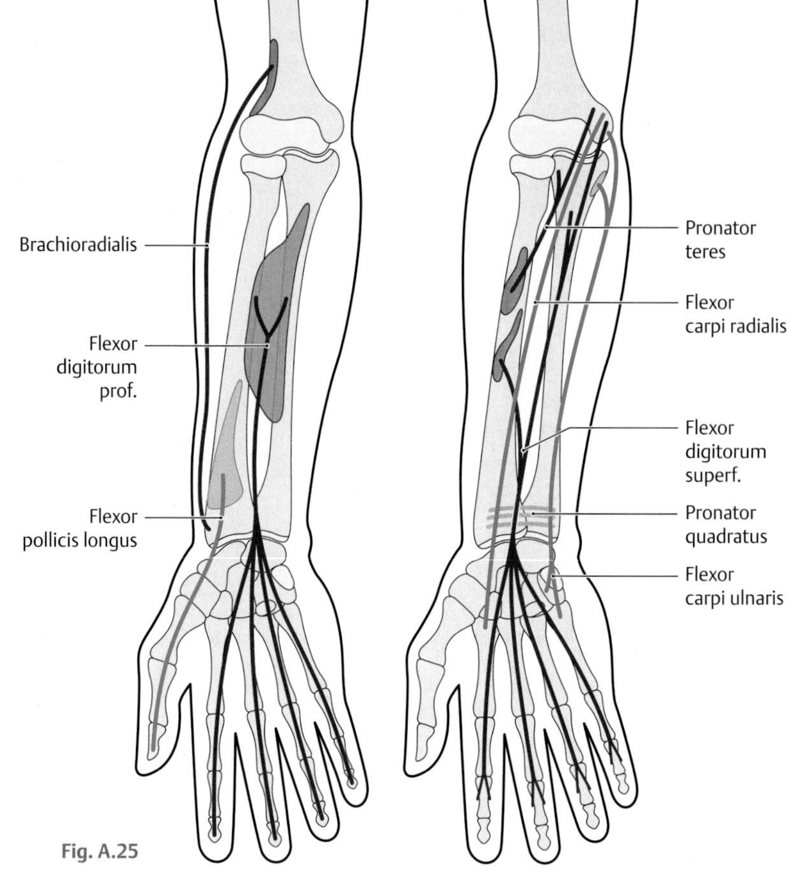


Fig. A.25

## Extensors of the Forearm and Hand

See also Pages: 106–107 / 140

**Tendon compartments in extensor retinaculum**

1 = Abductor pollicis longus and extensor pollicis brevis
2 = Extensor carpi radialis longus and brevis
3 = Extensor pollicis longus
4 = Extensor digitorum and extensor indicis
5 = Extensor digiti minimi
6 = Extensor carpi ulnaris

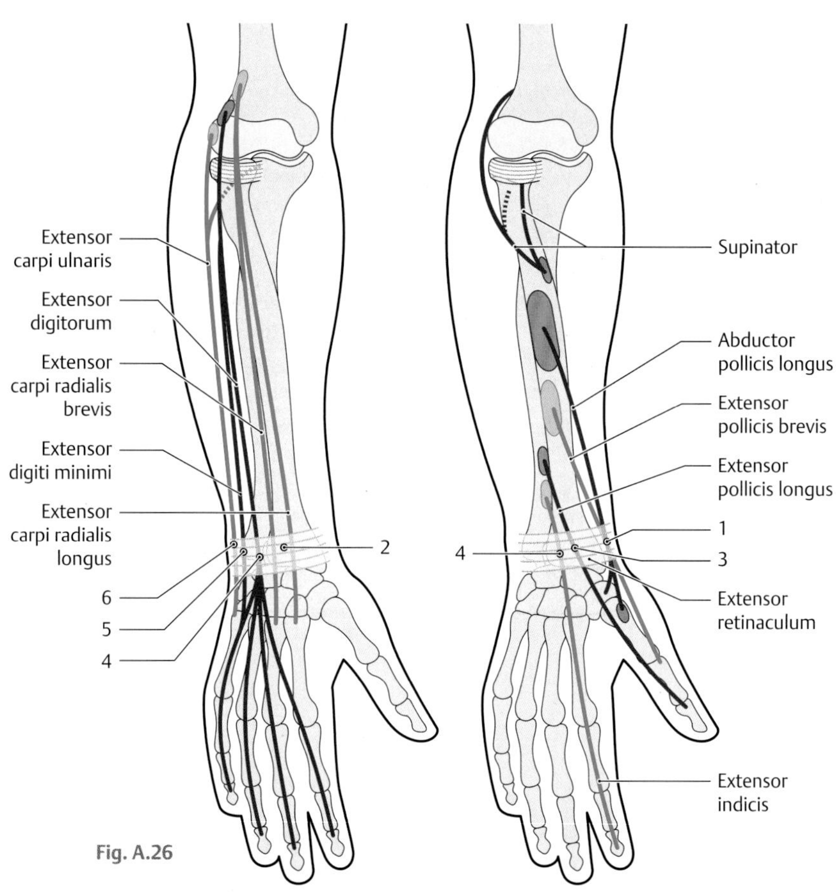


Fig. A.26

| Muscles | Origin | Insertion | Function | Innervation |
|---|---|---|---|---|
| **Brachioradialis** | Humerus (lateral border) | Radius (base of styloid process) | Flexion in the joint of the elbow, pro- and supination | Radial n. (C5–C6) |
| **Flexor digitorum profundus** | Ulna, interosseous membrane | Distal phalanges of the 2nd to 5th finger | Flexion of the interphalangeal joints, palmar flexion of the hand | Median n. and ulnar n. (C6–C8, T1) |
| **Flexor pollicis longus** | Radius | Thumb until end phalanx | Flexion of the thumb | Median n. (C6–C8) |
| **Pronator teres** | Humeral head: medial epicondyle of the humerus; ulnar head: coronoid process of the ulna | Radius | Pronation and flexion in the joint of the elbow | Median n. (C6) |
| **Flexor carpi radialis** | Medial epicondyle of the humerus | Base of metacarpal bone II | Radial abduction and palmar flexion of the hand, pronation and flexion in the joint of the elbow | Median n. (C5–C7) |
| **Flexor digitorum superficialis** | Humero-ulnar head: medial epicondyle of the humerus, coronoid process of the ulna; radial head: radius | Middle phalanges of the 2nd to 5th finger | Flexion of the middle phalanges and interphalangeal joints, palmar flexion of the hand | Median n. (C5–C7) |
| **Pronator quadratus** | Anterior side of the ulna | Anterior area of radius | Pronation | Median n. (C5–C7) |
| **Flexor carpi ulnaris** | Humeral head: medial: epicondyle of the humerus; ulnar head: olecranon | Hamate, metacarpal bone V | Ulnar abduction, palmar flexion of the hand, flexion in the joint of the elbow | Ulnar n. (C8–T1) |

| Muscles | Origin | Insertion | Function | Innervation |
|---|---|---|---|---|
| **Extensor carpi ulnaris** | Humeral head: lateral epicondyle of the humerus; ulnar head: ulna | Base of metacarpal bone V | Ulnar abduction, dorsal extension of the hand | Radial n. (deep branch) (C7, C8) |
| **Extensor digitorum** | Lateral epicondyle of the humerus | Extensor expansion of the 2nd to 5th finger | Extension in joints of the fingers and hands | Radial n. (deep branch) (C6–C8) |
| **Extensor carpi radialis longus and brevis** | Lateral epicondyle of the humerus, anular ligament of radius | Base of metacarpal bone II (longus) and III (brevis) | Radial abduction and dorsal extension of the hand, flexion in the joint of the elbow | Radial n. (C6, C7) |
| **Extensor digiti minimi** | Lateral epicondyle of the humerus | Extensor expansion | Extension of the 5th finger | Radial n. (C6–C8) |
| **Supinator** | Lateral epicondyle of the humerus, anular ligament, ulna | Radius | Supination | Deep branch of radial nn. |
| **Abductor pollicis longus** | Dorsal area of the radius and ulna, interosseous membrane | Base of metacarpal bone I, trapezium bone | Abduction of the thumb | Radial n. (deep branch) (C7, C8) |
| **Extensor pollicis brevis** | Radius and ulna, interosseous membrane | Base of proximal phalanx I | Extension of the thumb, radial abduction of the hand | Radial n. (deep branch) (C6, C7) |
| **Extensor pollicis longus** | Ulna, interosseous membrane | Distal phalanx of the thumb | Extension and abduction of the thumb | Radial n. (deep branch) (C6, C7) |
| **Extensor indicis** | Ulna | Extensor expansion of the 2nd finger | Extension of the 2nd finger | Radial n. (deep branch) (C7, C8) |

## Muscles of the Hand

See also Pages: 108–109 / 142–145

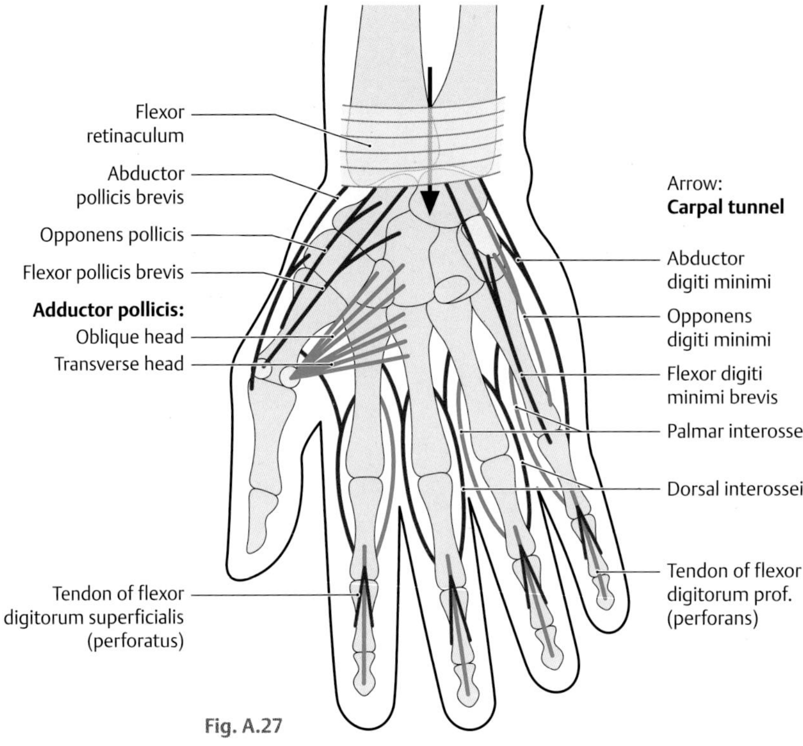


Fig. A.27

| Muscles | Origin | Insertion | Function | Innervation |
|---|---|---|---|---|
| **Abductor pollicis brevis** | Scaphoid bone, flexor retinaculum | Base of proximal phalanx I, lateral sesamoid bone | Abduction of the thumb | Median n. (C6, C7) |
| **Opponens pollicis** | Trapezium bone, flexor retinaculum | Lateral border of metacarpal bone I | Opposition of the thumb | Median n. (C6, C7) |
| **Flexor pollicis brevis** | Superficial head: flexor retinaculum | Lateral sesamoid bone of the main joint | Flexion and adduction of the thumb | Median n. (C6, C7) |
| | Deep head: trapezium bone, trapezoid bone, capitate bone, base of metacarpal bone I | Lateral sesamoid bone of the main joint | Flexion and adduction of the thumb | Ulnar n. (C8, T1) |
| **Adductor pollicis** | Oblique head: capitate bone, metacarpal bone II and III; transverse head: metacarpal bone III | Base of proximal phalanx I, ulnar sesamoid bone | Adduction and opposition of the thumb, flexion in the base joint of the thumb | Ulnar n. (C8, T1) |
| **Abductor digiti minimi** | Pisiform bone, flexor retinaculum | Base of proximal phalanx and dorsal aponeurosis of 5th finger | Adduction, flexion in the base joint, extension in middle and end joint of the 5th finger | Ulnar n. (C8, T1) |
| **Opponens digiti minimi** | Hook of hamate bone, flexor retinaculum | Outer area of metacarpal bone V | Opposition of the 5th finger | Ulnar n. (C8, T1) |
| **Flexor digiti minimi brevis** | Hook of hamate bone, flexor retinaculum | Base of proximal phalanx V | Flexion in base joint of the 5th finger | Ulnar n. (C8, T1) |
| **Palmar interossei** | Metacarpal bones II, IV, V (single headed) | Dorsal aponeurosis of 2nd, 4th and 5th finger | Adduction, flexion in the base joint, extension in middle and end joints of the fingers | Ulnar n. (C8, T1) |
| **Dorsal interossei** | Areas between the bones of metacarpal bones I–V (double headed) | Dorsal aponeurosis of 2nd, 4th and 5th finger | Abduction, flexion in base joint, extension in middle and end joints of the fingers | Ulnar n. (C8, T1) |

## Structure of the Segments and Cutaneous Innervation of the Arm

**See also Pages: 113–114 / 130–131 / 136–140 / 144**

*Left anterior aspect, right posterior aspect.*

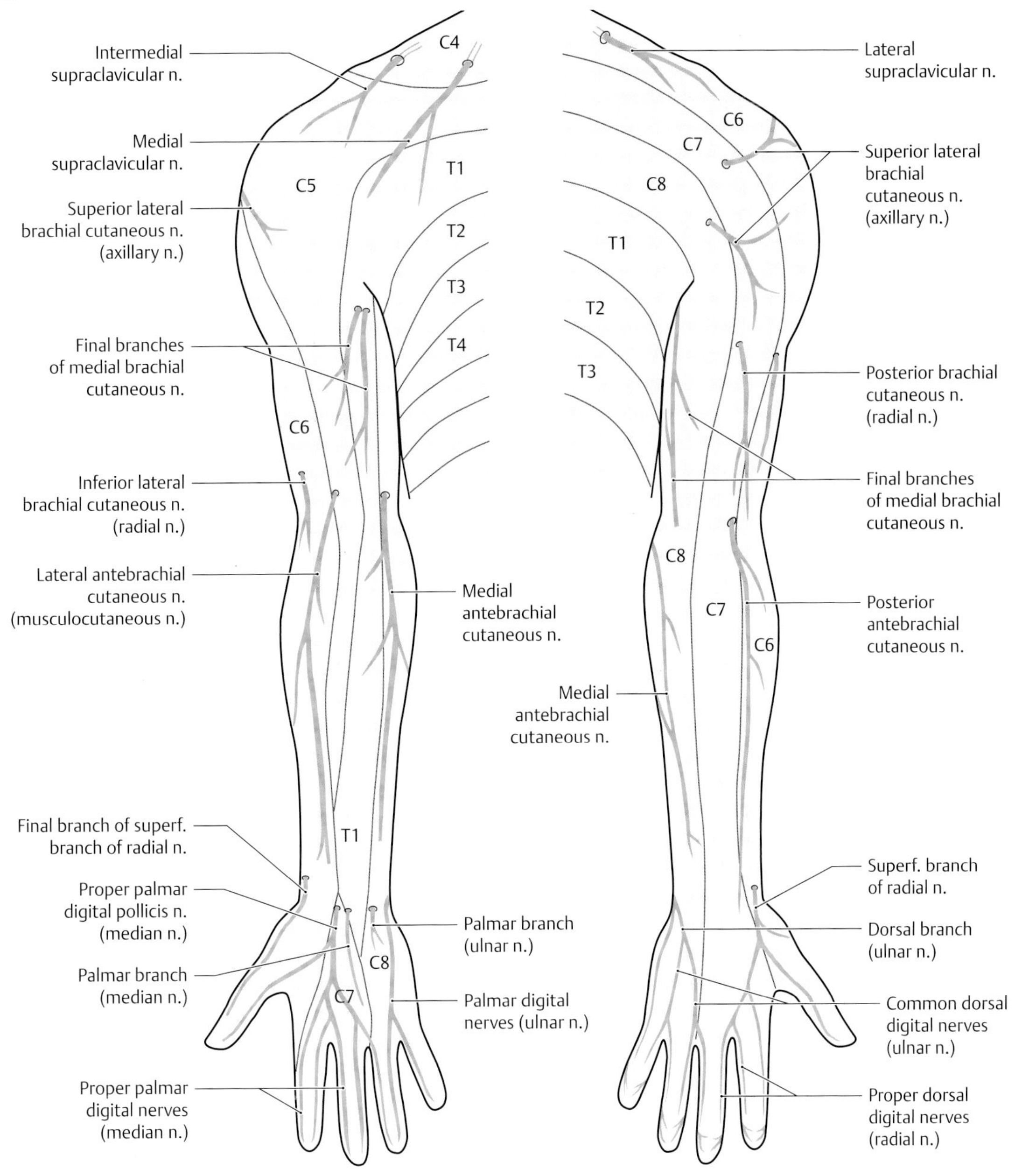


Fig. A.28

## Arteries of the Lower Limb

See also Pages: 184–185 / 204 / 215–216

**Femoral artery**

- **superf. epigastric artery** (to the anterior abdominal wall)
- **superf. circumflex iliac artery** (to the skin of the groin region)
- **ext. pudendal arteries** (to the external genitalia with anterior scrotal branches [or labial branches] and inguinal branches)
- **deep artery of thigh** (to the posterior side of the thigh)
  - **middle cirumflex femoral artery** with **superficial branch** and **deep branch** (for adductors and flexors)
  - **lat. circumflex femoral artery** with **ascending branch** and **descending branch** (for quadriceps muscle)
  - **perforating arteries I, II, III** (for adductors and flexors of the thigh)
  - **descending genicular artery** (to the genicular anastomosis)
- **Popliteal artery**
  - **superior lateral genicular artery**, **superior medial genicular artery** } to the genicular anastomosis
  - **middle genicular artery** (to the cruciate ligaments of the knee)
  - **inferior lateral genicular artery**, **inferior medial genicular artery** } to the genicular anastomosis
  - **sural arteries** (to gastrocnemius muscle, soleus muscle)
- **fibular artery** (for deep flexors and fibula)
  - **communicating branch** (anastomosis with posterior tibial artery)
  - **posterior and anterior lateral malleolar branch**
- **posterior tibial artery**
  - **medial malleolar branches**
  - **medial plantar artery**, **lateral plantar artery** } to the muscles of the sole
- **plantar arch**
  - **plantar metatarsal arteries**
  - **plantar, common** and **proper digital arteries**
  - **plantar artery of medial great toe**
- **anterior tibial artery**
  - **posterior tibial recurrent artery**
  - **anterior tibial recurrent artery**
  - **ant. lateral and medial malleolar arteries**
- **dorsalis pedis artery**
  - **lateral** and **medial tarsal arteries** (for the dorsal metatarsal arteries and the dorsal digital arteries at the back of the foot)
  - **deep plantar branch** (anastomoses with lat. plantar artery in plantar arch)

**Clinical**

**Femoral artery:** is accessible beneath the inguinal ligament for diagnostic or therapeutic purposes; in cases of emergency ligation through pressure against the iliac crest is possible.
**Popliteal artery:** must not be ligated, because collateral cycle through the arteries of the knee joint is not sufficient.
**Ant. tibial artery:** compression can lead to necrosis of the muscles (compartment syndrome).

## Veins of the Lower Limb

See also Pages: 186–187 / 192–193 / 202 / 205 / 208–209 / 215

**Femoral vein**
(gets blood from the genital region [external pudenal veins], from the inferior abdominal wall [superficial epigastric vein] and region of the pelvis [superficial circumflex iliac vein]) and from the

- **great saphenous vein** (from the back of the foot, lower leg and thigh; entrance through saphenous opening)
- **deep vein of the thigh** (from the posterior region of the thigh)
- **popliteal vein** (collection of the cutaneous veins of the lower leg [through the small saphenous vein] and of the deep veins of the lower leg [ant. and post. tibial vein])
- **ant. tibial vein** (of the extensors of the lower leg and of the back of the foot [dorsal venous arch of the foot, which forms the main drain of the sole and of the toes (dorsal digital veins)])
- **post. tibial vein** (from the flexors of the lower leg and the soles [plantar venous arch, receives blood from the plantar metatarsal veins and of the plantar digital veins])

**Clinical**

**Femoral vein:** can be accessed beneath the inguinal ligament for diagnostic or therapeutic reasons.
**Perforating veins:** flow from outside in; often form varicose veins on the interior side of the lower leg below the knee (Boyd's veins) or the distal lower leg (Cockett's veins). Circulatory disorders can lead to venous leg ulcers.
**Dorsal venous arch of foot:** responsible for "collateral edemas," e.g., through inflammation in the soles.

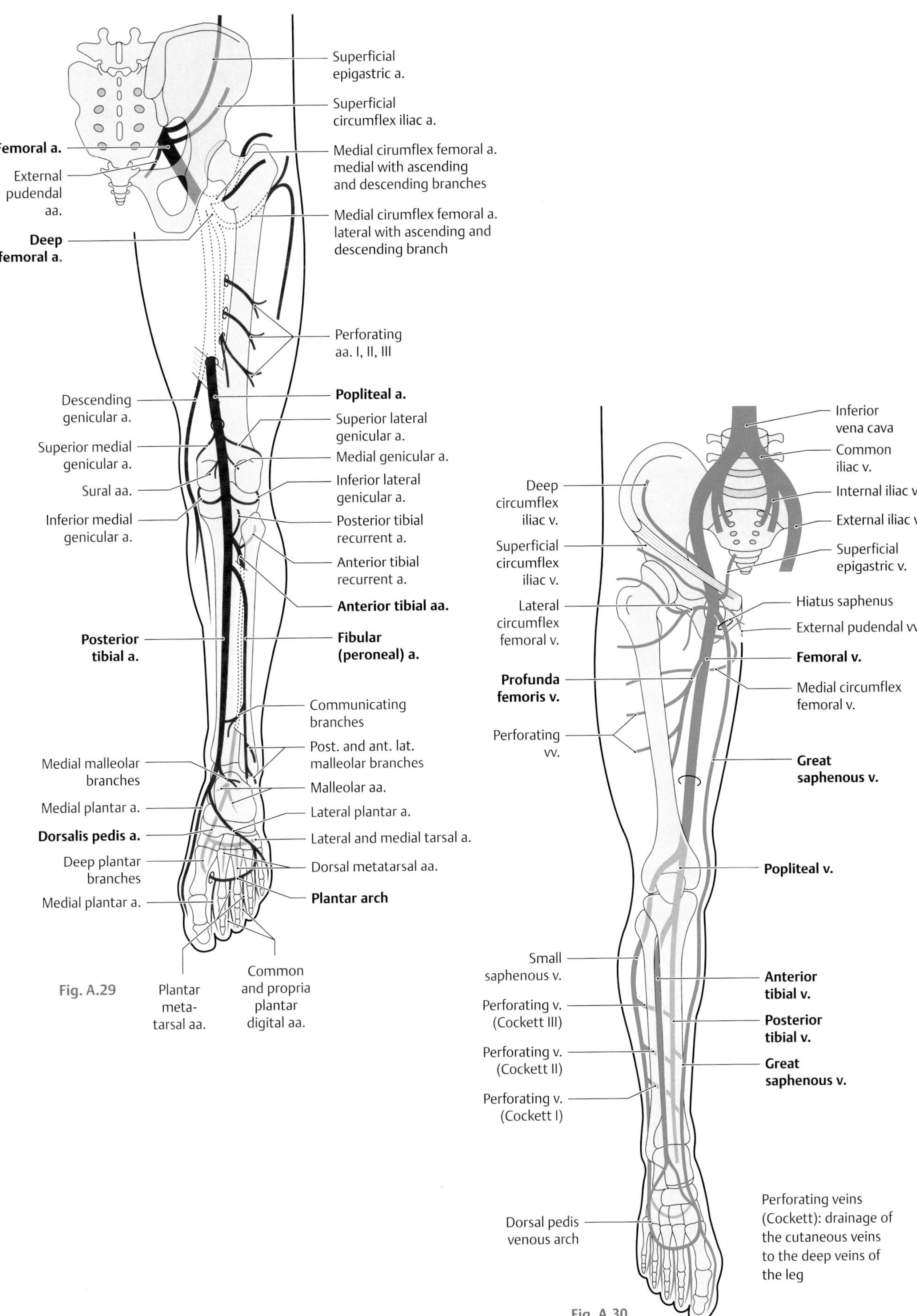
Superficial epigastric a.
Superficial circumflex iliac a.
Femoral a.
External pudendal aa.
Medial cirumflex femoral a. medial with ascending and descending branches
Medial cirumflex femoral a. lateral with ascending and descending branch
Deep femoral a.
Perforating aa. I, II, III
Descending genicular a.
Popliteal a.
Superior lateral genicular a.
Superior medial genicular a.
Medial genicular a.
Sural aa.
Inferior lateral genicular a.
Inferior medial genicular a.
Posterior tibial recurrent a.
Anterior tibial recurrent a.
Anterior tibial aa.
Posterior tibial a.
Fibular (peroneal) a.
Communicating branches
Post. and ant. lat. malleolar branches
Medial malleolar branches
Malleolar aa.
Medial plantar a.
Lateral plantar a.
Dorsalis pedis a.
Lateral and medial tarsal a.
Deep plantar branches
Dorsal metatarsal aa.
Medial plantar a.
Plantar arch
Plantar meta-tarsal aa.
Common and propria plantar digital aa.
Inferior vena cava
Common iliac v.
Deep circumflex iliac v.
Internal iliac v.
External iliac v.
Superficial circumflex iliac v.
Superficial epigastric v.
Lateral circumflex femoral v.
Hiatus saphenus
External pudendal vv.
Femoral v.
Profunda femoris v.
Medial circumflex femoral v.
Perforating vv.
Great saphenous v.
Popliteal v.
Small saphenous v.
Anterior tibial v.
Perforating v. (Cockett III)
Posterior tibial v.
Perforating v. (Cockett II)
Great saphenous v.
Perforating v. (Cockett I)
Dorsal pedis venous arch
Perforating veins (Cockett): drainage of the cutaneous veins to the deep veins of the leg

Fig. A.29

Fig. A.30

## Lymphatic Vessels of the Pelvis and Leg of the Female with the Accompanying Lymph Nodes

See also Pages: 310–311 / 340

The lymph vessels mainly follow the veins. Through the two lumbar lymphatic trunks the lymph reaches the cisterna chyli and therefore the thoracic duct. This runs in the posterior mediastinum upward until the left venous angle.

**Cisterna chyli**
(influx from both lumbar lymphatic trunks and intestinal lymphatic trunk)
**Left** and **right lumbar lymphatic trunk**
(to the posterior side of the thigh)
**Common iliac lymph nodes**
(influx from the pelvis [internal iliac lymph nodes] and the leg [external iliac lymph nodes])

**Leg:**
**External iliac lymph nodes**
(influx of the superficial and deep inguinal lymph nodes and popliteal lymph nodes)
**Superf.** and **deep popliteal lymph nodes**
(lymphatic drainage of the lower leg and foot)

**Organs of the pelvis:**
**Lumbar lymph nodes**
(influx of ovary and uterine tube through suspensory ligament of ovary and internal iliac lymph nodes from the organs of the pelvis)
**Internal iliac lymph nodes**
(influx of inguinal lymph nodes [through round ligament of uterus] and parauterine lymph nodes)
**Sacral lymph nodes**
(lymphatic drainage of rectum, vagina, cervix of uterus; drainage in common iliac lymph nodes)

> Clinical
>
> **Internal iliac lymph nodes:** often affected by metastases of the internal genital organs (testicles, uterus, prostate).
> **Superficial inguinal lymph nodes:** can be enlarged by tumors of the ovary or cervix of uterus. Swelling can also appear by inflammation of the outer genitalia (scrotum, penis, labia).

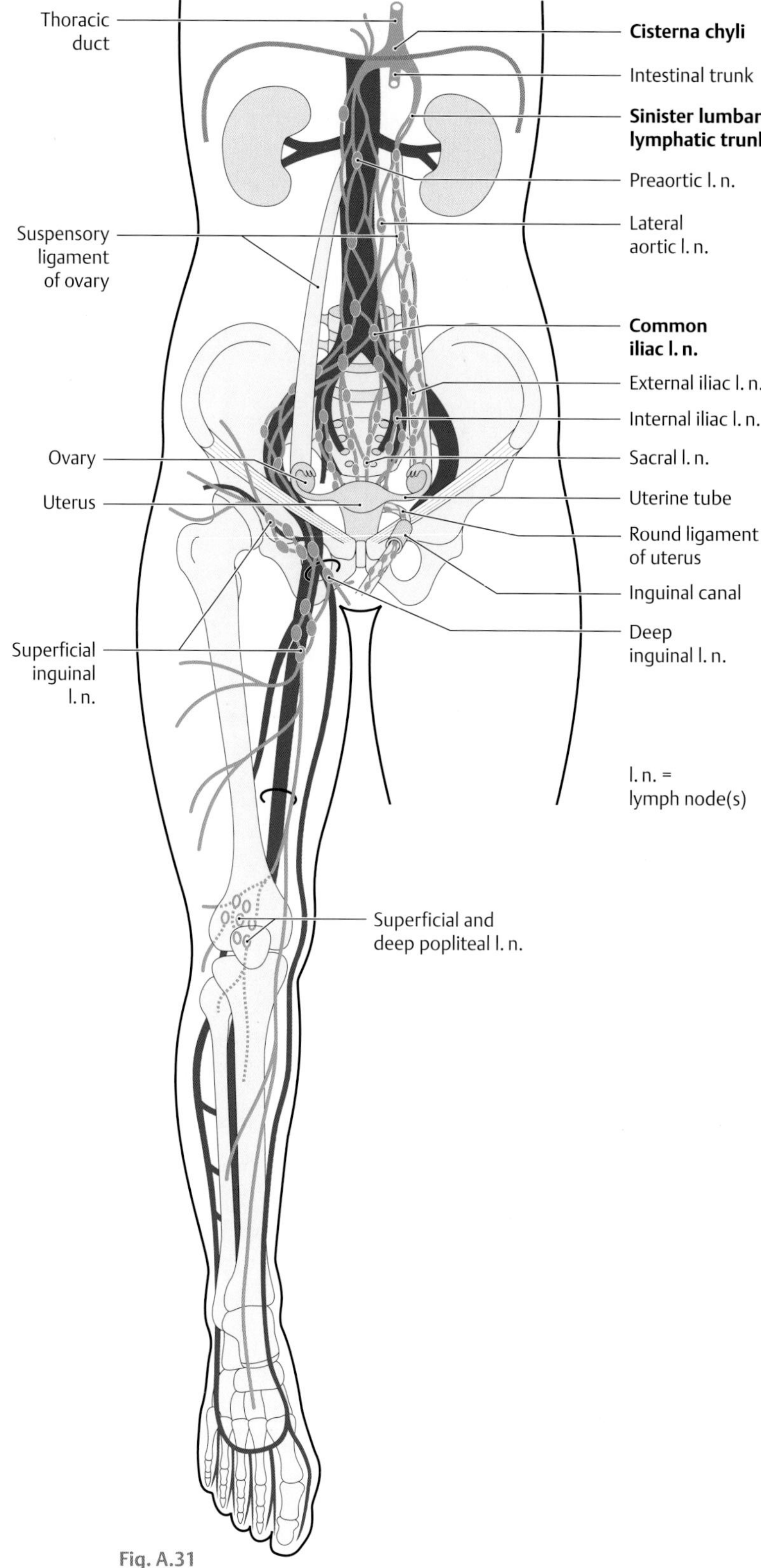


Fig. A.31

## Nerves of the Pelvis and Leg

See also Pages: 184 / 188–193 / 198–199 / 202 / 208–209 / 215 / 327 / 332–333

*Lateral aspect of the right leg.*

**Lumbar plexus** (T12–L4)
- **muscular branches** (for intertransversarii muscles, quadratus lumborum muscle, psoas major and minor muscle)
- **iliohypogastric nerve** (for skin of the region of the symphysis and the muscles of the stomach)
- **ilioinguinal nerve** (for the outer genitalia [scrotal or labial branches] and for the muscles of the stomach)
- **genitofemoral nerve** (with femoral branch and genital branch for the region of the groin and the coverings of the testicles or labia)
- **lateral femoral cutaneous nerve** (to the skin of the thigh)

**Obturator nerve** with anterior and posterior branch (for adductors, pectineus muscle and gracilis muscle; venous branch to the inner side of the thigh)

**Femoral nerve**
- **anterior femoral cutaneous branch** (to the anterior side of the thigh)
- **muscular branches** (for pectineus muscle, sartorius muscle and quadriceps femoris muscle)
- **saphenous nerve** (venous branches at the middle side of the lower leg [infrapatellar branch] and at the foot [medial crural cutaneous nerve])

**Sacral plexus** (L4–S3)
- **direct branches** (for the lateral rotator group, except the obturator externus muscle)
- **sup. gluteal nerve** (for gluteus medius and minimus muscle, tensor fasciae latae muscle)
- **inf. gluteal nerve** (for gluteus maximus)
- **posterior femoral cutaneous nerve** (cutaneous branches for posterior side of the thigh and the perineum)
- **sciatic nerve** (for quadratus femoris muscle, for the muscles of the hamstring and for all muscles for the lower leg and foot)
- **common fibular nerve**
  - **lateral sural cutaneous nerve** (cutaneous branch for the lower leg; confluence with the medial sural cutaneous nerve to the sural nerve)
  - **superficial fibular nerve** (for peroneus longus and brevis muscle and for the skin of the lower leg and foot)
  - **medial** and **intermedial dorsal cutaneous nerve** (to the skin of the back of the foot)
- **Deep fibular nerve** (for the extensors of the lower legs)
  - **dorsal digital nerves of the lateral great toe and medial second toe** (cutaneous branches for the inner side of the 1st and 2nd toe)

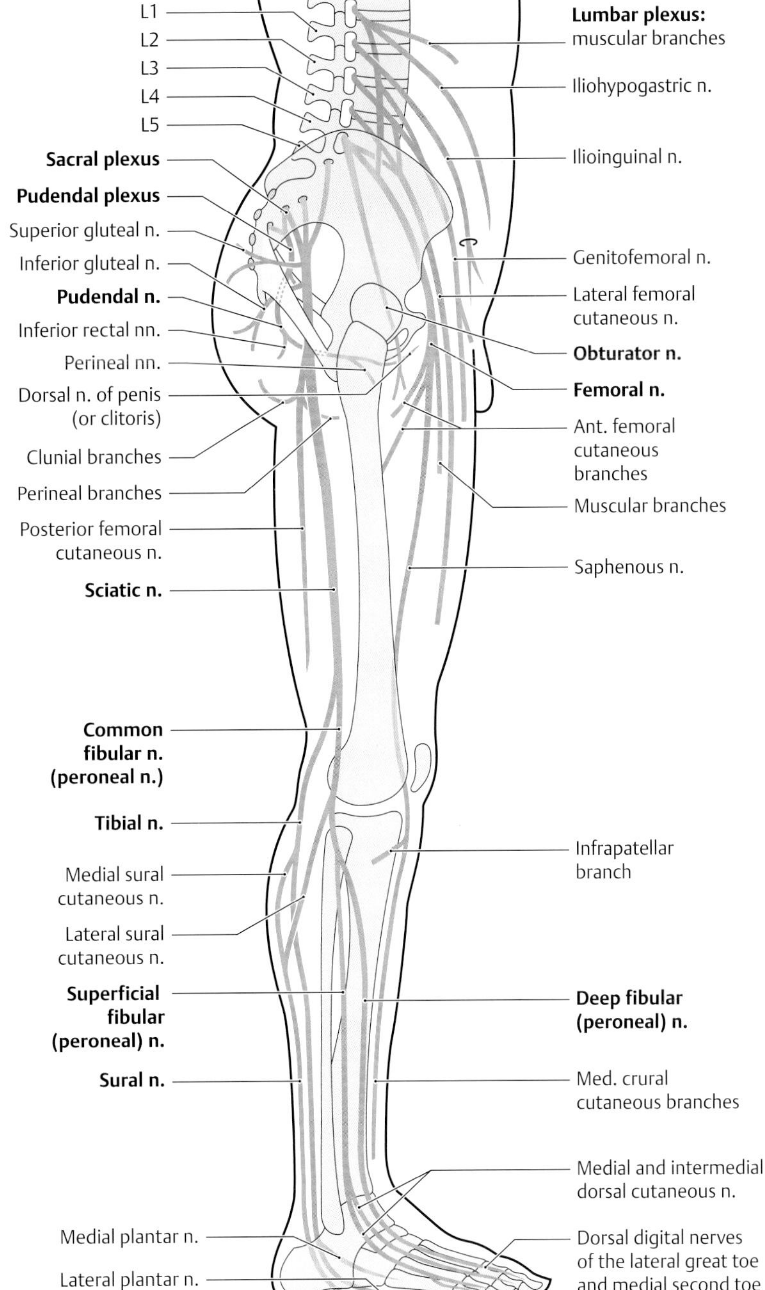


Fig. A.32

- **tibial nerve**
  - **medial sural cutaneous nerve** (cutaneous branch to the lower leg)

**Sural nerve** (formed by lateral and medial sural cutaneous nerve; to the skin of the lower leg and foot)
- **lateral plantar nerve** with superficial branch (for the skin of the lateral 1½ toes) and deep branch (for muscles of the small toe, adductor hallucis muscle, lumbrical muscles III and IV, quadratus plantae muscle, all interossei muscles and lateral head of the flexor hallucis brevis muscle)
- **medial plantar nerve** (for the muscles of the big toe; lumbrical muscles I and II, flexor digitorum brevis muscle and the skin of middle 3½ toes)

**Pudendal plexus** (S2–S4)
- **muscular branches** (for levator ani muscle and coccygeus)
- **pudendal nerve** (S2–S4)
  - **inferior rectal nerves** (to sphincter ani ext. muscle and to the skin of the anus)
  - **perineal nerves** (to the ischiocavernosus muscle and bulbospongiosus muscle, transversus perinei prof. and superf. muscle, to the skin of the region of the perineum)
  - **dorsal nerve of penis or clitoris** (for transversus perinei prof. muscle and outer genitalia)

**Coccygeal plexus** (S5, Co1–3)
- **anococcygeal nerves**

## Arteries and Nerves of the Lower Limb

See also Pages: 184 / 186 / 188 / 192 / 205

*The veins are not shown. They run parallel with the arteries.*

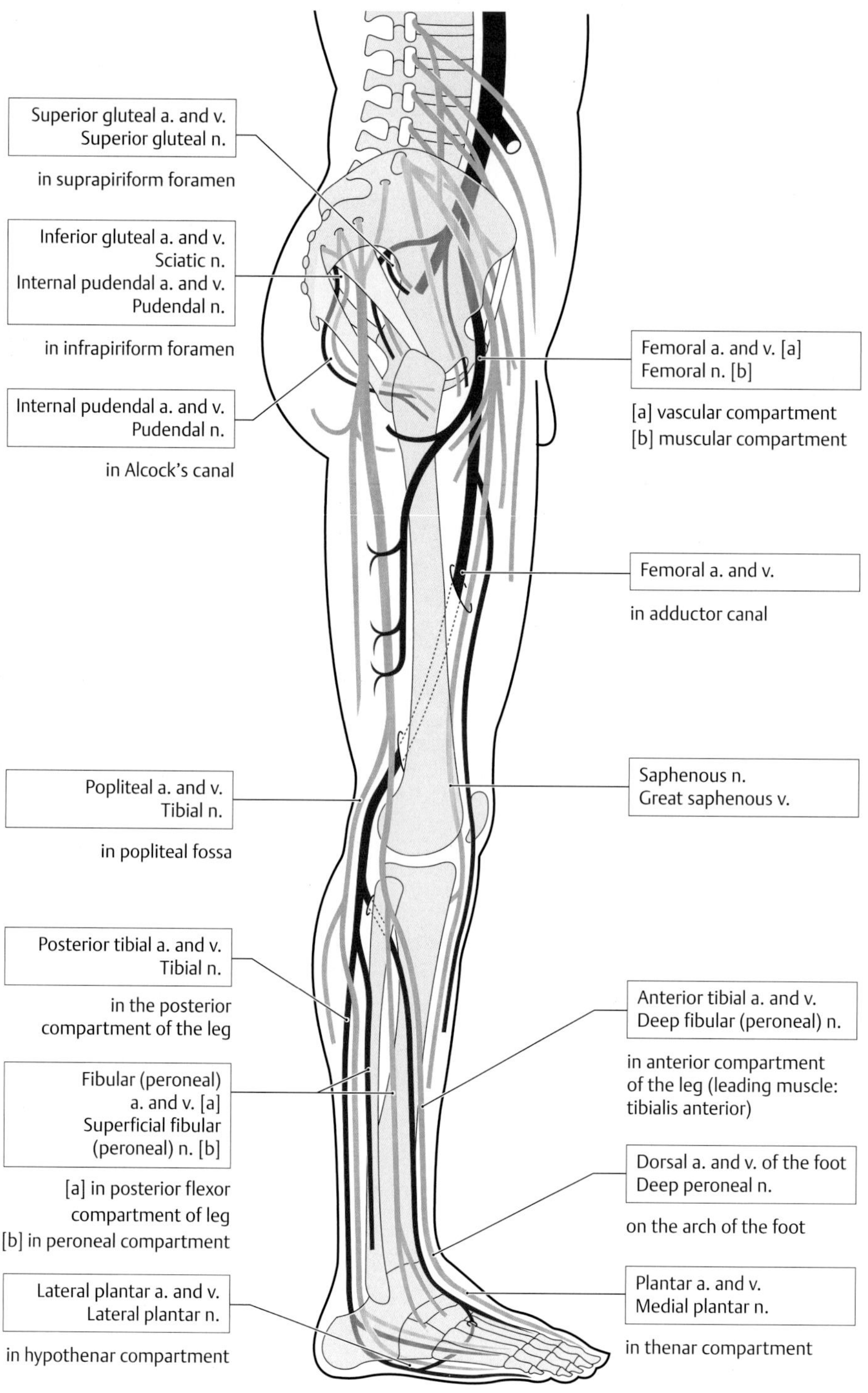


Fig. A.33

## Overview of the Main Muscle Functions of the Hip Joint

*The rotators are not shown.*

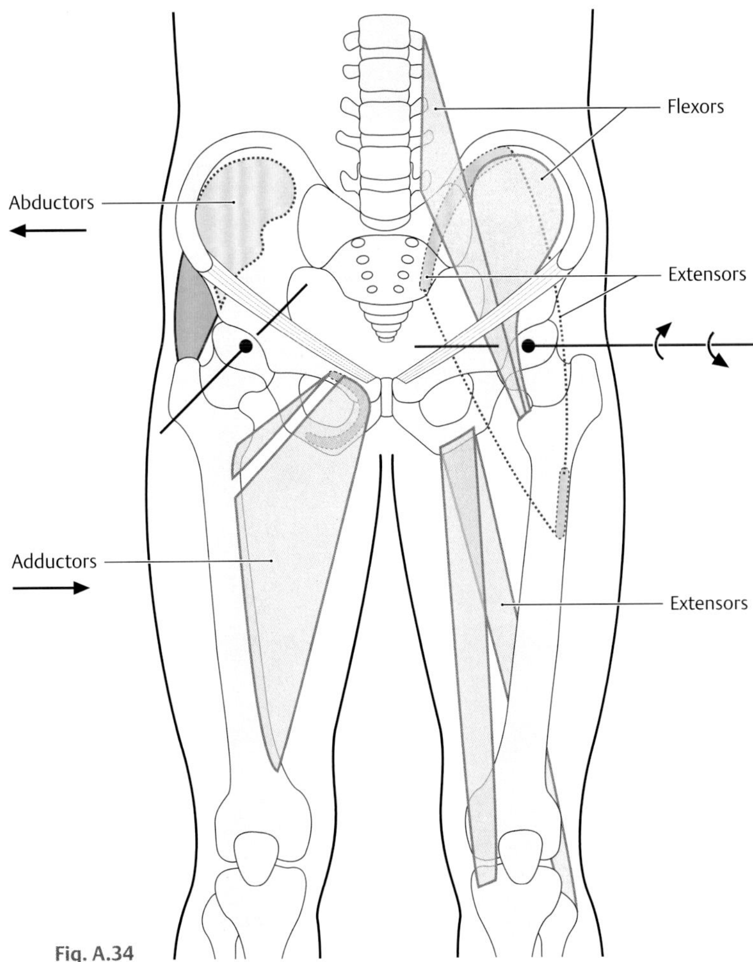


Fig. A.34

**Abductors**
- gluteus medius
- gluteus minimus

**Adductors**
- pectineus
- adductor brevis
- adductor longus
- adductor magnus

**Flexors**
- iliacus
- psoas major
- psoas minor
- rectus femoris
- adductor muscles

**Extensors**
- gluteus maximus
- biceps femoris
- gracilis
- semitendinosus
- semimembranosus
- adductor magnus

**Internal rotators**
- gluteus medius and minimus
- gracilis
- tensor fasciae latae

**External rotators**
- gluteus maximus
- gemellus muscles
- obturator internus and externus
- piriformis
- iliopsoas

## Anterior Muscles of the Pelvis and Thigh

See also Pages: 170–171 / 193–195

*Adductors and flexors of the hip joint, extensors in the knee joint.*

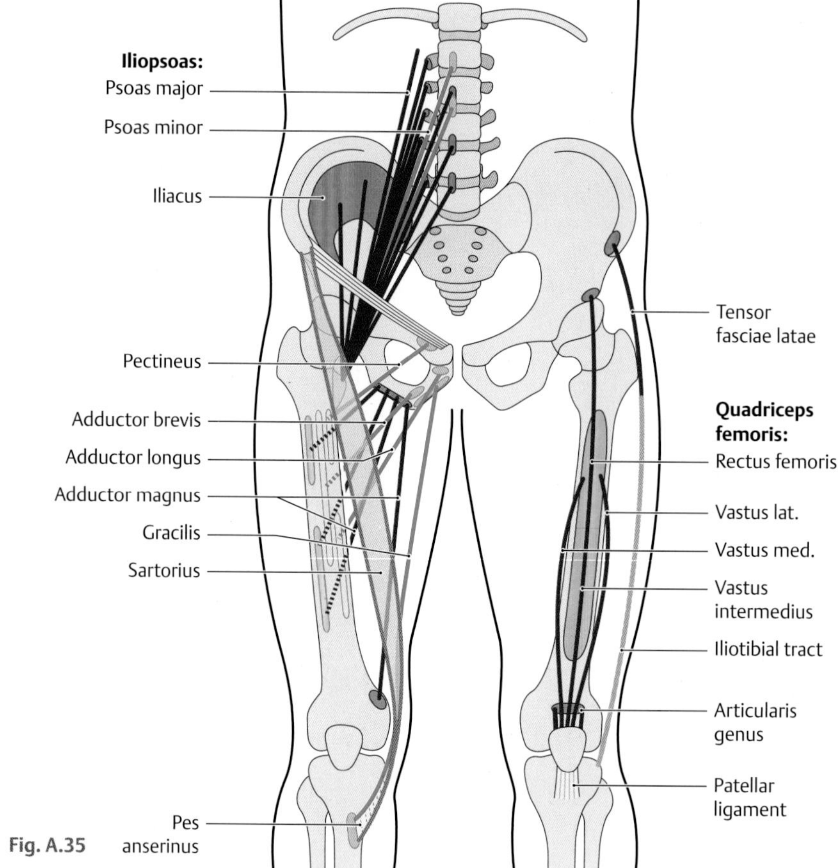


**Fig. A.35**

## Posterior Muscles of the Pelvis and Thigh

See also Pages: 172–174 / 196–199

Greater sciatic foramen with
a = suprapiriform foramen
b = infrapiriform foramen
c = lesser sciatic foramen

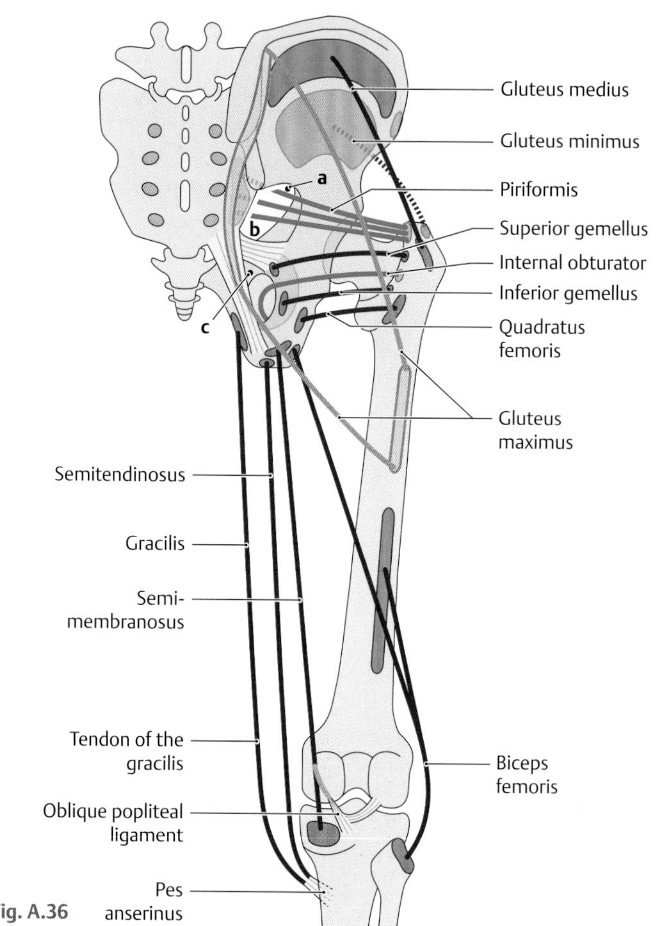


**Fig. A.36**

| Muscles | Origin | Insertion | Function | Innervation |
|---|---|---|---|---|
| **Iliopsoas** | | | | |
| • **psoas major** | Body of vertebra (T12–L4) | Lesser trochanter | Flexion of the hip joint, external rotation | Femoral n. (T12–L3) |
| • **psoas minor** | Costal processes (T12–L1) | | | |
| • **iliacus** | Iliac fossa | | | |
| **Pectineus** | Pecten pubis | Pectineal line of the femur | Adduction, flexion, external rotation of the thigh | Femoral n. and obturator n. |
| **Adductor brevis** | Pubis bone | Linea aspera of the femur | Adduction and external rotation of the hip joint | Obturator n. (L2–L4) |
| **Adductor longus** | Pubis bone | Linea aspera of the femur | Adduction, external rotation and flexion of the hip joint | Obturator n. (L2–L4) |
| **Adductor magnus** | Ischium bone, ischial tuberosity | Linea aspera, medial epicondyle of the femur | Adduction, extension, external and internal rotation of the hip joint, flexion | Obturator n., sciatic n. (tibial n.) (L3–L5) |
| **Gracilis** | Pubis bone | Tibia (pes anserinus) | Adduction of the hip joint, flexion and internal rotation of the knee joint | Obturator n. (L2–L4) |
| **Sartorius** | Anterior superior iliac spine | Tibia (pes anserinus) | Flexion, external rotation and abduction of the hip joint, flexion and internal rotation of the knee joint | Femoral n. (L2–L4) |
| **Tensor fasciae latae** | Anterior superior iliac spine | Iliotibial tract | Flexion and internal rotation of the hip joint, tension of fascia lata | Superior gluteal n. (L4–L5) |
| **Quadriceps femoris** | | | | |
| • **rectus femoris** | Anterior inferior iliac spine | Patellar ligament | Flexion of the hip joint, extension of the knee joint | Femoral n. (L2–L4) |
| • **vastus lateralis** | Femur | Tibial tuberosity | Extension of the knee joint | |
| • **vastus intermedius** | | | | |
| • **vastus medius** | | | | |
| • **articularis genus** | Femur | Joint capsule | Tension of the capsule of the knee joint | |

| Muscles | Origin | Insertion | Function | Innervation |
|---|---|---|---|---|
| **Gluteus medius** | Ilium bone (wing) (between anterior and posterior gluteal line) | Greater trochanter | Abduction, internal and external rotation (proportionally) of the thigh | Superior gluteal n. (L4, L5) |
| **Gluteus minimus** | Ilium bone (wing) (between anterior and inferior gluteal line) | Greater trochanter | Abduction, internal rotation of the thigh | Superior gluteal n. (L4–S1) |
| **Piriformis** | Sacrum bone (pelvic surface) | Greater trochanter | Abduction, external rotation of the thigh | Sacral plexus (L5–S2) |
| **Gemellus superior** | Ischial spine | Trochanteric fossa | External rotation | Sacral plexus |
| **Obturatorius internus** | Obturator membrane (inner side) | Trochanteric fossa | External rotation, adduction and retroversion | Sacral plexus (L5–S2) |
| **Gemellus inferior** | Ischial tuberosity | Trochanteric fossa | External rotation | Sacral plexus |
| **Quadratus femoris** | Ischial tuberosity | Intertrochanteric crest | External rotation, adduction | Inferior gluteal n. (L5–S2), sciatic n. |
| **Gluteus maximus** | Posterior gluteal line, sacrum bone, sacrotuberous ligament | Femur (gluteal tuberosity), iliotibial tract | Retroverison and external rotation, ab- and adduction of the leg | Inferior gluteal n. (L4–S2) |
| **Semitendinosus** | Ischial tuberosity | Tibia (pes anserinus) | (same as semimembranosus) | |
| **Semimembranosus** | Ischial tuberosity | Medial condyle of the tibia (oblique popliteal ligament) | Extension and adduction of the hip joint, extension and internal rotation of the knee joint | Tibial n. (L5–S2) |
| **Biceps femoris** | Long head: ischial tuberosity Short head: femur (linea aspera) | Head of fibula | Extension of the hip joint (only long head), flexion and external rotation of the knee joint | Tibial n. (S1, S2) (long head), common fibular n. (L5, S1) (short head) |
| **Obturatorius externus** | Obturator membrane | Trochanteric fossa | External rotation, flexion | Obturator n. |

## Extensors of the Lower Leg and Foot

**See also Pages: 176–177 / 180–181 / 210 / 212–213**

*Anterior aspect.*

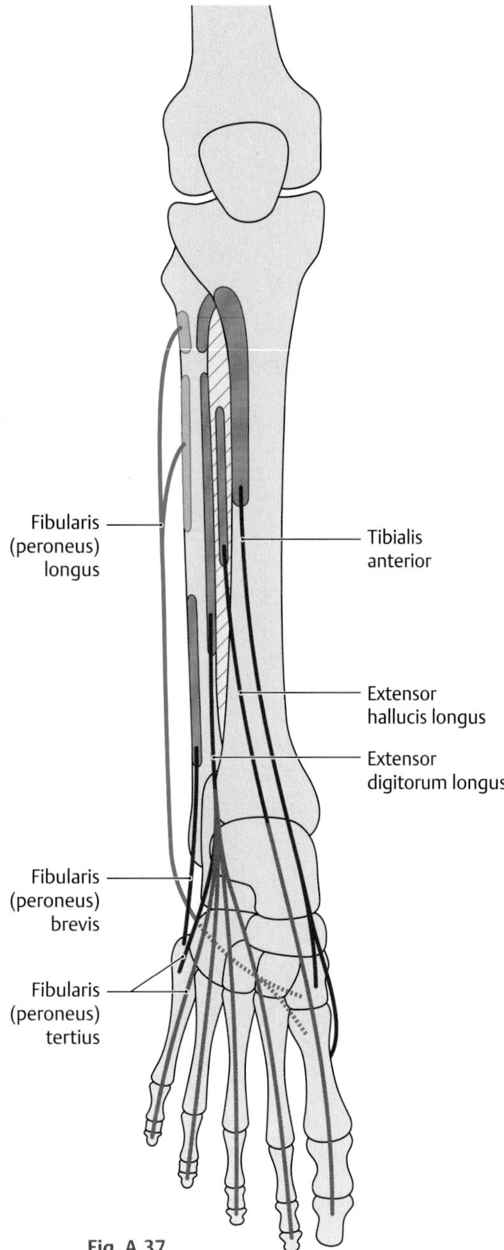


**Fig. A.37**

## Superficial Flexors of the Lower Leg and Foot

**See also Pages: 175 / 206–207 / 214–215**

*Posterior aspect.*

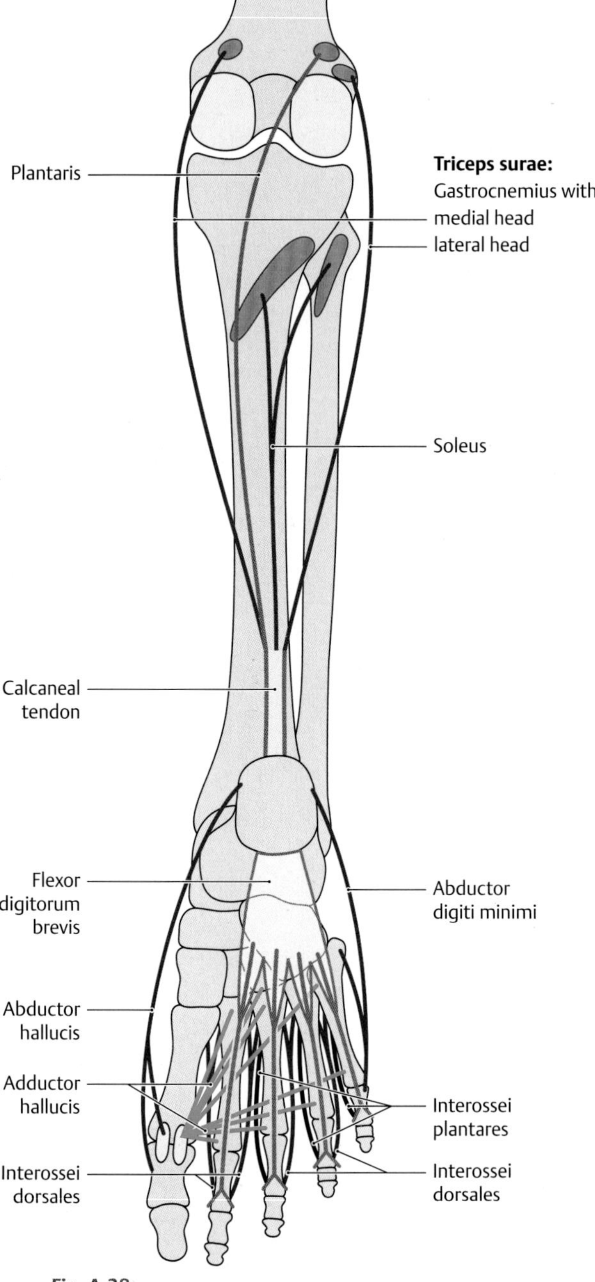


**Fig. A.38**

| Muscles | Origin | Insertion | Function | Innervation |
|---|---|---|---|---|
| **Tibialis anterior** | Tibia, interosseous membrane | Medial cuneiform bone, metatarsal bone I | Dorsal extension and supination of the foot | Deep fibular n. (L4, L5) |
| **Extensor hallucis longus** | Fibula, interosseous membrane | Distal phalanx of the 1st toe | Dorsal extension of the foot, extension of the 1st toe | Deep fibular n. (L5, S1) |
| **Extensor digitorum longus** | Tibia, fibula, interosseous membrane | Dorsal aponeurosis of the 2nd to 5th toe | Dorsal extension of the foot, extension of 2nd to 5th toe | Deep fibular n. (L5, S1) |
| **Fibularis (peroneus) longus** | Fibula, intermuscular septum | Medial cuneiform bone, metatarsal bone I | Pronation and plantar flexion of the foot, tension of the transverse arches of the foot | Superficial fibular n. (L5, S1) |
| **Fibularis (peroneus) brevis** | Fibula, intermuscular septum | Tuberosity of metatarsal bone V | Plantar flexion, pronation | Superficial fibular n. (L5, S1) |
| **Fibularis (peroneus) tertius** | Fibula, separation from extensor digitorum longus muscle (variable) | Metatarsal bone V | Dorsal extension, pronation | Deep fibular n. (L5, S1) |

| Muscles | Origin | Insertion | Function | Innervation |
|---|---|---|---|---|
| **Triceps surae**<br>• **Gastrocnemius** | Medial head: condyle of the femur | Calcaneal tuberosity (Achilles tendon) | Flexion of the knee joint | Tibial n. (S1, S2) |
| • **Soleus** | Lateral head: Condyle of the femur, tibia, head of fibula | | Plantar flexion and supination of the foot | |
| **Plantaris** | Lateral condyle of the femur | Calcaneal tuberosity (Achilles tendon) | (same as gastrocnemius) | Tibial n. (S1, S2) |
| **Abductor digiti minimi** | Calcaneal tuberosity | Proximal phalanx of the 5th toe | Abduction and flexion of the 5th toe | Lateral plantar n. (S1, S2) |
| **Interosseus plantaris muscles** (3 muscles) | Metatarsal bones III–V | Dorsal aponeurosis of 3rd to 5th toe | Adduction (apart from that same as interosseus dorsalis muscles) | Lateral plantar n. (S1, S2) |
| **Interosseus dorsalis muscles** (4 muscles) | Metatarsal bones I–V | Dorsal aponeurosis of 2nd, 3rd and 4th toe | Abduction of the toes (2nd toe as central axis), flexion in the base joints, extension in middle and end joints | Lateral plantar n. (S1, S2) |
| **Flexor digitorum brevis** | Calcaneal tuberosity | Middle phalanges of 2nd to 5th toe | Flexion of the middle joints of 2nd to 5th toe, tension of the longitudinal arch | Medial plantar n. (S1, S2) |
| **Abductor hallucis** | Calcaneal tuberosity | Proximal phalanx of the 1st toe, medial sesamoid bone | Abduction and flexion of the big toe | Medial plantar n. (S1, S2) |
| **Adductor hallucis** | Oblique head: long plantar ligament, cuboid bone, lateral cuneiform bone | Lateral sesamoid bone, proximal phalanx of the big toe | Abduction and flexion of the big toe | Lateral plantar n. (deep branch) (S1, S2) |
| | Transverse head: base joints of 2nd to 5th toe | | Adduction, tension of the transverse arch | |

## Deep Flexors of the Lower Leg and Foot

See also Pages: 178–179 / 182–183 / 214–217

*Posterior aspect.*

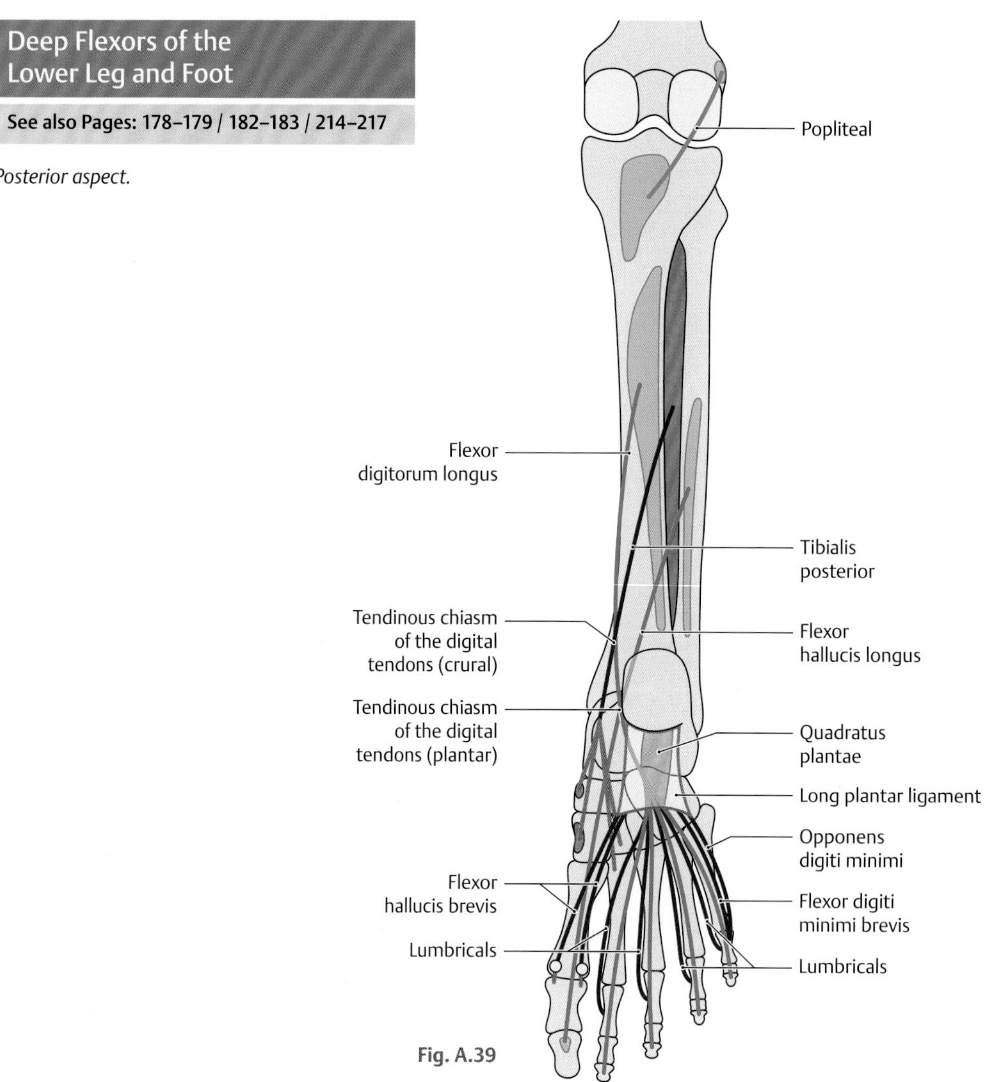


**Fig. A.39**

| Muscles | Origin | Insertion | Function | Innervation |
|---|---|---|---|---|
| **Popliteus** | Lateral epicondyle of femur | Tibia (above soleal line) | Internal rotation of the lower leg, withdrawal of the final rotation, stabilization of the posterior lateral areas of the knee joint | Tibial n. (L5, S1) |
| **Tibialis post.** | Tibia, fibula, interosseus membrane | Navicular bone, cuneiform bones, metatarsal bones II and III | Plantar flexion, supination and adduction of the foot | Tibial n. (L4–S1) |
| **Flexor hallucis longus** | Fibula, interosseus membrane | Distal phalanx of big toe | Flexion of the 1st toe, plantar flexion and supination of the foot | Tibial n. (S1, S2) |
| **Quadratus plantae** (flexor accessorius muscle) | Calcaneus | Tendon compartments of flexor digitorum longus | As flexor digitorum longus muscle, support of the longitudinal arch of the foot | Lateral plantar n. (S1, S2) |
| **Opponens digiti V** | Long plantar ligament | Metatarsal bone V | Abduction and opposition of the little toe | Lateral plantar n. (S1, S2) |
| **Flexor digiti V brevis** | Long plantar ligament, metatarsal bone V | Proximal phalanx V | Abduction and opposition of the little toe | Lateral plantar n. (S1, S2) |
| **Lumbrical muscles** | Tendon of flexor digitorum longus | Aponeurosis dorsalis digitalis II–V of foot | Flexion in the base joint and extension in middle and end joint of 2nd to 5th toe | Medial plantar n. (S1, S2); lateral plantar n. (S3, S4) (S1, S2) |
| **Flexor digitorum longus** | Tibia | Distal phalanx of 2nd to 5th toe | Flexion of the end joints of 2nd to 5th toe, plantar flexion and supination of the foot | Medial and lateral plantar n. |
| **Flexor hallucis brevis** | Long plantar ligament, cuneiform bones | Two-headed on both sesamoid bones, proximal phalanx I | Flexion of the big toe, support of the longitudinal arch | N. plantaris med. and lat. |

## Structure of the Segments and Cutaneous Innervation of the Leg

See also Pages: 188 / 190–193 / 198 / 202 / 205 / 208–209 / 212

*Left anterior aspect, right posterior aspect.*

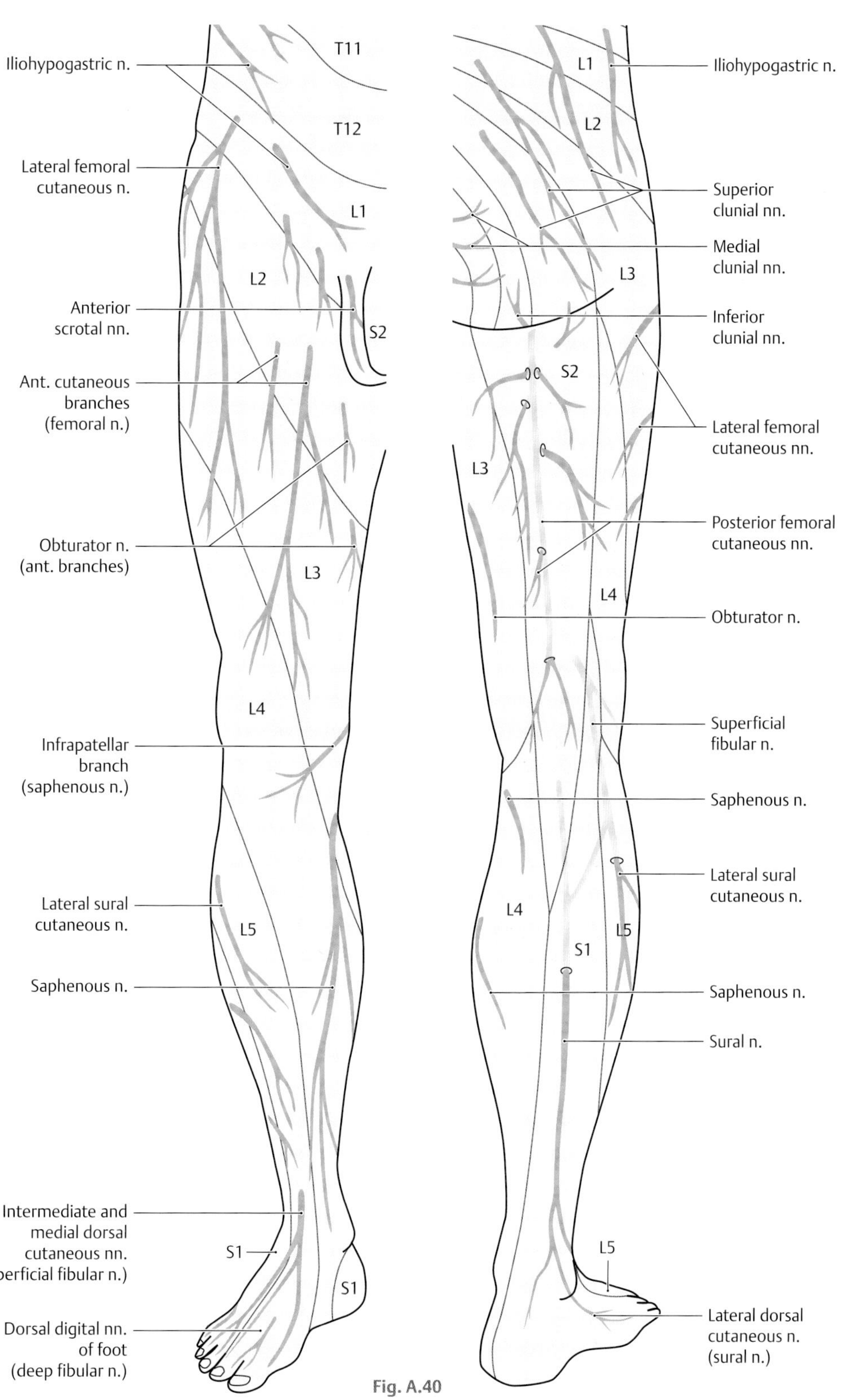


Fig. A.40

## Arteries and Blood Supply of the Brain

*Overview.*

Two large arteries supply the brain: the internal carotid artery (light red) and the vertebral artery (dark red). The main areas of blood supply are denoted by the various branches. The cerebral arterial circle (of Willis) connects both vascular areas.

**Internal corotid artery**
Runs through the carotid canal of the base of the skull to the brain; final branches are the **anterior cerebral artery** (over the corpus callosum; primary to the inner side of the hemispheres and to the parasagittal cortical zone [dark gray area]) and the **middle cerbral artery** (over the insular lobe in the lateral sulcus; mainly to the outer side of the frontal, parietal and temporale lobes [bright area])
**Vertebral artery**
Runs in the foramina transversaria of the cervical spine; transitions into the basilar artery at the base of the skull (supply of cerebellum [**cerebellar arteries**] and parts of the temporal and occipital lobe [**posterior cerebral artery**]) (light gray area)

Central sulcus
Anterior cerebral a.
Middle cerebral a.
**Cerebral arterial circle** (of Willis)
Posterior cerebral a.
Superior cerebellar a.
Anterior inferior cerebellar a.
Posterior inferior cerebellar a.
Basilar a.
**Internal carotid a.**
**Vertebral a.**

a = frontal lobe
b = parietal lobe
c = occipital lobe
d = temporal lobe
e = cerebellum

Fig. A.41

## Arteries of the Brain: Branches of the Internal Carotid Artery

See also Pages: 491–492 / 496

*From below.*

**Ophthalmic artery**
(for eye, forehead and anterior nasal cavity)

- **supratrochlear artery** (to the skin of the forehead)
- **dorsal nasal artery** (to the back of the nose, anastomoses with angular artery of the facial artery)
- **medial palpebral arteries** (to the eyelids)
- **supraorbital artery** (to the skin of the forehead)
- **ant. ethmoidal artery** (to anterior nasal cavity, dura and anterior ethmoidal cells) with branches
  - **ant. meningeal artery** (to dura of anterior cranial fossa) and
  - **anterior lateral nasal arteries and nasal septal arteries** (through cribriform plate to the nasal cavity)
- **ant. ciliary arteries** (to the conjunctiva and anterior uvea)
- **post. ethmoidal artery** (to the posterior ethmoidal cells)
- **lacrimal artery** (to the lacrimal gland and lateral skin of the eyelid)
- **short and long posterior ciliary arteries** (to the choroid of the eye)
- **central retinal artery** (in the optic nerve to the retina)

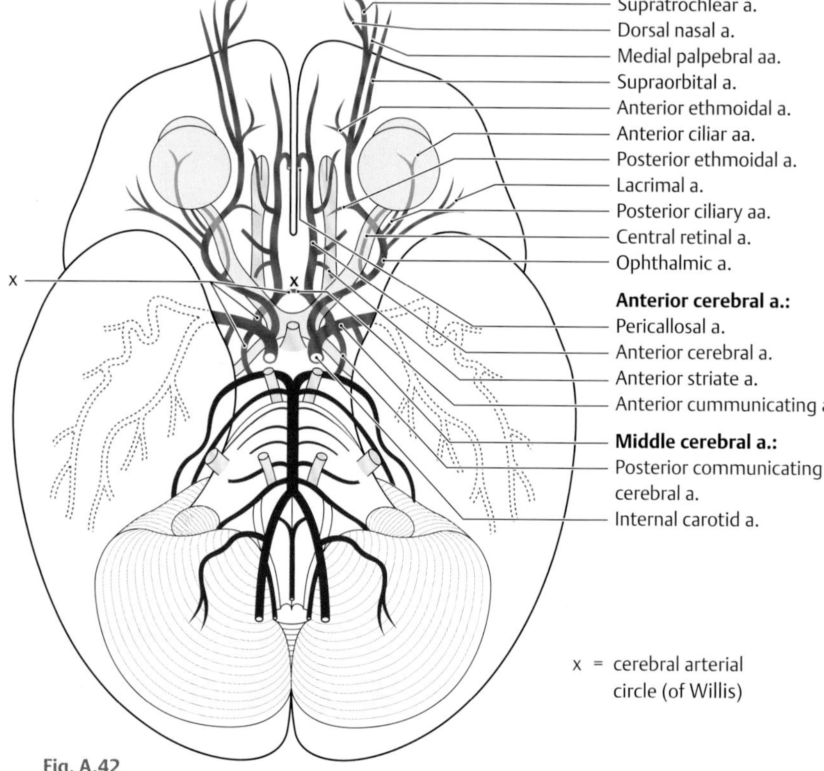


Fig. A.42

**Anterior cerebral artery**

- **pericallosal artery** (for cortical areas above the corpus callosum)
- **ant. striate artery** (so-called recurrent artery of Heubner to the basal ganglia)
- **anterior communicating artery**

**Middle cerebral artery**
(in lateral sulcus) divides into anterior and posterior branch to the cerebrum

## Branches of the External Carotid Artery

See also Pages: 110 / 418–420 / 495

Superficial temporal artery
- **parietal branch** } final branches to the regions
- **frontal branch** } of the forehead and temple
- **ant. auricular branches** and **parotid branches** (for auditory canal and parotid gland)
- **middle temporal artery** (to temporalis muscle)
- **transverse facial artery** (to the facial region)

Facial artery
- **angular artery** (anastomoses with ophthalmic artery)
- **sup. labial artery** (for upper lip)
- **inf. labial artery** (for lower lip)
- **ascending palatine artery** (to pharynx and soft palate)
- **submental artery** (to the muscles of the base of the mouth)

Lingual artery (for base of the mouth and tongue)
- **deep lingual artery** (final branch to the anterior muscles of the tongue)
- **sublingual artery** (to sublingual gland and to base of the mouth)
- **dorsal lingual branches** (to the back of the tongue)

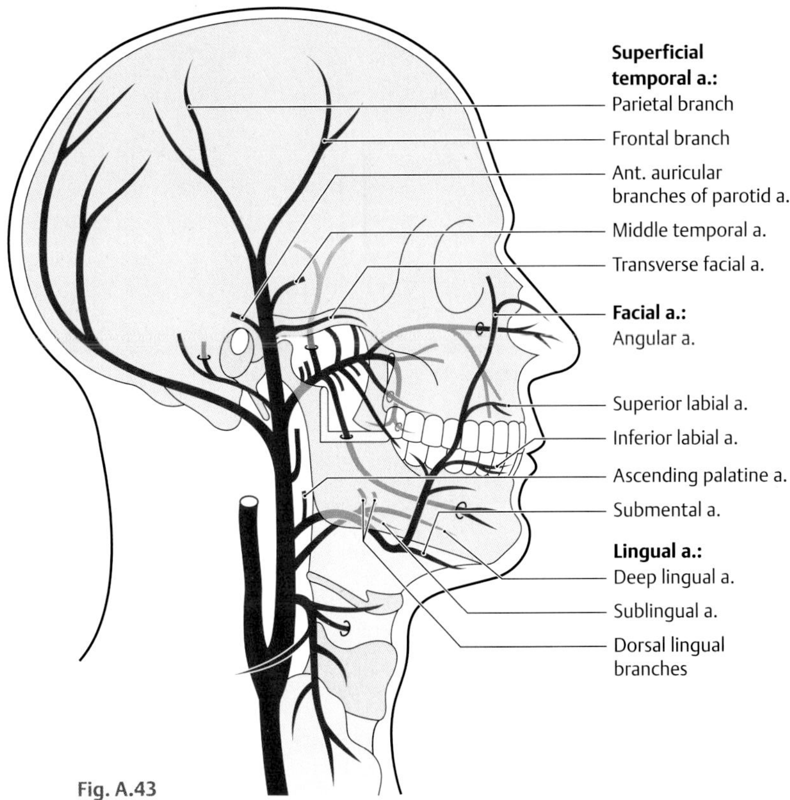


Fig. A.43

## Arteries of the Brain: Branches of Vertebral Artery and Basilar Artery

See also Pages: 491 / 493–496

*From below.*

Branches of vertebral artery and basilar artery (dark red), branches of internal carotid artery (light red), cranial nerves (yellow).

Basilar artery
- **posterior cerebral artery** (to basal surface of the temporal lobe, to the occipital lobe)
- **superior cerbellar artery** (to the upper surface of the cerebellum)
- **anterior inferior cerebellar artery** (to lower surface of the cerebellum)
- **branches to the pons**
- **labyrinthine artery** (to the inner ear)

Vertebral artery
- **posterior inferior cerebellar artery** (to the lower surface of the cerebellum)
- **posterior spinal artery** } (descending to
- **anterior spinal artery** } the spinal cord)

CN I
CN II
a
x
b
CN III
CN V
CN VI
Internal carotid a.
**Basilar a.**
Posterior cerebral a.
Superior cerebellar a.
Branches ad pontem
Labyrinthine a.
Anterior inferior cerebellar a.
**Vertebral a.**
Posterior inferior cerebellar a.
Anterior spinal a.
Posterior spinal a.

Fig. A.44

**Cranial nerves:**
CN I = olfactory bulb
CN II = optic nerve
CN III = oculomotor nerve
CN V = trigeminal nerve
CN VI = abducent nerve

x = **cerebral arterial circle** (of Willis) (anastomoses between middle cerebral artery and posterior cerebral artery)
a = anterior communicating artery
b = posterior communicating artery

## Arteries of the Head: Branches of the External Carotid Artery

See also Pages: 394 / 396 / 399–403 / 418–420 / 433–437

*Lateral aspect.*

**Superficial temporal artery** (see p. 557)
(to the parietal region and region of the ear)
- **posterior auricular artery** (for external and middle ear)
- **stylomastoid artery** (through stylomastoid foramen to the middle ear)

**Occipital artery** (to the occipital region)
**Maxillary artery** (see figure below)
- **ascending pharyngeal artery** (lateral ascending to the pharynx) with branches
  - **posterior meningeal artery**
  - **inferior tympanic artery**

**Facial artery** (see p. 557)
**Lingual artery** (see p. 557)
**Superior thyroid artery**
- **infrahyoid branch** (to the hyoid bone)
- **sup. laryngeal artery** (through thyrohyoid membrane to the inside of the larynx)
- **sternocleidomastoid branch** (to the muscle of the same name)
- **cricothyroid branch** (to the muscle of the same name)
- **glandular branches** (to thyroid gland)

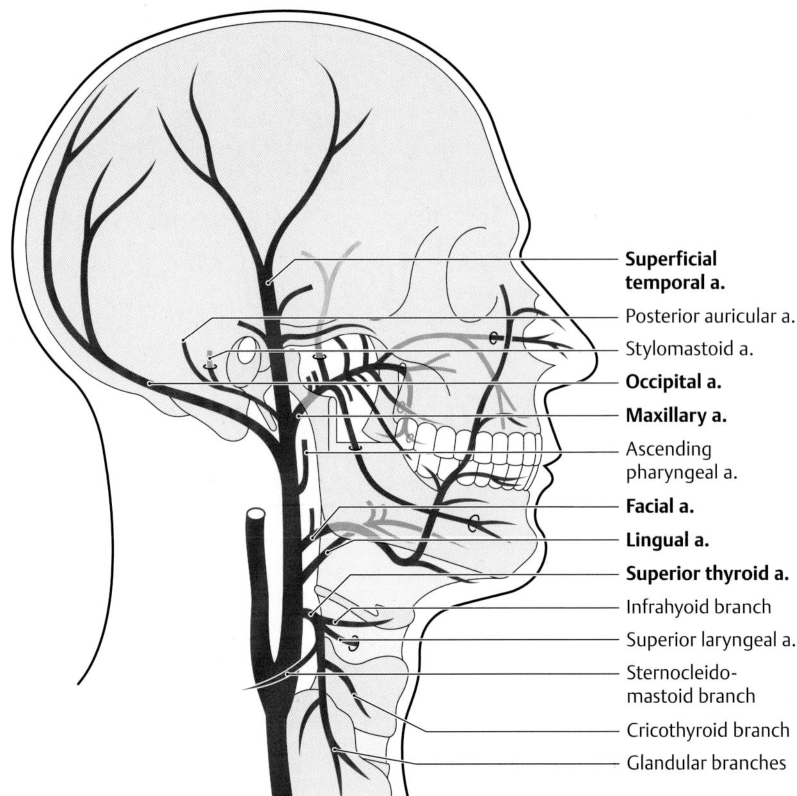


Fig. A.45

## Branches of the External Carotid Artery: Maxillary Artery

See also Pages: 394 / 399–403 / 418

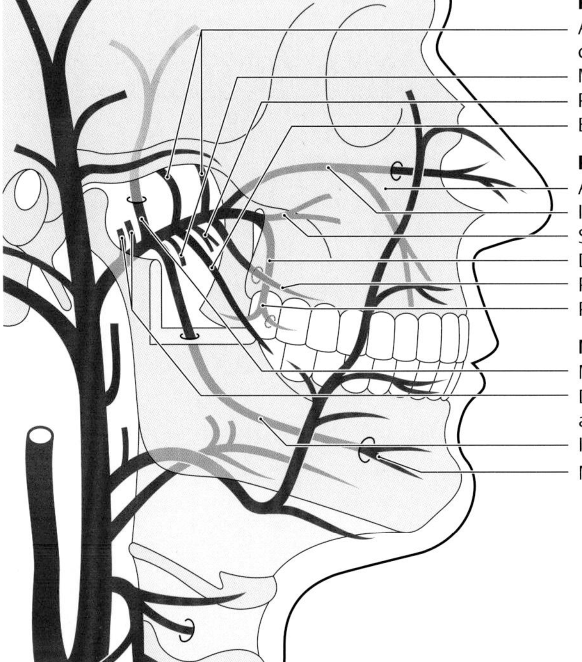


Fig. A.46

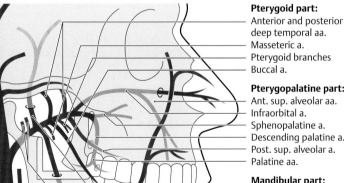

**Pterygoid part**
- **anterior** and **posterior deep temporal arteries** (to temporalis muscle)
- **masseteric artery** } to the masticatory muscles
- **pterygoid branches** } of the same name
- **buccal artery** (to the cheek, anastomoses with facial artery)

**Pterygopalatine part**
- **anterior superior alveolar arteries** (for upper jaw and anterior teeth) with final branches for nose, lower eyelid and upper lip
- **infraorbital artery** (in infraorbital canal to the facial region and to the anterior teeth)
- **sphenopalatine artery** (through sphenopalatine foramen to nasal cavity) with final branches
  - **posterior lateral nasal arteries** and **nasal septal arteries** (to the posterior nasal cavity)
- **descending palatine artery** (in pterygopalatine canal downward to the palatine) with final branches
  - **greater palate artery** (to the hard palate)
  - **lesser palatine arteries** (to the soft palate)
- **posterior superior alveolar artery** (through posterior alveolar foramina to the molars)

**Mandibular part**
- **middle meningeal artery** (through foramen spinosum to the middle cranial fossa)
- **deep auricular artery** (for the temporomandibular joint, auditory canal and tympanic membrane) and
- **anterior tympanic artery** (through petrotympanic fissure to the tympanic cavity)
- **inferior alveolar artery** (in mandibular canal to the lower jaw and to the chin)
- **mental artery**

## Veins of Head and Neck

See also Pages: 396–401 / 420–423

*Lateral aspect.*

**Superficial temporal vein**
(in the parietal region anastomoses with superior sagittal sinus [through parietal emissary vein]; connection behind the mandible with pterygoid plexus; drainage to internal jugular vein)
**Supraorbital vein** and **supratrochlear vein**
(drainage out of region of forehead [anastomoses with superior sagittal sinus through frontal emissary vein]; drainage to superior ophthalmic vein and facial vein)
**Occipital vein**
(connection through posterior emissary veins to superior sagittal sinus and sigmoid sinus; drainage through external jugular vein)
**Facial vein**
(through **angular vein** anastomoses with superior ophthalmic vein and cavernous sinus; in facial region confluence of inferior ophthalmic vein, superior and inferior labial vein and buccal vein [anastomoses with **pterygoid plexus**], in region of the jaw confluence of submental vein [from the base of the mouth])
**Internal jugular vein**
(main drainage of the veins of the head and of dural venous sinuses; confluence of subclavian vein [in venous angle] to brachiocephalic vein)

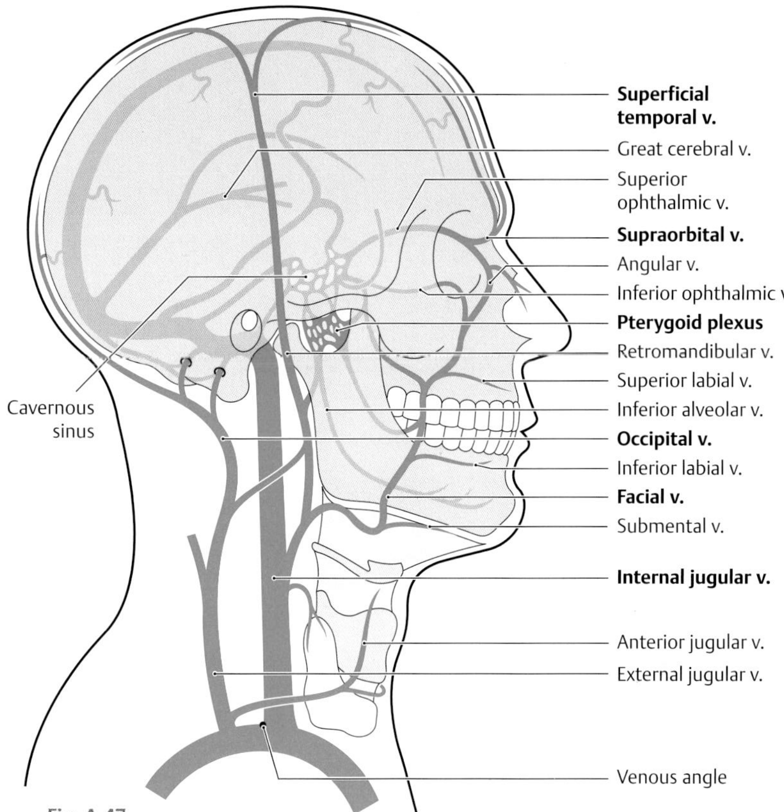


Fig. A.47

## Dural venous sinuses

See also Pages: 464 / 483–485

*Drainage of the blood of the cranial veins and of the cerebrospinal fluid.*

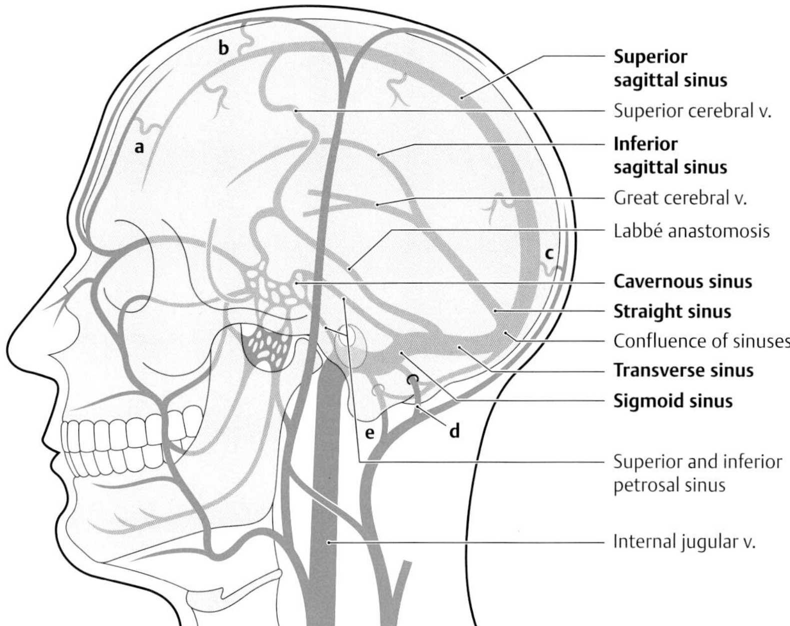


Fig. A.48

**Superior sagittal sinus**
(runs in falx cerebri; confluence of outer cerebral veins [**superior cerebral veins**]; connections with veins of the head through emissary veins)
**Inferior sagittal sinus** (at the lower edge of the falx cerebri; confluence of straight sinus)
**Cavernous sinus**
(surrounds sella turcica; connection with superior and inferior ophthalmic veins [of eye and orbit], with sphenoparietal sinus and with both petrosal sinuses; anastomoses through holes of the base of the skull with pterygoid plexus)
**Straight sinus**
(in tentorium cerebelli; collection of inferior sagittal sinus and great cerebral vein [drainage of the interior cerebral veins])
**Transverse sinus** – transition into
**Sigmoid sinus**
(confluence of superior and inferior petrosal sinus and sphenoparietal sinus; transition in internal jugular vein; connection through emissary veins [mastoid emissary vein and condylar emissary vein] to occipital vein)

**Emissary veins:**

**a** = **frontal emissary vein**
(anastomosis between supraorbital vein and superior sagittal sinus)
**b** = **parietal emissary vein**
(anastomosis between superficial temporal vein and superior sagittal sinus)
**c** = **occipital emissary vein**
(anastomosis between occipital vein and superior sagittal sinus)
**d** = **mastoid emissary vein** and
**e** = **condylar emissary vein**
(anastomosis between posterior auricular vein and occipital vein and sigmoid sinus)

## Lymphatic Vessels and Lymph Nodes of the Head and Neck

See also Pages: 422–423 / 432–437

**Superior deep cervical lymph nodes**
(confluence of the lymphatic vessels of the skin of the head [3 regions] and of the **parotid, retroauricular** and **occipital lymph nodes**)
**Submandibular lymph nodes**
(receives lymph from the lymphatic vessels of the tongue and base of the mouth [**submental lymph nodes**])
**Jugulodigastric lymph node**
(upper gathering point for lymphatic drainage of oral and nasal cavity; head and superior pharynx)
**Jugulo-omohyoid lymph node**
(lower gathering point for lymphatic drainage of the organs of the throat and neck; confluence of **jugular trunk** [left in **thoracic duct**; right in **right lymphatic duct**])
**Cervical trunk**
(of the lower regions of the neck)
**Subclavian trunk**
(of the region of the clavicle)

l. n. =
lymph node(s)
Retroauricular l. n.
Occipital l. n.
Parotid l. n.
Submental l. n.
**Submandibular l. n.**
**Superior deep cervial l. n.**
Superficial cervical l. n.
**Jugulodigastric l. n.**
**Jugulo-omohyoid l. n.**
Jugular lymph trunk
**Cervical lymph trunk**
Thoracic duct
**Subclavian lymph trunk**
Bronchomediastinal lymph trunk

**Fig. A.49**

## Oculomotor Nerve (CN III), Trochlear Nerve (CN IV) and Abducent Nerve (CN VI)

See also Pages: 361 / 443–445 / 455–457 / 466–467 / 512–513

**Nerves for the muscles of the eye**
**Trochlear nerve (CN IV)** for obliquus sup. muscle
**Oculomotor nerve (CN III)**

- **superior branch** (for rectus superior muscle and levator palpebrae sup. muscle)
- **inferior branch** (for rectus med. muscle, rectus inf. muscle, obliquus inf. muscle)
- **parasympathetic root** (oculomotor root) to ciliary ganglion

**Abducent nerve (CN VI)** for rectus lateralis muscle

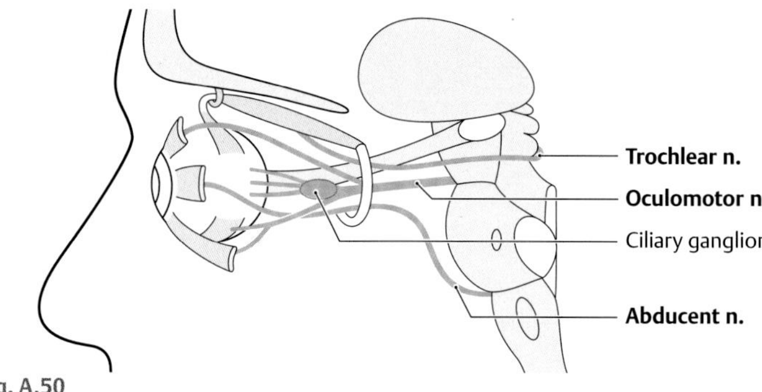


**Fig. A.50**

| Parts of the Brain | Nerve Type | Associated Cranial Nerve | Function |
|---|---|---|---|
| **Cerebrum** (telencephalon) | Sensory brain parts | CN I (olfactory n.) | Olfactory system |
| **Diencephalon** | | CN II (optic n.) | Optic system |
| **Midbrain** (mesencephalon) | Only motor cerebral nerves | CN III (oculomotor n.)<br>CN IV (trochlear n.) | Eye muscles |
| **Hindbrain** (rhombencephalon) | | CN VI (abducent n.) | |
| | Mixed nerves of the pharyngeal arch (1–4) | 1. CN V (trigeminal nerve, sensory root, motor root [only in CN $V_3$])<br>2. CN VII (facial nerve)<br>3. CN IX (glossopharyngeal n.)<br>4. CN X (vagus n.) | Sensibility of the head<br>muscles of mastication<br>mimic muscles<br>gustatory system, throat<br>larynx, organs of the chest and stomach |
| | Only motor cranial nerves | CN XI (accessory n.)<br>CN XII (hypoglossal n.) | Trapezius muscles, sternocleidomastoid muscle, muscles of the tongue |
| | Only sensory cranial nerves | CN VIII (vestibulocochlear n.) | Auditory and vestibular system |

## Trigeminal Nerve (CN V)

Overview of the three main branches of the trigeminal nerve and its supply areas (differently marked in gray). The three pressure points are marked with red circles.

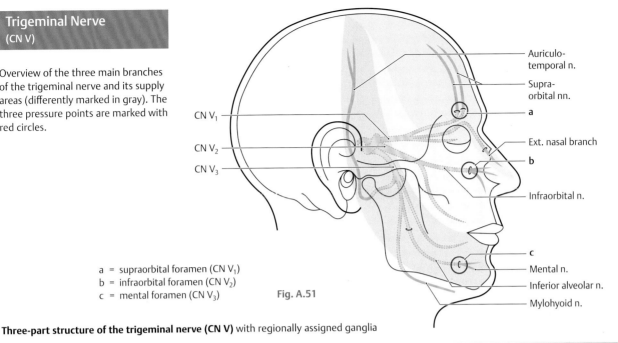

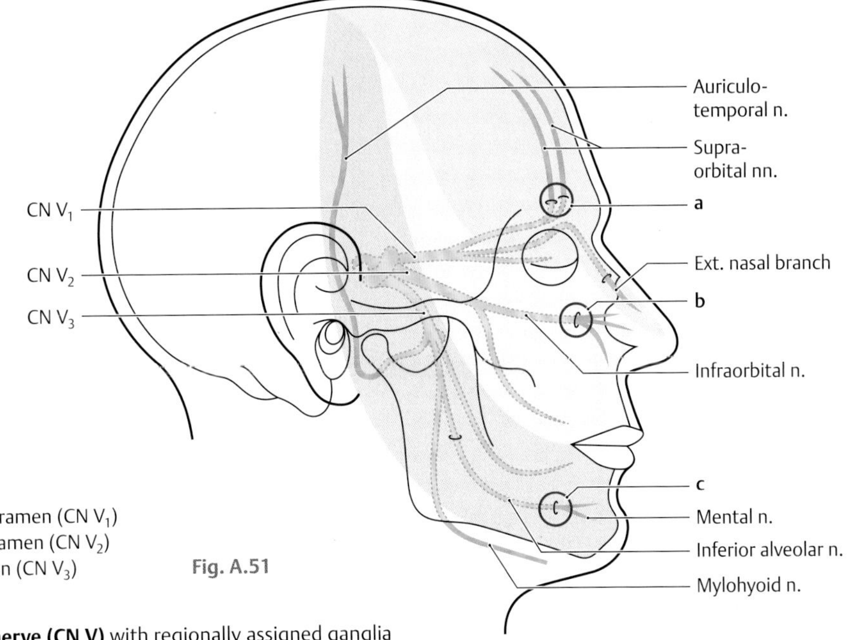


a = supraorbital foramen (CN $V_1$)
b = infraorbital foramen (CN $V_2$)
c = mental foramen (CN $V_3$)

Fig. A.51

**Three-part structure of the trigeminal nerve (CN V)** with regionally assigned ganglia

| Branches | External | Middle | Internal | Branches for Dura | Ganglion | Foramina |
|---|---|---|---|---|---|---|
| **Ophthalmic n.** (CN $V_1$) | Frontal n. (forehead skin, nose) | Lacrimal n. (lacrimal gland, conjunctiva) | Lacrimal nerve (lacrimal gland, conjunctiva) | Tentorial branch (dura, tentorium) | Ciliary ganglion | Superior orbital fissure |
| **Maxillary n.** (CN $V_2$) | Zygomatic n. (facial skin) | Infraorbital n. (teeth of upper jaw, etc.) | Pterygoplatine n. (nose, palate) | Middle meningeal branch (Dura) | Pterygopalatine ganglion | Foramen rotundum |
| **Mandibular n.** (CN $V_3$) | Auriculotemporal n. (skin of the temple) | Inferior alveolar n. (teeth of lower jaw, etc.) | Lingual n. (tongue) | Meningeal branch (Dura) | Otic ganglion, sub-mandibular ganglion | Foramen ovale |

## Trigeminal Nerve: Ophthalmic Nerve (CN $V_1$)

See also Pages: 361 / 443 / 455–457 / 462–463 / 465–467

**Ophthalmic nerve** runs through the superior orbital fissure to the orbit, skin of the forehead and nose.

Ophthalmic nerve
- **tentorial branch** (to the dura)

Frontal nerve
- **supraorbital nerve, medial branch** (through the frontal notch to the skin of the forehead)
- **supraorbital nerve, lateral branch** (through supraorbital notch to the skin of the forehead)
- **supratrochlear nerve** (to the middle corner of the eyelid)

Lacrimal nerve (to the lacrimal gland and to the lateral skin of the eyelid)
- **communicating branch with zygomatic nerve** (takes parasympathetic nerve fibers to the lacrimal gland)

Nasociliary nerve
- **infratrochlear nerve** (to the middle corner of the eyelid)
- **anterior ethmoidal nerve** (through **anterior ethmoidal foramen** and **cribriform plate** to the nose [internal nasal branches] and to the back of the nose [external nasal branches])
- **posterior ethmoidal nerve** (to ethmoidal cells and sphenoid sinus)
- **long ciliary nerves** (two delicate nerves to the uvea of the eye)
- **communicating branch** (sensible root of ciliary ganglion [c]), further in
- **short ciliary nerves** (to the choroid)

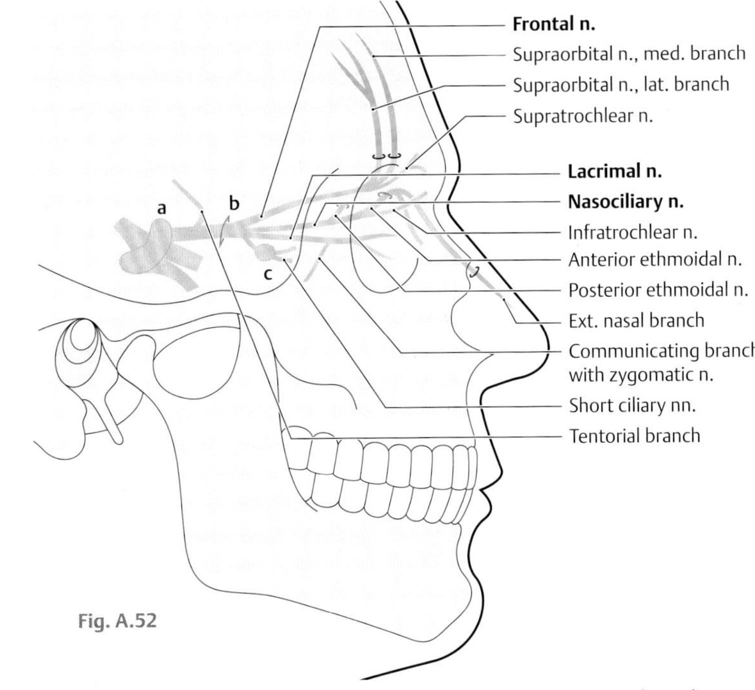


Fig. A.52

a = trigeminal ganglion
b = inferior orbital fissure
c = ciliary ganglion

## Trigeminal Nerve: Maxillary Nerve (CN $V_2$)

See also Pages: 361 / 403 / 443 / 449 / 455 / 463 / 466–467

The **maxillary nerve** runs through the foramen rotundum to the pterygopalatine fossa.

**Maxillary nerve**
- **meningeal branch** (middle) (to dura)
- **ganglionic nerves** (to pterygopalatine ganglion)
- **superior posterior nasal nerves** (through sphenopalatine foramen to nasal cavity and nasal concha) and **nasopalatine nerve** (to nasal septum and through incisive canal to the front teeth)
- **greater palatine nerve** (through greater palatine foramen to the palate)
- **lesser palatine nerves** (through lesser palatine foramina to soft palate)

**Zygomatic nerve** (through inferior orbital fissure to orbit and to skin of the region of the cheek bone; anastomoses with lacrimal nerve [communicating branch with lacrimal nerve])
**Infraorbital nerve** (through inferior orbital fissure and infraorbital foramen to the facial region)
- **inferior palpebral branches**
- **external nasal branches**
- **superior labial branches**

} to the skin of nose, upper lip and eyelids

- **ant. sup. alveolar branches**
- **middle sup. alveolar branch**
- **post. sup. alveolar branches**

} to the superior dental plexus

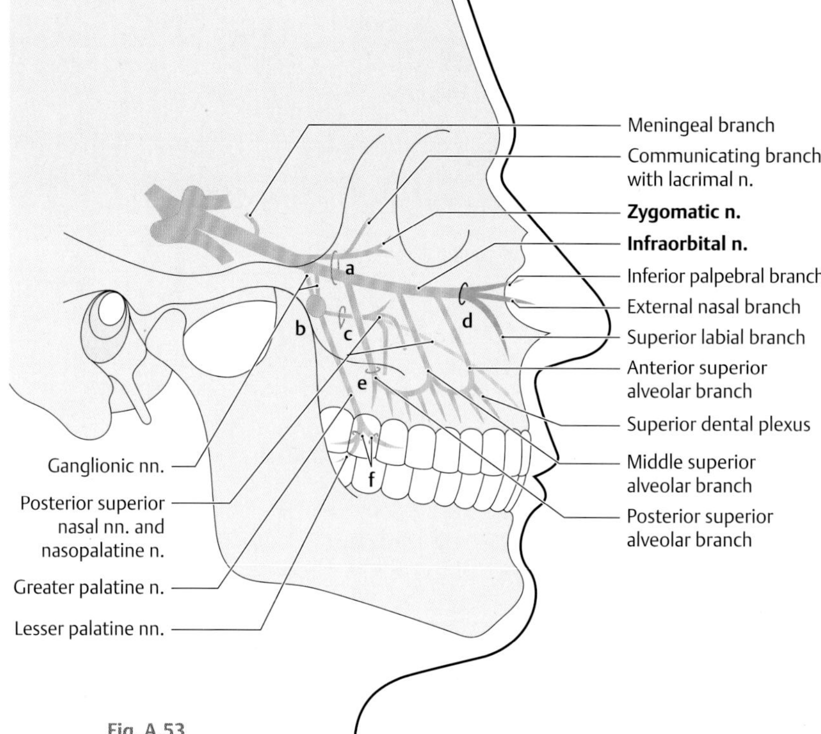


Fig. A.53

a = inferior orbital fissure
b = pterygopalatine ganglion
c = sphenopalatine foramen
d = infraorbital foramen
e = posterior alveolar foramina
f = greater palatine foramen, lesser palatine foramina

## Trigeminal Nerve: Mandibular Nerve (CN $V_3$)

See also Pages: 361 / 403 / 443 / 463 / 466–467

The **mandibular nerve** runs through the foramen ovale to the infratemporal fossa–to the region of the lower jaw and the base of the mouth.

**Mandibular nerve**
- **meningeal branch** (through the foramen spinosum to the dura)
- **deep temporal nerves, nerve to medial pterygoid; nerve to lateral pterygoid** (to the muscles of mastication of the same name)
- **masseteric nerve** (to the masseter muscle)
- **buccal nerve** (to the skin and mucosa of the cheek and gingiva)

**Auriculotemporal nerve** (to the skin of the temple) (final branches: superficial temporal branches)
- **nerves of external acoustic meatus** and **branches to tympanic membrane** (to the auditory canal and tympanum)
- **parotid branches** (to the parotid gland)
- **communicating branches** with **facial nerve** (parasympathetic nerve fibers for the parotid gland)

**Lingual nerve** (to the anterior ⅔ of the tongue; connections with submandibular glands)
**Inferior alveolar nerve** (through mandibular foramen to the lower jaw)
- **nerve to mylohyoid muscle** (to the mylohyoid muscle and anterior stomach of the digastric muscle)

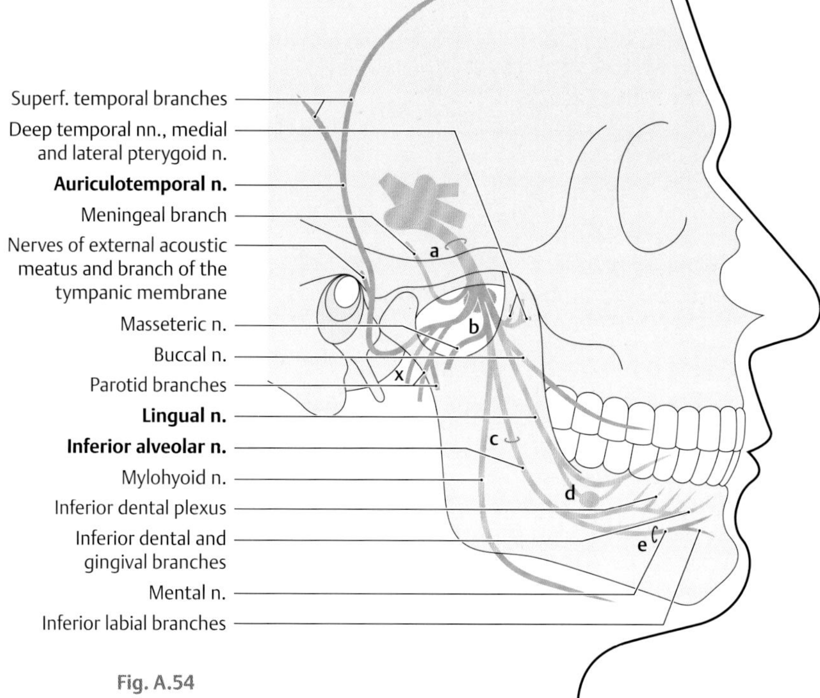


Fig. A.54

- **dental and inferior gingival branches** (to the inferior dental plexus)
- **mental nerve** (through the mental foramen to the skin of the chin)
- **inferior labial branches** (to the lower lip)

a = foramen ovale
b = otic ganglion
c = mandibular foramen
d = submandibular ganglion
e = mental foramen
x = communicating branches with facial nerve

## Facial Nerve (CN VII)

See also Pages: 361 / 396–401 / 443–445 / 464–465 / 467–469 / 480 / 512–513

Facial nerve (CN VII)
- **temporal branches** (to the facial muscles of the forehead and the eyelid)
- **zygomatic branches** (to the muscles of the palpebral and oral fissure)
- **greater petrosal nerve** (to pterygopalatine ganglion)
- **chorda tympani** (with lingual nerve [CN $V_3$] to the tongue)
- **posterior auricular nerve** (to the facial muscles of the ear and occipital head)

Parotid plexus
(network in the parotid gland)
- **stylohyoid branch**
- **digastric branch** (to the muscles of the same name)
- **buccal branches** (to the buccinator muscle and orbicularis oris muscle)
- **marginal mandibular branch** (to the muscles in the region of the lower jaw)
- **cervical branch** (for platysma; anastomoses with transverse cervical nerve)

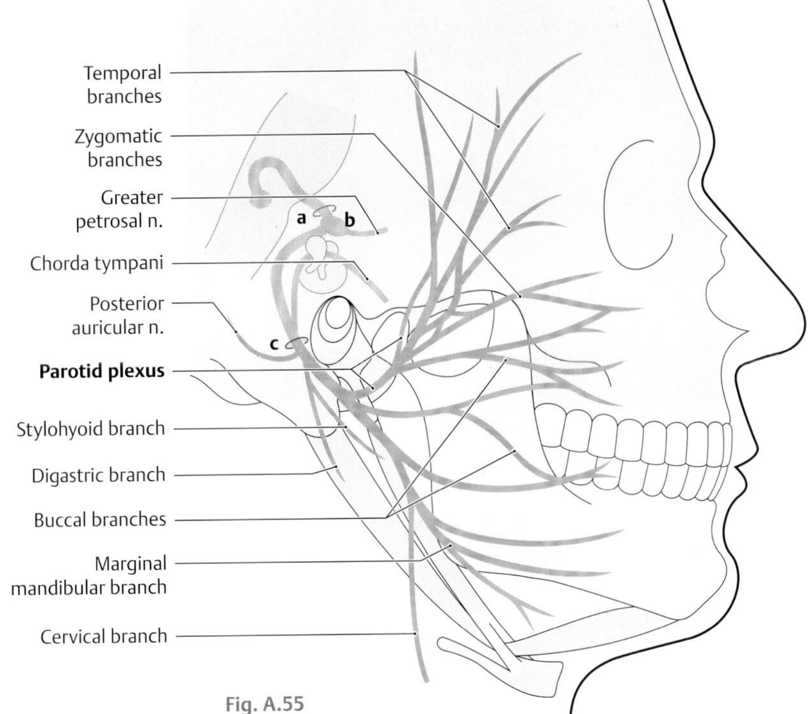


Fig. A.55

a = internal acoustic meatus
b = geniculate ganglion
c = stylomastoid foramen

## Glossopharyngeal Nerve (CN IX) and Hypoglossal Nerve (CN XII)

See also Pages: 361 / 404–405 / 412 / 429–431 / 443–445 / 467 / 469 / 480–481 / 491 / 495–496 / 512–513

Glossopharyngeal nerve (CN IX)
- **tympanic nerve** (to the tympanic cavity and auditory tube; further as lesser petrosal nerve to otic ganglion)
- **stylopharyngeal branch** and **pharyngeal branches** (to stylopharyngeus muscle and upper pharynx)
- **tonsillar branch** (to the region of the tonsils)
- **carotid branch** (carotid nerve to carotid body and carotid sinus)
- **lingual branches** (to posterior ⅓ of the tongue and taste region)

Hypoglossal nerve (CN XII)
- **lingual branches** (to the muscles of the tongue)
- **superior root of ansa cervicalis** (anastomoses with branches of spinal nerves of C2 and C3; to infrahyoid muscles)
- **geniohyoid branch** and **thyrohyoid branch** (to the muscles with the same name)

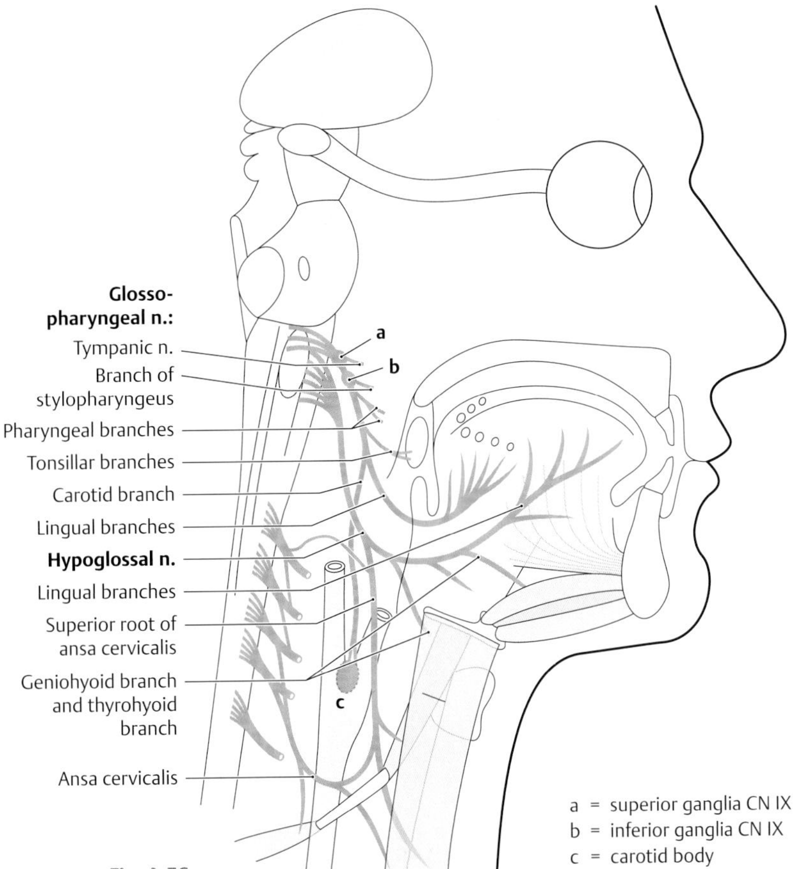


Fig. A.56

a = superior ganglia CN IX
b = inferior ganglia CN IX
c = carotid body

## Vagus Nerve (CN X) and Accessory Nerve (CN XI)

See also Pages: 242–259 / 361 / 404–405 / 412 / 429–431 / 443–444 / 467 / 469 / 472 / 480–481 / 496 / 509 / 512–513

**Vagus Nerve (CN X)**

- **meningeal branch** (through jugular foramen to dura of the posterior cranial fossa)
- **auricular branch** (to the exterior auditory canal)
- **pharyngeal branches** (to the middle and lower pharynx)
- **internal branch of superior laryngeal nerve** (through thyrohyoid membrane to the muscosa of the larynx)
- **external branch of superior laryngeal nerve** (to cricothyroid muscle)
- **recurrent laryngeal nerve** (to esophagus, trachea and inner muscles of the larynx)
- **superior cervical cardiac branches** (to cardiac plexus)
- **bronchial branches** (to bronchi and lungs)
- **inferior cervical cardiac branches** (to cardiac plexus)
- **anterior vagal trunk** (to the front wall of the stomach and to the intestines)
- **posterior vagal trunk** (to solar plexus, for back wall of the stomach, small and large intestine)

**Accessory nerve (CN XI)**

- **internal branch** (connections with vagus nerve)
- **external branch** (spinal root, C1–C6 for sternocleidomastoid muscle and trapezius muscle)

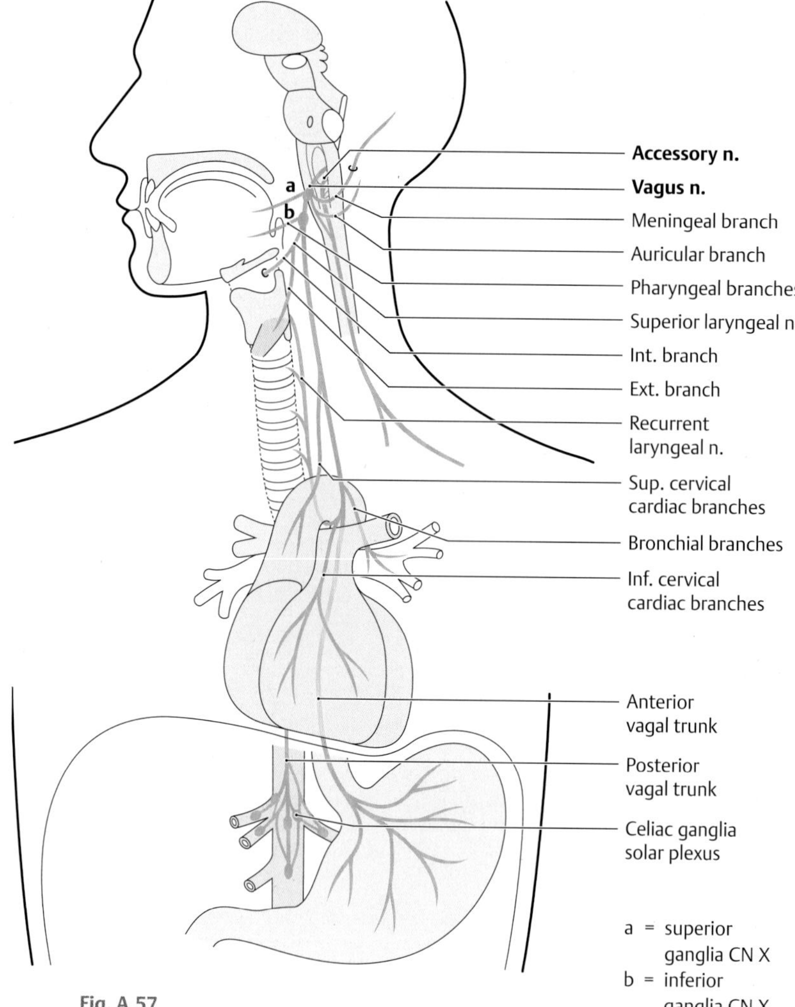


Fig. A.57

| No. | Cranial Nerves | Character | Function |
|---|---|---|---|
| I | Olfactory nerves | sensory | Olfactory system |
| II | Optic nerve | sensory | Optic system |
| III | Oculomotor nerve | somatic motor, visceral (parasympathetic) | Eye muscles, sphincter pupillae muscle, ciliaris muscle |
| IV | Trochlear nerve | somatic motor | Obliquus superior muscle |
| V | Trigeminal nerve | branchial motor (only CN $V_3$), somatic motor | Muscles of mastication, sensitivity of the head |
| VI | Abducent nerve | somatic motor | Rectus lateralis muscle |
| VII | Facial nerve | branchial motor | Facial muscles |
| VIII | Vestibulocochlear nerve | sensory | Auditory system, vestibular system |
| IX | Glossopharyngeal nerve | branchial motor and sensory, gustatoric | Stylopharyngeus muscle, upper pharynx, taste buds, carotid body |
| X | Vagus nerve | branchial motor and sensory, visceral (parasympathetic) | Larynx, dura mater, auditory canal, lower pharynx, esophagus, stomach, small and large intestine (⅔), pancreas, liver |
| XI | Accessory nerve | somatic motor | Sternocleidomastoid muscle, trapezius muscle |
| XII | Hypoglossal nerve | somatic motor | Muscles of the tongue |

## Muscles of Mastication

See also Pages: 384–386 / 388

*Mandible, fenestrated.*

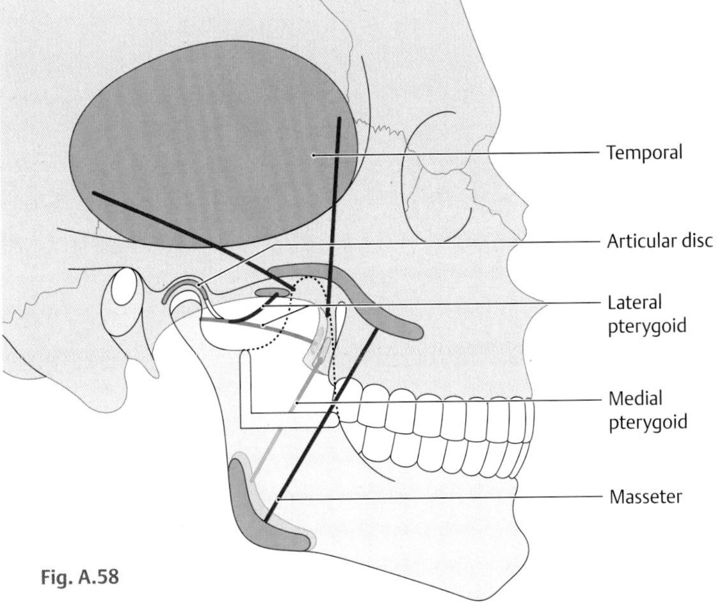


Fig. A.58

| Muscles | Origin | Insertion | Function | Innervation by CN $V_3$ |
|---|---|---|---|---|
| **Temporal** | Parietal bone (squamous part of temporal bone) | Coronoid process of mandible | Closing of the jaw, backward movement of the lower jaw | Deep temporal nn. |
| **Lateral pterygoid** • **superior part** | Infratemporal crest of sphenoid bone | Articular disc | Anterior movements of the disc, opening of the jaw | Lateral pterygoid n. |
| • **inferior part** | Lateral lamina (pterygoid process) | Condylar process of mandible | Protraction, rotation | Lateral pterygoid n. |
| **Medial pterygoid** | Pterygoid fossa | Mandibular angle (inner) | Closing of the jaw | Medial pterygoid n. |
| **Masseter** | Zygomatic arch | Mandibular angle (inner) | Closing of the jaw | Masseteric n. |

## Facial Muscles

See also Pages: 392–393 / 396–399

*Lateral aspect.*

Facial muscles are muscles of the skin, the tendons of which end in the dermis of the facial skin. The muscles originate at small areas of the bones of the skull (maxilla, zygomatic bone, mandible, etc.). Functionally, they are orientated to the orifices of the body (tarsal plate, nasal opening, oral opening, external ear).

The scalp (epicranial aponeurosis) is the common tendon of the facial muscles of the calvaria (epicranius muscle).

a = posterior auricular muscle
b = superior auricular muscle
c = anterior auricular muscle

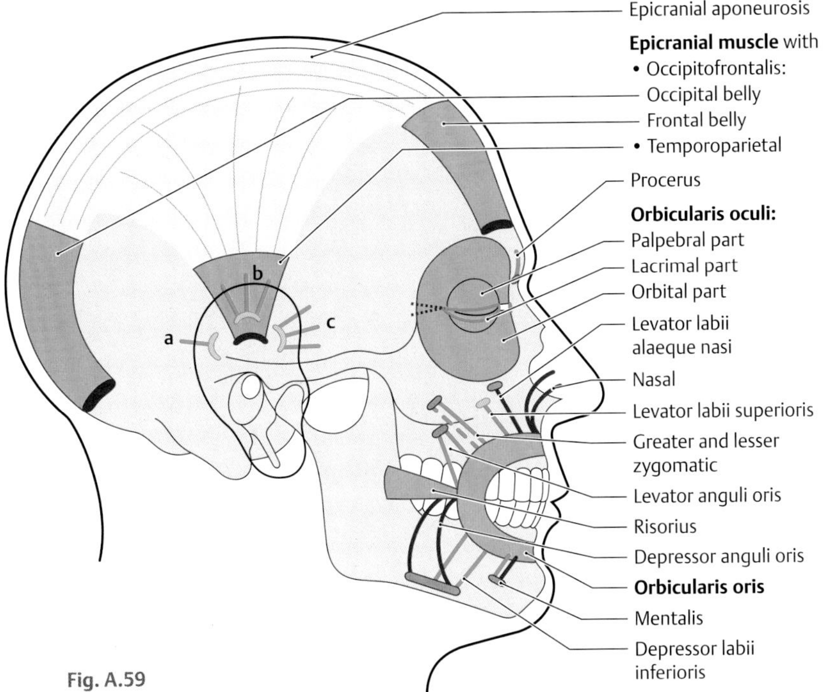


Fig. A.59

## Neck Muscles

See also Pages: 390–391 / 412 / 410 / 439 / 411 / 424–425 / 432–440

**Scalenus muscles, supra- and infrahyoid muscles**
*(lateral aspect).*

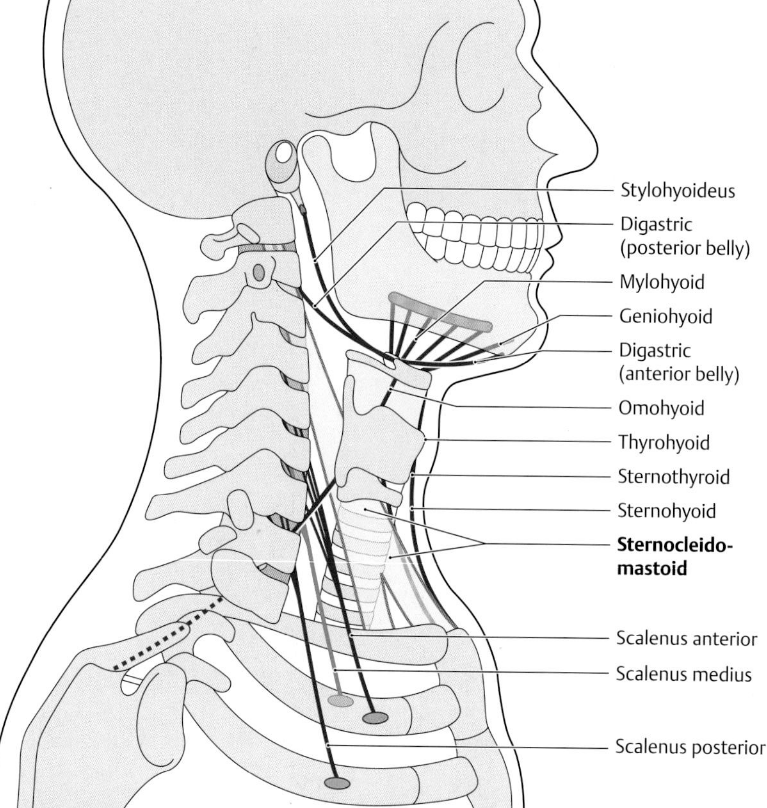


Fig. A.60

| Muscles | Origin | Insertion | Function | Innervation |
|---|---|---|---|---|
| **Sternocleidomastoid** | Manubrium of sternum, clavicle | Mastoid process | Flexion of the cervical spine, rotation of the head, inspiration | Accessory n. (CN XI) |
| **Suprahyoid Muscles** | | | | |
| **Geniohyoid** | Mental spine | Hyoid bone | Lowering of the lower jaw | Hypoglossal n. (cervical plexus) |
| **Stylohyoid** | Temporal styloid process | Hyoid bone (greater horn) | Raising of the hyoid bone | Facial n. (CN VII) |
| **Mylohyoid** | Mylohyoid line of mandible | Hyoid bone | Raising of the hyoid bone, lowering of the lower jaw | Mylohyoid n. (CN $V_3$) |
| **Digastric** (anterior and posterior muscle belly) | Mastoid process of the temporal bone | Digastric fossa of mandible (intermediate tendon at the hyoid bone) | Raising of the hyoid bone, lowering of the lower jaw | Mylohyoid n. (anterior belly), facial n. (posterior belly) |
| **Infrahyoid Muscles** | | | | |
| **Omohyoid** | Scapula (superior border) | Hyoid bone | Lowering of the hyoid bone, raising of the scapula, tension of the pre-vertebral layer of the cervical fascia | Cervical ansa (cervical plexus) |
| **Thyrohyoid** | Thyroid cartilage | Hyoid bone | Lowering of hyoid bone and larynx | Cervical plexus (C1 and 2) through hypoglossal n. |
| **Sternothyroid** | Manubrium of sternum, 1st rib | Thyroid cartilage | | Cervical ansa (cervical plexus) (C2–C3) |
| **Sternohyoid** | Manubrium of sternum, clavicle | Hyoid bone | Lowering of hyoid bone | Cervical ansa (cervical plexus) (C1–C3) |
| **Group of Scalenus Muscles** | | | | |
| **Scalenus anterior** | Transverse process, 3rd–6th cervical vertebrae | 1st rib | Lateral inclination of the cervical spine, inspiration | Ventral branches of the cervical spinal nerves |
| **Scalenus medius** | Transverse process, C3–C7 vertebrae | 1st rib | | |
| **Scalenus posterior** | Transverse process, C5–C6 vertebrae | 2nd rib | | |

## Vessels and Nerves of the Head and Neck

See also Pages: 396–403 / 418–423

In the head, arteries, veins and nerves essentially run parallel to each other. At the Erb's point the cutaneous branches of the cervical plexus come to the surface behind the sternocleidomastoid muscle, so that a targeted local anaesthetic is possible.

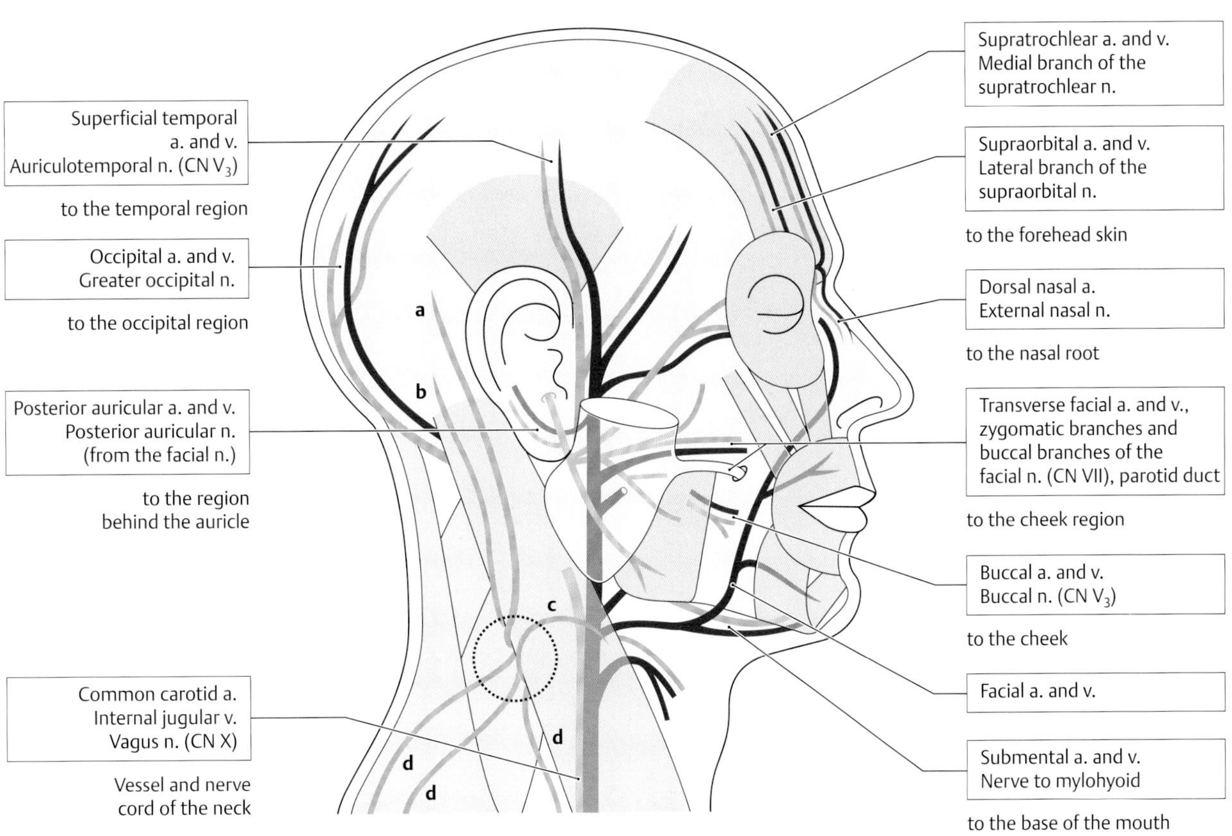


Fig. A.61 **Erb's point**
(dotted circle)
a = great auricular n.
b = lesser occipital n.
c = transverse cervical n.
d = medial, intermediate and lateral supraclavicular nn.

# Index

Page numbers in **bold** indicate main discussions, page numbers in blue refer to the appendix.

## A

## B

# D

# E



# F

## G



## H

# I

## J



## K



## L

# M

# N

## Q



## R

# S

# T

## W



## Z